D1396455

Veterinary Nursing

 NAPIER UNIVERSITY LEARNING INFORMATION SERVICES

STANDARD LOAN

NAPIER UNIVERSITY LIS

3 042 00535 6964

For Butterworth–Heinemann:

Senior Commissioning Editor: Mary Seager
Development Editor: Catharine Steers
Project Manager: Derek Robertson
Cover Design: Andy Chapman

Veterinary Nursing

Third Edition

Edited by

D. R. LANE
Trinity Court, York, UK

and

B. C. COOPER
College of Animal Welfare, Wood Green Animal Shelter, Huntingdon, UK

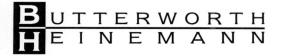

CA 636. 089073 LAN

BUTTERWORTH-HEINEMANN
An imprint of Elsevier Science Limited

First published 1994
Reprinted with corrections 1995
Reprinted 1996, 1997 (twice), 1998
Second edition 1999
Reprinted with corrections 1999, 2000
Third edition 2003

© BSAVA 2003

No part of this publication may be reproduced, stored in a retrieval
system, or transmitted in any form or by any means, electronic,
mechanical, photocopying, recording or otherwise, without either the
prior permission of the publishers (Permissions Manager, Elsevier
Science Limited, Robert Stevenson House, 1–3 Baxter's Place, Leith
Walk, Edinburgh EH1 3AF), or a licence permitting restricted copying
in the United Kingdom issued by the Copyright Licensing Agency,
90 Tottenham Court Road, London W1T 4LP.

ISBN 0 7506 55259

British Library Cataloguing in Publication Data
A catalogue record for this book is available from the British Library

Library of Congress Cataloging in Publication Data
A catalog record for this book is available from the Library of Congress

Veterinary knowledge is constantly changing. As new information becomes available, changes in treatment, procedures, equipment
and the use of drugs become necessary. The editors and the publishers have taken care to ensure that the information given in this
text is accurate and up to date. However, readers are strongly advised to confirm that the information, especially with regard to
drug usage, complies with the latest legislation and standards of practice.

The Publisher's policy is to use **paper manufactured from sustainable forests**

Contents

Foreword

This, the third edition of *Veterinary Nursing*, continues the tradition of being the most comprehensive textbook for veterinary nurses undergoing training, either in the practice environment or at college.

Just as the science of veterinary surgery is becoming ever more complex and technically advanced, so does the role of the veterinary nurse. This edition has been brought up to date and reflects the advances now taking place in general practice, both in terms of nursing care and the new occupational standards. However, the book never loses sight of the fact that it must also teach the veterinary nurse how to perform basic roles of animal care and nursing competently and conscientiously. For it is on the base of these elementary tasks that the more technical demands are made and the whole edifice of modern practice is built. Get the basics right and all else follows.

The British Small Animal Veterinary Association has a long tradition of working closely with Veterinary Nurses and in helping to train them. We are happy, and proud, to be associated with the continued publication of this book and feel sure it will find a well-deserved place in both the practice and the VN library, reflecting its central role in veterinary nursing training.

Richard G. Harvey
BSAVA President 2002–2003

Preface

The changing scene in veterinary nursing

The veterinary nurses of today are expected to be many things to many people and to function in a variety of settings. As an emerging profession it requires practice that is based on a systematic body of knowledge, recognition by the public, and a code of ethics regulating veterinary nurses with the public and their veterinary colleagues.

Veterinary nurses should have a framework upon which their own values, norms and symbols are clear. These values should have a body of specific knowledge that contributes to the welfare or needs of the owner and animals under their care and to reflective practice and advancement of the profession's own body of knowledge.

With the establishment of the RCVS Veterinary Nurse Council we can expect to see the move to regulation. Veterinary nurses will, however, still be subject to criminal law, employment law, civil law and public law. This new edition of *Veterinary Nursing* aptly incorporates a new chapter covering the basics of law, highlighting some of the important issues that should be considered by the newly qualified veterinary nurse.

To preserve the integrity of veterinary nursing and ensure that practice, which is the core of nursing, is developed and enhanced to levels of increasing excellence, the notion of theory, research and practice must be encompassed. Veterinary nurses must continue to meet the challenges that face them by:

- Establishing their profession further.
- Developing veterinary nurse theory.
- Integrating nursing research as a core component of their training.
- Continuing to educate veterinary nurses for senior and specialist positions.

This book possibly provides the answers to the foundation for all aspiring student veterinary nurses covering the knowledge required for the new occupational standards.

The role of the veterinary nurse is constantly changing and as veterinary practice becomes more sophisticated there will continue to be a need for further development of the occupational standards and thus preparation of veterinary nurses consistent with their changing role.

D. R. Lane and B. C. Cooper

Contributors

Mrs W. Adams, VN, Guide Dogs for the Blind, Tollgate House, Banbury Road, Bishops Tachbrook, Warwick, CV33 9QJ

Dr D. Anderson, MA VetMB PhD Cert SAS Diplomate ECVS MRCVS, Queen's Veterinary School Hospital, Madingley Road, Cambridge, CB3 0ES

Mrs V. Aspinall BVSc MRCVS, Principal, Abbeydale Veterinary Training, Gloucester

Ms T. Atkinson, Dip AS (CABC) VN, Bradford-on-Avon, Wiltshire

Ms Jackie Belle, BSc MSc VN, Veterinary Nurse, Durrell Wildlife Conservation Trust, Trinity, Jersey JE3 5BP, British Channel Isles

Dr P. A. Bloxham, MVB PhD MRCVS, Dawlish, Devon

Ms S. Bowden, Cert Ed, VN, Essex

Dr D. Brodbelt, Animal Health Trust, Lanwades Park, Kentford, Newmarket, Suffolk, CB8 7UU

Ms W. Busby, VN, Fife

Mr R. Butcher, MA VetMB MRCVS, Partner, The Wylie Veterinary Centre, Essex

Ms S. Chandler, DipAVN(Surg) VN, Senior nurse, Queens Veterinary School, Cambridge

Professor J. E. Cooper, DTVM FRCPath FIBiol FRCVS, Consultant Veterinary Pathologist, Durrell Wildlife Conservation Trust, Trinity, Jersey, JE3 5BP, British Channel Isles

Miss L. Daniels, Dip AVN(Surg) VN, Veterinary Nurse Course Organiser, Norton Radstock College, Ellsbridge House, Bath Road, Keynsham, Bristol

Miss R. Dennis, MA VetMB DRV DipECVDI MRCVS, Head of Diagnostic Imaging, Centre for Small Animal Studies, Animal Health Trust, Lanswade Park, Kentford, Newmarket, Suffolk, CB8 7UU

Dr C. J. Dutton, BSc BVSc MSc C Biol MIBiol MRCVS, 84 Glenview Avenue, Toronto, Ontario, M4R 1P8, Canada

Ms E. Earle, TD BA RN, Head of Veterinary Nursing, RCVS, Belgravia House, Horseferry Rd., London

Dr J. Elliott, MA VetMB PhD Cert SAC DipECVTP MRCVS, Reader in Veterinary Pharmacology, Royal Veterinary College, London

Dr G. C.W. England, BVetMed PhD DVetMed DVR CertVA DVRep, Guide Dogs for the Blind, Tollgate House, Banbury Road, Bishops Tachbrook, Warwick, CV33 9QJ

Mrs M. Fisher, BVetMed, MRCVS, C Biol, MI Biol, Independent Consultant in Veterinary Parasitology, Worcs

Ms C. France[†], DCR.

Mrs C. George, DipAVN(Surg) VN, Ashford, Kent

Ms J Goodwin, BSc VN, London Emergency and Referral Clinic, London

Ms N. Hill, VN, The Animal Health Trust, Centre for Small Animals, Suffolk

L. Jones, DipAVN (Surg) VN, Head Nurse, University of Glasgow Veterinary School, Glasgow

Ms E. Leece, BVSc Cert VA MRCVS, Anaesthetist, The Animal Health Trust, Suffolk

Dr S. E. Long, BVMS, PhD, DirECAR, MRCVS, Department of Clinical Veterinary Science, University of Bristol, Bristol

Dr C. May, MA VetMB Cert SAO PhD MRCVS, Grove Veterinary Hospital, 1 Hibbert Street, New Mills, Stockport SK12 3JS

Dr S. McCune BA PhD VN, Research Manager, Waltham Centre for Pet Nutrition (Animal Behaviour and Cognition), Leicestershire

Ms D. McHugh EVN DipAVN(Surg) VN, Head Nurse, Equine Practice, Newmarket

Mrs C. B. Mills, VN, Lincolnshire

Mr D. S. Mills, BVSc MRCVS, Principal Lecturer in Behavioural Studies and Animal Welfare, University of Lincoln

Dr H. Moreton, BSc PhD, The Royal Agricultural College, Gloucestershire

Mrs S. Morrissey, CVPM, Practice Manager, Cromwell Veterinary Group, Huntingdon, Cambs

Ms M. O'Reilly, BSc(Hons) Zoology, VN, College of Animal Welfare, London

Dr M. R. Owen, BVSc BSc PhD CertSAS MRCVS, Glasgow University Veterinary School, Bearsden Road, Bearsden, Glasgow G61 1QH

Ms E. Reubens, CertEd VN, St. John's Ambulance, London

Ms J. Seymour, VN, Stafford

Mrs L. Slater, DipAVN(Surg) VN, Queen Mother Hospital for Animals, Royal Veterinary College

J. Smith, Dip AVN(Surg), VN, Head Theatre Nurse, Queen's Veterinary School Hospital, Cambridge University.

Dr M. F. Stewart, DVM MRCVS, Senior Research Fellow, Glasgow Vet School, Glasgow

Ms J. Turner, VN, Middlesex

Mrs C. Van der Heiden, VN, Banffshire

Mrs J. Venturi-Rose, MSc BAEd(Hons) CertEd VN, West Sussex

Ms V. Walsh, VN, Worcester

Dr E. Welsh, PhD BVMS Cert VA Cert SAS MRCVS, Senior Lecturer, University of Edinburgh, Edinburgh

[†]Carol France died from cancer in October 2002. She was one of the longest-serving members of the clinical staff at The Royal Veterinary College and a cornerstone of the Radiology Service in the Queen Mother Hospital for Animals. During the 27 years she spent at the RVC, Carol touched the lives of a great many people, particularly student nurses and veterinary undergraduates, to whom she taught radiography. She is greatly missed. The installation of a second X-ray room in the QMHA was completed in November 2002 and this room has been dedicated to her memory.

Christopher R. Lamb MA, VetMB, MRCVS, DipACVR, DipECVDI
Senior Lecturer in Radiology, Head of Service, Anaesthesia and Radiology, Royal Veterinary College.

1

Handling and control

Trudi Atkinson

Learning objectives

After studying this chapter, students should be able to:

- Describe how the veterinary nurse should handle and restrain animals for examination or treatment.
- Recognise basic canine and feline 'body language' including signals indicating fear and potential aggression.
- Explain how to reduce fear and stress in veterinary patients during approach, handling and restraint.
- Identify the techniques used when handling aggressive or potentially aggressive animals, and list the equipment that may be required.
- Apply the principles of handling and restraint to everyday veterinary practice.

A frequent task for the veterinary nurse (VN) in practice is the handling and restraint of animals requiring treatment or examination. How an animal is handled can greatly affect the ease and efficiency by which procedures may be carried out. Inefficient or inappropriate handling can subject the patient to unnecessary stress and discomfort, which is not only damaging to patient welfare but may also result in the development of, or an increase in, defensive aggression towards the handler or practitioner. Proficiency in handling and control is one of the most essential and valuable skills for a VN to acquire.

The aims of the nurse when restraining an animal should be as follows:

- To allow an examination or procedure such as the application of dressings or the administration of medication to be carried out as efficiently as possible.
- To avoid injury or further injury to the patient. (For example, if sharp instruments such as scissors are used to cut the animal's hair or a scalpel blade is used to take a skin scrape for examination, injury may result if the animal moves excessively. Or further injury may be caused if a patient moves unexpectedly whilst attempts are made to examine or treat a fracture or open wound.)
- To prevent injury by the animal to the practitioner, handler or other persons.
- To achieve the above without causing additional or unnecessary pain or distress to the animal.

Canine and feline communication

Pain and fear may cause an animal to behave very differently in the veterinary surgery than it might do under other circumstances. An elementary knowledge of canine and feline communication can help the nurse to assess the possible reactions of an individual animal in its current situation and adapt means of handling and restraint accordingly.

Canine 'body language'

Figure 1.1 shows the typical range of canine body postures. (However, be aware that changes in body posture will also occur dependent on the dog's current activity.)

(a) Normal, relaxed. Tail is relaxed and down or held in whatever position is normal for the breed. Ears may orientate to sounds.
(b) Increased confidence and assertiveness is demonstrated by a forward body posture and elevated tail carriage.
(c–e) Reduced confidence is shown by a lowering of the body posture and tail position.
(f) The body posture of a fearful dog is normally low and backed away from the source of fear. The ears are held back and down and the tail held down between the back legs (Dunbar, 1979; Fox, 1971).

> A wagging tail can have several meanings including a willingness to interact (possibly aggressively) by an assertive dog, or a sign of appeasement by a nervous and potentially defensively aggressive dog. A handler should always consider other aspects of the dog's body language and never assume that a dog with a wagging tail is friendly and will not bite (Bradshaw and Nott, 1995).

Canine facial expressions

Figure 1.2 shows the typical range of a dog's facial expressions:

(a) Normal, alert. Face relaxed, ears orientating to sounds.
(b) Fearful, submissive. Ears back and down, lips drawn back into a 'submissive grin' face, averted to avoid direct eye contact.
(c) Fearful, potentially aggressive. Ears flat to head, 'submissive grin' with teeth bared as a warning. Eyes may dart back and forth as the dog tries to keep 'an eye on' the perceived threat whilst also trying to avoid prolonged direct eye contact. May growl or bark as a warning.
(d) Assertive, challenging, potentially aggressive. Ears forward, lips pushed forward with teeth bared as a warning. Direct eye contact maintained. May emit a low growl (Fox, 1971).

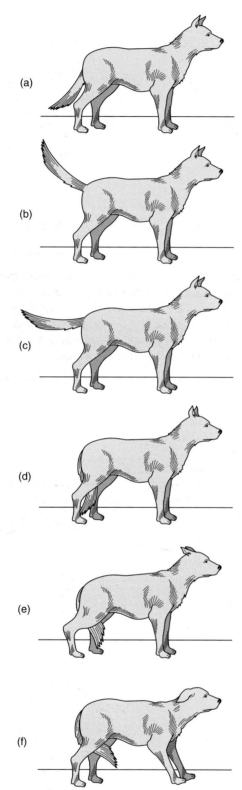

Fig. 1.1 Canine body language.

Be careful not to equate 'dominance' with aggression. Not only are the 'rules' of a canine hierarchy designed to reduce the risk of physical confrontation, but also conflicts or misunderstandings over hierarchy are more likely to occur with members of the dog's social group, i.e. the people or other animals that it lives with. Episodes of aggression towards people outside of that social group are more commonly due to fear, especially in a veterinary situation. However, a fearful dog may appear confident and assertive if it has had the opportunity previously to learn that aggression can be effective in making a potential threat 'back off' or keep its distance, even if only momentarily. However, it is important to realise that attempts to physically reprimand such a dog will only result in an increase in fear and consequently an increase in aggression (Heath, 2001; Overall, 1997).

Feline communication

Relaxed (Fig. 1.3a–c)

Body: If resting may be on back with belly exposed, or curled up. Feet may not be in contact with the ground. **Eyes:** May be half closed if cat is relaxed, pupil size dependent on available light. A 'slow eye blink' may be directed towards other animals including people as a signal of 'non-confrontation'. **Ears:** Normal 'relaxed'. **Tail:** Extended or loosely wrapped if cat is resting. If standing or if in motion tail may be held down in a 'U' shape away from the body or upright sometimes with a curl at the end as a friendly greeting. May purr while relaxed, or chirrup or meow as a friendly greeting.

Tense (Fig. 1.3d)

Body: May explore area looking for ways of escape or rest in 'ready' position with feet in contact with the ground so cat can move quickly if necessary. **Tail:** Usually wrapped around body. **Ears:** Slightly flattened sideways. **Eyes:** Open, pupils dilated.

Fearful (Fig. 1.3e)

Body: May be held low and away from source of fear with all four feet on the ground, or may attempt to hide. **Tail:** Very tight to body. **Ears:** Flattened sideways. **Eyes:** Wide with dilated pupils.

Fearful/defensively aggressive (Fig. 1.3f,g)

Body: Flattened and backed away from source of fear. If approached may 'lash out' with front feet, but with body held back. **Tail:** Tightly wrapped or 'lashing'. **Ears:** Fear and submission are signalled by the cat holding its ears down and to the side; however, to protect them from injury the ears are held back and down if an aggressive encounter becomes more likely. **Eyes:** Wide, pupils fully dilated, and focused on the source of fear. May growl, hiss or spit.

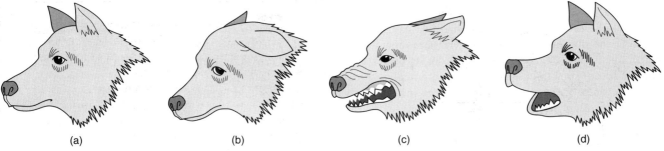

Fig. 1.2 Canine facial expressions.

A cat confronted by a sudden, unexpected danger, such as an unknown or unfriendly dog may arch its back and fluff out the hairs along the back and tail in an attempt to appear much larger than it really is (Bessant, 1992; Bradshaw, 1992; McCune, 1992).

> Cats often purr when relaxed or as a way of soliciting food or attention; however, cats may also purr when in extreme pain or distress. This could be one way that the cat tries to reduce its level of stress, in the same way that we might whistle or hum if anxious or frightened. Therefore do not always assume that a cat is not stressed or in pain because it is purring (Bradshaw, 1992).

Initial approach and handling

Dogs

Whenever possible, encourage a dog to approach you rather than directly approaching the dog. Try to avoid cornering a dog or leaning over it and avoid prolonged direct eye contact, which the dog may consider threatening. Crouching down to the dog's level can help with nervous individuals, but not so close that your face could be within 'biting' distance. Try to avoid grabbing a dog by the collar or scruff as this could frighten the dog and cause it to turn and bite.

Occasionally, dogs are reluctant to leave the safety of a hospital kennel and may become defensively aggressive if confronted or if attempts are made to enter the kennel in order to remove them. If a lightweight lead is left on the dog the end can be extracted using a broom handle or cat catcher allowing the handler to take hold of the lead safely without needing to confront the dog. In most instances once the handler has hold of the lead a dog will leave the kennel and walk willingly with the handler. **A lead must never be attached to a choke chain and the dog must be regularly supervised whilst in a kennel with a lead attached.**

Handling the animal with the owner present

> Always remember that, to the owner of a beloved pet, how they witness their animal being handled may reflect on the type and standard of care that they expect from the practice in general. If their pet is handled roughly or inefficiently they may choose to take their pet and their custom elsewhere.

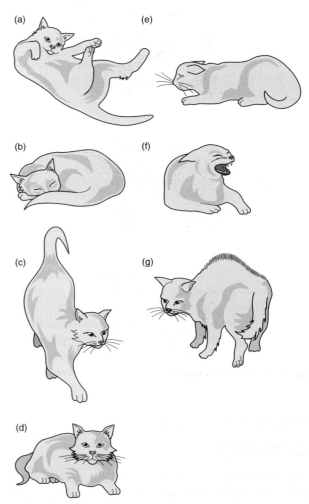

Fig. 1.3 Feline communication: (a–c) relaxed; (d) tense; (e–g) fearful.

Spend a little time 'chatting' with the owner before attempting to handle or approach a dog. This time can be spent watching the dog and making a general assessment of its temperament. The dog will take cues from its owner as to whether or not something or someone is a potential threat. A minute or so interacting with the owner in a 'friendly' manner can often help to convey the message to the dog that you are not a threat (McBride, 1995). It is not a good idea to attempt to shake the owner's hand, unless the client offers to shake your hand first, as the dog may regard this as a threatening gesture and then become aggressive towards you in order to protect its fellow 'pack member'.

Owners may unintentionally reinforce their pet's fear and aggression, therefore if a dog is difficult to handle it may be easier to deal with away from the owner.

When separating dog and owner it is often more successful to ask the owner to leave the room first and then lead the dog away.

Cats

Extracting a cat from a carrier

Top opening carriers:

(1) Lift the lid slowly. Most cats will prefer to stay in the carrier but some may try to jump out as soon as the lid is lifted, so be prepared.
(2) Stroke the cat to settle it and assess its temperament.
(3) Make sure the cat is well supported underneath (*see later on lifting and carrying*) and lift out and onto the examination table.

Front opening carriers:

(1) Open the front and try to encourage the cat out without putting a hand inside the carrier, which the cat may find threatening, making it less willing to leave the safety of the carrier.
(2) If the carrier can be separated into two halves, remove the top half and lift the cat out as you would with a top opening carrier. Some front-opening carriers have a tray in the base in which the cat sits. If so, this can be gently pulled out, bringing the cat out with it.
(3) If none of the above is possible, gently tilt the carrier, which may help to encourage the cat out.
(4) The cat should only be physically extracted from the carrier as a last resort; try to do so gently and be aware that the cat may become defensive. **Do not scruff the cat and pull it out unless it is absolutely necessary to do so and all other methods have been tried.**

Once the cat is out of the carrier, place the carrier on the ground away from the cat. If the carrier is left in sight of the cat it may repeatedly try to get back in and may become fractious when prevented from doing so.

Try to examine or carry out any procedures on cats as soon as possible. Cats often have a limited 'tolerance period', in other words they will put up with so much for so long and then suddenly decide that they've had enough and then try to escape or become defensively aggressive.

Cats and rabbits often feel very vulnerable in hospital kennels. Providing them with a box in which they can hide can often help them to feel more secure and therefore easier to approach and handle.

Moving, transporting and lifting animals

Dogs must be on a lead attached to a well-fitting collar if they are to be walked from one area of the surgery to another. Always check that the collar is not too tight or so loose that the dog could slip out of it. For added security it is often a good idea to also use a lightweight slip lead.

> If cats, rabbits or other small animals are to be transported from one area to another they must be securely contained in an appropriate carrier.

Be aware of any possible medical condition or injury that may be causing an animal pain or discomfort before attempting to lift or carry it. Try to keep points of pain away from your body as you carry the animal to reduce the risk of causing further discomfort.

Ensure that the animal is aware of your approach and your intent before you attempt to lift it.

Small to medium-sized dogs may be lifted by one person (Fig. 1.4). However, assistance may be required to carry drips, open doors, etc.

Large, heavy* or injured dogs should be lifted and carried by two people (Fig. 1.5).

Large, immobile or severely injured dogs are best carried by two or more people in a blanket or on a stretcher (Fig. 1.6).

Cats should be tucked in under the arm with the forearm supporting the underneath of the cat and hand gently holding the front legs (Fig. 1.7). The other hand can be used to stroke the cat over the head and neck, ready to take hold of the scruff if necessary.

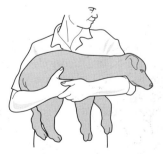

Fig. 1.4 Lifting a small/medium dog.

*Over 20 kg. See Chapter 5, 'Occupational Hazards'.

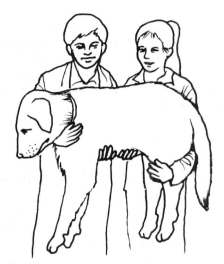

Fig. 1.5 Lifting a large dog.

Rabbits should be lifted by making sure the back end is well supported, holding the feet away from you and then securely but gently holding onto the scruff of the neck (Fig. 1.8). Never lift a rabbit by the ears or by the scruff alone *without* providing support underneath.

A rabbit should be carried with its head tucked under the handler's arm keeping the back and hindquarters well supported (Fig. 1.9).

> It is often a good idea to place a towel over a top opening carrier as you open it to prevent a frightened rabbit from jumping out.

> *MANUAL HANDLING*
> Always follow the health and safety rules when lifting: keep the back straight, legs slightly apart and bend at the knees. Always get assistance before attempting to lift a heavy or awkward weight. Keep the load close to the body.

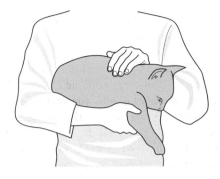

Fig. 1.7 Lifting a cat.

Restraint for examination or treatment

Restraint of pet animals should be firm but gentle, using no more than the minimum amount of restraint necessary. Care must be taken not to cause undue pain or discomfort by applying any more pressure than is required. It may be necessary to adjust the firmness of your hold momentarily, depending on the animal's reactions to the procedure being performed.

The means of restraint used is dependent on both the procedure to be performed and the reactions of the individual animal.

Restraint of dogs

Figure 1.10 shows methods of steadying a dog's head: (a) the hands are placed either side of the neck and the head is gently pushed forwards with the fingers; (b) the dog is held by the scruff on either side of the neck; (c) a rolled-up towel is held firmly but gently around the dog's neck. This method is particularly useful with small brachycephalic breeds and can be used to prevent a dog from turning round to bite when it is not possible to use a muzzle.

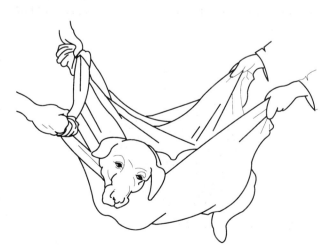

Fig. 1.6 Lifting – blanket/stretcher.

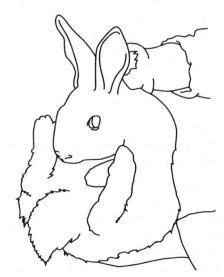

Fig. 1.8 Lifting a rabbit.

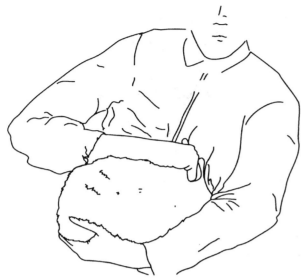

Fig. 1.9 Carrying a rabbit.

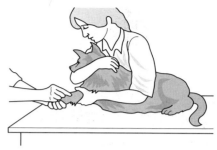

Fig. 1.11 Holding a dog for cephalic venepuncture.

Figure 1.11 shows a dog being held for cephalic venepuncture. It is often useful to have an additional person available to steady the back end of the dog if it starts to struggle. Figure 1.12 shows a dog being held for jugular venepuncture.

Figure 1.13 shows a dog being restrained on its side. It may be possible to manoeuvre a dog into this position by first getting the dog to lie down, on command if possible or by drawing the dog's legs forward whilst it is in a sitting position, and then gently rolling the dog over using the forearm to push the dog's head down whilst also holding onto the dog's legs. If the position cannot be achieved by the above method, the dog's legs that are closest to the handler are grasped and pulled away causing the dog to fall towards the handler (Fig. 1.14). The dog is then gently lowered down against the handler's chest and onto the surface. However, be aware that this manoeuvre and being held in this position can be frightening and may cause the dog to panic and attempt to bite. Gentle reassurance is essential and muzzling the dog beforehand may be advisable.

Restraint of cats

Figure 1.15 shows general restraint for examination or treatment of the head area. The cat's body should be held close to the handler to prevent the cat from backing away. A firm but gentle hold around the front legs prevents the cat using its front claws.

Figure 1.16 shows raising of the cephalic vein or restraint for examination or treatment of the foreleg. Figure 1.17 shows two methods of restraint for jugular venepuncture.

> It is sometimes necessary to hold a cat by the scruff of the neck if firmer restraint is required. Always try other methods first as many otherwise calm and tolerant cats can become fractious and difficult to handle as soon as attempts are made to handle them by the scruff.

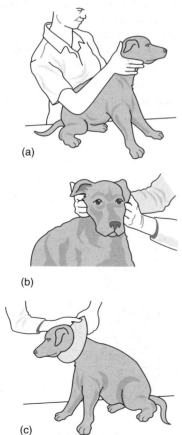

(a)

(b)

(c)

Fig. 1.10 Restraint of dogs.

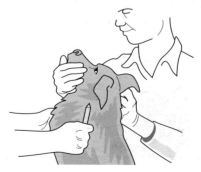

Fig. 1.12 Holding a dog for jugular venepuncture.

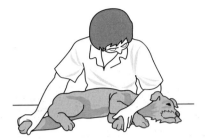

Fig. 1.13 Restraining a dog on its side.

Restraint of rabbits

Hold the rabbit around the shoulders with its back end held in close to your body to prevent the rabbit kicking out backwards (Fig. 1.18a). Wrapping the rabbit in a towel can also help the rabbit to feel secure and allow access to the ears, eyes and mouth. Covering a rabbit's eyes can often help to calm it (Fig. 1.18b). Rabbits can often be successfully restrained on their backs for examination or minor treatment of the ventral area (Fig. 1.18c).

Use of distractions

Gentle distractions can often help to calm an animal and allow procedures to be carried out more efficiently.

- Talking to the animal in a calm and friendly manner, especially if the animal's name is used, can often help to distract and calm a patient.
- Use the fingers to gently stroke, scratch or gently massage the animal.
- A short whistle can often 'still' a struggling dog, allowing a few moments to get a needle into a vein, take a radiograph or perform any other procedure that requires the animal to be still and distracted for a second or two.

Handling difficult or aggressive animals

> Remember that a frightened animal may use aggression as a defence. Therefore try to avoid any unnecessary actions that may cause an animal to be fearful or that may increase its fear.

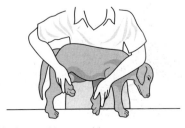

Fig. 1.14 Achieving position on side.

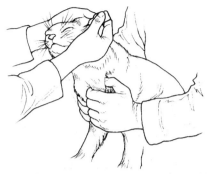

Fig. 1.15 Treatment of the head area.

Dogs
If a dog growls

- **Do not** attempt to punish the dog: a confrontation will only teach the dog that it has good reason to be defensive.
- **Do not** attempt to comfort or reassure the dog: this may actually reward and so reinforce the unwanted behaviour.
- **Do** muzzle the dog: a growl may not cause you to back off but a set of sharp teeth heading in your direction will. If this happens the dog will learn that direct aggression *is* effective even if a warning growl is not. Dogs that have already learnt this can be some of the most dangerous and unpredictable to handle.
- **Do** try to appear unconcerned by the growl: backing away, appearing fearful or angry, are all ways that the growling and potential aggression may be reinforced.
- **Do** try to understand *why* the dog may be growling: is it the dog in pain? Is it the way in which it is being handled? Is it the procedure being carried out? Unless the procedure is almost finished, or is one that will only take a few seconds, it is best to stop and continue once the dog is muzzled.

Muzzles

Whenever possible try to get a muzzle on a dog *before* it tries to bite. It can be far more difficult to get a muzzle on a dog

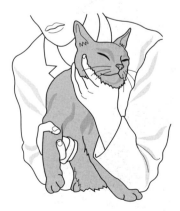

Fig. 1.16 Raising the cephalic vein or restraint for examination of the foreleg

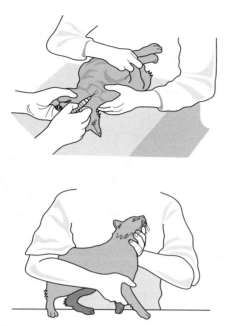

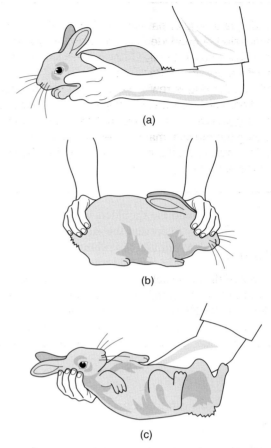

Fig. 1.17 Two methods of restraint for jugular venepuncture.

that has already decided that you are a threat and has discovered that trying to bite is effective in making you back off.

A variety of cloth, plastic and leather muzzles are available (Fig. 1.19). A good selection of different types and sizes should always be at hand. Be aware that open-ended muzzles may still allow a dog to 'nip' with its front teeth.

Fig. 1.18 Restraining rabbits: (a) holding rabbit; (b) covering eyes; (c) restrained on back.

> If a dog is to be muzzled for longer than a few minutes, always use a basket type muzzle that allows the dog to open its mouth enabling it to pant or vomit. Never leave a dog unattended for any length of time whilst muzzled.

Applying a tape muzzle (Fig. 1.20) Use a length of tape or non-stretch bandage at least 100 cm (40 in.) long for a medium-sized dog. Form a loop by tying a loose square knot without tightening. With the dog suitably restrained, drop the loop over the dog's nose, with the knot uppermost. Pull the ends quickly to tighten the knot and so 'muzzle' the dog. Cross the ends under the dog's jaw. Tie at the back of the dog's head using 'quick release' bow. The tape must be pulled tight in order for the muzzle to be effective; this can be uncomfortable for the dog and may even cause some slight injury. This muzzle should only be used in an emergency or if it is not possible to get close enough to the dog to use any other type of muzzle.

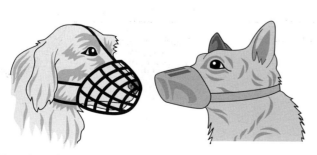
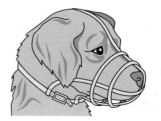
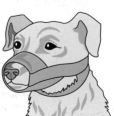

Fig. 1.19 Variety of muzzles.

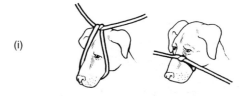

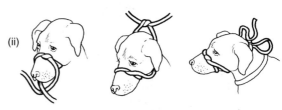

Fig. 1.20 Applying a tape muzzle.

Using a 'dog-catcher'

The noose of the dog-catcher (Fig. 1.21) is dropped over the animal's head and then tightened, thereby reducing the risk of injury to the handler when taking hold of a severely aggressive dog. The use of a dog-catcher can be highly traumatic for a dog, so it should only ever be used as a last resort.

Cats

Fractious cats can often be adequately restrained by wrapping them in a large towel. Figure 1.22 shows a cat being wrapped for cephalic venepuncture. An alternative is a 'cat-restraining bag' (Fig. 1.23).

Use of a 'crush cage' may be necessary with cats that cannot be handled; this is similar to a wire cat carrier but with a movable partition that is used to press the cat against one side of the cage, allowing an injection to be given through the mesh of the cage. If a crush cage is not available or if the cat cannot be moved from its carrier, the lid or door of the carrier can be opened just enough to allow thick towels to be pushed into the carrier, but not enough to allow the cat to escape. The towels are then used to press the cat against the side of the cage allowing an injection to be given.

If a dog is a regular patient and frequently needs to be muzzled, a good idea is to provide the owner with a suitable muzzle to take home. Advise that the muzzle is put on the dog frequently for short periods and that the dog is rewarded with food treats, play, affection, and even walks whilst wearing the muzzle. The dog will then make pleasant associations with wearing the muzzle, making it easier for the owner to put the muzzle on the dog before bringing the dog into the surgery.

KEY POINTS
- Be aware that frightened animals or animals in pain may use aggression to defend themselves.
- Do not scruff a cat unless it is absolutely necessary to do so.
- Always transport cats, rabbits or other small animals securely contained in an appropriate carrier. If dogs are to be walked from one place to another, ensure that they cannot slip out of their collar.
- Use correct lifting technique. Keep the back straight with legs slightly apart and bend at the knees. Always get assistance before trying to lift a heavy or awkward weight (20 kg or over).
- The means of restraint and the amount of control applied are dependent on both the procedure and the reactions of the individual animal. Be firm but gentle, using no more than the minimum amount of restraint necessary.

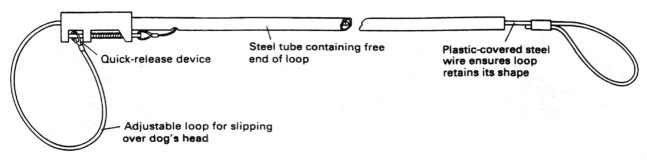

Fig. 1.21 A dog-catcher.

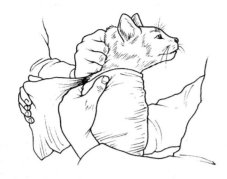

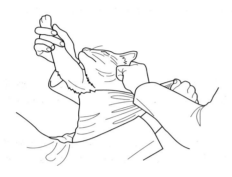

Fig. 1.22 Wrapping a cat for cephalic venepuncture.

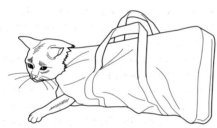

Fig 1.23 A cat-restraining bag.

Further reading

Anderson, R. S. and Edney, A. T. B. (eds) (1991) *Practical Animal Handling*, Pergamon Press, Oxford.

Bessant, C. (1992) *How to Talk to Your Cat*, Smith Gryphon, London.

Bradshaw, J. W. S. (1992) *The Behaviour of the Domestic Cat*, C.A.B. International, Wallingford, Oxon.

Bradshaw, J. W. S. and Nott, H. M. R. (1995) Social and communication behaviour of companion dogs. In Serpell, J. (ed.), *The Domestic Dog: its Evolution, Behaviour and Interactions with People*, Cambridge University Press.

BSAVA (2002) *Manual of Behaviour*, Cheltenham, Glos.

Dunbar, I. (1979) *Dog Behavior: Why Dogs Do What They Do*, T.F.H. Publications, New Jersey.

Fox, M. W. (1971) The comparative ethology of the domestic dog. In *Behaviour of Wolves, Dogs and Related Canids*, pp. 183–214, Jonathan Cape, London.

Heath, S. (2001) Understanding Dominance in Dogs. *Veterinary Nursing*, vol. 16. no. 4, pp. 124–126.

Malley, D. (2000) Handling, restraint and clinical techniques. In Flecknell, P. (ed.), *Manual of Rabbit Medicine and Surgery*, B.S.A.V.A. Quedgeley, Gloucester.

McBride, A. (1995) The Human–Dog relationship. In Robinson, I. (ed.), *The Waltham Book of Human–Animal Interaction: Benefits and responsibilities of pet ownership*, Pergamon, Oxford.

McCune, S. (1992) *Temperament and Welfare of Caged Cats*, PhD Thesis, University of Cambridge (unpublished).

Overall, K. L. (1997) Canine aggression. In *Clinical Behavioral Medicine for Small Animals*, pp. 88–137, Mosby, St. Louis.

2

Anatomy and physiology

Victoria Aspinall and *Melanie O'Reilly*

Learning objectives

After studying this chapter, students should be able to:

- Describe the basic tissues and fluids that make up the mammalian body.
- Describe how the body cavities are organised and their contents.
- Describe the structure of each of the component parts of the body systems.
- Describe the role played by each part of a system and how they interrelate to perform a cohesive function.
- Describe the anatomical relationship between one body system to another.
- Explain the methods by which the body systems contribute to maintaining the balance of the internal environment.

Reference should be made to the further reading list at the end of the chapter to complement this chapter.

Introduction

- **Anatomy** – the study of the structure of the body.
- **Physiology** – the study of how the body actually 'works'.

Dog and cats both belong to the class Mammalia, thus they are covered in hair and suckle their young; they are both carnivores, or flesh eaters. They have a similar anatomical structure, and any differences will be highlighted.

Directional terms

It is essential to understand the terms used to describe the position of the parts of the body in relation to each other (Fig. 2.1).

- **Dorsal** – towards or relatively near to the upper surface of the body, the head, neck, tail and the front surface of the paws.
- **Ventral** – towards or relatively near to the belly and to the corresponding surface of the neck and tail.
- **Lateral** – on the side or outer surface of the body, i.e. away from the median plane, which divides the body longitudinally into two halves.
- **Medial** – towards or relatively near to the median plane (i.e. the 'middle' of the body).
- **Cranial/anterior** – towards or relatively near to the head.
- **Caudal/posterior** – towards or relatively near to the tail.
- **Rostral** – structures on the head only; relates to those near to the nose.

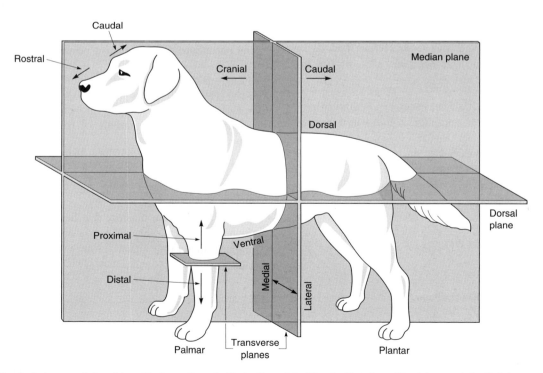

Fig. 2.1 Anatomical planes and directions. (Redrawn from L. Tartaglia and A. Waugh, *Veterinary Physiology and Applied Anatomy*, Butterworth–Heinemann, 2002.)

- **Proximal** – structures near to the main mass of the body or origin, e.g. in the limbs it is the attached end.
- **Distal** – away from the main body mass, e.g. in the limbs it is the free end.
- **Superficial** – relatively near the surface of the body or organ.
- **Deep** – relatively near the centre of the body or organ.

Body fluid compartments

Approximately 60–80% of the body is made of water. The water contains a variety of chemical compounds that are essential for life and it is usually described as 'fluid'. The function of this fluid is to maintain a constant environment in which the normal processes of the body can take place effectively.

Chemical compounds can be divided into two groups:

- **Inorganic compounds** – those that are **not** based on carbon, e.g. sodium, potassium and phosphate.
- **Organic compounds** – those containing **carbon**, e.g. proteins, carbohydrates and fats.

The most important inorganic compound in the body is **water**. The water content of the body is divided between two main compartments – **intracellular fluid** and **extracellular fluid** (Fig. 2.2).

- **Intracellular fluid** (ICF) consists of the fluid found within the **blood cells** and the fluid found within the rest of the **cells of the body.** It occupies 66% of the total body water.
- **Extracellular fluid** (ECF) consists of the fluid part of the blood or the **plasma,** the fluid around the cells or the **interstitial or tissue fluid** and **transcellular fluid** (lymph and cerebrospinal fluid). It occupies 33% of the total body water.

The water content of the body may vary – it is slightly *higher* in young and thin animals and slightly *lower* in overweight animals.

A healthy animal takes water into the body in food and drink and loses water from the body in a number of ways, such as in urine and faeces, and from the respiratory system. Typical daily water losses from a healthy animal are:

- 20 ml per kg bodyweight in **urine.**
- 20 ml per kg bodyweight from the **respiratory system** (i.e. panting etc.).
- 10–20 ml per kg bodyweight in **faeces.**

Under normal circumstances, an animal requires **50–60 ml of water per kg bodyweight per day** to replace the water loss over a 24-hour period.

Within the body, fluids and tissues there are a number of other inorganic compounds. These are called **minerals** and they exist in the body in the form of **ions.**

> An ion is a charged particle. An ion that has one or more *negative* charges is called an **anion**; an ion that has one or more *positive* charges is called a **cation.**

The mineral salts (e.g. sodium chloride) present in the body are ionic compounds, and when they are dissolved in water they split up into their constituent ions (e.g. sodium and chloride). These free ions allow the passage of electric currents and are classed as **electrolytes**.

- Within the **ICF** the main cation is **potassium**, although other cations such as sodium and magnesium are present in smaller amounts. The main anion is **phosphate** with smaller amounts of bicarbonate and chloride. ICF also contains protein.
- Within the **ECF** the main cation is **sodium**, although there are smaller amounts of potassium, calcium and magnesium. The anions present are **chloride, bicarbonate and phosphate.** ECF does not normally contain protein.

Inside the body there is constant movement of water, by osmosis and electrolytes, by diffusion, between the fluid compartments (Fig. 2.3). This movement is dependent on the **osmotic pressure or tonicity** of the ECF – mainly that of plasma and the ICF.

If a fluid has:

- the same tonicity as plasma, it is described as being **isotonic.**
- lower tonicity than plasma, it is described as being **hypotonic.**
- higher tonicity than plasma, it is described as being **hypertonic.**

> The **osmotic pressure or tonicity** of a fluid is the pressure needed to prevent osmosis from occurring and is dependent on the number of particles – both ions and undissolved molecules in a solution.

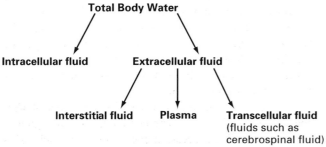

Fig. 2.2 Water distribution in the body.

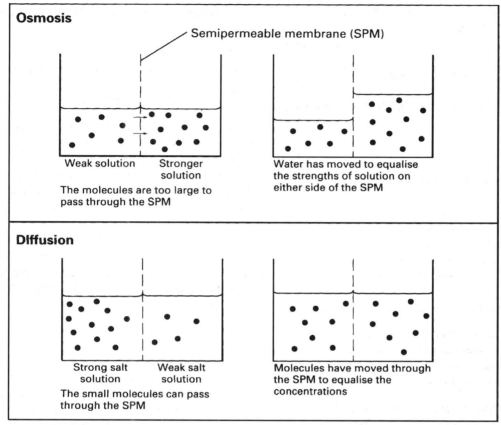

Fig. 2.3 Osmosis and diffusion.

Acid/base balance

> An **acid** is a substance that gives up hydrogen ions when it dissolves or dissociates in water. A **base** or **alkali** is a substance that can combine with the hydrogen ions liberated by the dissociation of an acid.
>
> The hydrogen ion concentration of a solution is expressed as its **pH** and is measured on a scale of 0–14. An **acidic solution** has a pH of less than 7, an **alkaline** (basic) **solution** has a pH that is greater than 7. A neutral solution has a pH of 7.

If the body is to function effectively it is vital that the pH of the blood and the body fluids remains within the normal range. The normal pH of blood is 7.4. Within the body there are several mechanisms that act to maintain this acid/base balance. They are:

(1) Respiration – this controls the levels of carbon dioxide dissolved in the blood. Excess carbon dioxide makes the blood more acid, i.e. it lowers the pH.

(2) Sodium and hydrogen ion exchange within the distal convoluted tubules of the renal nephrons. Excretion of hydrogen ions will raise the pH.

(3) The presence of buffers within the blood plasma.

> A buffer is a substance that can absorb or give up hydrogen ions to keep the pH of a solution within the normal range.

Cell structure

All living organisms are made of cells and these are arranged into tissues and organs.

In highly organised species such as the dog and cat, different types of cell are specialised to carry out separate functions. However, each cell type has certain features in common (Fig. 2.4).

- **Cell or plasma membrane** – this separates the cell from its surrounding environment and controls what enters and leaves the cell. It is said to be selectively permeable, allowing some substances to pass freely through the membrane while others are excluded. The cell membrane is formed by a phospholipid bilayer with protein molecules interspersed within it.

  Cells can take in solid particles by a process of **phagocytosis** or 'cell-eating'. The cell membrane invaginates to form a cup-like depression enclosing the particle. This then seals and pinches off the cell membrane to form a

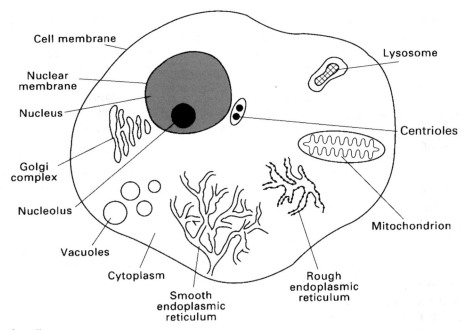

Fig. 2.4 The structure of a cell.

vacuole, which moves into the cell's interior. The vacuole then fuses with a lysosome containing enzymes which break down the contents of the vacuole. Pinocytosis or 'cell-drinking' is the process used for the intake of liquids.

- **Cytoplasm** – this is the aqueous material found within the interior of the cell. The cytoplasm contains the nucleus, organelles and numerous solutes, including glucose, ions and ATP.
- **Nucleus** – this controls the cell's activity and contains the hereditary information of the cell within the chromosomes. The nucleus is bounded by a double membrane that contains a number of pores to allow the entry and exit of molecules. Within the nucleus are one or more nucleoli, which manufacture ribosomes.

Lying within the cytoplasm are a number of **organelles**, which carry out the functions of the cell. They are the:

(1) **Centrioles** – a pair of structures that act as organisers of the nuclear spindle during cell division or mitosis.
(2) **Mitochondria** – these are the sites for cell respiration. They are responsible for the production of **energy** in the form of **ATP** (adenosine triphosphate). Mitochondria have a highly folded inner membrane that increases the surface area on which the processes of respiration take place. When a cell requires energy, a phosphate group is split off the ATP molecule liberating energy. The resulting molecule has only two phosphate groups and is called **ADP** (adenosine diphosphate). The ADP goes back into the respiratory cycle and is used to make ATP again. Mitochondria are found in abundance in cells, which are very active, e.g. skeletal muscle.

$$ATP \leftrightarrow ADP + energy$$

(3) **Ribosomes** – these spherical structures float free in the cytoplasm and are responsible for protein synthesis.
(4) **Endoplasmic reticulum** – an elaborate system of membranes and flattened sacs forming a series of sheets. There are two types:

- **Rough endoplasmic reticulum** has numerous ribosomes attached to its surface. Its function is to synthesise protein and transport it within the cell.
- **Smooth endoplasmic reticulum** has no ribosomes on its surface and its function is to synthesise and transport lipids and steroids.

(5) **Golgi apparatus or body** – consists of a stack of flattened sacs made of membrane. It modifies a number of cell products and plays a part in the formation of lysosomes.
(6) **Lysosomes** – these are membrane-bound sacs that contain digestive enzymes. They digest material phagocytosed by the cell, worn-out organelles and the cell itself when it dies.

Cell division

The cells of the body are able to reproduce and make copies of themselves, enabling the body to grow and repair tissues. There are two types of cell division that take place in the body:

- **Meiosis** – occurs in the germ cells of the ovary and testis (see Chapter 10 on genetics).
- **Mitosis** – occurs in the somatic cells of the body (i.e. all the other cells).

Mitosis (Fig. 2.5) involves the replication of the genetic 'information' or DNA that is carried by the chromosomes in every cell. The cell then divides into two new ones by a process known as binary fission. The resulting 'new' cells are called the **daughter cells** and are identical to each other. When the cell is resting between divisions it is said to be in **interphase**, and it is during this stage that the DNA replicates in preparation for mitotic division.

There are four stages of mitosis:

- **Prophase** – the nuclear membrane breaks down and the chromosomes become shorter and fatter and more visible. The chromosomes consist of two **chromatids** held together at the centre by a **centromere**. The centrioles of the cell migrate, one to each pole of the cell, and from them **spindle fibres** form.
- **Metaphase** – the chromosomes arrange themselves along the equator of the cell and attach to the spindle fibres, which start to pull the chromatids apart.
- **Anaphase** – the spindle fibres contract and pull the chromatids apart, moving them to the opposite ends of the cell.
- **Telophase** – the spindle fibres disintegrate and a nuclear membrane forms around the chromosomes. The cytoplasm divides forming two new 'daughter' cells, each containing an identical set of chromosomes. The nuclear membrane reforms, the chromosomes then unravel and the cell goes into **interphase** again.

A **tissue** is a collection of cells and their products in which one cell predominates. An **organ** is a collection of tissues, which performs or is adapted for a specific purpose. A **system** is a collection of parts, structures, tissues and organs, which are related by function.

Basic tissue types

The body contains four types of tissue, each of which is highly specialised to carry out a particular function. They are:

- **Epithelial.**
- **Connective.**
- **Muscular.**
- **Nervous.**

Muscular and nervous tissues will be discussed later in this chapter, in the sections on muscles and the nervous system.

Epithelial tissue

Epithelial tissue covers the inner and outer surfaces of the body, e.g. skin, organs, body cavities and blood vessels (Table 2.1). Epithelial tissue consists of single or layered sheets of cells held together by an intercellular substance.

The bottom layer of cells sits on a basement membrane. A single sheet of epithelium is described as **simple**; when it is layered it is described as **stratified**. Epithelial cells may be further described by their cell shape:

- **cuboidal** – cube shaped.
- **squamous** – flattened.
- **columnar** – tall and column-like.

Epithelial tissue may also contain specialised cells, called **goblet cells**, which produce **mucus.** It may also possess hair-like structures or **cilia** on its surface, which project from the free edge of the epithelial layer and waft the mucus along the surface of the epithelium. Mucus is a proteinaceous secretion that serves to protect the surface of the tissue.

All glandular tissue in the body is derived from epithelial tissue and they may be unicellular (e.g. goblet cells) or multicellular (Fig. 2.6).

Connective tissue

Connective tissue is responsible for supporting and binding together all the tissues and organs of the body. It also acts as a transport system carrying nutrients around the body and removing waste materials.

Connective tissue consists of a **ground substance or matrix** that has cells and fibres embedded within it. There are five categories of connective tissue in the body:

- **Loose connective tissue** – areolar and adipose tissue.
- **Dense connective tissue** – tendons and ligaments.
- **Cartilage.**
- **Bone.**
- **Blood.**

Loose connective tissue (Fig. 2.7)

Areolar tissue is found all over the body – beneath the skin, connecting organs and as the 'packing' material in the spaces between tissues. It consists of a ground substance containing cells known as fibroblasts and macrophages, and collagen and elastic fibres.

Adipose (fatty) tissue is similar to areolar tissue but it contains numerous closely packed **fat cells**. Fat is important for the storage of energy and for the insulation of the body.

Dense connective tissue (Fig. 2.7)

This contains a large number of fibres in proportion to cells in the matrix and may be known as fibrous connective tissue. In **tendons** the matrix contains densely packed collagen fibres arranged in parallel, giving great tensile strength. **Ligaments** (yellow elastic tissue) contain a large number of elastic fibres, giving them strength and elasticity.

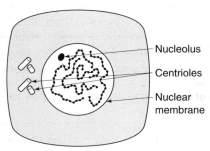

A Interphase

Cell has normal appearance of
non-dividing cell condition:
chromosomes too threadlike
for clear visibility.

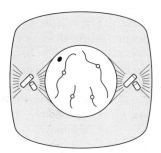

B Early prophase

Chromosomes become visible as
they contract, and nucleolus shrinks.
Centrioles at opposite sides of the
nucleus. Spindle fibres start to form.

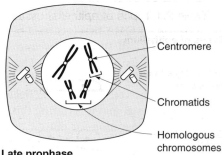

C Late prophase

Chromosomes become shorter and
fatter—each seen to consist of a pair
of chromatids joined at the centromere.
Nucleolus disappears. Prophase ends
with breakdown of nuclear membrane.

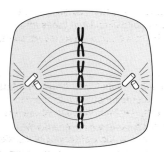

D Early metaphase

Chromosomes arrange themselves
on equator of spindle. Note that
homologous chromosomes do
not associate.

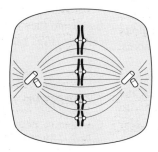

E Late metaphase

Chromatids draw apart at the
centromere region. Note that
the daughter centromeres are
orientated toward opposite
poles of the spindle.

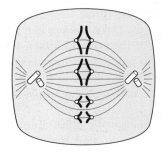

F Early anaphase

Chromatids part company and
migrate to opposite poles of cell,
the centromeres leading.

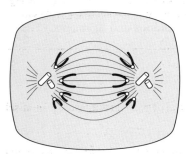

G Late anaphase

Chromosomes reach their destination.

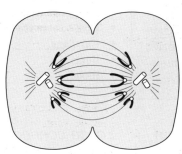

H Early telophase

The cell starts to constrict across the middle.

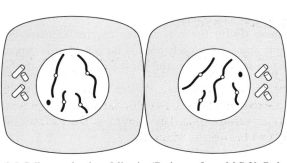

I Late telophase

Constriction continues. Nuclear membrane
and nucleolus reformed in each daughter
cell. Spindle apparatus degenerates.
Chromosomes eventually regain their
threadlike form and the cells return to
resting condition (interphase).

**Note that the daughter cells have
precisely the same chromosome
constitution as the original parent cell.**

Fig. 2.5 Cell reproduction: Mitosis. (Redrawn from M.B.V. Roberts, *Biology: a Functional Approach*, 4th edn, Nelson, 1986.)

Table 2.1 Types of epithelial tissue		
Types of epithelium		**Description/function**
Simple squamous epithelium	cells basement membrane	Composed of a single sheet of very thin, flat cells. The sheet of cells is thin and delicate, and is found in areas where diffusion occurs (e.g. **alveoli of lungs, lining blood vessels, Bowman's capsule**)
Simple cuboidal epithelium		This type of epithelium is found lining many of the **glands** and their **ducts**, and also lining parts of the **kidney tubules**
Simple columnar epithelium		This type of epithelium is found lining the **intestine** allowing the absorption of soluble food material
Ciliated epithelium	cilia goblet cells	Usually columnar in shape. It has numerous cilia on the free surface of each cell. This type of epithelium lines tubes and cavities where materials must be moved (e.g. **respiratory tract, oviducts**)
Stratified epithelium		Comprises a series of layers making it tough and it therefore has a protective function. It is found in areas that are subjected to friction (e.g. **oesophagus, mouth, vagina**). In areas where it is subject to considerable abrasion the cells are infiltrated with a tough protein called **keratin**, as seen in the **epidermis** of the skin
Transitional epithelium		A modified form of stratified epithelium. Found in structures that must be able to stretch (e.g. **bladder, urethra**)
Glandular epithelium	 Mucus-secreting cell	This type of epithelium has interspersed secretory cells, which secrete materials into the cavity or space they are lining. Folding of glandular epithelium results in the formation of a gland (see Fig. 2.6 for examples)

Cartilage (Fig. 2.8)

Cartilage consists of a matrix called **chondrin** with cells or **chondrocytes** and collagen fibres embedded within it. Cartilage is strong but resilient and flexible. It has no blood supply but its nutrition is supplied by the fibrous connective tissue **perichondrium** covering its surface. There are three types of cartilage:

- **Hyaline cartilage.**
- **Elastic cartilage.**
- **Fibrocartilage.**

Hyaline cartilage is the simplest form of cartilage and forms the **articular surfaces** of bones within joints, and the **rings of the trachea.**

Elastic cartilage has a higher number of elastic fibres and is found in areas where support with flexibility is required, e.g. **external ear** and **epiglottis of the larynx.**

Fibrocartilage has a higher number of collagen fibres within its matrix than hyaline cartilage and is very strong. It occurs where tough support or tensile strength is required. Fibrocartilage contributes to the structure of the **interverteb-** **ral discs** and forms the **intra-articular cartilages,** e.g. menisci in stifle joint.

Bone and blood will be discussed later in the skeletal and blood vascular systems.

The body cavities

The body is divided into three separate cavities, which are only potential spaces as they are filled with the visceral structures and a little fluid. All the body cavities are lined with a **serous membrane** – an epithelial lining that produces a watery or serous fluid. This lubricates the surfaces of the cavity and the organs within it.

- The serous membrane lining the boundaries of the cavity is described as **parietal,** e.g. parietal pleura.
- The serous membrane covering the organs within the cavity is described as **visceral,** e.g. visceral peritoneum.

The three body cavities are as follows.

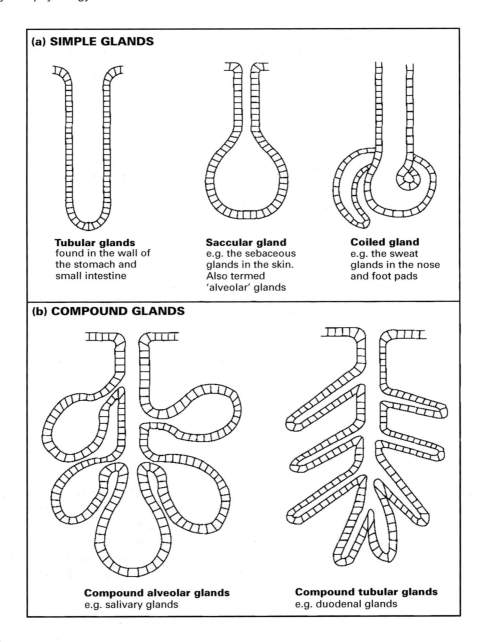

Fig. 2.6 Glands.

The thoracic cavity

This is contained within the bony thoracic cage (Fig. 2.9). The serous membrane lining the thoracic cavity is called the **pleura**. The different regions of the pleura are named according to their position within the thoracic cavity – the **diaphragmatic pleura** covers the diaphragm, the **costal pleura** covers the inside of the ribs and the **pulmonary pleura** covers the lungs.

The boundaries of the thoracic cavity are:

- *Cranially* – the thoracic inlet.
- *Caudally* – the diaphragm.
- *Dorsally* – the bodies of the thoracic vertebrae and hypaxial muscle.
- *Ventrally* – the sternum.
- *Laterally* – the ribs and intercostal muscles.

The thoracic cavity (Fig. 2.9) is divided into right and left **pleural cavities** by a double layer of pleura called the **mediastinum**. The mediastinum contains the pericardial cavity surrounding the heart. Each pleural cavity contains one of the lungs and a small amount of **pleural fluid** to prevent the organs rubbing each other. The lungs are covered in visceral pleura called the **pulmonary pleura.**

The abdominal cavity

The abdominal cavity is lined by a serous membrane called the **peritoneum**, which is a continuous sheet forming a closed cavity – the **peritoneal cavity**. The abdominal cavity is filled with the abdominal viscera or organs and the peritoneal cavity is the potential space between the layers of the peri-

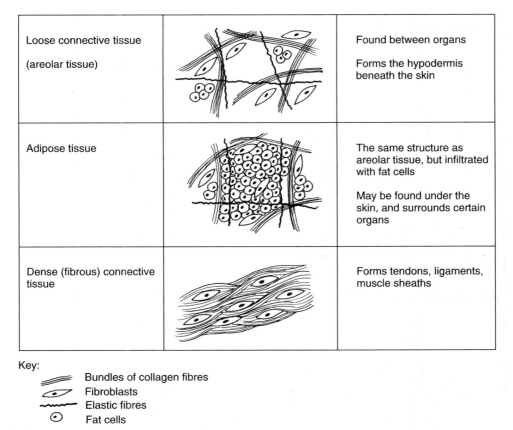

Loose connective tissue (areolar tissue)		Found between organs Forms the hypodermis beneath the skin
Adipose tissue		The same structure as areolar tissue, but infiltrated with fat cells May be found under the skin, and surrounds certain organs
Dense (fibrous) connective tissue		Forms tendons, ligaments, muscle sheaths

Key:
≡ Bundles of collagen fibres
⬭ Fibroblasts
∿ Elastic fibres
⊙ Fat cells

Fig. 2.7 Connective tissues.

toneum covering the body wall and the organs in the abdomen. The peritoneal cavity is filled only with a little serous fluid called **peritoneal fluid** (i.e. it contains no organs). This acts as a lubricant and prevents adhesions forming between the layers of the peritoneum and the organs. The boundaries of the abdominal cavity are:

- *Cranially* – the diaphragm.
- *Caudally* – the pelvic inlet (the abdominal and pelvic cavities are continuous and not separated by a physical barrier).
- *Dorsally* – lumbar vertebrae and hypaxial muscle.
- *Ventrally* – ventral abdominal wall muscle.
- *Laterally* – lateral abdominal wall muscle.

The **parietal peritoneum** lines the abdominal cavity, while the **visceral peritoneum** covers the surface of the organs within the abdomen. The peritoneum has folds that separate the organs and carry blood vessels and nerves to and from the viscera. There are different names for these folds depending on their position, for example **mesentery** and **omentum**.

The pelvic cavity

The pelvic cavity is continuous with the abdominal cavity and the cranial part is also lined with **peritoneum**. The boundaries of the pelvic cavity are:

- *Cranially* – the pelvic cavity is continuous with the abdominal cavity but a bony ring referred to as the pelvic inlet forms the entrance to it.
- *Caudally* – the pelvic outlet (bony ring that forms the caudal border of the pelvic cavity) and pelvic diaphragm (consists of the set of muscles that closes the caudal end of the pelvic cavity).
- *Dorsally* – the sacrum.
- *Ventrally* – floor of the pelvis.
- *Laterally* – lateral walls of the pelvis.

The skeletal system

The skeletal system consists of bones, cartilages and joints, and is the supportive 'frame' of the body. The functions of the skeletal system are to:

1. Provide attachment for the muscles enabling the animal and its parts to move – **locomotion.**
2. Provide **protection** for the organs and the soft parts of the body.
3. Form blood cells by the bone marrow in the long bones – known as **haemopoiesis.**
4. Provide a **reservoir** of some of the body's essential minerals, e.g. calcium and phosphorus.

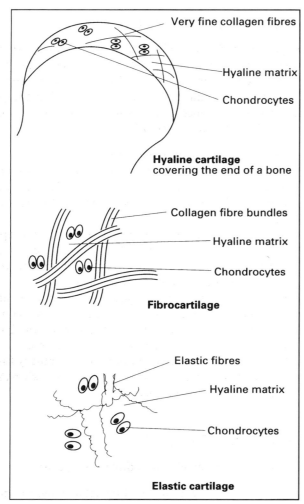

Fig. 2.8 Types of cartilage.

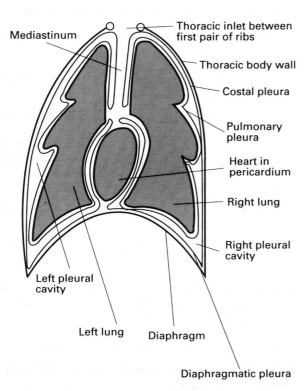

Fig. 2.9 Horizontal section through the thorax.

Bone tissue

Bone is a specialised type of rigid connective tissue consisting of cells or **osteocytes** in a matrix composed mainly of **calcium phosphate**, which gives bone its distinctive rigidity and hardness (Fig. 2.10). **Collagen** fibres are also found in bone tissue, contributing to its strength and resilience. These components are arranged in concentric circles, called **lamellae**, around a central channel or **Haversian canal** containing the blood vessels, nerves and lymphatic vessels. There are spaces in the lamellae called **lacunae** that contain the osteocytes. The whole system is referred to as a **Haversian system** (Fig. 2.10).

There are two types of bone tissue:

- **Compact bone** – the Haversian systems of compact bone are densely packed together. Compact bone is found in the outer edge or **cortex** of all types of bone (Fig 2.10).
- **Cancellous or spongy bone** – this is lighter than compact bone and has a network of interconnected 'bars', called **trabeculae**, providing a 'honeycomb' appearance.

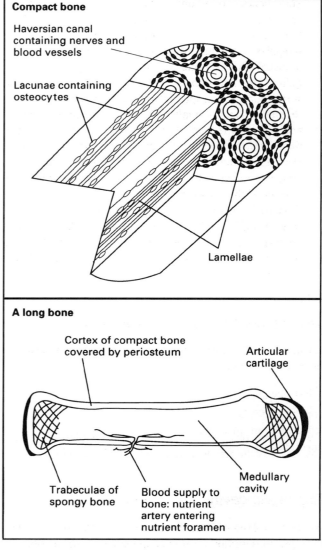

Fig. 2.10 The structure of bone.

Cancellous bone is found at the ends of long bones and in the core of all other types of bone (e.g. flat, irregular) (Fig. 2.10).

All bones are covered by a fibrous connective tissue layer – the **periosteum**. Blood reaches the bone via a **nutrient artery**, which enters through a **nutrient foramen**.

Classification of bone

Bones can be classified according to their shape:

1. **Long bones** – most of the bones of the limbs. They act as levers to facilitate movement and have a long cylindrical shape with a shaft (**diaphysis**) containing a **medullary cavity**. The two ends of a long bone (**epiphyses**) consist of cancellous bone, with a layer of compact bone at the edges (Fig. 2.10).
2. **Flat bones** – many of the bones of the skull, the ribs and scapula. These bones have broad flat surfaces. They consist of compact bone at their outer edges, with a core of cancellous bone.
3. **Short bones** – found only in the carpus and tarsus. These are small 'cubes' of bone that have a core of cancellous bone covered by a layer of compact bone on the surface.
4. **Irregular** – includes vertebrae and some of the more 'unusual' shaped bones of the skull. They have an irregular form and consist of a core of cancellous bone surrounded by compact bone on their surface.
5. **Sesamoid bones** – small bones that develop in tendons and are 'sesame-seed' shaped. The function is to reduce the friction and wear on a tendon, by altering the angle at which the tendon passes over a joint, e.g. the **patella**, which contributes to the stifle joint and is found in the tendon of the quadriceps femoris muscle.
6. **Pneumatic bones** – bones that contain air, e.g. the frontal and maxillary bones of the skull contain air-filled cavities called **sinuses**. These enable the bone to maintain its strength while remaining lightweight.

Development of bone – ossification

The process by which bone develops is called **ossification.** There are two types:

- **Intramembranous**.
- **Endochondral**.

The cells that produce bone are called **osteoblasts**, the cells that reabsorb or remodel bone are called **osteoclasts**.

Intramembranous ossification

Many of the bones of the skull develop by this process. The bone develops within a fibrous connective tissue membrane, without a cartilage model.

Endochondral ossification

This type of ossification (Fig. 2.11) is the means by which the long bones develop and involves the replacement of a cartilage model within the embryo, by bone. The process is not fully completed until the animal has reached maturity.

The process of endochondral ossification in a long bone occurs in the following stages (Fig. 2.11):

(a) The cartilage model forms in the foetus.
(b) Primary centres of ossification appear in the diaphysis of the bone as the osteoblasts start to replace the cartilage with bone. This progresses towards the ends of the bone.
(c) Secondary centres of ossification appear in the epiphyses or ends of the bone. The medullary cavity is formed by the action of osteoclasts reabsorbing the bone tissue in the centre of the diaphysis.
(d) Between the developing diaphysis and epiphyses are two bands of cartilage – one at each end of the bone. These are the epiphyseal or growth plates, which allow for elongation of the bone as the animal grows.
(e,f) The epiphyses are replaced by bone and eventually fuse after which no further growth is possible – i.e. when the animal reaches its adult size.

The skeleton (Fig. 2.12)

The skeleton can be divided into three main parts:

- **Axial** – bones of the head, vertebral column and the ribs and sternum.
- **Appendicular** – bones of the limbs.
- **Splanchnic** – bones that develop within soft tissues.

In order to describe bones it is important to understand the descriptive terminology of the skeletal system.

- **Foramen** (pl. foramina) – a hole in a bone to allow the passage of blood vessels and nerves.
- **Fossa** – a hollow or depressed area on the surface of a bone.
- **Head** – a spherical articular surface on the proximal end of a long bone. The head is joined to the **shaft** of the bone by a narrowed region called the **neck.**
- **Condyle** – a rounded articular surface on a bone.
- **Epicondyle** – a prominence on a bone, lying above a condyle.
- **Trochlea** – a bony structure through or over which tendons pass; e.g. a groove in a bone in which a tendon, acting as a pulley, runs.
- **Tuberosity/trochanter/tubercle** – names given to the various protuberances on bones. They are usually sites for muscle attachment.

A **tendon** attaches a muscle to a bone; a **ligament** connects bone to bone.

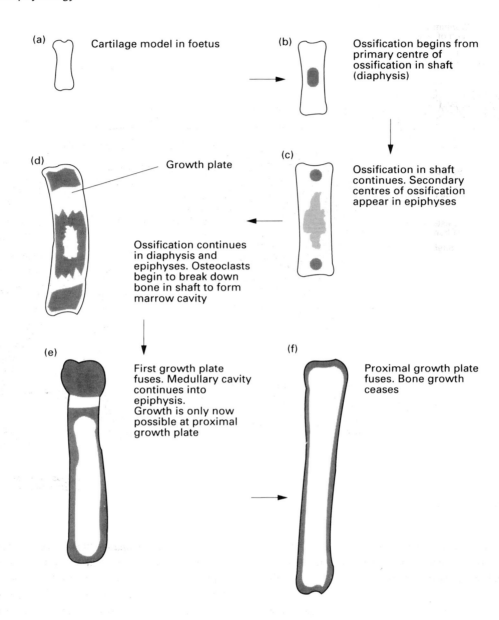

(a) Cartilage model in foetus

(b) Ossification begins from primary centre of ossification in shaft (diaphysis)

(c) Ossification in shaft continues. Secondary centres of ossification appear in epiphyses

(d) Growth plate

Ossification continues in diaphysis and epiphyses. Osteoclasts begin to break down bone in shaft to form marrow cavity

(e) First growth plate fuses. Medullary cavity continues into epiphysis. Growth is only now possible at proximal growth plate

(f) Proximal growth plate fuses. Bone growth ceases

Fig. 2.11 Endochondral ossification of a long bone.

The axial skeleton (Fig. 2.12)

This forms the axis of the body and runs from the skull to the tip of the tail. It consists of the skull, the vertebral column, the ribs and the sternum.

The skull

This consists of a bony **cranium** that houses and protects the brain, and the **maxilla**, which forms the upper jaw containing the teeth and **nasal chambers**. The skull houses the sense organs and provides attachment for the lower jaw or **mandible,** and the **hyoid apparatus**.

The skull consists of a number of bones joined together by immovable fibrous joints called **sutures.** The bones of the skull, some paired and some single, fit very closely together forming a single rigid structure. In the adult the suture lines are almost invisible.

The **shape** of an animal's skull varies between species, and in the case of the dog, even between breeds. There are three morphological forms that are generally recognised, with the difference mainly being expressed in the facial region of the skull:

- **Mesaticephalic** – the 'normal' type of skull, i.e. that which has changed the least from the 'wild type' of skull seen in the ancestor of the dog, the wolf. This type of skull is seen in the labrador and beagle.
- **Doliocephalic** – this skull is long and narrow and is seen in the greyhound, borzoi and afghan hound.
- **Brachycephalic** – this skull is short, broad and 'flat' in the facial region and is seen in the boxer, pug and pekingese.

Skull bones

- **Cranium** – two **parietal** bones form the dorsolateral walls and meet the **occipital** bone which forms the caudoventral surface of the skull (Fig. 2.13). Within the occipital bone is a large hole – the **foramen magnum,**

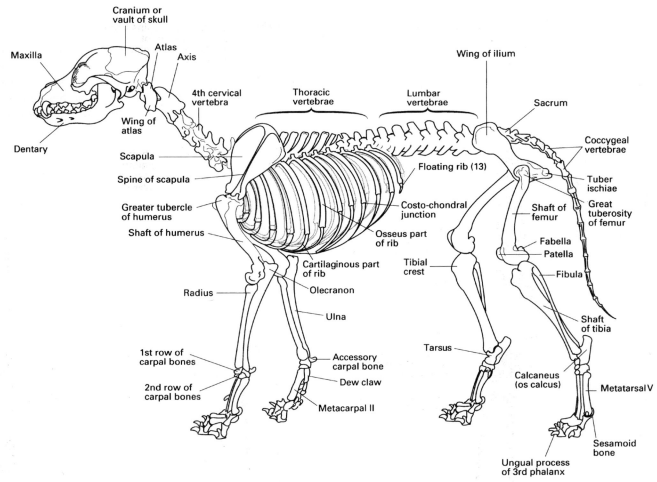

Fig. 2.12 The skeleton of a dog.

which allows the spinal cord to leave the cranium. On either side of the foramen magnum are the **occipital condyles**, which articulate with the first cervical vertebra – the **atlas**.

The front of the cranium is formed by the **frontal** bones, which contain the air-filled **frontal sinus.** The two **temporal** bones lie ventral to the parietal bones on the lateral surface. On the ventral aspect of the temporal

bones are the **tympanic bullae**, which house the middle ear. The **external acoustic meatus** is an opening in the tympanic bulla that is covered by the **tympanic membrane**, or ear drum, in life, and is the point to which the external ear canal attaches to the skull.

The ventral surface (Fig. 2.14) of the cranium is formed by the **sphenoid** bone with the **ethmoid** bone lying rostral to it.

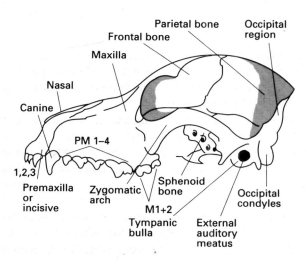

Fig. 2.13 Lateral view of a dog skull.

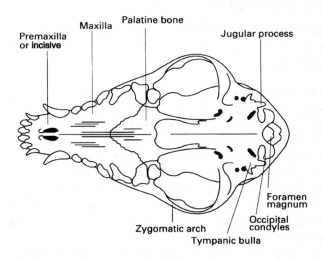

Fig. 2.14 Ventral view of a dog skull.

The **zygomatic** bones form the arch on either side of the skull often called the 'cheekbones'. The **orbit** is the socket in which the eyeball sits. The **lacrimal** bone lies at the base of the orbit and is penetrated by a foramen through which the nasolacrimal duct runs from the eye into the nasal chamber.

- **Nasal chambers** – the **nasal** bones form the roof of the two chambers, which are divided by the **nasal septum**. Each chamber is filled with fine scrolls of bone covered in ciliated mucous epithelium – the **ethmoturbinates**, or **conchae**. The floor of the chambers is formed by the **maxilla**, the **palatine** and the **incisive** bones, which also form the roof of the mouth.

The whole structure is penetrated by many foramina to allow for the passage of the numerous nerves and blood vessels that enter and leave the skull.

- **Mandible** (Fig. 2.15) – this is the lower jaw which attaches to the temporal region of the skull at the **temporomandibular joint**. The right and left mandibles are joined together by a cartilaginous joint called the **mandibular symphysis**. Each mandible consists of a horizontal **body** that houses the **alveoli or sockets** for the teeth and a vertical **ramus** to which the jaw muscles attach. Caudally, an articular surface, the **condylar process**, forms part of the temporomandibular joint.
- **Hyoid apparatus** – this is composed of a number of fine bones joined together in a trapeze-like structure by cartilage. It lies in the neck and is attached to the temporal bone by a cartilaginous joint. The tongue is attached to one side and the larynx to the other side (see Fig. 2.39 in the section on the respiratory system).

The vertebrae   The **vertebral column** or spine consists of a number of **vertebrae** arranged in series in the midline of the body. Its function is to provide a stiff but flexible rod to support the body. It is divided into a number of regions, each of which has a constant number of vertebrae:

- **Cervical or neck** – always seven vertebrae.
- **Thoracic or chest** – 13 or 14 vertebrae in the dog and cat.
- **Lumbar or lower back** – six or seven vertebrae.
- **Sacral** – three fused vertebrae.
- **Coccygeal or caudal** – varies according to length of tail.

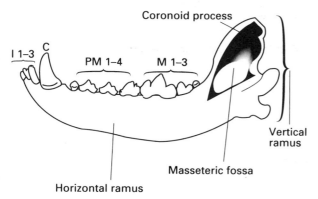

Fig. 2.15 Lateral view of the mandible.

All vertebrae share a basic structural plan. On the ventral aspect of a typical vertebra is the **body** that makes up the bulk of the vertebrae. Above it is the **neural arch** forming the **vertebral foramen**. When the vertebrae are linked together, the vertebral foramina form the **spinal canal** through which the spinal cord passes. Projecting dorsally from the neural arch is a **spinous process**, and projecting laterally are two **transverse processes**. These processes act as sites for muscle attachment and vary in size in the different regions. On the cranial and caudal ends of the neural arch are **articular processes** that form joints with the adjacent vertebrae.

Lying between the bodies of each vertebra are fibrocartilaginous 'shock-absorbers', called **intervertebral discs**. The outer part of the disc is fibrous, the **annulus fibrosus**, while the inner part contains a gelatinous material called the **nucleus pulposus** (Fig. 2.16).

The vertebrae of each region (Fig. 2.17) of the vertebral column show distinguishing features:

- **Cervical vertebrae**:
  - **Atlas**, or first cervical vertebra, consists only of two large lateral wing-like processes, joined by ventral and dorsal arches. The atlas articulates with the occipital condyles of the skull in a synovial joint which allows the head to nod.
  - **Axis**, or the second cervical vertebra has a blade-like spinous process and a cranial projection – the **dens**, or **odontoid process**. This articulates with the atlas and allows a rotating movement.
  - The remaining five cervical vertebrae are similar to each other and follow the basic plan.

- **Thoracic vertebrae**: each thoracic vertebra has a short body and a distinctively tall spinous process. They have short transverse processes that have **fovea** for articulation with the **tubercle** of the rib. The bodies of thoracic vertebrae also have fovea for articulation with the **head** of the rib (Fig. 2.18).
- **Lumbar vertebrae**: lumbar vertebrae have longer bodies than thoracic vertebrae and their transverse processes are large and angled cranioventrally.
- **Sacral vertebrae**: there are **three** sacral vertebrae fused to form the **sacrum**. This articulates with **ilium** of the pelvis forming the **sacroiliac joint**.
- **Coccygeal vertebrae**: the first few coccygeal vertebrae have a regular shape but they get progressively smaller and simpler towards the tip of the tail.

The ribs   There are **thirteen pairs** of ribs in the cat and dog, which articulate with the thoracic vertebrae (Fig. 2.18). Each rib has a dorsal **bony** part, which articulates with the appropriate vertebra, and a ventral **cartilaginous** part – the **costal cartilage**. The costal cartilages of ribs 1–8 articulate with the sternum and are called **sternal ribs**. The costal cartilages of ribs 9–12 touch the cartilage of the rib in front forming the **costal arch** – these are called **asternal ribs**. The last pair of ribs

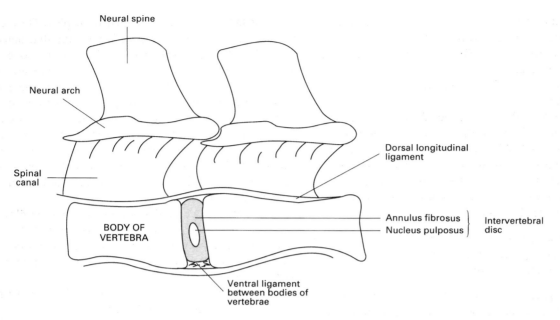

Fig. 2.16 Section through two lumbar vertebrae.

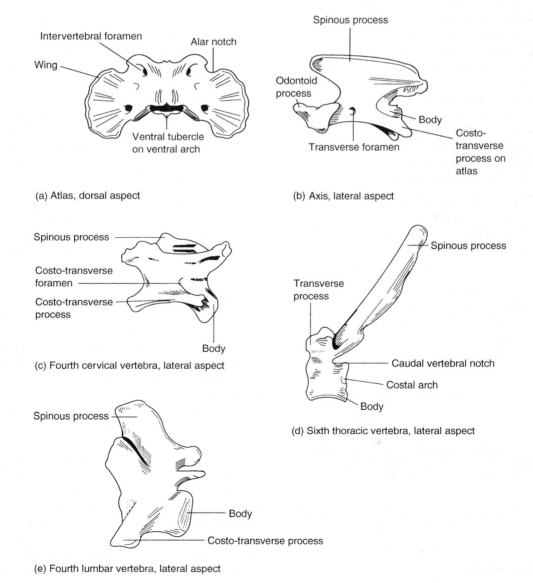

(a) Atlas, dorsal aspect

(b) Axis, lateral aspect

(c) Fourth cervical vertebra, lateral aspect

(d) Sixth thoracic vertebra, lateral aspect

(e) Fourth lumbar vertebra, lateral aspect

Fig. 2.17 Regional differences in vertebrae structure.

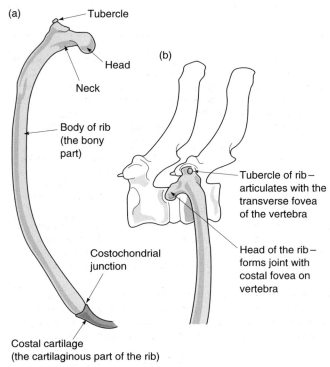

(a)

— Tubercle

Head

Neck

Body of rib
(the bony
part)

(b)

Costochondrial
junction

Tubercle of rib –
articulates with the
transverse fovea
of the vertebra

Head of the rib –
forms joint with
costal fovea on
vertebra

Costal cartilage
(the cartilaginous part of the rib)

Fig. 2.18 Structure of a rib and rib articulation. (Redrawn from Dyce, Sack and Wensing, *Textbook of Veterinary Anatomy*, 2nd edn, W.B. Saunders, 1996.)

(13) do not articulate with the cartilages of the other ribs and their cartilaginous ends lie free in the muscle wall – these are referred to as the '**floating ribs**'. This arrangement creates the rib cage.

The sternum   This is composed of eight bones called the **sternebrae**. The most cranial sternebra is called the **manubrium** and lies in the cranial thoracic inlet. The most caudal sternebra is called the **xiphoid process**, which has a flap of cartilage called the **xiphoid cartilage** attached to it.

The appendicular skeleton

This consists of the fore and hind limbs and the pectoral and pelvic girdles, which attach the limbs to the axial skeleton (Tables 2.2 and 2.3).

The splanchnic skeleton

The only example of a splanchnic bone in the dog and cat is the bone of the penis – the **os penis**. The urethra lies in the **urethral groove** on the ventral surface of the os penis in the dog. In the cat the urethral groove is on the dorsal surface of the os penis, due to the different orientation of the penis (see Reproductive System, p. 72).

Joints

A joint or **arthrosis** is the point where two or more bones join together. Joints allow varying degrees of movement and can be classified according to their structure:

- Fibrous joints.
- Cartilaginous joints.
- Synovial joints

Table 2.2 The bones of the forelimb

Name	Description
Scapula	A flat bone, roughly triangular in shape. Has a prominent **spine** dividing the lateral surface into two fossae (the (**supraspinous fossa** and **infraspinous fossa**). At the distal end of the spine is a projection called the **acromion**. The articular socket at the end of the bone is the **glenoid cavity**
Clavicle	Most usually absent in the dog and when present is just a remnant of bone in the muscle cranial to the shoulder. The clavicle is normally present in the cat but does not articulate with any other bones.
Humerus	A long bone. Has an articular **head** proximally and a long **body** or shaft. At the proximal end are two prominences, the **greater** and **lesser tubercles**, which are sites for muscle attachment. The distal articular surface is the **condyle**, which has a depression, called the **olecranon fossa** and a hole in the centre called the **supratrochlear foramen**
Radius	A long bone that lies alongside the ulna in the forearm. Proximally the depressed articular surface is called the **fovea capitis** (articulates with the humerus). At the distal end there is a rounded projection called the **styloid process** that articulates with the carpus
Ulna	Longer than the radius and has an irregular shape, tapering from its proximal to its distal end. Proximally there is a half-moon-shaped articular surface called the **trochlear notch**, with a hooked projection called the **anconeal process** at its proximal end. At the distal end of the notch are the **medial** and **lateral coronoid processes**). The 'point' of the elbow is formed by the **olecranon**
Carpals	Consists of seven short bones arranged in two rows. The proximal row contains three bones, one of them, the **accessory carpal bone**, projects caudally
Metacarpals	There are five metacarpal bones (I–V), which are small rods of bone. The most medial, metacarpal I, differs from the others as it is shorter and non-weight-bearing (forms part of **dew claw**)
Digits	Digits II–V are composed of three phalangeal bones – a proximal, middle and distal phalanx. Digit I (the dew claw) has only two phalangeal bones. The distal phalanx of each digit bears the **ungual process** that extends into the claw

Table 2.3 Bones of the hindlimb	
Name	**Description**
Pelvis	The pelvis consists of two hipbones joined together ventrally at the **pelvic symphysis**. The pelvis articulates with the sacrum dorsally at the **sacroiliac joints**. Each hipbone is composed of three fused bones – the **ilium**, the **ischium** and the **pubis**. The ilium is the largest bone and has a cranial expansion called the **iliac wing**. The ischium is the most caudal pelvic bone and has a prominent caudolateral margin called the **ischiatic tuberosity**. The pubis is the smallest of the bones and forms the cranial portion of the pelvic floor. The three bones unite at the articular socket of the pelvis, called the **acetabulum**, which articulates with the head of the femur via a ball and socket joint. On either side of the pelvic symphysis are two large holes, each being called the **obturator foramen**
Femur	The thigh bone is a typical long bone. Proximally it has an articular **head**, which attaches to the shaft by the **neck**. There is a projection on the proximal femur, lateral to the head, called the **greater trochanter**, and another lies medial to the head, called the **lesser trochanter**. These are sites for muscle attachment. The distal end of the bone has three articular surfaces – the **medial condyle** and **lateral condyle** articulate with the **tibia**, and between them is a smooth groove called the **trochlea** that articulates with the **patella**
Patella and fabellae	These sesamoid bones are associated with the stifle joint. The **patella** is the largest sesamoid bone in the body and is incorporated into the tendon of the quadriceps femoris muscle that runs down the front of the thigh. The patella articulates with the trochlea of the distal femur. The **fabellae** are two smaller sesamoid bones that articulate with the femoral condyles caudally in the stifle joint. The fabellae are located in the tendons of the gastrocnemius muscle
Tibia	The tibia is a long bone and is the main weight-bearing bone of the lower leg. The tibia is expanded proximally providing a wide articular surface for the femur at the stifle joint. Proximally there is a cranially projecting process called the **tibial tuberosity**, which is the point of insertion of the quadriceps femoris muscle. The tibial tuberosity continues distally as a ridge called the **tibial crest**. At the distal end of the tibia is an articular surface and a palpable process called the **medial malleolus**
Fibula	This is a thin long bone that lies lateral to the tibia. At the distal end there is a prominent bony bulge on the lateral surface of the ankle called the **lateral malleolus**
Tarsals	The **tarsus** (hock) comprises seven **tarsal bones** arranged in three rows. The proximal row contains the **talus** medially and the **calcaneus** laterally. The calcaneus is extended caudally to form the 'point' of the hock (**tuber calcis**) and serves as a site for the attachment of muscles
Metatarsals	Similar to the metacarpus except that there are only four metarsal bones (although some breeds have a small metatarsal I forming the hind dew claw)
Digits	Similar to the digits in the forepaw but only four digits (II–V) present

Fibrous joints

The bones forming fibrous joints are united by dense fibrous connective tissue which allows very little movement. Most fibrous joints are found in the skull, between the flat bones, and are called **sutures**. They are also responsible for attaching the tooth to the bone of its socket.

Cartilaginous joints

The bones forming cartilaginous joints are connected by cartilage and allow little or no movement. They are seen in joints connecting opposite sides of the body and include the **pelvic symphysis** between the two hip bones, and the **mandibular symphysis** between the two halves of the mandible.

Synarthrosis – a joint that allows little or no movement. Includes fibrous and cartilaginous joints.
Amphiarthrosis – a joint that allows some movement. This type of joint is found between the bodies of the vertebrae.

Synovial joints

Synovial joints (or **diarthroses**) allow a wide range of movement (Fig. 2.19). A fluid-filled space – the **joint cavity**, which is filled with synovial fluid, separates the bones. A dense

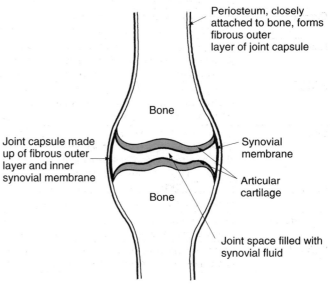

Periosteum, closely attached to bone, forms fibrous outer layer of joint capsule

Bone

Joint capsule made up of fibrous outer layer and inner synovial membrane

Synovial membrane

Articular cartilage

Bone

Joint space filled with synovial fluid

Fig. 2.19 A synovial joint.

fibrous connective tissue **capsule** surrounds the whole joint. The outer layer serves as protection, while the inner layer, or **synovial membrane**, lines the joint cavity and secretes synovial fluid, which lubricates the joint. The articular surfaces of the bones are covered by **hyaline cartilage**.

Synovial joints may be stabilised by **ligaments**. The most common are found on either side of the joint – **collateral ligaments**. Some synovial joints have stabilising ligaments attached to the articulating bones within the joint – **intracapsular ligaments**, e.g. the cruciate ligament within the stifle joint (Fig. 2.20).

Inside a few synovial joints are one or more fibrocartilaginous **menisci**, e.g. the stifle joint has two, while the temporomandibular joint has one (Fig. 2.20). These structures help to increase the range of movement of the joint and act as 'shock absorbers'.

Synovial joints allow a wide range of movement between the articulating bones. The motion may be in a single plane or in multiple directions. The types of movement that can occur at synovial joints are:

- **Gliding** – one articular surface slides over the other.
- **Flexion** – reduces the angle between the bones (i.e. bends the limb).
- **Extension** – increases the angle between the bones (i.e. straightens the limb).
- **Abduction** – carries the moving part away from the median plane of the body, e.g. when a dog 'cocks' its leg to urinate.
- **Adduction** – brings the body part back towards the median plane of the body.

- **Rotation** – the moving bone rotates about a longitudinal axis.
- **Circumduction** – allows one end of a bone, e.g. the extremity of a limb, to move in a circular pattern.
- **Protraction** – moves a structure away from the body cranially, e.g. moves the foreleg forwards when walking.
- **Retraction** – moves a structure back towards the body, e.g. moves the foreleg back to original position when walking.

Synovial joints can be further classified according to the types of movement that they allow:

- **Plane or gliding joint** – allows sliding of one bone's surface over the other, e.g. joints between the rows of carpal and tarsal bones.
- **Hinge joint** – allows movement in one plane only, e.g. elbow and stifle joints, which allow just flexion and extension.
- **Pivot joint** – consists of a 'peg' fitted within a 'ring' and allows rotation, e.g. atlanto-axial joint between the first and second cervical vertebrae.
- **Condylar joint** – formed by a convex surface (condyle) that fits into a corresponding concave surface and allows movement in two planes, i.e. flexion, extension, and over extension, e.g. the hock joint.
- **Ball-and-socket joint** – consists of a portion of a sphere or ball received within a corresponding socket. Allows the greatest range of movement, e.g. hip and shoulder joints.

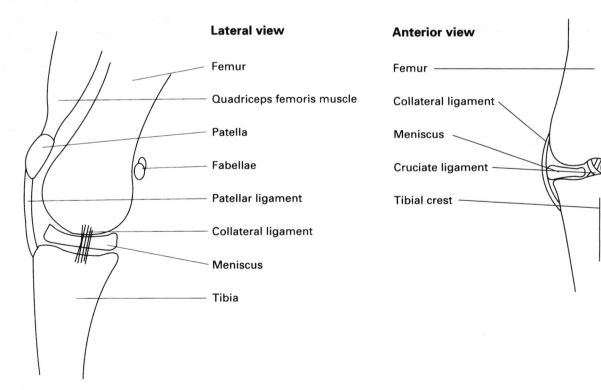

Fig. 2.20 A stifle joint.

The muscular system

Muscle tissue

There are three types of muscle tissue in the body (Fig. 2.21):

- **Skeletal (striated/voluntary) muscle** – attached to the skeleton, is concerned with locomotion. It is under the conscious or voluntary control of the brain. The cells of skeletal muscle are cylindrical and are called **muscle fibres**. They are arranged in parallel bundles. The muscle fibres are composed of protein filaments called **actin** (thin filaments) and **myosin** (thick filaments), arranged in a way that gives the muscle its striped or striated appearance.
- **Smooth (non-striated/involuntary) muscle** – found throughout the body, e.g. within the walls of the blood vessels, oesophagus and bladder. Its cells are spindle-shaped and arranged in sheets or bundles. Contraction of smooth muscle is under the involuntary control of the autonomic nervous system.
- **Cardiac muscle** – specialised type of involuntary muscle that is only found in the heart. It contracts rhythmically and automatically, i.e. the contraction is stimulated from within the muscle tissue itself (myogenic). Its fibres are branched and linked by **intercalated discs** and the tissue appears striated.

The muscular system is primarily concerned with skeletal muscle, i.e. those muscles attached to the skeleton.

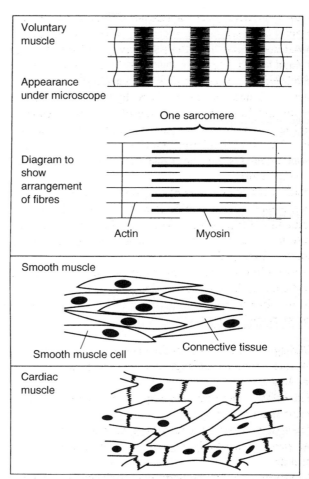

Fig. 2.21 Structure of muscle tissue.

Muscle contraction

The unit of muscle contraction is called a **sarcomere** (Fig. 2.21). A sarcomere consists of two types of longitudinal protein molecules – **myosin** (thick filaments) and **actin** (thin filaments). Muscle contraction is achieved when the myosin molecules form 'cross-bridges' with the actin molecules. The myosin and actin then slide over one another and the muscle shortens or contracts. This process requires a plentiful supply of energy, in the form of ATP, and free calcium ions.

The cells of skeletal muscle are stimulated to contract by nerve impulses to the muscle fibres. The number of muscle fibres supplied by an individual nerve varies according to the type of movement that the muscle makes. A group of muscle fibres supplied by the one nerve fibre is called a **motor unit**. The size of the motor unit varies – some nerves supply only a few muscle fibres, whereas others may supply as many as 200 muscle fibres.

Muscles are always in a slight state of tension – nerve impulses are constantly being sent to the muscle to keep it prepared for action. This is called **muscle tone**, and it is responsible, for example, in maintaining posture. When an animal is anxious the number of nerve impulses being sent to a muscle increases. Muscle tone increases and the muscles become 'twitchy' to prepare them for action. The converse is seen when an animal is asleep and fully relaxed. Only a few nerve impulses are sent to the muscle and the animal is more 'floppy'.

Skeletal muscles

These are the muscles responsible for bringing about movement of part or the whole animal (Tables 2.4, 2.5 and 2.6).

Table 2.4 Muscles of the axial skeleton

Muscle	Origin	Insertion	Action
Muscles of facial expression	Intrinsic muscles found on the face, around the ears, lips, eyes, mouth and nose. Innervated by cranial nerve VII (facial)		Move the lips, cheeks, nostrils, eyelids and external ears
Muscles of mastication			
Temporalis	Fills temporal fossa of skull	Coronoid process of mandible	Closes the jaw
Masseter	Zygomatic arch (lies lateral to mandible)	Masseteric fossa of mandible	Closes the jaw
Digastricus	Jugular process of occipital bone	Angle and ventral surface of mandible	Opens the jaw
Muscles of the eye			
Dorsal, ventral, medial and lateral rectus muscles	The extra-ocular muscles that move the eye in the socket. They insert on the sclera at the equator of the eye		Move the eye up, down, inwards and outwards
Dorsal and ventral oblique muscles			Rotate the eye about the visual axis
Retractor bulbi	Forms a muscular cone around the optic nerve		Pulls the eyeball back into the socket
Muscles of the vertebral column	Lie in two groups		
Epaxial group	This group of muscles lies dorsal to the transverse processes, i.e. *above* the vertebral column		Support the spine, extend the vertebral column
Hypaxial group	This group lies ventral to the transverse processes, i.e. *below* the vertebral column		Flex the head, neck, tail and vertebral column
Muscles of the thorax	The muscles involved in respiration		
External intercostals	These muscles run from an origin on one rib to a termination on the next, i.e. fill one intercostal space		Draw the ribs together during inspiration
Internal intercostals	Lie more deeply within the intercostal space, but as with the above they run from one rib to the next		Assist in expiration
Diaphragm	The muscle that separates the thoracic cavity from the abdominal cavity. Has three openings to allow the passage of structures from the thorax to the abdomen: ● **Oesophageal hiatus** transmits the oesophagus and vagal nerves ● **Aortic hiatus** transmits the aorta, the azygous vein and thoracic duct ● **Caval foramen** transmits the posterior vena cava		Inspiration – it contracts to enlarge the thoracic cavity, thus drawing air into the lungs
Muscles of the abdominal wall	Three muscles make up the lateral wall of the abdomen and one that forms the ventral floor of the abdominal wall		
External abdominal oblique	Form the lateral abdominal wall. All three muscles insert on the **linea alba**, a 'white line' that runs midventrally on the abdomen		The fibres run in different directions giving the lateral wall great strength to protect the contents of the abdomen
Internal abdominal oblique			
Transversus abdominis	The deepest of the lateral abdominal muscles		
Rectus abdominus	Runs in a band either side of the linea alba and inserts on the pubis via the **prepubic tendon**		Supports the ventral floor of the abdomen

Table 2.5 Muscles of the forelimb			
Muscle	**Origin**	**Insertion**	**Action**
Trapezius	Dorsal midline (level of 2nd cervical to 9th thoracic vertebrae)	Spine of scapula	Protracts the limb (draws the leg forward)
Latissimus dorsi	Broad origin on dorsal midline	Humerus	Retracts the limb (pulls the leg backwards)
Brachiocephalicus	Base of the skull	Cranial aspect of humerus	Bends neck laterally (side to side)
Supraspinatus	Supraspinous fossa of scapula	Greater tubercle of humerus	Extends the shoulder and stabilises the joint
Infraspinatus	Infraspinous fossa of scapula	Greater tubercle of humerus	Flexes the shoulder and stabilises the joint
Triceps brachii	Proximal humerus and scapula	Olecranon of ulna	Extends the elbow joint
Biceps brachii	Supraglenoid tubercle of scapula	Radius and ulna	Flexes the elbow joint
Brachialis	Humerus	Radius and ulna	Flexes the elbow joint
Carpal extensor muscles (2)	Humerus (muscle group that runs on the front of carpus)	Carpal bones	Extend the carpus
Carpal flexor muscles (2)	In the group of muscles that run behind the carpus	Carpal bones	Flex the carpus
Digital extensor muscles (2)	Humerus	3rd phalanx	Extend the digits (toes)
Digital flexor muscles (2)	In the group of muscles that run behind the paw	Digits	Flex the digits

Table 2.6 Muscles of the hindlimb			
Muscle	**Origin**	**Insertion**	**Action**
Quadriceps femoris	Ilium and femur, runs down the front of the thigh	Consists of four parts, all inserting on the tibial tuberosity	Extends the stifle (tendon contains the **patella** which articulates with the femur at stifle joint)
Hamstring group			
Biceps femoris	Pelvis (ischium)	Tibia and calcaneus	Extends hip, stifle and hock
Semitendinosus	Ischiatic tuberosity (pelvis)	Tibia and calcaneus	Extends hip and hock Flexes stifle
Semimembranosus	Ischiatic tuberosity	Femur and tibia	Extends hip and stifle
Pectineus	Pubis	Distal femur	Adducts the limb
Gastrocnemius	Caudal femur	Calcaneus	Extends hock Flexes stifle
Cranial (anterior) tibial	Tibia	Tarsus	Flexes hock
Digital flexors (2)	Run on the caudal surface of the leg	Digits (phalanges)	Flex the toes (digits)
Digital extensors (3)	Run on the cranial surface of the leg	Digits	Extend the toes (digits)

The nervous system

The function of the nervous system is to:

- Receive stimuli from the environment.
- Analyse and integrate the stimuli.
- Initiate the correct response.

Within the body, the nervous system functions as a well-integrated unit, but for descriptive purposes, it can be divided into:

- The central nervous system (CNS) – brain and spinal cord.
- The peripheral nervous system – all nerves leading away from the central nervous system.

Nervous tissue

The nervous system consists of nervous tissue. The main cell of nervous tissue is the **neuron**. Neurons are responsible for the transmission of nerve impulses from one area to another (Fig. 2.22).

Each neuron consists of:

(1)   A **cell body** containing the nucleus.
(2)   Many fine **dendrites** or thicker **dendrons**, which carry impulses *towards* the cell body.
(3)   A single **axon** which carries impulses *away* from the cell body.

> Each neuron is only a few micrometres in diameter but the length may vary from a few millimetres to a metre. A 'nerve' is made of many neurons held together by connective tissue.

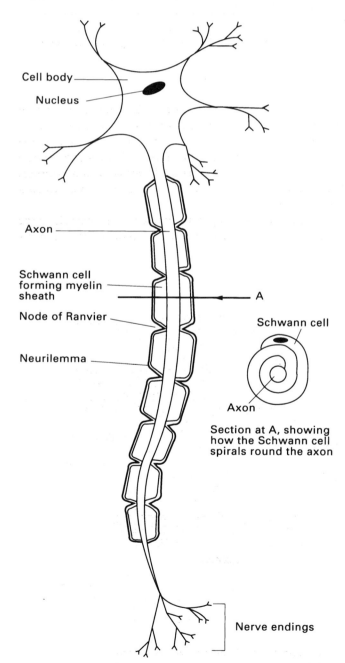

Section at A, showing how the Schwann cell spirals round the axon

Fig. 2.22 Structure of a neuron.

Most axons are covered in a sheath of **myelin**, a white lipoprotein material produced by **Schwann cells** and wrapped like a 'Swiss roll' around the central nerve fibre (Fig. 2.22). Between the cells are gaps known as the **nodes of Ranvier**, and it is through these that nutrients are able to reach the axon fibre. Myelinated axons conduct nerve impulses faster than non-myelinated axons. Non-myelinated fibres are rare, and may be found in sites such as the retina of the eye and in the grey matter of the central nervous system.

Each neuron terminates in a specialised ending whose function is to conduct nerve impulses from:

* One neuron to another – the ending is called a **synapse.** A single cell body may receive as many as 6000 synaptic endings.
* A neuron to a muscle fibre – the ending is called a **neuromuscular junction.**

> Each nerve pathway consists of neurons and synapses. Nerve impulses travel along the pathway at rates of approximately 100 m/s.

Each synapse consists of a button-like swelling containing vesicles of a **chemical transmitter** (Fig. 2.22). The most common transmitter is acetyl choline, but others include noradrenaline and adrenaline. As the nerve impulse travels towards the synapse the chemicals are released and stimulate the muscle fibre or cell body with which they are in contact. This process conducts the impulse across the synaptic ending to the next neuron or brings about contraction of the muscle fibre. The presence of calcium ions is essential for the transmission of a nerve impulse.

A nerve impulse is an 'all or nothing' phenomenon – i.e. each neuron is either stimulated or it is not. A graduated effect is achieved by the relative numbers of neurons in a nerve pathway having an inhibitory effect, compared to the numbers having an excitatory effect.

Nerve definitions

The various nerve types are defined in Table 2.7.

The central nervous system

This consists of two structures:

* Brain.
* Spinal cord.

Control by the CNS is voluntary or conscious – the animal is aware of its actions.

Within the embryo the CNS develops as a hollow **neural tube** from the ectodermal layer of the inner cell mass. It runs along the dorsal surface of the embryo and gives off nerves, which eventually extend to all parts of the body. The ante-

Table 2.7 Definition of nerve types

Nerve type	Definition
Sensory nerve	Carries nerve impulses towards the CNS
Motor nerve	Carries nerve impulses away from the CNS
Intercalated neuron	Lies between a sensory neuron and a motor neuron. May not always be present within a nerve pathway
Mixed nerve	Carries both sensory and motor nerve fibres
Afferent nerve	Carries impulses towards a structure
Efferent nerve	Carries impulses away from a structure
Visceral sensory nerve	Carries information from blood vessels, mucous membranes and visceral body systems, i.e. respiratory, digestive and urinogenital systems and the heart to the CNS
Visceral motor nerve	Carries information from the CNS to smooth muscle and glandular tissue within the visceral body systems
Somatic sensory nerve	Carries information from skin, skeletal muscles, tendons, joints and special sense organs to the CNS
Somatic motor nerve	Carries information from the CNS to skeletal muscle
Ganglion	Collection of cell bodies

NB: *The terms efferent/afferent are not restricted to the nervous system and may be applied to blood or lymphatic vessels. Motor nerves are also efferent nerves; sensory nerves are also afferent nerves*

rior part of the tube becomes the brain, while the remainder becomes the spinal cord.

The nervous tissue of the CNS is described as:

- **White matter** – contains a high proportion of white myelinated fibres.
- **Grey matter** – aggregations of cell bodies, with little or no myelin.

In the brain, the white and the grey matter are mixed up, creating an outer grey layer and an inner white layer. Distributed within the white matter are islands of grey matter referred to as **ganglia** or **nuclei**. Each one acts as a relay centre where information, in the form of nerve impulses, is gathered and sent out. In the spinal cord, the grey matter forms a butterfly-shaped core surrounded by white matter.

The brain (Fig. 2.23)

The anterior end of the neural tube lying within the cranial cavity, swells to form a hollow organ with three distinct regions:

- Forebrain – cerebrum, thalamus, hypothalamus and associated structures.
- Midbrain – linking pathway between the fore and hindbrain.
- Hindbrain – cerebellum, pons and medulla oblongata.

Forebrain The **cerebrum** occupies the greater part of the forebrain and consists of the **right and left cerebral hemispheres**. The surface is deeply folded, which enables a large surface area to be fitted into the relatively small cranial cavity. The folds of the cerebrum are called **gyri** (upfolds) and **sulci** (downfolds). Ninety per cent of all the neurons in the nervous system are found in the cerebral hemispheres.

A central **longitudinal fissure** divides the two cerebral hemispheres. They are linked across the midline by a tract of white matter known as the **corpus callosum**, forming the roof of the third ventricle. Each hemisphere is divided into four lobes – the **frontal, parietal, occipital** and **temporal lobes**, each of which contributes in a different way to conscious thought.

The **thalamus** lies deep in the tissue of the forebrain at the base of the cerebral hemispheres. Its function is to process

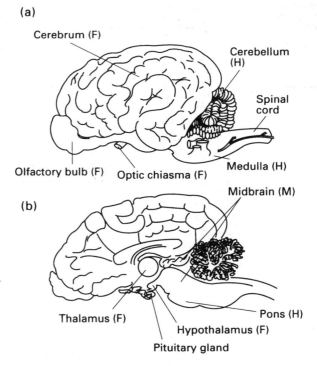

(a)

Cerebrum (F)

Cerebellum (H)

Spinal cord

Olfactory bulb (F) Optic chiasma (F) Medulla (H)

Midbrain (M)

(b)

Thalamus (F)

Hypothalamus (F)

Pituitary gland

Pons (H)

F = Forebrain   M = Midbrain   H = Hindbrain

Fig. 2.23 The dog's brain.

information from the sense organs and relay it to the cerebral cortex.

The **hypothalamus** lies ventral to the thalamus and dorsal to the pituitary gland and is one of the most vital regions of the brain. Its function is to:

- Link the nervous and endocrine systems by secreting a series of releasing hormones which are stored in the pituitary gland, e.g. gonadotrophin releasing hormone (GRH).
- Help control the autonomic nervous system affecting activities such as sweating, shivering, vasodilation and vasoconstriction.
- Exert a major control on the homeostatic mechanisms of the body, e.g. osmotic balance of fluids, regulation of body temperature, thirst and hunger.

On the ventral surface of the forebrain (Fig. 2.23) are:

- A pair of **olfactory bulbs** – responsible for the sense of smell or olfaction. They receive sensory nerve fibres from the mucosa lining the nasal chambers.
- **Pituitary gland** – endocrine gland which secretes and stores a wide range of hormones.
- The **optic chiasma** – information from both eyes goes to both the right and left sides of the brain via this crossover point.

Midbrain This short length of brain is difficult to see as it is overhung by the large cerebral hemispheres. Its function is to conduct nerve impulses from the forebrain to the hindbrain and in the opposite direction.

Hindbrain The **cerebellum** is a globular organ consisting of two hemispheres folded into deep fissures. It lies dorsal to the medulla oblongata and is attached by three pairs of peduncles through which run tracts of nerves. The function of the cerebellum is to coordinate balance and muscular movement. Nerve impulses initiating voluntary movements begin in the cerebral hemispheres. Fine adjustments are made in the cerebellum and the nerve impulses are sent down the spinal cord to the skeletal muscles and movement results.

The **pons** lies ventral to the cerebellum, forming a bridge of fibres from one cerebellar hemisphere to the other. Contains centres involved in the control of respiration.

The **medulla oblongata** extends from the pons to the point where the spinal cord passes through the foramen magnum of the skull. Contains centres responsible for the control of respiration and blood pressure.

All the cranial nerves, apart from the olfactory (I) and optic (II) nerves arise from the ventral surface of the midbrain and hindbrain (Fig. 2.23).

Protection of the central nervous system

If an animal is to survive, it is vital that the brain is able to function normally. The brain is protected from mechanical damage externally by the bony cranial cavity of the skull and internally by the meninges and the ventricular system.

Meninges The entire CNS is surrounded by three membranes (Fig. 2.24). From the outside to the inside these are:

- **Dura mater** – tough fibrous layer. In the cranial cavity this is interwoven with the periosteum of the overlying bones; in the vertebral canal there is a fat-filled **epidural space** between the vertebrae and the dura mater – this is used as a site for local anaesthesia.
- **Arachnoid mater** – a network of collagen fibres and large blood vessels. Between the dura mater and the arachnoid mater is the **subdural space**. Below the arachnoid mater is the **subarachnoid space** – this is filled with **cerebro-spinal fluid (CSF)**.
- **Pia mater** – a fine membrane closely applied to the surface of the brain following the gyri and sulci. It contains many small blood capillaries, which supply the underlying nervous tissue.

Ventricular system In the embryo, the CNS forms from a hollow neural tube and the central lumen develops into a system of interconnecting cavities or ventricles, and canals (Fig. 2.24).

A **central canal** runs along the entire length of the spinal cord, surrounded by grey matter. Within the brain, this canal continues as the:

- **Fourth ventricle** – in the hindbrain.
- **Cerebral aqueduct** – narrow canal in the midbrain.
- **Third ventricle** – in the forebrain. This gives off two **lateral ventricles**, one inside each cerebral hemisphere.

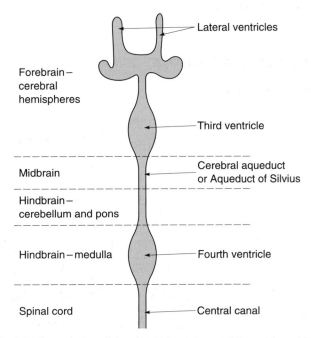

Forebrain – cerebral hemispheres

Lateral ventricles

Third ventricle

Midbrain

Cerebral aqueduct or Aqueduct of Silvius

Hindbrain – cerebellum and pons

Hindbrain – medulla

Fourth ventricle

Spinal cord

Central canal

Fig. 2.24 General plan of the ventricular system and its position within the brain, dorsal view. (Adapted from Frandson and Spurgeon, *Anatomy and Physiology of Farm Animals*, 5th edn, Lea and Febiger, Philadelphia, 1992, p. 140.)

Cerebrospinal fluid (CSF) formed by **choroid plexuses** – capillary networks – in the roof of the ventricles, circulates in the ventricular system and bathes the outer surface of the CNS in the subarachnoid space. It is a clear yellowish fluid resembling plasma, but without protein. The function of CSF is to protect the CNS from sudden movement and knocks and to supply the nervous tissue with nutrients.

Spinal cord (Fig. 2.25)

This is a glistening white structure extending from the medulla oblongata to the lumbar region of the vertebral column. It leaves the cranial cavity via the **foramen magnum** in the occipital bone of the skull and runs in the vertebral canal formed from the interlinked vertebrae. At approximately L6–L7 the cord narrows and breaks up into a group of spinal nerves known as the **cauda equina**. These run towards the hindlimbs and tail. The spinal cord is protected by the surrounding meninges and by the bony vertebral column. Along its length the spinal cord gives off pairs of **spinal nerves**.

In cross-section (Fig. 2.25), the tissue of the spinal cord consists of:

- **Central canal** containing CSF.
- Butterfly-shaped area of **grey matter** made of non-myelinated neurons. Most of the synapses in the spinal cord are in this area.
- Outer layer of **white matter** consisting of organised tracts of myelinated nerve fibres running towards (ascending) and away from (descending) the brain. Each tract has a definite origin and destination so that transmission of nerve impulses is fast and efficient.

The peripheral nervous system

This consists of the:

- **Cranial nerves** – leaving the brain.
- **Spinal nerves** – leaving the spinal cord.
- **Autonomic nervous system** – contains some nerve fibres from the brain, but the majority arise from the spinal cord.

Cranial nerves (Table 2.8)

There are twelve pairs of cranial nerves, which leave the brain via various foramina in the skull. Most supply structures on or around the head, so they are short – the longest cranial nerve is the vagus (X). Cranial nerves may be sensory, motor or mixed (Table 2.7). They are always numbered using Roman numerals.

Spinal nerves

The spinal cord is described as being segmented. Each segment corresponds to a vertebra and gives off a pair of spinal nerves, which leave the vertebral canal by the intervertebral **foramina** – one to the left side of the body and one to the right side (Fig. 2.25). The spinal nerves then travel towards the organs they supply.

Each spinal nerve is divided into:

- **Dorsal root** – carries sensory fibres from the body towards the spinal cord. A few millimetres from the cord is the **dorsal root ganglion** – a swelling containing all the cell bodies of these neurons.
- **Ventral root** – carries motor fibres away from the spinal cord towards the organs. There is no ganglion.

Linking the sensory and motor fibres in the grey matter of the cord there may be one or more **intercalated neurons**.

Once outside the vertebral canal, the sensory nerve fibres entering the dorsal root and the motor nerve fibres leaving the ventral root run together in the same myelin sheath, forming a **mixed nerve**.

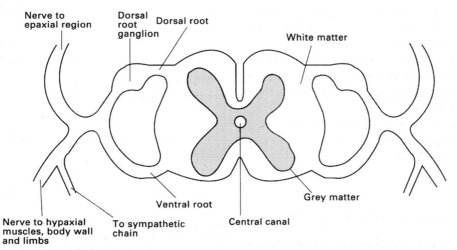

Fig. 2.25 Cross-section through the spinal cord.

Table 2.8 Cranial nerves

Cranial nerve	Type of nerve fibre	Function
I. Olfactory	Sensory	Carries the sense of smell or olfaction from the olfactory bulbs to the brain
II. Optic	Sensory	Carries information about sight from the eyes to both sides of the brain via the optic chiasma
III. Oculomotor	Motor	Supplies the extrinsic muscles of the eye enabling it to make delicate and accurate movements
IV. Trochlear	Motor	Supplies the extrinsic muscles of the eye
V. Trigeminal	Mixed	Carries sensory fibres from the skin around the face and eyes and motor fibres to the muscles of mastication – mainly the temporal and masseter
VI. Abducens	Motor	Supplies the extrinsic muscles of the eye
VII. Facial	Motor	Supplies the muscles of facial expression including those associated with the movement of the lips, ears and skin around the eyes
VIII. Vestibulocochlear (auditory)	Sensory	Vestibular branch carries sensation of balance from the semicircular canals in the inner ear. Cochlear branch carries sensation of hearing from the cochlear of the inner ear
IX. Glossopharyngeal	Mixed	Carries the sensation of taste or gustation from the taste buds on the tongue and pharynx. Supplies motor fibres to the muscles of the pharynx
X. Vagus	Mixed	Carries sensory fibres from the pharynx and larynx. Supplies motor fibres to the muscles of the larynx. Parasympathetic visceral motor fibres to the heart and various thoracic and abdominal organs including the gastrointestinal tract as far as the descending colon
XI. Accessory (spinal accessory)	Motor	Supplies the muscles of the neck and shoulder
XII. Hypoglossal	Motor	Supplies the muscles of the tongue

Spinal nerves supply the whole musculoskeletal system. In the area of the pectoral and pelvic girdles the spinal nerves are thicker and form a network or **nerve plexus,** which supply the limbs.

Reflex arcs   A reflex arc may be defined as a fixed involuntary response to certain stimuli. Reflexes are rapid, automatic, always the same and only involve pathways in the spinal cord.

Sensory nerves carry nerve impulses, received from sensory receptors in organs such as the skin, joints and muscles, to the spinal cord. Here they synapse with motor nerves in that segment of the spinal cord and an impulse is sent out to skeletal muscle, which brings about a response. Thus in the pedal reflex, the paw is pinched, pain receptors in the skin send sensory impulses to the spinal cord and a motor impulse is sent to the muscles of the leg, and the paw is withdrawn.

Reflex arcs may be described as being:

- **Monosynaptic** or **simple** – involving only one synapse in the pathway.
- **Polysynaptic** – involving at least one intercalated neuron in the pathway.

Reflex arcs use pathways within a relevant segment of spinal cord but their presence does not indicate that the spinal cord is intact. However, if the animal cries out or bites when a reflex is tested it indicates that nerve impulses have also travelled up the spinal cord towards the brain where they have been consciously perceived – this indicates that the cord is intact.

Reflex arcs are modified by neurons in other segments above (**upper motor neurons**) or below (**lower motor neurons**) that particular segment. If a reflex is extravagant or abnormally suppressed, this could indicate that the cord is severed above or below the area and the modifying effect has been lost.

The brain can override reflex arcs. For example, you can force yourself to hold your hand on a hot iron even though your reflex would be to pull your hand away – this is a **conditioned reflex.**

The reflex arcs commonly tested include the pedal, panniculus, palpebral, pupillary light response, patella and anal reflexes.

Autonomic nervous system

This can be considered to be a visceral motor system, i.e. it supplies motor nerves to cardiac muscle, smooth muscle and to glands within the visceral body systems and the heart. Control of the autonomic nervous system is involuntary or unconscious.

The system can be divided into two parts:

- Sympathetic.
- Parasympathetic.

They occupy different areas of the body and have opposite effects (Fig. 2.26). Most organs receive a nerve supply from both systems and control is achieved by balancing the effects (Table 2.9).

Special senses

The body has evolved specialised sensory receptor cells, each adapted to respond to particular stimuli in the external environment and housed within organs known as the special sense organs. The special senses are:

- Taste.
- Smell.
- Sight.
- Hearing.
- Balance.

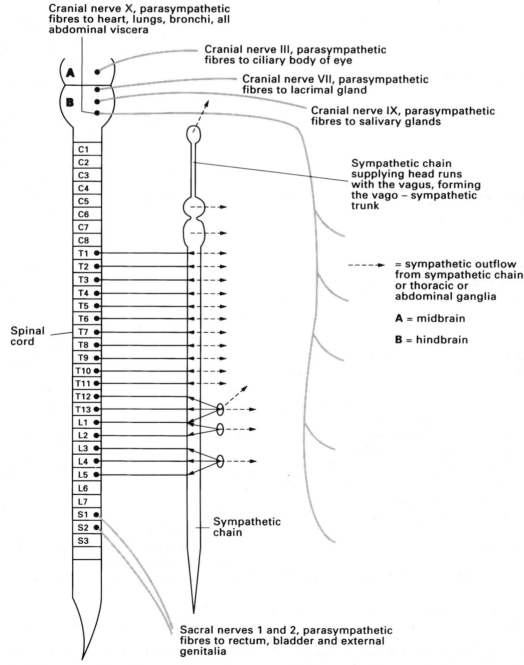

Cranial nerve X, parasympathetic fibres to heart, lungs, bronchi, all abdominal viscera

Cranial nerve III, parasympathetic fibres to ciliary body of eye

Cranial nerve VII, parasympathetic fibres to lacrimal gland

Cranial nerve IX, parasympathetic fibres to salivary glands

Sympathetic chain supplying head runs with the vagus, forming the vago – sympathetic trunk

----→ **= sympathetic outflow from sympathetic chain or thoracic or abdominal ganglia**

A = midbrain

B = hindbrain

Spinal cord

Sympathetic chain

Sacral nerves 1 and 2, parasympathetic fibres to rectum, bladder and external genitalia

Fig. 2.26 The autonomic nervous system.

Table 2.9 Autonomic nervous system		
	Sympathetic	**Parasympathetic**
Origin of nerve fibres	Arise from spinal cord from T1 to L4 or L5. Nerve fibres run to ganglia arranged in two chains along the dorsal body wall on either side of the vertebral column – sympathetic chains	Arise from brain in cranial nerves – III, VII, IX and X. Also from spinal cord at S1 and S2
Organs supplied	Eye, salivary glands, heart and lungs. Unpaired ganglia are: • Coeliac – stomach, small intestine, pancreas, large intestine, and adrenal medulla • Cranial mesenteric – large intestine • Caudal mesenteric – bladder and genitals	Eye, salivary glands. Vagus X supplies heart, lungs, stomach, small intestine, pancreas, large intestine. Fibres from S1/S2 supply bladder and genitals
Length of preganglionic fibres	Short – run to sympathetic chain	Long
Length of postganglionic fibres	Long – ganglia are close to the organ they supply	Short
Transmitter substance at: 1. Synapses within the system 2. Terminal synapses	Acetyl choline Noradrenaline	Acetyl choline Acetyl choline
General effect	Prepares body for 'fear, flight, fight'. Increases respiratory and heart rates, vasodilation, dilates bronchioles, increases levels of stress, reduces gastrointestinal activity, dries salivary secretions, dilates the pupil	Slows the heart and respiratory rates, increases gastrointestinal activity, constricts the pupil, reduces stress levels

Taste (gustation)

Receptor cells (gustatory cells) lie within discrete organs known as **taste buds.** These are distributed over the dorsal surface of the tongue, the epiglottis, and the soft palate. Chemicals, responsible for taste, dissolve in mucus covering the oral cavity and stimulate the taste buds. The resulting nerve impulses travel along fine nerve fibres associated with the receptor cells to cranial nerves VII, IX and X and so to the brain where the information is interpreted as taste.

Smell (olfaction)

Receptor cells lie within the mucous membrane lining the nasal cavities. Chemicals responsible for smell dissolve in mucus and stimulate the fine nerve fibres of the **olfactory nerve (I)** in close contact with the mucosa. These fibres carry nerve impulses through the cribriform plate of the ethmoid bone at the back of the nasal cavity to the olfactory bulbs of the forebrain where they are interpreted as smell.

Gustatory and olfactory cells are known as chemoreceptors. Gustation is closely allied to olfaction and they often work together.

Sight

The eye houses receptor cells (photoreceptors) adapted to respond to light and so bring about sight. Each eye lies within a bony **orbit** in the skull, lateral to the nasal cavities and rostral to the cranium. In the dog and cat the eyes are directed forwards providing a wide field of binocular or 3D vision. This enables the animal to locate objects accurately, which is important in predatory species.

The eye (Fig. 2.27) comprises three main parts:

- **Eyeball**.
- **Extrinsic muscles**.
- **Eyelids**.

The eyeball

This is a globe-shaped structure made of three layers:

- Sclera.
- Uvea.
- Retina.

Sclera   A tough fibrous outer coating whose function is to protect the inner structures. The anterior sixth of the sclera is the transparent **cornea**, which allows light into the eye and plays a part in focusing light rays onto the retina. The cornea is covered in a thin layer of epithelium called the **conjunctiva.** The junction between the sclera and cornea is known as the **limbus**.

Uvea   A vascular pigmented middle layer consisting of the following structures:

- **Choroid** – darkly pigmented, containing blood vessels which supply all the internal structures.
- **Tapetum lucidum** – area of yellow-green iridescent cells lying in the dorsal part of the choroid above the exit of the optic nerve. Its function is to reflect light back to the retina making use of low light levels and improving night

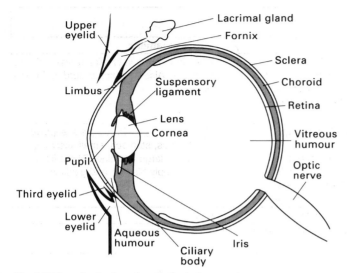

Fig. 2.27 Longitudinal section through the eye.

vision. Most mammals, except man, have a tapetum lucidum.

- **Ciliary body** – thickened part of the uvea which projects towards the centre of the eye. It consists of the **ciliary muscle** which is linked to the lens by the **suspensory ligament**. This arrangement is responsible for controlling the thickness of the lens.
- **Iris** – continues anteriorly from the ciliary body. The iris contains pigment cells and smooth muscle fibres whose function is to constrict and dilate the pupil in response to changes in light intensity.
- **Pupil** – formed by the free edge of the iris and allows light to reach the lens. Its shape is characteristic of the species – cats have vertical slits and dogs have round pupils.
- **Cornea** – clear, transparent anterior segment of the fibrous tissue of the eye.

Retina   This innermost layer contains the photoreceptor or light sensitive cells. It consists of the following layers:

- Ganglion cells – transmit nerve impulses to the optic nerve (II).
- Bipolar receptor cells.
- Photoreceptor cells – consist of two types named according to their shape:

  (1)   **Rods** – black/white vision and night vision.
  (2)   **Cones** – colour vision.

- Pigmented cells lying close to the choroid.

Light focused on to the retina by the lens travels through the layers of cells and stimulates the photoreceptors. The resulting nerve impulses pass back to the ganglion cells, which transmit them via the fibres of the optic nerve (II) to the brain. At the exit of the optic nerve is the **optic disc** (Fig. 2.27) – this area contains no photoreceptors.

The central cavity of the eye is divided into two chambers by the crystalline biconvex **lens** surrounded by the suspensory ligament and the ciliary body (Fig. 2.27).

- **Anterior chamber** – contains transparent watery fluid called **aqueous humour** which is secreted by the ciliary body and drains out of the eye back into the circulation at the **limbus**.
- **Posterior chamber** – contains transparent jelly-like fluid called **vitreous humour.**

The function of these fluids is to maintain the shape of the eye and to provide nutrients to the structures of the eye.

The extrinsic muscles

The eyeball is well supplied with extrinsic muscles. These are striated muscles which originate on the sclera and insert on the periosteum of the bones of the orbit. They are responsible for the fine movements of the eyeball. These movements are coordinated to provide 3D or binocular vision. The nerve supply to these muscles is from cranial nerves III, IV and VI.

The eyelids (Fig. 2.27)

The eyes are essential to the survival of an animal and they must be protected from mechanical damage. The posterior two-thirds of the eyeball lies within the bony orbit, while the eyelids protect the anterior third formed by the cornea and conjunctiva.

Each eye has an **upper** and **lower eyelid** which are joined at the **medial canthus**, close to the nose, and the **lateral canthus**. Both eyelids consist of **palpebral muscle** covered in hairy skin. The inner surface is lined with a continuation of the epithelium forming the conjunctiva. On the outer edge of the more mobile upper eyelid is a row of **cilia**, or **eyelashes**. Lying within the tissue of the eyelids are the **Meibomian glands**, which secrete fluid to lubricate and protect the eyes.

Deep to the upper and lower eyelids and lying within the medial canthus is the **third eyelid**, or **nictitating membrane**. This is a T-shaped piece of cartilage with associated smooth muscle and glandular and lymphoid tissue. The eyelid moves across, providing a third protective layer as the other eyelids close and the eyeball retracts into the orbit.

> The eyelids and associated eyelashes of the dog may be affected by several inherited conditions. These are **entropion** – inturning eyelids, **ectropion** – drooping of the lower eyelids and **distichiasis** – ectopic eyelashes. Affected dogs should not be used for breeding.

The cornea is kept clean, moist and supple by secretions or **tears** from the **lacrimal gland** on the dorsolateral surface of the eye beneath the upper eyelid. Tears flow across the eye, drain into a pair of openings at the medial canthus and

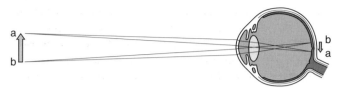

Fig. 2.28 Formation of the image on the retina. (Redrawn from Phillips and Chilton, *A-Level Biology*, OUP, 1991.)

then into the **nasolacrimal duct** which runs through the nasal cavity to open into the nostril.

Formation of the image (Fig. 2.28)

Light rays from an object pass:

(1) Through the **cornea** and the **pupil** and hit the **lens.**

- The cornea plays a part in focusing the light onto the retina.
- The iris alters in size and controls the amount of light entering the eye.
- The curvature of the lens is altered by the ciliary muscles and focuses the light rays onto the retina.

(2) Through the lens and are focused onto the **retina.**
(3) Through the layers of the retina and hit the **photoreceptor cells**; some light is reflected back to the retina by the **tapetum lucidum** to stimulate more receptor cells.
(4) Resulting nerve impulses, generated by the photoreceptors, travel along the nerve fibres of the **optic nerve (II)** to the **brain.**
(5) On the ventral surface of the brain, a proportion of nerve fibres cross via the **optic chiasma** to opposite sides of the brain so that each cerebral hemisphere receives information from both eyes.
(6) Information is carried to the **visual cortex** of the cerebral hemispheres where it is interpreted as an image. The image formed on the retina is inverted but the brain automatically modifies it.

Hearing and balance

The ear (Fig. 2.29) contains receptors adapted to respond to sound waves and to the movement of the body. All mammals have two ears comprising three parts:

- **External ear.**
- **Middle ear.**
- **Inner ear.**

The external ear

Pinna　Also called the ear flap (Fig. 2.29). Each pinna consists of a funnel-shaped flap of elastic cartilage covered

in hairy skin. There are fewer hair follicles on the inner surface of the flap.

The shape of the pinna is characteristic of the breed. The wolf, from which the domestic dog evolved, has upright V-shaped ears, but years of selective breeding have led to the development of a variety of different ear shapes. Most cats have pointed upright ears.

Both pinnae are very mobile and can move independently, which allows them to pick up sound waves from the environment and to be used as a means of facial expression and communication.

External ear canal　Also called the external auditory meatus (Fig. 2.29). This is formed by an incomplete tube of cartilage connecting to the pinna and at its distal end to the acoustic process of the **tympanic bulla** of the skull. The canal runs down the side of the head and then turns inwards to run horizontally. It terminates in the **tympanic membrane**.

The canal is lined by modified skin with few hair follicles and many **ceruminous glands,** which secrete wax to protect the ear canal from damage.

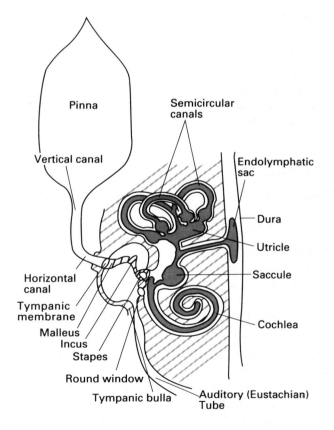

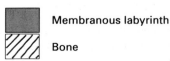

Fig. 2.29 Cross-section through the ear.

Inflammation of the ear is common in both dogs and cats. Otitis externa is inflammation of the external ear, otitis media is inflammation of the middle ear and otitis interna, which may involve loss of balance, is inflammation of the inner ear.

The middle ear

This lies mainly within the **tympanic bulla** of the petrous temporal bone of the skull, and is filled with air.

Tympanic membrane Also called the eardrum (Fig. 2.29). This is a thin semitransparent membrane whose function is to convey the vibrations caused by sound waves from the external to the middle ear.

Auditory ossicles Three small bones (Fig. 2.29) linked by synovial joints to form a flexible chain lying across the dorsal part of the middle ear. They are the:

- **Malleus** or **hammer** – in contact with the tympanic membrane.
- **Incus**, or **anvil.**
- **Stapes**, or **stirrup** – in contact with the oval window of the inner ear.

Their function is to transmit the vibrations caused by the sound waves from the tympanic membrane to the inner ear.

Eustachian tube Also called the auditory tube. This is a short tube connecting the middle ear to the nasopharynx. Its function is to equalise the air pressure on either side of the tympanic membrane, enabling it to vibrate freely and so transmit the sound waves.

The inner ear

This lies within the temporal bone and consists of an inner membranous labyrinth surrounded by an outer bony labyrinth (Fig. 2.29).

Bony labyrinth This is 'carved out' of the bone and closely follows the shape of the membranous labyrinth. It contains **perilymph**, which flows around the outside of the membranous labyrinth. It is linked to the middle ear by two membranes – the round and oval windows.

Membranous labyrinth This is a system of interconnecting tubes filled with **endolymph.** Inside the labyrinth are groups of sensory receptor cells adapted to respond to sound and movement. Projecting from each cell is a hair-like structure and touching the base is a nerve fibre from the **vestibulocochlear nerve (VIII).**

The membranous labyrinth has three parts.

Cochlea This is responsible for the perception of sound and consists of a tube arranged in a ventral spiral similar to a snail shell. Inside is a group of sensory receptor cells known as the **organ of Corti.**

Sound waves are picked up by the **pinna**, travel down the **external auditory meatus** and cause the **tympanic membrane** to vibrate. This starts the **auditory ossicles** vibrating. The third ossicle, the **stapes**, vibrates against the **oval window** of the inner ear causing first the **perilymph** and then the **endolymph** to move. Movement of the endolymph 'tweaks' the hair cells of the **organ of Corti** and initiates nerve impulses, which travel along the fibres of the **cochlear branch** of the vestibulocochlear nerve to the brain where they are interpreted as sound.

Utricle and saccule These are responsible for maintaining the position of the body when standing still. They are two sac-like structures in the centre of the membranous labyrinth (Fig. 2.29). Each contains a group of receptor cells or **maculae** surrounded by jelly. As the head moves, the jelly responds to the pull of gravity, moving the hairs of the receptor cells and initiating nerve impulses, which travel along the **vestibular branch** of the vestibulocochlear nerve to the brain.

Semicircular canals These are responsible for maintaining balance when moving. They are three canals, each one describing two-thirds of a circle and lying approximately at right angles to each other. Each canal is attached to the utricle by a swelling known as an **ampulla**, inside of which is a group of receptor cells. As the animal moves, endolymph in the semicircular canals moves, tweaking the hairs of the receptor cells and initiating nerve impulses. These are carried to the brain by the **vestibular branch** of the vestibulocochlear nerve. Within the brain they are interpreted and relayed to the **cerebellum**. Impulses are then sent to the skeletal muscles, bringing about the appropriate muscle movements necessary to maintain balance.

The endocrine system

The endocrine system forms part of the regulatory system of the body. A series of **endocrine glands** secrete chemical messengers known as **hormones** which are carried by the blood to their **target organs**. These may be some distance away from the gland.

Hormones regulate the activity of the target organ, which responds only to that particular hormone, leaving all other organs unaffected. The response produced by hormones is slower and lasts longer, and complements the rapid and relatively short-lived responses of the nervous system.

The endocrine glands are distributed throughout the body and may secrete more than one hormone (Fig. 2.30).

The endocrine glands are:

- Pituitary gland.
- Thyroid gland.
- Parathyroid gland.
- Pancreas.
- Ovary.
- Testes.
- Adrenal glands.

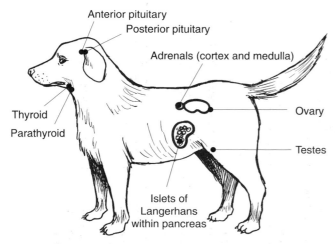

Fig. 2.30 Components of the endocrine system.

Not all hormones are secreted by endocrine glands – some are produced from tissue within another organ. These include:

(1) **Gastrin** – produced by the wall of the stomach. As food enters the stomach, gastrin stimulates the release of gastric juices from the gastric glands and digestion begins.
(2) **Secretin** – produced by the wall of the small intestine. As food enters the duodenum from the stomach, secretin stimulates the secretion of intestinal and pancreatic juices, which continue the process of digestion.
(3) **Chorionic gonadotrophin** – produced during pregnancy by the ectodermal layer of the chorion surrounding the conceptus. It helps to maintain the corpus luteum in the ovary throughout gestation.
(4) **Erythropoietin**, or **erythropoietic stimulating factor** – produced by the kidney in response to low levels of blood oxygen. It stimulates the bone marrow to produce erythrocytes or red blood cells.

For details of endocrine glands and their associated hormones, see Table 2.10.

The blood vascular system

This consists of the following parts:

- **Blood.**
- **The heart.**
- **Circulatory system.**
- **Lymphatic system.**

Blood

The functions of the blood are:

(1) **Transport** – blood carries:

- Oxygen to and carbon dioxide away from the tissues.
- Nutrients to the tissues and waste products of metabolism away from the tissues.

- Hormones secreted by endocrine glands to their target organs.
- Enzymes to their site of reaction.

(2) **Regulation** – blood is responsible for controlling:

- Volume and osmotic balance of the body fluids.
- Body temperature by constriction or dilation of peripheral blood vessels.
- Acid/base balance of fluids – the presence of buffers, e.g. bicarbonate in the blood regulate levels of hydrogen ions in plasma.
- Blood loss by the clotting mechanism.

(3) **Defence** – the white blood cells are responsible for the body's defence against disease and foreign particles such as bacteria and viruses.

Composition of blood

Blood is a specialised type of liquid connective tissue consisting of several types of **blood cells** suspended in a fluid matrix called **plasma** (Fig. 2.31). The pH of blood is 7.4 and it occupies about 7% of the total bodyweight.

Plasma   This is the fluid part of blood and takes up approximately 55–70% of blood. It consists mainly of water containing dissolved substances that are in the process of being transported around the body.

Plasma contains:

- **Water** – about 90%.
- **Plasma proteins** – albumin, prothrombin, fibrinogen and globulins. These are too large to pass out of the blood so they help to maintain the osmotic pressure, i.e. they prevent excessive fluid leaving the blood.
- **Gases** – oxygen and carbon dioxide – the majority of oxygen is carried by the red blood cells.
- **Electrolytes** – sodium, potassium, calcium, magnesium, chloride and bicarbonate ions.
- **Nutrients** – the products of digestion, i.e. amino acids, fatty acids and glucose are transported to the cells in the plasma.
- **Waste products** – the waste products of the many metabolic processes, such as urea and creatinine, are transported in the plasma to the kidney and to the liver for excretion.
- **Hormones and enzymes** – the hormones are secreted by endocrine glands directly into the bloodstream and are transported in the plasma to their target organs.
- **Antibodies and antitoxins** – form part of the body's defence system.

Blood cells   There are three types of cells (Fig. 2.31) suspended within the plasma:

- **Erythrocytes**, or **red blood cells.**
- **Leucocytes**, or **white blood cells.**
- **Thrombocytes**, or **platelets.**

Erythrocytes   These are responsible for transporting oxygen from the lungs to the tissues of the body. They are the

Table 2.10 The endocrine glands and their associated hormones

Endocrine gland	Location	Hormone	Function	Control of secretion
Anterior pituitary	Ventral to the forebrain	1. Thyrotrophic stimulating hormone (TSH)	Stimulates the release of thyroid hormone	Hypothalamus
		2. Growth hormone or somatotrophin	Controls epiphyseal growth; protein production; regulates the use of energy	Hypothalamus
		3. Adrenocorticotrophic hormone (ACTH)	Controls the release of adrenocortical hormones	Hypothalamus
		4. Prolactin	Stimulates the development of mammary glands and secretion of milk	—
		5. Follicle stimulating hormone (FSH)	Female – stimulates the development of the ovarian follicles. Male – stimulates development of seminiferous tubules and spermatogenesis	Gonadotrophin releasing hormone from the hypothalamus (GRH)
		6. Luteinising hormone (LH)	Female – brings about ovulation of the ovarian follicles and development of the corpus luteum	Oestrogen secreted by Graafian follicles
		7. Interstitial cell stimulating hormone (ICSH)	Stimulates secretion of testosterone from the interstitial cells in the testis	Gonadotrophin releasing hormone from the hypothalamus (GRH)
Posterior pituitary	Ventral to the forebrain	1. Antidiuretic hormone (ADH) – vasopressin	Acts on the collecting ducts of the renal nephrons – changes the permeability to water	Status of the ECF and blood plasma
		2. Oxytocin	Stimulates uterine contractions during parturition and milk 'let down'	Suckling by the neonate initiates a reflex arc
Thyroid	Midline on the ventral aspect of the first few rings of the trachea	1. Thyroxin	Controls metabolic rate Essential for normal growth	TSH
		2. Thyrocalcitonin	Decreases the resorption of calcium from bones	Raised blood calcium levels
Parathyroid	On either side of the thyroid gland	Parathormone	Stimulates calcium resorption from bones. Promotes calcium uptake from the intestine	Low blood calcium levels
Pancreas	Within the loop of the duodenum in the peritoneal cavity	1. Insulin – from the β cells in the islets of Langerhans	Increases uptake of glucose into the cells. Stores excess glucose as glycogen in the liver – glycogenesis	Raised blood glucose levels after eating
		2. Glucagon – from the α cells in the islets of Langerhans	Breaks down glycogen stored in the liver to release glucose into the blood – glycogenolysis	Low blood glucose levels

Table 2.10 (*continued*)

Endocrine gland	Location	Hormone	Function	Control of secretion
		3. Somatostatin – from the δ cells in the islets of Langerhans	Mild inhibition of insulin and glucagon preventing swings in blood glucose levels. Decreases gut motility and secretion of digestive juices	–
Ovary	One on either side of the midline in the dorsal peritoneal cavity	1. Oestrogen – from the Graafian follicles	Signs of oestrus; preparation of the reproductive tract and external genitalia for coitus	FSH
		2. Progesterone – from the corpus luteum	Preparation of the reproductive tract for pregnancy; development of the mammary glands; maintains the pregnancy	LH
Testis	Outside the body cavity within the scrotum	Testosterone from the cells of Leydig	Spermatogenesis. Male secondary sexual characteristics and behaviour	ICSH
Adrenal cortex	Cranial to the kidney in the peritoneal cavity – outer layer	1. Glucocorticoids	Raise blood glucose levels Reduce the inflammatory response	ACTH
		2. Mineralocorticoids, e.g. aldosterone	Acts on the distal convoluted tubules of the renal nephrons – regulates uptake of sodium and acid/base balance	Status of the ECF and blood plasma
		3. Sex hormones	Very small quantities	–
Adrenal medulla	Cranial to the kidney in the peritoneal cavity – inner layer	Adrenaline and noradrenaline	Fear, flight, fright syndrome	Sympathetic nervous system

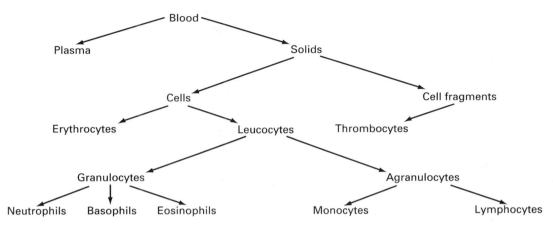

Fig. 2.31 The cells of the blood.

most numerous of the blood cells (about 5–8 million per ml). Erythrocytes are small (seven μm diameter) biconcave discs with no nuclei. They contain a complex protein pigment containing iron, called **haemoglobin**, which gives them their red colour. Haemoglobin combines with oxygen in the lung capillaries, which is then transported around the body by the red blood cells.

Erythropoiesis is the formation of erythrocytes. This takes place in the bone marrow and is controlled by the hormone **erythropoietin** secreted by the kidney in response to low blood oxygen levels.

Erythrocytes are formed from nucleated cells known as **erythroblasts**. As the nucleus begins to shrink, the cell takes up haemoglobin and is then called a **normoblast.** The nucleus continues to shrink until only fine threads remain – these are known as Howell–Joly bodies and the cell is called a **reticulocyte.** Reticulocytes may be seen in the circulation if there is a shortage of mature red blood cells, e.g. in some types of anaemia. As the nucleus completely disappears the cell becomes a mature erythrocyte and passes into the circulation. Circulating erythrocytes have a lifespan of about 120 days after which they are destroyed in the spleen or liver.

Erythroblast → Normoblast → Reticulocyte → Erythrocyte

Leucocytes These are nucleated cells and are far less numerous in the blood than erythrocytes. Each type of leucocyte has a specific function but they are all involved in the body's defence system. Leucocytes can be classified according to whether they have granulated or clear cytoplasm when stained by Romanowsky stains:

- **Granulocytes** – neutrophils, eosinophils and basophils. These make up 70% of the leucocytes and have visible granules in the cytoplasm when stained. They have irregularly shaped nuclei and are referred to as polymorphonucleocytes (PMNs) or 'polymorphs'. Granulocytes have a lifespan of about 21 days.

  Granulocytes can be further classified according to which type of stain they take up, i.e. neutral, acidic or basic (Table 2.11).
- **Agranulocytes** – monocytes and lymphocytes. Agranulocytes do not have visible granules, so have clear cytoplasm. Their nuclei are more uniform in shape (Table 2.12).

Thrombocytes These are cell fragments produced from cells in the bone marrow called **megakaryocytes**. They are numerous in the blood (2000–5000 per ml) and are involved in the **blood clotting mechanism.**

Table 2.11 Types of granulocyte

Granulocyte	Numbers present	Appearance	Function
Neutrophils	Most abundant WBC 60–75% of leucocytes (5000–9000 per ml)	Cytoplasmic granules do not stain (remain clear). Nuclei have many shapes and are segmented	Phagocytes (i.e. engulf micro-organisms and foreign particles). Can move from blood into tissues
Eosinophils	2–10% of leucocytes	Cytoplasmic granules stain with an acidic dye (eosin) and appear red	Inhibit the allergic responses and secrete anti-inflammatory substances. They are also involved in the response to parasitic infections
Basophils	Rare (0.5–1% of leucocytes)	Cytoplasmic granules stain with an alkaline (basic) dye and appear blue	Contain histamine which is involved in inflammation and allergic reactions. Also contain heparin (anticoagulant)

Table 2.12 Types of agranulocyte

Agranulocyte	Numbers present	Appearance	Function
Lymphocytes	Make up about 30% of circulating leucocytes	Large nucleus surrounded by a narrow rim of cytoplasm	*Immunity.* There are two types: **B-lymphocytes** produce antibodies; **T-lymphocytes** are involved in the cellular immune response
Monocytes	5–6% of circulating leucoytes	Largest leucocyte. Clear cytoplasm with a large bean-shaped nucleus	*Phagocytic.* Spend a short time in circulation before moving into tissues where they mature into **macrophages**.

- **Haemopoiesis** is the formation of blood cells.
- **Erythropoiesis** is specifically the production of red blood cells. There are two types of haemopoietic tissue in the body:
- **Myeloid tissue** – in the red bone marrow. Produces **erythrocytes** and **granular leucocytes**.
- **Lymphoid tissue** – in lymphatic tissues such as the lymph nodes and spleen produces **agranular leucocytes**.

Blood clotting mechanism

When a blood vessel is damaged, the body is able to 'plug' the wound with a clot of blood, preventing excessive blood loss and the entry of micro-organisms. The blood clotting process involves a complicated cascade of events involving several **clotting factors**. A brief summary of the events that take place is as follows:

(1) At the site of a wound the **thrombocytes** release an enzyme called **thromboplastin**.
(2) In the presence of **vitamin K** and **calcium ions** thromboplastin converts the inactive plasma protein **prothrombin** to the active form, **thrombin**.
(3) Thrombin converts the soluble plasma protein **fibrinogen** to the insoluble **fibrin**.
(4) The fibrin forms a meshwork of fibres across the site, which trap red blood cells, forming a clot.

Substances that interfere with the blood clotting mechanism are called **anticoagulants**. Some, such as heparin, occur naturally in the body, while others, e.g. citrate and ethylene diamine tetra acetic acid (EDTA), can be used to prevent blood samples from clotting.

If a blood sample is allowed to clot naturally, the clot will form a compact mass leaving a clear yellow liquid called **serum**. Serum is the same as plasma but without the clotting factors – fibrinogen and prothrombin.

The immune system

The immune system is responsible for protecting the animal from disease or damage from foreign materials. It has the ability to recognise anything that is 'foreign' to the body, i.e. 'not self', and it then produces a specific response to the particular invader (called **antigens**) that is causing the threat. The immune system employs a number of mechanisms to deal with the problem; some, such as phagocytosis and blood clotting, have already been mentioned. However, one very specific response is the production of proteins called **antibodies** or **immunoglobulins**, which act to neutralise a specific antigen.

Antibodies are produced by lymphocytes. There are two types:

- **T-lymphocytes** are formed in the bone marrow and mature in the thymus.
- **B-lymphocytes** are formed and mature in the bone marrow.

Thus there are two types of immune response:

- **Humoral immune response** – **B-lymphocytes** produce specific **antibodies** that combine with the antigen and 'neutralise' it, preventing it from causing harm.
- **Cell-mediated immune response** – **T-lymphocytes**. These are able to recognise foreign cells and the body's own cells that have been invaded by viruses or are cancerous. T-lymphocytes are not confined to lymphoid tissue but are able to move around in the blood.

The heart

The heart is a four-chambered muscular organ that pumps the blood around the body (Fig. 2.32). The heart lies in the mediastinum within the thoracic cavity. It is conical in shape and it lies at a slight angle in the thorax with its base situated craniodorsally above its apex. The heart lies just to the left of the midline with its apex near the sternum.

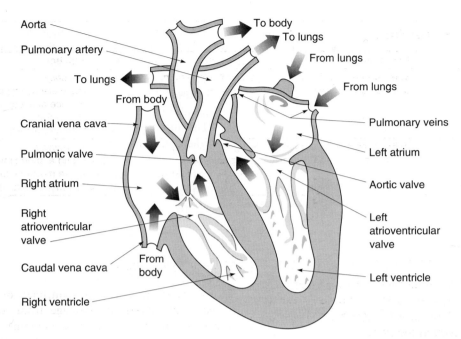

Aorta

Pulmonary artery

To lungs

From body

Cranial vena cava

Pulmonic valve

Right atrium

Right atrioventricular valve

Caudal vena cava

From body

Right ventricle

To body

To lungs

From lungs

From lungs

Pulmonary veins

Left atrium

Aortic valve

Left atrioventricular valve

Left ventricle

Fig. 2.32 The structure of the heart and the direction of blood flow. (Redrawn from B. J. Smith, *Canine Anatomy*, Lippincott, Williams & Wilkins, 1999.)

Heart structure

The heart is completely enclosed by a double-layered membrane called the **pericardium**. The inner layer of this, the **epicardium**, is a serous membrane and directly covers the heart wall. Within the pericardial cavity is a little serous fluid, which lubricates the heart as it beats.

The wall of the heart consists of a layer of cardiac muscle – the **myocardium**, and a thin inner epithelial layer that lines the heart – the **endocardium**. This layer is continuous with the endothelium lining the blood vessels.

The heart is divided into right and left sides by a partition called the **septum**. Each side is divided into two chambers – the thin-walled collecting chamber is called the **atrium** and the thicker-walled pumping chamber is the **ventricle** (Fig. 2.32). The right side of the heart pumps blood into the **pulmonary circulation** (carries blood from the heart to the lungs and back), the left side of the heart pumps blood into the **systemic circulation** (carries blood all around the body).

Heart valves

Within the heart there are two sets of valves whose function is to prevent backflow of blood (Fig. 2.32).

(1) Between the atria and ventricles are valves, which prevent the backflow of blood into the atria when the ventricles contract – these are called the **atrioventricular valves**. They are attached to the **papillary muscles** of the ventricular wall by fibres called the **chordae tendinae** which prevent the valves being turned inside out by the pressure of the blood flow.

- **The right atrioventricular valve** lies between the **right atrium** and **right ventricle** and comprises

three fibrous tissue cusps. Also called the **tricuspid valve**.
- **The left atrioventricular valve** lies between the **left atrium** and **left ventricle** and comprises two cusps. Also called the **bicuspid** or **mitral valve**.

It is the atrioventricular valves closing that can be heard in the **first** heart sound – **lubb.**

(2) At the base of the two major vessels leaving the heart are the **semilunar valves**.

- **The pulmonary valve** lies at the base of the pulmonary artery and prevents the backflow of blood from the pulmonary artery to the right ventricle.
- **The aortic valve** lies at the base of the aorta and prevents backflow of blood from the aorta to the left ventricle.

It is the semilunar valves closing that can be heard in the **second** heart sound – **dub.**

Circulation of blood through the heart (Fig. 2.32)

Deoxygenated blood is carried back to the heart in the veins. Two major veins collect all the blood and enter the right side of the heart – the **cranial vena cava** and **caudal vena cava**.

- The venae cavae empty into the **right atrium**, which when full contracts, sending deoxygenated blood into the **right ventricle** via the right atrioventricular valve.
- The right ventricle contracts, pumping blood into the **pulmonary artery** via the pulmonary valve. The deoxygenated blood is carried in the pulmonary circulation to the **lungs**.

- The blood is oxygenated in the lungs and is then carried back to the left side of the heart in the **pulmonary veins**, which enter the **left atrium**.
- When the left atrium is full it contracts, forcing oxygenated blood into the **left ventricle** via the left atrioventricular valve.
- The left ventricle contracts and pumps blood into the **aorta** via the aortic valve, which carries the oxygenated blood all around the body in the systemic circulation.

Oxygenated blood is delivered to the tissues and the deoxygenated blood is collected up by the veins and transported back to the heart.

(**NB**: the two atria, i.e. the left and right, contract in unison, as do the two ventricles.)

Control of the heartbeat (cardiac cycle)

The heart is made of cardiac muscle, which is a specialised type of muscle tissue that has the ability to initiate a contraction from within the muscle itself (i.e. without a nervous impulse). The mechanism that is responsible for controlling the **rate** of contraction of heart muscle (i.e. the heartbeat) is called the **conduction mechanism** (Fig. 2.33).

Within the wall of the right atrium is an area of modified cardiac muscle called the **sinoatrial (SA) node** (Fig. 2.33). This node determines the basic rate of the heartbeat and is referred to as the 'pacemaker'. If the muscles require more oxygen, e.g. during exercise, the SA node will increase the basic rate of contraction so that more oxygenated blood reaches the muscles; during sleep, the SA node will slow the basic heart rate.

(1) The SA node initiates a wave of contraction, which passes over the walls of the atria. The myocardium of the atria and of the ventricles although physically joined, is not in electrical continuity. It is separated, which prevents the wave of contraction in the atria spreading into the ventricles.

(2) The impulse is passed to another specialised group of cells called the **atrioventricular (AV) node** lying at the top of the interventricular septum.

(3) The wave of excitation passes down a specialised group of fibres called the **bundle of His**, within the interventricular septum.

(4) The impulse is then conducted to the apex of the heart where it spreads out into the ventricles in specialised nerve cells called **Purkinje fibres**. Thus, the wave of contraction in the myocardium of the ventricles starts at the apex and spreads upwards, forcing blood into the arteries that are situated at the top of the ventricles.

This is called the **cardiac cycle**.

- The period of **contraction** within the heart is called **systole** and is when the blood is being pumped into the ventricles or the pulmonary and systemic circulations.
- The period of **relaxation** in the heart is called **diastole** and is when the atria are filling with blood.

The circulatory system

This is a branching network of channels that transport the blood from the heart to the tissues, where oxygen and nutrients are delivered, and then transport it back again to the heart.

The network consists of:

- **Arteries.**
- **Capillaries.**
- **Veins.**

Arteries

An **artery** is a relatively large vessel that carries blood under pressure **away** from the heart. Most arteries carry oxygenated blood; however, the pulmonary artery carries deoxygenated blood from the heart to the lungs. Arteries have

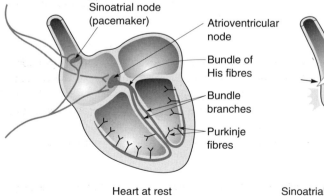
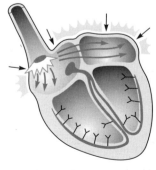
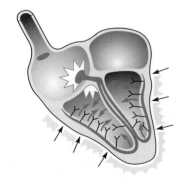

Heart at rest

Sinoatrial node fires, action potentials spread through atria which contract

Atrioventricular node fires, sending impulses along conducting fibres; ventricles contract

Fig. 2.33 The conduction mechanism of the heart. (Redrawn from Purves, Orians and Keller, *Life, the Science of Biology*, 3rd edn, Sinauer/Freeman, 1992.)

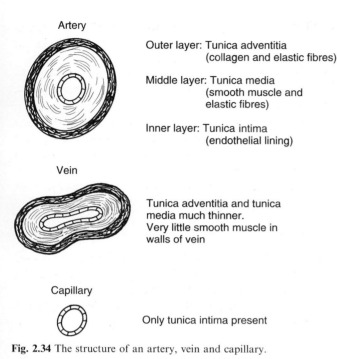

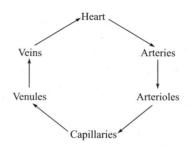

Fig. 2.34 The structure of an artery, vein and capillary.

thick muscular walls (Fig. 2.34) to enable the vessel to dilate or constrict, thus changing the volume of blood flowing through it. Blood travels along the arteries in pulses reflecting the heart beat, and this is felt in the more superficial arteries as the pulse.

As the arteries enter the tissues they branch and get smaller – these are the **arterioles**, which then flow into the capillary networks.

Capillaries

The capillaries form a branching network in all tissues and link the arteries and the veins. They are narrow with thin walls consisting of a single layer of endothelial cells with no muscle or elastic tissue (Fig. 2.34). This means that they are permeable to gases, nutrients and waste products, which diffuse between the blood and tissues and from the tissues back into the blood.

Veins

A **vein** is a relatively large vessel, which carries blood **towards** the heart (Fig. 2.34). The walls are thinner than those of arteries and they contain less muscle and elastic tissue. Blood flows slowly under low pressure and **valves** may be present in some veins, e.g. the leg, to prevent pooling of blood in the extremities. Most veins carry deoxygenated blood from the tissues; however, the pulmonary veins carry oxygenated blood from the lungs back to the heart.

The capillaries collect together to form **venules** or small veins which eventually drain into the larger veins.

The circulation

The circulation in the mammal is described as being double as blood passes through the heart twice during one complete circuit (Fig. 2.35). There are two parts to the circulatory system:

- **Systemic circulation** – carries oxygenated blood around the body and returns deoxygenated blood to the heart.
- **Pulmonary circulation** – carries deoxygenated blood from the heart to the lungs where it is oxygenated and returned to the heart.

Systemic circulation

Arterial supply Oxygenated blood leaves the left ventricle of the heart in the major artery known as the **aorta**. This gives off a number of **arteries** that supply the various parts of the body (Fig. 2.36). In the order that they leave the aorta they are the:

(1) Arteries that supply the heart muscle – **coronary arteries**.
(2) **Brachiocephalic trunk**, which gives rise to the arteries that supply the head – the **common carotid arteries**. The brachiocephalic trunk then supplies the right forelimb as it becomes the **right subclavian artery**, continuing as the **right axillary artery** and then the **right brachial artery** as it passes down the limb.
(3) **Left subclavian artery** supplies the left forelimb with blood, becoming the **left axillary artery** and then the **left brachial artery**.
(4) The aorta continues through the thorax, passing through the diaphragm into the abdomen and pelvis, giving off branches that supply the bones, muscles and organs of the body. These include:

- A pair of **renal arteries** that supply the kidney.
- **Ovarian/testicular arteries** that supply the gonads.
- **Coeliac artery** that has branches supplying the stomach, spleen and liver.
- **Cranial mesenteric artery** that supplies the small intestine.
- **Caudal mesenteric artery** that supplies the large intestine.

(5) The hind limb is supplied by the **external iliac artery**, which branches into the **femoral artery** in each of the hind limbs.
(6) A branch of the aorta called the **internal iliac artery** supplies the pelvic organs.

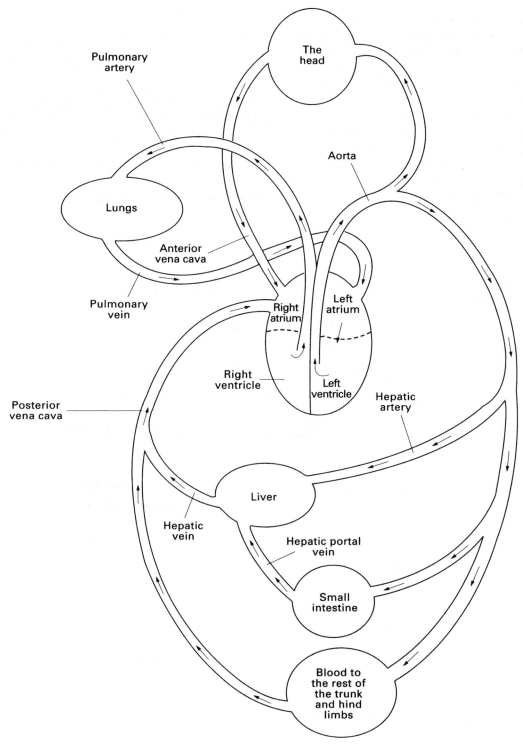

Fig. 2.35 Circulation of the blood around the body.

Venous return Deoxygenated blood returns to the heart from the tissues in the **veins**, which follow a similar pattern to those of the arteries and often have the same name, e.g. renal artery and renal vein. The veins of the pelvis, hind limbs and abdominal viscera all drain into one of the two major veins of the body, the **caudal vena cava**. This empties into the right atrium of the heart.

Venous blood returns:

- From the head in the **jugular veins.**

- From the neck and forelimbs in the **cephalic veins, brachial veins** and then **subclavian veins.**

It then drains into the **cranial vena cava**, which empties into the right atrium of the heart.

The **azygous vein** carries deoxygenated blood from the thoracic body wall and either joins the cranial vena cava or drains directly into the right atrium.

The deoxygenated blood from the heart muscle drains into the **coronary veins**, which join to form the **coronary sinus**.

The hepatic portal system This is a modified circulatory system within the systemic circulation (Fig. 2.35). Its function is to carry blood straight from the digestive system to the liver so that the products of digestion can be utilised immediately, rather than having to transport them all round the rest of the body.

Veins draining the small intestine empty into the **hepatic portal vein**, which supplies blood to the liver. The liver thus receives the products of digestion in the hepatic portal vein and oxygenated blood in the **hepatic artery**. Waste products from the liver are drained by the **hepatic vein,** which then flows into the caudal vena cava.

Pulmonary circulation Deoxygenated blood is pumped from the right ventricle of the heart and is carried to the lungs in the **pulmonary artery** (Fig. 2.36). Within the lung tissue the artery divides into numerous fine capillaries which wrap around the thin-walled alveoli of the lungs. Oxygen in the inspired air diffuses into the blood and carbon dioxide in the blood diffuses into the air in the alveoli.

The newly oxygenated blood is carried to the left atrium of the heart by the **pulmonary veins** and is pumped around the body in the systemic circulation.

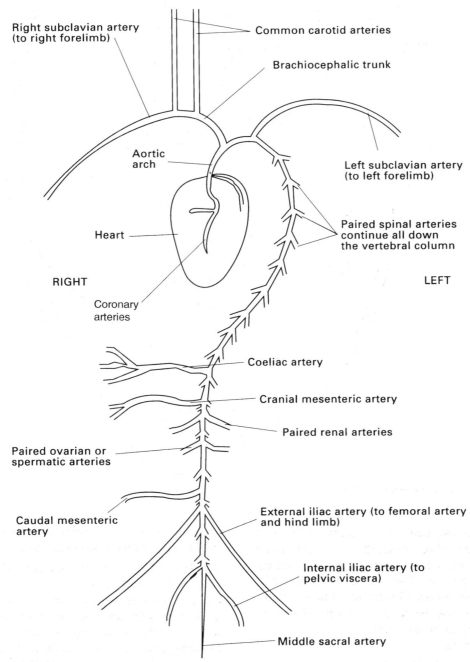

Fig. 2.36 The main branches of the aorta.

NAPIER UNIVERSITY L.I.S.

The lymphatic system

The lymphatic system is responsible for the circulation of **lymph**, the tissue fluid that leaks out of the blood capillaries and bathes the cells in the interstitial spaces. Lymph is similar to plasma but contains more lymphocytes.

The functions of the lymphatic system are to:

(1) Return excess tissue fluid to the circulation
(2) Filter out foreign materials, e.g. bacteria from the lymph by the lymph nodes before being returned to the venous circulation.
(3) Produce lymphocytes as part of the immune system.
(4) Transport digested fats. The products of fat digestion and fat-soluble vitamins are collected by the **lacteals** of the intestinal villi.

The lymphatic system consists of:

- **Lymphatic capillaries.**
- **Lymphatic vessels**.
- **Lymph nodes**.
- **Lymphatic ducts.**
- **Lymphatic tissues.**

Lymphatic capillaries

The lymphatic capillaries are small, thin-walled vessels that are widely distributed throughout all the tissues of the body except the central nervous system. These capillaries are responsible for draining the excess tissue fluid from the interstitial spaces. In the intestinal villi the lymphatic capillaries are called **lacteals** and they collect the majority of the digested fats.

Lymphatic vessels

The lymphatic capillaries in the tissues merge to form larger lymphatic vessels. These are similar in structure to veins and contain valves that prevent backflow of the lymph. The movement of lymph is passive and is dependent upon contraction of the surrounding muscles and the non-return valves.

Lymph nodes

Lymph nodes are bean-shaped structures located at points along the lymph vessels. Each lymph node is enclosed within a connective tissue capsule and is divided into two regions – the cortex and medulla. The cortex contains germinal centres where lymphocytes are produced. There are also phagocytic cells within the lymph node, which remove bacteria and foreign particles as the lymph filters through the node.

Afferent lymphatic vessels carry lymph towards the node and enter it all over its surface. A single **efferent** vessel carries lymph away from the node at an indented area called the **hilus.**

Lymph must pass through at least one lymph node before entering the lymphatic ducts that return it to the venous circulation. Some of the lymph nodes are quite superficial and can be palpated (Fig. 2.37). When the body is fighting an infection the lymph node that lies closest to the source of the infection may become enlarged. If the disease or infection is generalised all the lymph nodes may become enlarged.

The superficial lymph nodes include the:

- **Submandibular** – located on the caudal edge of the mandible at the angle of the jaw.
- **Parotid** – caudal to the temporomandibular joint.

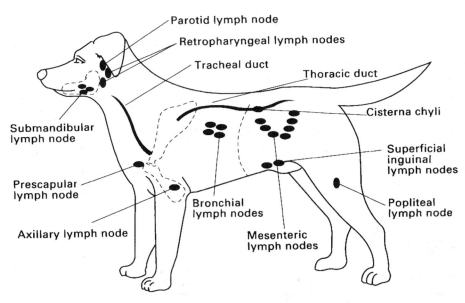

Fig. 2.37 The lymphatic system: major nodes and ducts.

- **Superficial cervical or prescapular** – just cranial to the scapular.
- **Superficial inguinal nodes** – in the groin, between the inner thigh and the abdomen.
- **Popliteal** – caudal to the stifle joint within the gastrocnemius muscle.

Lymphatic ducts

After lymph has passed through a lymph node it drains into a larger lymphatic duct. The main lymphatic ducts are:

- **Right lymphatic duct** – collects lymph from the right forelimb and the right side of the head and neck.
- **Cisterna chyli** – lies within the dorsal abdomen and collects lymph from the hind limbs, pelvis and abdomen including the lacteals.
- **Thoracic duct** – collects the lymph from the cisterna chyli, from the left forelimb and left side of the upper body.

Both the right lymphatic duct and the thoracic duct empty into either the jugular vein or the cranial vena cava near the heart.

Lymphatic tissues

These are large accumulations of lymphoid tissue, which play an important part in the body's defence system.

The spleen This is a haemopoietic lymphoid organ found closely attached to the greater curvature of the stomach. The functions of the spleen are:

- Storage of blood.
- Removal of old red blood cells.
- Production of lymphocytes.
- Removal of bacteria and foreign material by the action of the phagocytic cells.

Though the spleen has these important functions it is not essential to life and can be surgically removed if necessary.

The thymus This lies in the thorax, cranial to the heart. It is an important site for lymphocyte production in the young animal and plays an essential role in their immune system. As the animal grows older the thymus atrophies.

The tonsils These form a ring of lymphoid tissue in the subepithelial layer of the pharynx. They provide a defence against the introduction of infection into the digestive and respiratory systems.

The respiratory system

The function of the respiratory system is to extract oxygen from atmospheric air and excrete carbon dioxide, formed by the tissues, out into the air again.

Respiration is the exchange of gases between a living organism and its environment. It can be considered to occur in two stages:

- **External respiration** is the gaseous exchange between the air and the blood.
- **Internal or tissue respiration** is the gaseous exchange between the blood and the tissues.

The parts of the respiratory system are:

- The nasal chambers.
- The pharynx.
- The larynx.
- The bronchi and bronchioles.
- The alveoli

Nasal chambers

Air enters the respiratory system through the **external nares** or nostrils to reach the **nasal chambers** (Fig. 2.38). The nostrils are surrounded by the **rhinarium** or nosepad. The nasal chambers are divided by a cartilaginous nasal **septum** and are filled with fine scrolls of bone called **ethmoturbinates** or **conchae.** The entire cavity and the ethmoturbinates are covered by **ciliated mucous epithelium**, which is well supplied with capillaries and sensory nerve fibres. These nerve fibres travel the short distance to the olfactory bulbs of the forebrain, carrying the sensation of smell, or **olfaction.**

Leading from the nasal cavities are small air-filled diverticuli in the surrounding facial bones – the **paranasal sinuses** (Fig. 2.38). They are lined with ciliated mucous epithelium and communicate with the nasal cavity through narrow openings:

- **Maxillary sinus** – this is not a true sinus in the dog but a recess at the caudal end of the nasal cavities.
- **Frontal sinus** – this sinus lies within the frontal bone of the skull.

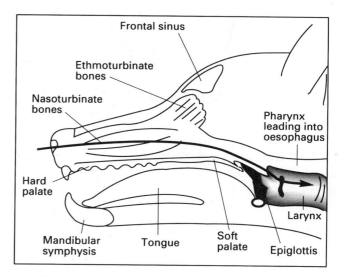

Fig. 2.38 Midline section through dog's head.

The paranasal sinuses lighten the weight of the skull allowing the surface area to be used for the attachment of larger muscles. They also act as an area for thermal exchange and for mucus secretion.

The **function** of the nasal cavities is to:

(1) Warm and moisten incoming air.
(2) Trap dust and foreign particles in the covering of mucus. The cilia waft them to the back of the nasal cavity where they pass to the pharynx and are swallowed or coughed out.
(3) Olfaction.

Pharynx

Inspired air passes into the pharynx (Fig. 2.38). This structure at the back of the oral and nasal cavities is shared by the respiratory and digestive systems. The entrance from the nasal cavity into the pharynx can be sealed off by a musculomembranous partition – the **soft palate**, which prevents food from entering the nasal cavities when the animal swallows (see Digestive System). The soft palate is the caudal extension of the hard palate and divides the pharynx into the **nasopharynx**, which conducts air from the nasal cavity to the larynx, and the **oropharynx**, which conducts food from the mouth to the oesophagus. During respiratory difficulty, or strenuous exercise, 'mouth breathing' may occur and air may enter the pharynx from the mouth as well as the nose, allowing a greater volume of air to reach the lungs.

In addition to these openings there are paired openings into the **Eustachian or auditory tubes** that connect the pharynx to the middle ear.

Larynx

The larynx leads from the pharynx and is a complex, mobile structure consisting of a number of cartilages and muscle. It lies in the space between the two mandibles and is suspended from the skull by the bony **hyoid apparatus,** which allows it to swing forwards and backwards like the seat of a swing (Fig. 2.39).

The opening to the larynx, the **glottis**, is closed off by a flap of elastic cartilage, the **epiglottis**, during swallowing (Fig. 2.38) (see Digestive System). When the larynx moves back to its resting position the epiglottis falls open and air is able to enter the glottis.

Within the lumen of the larynx is a pair of **vocal ligaments**. The mucous membrane covering their inner surface forms the **vocal folds**, which project into the larynx. Sound is produced when air rushes past the vocal folds, causing them to vibrate.

The function of the larynx is to:

(1) Prevent entry of anything other than gases into the respiratory tract.
(2) Regulate the flow of gases into the tract.
(3) Produce sounds.

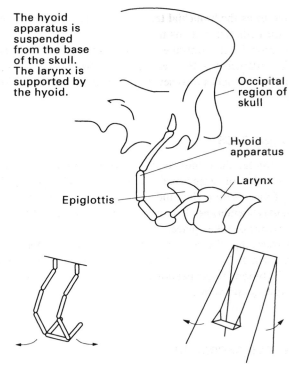

The hyoid apparatus is suspended from the base of the skull. The larynx is supported by the hyoid.

Occipital region of skull

Hyoid apparatus

Larynx

Epiglottis

The movement of the hyoid apparatus – and so of the larynx – is like a swing

Fig. 2.39 The hyoid apparatus.

Trachea

The trachea is a permanently open tube attached to the caudal laryngeal cartilages. It lies on the ventral aspect of the neck and extends the full length of the neck. It passes through the thoracic inlet and is carried in the **mediastinum** of the thoracic cavity. It bifurcates into the **right** and **left bronchi** above the heart.

The lumen of the trachea is kept open by a series of C-shaped incomplete rings of hyaline cartilage joined by smooth muscle and connective tissue. The trachea is flexible to allow movement of the head and neck. It is lined with **ciliated mucous epithelium** which traps and wafts any foreign particles towards the larynx where they are coughed up and swallowed. Any irritation of the tracheal lining causes coughing, which serves to expel substances from the respiratory tract.

Bronchi and bronchioles

The trachea bifurcates into the **right** and **left bronchi** – one leading to each lung. These divide into smaller and smaller branches as they enter the lung tissue.

The bronchi are similar in structure to the trachea, but the cartilage rings are complete and gradually reduce as the branches of the bronchi decrease in size. The bronchi branch and give off smaller branches – the **bronchioles.** Within the bronchioles the cartilage support reduces and disappears. This arrangement of tubes creates a 'tree-like' pattern referred to as the **bronchial tree**. The whole bronchial tree is lined with ciliated mucous membrane.

The bronchioles continue to branch until they reach their smallest diameter – the **respiratory bronchioles**, at which point each branches into several **alveolar ducts** (Fig. 2.40).

Alveolar sacs

Each alveolar duct ends as an **alveolar sac** consisting of a large number of 'grape-like' **alveoli** (Fig. 2.40). The epithelium of the alveoli is thin and non-ciliated and known as the **pulmonary membrane.** It is across this membrane that gaseous exchange takes place.

Surrounding the alveoli are thin-walled **capillary networks**, which bring air in the alveoli into close contact with the blood. These networks are branches of the pulmonary arteries and veins.

Gaseous exchange

Oxygen diffuses across the pulmonary membrane into the blood within the capillaries, while carbon dioxide diffuses out of the blood and into the alveoli. There are millions of alveoli in each lung and they provide a large surface area for gaseous exchange. Gaseous exchange takes place **only** in the alveoli. The rest of the respiratory tract conducts the air to the site of gaseous exchange in the alveoli and is called the conducting system. Because the component structures of the conducting system have no part in gaseous exchange they are sometimes collectively referred to as the **dead space**.

The lungs

The right and left lungs lie within the thoracic cavity, on either side of the mediastinum. Each lung consists of the air passages, blood vessels and surrounding connective tissue, all enclosed within a membrane called the **pulmonary pleura.**

Each lung (Fig. 2.41) is divided by deep furrows into lobes – the left lung has three lobes; the right lung has four. These lobes are called the **cranial (apical) lobe**, the **middle (cardiac) lobe** and the **caudal (diaphragmatic) lobe**. The fourth lobe of the right lung lies on the medial surface of the caudal lobe and is small and irregularly shaped – this is called the **accessory lobe**.

The mechanics of breathing

Breathing, or pulmonary ventilation, is achieved by the action of muscles that alternately increase and decrease the volume of the thoracic cavity. The muscles that are responsible for breathing are the **diaphragm** and the **external intercostals**.

The lungs lie within the thoracic cavity, lined by the pleural membranes, which divide the cavity into the right and left pleural cavities. These cavities are closed spaces and there is a vacuum between the lung and the chest wall. Any change in the volume of the thoracic cavity will result in a change in pressure and air will be sucked in or forced out.

(1) **Inspiration** – contraction of the external intercostals causes the upward and outward movement of the ribs. The diaphragm contracts, flattens and moves downwards. The volume of the thoracic cavity is increased creating a negative pressure in the lung tissue and air is drawn down into the lungs.
(2) **Expiration** is mainly passive – the diaphragm and intercostal muscles relax, causing the thoracic cavity to decrease in size. Pressure is put on the lungs and air is pushed out of the lungs.

The internal intercostal muscles are mainly used in **forced expiration** in conjunction with the abdominal muscles which

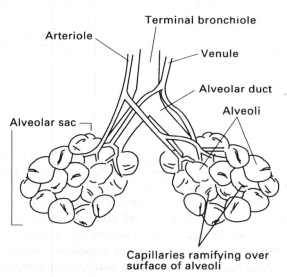

Fig. 2.40 The terminal air passages.

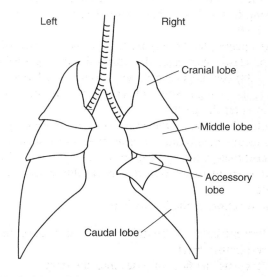

Fig. 2.41 The lobes of the lung.

contract and raise the pressure in the abdominal cavity and force the diaphragm upwards.

Control of respiration

Respiration is an automatic process that must be constantly adjusted to meet the demands of the body. It is controlled by a system involving receptors, which send information about the status of the body to a central controller.

(1) **Respiratory centres** in the pons and medulla of the hindbrain affect the basic **rhythm** of respiration:

- **Apneustic and pneumotaxic** centres control expiration.
- **Inspiratory centre** controls inspiration.

These centres inhibit each other and cannot work simultaneously.

(2) **Receptors** within the tissues of the body affect the **rate** and **depth** of respiration:

- **Stretch receptors** within the lung tissue, e.g. the **Hering–Breuer** reflex, which prevents overinflation of the lungs. As the lung inflates, the stretch receptors send impulses via the **vagus nerve** to the inspiratory centre within the hindbrain and prevent further inspiration. They also stimulate the expiratory centres and the animal breathes out.
- **Chemoreceptors** monitor the pH of the blood and the carbon dioxide/oxygen levels in the blood. They are found in the walls of the aorta and carotid arteries. For example, if carbon dioxide builds up in the blood it lowers the pH. This is detected by the chemoreceptors, which send the information to the expiratory centres. The carbon dioxide is exhaled and the pH of the blood returns to normal.

LUNG VOLUMES

Tidal air – air passing in and out of the lungs.

Tidal volume – volume of air passing in and out of the lungs during normal respiration.

Residual volume – volume of air left in the lungs after forceful expiration.

Total lung capacity – volume of air breathed in with maximum inspiration or out with maximum expiration.

Vital capacity – total amount of air that can be expired after a minimum respiration.

Functional residual capacity – volume of air left in the lungs after normal respiration.

Dead space – volume of air in the respiratory tract that never reaches the area of gaseous exchange.

Respiratory rate – number of breaths per minute.

The digestive system

The digestive tract (Fig. 2.42) comprises the:

- Oral cavity.
- Pharynx.
- Oesophagus.
- Stomach.
- Small intestine – duodenum, jejunum, ileum.
- Large intestine – caecum, colon, rectum.
- Anus.

Associated with the tract are several accessory glands:

- Salivary glands.
- Pancreas.
- Gall bladder.
- Liver.

The different parts of the system work together to produce energy from the food eaten by the animal (Table 2.13). The dog and the cat are carnivorous species, i.e. flesh eaters, and the structure of the digestive tract is adapted to deal with a diet which is relatively easily digested.

Oral cavity

This is the external opening of the digestive tract and is also called the buccal cavity or the mouth. It contains the tongue, teeth and salivary glands and its function is to:

(1) Pick up food – prehension.
(2) Break up the food and manipulate it into boluses – mastication.
(3) Lubricate the food to aid swallowing.

The oral cavity is supported by the upper jaw, formed by the **maxillary** and **incisive bones**, and the lower jaw, formed by the **left and right mandibles**. The **palatine bone** forms the roof of the mouth and is known as the **hard palate.** An outer layer of skin, which forms the **cheeks**, connects the jaws. Beneath the skin is the main muscle of mastication – the **masseter muscle**. The external entrance to the oral cavity is marked by the **lips** composed of muscle. The upper lip has a central vertical cleft known as the **philtrum**.

The entire cavity is lined by mucous membrane, which reflects on to the jawbones forming the **gums** and is pierced by the teeth.

Tongue

This lies on the floor of the oral cavity and is made of striated muscle fibres running in all directions. The tip of the tongue is unattached and very mobile, while the root of the tongue is continuous with the larynx and is attached to the hyoid apparatus and to the mandibles.

The tongue is covered in mucous membrane arranged in backward pointing papillae, giving it a rough surface useful for grooming and for ingestion and manipulation of food.

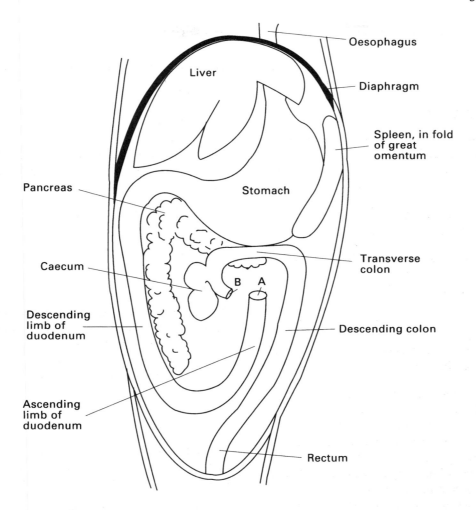

A. **Junction of duodenum and jejunum**
B. **Junction of ileum and ascending colon (ileo-caeco-colic junction)**

Fig. 2.42 Position of gastrointestinal tract in the abdomen.

Embedded among the papillae particularly at the back of the tongue are the taste buds (see Special Senses). Underneath the tongue is the **lingual vein**, which may be used for venepuncture in an anaesthetised patient.

In the dog the tongue is the main method of thermoregulation. Saliva on the tongue evaporates as the animal pants, causing cooling.

Table 2.13 Processes occurring in the digestive system		
Process	**Definition**	**Parts of the tract involved**
Ingestion	Food is taken into the body	Lips, teeth, tongue
Mastication (chewing)	Food is mixed with saliva and formed into a bolus ready for swallowing	Lips, cheeks, tongue, salivary glands
Digestion	Food is broken down by digestive enzymes into small soluble chemical units	Stomach and small intestine
Absorption	Small units pass through the intestinal wall into the bloodstream	Small intestine
Metabolism	Small units are processed to produce energy and material necessary for normal body functions	Liver and all cells of the body
Excretion	Remaining insoluble material passes out as faeces	Large intestine, anus

Salivary glands

These are paired glandular structures embedded in the soft tissues of the oral cavity whose secretions enter the cavity by means of ducts. The position of the ducts is shown in Fig. 2.43.

Saliva produced by the dog and cat contains 99% water and 1% mucus. There are no enzymes as food spends little time in the oral cavity before being swallowed. Its main function is to aid mastication and swallowing and in thermoregulation.

Sight and/or smell of food, fear, irritant smells and tastes, vomiting, pain and poisoning by certain chemicals, e.g. organophosphates, may all stimulate salivation.

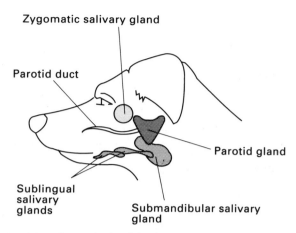

Fig. 2.43 The salivary glands of the dog.

Teeth

These are hard structures embedded in sockets or **alveoli** in the upper and lower jaw. Each jaw forms a **dental arch** of which there are four. The mucous membrane covering the gums is called the **periodontal membrane** or the **gingival membrane.**

- Structure: all teeth have the same basic structure, as shown in Fig. 2.44.
- Function: the teeth of the cat and dog are adapted to tearing flesh from the bones of prey. There are four types, each with a different position in the jaw (Fig. 2.45) and a different function (Table 2.14).

Dogs and cats have two sets of teeth during their lives. These are the:

(1) **Deciduous, temporary or 'milk' dentition** – present in the jaw at birth and erupt during the first few months of life. Smaller and whiter than adult teeth.

(2) **Permanent or adult dentition** – replaces the milk teeth and last for the whole of adult life. Larger and show signs of wear as the animal ages.

Eruption times for each dentition are shown in Table 2.15.

The number and type of teeth are written as a **dental formula**:

- **Dog**

  (a) Deciduous teeth: I3/3 C1/1 PM3/3 × 2 = 28.
  (b) Permanent teeth: I3/3 C1/1 PM4/4 M2/3 × 2 = 42.

- **Cat**

  (a) Deciduous teeth: I3/3 C1/1 PM3/2 × 2 = 26.
  (b) Permanent teeth: I3/3 C1/1 PM3/2 M1/1 × 2 = 30.

Pharynx

This is short muscular tube lined with mucous membrane, which acts as a crossover point between the respiratory and

Table 2.14 Tooth type and function

Type	Shape	Function
Incisor (I)	Lie in the incisive bone of the upper jaw and in the mandible of the lower jaw. Small pointed with a single root	Fine nibbling and cutting flesh. Often used for delicate grooming
Canines (C) – 'eye teeth'	One on each corner of the upper and lower jaws. Pointed with a simple curved shape, single root deeply embedded in the bone	Holding prey firmly in the mouth
Premolars (PM) – 'cheek teeth'	Flatter surface with several points known as cusps or tubercles. Usually have 2 or 3 roots arranged in a triangular position to give stability in the jawbone	Shearing meat off the bone using a scissor-like action. Flattened surface helps to grind up the meat to facilitate swallowing and digestion
Molars (M) – 'cheek teeth'	Similar shape to premolars. Usually larger with at least 3 roots	Shearing and grinding flesh (**NB**: There are no molars in the deciduous dentition)
Carnassials	Largest teeth in the jaw. Similar shape to other cheek teeth **These are the first lower molar and the last upper premolar on each side**	Very powerful teeth sited close to the angle of the lips and used for bone crunching. Only found in carnivores

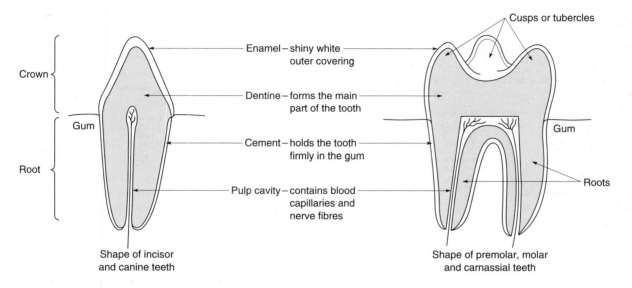

Fig. 2.44 Tooth structure. (Redrawn from Masters and Bowden, *Pre-Veterinary Nursing Textbook*, Butterworth–Heinemann, 2001.)

digestive systems. The **soft palate** extends caudally from the hard palate towards the epiglottis of the larynx and divides the pharynx into **nasopharynx** at the back of the nasal cavity and the **oropharynx** at the back of the oral cavity (see Respiratory System).

The pharynx conveys food from the oral cavity to the oesophagus by a process known as **swallowing** or **deglutition**. This occurs in the following steps:

(1) Food is formed into a bolus and passed to the back of the mouth.
(2) The walls of the pharynx contract and push the bolus towards the oesophagus.
(3) Simultaneously the epiglottis closes to prevent food from entering the larynx.
(4) A wave of contraction – peristalsis – pushes the food down the oesophagus.
(5) As the food leaves the pharynx the epiglottis falls open, allowing air to pass down the larynx and trachea.

Oesophagus

This simple muscular tube conveys food by a series of organised muscular contractions known as **peristalsis** from the pharynx through the thorax and diaphragm to the stomach (Fig. 2.42). In the neck, it lies dorsal to and slightly to the left of the trachea. It is lined with stratified squamous epithelium arranged in longitudinal folds, which allow widthways expansion as food passes down. Beneath this are layers of smooth muscle well supplied with nerves and blood capillaries.

The average time for food to pass down the oesophagus is 15–30 s, but this depends on the nature of the food. Food is able to pass back up the oesophagus during vomition.

Stomach

This is a C-shaped sac-like organ lying mainly on the left side of the cranial abdominal cavity. Its functions are to:

Tooth type	Dog	Cat
Deciduous dentition		Entire dentition starts to erupt at 2 weeks and is complete by 4 weeks
Incisors	3–4 weeks	
Canines	5 weeks	
Premolars	4–8 weeks	
Molars	Absent	
Permanent dentition		Variable. Full dentition present by 6 months
Incisors	3.5–4 months	12 weeks
Canines	5–6 months	
Premolars	1st premolars 4–5 months	
	Remainder 5–7 months	
Molars	5–7 months	

Table 2.15 Eruption times for the deciduous and permanent dentitions

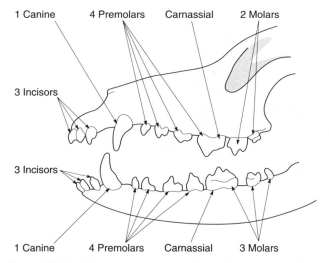

1 Canine   4 Premolars   Carnassial   2 Molars

3 Incisors

3 Incisors

1 Canine   4 Premolars   Carnassial   3 Molars

Fig. 2.45 Skull of dog to show tooth position. Redrawn from Masters and Bowden, *Pre-Veterinary Nursing Textbook*, Butterworth–Heinemann, 2001.)

(1)   Act as a reservoir for food prior to digestion.
(2)   Break up the food and mix it with gastric juices.
(3)   Begin protein digestion.

Food in the oesophagus enters the stomach via the **cardiac sphincter** and leaves via the **pyloric sphincter**. These muscular structures control the rate of flow of material into and out of the stomach. The outer curve of the stomach is called the **greater curvature** and the inner curve is called the **lesser curvature.** The entire organ is covered in a layer of visceral peritoneum or mesentery – the mesentery attached to the lesser curvature is the **lesser omentum** and that attached to the greater curvature is the **greater omentum. The spleen** is closely applied to the greater curvature and lies within the greater omentum.

The walls of the stomach are thick and very distensible. When empty it lies under the ribs, but when full the stomach may occupy as much as half of the abdomen and can easily be seen from the outside.

Structure of the stomach wall (Fig. 2.46)

The stomach can be divided into three regions:

- Cardia – close to the cardiac sphincter.
- Fundus – forms the largest region and contains most of the gastric glands.
- Pylorus – close to the pyloric sphincter.

The walls are lined in mucous membrane – the **gastric mucosa** which is arranged in deep folds or **rugae.** These enable the stomach to stretch when filled with food. Within the mucosa are the **gastric pits,** which consist of three types of cells responsible for the production of gastric juices:

(1)   **Goblet cells** – secrete mucus to aid lubrication of the food and protect the stomach wall from autodigestion.

(2)   **Chief cells** – secrete pepsinogen, the precursor of the enzyme pepsin.
(3)   **Parietal cells** – secrete hydrochloric acid. This creates an acid pH, which protects against infection and converts pepsinogen to the active pepsin. Pepsin digests protein to form peptides.

The secretion of gastric juices is initiated by the hormone **gastrin** produced by the stomach walls in response to the distension of the stomach by food.

Beneath the gastric mucosa are three layers of **smooth muscle fibres** lying in all directions. These are responsible for peristaltic contractions, which push the food onwards, and rhythmic segmentation, which mixes the food with the gastric juices.

Within the stomach, food is changed into partially digested **chyme** with an acid pH. This is released in spurts through the pyloric sphincter into the duodenum. The time taken to pass through the stomach depends on food type – liquids may take up to 30 minutes, while more solid or fatty foods may take as long as 3 hours.

Vomiting

This is the return of ingesta and fluids against the normal direction of swallowing and peristalsis. There are three types:

(1)   True vomiting – involves active abdominal contractions and expulsion of the vomitus, preceded by a feeling of nausea and salivation.
(2)   Passive vomiting or regurgitation – overflow of oesophageal contents. No muscle contractions involved.
(3)   Projectile vomiting – violent ejection of the stomach contents.

Small intestine

This is the main site for the enzymatic digestion of food and its subsequent absorption. The small intestine is a long narrow tube divided into three parts, each of which has a similar structure with certain functional differences.

(1)   **Duodenum** – this relatively short tube lies in the dorsal abdomen and is held in a U-shaped loop by a short piece of mesentery – the **mesoduodenum. The pancreas** lies within the loop. Its secretions enter the duodenum via the **pancreatic duct** near to the pyloric sphincter and close to the opening of the **common bile duct** leading from the gall bladder.
  Within the walls of the duodenum are **Brunner's glands.** These are digestive glands, which secrete a mixture of enzymes referred to as **succus entericus.**
(2)   **Jejunum and ileum** – these are difficult to distinguish externally and form a long thin tube suspended by the **mesojejunum** and **mesoileum.** This is long and mobile and enables the intestine to fill any free space within the peritoneal cavity.

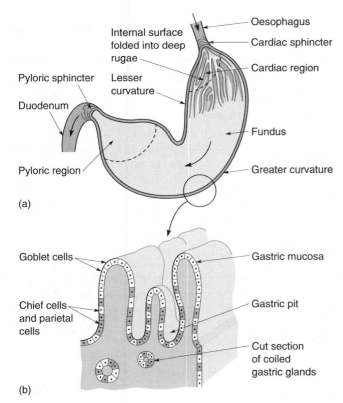

Fig. 2.46 (a) Cross-section through the stomach wall. (b) Section showing gastric pits.

Within the walls are digestive glands known as the **crypts of Lieberkühn.** The ileum terminates at the **ileo-caecal junction.**

Structure of the intestinal wall

Each part of the intestinal wall has a similar structure (Fig. 2.47). The epithelium is folded into numerous tiny folds called **villi** (sing. villus). Extending from each epithelial cell is a border of minute microvilli forming a 'brush border'. Both these structures increase the surface area for the absorption of digested food.

Inside each villus is:

- A capillary network, which carries digested proteins and carbohydrates to the liver via the **hepatic portal vein.**
- A lymphatic capillary known as a **lacteal** which carries **chyle,** a milky liquid containing digested fat, to the **cisterna chyli** in the dorsal abdomen.

Pancreas

This is a pale pink lobulated gland lying in the loop of the duodenum. It is described as a mixed gland as it has an endocrine part (see Endocrine System) and an exocrine part. The exocrine secretions, consisting of several digestive enzymes and bicarbonate, enter the duodenum via the **pancreatic duct.**

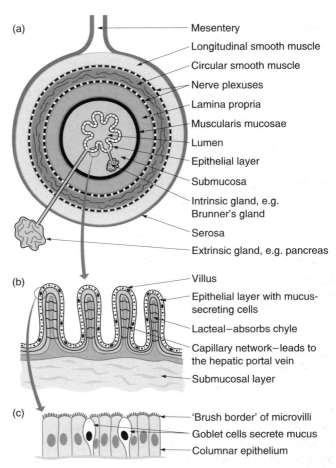

Fig. 2.47 (a) Cross-section through the intestine wall. (b) Detail of villus structure. (c) Detail of epithelium.

Gall bladder

Lies between the lobes of the liver and collects bile formed by the liver. Bile is coloured yellow-green by the pigment **bilirubin** and contains **bile salts** needed for the emulsification of fats. It enters the duodenum via the **common bile duct.**

Digestion

Digestion is the process by which proteins (polypeptides), carbohydrates (polysaccharides) and fats (lipids) are broken down into small soluble units, which can then be absorbed by the blood capillaries and the lacteals.

An **enzyme** is a protein, which acts as a catalyst, increasing the speed of a reaction. They are specifically structured to act on particular materials or substrates and do not affect any other substrates. Some enzymes are produced as precursors – an inactive form, which must be activated by another enzyme before it can work.

Chemicals known as enzymes are secreted by digestive glands and begin to break down the food as it enters the stomach and small intestine. Details of digestion can be found in Table 2.16.

The result of the digestive process is that the basic constituents of food are converted to small soluble molecules thus:

Protein (polypeptides) ⟶ Amino acids

Carbohydrates ⟶ Glucose and other simple
(polysaccharides and disaccharides) sugars (monosaccharides)

Fats ⟶ Fatty acids and glycerol
(monoglycerides)

Absorption

Absorption is the process by which small soluble units are taken into the circulation. The site of absorption is the small intestine and its efficiency is increased by the tube length and by the lining of villi (Fig. 2.47), which provide a large surface area with a good supply of blood capillaries and lacteals.

During absorption:

- Amino acids and simple sugars pass into the **blood capillaries** and are carried to the liver by the **hepatic portal vein**.
- Fatty acids and glycerol pass into the **lacteals** as a milky liquid called **chyle**, which is carried to the **cisterna chyli** in the dorsal abdomen. Here it mixes with lymph and is carried to the heart by the thoracic duct, where it joins the blood circulation.

Large intestine

This is a relatively short tube with a large diameter. The lining is not folded into villi and there are no digestive glands, although there are more goblet cells, which secrete mucus to lubricate the passage of faeces. It consists of the following parts:

(1) **Caecum** – short blind-ending sac which joins the ileum at the **ileocaecal junction.** It has very little function in the carnivore.
(2) **Colon** – divided into the ascending, transverse and descending colon according to its position in the peritoneal cavity. It is suspended by the short **mesocolon.** Water and electrolytes are absorbed from the remaining indigestible food within the colon.
(3) **Rectum** – the part of the colon running through the pelvic cavity. It is held in place by the surrounding connective tissue and muscle.
(4) **Anus** – the external opening of the digestive tract. It forms a muscular sphincter which controls the passage of faeces out of the body. It has two parts:

- Internal anal sphincter – ring of smooth muscle under involuntary control.
- External anal sphincter – outer ring of striated muscle under voluntary control.

The lumen of the anus and the rectum is folded longitudinally enabling the lining to stretch during the passage of bulky faeces. Between the two anal rings in the '20 to 4' position is a pair of **anal sacs**. These are modified cutaneous glands whose size is approximately that of a pea. They secrete a pungent smelling paste-like material, which coats the faeces as it passes through the sphincter. The characteristic smell is used as a means of territorial marking by the dog and the cat.

Defecation

The faecal mass passes along the colon and rectum by means of peristalsis and by slower stronger but infrequent contractions known as mass movements. As the faeces enter the pelvic cavity the wall of the rectum is stretched which stimulates voluntary straining. The anal sphincter, normally held tightly closed, relaxes, the abdominal muscles contract, the animal adopts the correct position and the mass is forced out.

Composition of faeces

Normal faeces has a smell, colour and shape that is characteristic of the species. Faeces consists of:

- Water and fibre – the relative proportions affect the consistency and shape.
- Dead and living bacteria – these are normal commensals and may contribute to the smell and help to breakdown any remaining protein.
- Mucus – adds bulk and aids lubrication.
- Stercobilin – derived from bile. Gives faeces its colour.
- Sloughed intestinal cells.
- Secretion from anal sacs.

The liver

The liver lies in the cranial abdominal cavity and is the largest gland in the body. The cranial aspect is convex, conforming to the abdominal side of the diaphragm. The caudal aspect is concave and in contact with the stomach, duodenum and right kidney. A normal liver is deep red in colour.

The remnants of the fetal blood vessels from the umbilicus, the **falciform ligament**, is found in the centre of the caudal aspect of the liver and is of no significance in the adult.

Microscopically, the liver consists of millions of cells known as **hepatocytes** arranged in hexagonal **lobules**. Running between the hepatocytes is an interconnecting network of tiny **bile canaliculi** into which bile is secreted.

Table 2.16 Processes involved in digestion

Digestive juice	Contents	Action	Comments
Stomach secretes gastric juices			The hormone gastrin is produced as food enters the stomach and stimulates the gastric pits to secrete gastric juices
1. Goblet cells	Mucus	No enzyme action. Lubricates food. Protects gastric mucosa from autodigestion	
2. Parietal cells	Hydrochloric acid (HCl)	Denatures protein. Creates a pH of 1.3–5. Converts pepsinogen to active pepsin	Protein digestion is made easier. Acid pH kills most pathogenic bacteria
3. Chief cells	Pepsinogen	When activated by HCl, pepsin converts protein to peptides	Peptides are smaller molecules
Small intestine:			
1. Bile from the liver	Bile salts	Emulsifies fats to produce small globules. Activates lipases	As chyme enters the duodenum, the gall bladder contracts forcing bile along the bile duct
2. Pancreatic juices from exocrine part of the pancreas			Produced in response to gastrin and to the hormone cholecystokinin secreted by duodenal cells as chyme passes through the pyloric sphincter
	a. Bicarbonate	No enzyme action. Neutralises the acid pH	Neutral pH stops action of pepsin and enables intestinal digestive enzymes to act
	b. Trypsinogen	Inactive	Converted to active trypsin by enterokinase present in succus entericus. Spontaneous conversion is prevented by a trypsin inhibitor
	c. Trypsin	Activates other enzyme precursors. Converts peptides and other proteins to amino acids	Amino acids are absorbed into the bloodstream
	d. Lipase	Converts fats to fatty acids and glycerol	Activated by bile salts
	e. Amylase	Converts starches to maltose	Starches are plant carbohydrates
3. Intestinal juices from Brunner's glands as succus entericus and from the crypts of Lieberkuhn			Produced in response to the hormone secretin, secreted as the chyme passes through the pyloric sphincter
	a. Maltase	Converts maltose to glucose	Glucose is absorbed by the blood capillaries
	b. Sucrase	Converts sucrose to glucose and fructose	Glucose and fructose are absorbed by blood capillaries
	c. Lactase	Converts lactose to glucose and galactose	Glucose and galactose are absorbed by blood capillaries
	d. Enterokinase	Converts trypsinogen to trypsin	Trypsin is activated
	e. Aminopeptidase	Converts peptides to amino acids	Amino acids are absorbed into the bloodstream
	f. Lipase	Converts fats to fatty acids and glycerol	Fatty acids and glycerol are absorbed into the lacteals

The bile eventually drains into the gall bladder, which lies between the central lobes of the liver on the caudal aspect.

Arterial blood reaches the liver tissue via the **hepatic artery.** The products of digestion reach the liver from the small intestine via the **hepatic portal vein** (Fig. 2.35). Blood from these two vessels bathes the hepatocytes, permeating through the liver lobules in minute **sinusoids** and draining into a **central vein** in the middle of each lobule. The central veins flow into the **hepatic vein** and so to the caudal vena cava. There is no contact between the bile canaliculi and the sinusoids.

The liver has many functions and is essential to normal health:

(1) Carbohydrate metabolism – excess glucose is stored as glycogen (glycogenogenesis) in the presence of insulin from the pancreas. When the body requires extra energy, glycogen is broken down to release energy (glycogenolysis) in the presence of glucagon from the pancreas.

(2) Protein metabolism:

- Formation of plasma proteins – albumin, pro-thrombin, fibrinogen.
- Amino acids from the digestion of protein in food are converted into the amino acid of body protein for maintenance and growth – a process known as **transamination.**
- Production of urea – surplus amino acids are converted to ammonia and urea in a process known as **deamination.** Urea is excreted in the urine.

(3) Fat metabolism – fat is the main energy source for the body. Excess fat is deposited around the body. Fatty acids and glycerol resulting from fat digestion are converted into phospholipids for cell membranes and cholesterol for bile salts.

(4) Formation of bile – stored in the gall bladder and used in digestion.

(5) Destruction of old red blood cells – haemoglobin is excreted as bilirubin in the bile.

(6) Formation of new red blood cells – only in the foetus.

(7) Storage of vitamins – mainly the fat-soluble vitamins (A, D, E, K), but may store some water-soluble ones.

(8) Storage of iron.

(9) Thermoregulation.

(10) Detoxification of certain substances such as alcohol.

(11) Detoxification and conjugation of steroid hormones.

The urinary system

The system is made up of:

- Kidney.
- Ureter.
- Bladder.
- Urethra.

The urinary system is anatomically linked with the reproductive system as the penis (male) or vagina and vulva (female) is common to both – the system may be referred to as the urinogenital system.

The functions of the urinary system are to:

(1) Remove nitrogenous waste products and excess water from the body.

(2) Regulate the chemical makeup of the body fluids – plays an important role in homeostasis.

(3) Secrete the hormone erythropoietin or erythropoietic stimulating factor (see Endocrine System).

Kidney

Structure

Position In the normal mammal there are a pair of kidneys. One lies on each side of the major blood vessels, the dorsal aorta and caudal vena cava in the cranial dorsal abdomen. They are closely attached to the lumbar hypaxial muscles by the parietal peritoneum and are described as being **retroperitoneal** (Fig. 2.48). The right kidney lies cranial to the left as the stomach occupies the left side of the cranial abdomen. The kidneys lie cranial to the right

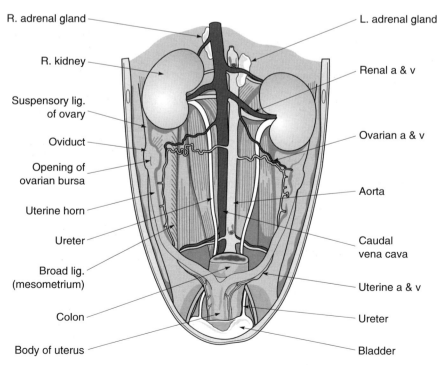

Fig. 2.48 Ventro-dorsal view of the urinary system of the bitch. (Redrawn from H. E. Evans, *Miller's Anatomy of the Dog*, W. B. Saunders, 1993.)

and left ovaries and caudal to the right and left adrenal glands (Fig. 2.48).

Shape and size   Kidney-bean shaped with a smooth outline. Normally browny-red in colour. When examining the kidneys on a lateral radiograph, the normal kidney measures approximately 2.5 lumbar vertebrae.

Blood supply   A single **renal artery** from the dorsal aorta carries arterial blood to each kidney, entering via the **hilus**. Blood carried by the renal arteries may be as much as 20% of cardiac output (Fig. 2.48). Within the kidney the renal artery divides into several **interlobar arteries** which give off capillary networks to supply the tubules and to form the **glomeruli** (sing. glomerulus). The capillaries then recombine to form **interlobar veins**, which enter the single **renal vein**. Venous blood then drains into the caudal vena cava.

Macroscopic appearance.   If the kidney is cut longitudinally (Fig. 2.49) it is possible to identify the following layers:

- **Fibrous tissue capsule** – tough outer coat closely attached to the cortex but may be peeled away from the kidney itself. It protects the kidney from mechanical damage and may be surrounded by deposits of fat in obese animals.
- **Cortex** – outer layer of the kidney tissue containing the renal corpuscles and convoluted tubules of the nephrons. Its good blood supply gives it a dark red colour.

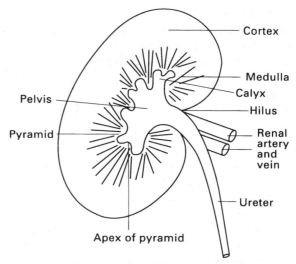

Fig. 2.49 Longitudinal view of the kidney.

- **Medulla** – paler than the cortex. May be able to see triangular areas called **pyramids**, which contain the collecting ducts of the nephrons. The remainder contains the loops of Henle.
- **Pelvis** – basin-shaped structure made of dense connective tissue. Collects urine formed by the nephrons and is drained by a single **ureter**, which leaves by the **hilus**.

Microscopic appearance   The functional unit of the kidney is the **nephron** (Fig. 2.50). Each kidney contains around a million nephrons. Each nephron consists of several parts:

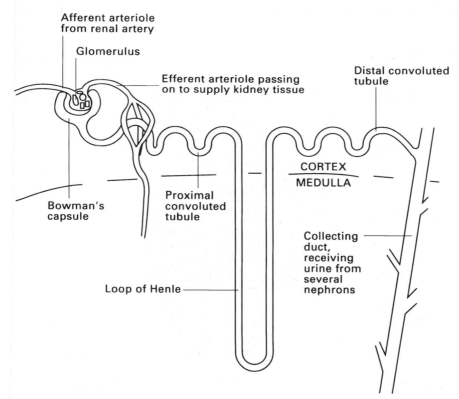

Fig. 2.50 A kidney nephron.

- **Glomerular capsule** – also called Bowman's capsule. A cup-shaped structure enclosing a network of blood capillaries known as the **glomerulus**. A capsule and a glomerulus together form a **renal corpuscle**. The glomerular capsule is hollow and its inner surface forms a **basement membrane** perforated by microscopic pores. This membrane is in close contact with the endothelium of the glomerulus and allows the free flow of fluid from the blood into the lumen of the capsule, but restricts the passage of large molecules, e.g. protein.
- **Proximal convoluted tubule** – long twisted tubule lying within the cortex. Lined with cuboidal epithelium with a brush border of microvilli which increases the surface area for reabsorption of water and electrolytes.
- **Loop of Henle** – U-shaped tube which extends into the medulla. It has a descending part lined by a thin squamous epithelium and an ascending part lined by a thicker squamous epithelium.
- **Distal convoluted tubule** – lies within the cortex and is lined by cuboidal epithelium without a brush border.
- **Collecting duct** – each duct collects urine from several nephrons, runs through a pyramid area and empties into the pelvis of the kidney.

Function – urine formation

The kidneys filter the blood and the filtrate undergoes a series of modifications within the renal tubules to form urine. The urine is very different in composition and volume from the original filtrate – for every 100 litres of fluid removed from the blood, only 1 litre is excreted as urine. The changes to the filtrate reflect the status of the extracellular fluid (ECF) and in particular that of the blood plasma. They are made by different parts of the nephron and make use of different physiological processes (Table 2.17).

Blood enters the kidneys via the renal artery and reaches the capillaries of the glomerulus.

Glomerular capsule   Here the blood is under high pressure because:

- Blood comes straight from the heart via the dorsal aorta and the renal artery.
- The arteriole leaving the glomerulus is able to constrict under the control of the hormone **renin** (Table 2.18) which regulates the pressure in the glomerulus.

This high pressure forces fluid and small molecules out of the glomerulus, through the pores of the basement membrane into the lumen of the capsule. Larger molecules, e.g. protein are retained in the blood. This process is known as **ultrafiltration** and results in a dilute glomerular filtrate or primitive urine.

Proximal convoluted tubule   Eighty-five per cent of all the resorptive processes take place here. These are:

- Sodium ions (Na^+) are reabsorbed.
- Sixty-five per cent of the water is reabsorbed by osmosis.
- All glucose in the filtrate is reabsorbed. Normal urine does not contain glucose.
- Concentration of nitrogenous waste by the reabsorption of water. This is mainly urea from protein metabolism in the liver. Some urea also diffuses back into the blood from the tubules.
- Secretion of toxins and certain drugs, e.g. penicillin.

Loop of Henle   The **concentration and volume** of the urine is regulated here according to the status of the ECF. The filtrate flows into the descending loop and then into the ascending loop both of which lie in the renal medulla.

- **Descending loop** – the lining cells are *permeable* to water but do not have the mechanism to reabsorb Na^+ ions. Water is drawn out of the filtrate by osmosis – pulled by the high concentration of Na^+ ions in the surrounding medulla. The concentration of the filtrate increases as it travels towards the tip of the loop.
- **Ascending loop** – the lining cells are *impermeable* to water but are able to reabsorb Na^+ ions into the tissue of the medulla and the capillaries. As water cannot leave the filtrate it becomes less concentrated as it passes upwards.

The result of this mechanism is that the filtrate is the same concentration when it enters the loop as it is when it leaves, but the volume is reduced – water has been conserved in the body. If an animal is dehydrated more water is reabsorbed; if it is overhydrated more water is excreted in the urine.

Distal convoluted tubule   The final adjustments are made to the **electrolyte content** of the urine according to the status of the ECF.

- Na^+ is reabsorbed and is replaced in the urine by potassium (K^+) ions.

Table 2.17 Physiological processes occurring in the renal tubules	
Process	**Description**
Osmosis	Passage of water through a semipermeable membrane from a weaker to a stronger solution
Diffusion	Passage of a solute from an area of high concentration to an area of low concentration
Reabsorption	Passage of a substance from the lumen of the renal tubules into the surrounding capillaries and back into the circulation. This is an active process and requires expenditure of energy
Secretion	Passage of a substance from the surrounding capillaries into the lumen of the renal tubules and out of the body in the urine. This is an active process and requires expenditure of energy

Table 2.18 Factors involved in osmoregulation	
Controlling factor	**Function**
Renin–hormone	Produced by the glomeruli of the kidney in response to low arterial pressure
Angiotensinogen – plasma protein	Converted to angiotensin by the action of renin
Angiotensin – protein	Causes vasoconstriction. Stimulates the release of aldosterone from the adrenal cortex
Aldosterone – hormone – mineralocorticoid	Secreted by the cortex of the adrenal gland. Acts mainly on the distal convoluted tubules but has a lesser effect on the collecting ducts. Regulates the reabsorption of Na^+ ions
Antidiuretic hormone, ADH (vasopressin)	Secreted by the posterior pituitary gland. Mainly affects the collecting ducts by changing their permeability to water. Also has an affect on the distal convoluted tubules
Baroreceptors	Found in the walls of the blood vessels. Monitor arterial blood pressure
Osmoreceptors	Found in the hypothalamus. Monitor the osmotic pressure of the plasma. Affect the thirst centre of the brain and influence the secretion of ADH

- Reabsorption of water varies and is controlled by the hormone **aldosterone** (Table 2.18).
- Regulation of **acid/base balance** by excretion of hydrogen (H^+) ions. Normal pH of blood is 7.4. If there are excess H^+ ions in the blood the pH falls (more acid) and the excess ions are excreted in the urine, returning the pH to normal, and vice versa.

Collecting duct Final adjustments are made to the **volume of water** in the urine. **Antidiuretic hormone (ADH)** (Table 2.18) is able to alter the permeability of the walls of the collecting ducts to water to control the volume. If the animal is dehydrated, the walls become more permeable, so water is reabsorbed from the urine into the blood capillaries, and vice versa.

The urine produced by repeated reabsorption and secretion leaves the kidney via the ureter.

Control of kidney function – osmoregulation

Osmoregulation ensures that the volume of the ECF – principally plasma volume – and the concentration of dissolved chemicals in the fluid remains constant so that homeostasis is maintained and the body functions normally.

Osmoregulation is controlled by various factors (Table 2.18) and occurs in two ways:

- Control of water loss.
- Control of salt (Na^+) levels.

Control of water loss Water is taken into the body in food and drink and is excreted in urine, faeces, sweat and respiration. Small amounts may be lost in vaginal secretions and tears. If intake is reduced or output is excessive, e.g. vomiting and diarrhoea, the total volume of

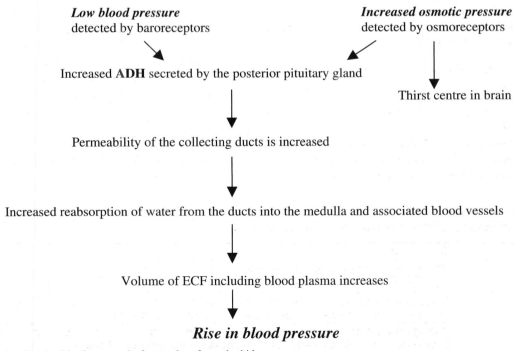

Fig. 2.51 Mechanism involved in the control of water loss from the kidney.

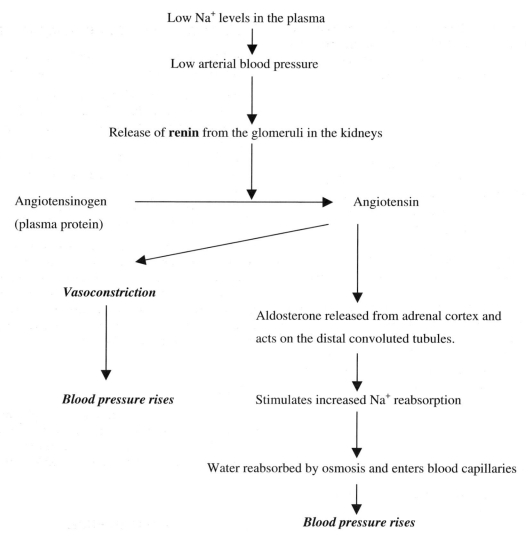

Low Na$^+$ levels in the plasma

Low arterial blood pressure

Release of **renin** from the glomeruli in the kidneys

Angiotensinogen
(plasma protein)　　　　　　　　　　　　Angiotensin

Vasoconstriction

Aldosterone released from adrenal cortex and
acts on the distal convoluted tubules.

Blood pressure rises　　　Stimulates increased Na$^+$ reabsorption

Water reabsorbed by osmosis and enters blood capillaries

Blood pressure rises

Fig. 2.52 Mechanism involved in the control of sodium by the kidney.

the ECF falls and the animal becomes dehydrated. This will present as:

- Lowered blood pressure – plasma volume falls and exerts less pressure on the blood vessel walls.
- Raised Na$^+$ ions concentration – a fall in volume concentrates the Na$^+$ ions increasing the osmotic pressure of the plasma.

Osmotic pressure – the pressure needed to prevent osmosis from occurring. It depends on the number of undissolved molecules and ions in the solution. Detected by **osmoreceptors**.
Blood pressure – the pressure exerted on the walls of the blood vessels by the blood. It depends on the blood volume. Detected by **baroreceptors**.

Osmoregulatory mechanisms (Fig. 2.51) now begin to work and result in a rise in blood pressure and a fall in urine output. The hormone ADH controls water reabsorption from the collecting ducts (Table 2.18). Raised blood pressure will have the opposite effect and the animal will excrete increased quantities of urine.

Control of salt levels
Sodium (in the form of NaCl) is taken into the body in food and is normally lost in urine, faeces and sweat. It is found in the ionised form Na$^+$ in all the body fluid compartments and plays an important part in determining blood pressure. High levels of Na$^+$ in the diet increase osmotic pressure, which draws fluid into the plasma by osmosis, increasing blood volume and thus blood pressure; conversely, low Na$^+$ draws less fluid in and blood volume and pressure fall (Fig. 2.52).

Regulation of Na$^+$ in the plasma occurs mainly in the distal convoluted tubule and is under the control of the hormone **aldosterone** (Table 2.18).

The ureter

Urine formed by each kidney is conveyed to the bladder along a single ureter by means of peristaltic waves brought about by contraction of smooth muscle. Each ureter is a narrow muscular tube lined by transitional epithelium, running caudally towards the bladder, one on each side of the dorsal abdomen (Fig. 2.48). Each is suspended in a fold of visceral peritoneum – the **mesoureter.**

The bladder

This is a pear-shaped hollow organ lying in the midline and used for the storage of urine – the rounded end points cranially (Fig. 2.48). The size varies according to the volume it contains – when full the ventral surface may touch the abdominal floor; when empty it lies entirely within the pelvic cavity.

Each ureter enters the bladder in an area known as the **trigone,** at an oblique angle which helps to prevent backflow of urine up the ureter.

The bladder is lined with transitional epithelium, and the walls contain elastic tissue and layers of smooth muscle. This structure allows expansion as the bladder fills with urine. Flow of urine out of the bladder is controlled by a **sphincter** at the **neck** of the bladder. This has an inner layer of smooth muscle under involuntary control and an outer layer of striated muscle under voluntary control.

The urethra

This carries urine caudally from the neck of the bladder to the outside of the body.

Female This is a short tube entering the floor of the reproductive tract at the junction of the vestibule and vagina known as the **external urethral orifice.** A small swelling called the **urethral tubercle** marks the opening.

Male The urethra can be divided into a pelvic and a penile part. There is a difference between the dog and the tomcat:

- **Dog** – as the urethra leaves the bladder the **prostate gland** and the **deferent ducts** from the testes open into it. The urethra runs caudally through the pelvis and curves over the edge of the ischial arch where it is surrounded by cavernous erectile tissue to form the **penis.** It continues as the penile urethra and opens to the outside at the tip of the penis.
- **Tomcat** – there is a short length of urethra cranial to the opening of the prostate gland, the **preprostatic urethra.** The urethra runs caudally and opens to the outside ventral to the anus in the perineum. Close to the end of the urethra are the openings from the paired **bulbo-urethral glands.**

From the point at which the deferent ducts join the urethra it conveys both urine and sperm to the outside of the body.

Micturition – the act of passing urine

This is normally a reflex activity but can be overridden by voluntary control from the brain. The steps are:

- The bladder is distended by urine formed by the kidneys.
- Stretch receptors within the smooth muscle of the bladder wall are stimulated and nerve impulses are sent to the spinal cord.
- Nerve impulses are transmitted back to the smooth muscle by parasympathetic nerves and contraction is initiated.
- Other nerve impulses trigger relaxation of the internal bladder sphincter and urine is expelled.

If it is inappropriate for the animal to micturate, the brain overrides this reflex pathway and prevents the bladder sphincter from relaxing. At a more appropriate time the brain stimulates the internal and external sphincters and urine is released. Voluntary control develops as the young animal matures and is not fully developed in puppies and kittens until about 10 weeks of age.

Urinalysis

Urine is derived from the ultrafiltrate of plasma and reflects the health status of the animal. Normal urine contains only water salts and urea. The clinical parameters used to evaluate a sample of urine are shown in Table 2.19.

The reproductive system

The reproductive system shares part of its structure with the urinary system and together they may be referred to as the urinogenital system.

Male

The reproductive systems of the dog and the tomcat are similar – any differences will be described as appropriate (Figs 2.53 and 2.54). The parts of the tract are:

- Testis.
- Epididymis.
- Deferent duct.
- Urethra.
- Penis.
- Prostate – accessory gland.
- Bulbo-urethral glands – accessory gland seen only in the tomcat.

Testis

This is the male gonad. Its functions are to:

(1) Produce spermatozoa (sperm) by spermatogenesis (Fig. 2.55).

Table 2.19 Normal values shown by the urine of the dog and cat		
Clinical parameter	**Normal value**	**Comments**
Daily volume	Dog: 20–100 ml/kg body weight Cat: 10–12 ml/kg body weight	Polydipsia – increased volume of urine Oliguria – reduced volume or urea Anuria – absence of urine
Appearance	Clear, yellow, characteristic smell	Tomcat urine has an unpleasant strong smell. Old samples smell ammoniacal
pH	5–7	Carnivorous diet produces acid urine. Herbivorous diet produces alkaline urine
Specific gravity (SG)	Dog: 1.016–1.060 Cat: 1.020–1.040	Reflects the concentration of urine. Exercise, high environmental temperatures and dehydration will cause a rise in SG
Protein	None	Proteinuria – presence of protein, may indicate damage to nephrons, chronic renal failure, inflammation of the urinary tract
Blood	None	Haematuria – presence of blood Haemoglobinuria – presence of haemoglobin; due to rupture of red cells May indicate damage or infection to the tract
Glucose	None	Glucosuria – presence of glucose. May indicate diabetes mellitus. Levels of glucose in the filtrate exceed the renal threshold and excess is excreted in the urine
Ketones	None	Ketonuria – presence of ketones. May be accompanied by acid pH and smell of 'peardrops' in urine and on the breath
Bile	None	Bilirubinuria – presence of bile. Indicator of some form of liver disease
Crystals and casts	In small quantities, these may be considered to be normal	Crystalline or colloidal material coalesce to form a cast of the renal tubules and are flushed out by the urine. In large quantities, crystals may form calculi or uroliths and block the tract

(2) Secrete the hormone testosterone.

(3) Produce fluids, which transport sperm from the testes and aid their survival.

There is a pair of oval testes, which in the adult animal lie in a small almost hairless sac known as the **scrotum.** The scrotum hangs ventral to the pelvis outside the body cavity where the lower temperature promotes more efficient spermatogenesis. The position of the testis can be altered in response to changes in temperature by smooth muscle within the connective tissue of the scrotum known as the **Dartos muscle** and by smooth muscle in the spermatic cord called the **cremaster muscle.**

The testicular tissue consists of numerous coiled **seminiferous tubules.** These lead into wider **efferent tubules** draining into the **epididymis,** which runs along the dorsolateral border of the testis. The tail or **cauda epididymis** is attached to the caudal extremity and is the site for the storage and final maturation of sperm ready for fertilisation. The epididymis continues as the **deferent duct** (or the vas deferens or ductus deferens) which conveys sperm out of the scrotum into the

urethra within the pelvic cavity (Figs 2.53 and 2.54). A spermatic artery and vein and the spermatic nerve accompany the deferent duct – together they form the **spermatic cord.**

Microscopically, the seminiferous tubules are lined by two cell types:

- **Spermatogonia** – responsible for producing immature sperm or spermatids by meiosis.
- **Sertoli cells** – secrete the hormone **oestrogen** and nutrients to aid the survival of the spermatids as they travel along the seminiferous tubules.

Lying between the tubules are **interstitial cells,** or **cells of Leydig.** These are stimulated by the hormone interstitial cell stimulating hormone (ICSH) produced by the anterior pituitary gland and secrete the hormone testosterone. **Testosterone** affects:

- Spermatogenesis – the formation of spermatozoa.
- Development of the male reproductive tract.
- Development of male secondary sexual characteristics, e.g. muscle development, size, male behaviour.

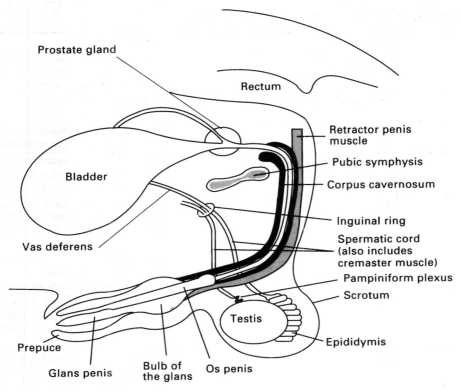

Fig. 2.53 Reproductive tract of the dog.

Testicular development   In the embryo, the testes develop within the abdominal cavity close to the kidney. During late fetal and early neonatal life, a band of tissue attached at one end to the tail of the testis and at the other to the inside of the scrotal sac contracts, pulling the testis caudally through the abdomen. It passes out of the abdominal cavity into the scrotum via the **inguinal ring** – a split in the abdominal oblique muscle in the groin of the animal. As it does so, the testis and its associated nerves and blood vessels and deferent duct become wrapped in a fold of peritoneum called the **tunica vaginalis**.

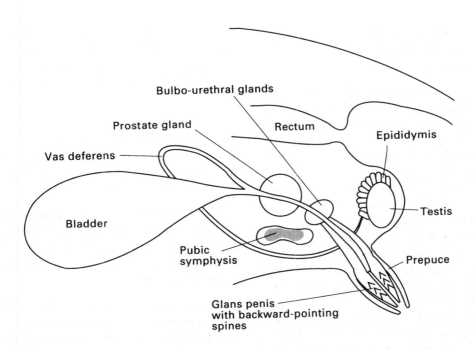

Fig. 2.54 Reproductive tract of the tomcat.

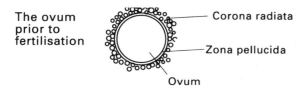

The ovum prior to fertilisation

- Corona radiata
- Zona pellucida
- Ovum

The sperm prior to fertilisation

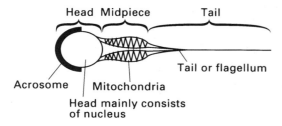

Head Midpiece Tail

Tail or flagellum

Acrosome Mitochondria

Head mainly consists of nucleus

(Not to same scale)

Fig. 2.55 Structure of ovum and sperm.

During castration, the tunica vaginalis is incised to expose the testis and the spermatic cord. The contents of the spermatic cord are then ligated.

The testes should be palpable within the scrotum of the dog and tomcat at about 12 weeks of age. Failure of the testes to descend into the scrotum is known as **cryptorchidism** – if one testis is retained in the abdominal cavity this is called **monorchidism**, and if both are retained this is called **bilateral cryptorchidism**. This may be an inherited characteristic.

Accessory glands

There are two types of gland:

- **Prostate gland** – bilobed structure surrounding the urethra. In the dog it lies close to the neck of the bladder, while in the tomcat, there is a short preprostatic urethra cranial to the gland (Figs 2.53 and 2.54). Secretions of prostatic fluid enter the urethra by short ducts.
- **Bulbo-urethral gland** – found only in the tomcat. Lies on either side of the urethra close to the tip of the penis.

The accessory glands produce **seminal fluid** which:

(1) Increases the volume of the ejaculate to flush sperm through the penis into the female tract during mating.
(2) Aids sperm survival.
(3) Neutralises the acidity of the urine within the urethra.

Penis

During ejaculation, spermatozoa produced within the seminiferous tubules are conducted along the **epididymis** and up the **deferent duct** to enter the **urethra** at a point close to the neck of the bladder and to the prostate gland. The urethra runs through the centre of the **penis** and is shared by both the urinary system and reproductive systems (see Urinary System).

The functions of the penis are to:

(1) Conduct sperm and seminal fluid into the female reproductive tract during mating.
(2) Conduct urine from the bladder out of the body.
(3) Direct urine for territorial marking.

The penis of the dog and the tomcat are anatomically different.

Dog   The penis runs from the ischial arch of the pelvis, passing cranioventrally along the perineum and between the hind legs. The urethra runs along the centre of the penis and is surrounded by cavernous erectile tissue known as the **corpus cavernosum penis**. During sexual excitement the erectile tissue becomes engorged with blood under pressure. At the proximal end this expands into the **bulb of the penis** and towards the distal end as the **glans penis**. A pair of connective tissue **crura** (sing. crus) attaches the penis to the ischial arch – these form the **root of the penis.**

Within the glans penis is a small tunnel-shaped bone – the **os penis**, which aids entry of the penis into the female's vagina during mating. The urethra runs *ventral* to the os penis through the 'tunnel', which may restrict its ability to dilate and may be a site for blockage with urethral calculi.

The distal part of the penis is enclosed within and suspended from the ventral body wall by a fur-covered **prepuce**. This is lined with mucous membrane and well supplied with lubricating glands. During mating the prepuce is pushed back to reveal the glans penis.

Tomcat   The penis is shorter than that of the dog and points caudally – the external opening lies ventral to the anus under the tail. The tip of the **glans penis** is covered in tiny barbs, which elicit a pain response from the female during mating. This stimulates a nerve pathway inducing ovulation within 36 hours of mating. The urethra lies *dorsal* to the **os penis** at a point close to the bulbo-urethral glands.

During sexual excitement, the penis engorges and points cranioventrally allowing the tomcat to mate in a similar position to the dog.

Female

The reproductive systems of the bitch and the queen are similar, varying only in size. The tract is adapted to bear several foetuses in a single pregnancy and is described as **bicornuate**. Species that bear litters of young are said to be **multiparous** (Fig. 2.56).

The parts of the tract are:

- Ovary.
- Uterine tube.
- Uterus – uterine horn and uterine body.
- Cervix.

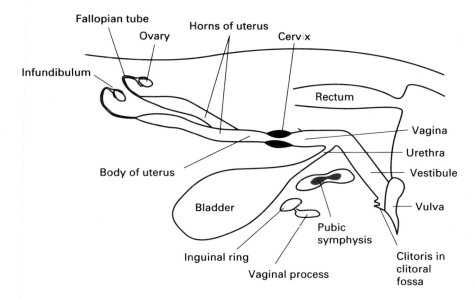

Fig. 2.56 Reproductive tract of the bitch.

- Vagina.
- Vestibule.
- Vulva.

Ovary

The ovary is the female gonad. Its functions are to:

(1) Produce ova, or eggs, ready for fertilisation by the male sperm.
(2) Secrete the hormones oestrogen and progesterone.

There is a pair of ovaries, each one lying on either side of the midline, close to the dorsal abdominal wall. Each ovary lies caudal to the kidney on that side and is held in place by a suspensory ligament containing smooth muscle – the **ovarian ligament.**

The ovary is suspended from the abdominal wall by a fold of the visceral peritoneum – the **mesovarium**, which also carries part of the uterine tube. Part of the mesovarium is folded to form a pouch-like **ovarian bursa**. This completely encloses the ovary and within it is a small opening into the peritoneal cavity.

The ovary consists of a framework of connective tissue, blood capillaries and smooth muscle within which are a large number of germ cells and developing follicles.

Ovulation At birth, the ovary contains all the **germ cells** that will ever be needed. These form a reservoir from which the **primary follicles** develop. At the onset of sexual maturity some of the primary follicles begin to develop into ripe **Graafian follicles,** each one consisting of an ovum surrounded by follicular fluid and an outer layer of cells. The Graafian follicle secretes the hormone **oestrogen.** When the follicle is mature, it ruptures to release the ovum – **ovulation**. The ovum passes down the uterine tube, while the remaining follicular tissue becomes restructured to

form the **corpus luteum**. This secretes the hormone **progesterone.**

Hormonal control Ovulation is associated with a series of interrelated hormonal changes in the ovary and the pituitary gland.

(1) External stimuli, e.g. daylength, environmental temperature, presence of other animals, stimulate the hypothalamus at the base of the brain (see Nervous System). This initiates the release of **gonadotrophin releasing hormone (GRH)** which stimulates the anterior pituitary gland.
(2) The anterior pituitary gland secretes **follicle stimulating hormone (FSH)** which stimulates a few primary follicles to develop into Graafian follicles.
(3) The Graafian follicles secrete increasing levels of **oestrogen** which:

- Initiate pro-oestrous behaviour of the female.
- Prepare the reproductive tract for mating.
- Stimulate the secretion of **luteinising hormone (LH)** from the anterior pituitary gland.
- Inhibit further secretion of FSH.

(4) As a result of FSH inhibition the levels of oestrogen begin to fall. LH acts on the Graafian follicles and they ovulate. The ovum passes down the uterine tube and the remains of the follicle changes into the corpus luteum – it becomes luteinised.
(5) The corpus luteum starts to secrete **progesterone**. The reducing levels of oestrogen and increasing levels of progesterone cause the mating behaviour of the female – she will stand still and allow the male to mount her.
(6) Progesterone is the dominant hormone during pregnancy. It:

- Prepares the reproductive tract to receive the fertilised ova.

- Causes enlargement of the mammary glands.
- Inhibits secretion of GRH, which stops the production of FSH, so preventing further development of any more follicles

If the female has not conceived, the corpus luteum will regress within a period characteristic of the species and the cycle will begin again.

NB: As the queen is an induced ovulator, the corpus luteum is only formed if she is mated and conceives.

Pseudopregnancy   This is also called false or phantom pregnancy, or pseudocyesis. This condition is relatively common in the bitch and may occur at about 6 weeks after the start of the oestrous cycle. The symptoms, which are linked to the high levels of progesterone at this stage of the cycle, include maternal behaviour, enlargement of the mammary glands and lactation.

Full details of the oestrous cycle of the bitch and the queen are included in Chapter 18, 'Obstetric and Paediatric Nursing of the Dog and Cat'.

Uterine tube

This is also called the oviduct or the Fallopian tube. Its function is to:

(1) Collect ova as they are released from the Graafian follicles.
(2) Convey the ova from the ovaries to the uterine horns.
(3) Provide the correct environment for the survival of ova and sperm.

The uterine tube is a narrow convoluted structure lying close to the ovary and suspended in a fold of peritoneum known as the **mesosalpinx.** The proximal end called the **infundibulum.** It is funnel-shaped and the opening is fringed by finger-like processes known as **fimbriae.** The infundibulum is able to move over the surface of the ovary to trap the ova as they ovulate. A lining of ciliated columnar epithelium helps the passage of the ova down the tube.

Uterus

This is a Y-shaped structure lying in the midline of the dorsal abdomen. In the pregnant animal, the weight of the conceptuses pulls the uterus ventrally and at full term it occupies most of the abdominal cavity. Its function is to:

(1) Contain the fertilised ova until they develop into full-term foetuses.
(2) Provide the correct environment for the survival of the developing embryos.
(3) Provide the means by which the developing foetuses are supplied with nutrients – the **placenta**.

The uterus (Fig. 2.56) comprises two parts:

- A pair of **uterine horns** – each one leads from a uterine tube and is up to five times longer than the uterine body. During pregnancy they contain the developing embryos.
- A short central **body**.

In cross-section, the uterine wall consists of:

(1) **Endometrium** – inner layer of columnar mucous membrane, blood vessels and glandular tissue. This layer thickens during pregnancy to provide nutrition for the embryo before implantation and to support the placenta.
(2) **Myometrium** – smooth muscle fibres which contract strongly during parturition.
(3) **Mesometrium** – or broad ligament. Fold of visceral peritoneum, which suspends the uterus and is continuous with the mesosalpinx and the mesovarium.

Blood supply to the tract   The blood vessels run in the mesometrium, mesosalpinx and the mesovarium. They are:

- **Ovarian artery** – arises from the dorsal aorta caudal to the renal artery, and supplies the ovary.
- **Uterine artery** – anastomoses with the ovarian artery and supplies the caudal part of the tract.

Cervix

This is a short thick-walled muscular sphincter connecting the uterus with the vagina. In the centre of the cervix is a narrow **cervical canal**, which relaxes only to allow the passage of foetuses during parturition.

Vagina and vestibule

Together these form a highly dilatable channel leading from the cervix to the outside at the vulva. The vagina extends from the cervix to the **external urethral orifice** – the point at which the urethra joins the reproductive tract, while the vestibule runs from the external urethral orifice to the outside at the **vulva** and is shared by both the urinary and reproductive systems. The function is to:

(1) Convey sperm from the penis of the male into the female tract – sperm is usually deposited at the entrance to the cervix.
(2) Convey the foetuses from the uterus to the outside.
(3) Convey urine from the bladder to the outside of the body – the vestibule performs this.

The lumen is lined with stratified squamous epithelium, which shows hormonally induced changes during the oestrous cycle. Study of the epithelial debris known as **exfoliative vaginal cytology** can be used to assess the stages of the cycle and to gauge the correct time for mating. The walls are arranged in longitudinal folds enabling the vagina and vestibule to expand widthways during parturition.

Vulva

This is the external opening of the female tract. It consists of two parts:

- **Labiae** – two vertical lips joined ventrally and dorsally and made of fibrous and elastic connective tissue, smooth muscle and fat. The **vulval cleft** lies between them. The vulva may be enlarged during pro-oestrus and oestrus in the bitch.
- **Clitoris** – small knob of cavernous erectile tissue lying in the **clitoral fossa** just inside the ventral part of the vulval cleft.

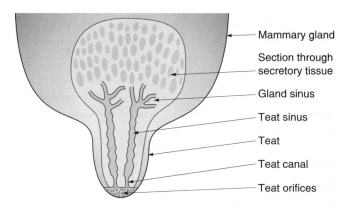

Mammary gland

Section through secretory tissue

Gland sinus

Teat sinus

Teat

Teat canal

Teat orifices

Fig. 2.57 Section through a mammary gland.

Mammary glands

Although these are not strictly part of the reproductive tract, the mammary glands are the defining feature of the class Mammalia. All mammals feed their young on milk from the mammary glands produced by a process known as **lactation.**

Mammary glands are modified cutaneous glands, which lie on either side of the midline on the external ventral wall of the abdomen and the thorax. The bitch has five pairs and the queen has four pairs. The glands are present in both sexes.

Each gland (Fig. 2.57) consists of glandular tissue lined with secretory epithelium. The secreted milk drains through a network of sinuses into **teat canals**, which open onto the surface of the teat as **teat orifices.** Each gland has one teat, but each teat has several orifices.

Lactation is influenced by three hormones:

(1) **Progesterone** – from the corpus luteum. Causes the glands to enlarge during pregnancy. Sometimes seen in false pregnancies.
(2) **Prolactin** – secreted by the anterior pituitary gland. Stimulates milk production near the end of the pregnancy.
(3) **Oxytocin** – secreted by the posterior pituitary gland in the few hours around parturition. Enables the release or 'let down' of milk in response to suckling by the neonate.

Composition of milk This varies between species – milk produced by the bitch and the queen is more concentrated, contains more protein and twice as much fat as cow's milk. The average composition of milk is shown in Table 2.20.

The first milk produced by the dam after parturition is known as **colostrum**. It is rich in maternal antibodies, which are responsible for providing the neonate with immunity to diseases to which the bitch has been exposed. The neonate must receive colostrum during the first 24 hours of life, as at this time, the protein antibodies can be absorbed without being broken down by digestion. After 24 hours normal protein digestion will destroy the antibodies. Production of colostrum ceases after a few days.

Embryonic and fetal development

It is important to understand the terms applied to the stages of development (Table 2.21).

Fertilisation and cell division During ovulation ova are released from the ovary. The bitch and the queen are **multiparous** species, so several ova are released at one time. An outer layer of follicular cells, the **corona radiata**, and an inner layer of glycoprotein, the **zona pellucida**, surrounds each ovum. The ova enter the uterine tube and are carried along by movement of the cilia of the lining epithelium.

Table 2.20 Average composition of milk	
Constituent	**Quantity**
Water	70–90%
Fat	0–30%
Protein	1–15%
Carbohydrate	3–7%
Minerals	0.5–1% calcium phosphate, magnesium, sodium, potassium and chloride. Deficient in iron and copper. Traces of iodine, cobalt, tin and silica
Vitamins	A, B_2, B_5, E, K. Low in C and D

Table 2.21 Terminology used to describe embryonic and fetal development	
Term	**Definition**
Gestation period	Interval between fertilisation of the ovum and birth of the offspring. Approximately 63 days (range 60–70 days) in dog and cat
Embryology	The study of the development of the embryo
Gamete	Male or female germ cell – sperm or ovum
Zygote	Fertilised ovum
Embryo	Stage during which the major organs are forming
Foetus	Stage from that where the formation of the major external and internal organs is complete until parturition fetal membranes present
Conceptus	Embryo or foetus, the extra embryonic membranes and the placenta
Organogenesis	Period during which the internal organs are developing. Takes about 35 days in the dog and cat
Neonate	A newborn animal

After mating, sperm travel up the female reproductive tract and fertilisation takes place in the uterine tube. During fertilisation, enzymes are released by the **acrosome** of the sperm (Fig. 2.55), breaking down the zona pellucida of the ovum and enabling one sperm to penetrate the ovum. This results in a **fertilisation reaction** preventing fertilisation by any other sperm. The fertilised ovum – now called a **zygote** – begins to divide within a few hours of fertilisation.

Cell division occurs by **mitosis** – one cell becomes two and so on (Fig. 2.58). When the cells become too numerous to count, the ball of cells is called **a morula.** A fluid-filled cavity forms and the structure becomes a **blastocyst.** At this stage the blastocysts are floating free in the uterine tube relying on secretions from the tube walls to survive.

The blastocysts move slowly down the tract into the uterine horns where they become attached to the walls at equal distances – **implantation.** Equal spacing between the blastocysts enables each conceptus to have the maximum amount of space for growth. Implantation occurs at 14–20 days after ovulation in the bitch and at 11–16 days in the queen.

Within the blastocyst, the majority of the cells lies to one side of the fluid-filled cavity and are known as the **inner cell mass** – this becomes the embryo. The remaining cells form a thinner layer – the **trophoblast,** which forms the extra embryonic membranes. The cells begin to differentiate into three **germ cell layers**, which eventually develop into different parts of the embryo and its membranes.

Development of the embryo from the inner cell mass

In the early stages the **inner cell mass** is a flat plate of cells. As it grows, it curls around to enclose the organs (Fig. 2.58). The germ cell layers differentiate into:

- Outer layer, or **ectoderm** – the nervous system and the skin.
- Middle layer, or **mesoderm** – the musculoskeletal system and the internal organs.

- Inner layer, or **endoderm** – the lining of the digestive tract and the other visceral systems. Endodermal cells also line the trophoblast and form the **yolk sac** (Fig. 2.58) – in mammals this does not contain yolk.

As the inner cell mass grows, it forms the head and trunk, while internally the body cavity or **coelom** forms and is later divided into the thoracic and abdominal cavities by the diaphragm. **Organogenesis** is complete by 35 days and after this the foetus grows rapidly until it reaches its final size prior to parturition. The later stages of development in a medium-sized breed of dog are summarised in Table 2.22. Kittens are often slightly more advanced than puppies.

Development of the extra-embryonic membranes

The **trophoblast** forms the outer part of the fluid-filled cavity and later develops into the extra-embryonic membranes whose function is to protect the embryo during the gestation period.

Mesodermal cells between the yolk sac and the trophoblast split into two layers, forming a cavity between them. One layer lies adjacent to the trophoblast and later becomes the **chorion,** while the other lies close to the yolk sac. The extra embryonic membranes now begin to develop as follows:

- **Yolk sac** – formed from endodermal cells. Disappears some time before birth.
- **Chorion** – formed from the trophoblast and the outer layer of mesodermal cells.
- **Amnion** – the trophoblast and mesoderm grow and eventually form a fluid-filled cavity around the developing embryo – **the amniotic cavity.** The outer layer is the **amnion** and it is in this membrane that the foetus is delivered. The amniotic cavity is entirely separate from all the other cavities.
- **Allantois** – a balloon-like diverticulum develops from the endoderm forming the primitive gut and pushes out from the caudal end of the embryo (Fig. 2.58). This sac collects urine from the fetal bladder via a tube known as the **urachus.** As the allantois expands with fetal urine it encir-

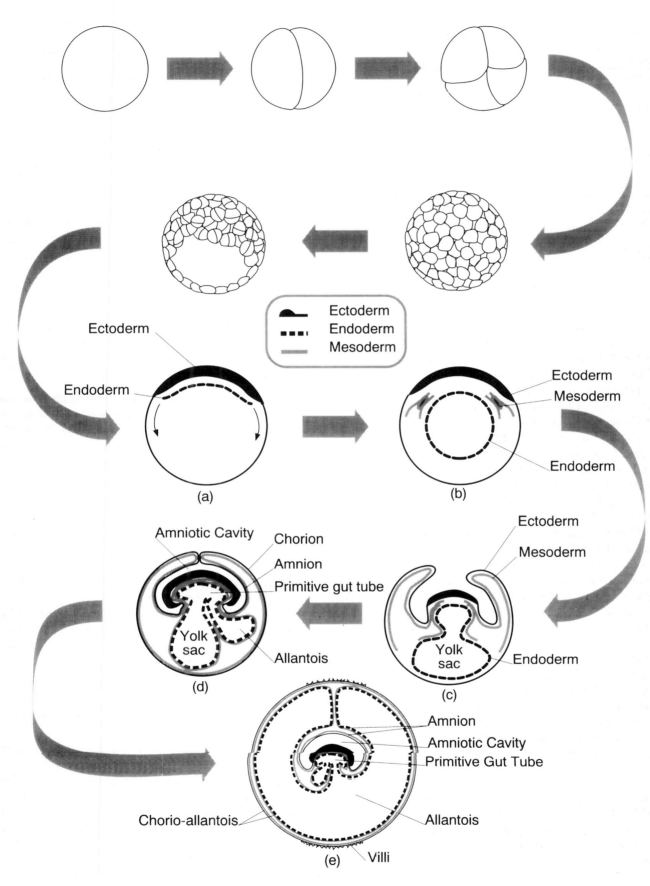

Fig. 2.58 Early embryonic development.

Table 2.22 Developmental stages of the canine embryo and foetus	
Timescale	**Stage of development**
3 weeks	5 mm long. Fore and hindlimbs are small buds sticking out from the trunk. Amnion is complete and the allantois is formed
4 weeks	20 mm long. Limbs are small cylinders with evidence of a paw shape. Eyes are pigmented. External ear has a ridge of visible skin
5 weeks	35 mm long. Ear flap is distinct. Eyelids partly cover the eyes. Digits can be seen on the paws. External genitalia are near to final positions. Tactile (sinus) hairs are present on the upper lip. Formation of internal organs (organogenesis) is complete
6 weeks	60 mm long. Prominent scrotal or vulval tissues. Digits widely spread. Eyelids are fused. Hair follicles and tactile follicles present on the body. Claws present. Ossification of skeleton at 45 days
7 weeks	100 mm long. Body hair and colour markings are developing
8 weeks	150 mm long. Hair covering is complete. Pads have developed
9 weeks	Ready for birth

cles the foetus. Eventually its inner surface becomes part of the amnion and its outer surface fuses with the chorion to become the **chorioallantois**. During parturition the chorioallantois may be identified as the first 'water-bag' which ruptures to release the foetus in the amnion.

The placenta The placenta is a vascular band, which develops from the chorioallantois around the centre of the conceptus (Fig. 2.59). At implantation, small finger-like villi emerge from the chorioallantois and burrow into the endometrium of the uterine horn. Blood capillaries covering the membrane penetrate through the villi and come to lie in close apposition to the capillaries of the endometrium. These form the fetal and maternal parts of the placenta – they are *not* continuous with each other. The villi thicken into broad bands forming a belt-like or **zonary placenta** around the middle of the conceptus.

At the edge of the placenta, between it and the membranes, is an area known as the **marginal haematoma** where blood escapes from broken capillaries and becomes trapped. The blood gradually breaks down and later stains the parturient discharges – green in the bitch and brown in the queen – this is normal!

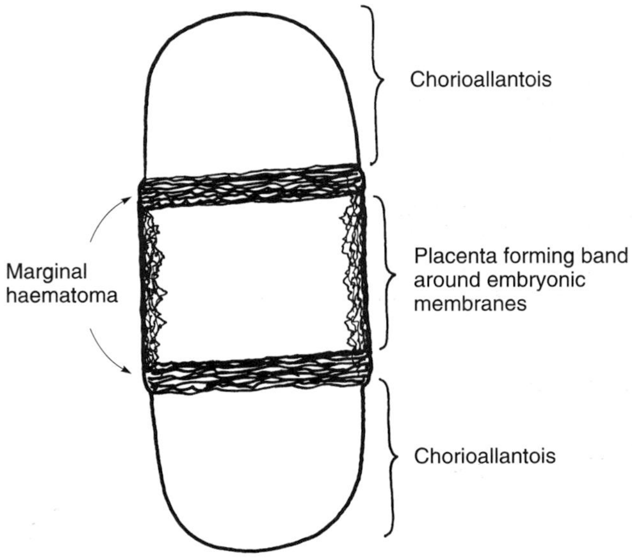

The placenta anchors the conceptus to the uterine wall and provides the foetus with all it needs for growth and development. Nutrients and oxygen pass from the maternal placenta into the foetus via the **umbilicus**, which contains the umbilical artery and vein, the remains of the yolk sac and the stalk of the allantois connected to the urachus. Waste materials pass in the opposite direction.

The processes involved in mating and parturition are described in Chapter 18, 'Obstetric and Paediatric Nursing of the Dog and Cat'.

The integument

The integument is said to be the largest organ of the body and includes the:

- **Skin.**
- **Hair.**
- **Footpads.**
- **Claws.**

The skin

The skin completely covers the external surface of the body and blends with the mucous membranes at the various natural openings. The functions of the skin are as follows.

(1) **Protection**:

- Protects the underlying structures of the body from physical damage.
- Prevents invasion by micro-organisms by creating an intact barrier and by the secretion of sebum

Fig. 2.59 The extra-embryonic membranes.

Chorioallantois

Placenta forming band around embryonic membranes

Marginal haematoma

Chorioallantois

from the sebaceous glands which has antibacterial properties.

- Creates a waterproof barrier, which prevents the body from drying out and from becoming waterlogged.
- Prevents damage by ultraviolet radiation by the presence of pigments in the skin and hair.

(2) **Sense organ** – the skin contains numerous nerve endings to detect temperature, pain and touch, which provide sensory information to assist the body to monitor its external environment.

(3) **Secretory organ** – secretions are produced by various skin or cutaneous glands. These include:

- **Sebaceous glands** – associated with the hair follicles and secrete sebum, which waterproofs the coat, has an antibacterial action and contains the precursor to vitamin D. This is activated by the action of ultraviolet light.
- **Sweat glands** – also called sudoriferous glands. Only found on the nose and the footpads of the dog and cat. Secrete sweat, which cools the body by evaporation.
- **Ceruminous glands** – modified sebaceous glands which secrete protective wax (cerumen) on to the skin lining the ear canal.
- **Mammary glands** – modified sweat glands that secrete milk.
- **Glands of the anal sacs** – produce a secretion with a characteristic smell used for territorial marking.

(4) **Storage** – fat is stored under the skin as adipose tissue and acts as an energy store and as a thermal insulating layer.

(5) **Thermoregulation** – heat loss is prevented by:

- Constriction of surface blood capillaries, which diverts blood away from the skin's surface.
- Erecting the hairs and trapping a layer of insulating air between the body and the outer surface.
- Layer of adipose tissue insulates the body.

(6) **Communication** – specialised glands produce **pheromones**, which are natural scents used for intraspecific communication. Other scents used for communication include those secreted by the **circum-anal glands** and glands of **the anal sacs**. The integument also provides **visual communication**, e.g. a dog raises its hackles when threatened.

Structure of skin (Fig. 2.60)

The skin is composed of three layers:

- **Epidermis.**
- **Dermis.**
- **Hypodermis.**

Epidermis The epidermis is composed of **stratified squamous epithelium** arranged in multiple layers (or strata) of cells. Cells are constantly being produced to replace the cells that are lost or damaged by injury and wear. The epidermis is avascular and receives nutrients from the underlying dermis. The layers of the epidermis are, from deep to superficial:

(1) **Stratum basale (germinativum)** – a single layer of cells which divide by **mitosis**. As the new cells are produced they push those above into the next layer of the epidermis. **Melanocytes** containing granules of the pigment melanin are also present. This pigment gives skin and hair its characteristic colour.

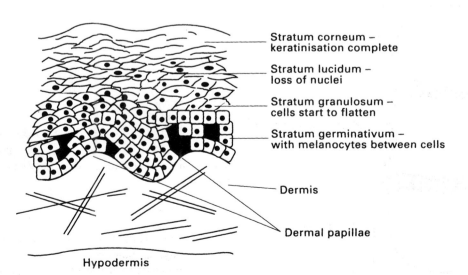

Stratum corneum – keratinisation complete

Stratum lucidum – loss of nuclei

Stratum granulosum – cells start to flatten

Stratum germinativum – with melanocytes between cells

Dermis

Dermal papillae

Hypodermis

Fig. 2.60 The structure of the epidermis.

(2) **Stratum granulosum** – the cells are flattened and the process of **keratinisation** or infiltration of the cells by the structural protein **keratin,** begins.

(3) **Stratum lucidum** – the cells lose their nuclei.

(4) **Stratum corneum** – the most superficial layer. The cells have no nuclei (they are dead), are fully keratinised and are flattened in shape. They are known as **squames** and flake off from the skin surface.

Dermis   The dermis is composed of dense connective tissue with collagen and elastic fibres. It has a generous supply of blood vessels and nerves. Also found in the dermis are the **hair follicles, sebaceous glands** and **sweat glands** which are only active in the hairless skin of the nose and footpads of the dog and cat, are also found in the dermis.

Hypodermis   The hypodermis, or subcuticular layer is not actually part of the skin, but is a layer of loose connective tissue and fat that lies beneath the dermis. It also contains elastic fibres, which gives the skin of the dog and cat its ability to move and return to its original position.

The nose pad

The **rhinarium**, or nose pad, is covered by thickened, hairless pigmented skin and surrounds the nares or nostrils. The epidermis on a dog's nose has a unique patterning that is much like a human 'fingerprint'. The nose also has active sweat glands.

Hair

Hair is a keratinised structure and is a distinctive characteristic of mammals. It covers the entire body of the dog and cat with the exception of a few areas such as the nose and footpads.

The visible part of the hair above the skin's surface is called the **hair shaft** and the part that lies within the skin is called the **hair root**. Each hair grows from a **hair follicle,** which develops from epidermal cells. These grow down into the underlying dermis and form a 'hair cone' over a section of dermis called the **dermal papilla**. From the hair cone, the cells keratinise and form a hair. As the hair grows up through the epidermis to the skin's surface the cells at the point of the cone die, forming a channel – the hair follicle. The hair continues to grow until it eventually dies and becomes detached from the follicle. Hair growth is cyclic and once the hair is shed a new hair will start to grow from a new follicle.

Moulting

Moulting or the shedding of hair is influenced by seasonal factors, e.g. temperature and daylength. Most dogs moult more heavily in the spring and autumn. Cats moult most heavily in spring and this is followed by a less heavy hair loss throughout the summer and autumn. However, pet cats and dogs are usually kept inside centrally heated houses with electric lighting and this disrupts the natural seasonal triggers, so they may moult all year round.

Hair types

There are three main types of hair:

(1) **Guard hairs** – these are the thicker and longer hairs that form the outer protective coat of the animal. The nature of the guard hairs gives the coat its waterproof quality so water 'runs off', preventing it from penetrating the coat. One guard hair grows from each follicle and is associated with an involuntary muscle called the **arrector pili muscle** (Fig. 2.61). This raises the hair from its resting position trapping a layer of warm air close to the body. The muscle contracts in response to cold, but can also be stimulated by fear or threat, e.g. the hairs of the tail (bottlebrush effect) in the cat as a response to threat.

(2) **Wool hairs** – these form the soft undercoat. They are thinner, softer and shorter than guard hairs and are more numerous. Their number fluctuates with the seasons – in winter they serve to keep the body warm by providing an insulating layer. The thickness of the wool hairs also varies between breeds, e.g. huskies have a very thick undercoat and are well adapted to extreme cold; Dobermans have a very short outer coat and no undercoat so they do not tolerate cold weather. There may be a number of wool hairs growing from one follicle with one guard hair.

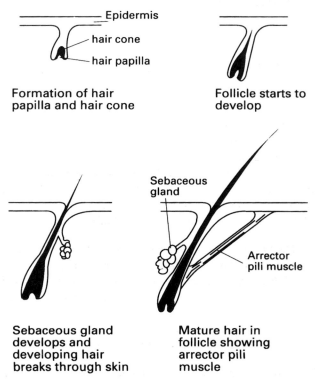

Fig. 2.61 The formation of hair.

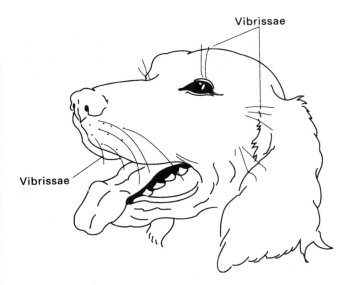

Fig. 2.62 Vibrissae.

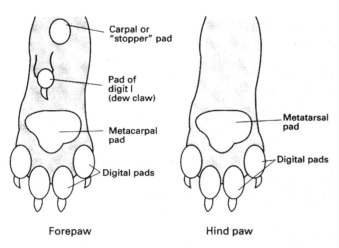

Fig. 2.63 Ventral view of dog's (a) forepaw and (b) hindpaw, showing footpads.

(3) **Tactile hairs (vibrissae)** (Fig. 2.62) also called 'whiskers' or sinus hairs. They are much thicker than guard hairs and protrude outwards beyond the rest of the coat. They are specialised hairs that grow from follicles found deep in the hypodermis. Each follicle is surrounded by nerve endings that are responsive to mechanical stimuli and provide sensory information from the environment. Tactile hairs are mostly found on the face – principally on the upper lip and near the eyes. However, they are found in other areas such as the cluster of tactile hairs on a cat's carpus and the tuft of whiskers on a dog's cheek. In the foetus they are the first hairs to be formed.

Footpads

The footpads are covered by thick, keratinised, hairless epidermis. The surface is roughened by conical **papillae**, which provide traction when the dog walks. The surface of the cat's pads is smoother.

The dermis is also thickened, contains fatty tissue and is very vascular. This forms the **digital cushion**, which acts as a shock absorber as the animal walks and runs. Active sweat glands are found in the footpads of dogs and cats.

There are three types of pad (Fig. 2.63):

(1) **Digital pads** – protect the distal interphalangeal joints; one pad per digit including the 'dew' claw.
(2) **Metacarpal/metatarsal pad** – protect the phalangeal/metacarpal or metatarsal joint; heart-shaped in the dog, rounder in the cat.
(3) **Carpal pad** – also called the **stop pad**; found only on the forepaw and lies just distal to the carpus.

There are seven pads on each forepaw and five on each hind paw.

Claws

The claws are modified epidermal structures (Fig. 2.64), and form the outer layer of the distal or third phalanx where they cover the **ungual process**. The epidermal cells contain a high proportion of keratin, which makes them hard and protective, and the tissue is referred to as **horn**.

Each claw grows from a specialized region of epidermis – the **coronary border**, which lies underneath a fold of skin called the **claw fold**. The claw consists of two hard, laterally compressed **walls**. In a groove between the walls on the ventral surface, is the softer horn of the **sole**. The **dermis** or 'quick' lies at the base of the claw and contains blood capillaries and nerve fibres.

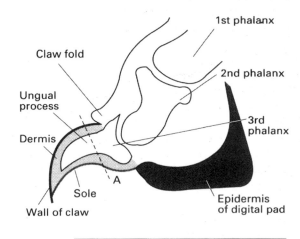

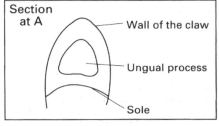

Fig. 2.64 Longitudinal section of dog's toe, showing claw.

Dog claws are non-retractable. Cat claws are held retracted by means of elastic ligaments that run from the second and third phalanges. When the cat unsheathes its claws, the digital flexor muscle overcomes the tension in the elastic ligaments.

KEY POINTS

- Anatomy is the study of the body's structure; physiology is the study of how it works.
- All living organisms are made of cells which have a basic structure with specific anatomical features which adapt them to a particular function.
- Cells are arranged into four basic tissue types. These are epithelial, connective, muscle and nervous tissues.
- The four tissue types combine to form the organs of the body, each of which is adapted to perform a specific function or range of functions.
- The body comprises a series of body systems, each of which is made up of organs which work together to perform a particular function, for example the respiratory system takes in oxygen and expels carbon dioxide, while the reproductive system produces offspring to ensure the survival of the species.
- The body is divided into three cavities – the thorax, the abdomen and the pelvis. Each of these contains one or more of the body systems.
- Although each system works individually to perform a range of functions, the systems also work together to maintain the body in a balanced state – a process known as homeostasis.
- The body must be maintained in a state of balance, e.g. normal temperature and normal pH of blood, so that the body systems can work effectively and efficiently.
- If the homeostatic mechanisms fail, the body systems start to malfunction and the animal becomes ill.

Further reading

Aspinall, V. and O'Reilly, M. (2003) *Introduction to Veterinary Anatomy and Physiology*, Butterworth-Heinemann, Oxford.

Boyd, J. S. (2001) *Colour Atlas of Clinical Anatomy of the Dog and Cat*, 2nd edn, Mosby, London.

Dyce, K. M., Sack, W. O. and Wensing, C. J. G. (1996) *Textbook of Veterinary Anatomy* 2nd edn W. B. Saunders, Philadelphia.

Evans, H. E. (1993) *Miller's Anatomy of the Dog*, 3rd edn, W. B. Saunders, Philadelphia.

Phillips, W. D. and Chilton, T. J. (1991) *A-Level Biology* Oxford University Press, Oxford.

Smith, B. J. (1999) *Canine Anatomy*, Lippincott, Williams and Wilkins, Philadelphia.

Tartaglia, L. and Waugh, A. (2002) *Veterinary Anatomy and Applied Physiology*, Butterworth Heinemann, Oxford.

Vetlogic series of CD ROMS on Anatomy and Physiology for Veterinary Nurses, Keyskill Co. Ltd.

3

Observation and care of the patient

J. S. Seymour

Learning objectives

After studying this chapter, students should be able to:

- Describe the procedure for performing a general health check on a hospitalised patient.
- Recognise the possible causes of abnormalities observed in hospitalised patients.
- Apply the knowledge of normal and abnormal appearance of animals to evaluate the condition of patients in the veterinary practice.
- Apply the principles of bandaging and administration of medicines to practical nursing situations.
- Discuss the various types of bandage materials available in veterinary practice.

Observation

During the course of a working day veterinary nurses will come into contact with a range of patients. They will have to deal with healthy animals of many species and temperaments and care for in-patients whose needs will vary from basic tender loving care to intensive treatment and nursing procedures. They must recognise the normal and abnormal appearance and behaviour patterns of those in their care, and report all relevant information to the veterinary surgeon. The nurse's observations can give valuable input to the case history of the patient and may assist the veterinary surgeon's diagnosis and treatment. All observations should be noted and any abnormalities reported immediately.

Dogs and cats in the hospital environment

It should be remembered that every patient is an individual. Signs considered normal for one patient may be abnormal for another. It is necessary, therefore, to become familiar with each animal and to recognise its normal appearance and behaviour patterns.

The veterinary hospital is not usually a relaxed environment for dogs, cats or small animals. They will be surrounded by faces, smells and sounds unfamiliar to them, and therefore may be expected to behave in an abnormal fashion. Normally placid animals may become nervous and exhibit signs of aggression or submission.

Furthermore, these patients are often required to be secured in a small enclosed space from which there is no visible means of escape. When approached by an unfamiliar person the animal may feel threatened and react to the "flight or fight" response by growling or snapping at the perceived threat. Cats, being solitary animals, are particularly inclined to feel stressed away from their home territory and will often resort to attack as their only means of defence.

Fear and anxiety are not conducive to a smooth and speedy recovery. By considering the natural environment and routine of patients, many simple measures may be implemented by the veterinary nurse to alleviate stress in the hospitalised patient.

The following guidelines for stress reduction should be followed:

- Wherever possible avoid placing cats in cages where they can see and be seen by other patients. If necessary, cover the cage with a blanket, but ensure that regular observation of the patient is maintained.
- Provide cats with the security of somewhere to hide. This is easily achieved by the inclusion of an igloo or cardboard box in the pen.
- Dogs may enjoy the stimulation of everyday activity around them but try to avoid potentially confrontational situations.
- Direct eye contact may be perceived by a dog as a challenging gesture and one that demands an aggressive response. This should be avoided.
- Noise levels should be kept to a minimum and any sudden loud noises should be avoided. Barking dogs should be isolated if practical and returned home as soon as possible.
- Ample provision should be made for urination and defecation. Animals easily become agitated if this is not allowed and often are mortified if they soil their kennel. Cats should always be provided with a litter tray unless specifically told otherwise by the veterinary surgeon.
- Male dogs can become extremely agitated if kennelled in close proximity to a bitch in season. It is advisable therefore not to admit bitches in oestrus to the veterinary hospital unless absolutely necessary.
- A stressed nurse will increase the anxiety of a nervous animal. Providing a calm environment and using a quiet, gentle voice can do much to soothe a frightened patient.
- Ideally, each patient should be monitored and cared for by a specific nurse. This will provide continuity and allow mutual trust to develop.

Normal appearance of the dog and cat

A routine health check of the patient should be performed on admission and regularly throughout its stay in the hospital.

The general demeanour, temperament and overall condition of the animal should be assessed before performing a physical examination.

Examination of the patient should be carried out starting at the external nares and progress methodically, caudally to the tail. All findings should be recorded and reported.

A normal, healthy dog or cat will exhibit the following signs:

- Keen reflexes with sharp reaction to stimuli.
- Clear, bright eyes that are free of discharge.
- Clear nasal orifices with no discharge.
- Clean and odour-free ears.
- Glossy coat with skin that is supple and free of wounds and parasites.
- Suitable weight for breed and size with no signs of obesity or wastage.
- Free limb movement with no signs of stiffness or pain.
- Temperature, pulse and respiration within the normal range, although these may increase slightly under the stress of hospital conditions.
- Pink mucous membranes with a capillary refill time of 1–2 seconds (Fig. 3.1).
- Clear, pale yellow urine passed without pain or difficulty.
- Firm, brown faeces passed freely without undue straining or pain.
- Interest shown in food if offered, with an ability to eat and drink comfortably.

Abnormal appearance of the dog and cat

Any abnormality, however minor, may be significant to the case history of the patient and therefore to the veterinary surgeon in charge. It is vital that all abnormal signs are reported by the veterinary nurse as soon as possible. It is recommended that hospital charts are utilised for all

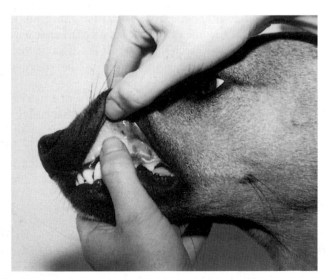

Fig. 3.1 Assessing capillary refill time by applying pressure to the mucous membranes of the gum. (Photograph courtesy of R. Hancocks and R. Meredith.)

patients and that vital signs are monitored and recorded routinely.

Abnormal signs and their possible significance

Appetite changes

Many animals, especially cats, have a normally capricious appetite. However, alterations in feeding patterns may occur in the hospital situation as a result of a change in environment or diet.

Loss of appetite is often the first sign that an animal is unwell. This may be due to a number of factors, including:

- Mouth ulcers.
- Pain in the mouth or dysphagia.
- Nasal congestion, causing impaired olfactory function.
- Infectious diseases
- Pyrexia.
- Metabolic diseases.
- Anxiety or fear in the hospital environment.
- Cats in season.

Voracious appetite with subsequent loss of weight and condition may be a symptom of pancreatic insufficiency or worms. **Pica** (craving for unnatural foodstuffs) may occur as a result of dietary imbalance, but is often merely an undesirable habit. **Coprophagia** (eating of faeces) is an example of this condition.

Changes in urination patterns

Polyuria (increased urine production) and **polydipsia** (increased thirst) are symptoms of many conditions, including:

- Nephritis.
- Diabetes mellitus.
- Diabetes insipidus.
- Pyometra.
- Hyperadrenocorticalism (Cushing's disease).
- Pro-oestrus.

Dysuria describes painful or difficult urination and may be seen in a patient suffering from:

- Cystic calculi.
- Feline urological syndrome (FLUD).
- Prostatic enlargement.
- Obstruction of the urinary tract.
- Trauma to the pelvis or urinary tract.

Haematuria indicates the presence of blood in the urine.

Anuria (total inability to pass urine) and **oliguria** (passage of decreased volume of urine) are potentially emergency situations and may be caused by:

- FUS.
- Obstruction or trauma to the urinary tract.

- Infection.
- Renal failure.
- Shock.

All changes in urination patterns should be monitored and water intake and urine output accurately measured. (The normal urine output for a dog is 2 ml/kg/hour.) The colour, smell and consistency of the urine passed should be assessed and reported.

Unless otherwise instructed by the veterinary surgeon, clean, fresh water should be available to patients at all times.

Changes in defecation patterns

Constipation (the failure to evacuate faeces, which may cause straining) may be caused by a number of factors, including:

- Ingestion of foreign material such as bones or fur balls.
- Tumours in the rectum or colon.
- Environmental factors such as soiled litter trays or confinement.
- Enlargement of the prostate gland.
- Lack of exercise.
- Key–Gaskell syndrome in cats.
- Diverticulum.

Diarrhoea (the frequent evacuation of watery faeces from the bowel) may be caused by:

- Canine parvovirus.
- Bacterial infections including Leptospirosis, Campylobacter, etc.
- Distemper.
- Feline panleucopenia.
- Colitis.
- Tumours of the intestine.
- Intussusception.
- Endoparasites.
- Unsuitable diet.
- Ingestion of placental membranes by post-parturient bitch.

The volume and frequency of faecal material passed should be monitored and recorded. The faeces should be assessed for colour, smell and texture and examined for the presence of blood, mucus or parasitic worms. Microscopic examination may also be carried out.

Vomiting

This is the emission from the mouth of stomach contents and may be caused by:

- Ingestion of foreign material such as poisons, decaying food or small prey.
- Gastritis.
- Diabetes mellitus.
- Nephritis.

- Pancreatitis.
- Pyometra.
- Foreign body in digestive tract such as plastic or stone.
- Endoparasites.
- Viral infections (hepatitis, canine parvovirus, feline panleucopenia, feline infectious peritonitis).
- Anaesthesia.

The volume and frequency of vomitus should be monitored and recorded and the specimen examined for blood, mucus or evidence of poisons. The incidence of vomiting related to feeding patterns is of great relevance and should be monitored, with recording of the times that sickness occurs.

TYPES OF VOMITING
The veterinary nurse should be able to recognise the various types of vomiting that may be seen in the cat and dog. These include:
- **Projectile vomit** – forceful vomiting of stomach contents usually without retching.
- **Regurgitation** – the backflow of food from the oesophagus.
- **Stercoraceous vomit** – vomit containing faeces.
- **Haematemesis** – vomit containing blood.
- **Bilious vomit** – vomit containing bile.
- **Cyclic vomiting** – recurring acts of vomiting.
- **Retching** – ineffectual attempts to vomit. (This may be confused with coughing, especially in cats.)

Nasal discharge

This is commonly accompanied by sneezing and may be caused by:

- Foreign bodies such as grass seeds, tumours or polyps.
- Distemper virus.
- Feline calicivirus.
- Feline viral rhinotracheitis.

The nasal passages should be examined for any evidence of foreign bodies and the discharge examined for presence of blood or pus. Patients, especially cats, may be reluctant to eat when their nasal passages are congested due to diminished olfactory function.

Aural discharge

This is most commonly seen in long-eared breeds such as the spaniel. It is often accompanied by vigorous head shaking and frantic scratching of the ears, causing considerable irritation and distress. It may be caused by:

- Foreign bodies such as grass seeds.

- Ear mite infestation.
- Infection.

The ears should be examined for evidence of obvious foreign body. The use of an auroscope may be required.

Ocular discharge

This can cause considerable distress to a patient and signs such as pawing at the face and rubbing the head against the floor may be seen. This may be a symptom of:

- Distemper.
- Feline upper respiratory tract infection.
- Foreign body such as grass seed.
- Abnormal eyelid or eyelash structure.
- Allergic responses.

The eyes should be examined carefully, taking care not to touch the surface of the cornea.

Vaginal discharge

This is associated with the reproductive cycle of the bitch or queen and may be normal or abnormal. Indications include:

- **Pro-oestrus** – blood-red discharge.
- **Oestrus** – straw-coloured discharge.
- **Imminent parturition** – dark green/brown discharge.
- **Metritis** – brown/black discharge.
- **Abortion** – foul-smelling, black discharge.
- **Pyometra** – purulent discharge, often green or pale coffee colour.

An accurate history should be obtained to help establish the cause of the discharge and ensure the correct course of action is taken.

Coughing

This may be heard in the hospitalised patient and may vary from a dry, harsh cough to one that is fluid and productive. Coughing may be caused by:

- Congestive heart failure.
- Roundworm infestation in young animals.
- Canine contagious respiratory disease.
- Bronchitis.
- Distemper virus.
- Inhalation of chemicals or irritant gases.
- Placement and subsequent removal of endotracheal tube.
- Asphyxia.
- Trauma to the respiratory tract.
- Malformation of the respiratory tract.
- Laryngeal paralysis.

Any method of restraint that may aggravate the situation should be avoided.

Changes in colour of mucous membranes

The colour of mucous membranes is a good indicator of the general health of an animal and will sometimes signal the need for emergency action:

- **Pale mucous membranes** – may indicate haemorrhage, shock, anaemia or circulatory collapse.
- **Blue tinged (cyanotic) membranes** – may indicate respiratory obstruction leading to hypoxia.
- **Yellow (icterus) membranes** – may indicate liver disease.
- **Petechiae** – this refers to small pinpoint red haemorrhages on the mucosae. This may be seen in patients suffering from clotting disorders. Particularly indicative of animals poisoned with anticoagulant rodenticides.

Restlessness

Any animal that appears to be unduly restless should be examined to establish the cause, and steps should be taken if possible to alleviate its distress. Signs of restlessness include:

- Panting.
- Whining.
- Pacing.
- Scratching at bedding.
- Barking.
- Inability to settle.
- Cowering.

These signs may be caused by:

- Pain or discomfort.
- Fear.
- Excess heat or cold.
- Need to urinate or defecate.
- Hunger or thirst.
- Loneliness or boredom.
- Dressings too tight.
- First-stage parturition.

Temperature, pulse and respiration

These vital signs should be monitored routinely in every hospitalised patient. See Table 3.1.

Temperature

Thermometers

The most common type of clinical thermometer is the veterinary **mercury thermometer**. This consists of a graduated glass tube with a stubby bulb at one end containing mercury. When the temperature rises, the mercury expands causing it to travel along the tube. The thermometer has a kink in the bulb end which prevents the backflow of mercury

Table 3.1 Normal range of vital signs in the cat and dog			
	Temperature °C (°F)	Pulse beats/min	Respiration breaths/min
Dog	38.3– 38.7 (100.9–101.7)	60–180[a]	10–30
Cat	38.0– 38.5 (100.4–101.6)	110–180	20–30

[a] *Depending on size*

when it is removed from the animal. This allows an accurate reading of body temperature.

The thermometer may be calibrated in degrees Celsius (°C) or Fahrenheit (°F). Although the veterinary nurse should be familiar with both readings, degrees Celsius is now the standard unit for measurement of temperature. A Fahrenheit reading may be converted to Celsius by use of the formula:

$$°C = (°F - 32) \times 5/9$$

The **electronic thermometer** is now widely used and is designed for rectal or oesophageal use. It allows continual monitoring of body temperature. The temperature may be read from a digital readout. The **subclinical thermometer** may be used to record subnormal temperatures and is valuable for anaesthetised patients and those that are critically ill.

Care and storage of the mercury thermometer The mercury thermometer should be stored in a glass jar with a pad of cotton wool at the bottom. The jar should be filled with antiseptic solution. Both the cotton wool and the antiseptic should be changed daily. The thermometer should be cleaned with cool water and antiseptic. The use of hot water will cause the mercury to expand and the glass to break and should therefore not be used.

Thermometers should not be shared between infectious and non-infectious patients.

Great care should be taken when using and storing the mercury thermometer as both broken glass and the mercury can be hazardous.

Taking the temperature

It is usual and preferable to take the temperature of an animal via the rectal route. However, if this is not possible due to pain or trauma, the axilla or the external ear canal may be used. Generally, the reading can be expected to be 2°C lower than the rectal reading in these areas.

Pyrexia (high body temperature) may be caused by:

- Infection.
- Heat stroke.
- Convulsions.
- Pain.
- Excitement.

PROCEDURE FOR TAKING THE TEMPERATURE VIA THE RECTAL ROUTE USING THE MERCURY THERMOMETER

(1) The patient should be restrained by an assistant.
(2) Shake down the thermometer to ensure the mercury returns to the bulb. (To avoid the possibility of breakage, this should never be done near hard surfaces.)
(3) Lubricate the stubby bulb end of the thermometer with Vaseline, K-Y jelly or similar lubricant.
(4) Gently insert the thermometer into the rectum with a twisting motion. The anal sphincter of the dog will relax easily but slightly more pressure will be required in the cat to relax its inner sphincter muscle. The thermometer should be directed against the upper surface of the rectum to avoid insertion into a faecal mass.
(5) Hold the thermometer in the rectum for the stated time (30 seconds to 1 minute).
(6) Gently remove the thermometer and wipe it clean with cotton wool. Avoid touching the bulb. Dispose of cotton wool in clinical waste.
(7) Hold the thermometer horizontally and rotate it until the mercury level is visible.
(8) Read and record the temperature.
(9) Report any abnormalities to the veterinary surgeon.
(10) Clean thermometer using antiseptic solution.

Low body temperature may be caused by:

- Shock.
- Circulatory collapse.
- Impending parturition.
- General anaesthetic.
- Hypothermia.

Fluctuating temperature is known as diphasic and is a symptom of canine distemper.

Pulse

The pulse rate of an animal can be palpated at any point where an artery runs close to the body surface. Each pulsation corresponds with the contraction of the left ventricle of the heart. In the dog and cat, suitable sites for monitoring the pulse include:

- The femoral artery, on the medial aspect of the femur (see Fig. 3.2).
- The digital artery, on the palmar aspect of the carpus.
- The coccygeal artery, on the ventral aspect of the base of the tail.
- The lingual artery, on the underside of the tongue (in anaesthetised patients).

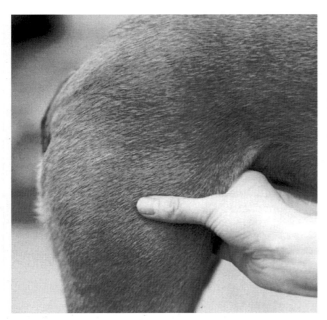

Fig. 3.2 Taking the pulse, using the femoral artery. (Photograph courtesy of R. Hancocks and R. Meredith.)

PROCEDURE FOR PULSE-TAKING (FIG. 3.2)
(1) The patient should be restrained by an assistant.
(2) Locate the artery with the fingers.
(3) Count the pulsations for exactly one minute. (With very rapid pulse rates, a shorter period may be all that is possible.)
(4) Record the rate.

Respiration

The rhythm and rate of respiration can be assessed by careful observation of the patient or by gently resting the hands on either side of the chest cavity.

POSSIBLE CAUSES OF ABNORMAL PULSE RATES
Raised (tachycardia)
- Fever.
- Exercise.
- Hypoxia.
- Pain.
- Fear.

Lowered (bradycardia)
- Unconsciousness.
- Anaesthesia.
- Debilitating disease.
- Sleep.
- Hibernation.

Weak
- Shock.
- Diminished cardiac output.

Strong and jerky ('water hammer' pulse)
- Valvular insufficiency.
- Congenital heart defects such as patent ductus arteriosus.

POSSIBLE CAUSES OF ABNORMAL RESPIRATION
Tachypnoea (increased respiratory rate)
- Heat.
- Exercise.
- Pain.
- Fear.
- Poisons.

Bradypnoea (decreased respiratory rate)
- Poisons (narcotic or hypnotic).
- Metabolic alkalosis.
- Sleep.
- Hibernation.

Dyspnoea (difficult breathing)
(1) Inspiratory dyspnoea:
- Obstruction or stenosis of the respiratory tract.
(2) Expiratory dyspnoea:
- Bronchitis and emphysema of the lungs.
- Pleural adhesions.
(3) Mixed dyspnoea:
- Pneumonia.
- Pneumothorax.
- Hydrothorax.
- Pyothorax.

Although the rate of pulse is important, the character of the pulse should also be assessed. In a normal patient, the pulse rate increases on inspiration and decreases on expiration; this variation is known as **sinus arrhythmia**.

A pulse rate that is lower than a corresponding heart rate is known as a **pulse deficit** and is indicative of **dysrhythmia**.

Cheyne–Stokes respiration often occurs shortly before death and is characterised by alternating periods of deep, rapid and shallow breathing followed by **apnoea** (cessation of breathing).

The respiratory rate should be taken when the patient is at rest but not sleeping or panting. Count either inspirations *or* expirations for exactly 1 minute. Also assess the depth of respiration, which indicates the volume of air inspired with each breath.

General care of the patient

The specific needs of the hospitalised patients will obviously be dependent on their condition. However, all patients have a basic requirement for nutrition, warmth, comfort, hygiene and mental stimulation.

Nutrition

Correct nutrition is of vital importance to the hospitalised patient. A palatable, high-energy diet is required to support the animal during its recovery.

Easily digested foods such as scrambled eggs and chicken may be offered to the inappetent patient. Alternatively, a wide range of commercial diets are available. Strong-smelling foods such as pilchards or meat extract are useful for encouraging animals (especially cats) to eat.

All food should be warmed to blood temperature before feeding. Meals should be fed little and often and any food not eaten after 15 minutes removed.

There are various ways of ensuring that hospitalised patients are encouraged to eat and receive sufficient nutrients. These include:

- Placing food on nose and paws of patient.
- Spoon feeding.
- Syringe feeding.
- Orogastric tubing.
- Nasogastric tubing.
- Pharyngostomy tubing.
- Percutaneous endoscopically placed gastrostomy tubing (PEG).

Warmth

It is important that all patients are kept warm and free from draughts. The temperature of the hospital ward should be kept constant with adequate ventilation. A temperature of 18–20°C is recommended. Additional warmth may be provided by several means:

- **Blankets and towels** are often used in the veterinary hospital, but care should be taken that they do not become soaked with urine, which could lead to urine scalds in a recumbent or weak patient.
- **Vetbeds** are ideal for use in the ward. They are comfortable, warm and easily washed. Their main advantage is that the base of the vetbed absorbs any fluid, thereby ensuring that the patient remains dry.
- **Bubblewrap** is a cheap, readily available material which is particularly suitable for cats, small mammals and birds.
- **Heat lamps** should be used with great care. Animals that are unable to move can easily become overheated and possibly burnt if a lamp is used injudiciously. The heat lamp should be set at a minimum height of 61 cm (24 inches) from the patient and constant observation should be maintained.

- **Hot water bottles** are a good source of heat for weak patients, although they do have certain disadvantages. They will require refilling at regular intervals and should always be covered with a towel or blanket. It is possible that the stopper may become loose or that patients may chew the rubber, and scalding may occur as a result. Boiling water should never be used.
- **Microwave pads** are now commonly used in veterinary practice. They are quick and easy to use and have the advantage of staying warm longer than hot water bottles and having no flex.
- **Heated pads** are useful, but must be used with care. They should be covered with a towel and the patient checked and turned at regular intervals. Animals with a tendency to chew should not be allowed heated pads as chewing the flex could lead to electrocution.
- **Incubators** are ideal for smaller critical patients and for newborn puppies and kittens. The environment can be automatically maintained at the desired temperature. Newborn animals are **poikilothermic** (body temperature varies with ambient temperature) and therefore a constant temperature of 30–33°C should be maintained for these patients.

Comfort

Patients should be provided with adequate bedding materials. They should be allowed to assume a position that they find comfortable. Fractured limbs, open wounds and dressings should be kept uppermost. Familiar bedding brought in by the owner may provide extra comfort and security.

Recumbent animals should be provided with extra padding, such as foam wedges, to prevent the occurrence of decubitus ulcers. Bony prominences such as the hock, elbow and sternum should be especially protected. The application of a bandage or Vaseline to these areas may be beneficial. The recumbent patient should be turned regularly every 2–4 hours.

Various physiotherapy techniques may be beneficial for the recumbent patient. These include massage, coupage, application of cold or warmth and hydrotherapy.

Hygiene

A high standard of hygiene must be maintained on the hospital ward. All faeces, urine, vomit and discharge should be removed from the kennel immediately and the patient cleaned thoroughly. Suitable disinfectants, diluted correctly, should be used when cleaning. Protective clothing should be worn when using these solutions to comply with COSHH regulations. Uneaten food should not be left in the kennel as it will be unpleasant for the patient and may attract flies in hot weather.

The mouth, eyes and nose of patients should be kept free of discharge by wiping with damp cotton wool.

Mental stimulation

It is important to maintain the morale of the hospitalised patient. This can be achieved by talking, fussing and stroking with constant use of the animal's name. It should, however, be allowed periods when it can sleep and rest without distraction.

Regular grooming should be carried out, especially in long-haired breeds. This will remove dead hairs, assist in the detection of ectoparasites and most importantly promote a feeling of well-being.

Long-stay patients may benefit from visits by the owner, although this may not be advisable in all cases as patient and owner alike may become distressed when parting.

Toys and other belongings from home may be allowed at the veterinary surgeon's discretion.

Whenever possible, the patient should be taken outside to enjoy fresh air and a change of environment.

Transport of the patient

Animals should be suitably restrained when they are moved to and from the hospital ward. Dogs that are able to walk should be held on leads and cats confined to a secure basket or carrier.

Anaesthetised or unconscious patients should be supported by stretcher or trolley and observed constantly for struggling, vomiting or respiratory distress. A patent airway must be maintained by extending the head and neck and pulling the tongue forwards. Body temperature of the patient must be maintained during transport and subsequent recovery.

Emesis

Emetics are used to induce vomiting in order to empty the stomach contents. This may be required prior to surgery or more often as a means of eliminating poisonous substances following accidental ingestion. The veterinary nurse may be required to carry out this procedure or may need to advise clients on how to give an emetic in an emergency. Methods for emesis are given in Chapter 4.

WARNING
Emesis is contraindicated in cases of corrosive poisoning or for unconscious or convulsing patients.

Bandaging

The veterinary nurse should be:

- Competent in carrying out routine bandaging procedures.
- Familiar with the more specialised techniques.
- Capable of advising the client on care and protection of the bandage.
- Able to recognise the need for attention to or removal of the bandage.

REASONS FOR BANDAGING
Support for:
- Fractures or dislocations.
- Sprains or strains.
- Healing wounds.

Protection against:
- Self-mutilation.
- Infection.
- Environment.

Pressure to:
- Arrest haemorrhage.
- Prevent or control swelling.

Immobilisation to:
- Restrict joint movement.
- Restrict movement at fracture site.
- Provide comfort and pain relief.

Dressing materials

Various types of dressings are available. They are applied in direct contact with the surface of the skin:

- **Dry dressings** absorb pus or fluid from the wound.
- **Impregnated gauze dressings** may be applied to wounds that need to be kept moist, e.g. burns and scalds.
- **Occlusive dressings** such as hydrocolloids retain moisture within the wound. This stimulates the shedding of necrotic tissue and exposes new healthy tissue below.
- **Haemostatic dressings** such as alginates are used to control haemorrhage or absorb excessive exudate.

Padding materials

These provide the intermediate layer of many dressings. They cushion and support the wound, and they also provide protection to bony prominences and prevent excoriation. They may be made from natural or man-made fibres, including:

- **Cotton wool**, a natural fibre which is cheap and has good absorptive properties.
- **Softban**, a soft, natural padding material available on rolls of varying width and thickness.
- **Foam**, a useful padding material also available on rolls.

Bandaging materials

These are applied to protect the wound and to hold dressings in place. They include:

- **White open weave**, a natural bandage which is strong and firm, but has the disadvantage of not conforming to the patient's body and a tendency for the cotton fibres to fray.
- **Conforming bandage**, the bandage of choice for most dressings, provides a strong neat bandage that conforms to the patient's body.
- **Cohesive bandage** has self-adhering properties but does not stick to hair or skin. It is strong, flexible and conforming.
- **Tubular bandage**, an elasticated cotton or nylon bandage applied with the use of an applicator, is particularly useful for bandaging limbs or the tail.
- **Crepe bandage**, not frequently used in veterinary practice but it has the advantage of being washable and therefore may be reused. It conforms to the larger parts of the animal's body and is useful for head and thorax bandaging.

Covering materials

These form the outer or tertiary layer of the dressing and provide support and protection:

- **Zinc oxide tape**, an adhesive, inelastic, relatively nonconforming material with a tendency to fray. Most commonly used as a traction tape.
- **Elastoplast**, an adhesive, elastic material which provides a neat, conforming protective layer.
- **Non-adhesive tape**, a material that will adhere to itself but not to the patient.

Casting materials

- **Fibreglass cast**, a rigid, lightweight material that provides a strong, fast-setting cast.
- **Plaster of Paris**, a roll of gauze impregnated with calcium sulphate dihydrate. It is applied by immersing the roll in hot water and winding around the affected part in the manner of a bandage. Once dry, it sets to a hard supportive conforming cast.

NB: Protective clothing should be worn when preparing and applying casting materials.

Common bandaging techniques

Limbs

Limbs are frequently bandaged in veterinary practice to provide protection and support for cuts, torn dew claws and surgical procedures. Various materials may be utilised, including narrow open-weave bandage, conforming bandage or elasticated tubular gauze.

STANDARD PROCEDURE FOR LIMB BANDAGE (FIG. 3.3)

(1) The patient is suitably restrained.
(2) In order to absorb sweat and prevent irritation, cotton wool is placed between the patient's toes, pads and dew claws.
(3) Apply a layer of cotton wool or softban around the foot.
(4) Apply the conforming bandage longitudinally to the cranial and caudal surface of the limb and then turn it to wind around the limb in a figure-of-eight pattern. This ensures an even tension throughout the bandage. The bandage is anchored over the hock or carpus.
(5) Apply an external layer of adhesive tape in the same manner.

Ear

One or both ears are often bandaged following trauma, bleeding from ulcerated ear tips or surgical procedures such as aural haematoma or resection.

It is important that the ear bandage is not applied too tightly. The patient should be able to open its mouth normally and its respiration must not be obstructed.

PROCEDURE FOR SINGLE EAR (FIG. 3.4)

(1) Place a pad of cotton wool on the top of the patient's head. Fold the ear back onto the pad.
(2) Apply a dry dressing and place a further pad of cotton wool over the ear.
(3) Apply conforming bandage over the ear and then under the chin; anchor it on either side of the free ear.
(4) The bandage may be covered with adhesive tape.

Abdomen

The abdomen is occasionally bandaged following trauma or surgery. Apply conforming bandage around the abdomen and secure with adhesive tape or tubular gauze. The bandage may have to be extended forwards to the axilla to stop it 'bunching up' later. Care should be taken to prevent the bandage rubbing on the exposed ventral surface of the abdomen – use cotton wool padding or apply Vaseline.

Chest

The procedure for bandaging the abdomen also applies to the chest. The bandage may be anchored between the front legs in figure-of-eight fashion. See Fig. 3.5.

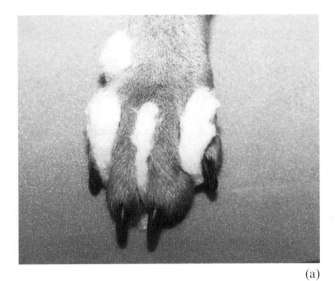

(a)

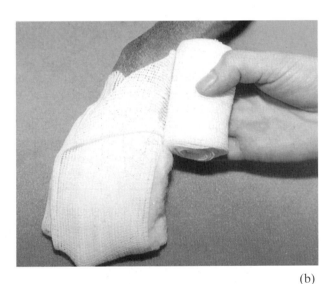

(b)

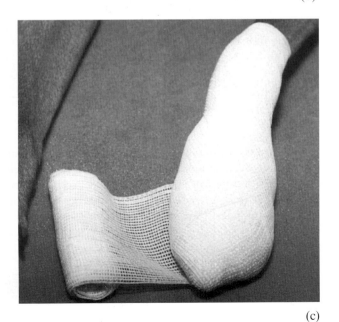

(c)

Fig. 3.3 Procedure for limb bandage: (a) padding between the toes; (b) applying the conforming bandage longitudinally; (c) winding the conforming bandage in a figure-of-eight. (Photographs courtesy of R. Hancocks and R. Meredith.)

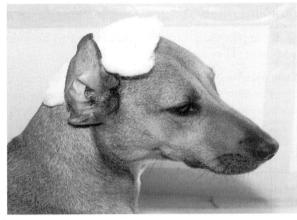

(a)

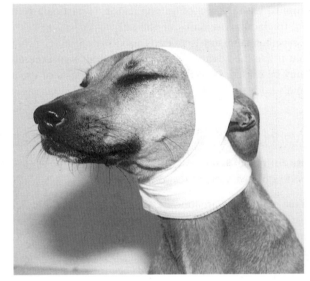

(b)

Fig. 3.4 Procedure for ear bandage: (a) padding the top of the head; (b) the conforming bandage in place. (Photographs courtesy of R. Hancocks and R. Meredith.)

Tail

A light bandage may be required following trauma to the tail or amputation of vertebrae. This can be one of the most difficult areas for keeping a bandage in place. See Fig. 3.6.

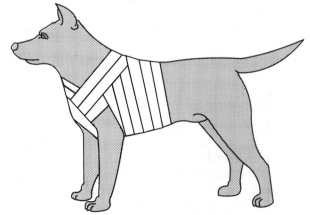

Fig. 3.5 Chest bandage.

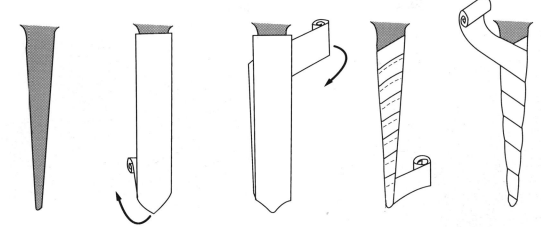

Fig. 3.6 Tail bandage.

Specialised bandaging techniques

The three most common special techniques are:

- **Ehmer sling**, to support the hind limb following reduction of hip luxation.
- **Velpeau sling**, to support the shoulder joint following luxation or surgery.
- **Robert Jones bandage**, to provide support and immobilisation to fractured limbs in a first aid situation or following surgery.

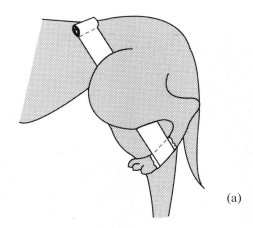

(a)

Care of bandages and dressings

Once the bandage has been applied, constant checks should be maintained until it is removed. Any evidence of odour, oedema, discharge or skin irritation should be reported to the veterinary surgeon. The bandage should be checked to ensure it is not too tight or uncomfortable.

It is important that the dressing does not become soiled or wet. This may be prevented by covering it with a plastic bag when the patient is taken outside.

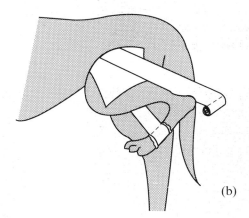

(b)

> **PROCEDURE FOR EHMER SLING (FIG. 3.7)**
> (1) Apply padding material to the metatarsus and stifle.
> (2) Flex the leg and rotate the foot inwards. This will force the hip joint into the acetabulum.
> (3) Apply conforming bandage to the metatarsus, bringing it medial to the stifle joint.
> (4) Continue the bandage over the thigh and back to the metatarsus in a figure-of-eight motion.
> (5) Repeat until full support of the hip is achieved.
> (6) The bandage is then held in place with adhesive tape.
> This dressing is usually kept in place for 4–5 days.

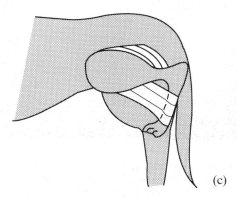

(c)

Fig. 3.7 Ehmer sling.

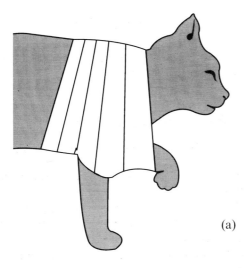

(a)

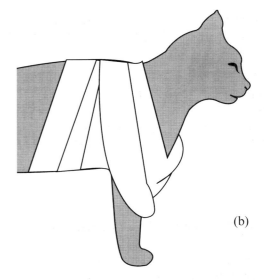

(b)

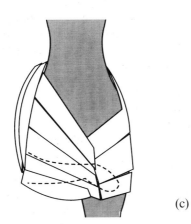

(c)

Fig. 3.8 Making a Velpeau sling.

PROCEDURE FOR VELPEAU SLING (FIG. 3.8)
This is applied to support the shoulder joint following luxation or surgery.
(1) Apply a layer of padding material to the foreleg.
(2) Apply conforming bandage to the paw.
(3) Hold the leg in flexion and apply the bandage over the elbow, then over the shoulder and round the chest.
(4) Repeat until full support of the shoulder is achieved.
(5) The dressing is then secured using adhesive tape.

PROCEDURE FOR ROBERT JONES BANDAGE (FIG. 3.9)
(1) Apply zinc oxide traction tapes to the dorsal and ventral surfaces of the foot.
(2) Take cotton wool from the roll and wrap it tightly around the leg and foot. A large quantity should be used to support the limb.
(3) Apply conforming bandage firmly to the padded leg.
(4) Incorporate the traction tapes into the bandage to prevent slipping.
(5) Cover the bandage with adhesive tape for protection and extra support.
On completion, the foot should be visible so that checks may be made for oedema and temperature. This bandage may be kept in place for up to 2 weeks. Occasionally the toes are included in the bandage.

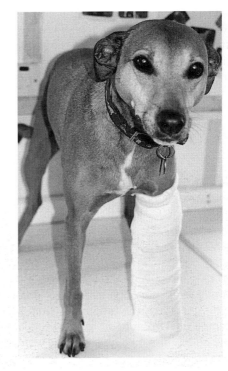

Fig. 3.9 Robert Jones bandage in place. (Photograph courtesy of R. Hancocks and R. Meredith.)

Constant chewing or licking at the bandage by the patient should be discouraged. If this persists, try one of the following measures:

- Discipline.
- Elizabethan collar (Fig. 3.10).
- Muzzle.
- Application of foul-tasting substance to dressing.
- Sedation at veterinary surgeon's direction.

Local applications of heat and cold

Heat may be provided by applying cotton wool soaked in hot water or by means of a poultice prepared with medicants such as kaolin. The hot application will cause vasodilation and therefore increased blood supply to the affected area. This will provide white blood cells for wound healing and assist in fluid removal from the area. The application of heat is indicated in cases of:

- Oedema.
- Infected wounds.
- Abscesses.

Cold may be provided by applying gauze soaked in cold water or an ice pack. Burns and scalds should be flushed with cold water from the tap. The cold application will cause vasoconstriction, therefore reducing heat and blood loss. The application of cold is indicated in cases of:

- Pain.
- Haemorrhage.
- Minor burns and scalds.
- Heatstroke.

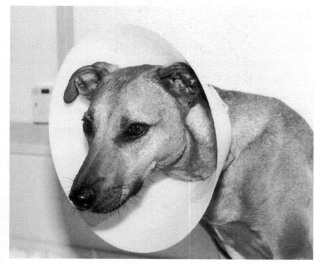

Fig. 3.10 Elizabethan collar. (Photograph courtesy of R. Hancocks and R. Meredith.)

Administration of medicines

Drug classification, dosage and administration are considered in depth in Chapter 12.

Routes for the administration of drugs

Medicines may be administered via various routes:

- **Orally** in the form of tablets, capsules, liquids, pastes or powders.
- **Rectally** in the form of an enema or suppository.
- **Parenterally** by, e.g. intravenous, subcutaneous or intramuscular injection.
- **Topically** to the skin, eyes, ears, nose or mucous membranes.

Systemic routes are those by which the drug affects the body as a whole. They include oral, rectal and parenteral routes.

Choose the route that is the most appropriate for the patient and for the drug. The following factors should be considered before drugs are administered:

- Pharmacological properties.
- Rate of absorption.
- The patient.
- Convenience for the administrator.

Pharmacological properties   It is essential that the drug to be administered is compatible with the chosen route. Some drugs will not be adequately absorbed from the gastrointestinal tract if given orally, whereas others (e.g. pancreatic enzymes extract) must be given via this route as they act on the digestive system. Some drugs may be dangerous if not administered via the recommended route. If thiopentone sodium is injected subcutaneously, it causes irritation and sloughing of the skin.

Rate of absorption   The requirements for the onset of action of the administered drug should be considered. Generally an intravenous injection will have the fastest action, followed (in descending order) by intramuscular injection, subcutaneous injection and the oral route.

The patient   The condition and temperament of the patient will influence the route of drug administration. It may not be possible to administer drugs to an aggressive patient via the oral, topical or intravenous routes, and therefore an alternative route should be used. Administration of oral drugs to patients with respiratory embarrassment or mouth trauma such as a fractured jaw may cause pain or distress and should be avoided. Continued use of the same injection site may cause soreness and pain and should be minimised if possible.

Convenience for the administrator   Most clients will be able to give drugs orally to their animals and this will allow treatment to be given in the familiar surroundings of home. For the veterinary surgeon or nurse, however, it may be more convenient to administer drugs parenterally.

Oral

Drugs are administered orally in the form of tablets, capsules, liquids, pastes or powder/granules.

It is important to take precautions and wear personal protective clothing (PPC) when administering cytotoxic drugs as the drug may be inhaled or absorbed through the skin, causing irritation or carcinogenic effects.

RECOMMENDATIONS FOR ADMINISTERING CYTOTOXIC DRUGS
(1) Wear gloves, apron and mask.
(2) Do not dispense on surfaces where food is prepared.
(3) Protect work surfaces with disposable absorbent sheets.
(4) Dispose of packaging in a safe manner to comply with COSHH regulations.
(5) Wash hands thoroughly after handling.

PROCEDURE FOR ORAL ADMINISTRATION OF TABLETS OR CAPSULES (FIG. 3.11)
(1) The patient should be restrained as gently as possible.
(2) The tablet may be lubricated with butter or oil for ease of swallowing.
(3) Open the animal's mouth by placing one hand over the muzzle, while the other hand is used to hold the tablet and also to pull down the lower jaw.
(4) Place the tablet on the base of the patient's tongue.
(5) Close the mouth and stroke the neck to ensure swallowing.

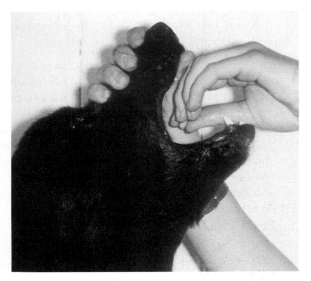

Fig. 3.11 Administration of a tablet via the oral route. (Photograph courtesy of R. Hancocks and R. Meredith.)

PROCEDURE FOR ORAL ADMINISTRATION OF LIQUID MEDICATION
(1) The liquid should be placed in a syringe for ease of administration.
(2) The patient's head should be tilted back.
(3) Place the syringe into the side of the mouth behind the canine teeth.
(4) Slowly administer the liquid to the back of the throat.
(5) Stroke the neck to ensure swallowing.

Rectal

The rectal route is not commonly used in small-animal practice, but drugs such as liquid paraffin or glycerine may be administered in the form of an enema or suppository. Details of enemata are given in Chapter 16 (General Nursing), p. 401.

Parenteral (see p. 629)

This term describes the administration of medicines via routes not involving the alimentary canal. This may be achieved using hypodermic injections given via the following routes:

- Subcutaneous.
- Intramuscular.
- Intravenous.
- Intracardiac.
- Intraperitoneal.
- Intrapleural.
- Intra-articular.
- Epidural.

The choice of route should be decided by considering the condition and temperament of the patient, the properties and volume of the drug to be administered, and the desired speed of effect. Hypodermic injections are most commonly administered via the subcutaneous, intramuscular and intravenous routes.

Subcutaneous injections   The loose skin from the back of the neck to the rump is the most common site for the administration of this injection (Fig. 3.12). This area is suitable because of its poor supply of nerves and large blood vessels. Only non-irritant drugs should be administered via this route as there may be irritation or necrosis of tissues. Action following subcutaneous injection will take effect after 30–45 minutes.

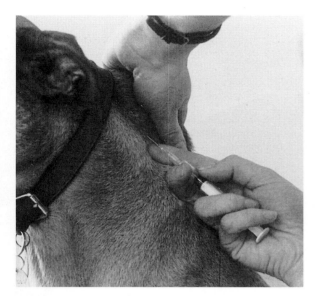

Fig. 3.12 Subcutaneous injection in the scruff. (Photograph courtesy of R. Hancocks and R. Meredith.)

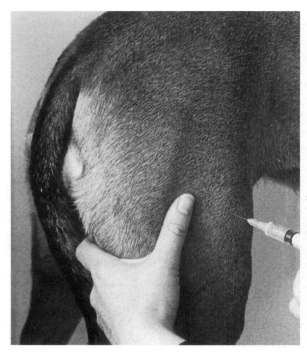

Fig. 3.13 Intramuscular injection in the quadriceps. (Photograph courtesy of R. Hancocks and R. Meredith.)

PROCEDURE FOR SUBCUTANEOUS INJECTION (FIG. 3.12)

(1) Select a sterile needle and syringe. Draw up the required volume of drugs.
(2) The patient should be suitably restrained.
(3) Raise a fold of skin from a suitable area.
(4) Moisten the skin with a spirit swab to flatten the hair and remove surface dirt. (Spirit should not be used when injecting a vaccine, as it may inactivate the drug.)
(5) Insert the needle under the skin and withdraw the syringe plunger slightly. If blood appears in the syringe, a blood vessel has been punctured and a new site must be selected.
(6) If no blood appears, the drug may be injected into the patient.
(7) Massage the injection site gently to disperse the drug.
(8) Make detailed records of the medication given.
(9) Dispose of needle and syringe safely.

Action following intramuscular injection will take effect after 20–30 minutes.

The technique is similar to that for the subcutaneous route except that the needle should be inserted at right angles into the muscle mass.

PROCEDURE FOR A CEPHALIC VEIN INJECTION (FIG. 3.14)

(1) The patient, either sitting or in sternal recumbency, should be restrained by an assistant.
(2) The assistant should restrain the patient's head with one hand and use the other hand to extend the leg and 'raise' the vein by applying pressure around the elbow joint with the thumb.
(3) The operator should stabilise the vein and insert the needle through the sterilised and alcohol-cleaned skin into the vein. Blood should flow gently into the syringe.
(4) The assistant should then release the pressure on the vein and the operator may gently introduce the drug into circulation. If large volumes of fluid are to be injected, regular checks should be made to ensure that the needle remains in the vein (by occasionally drawing back a little blood).
(5) Once the injection has been administered, the needle may be removed from the vein and pressure applied to the injection site for a minimum of 30 seconds, to prevent haemorrhage.

Intramuscular injections The most common site for intramuscular injections is the quadriceps group of muscles in front of the femur (Fig. 3.13). The lumbodorsal muscles and triceps muscles may also be used. The gluteal muscles of the buttocks and the hamstring muscle group should be avoided, as there is a danger of bone or sciatic nerve damage.

Because of the density of muscle tissue, large amounts of fluid may be very painful if injected via this route. The maximum administration should be 2 ml in the cat and 5 ml in the dog.

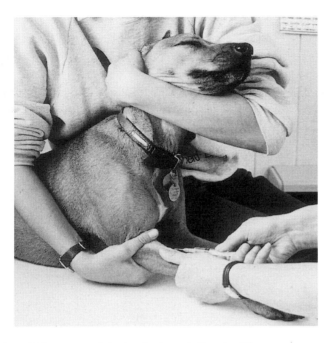

Fig. 3.14 Intravenous injection in the cephalic vein. (Photograph courtesy of R. Hancocks and R. Meredith.)

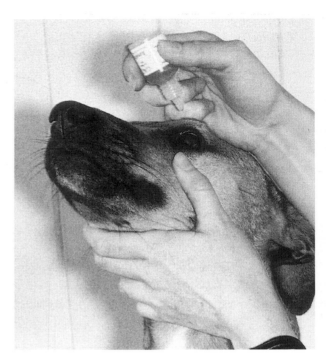

Fig. 3.15 Application of drops to the eye. (Photograph courtesy of R. Hancocks and R. Meredith.)

Intravenous injections   The common sites for intravenous injection are the cephalic vein in the forelimb, the lateral saphenous vein in the hindlimb and the jugular vein in the neck. The sublingual vein may be used in an anaesthetised or unconscious patient.

Action following intravenous injections will take effect in 0–2 minutes.

Topical

This refers to the application of medication to the external surfaces of the body, e.g. the skin, the eyes and the ears.

The skin   Skin treatment may be applied in the form of shampoo, ointment and cream.

The eyes   Eye medication may be applied in the form of drops or ointment. For either medium, the animal's head is tilted back and its eye is held open with the fingers. When applying any substance to the eye, the surface of the cornea should never be touched by the fingers or the nozzle of the applicator.

Drops are applied by dropping liquid onto the centre of the eyeball (Fig. 3.15).

Ointment is applied by gently squeezing a line of the drug onto the inner canthus of the eye, taking care not to touch the surface of the eye with the nozzle or finger. It is often best to approach the patient from the side when using eye ointment, rather than a face-to-face confrontational approach.

After the medication has been applied, the patient should be allowed to blink to disperse the drug evenly over the eye.

The ears   Ear medication may be applied in the form of drops or ointment. The ear should be free from wax and discharge before application. The patient should be restrained and its pinna held firmly. Introduce the nozzle of the applicator into the ear canal and apply the contents gently (Fig. 3.16). Gently massage the external auditory meatus to ensure maximum coverage by the medication.

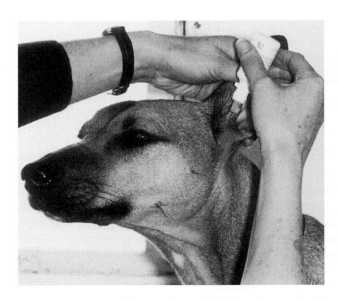

Fig. 3.16 Application of drops to the ear. (Photograph courtesy of R. Hancocks and R. Meredith.)

KEY POINTS
- Observation and care of hospitalised patients should be considered a major and important role of the veterinary nurse.
- The veterinary nurse should provide all patients with the care and attention they deserve.
- All relevant information should be recorded and reported.

Further reading

BSAVA (2000) *Manual of Veterinary Nursing*, BSAVA, Gloucester.

Houlton, J. E. F. and Taylor, P. M. (1987) *Trauma Management in the Dog and Cat*, Blackwell Science, Oxford.

4

First aid

J. Goodwin

Learning objectives

After studying this chapter, students should be able to:

- Apply the four basic rules of first aid to emergency situations.
- Recognise different types of emergencies, and distinguish between those that are life threatening, those requiring prompt attention, and those that are minor emergencies.
- Describe the necessary steps used to evaluate injured or critically ill animals.
- Discuss the different handling, restraining and transportation considerations employed in all types of veterinary emergencies.
- Explain the veterinary nurse's role in first aid situations and recognise professional limitations.
- Apply the principles of emergency nursing care to injured or critically ill animals in a first aid situation.

Introduction

In veterinary medicine an emergency can be classified as any illness or injury which the owner or guardian perceives as requiring urgent medical attention.

The Royal College of Veterinary Surgeons Guide to Professional Conduct (2000) stipulates that if an animal is presented at a veterinary surgery requiring emergency treatment, the surgery staff are committed to provide first aid care and pain relief regardless of the species or financial circumstances of the owner or guardian.

First aid is the immediate treatment of injured animals or those suffering from sudden illness.

In this chapter you will find the aims, rules and limitations of first aid that relate to veterinary nursing and the provision of care and treatment in an emergency situation. The first part of the chapter concentrates on familiarising the reader with the general first aid and emergency nursing skills necessary to:

- Recognise and prioritise different types of emergency (triage).
- Handle, restrain and transport injured animals.
- Take clinical details and perform a thorough clinical examination.
- Differentiate between the states of collapse, unconsciousness, coma and death.
- Perform the stages of cardiac and pulmonary resuscitation (CPR).

The second part of the chapter focuses on the different conditions a veterinary nurse may be faced with in an emer-

gency situation. Although some of these treatments are beyond the scope of veterinary nursing, they have been included to give some idea as to what may be required by the veterinary surgeon.

FIRST AID

Aims
- Preserve life.
- Prevent suffering.
- Prevent the situation deteriorating.

Rules
- Remain calm (do not panic).
- Maintain airway.
- Control haemorrhage.
- Contact veterinary surgeon as soon as possible.

Types of emergency

First aid care covers a wide scope of emergency nursing procedures. All first aid situations will benefit from experience, a calm rational approach and common sense. As it is often the veterinary nurse who is the first point of contact for the owner (either through the telephone or face to face in the veterinary clinic) it is important for him/her to be able to classify the emergency into one of three categories:

(1) **Life-threatening** emergency – requires immediate action at home and on arrival at the surgery. Examples: **unconsciousness, conscious collapse with dyspnoea/cyanosis, severe haemorrhage, severe burns, prolapsed eye, poisoning**.

(2) **Serious** emergency – requires immediate attention at the surgery – not life threatening in itself. Examples: **conscious collapse, dyspnoea, fractures, dislocations, haemorrhage, gaping wounds, severe dysuria, dystocia**.

(3) **Minor** emergency – requires advice to enable the owner to alleviate suffering until a veterinary surgeon can attend the patient. Examples: **insect stings, minor wounds, minor burns, abscess, weight bearing lameness, haematuria, aural haematoma**.

Telephone calls

Immediate classification of an emergency may not be easy over the telephone as owners are often in a panic and unable to judge the severity of the situation. Owners may resent questioning by the veterinary nurse and regard it as a waste of valuable time. It is important to bear this in mind and always remain calm, sympathetic and patient. If possible it is best to speak directly to the owner of the animal, as second-hand information leads to inaccuracies, confusion and frustration. Questions should be specific, clear and concise. There are eight basic questions that should be asked.

(1)   What is the nature of the injury or illness?
       (*Scalding due to household accident? Haemorrhage from a deep cut? Insect sting? Poisoning?*)
(2)   What is the extent or degree of the injury or illness?
       (*Is the animal conscious or unconscious? Is it able to breathe freely? How severe is any haemorrhage? What is the general appearance of the animal?*)
(3)   When was the onset of the injury or illness?
       (*When was it first noticed? Was the accident witnessed? Has the animal's condition deteriorated or improved? How rapidly have any symptoms changed?*)
(4)   What age, sex and breed is the patient?
(5)   Does the animal usually attend a veterinary surgery? If so which one?
(6)   Is the patient receiving current veterinary treatment?
       (*For example, insulin injections if a diabetic, NSAIDs if a gastric haemorrhage is reported.*)
(7)   If injured or taken ill away from home, where exactly is the animal?
(8)   What is the owner's name, address and telephone number?
       (*Important in case the veterinary surgeon needs more information before deciding on a course of action.*)

It is often best to ask these questions in the order set out above because it immediately allows the owner to talk about the problem. It shows that the nurse receiving the phone call is experienced and this in itself gives the owner confidence. There is nothing more frustrating and upsetting for an anguished owner than someone insisting on taking their name and address whilst refusing to listen to details of their pet's illness. Once they have talked to the veterinary nurse and received some reassurance, or been told what to do, they very often calm down and can lucidly give their names, addresses and phone numbers. These can be repeated back to the caller to confirm the accuracy of the details.

After the type of emergency has been decided, the veterinary nurse should give the owner all the relevant information. If immediate first aid measures need to be carried out in the home, step-by-step instructions should be clearly communicated (*e.g. how to maintain the airway of an unconscious pet*).

The nurse should then make the necessary preparations to receive the patient at the surgery (*e.g. prepare dressings, fluids, oxygen, etc.*).

Handling and transportation

Owners often require advice regarding handling and transportation of their ill or injured animal. General advice on handling and transport is given in Chapter 1 but emergency situations away from the surgery often call for different techniques and a degree of ingenuity.

Unless life is endangered by road traffic, falling masonry, fire, poisonous atmosphere, etc., no attempt should be made to move an immobile or collapsed accident victim until it has been given a brief examination. This will ensure that injuries can be adequately protected during handling. The walking wounded may be handled as described later.

Approaching the injured animal

An injured animal is usually frightened and shocked which means that it is liable to bite and scratch viciously if cornered or approached too quickly. The gentle approach is usually best but it should not be hesitant. Slow, deliberate movements accompanied by the continuous gentle reassurance of the human voice can do much to calm the anxious patient.

Handling and restraining cats

Shocked and injured cats are not usually aggressive when approached. Observe the animal closely whilst extending the hand to stroke it under its chin. If this is permitted, slide the hand around the cat's face to stroke its neck and then gently grasp its scruff. The animal is now restrained and an examination can be made.

If the animal reacts aggressively when approached, do not attempt to grasp it as this may only provoke an attack or an attempted escape. In these cases an inverted box or basket should be lowered gently over the cat to confine it and a thin piece of hardboard or strong cardboard slid slowly under the inverted box so that the cat comes to lie on it. The whole may then be lifted and made secure for transport to the surgery.

If no box or basket is available, a thick coat or blanket can be thrown gently over the patient but the nurse should be very careful to ensure the head is restrained by grasping the scruff through the material before attempting to lift the animal. Canine teeth can puncture thick material and leather gloves, so this approach must only be used in dire situations.

Handling and restraining dogs

Frightened injured dogs are much more inclined to snap at approaching humans, especially strangers. Even the dog's owner may be bitten if a normally placid pet is in pain from its injuries. If there is any indication of aggression, form a looped lead as a running 'noose' and try to drop it over the dog's head. Leather leads are better than chain or material ones because the noose tends to hang as an open loop and it is easier to position it around the dog's neck.

Some dogs react to the lead, biting and snapping at the noose as it is lowered towards the head. This makes restraint difficult and, unless there is a 'dog-catcher' available, it is often necessary to ask someone else to stand in front of the dog (at a safe distance), talking to it and **maintaining constant eye contact**. The veterinary nurse can then approach the dog from behind and lower the lead over its head.

Many dogs immediately feel more secure if they are on a lead with a human in control but they still might bite. A muzzle should therefore be tied in place before handling **unless the dog is dyspnoeic or the dog's face is injured**.

Once the animal is under control, a brief but thorough examination should be carried out:

- **Airway** must be patent (see Resuscitation).
- **Haemorrhage** must be controlled (see Haemorrhage).
- **Fractures** should be immobilised (see Fractures).
- **Wounds** should be dressed (see Wounds).

The patient should then be restrained as gently as possible until it can be transported to the surgery or until a veterinary surgeon can attend the animal. The patient should be allowed to assume the position that it finds most comfortable and most injured animals will lie on the wounded side. This distresses owners but the patient should not be interfered with if it seems to be comfortable. The owner should be asked to stay with the animal to reassure and comfort it.

Transporting animals

The aim is to move the injured animal to the surgery with minimum discomfort and without disturbing any dressings that have been applied. There are two groups of animals: the ambulatory (able to walk) and the non-ambulatory.

Ambulatory

An ambulatory animal is one that can rise to its feet and is able to walk, even if only to limp slowly.

Cats The best way to transport cats is to have them contained in a basket or box. Types range from wire, wicker or wooden cages to cardboard boxes, laundry baskets, washing baskets and any other containers that may be at hand in an emergency. There are three important criteria:

(1) Escape proof.
(2) Adequately ventilated.
(3) Observation possible.

Dogs Ambulatory dogs are often transported less painfully and with less stress if they are allowed to move themselves. Gentle encouragement should be used to guide the animal to the transport vehicle. Assistance may be required to help the animal climb in.

Large dogs that have difficulty supporting their weight on their hind limbs can be assisted by the use of a towel or blanket acting as a sling under their abdomen.

Non-ambulatory

A non-ambulatory animal is unable to rise to its feet and walk. If the animal is collapsed and severe injuries are suspected, it should be lifted with great care to lessen the pain and distress and to prevent further injury.

In any (suspected) cases of the following, it is best to advise the use of a stretcher for transportation.

(1) Spinal fracture.
(2) Collapse with dyspnoea.
(3) Collapse with thoracic/abdominal injuries.
(4) Collapse and unconsciousness.
(5) Other severe injuries (multiple fractures/wounds).

Most people do not have access to an animal stretcher, but the principles of using a stretcher can be applied to any flat rigid object large and strong enough to accommodate the animal in lateral recumbency, yet small enough to fit into the transport vehicle. Stretchers can be improvised from:

(1) Wood or hardboard sheets.
(2) Wire mesh or plastic-coated fencing wire (*needs to have handles so it can be pulled taut*).
(3) Sacks or coats mounted on wooden poles.
(4) Blankets (*these offer little support for spinal injuries, but are readily available, and easily slid underneath the collapsed patient*).

Transferring patients to stretchers may contribute to their pain. The use of a tape muzzle is advisable to avoid being bitten in this situation. Several people should help with the transfer so the animal can be moved as a unit.

If spinal damage or multiple fractures are suspected then the best way to transfer a patient to a stretcher is as follows:

(1) Lay the stretcher on the floor behind the animal.
(2) Grasp the skin along the back (*above the scapula, midway along the back*).
(3) Pull the animal slowly and steadily on to the stretcher.
(4) Avoid any twisting of the spine.

If spinal damage is not suspected then the animal can be rolled on to the stretcher as follows:

(1) Lay the stretcher on the floor behind the animal.
(2) Roll the animal half on to its chest.
(3) Push the stretcher underneath the animal as far as possible.
(4) Allow the animal to relax back into lateral recumbancy, and thus onto the stretcher.

Cats Non-ambulatory cats can be lifted in the owner's arms. They may be held firmly round the neck with one hand (taking care not to obstruct the breathing) whilst the other hand and arm are slid around the sternum to scoop the body up, supporting the weight along the length of the forearm (Fig. 4.1). Both forelegs can then be held firmly in the left hand, to prevent the animal scrabbling to get free, whilst the handler's right hand continues to hold the neck gently in extension, like a wide collar, so that the animal is

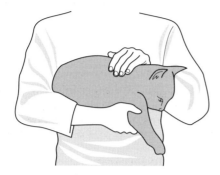

Fig. 4.1 Carrying a cat.

unable to turn its head round or down to bite the handler. It is advisable to contain these animals in a secure basket for transit. Alternatively the owner can be advised to find a small sheet of hardboard or thick cardboard (which is the same size or smaller than the basket or box) and slide this gently under the patient. The animal can then be picked up on the support and placed in the container with minimal disturbance.

If the patient is too aggressive to allow either procedure, it may be less distressing and painful if it is lifted up bodily by the scruff in one hand, with minimal gentle support of the hindquarters by the other hand, and placed gently and carefully in the basket, accomplishing the manoeuvre as smoothly and as quickly as possible to minimise the length of painful handling.

Dogs **Small dogs** can be handled in a similar manner to cats. **Medium-sized dogs** may be lifted with one arm encircling the front of the sternum, the other around the back of the pelvis to support the hindquarters. The animal is then held against the handler's chest. To prevent injury to the human back, always lift the dog with an almost straight back, using bent knees to provide most of the lifting effort and always ask for help if the dog seems too heavy for one person.

Large and heavy dogs must be lifted by two (or more) people. One person stands at the dog's shoulder with one arm curled around the dog's neck, holding its head against the handler's shoulder to control it, with the other arm under and around its thorax, just behind its forelegs. The second person stands by the hindquarters and places one arm under the abdomen, just in front of the hind legs, and the other around the pelvis.

Care in transit

Within the vehicle, the patient needs to be observed constantly and restrained to ensure that:

(1) The condition does not deteriorate.
(2) Any first aid treatments (*dressings/ice packs*) are not disturbed.

(3) The animal does not escape from its container.
(4) The animal does not fall off the seat.
(5) The animal cannot interfere with the driver of the vehicle.

It is important to have a second person in the vehicle (preferably the owner) who will be able to give a full case history at the surgery and who will want to be with the pet anyway. The owner's presence may also help to calm the patient.

If it is impossible or impractical for a second person to accompany the animal, the patient must be securely restrained (*either on a lead which is securely fastened – inside the vehicle or shut in the car door, or in a basket which is fastened in place by a seat belt*).

Arrival at the surgery

It is important to have any necessary paperwork (*e.g. consent form*) previously prepared and ready for signatures, enabling first aid procedures and emergency treatments to be top priority. The first procedure on arrival at the surgery should be the attachment of an identification collar or label to the patient.

Case history

If the owner has already answered the questions previously outlined then the veterinary nurse should have a clear case history. If not then these questions need to be answered on arrival at the surgery. Previous health and veterinary treatments may hold the key to a correct diagnosis (*e.g. an unconscious bitch may be in a hypoglycaemic coma if she is a known diabetic; or a bitch which has recently had pups may have collapsed because she is hypocalcaemic*). Further questioning may be needed in cases of suspected poisoning (*see Poisoning*).

Primary clinical examination

The patient should be observed closely before any attempt is made to touch it. The state of consciousness, the general behaviour and the respiration should be observed before any external stimuli interfere with the evaluation. If the animal is stable, then a thorough physical examination should be performed (Table 4.1). A common mnemonic (A CRASH PLAN) is useful for ensuring nothing is excluded from the physical examination. **All information should be recorded**.

Table 4.1 Stages of a detailed examination

Area	Examination
Nose	Note any haemorrhage (*epistaxis*) and whether it comes from one or both nostrils. Note any swellings which may suggest fracture of the nasal bones
Mouth	**Odours**. Carefully open the mouth and smell the breath. Note any unusual smell: e.g. ketones ('pear drops') in cases of untreated diabetics; creosote or phenol in cases of poisoning; urine odour in cases of kidney failure **Haemorrhage**. Check for signs of haemorrhage and locate its source, e.g. gums, tongue (dorsal and ventral surfaces), palate, etc. If no injuries are apparent, the blood may have been coughed up from the lungs or issued from wounds in the throat area. **Tongue**. Check for signs of redness or ulceration, which often occur after licking corrosive poisons **Fractures**. Examine the bony structure for signs of fracture: splitting of the hard palate down its centre, jaw fractures **Teeth**. Look for any signs of food caked in the crevices. Pesticides are often highly coloured and some evidence may be seen on the teeth if the animal has eaten poisoned bait **Mucosa**. Note the colour of the mucosa, which may be: (a) Normal (pale pink) (b) Congested (brick-red) (toxic or septicaemic animals and heatstroke patients) (c) Pale (may appear white) (severe shock or severe haemorrhage) (d) Cyanosed (purple) (e.g. patients with severe dyspnoea) (e) Jaundiced (orange or yellow) (acute liver damage) Note whether the mucosa is dry or normally moist, or if the animal is salivating so profusely that it drools. Certain poisons affect the rate of production of saliva. If the gums or lips are not darkly pigmented, test the capillary refill by pressing the mucosa to blanch it. In an animal with normal blood pressure, the pink colour returns rapidly within 1–2 seconds of the pressure being removed. In an animal with a low blood pressure, it may take up to 5 seconds before the capillaries refill with blood and the mucosa becomes pink again. This simple test is very helpful in assessing whether the animal has suffered a severe haemorrhage
Eyes	The eye is a very delicate and sensitive organ and must be treated gently. It is best to examine the animal in a dimly lit or darkened room, where the patient is more likely to open its eye. For detailed examination, an auroscope head or torch may be used to illuminate the eye. Note any discharges of fluid and their appearance and quantity. Clear fluid may indicate that the eyeball has ruptured; purulent discharges could be evidence of a foreign body Eyelids can easily be examined for signs of injury and may be opened gently and everted slightly to allow examination of the conjunctiva and nictitating membrane (third eyelid) Check the palpebral reflex Examine the colour of the conjunctival mucosa for an indication of anaemia (pale pink or white), jaundice (yellow) or cyanosis (mauve) Check the eyeball for bruising to the sclera or conjunctiva and note any sign of jaundice. Note any injuries to the eyeball, haemorrhage into the anterior chamber, collapsed eyeball or corneal opacity Note the position of the eyeball in the socket in cases of unconsciousness and any *nystagmus* (involuntary flicking movement of the eyeball from side to side) Note the size of the pupil in each eye and check for response to light. Brain-damaged patients often show a difference in the size of the two pupils; poisoned patients may have very constricted or very dilated pupils that do not respond normally to light
Skull	Look for signs of depressed fractures, swelling, pain or crepitus. Be very gentle when checking for a suspected fracture of the cranium as heavy handling could depress the bone fragments into the brain cortex and cause enormous damage to the cerebral hemispheres
Ears	Examine for signs of haemorrhage from the ear canal as this can occur with brain damage
Limbs	Palpate all limbs, bones and joints, for signs of swelling or pain. In cases of suspected deformity, it is useful to compare the injured leg with its normal partner. If a fracture is suspected, treat it as such pending diagnosis by the veterinary surgeon Record the way the limb is held and note any obvious *paralysis*: (a) **Flaccid**. The muscles are totally relaxed (b) **Spastic**. The muscles are contracted to fix the limb rigidly in extension or flexion. Note any loss of feeling, which may be tested by pinching the toes. If the animal is able to feel this stimulus, it will look round at the foot, try to move away or attempt to bite the cause of its discomfort as well as flexing the leg to draw it away from the painful stimulus. This is known as conscious proprioception and should not be confused with the simple withdrawal reflex when the limb is simply flexed to remove it from the pinching stimulus without the animal showing any signs that it is aware of the pain.
Rib cage	Gently palpate for signs of fractured ribs. Listen to any wounds to detect a 'hiss' sound on inspiration indicating penetration of the pleural cavity
Abdomen	Palpation of the abdomen is a skilled procedure and can cause considerable harm if attempted by the inexperienced: do not attempt it. Haemorrhage from the penis or bruising or swellings of the abdomen wall should be noted
Spine	Note any obvious deformities in the spinal column and gently palpate to detect any gross abnormalities. The spinal column is covered by a large muscle trunk and severe spinal fractures are not always obvious. Always assume a fracture is present if there is any doubt. Fractures or dislocations in the cervical region may cause paralysis of all four

Area	Examination
	legs, *quadriplegia*, or, more rarely, paralysis of one side of the body, *hemiplegia*. Fractures or dislocations of the thoracolumbar region may cause paralysis of the hindlegs, *paraplegia*, and many cases show rigid extension of the forelegs and flexion of the hindlegs, with the back arched at the fracture site. It is important to realise that the spinal cord may continue to function normally above and below the fracture site. Thus limb withdrawal reflexes are often unaffected as they are a local reflex arc and do not require input from the brain. However, conscious proprioception may be absent from areas caudal to the spinal injury if nerve impulses are unable to pass to the brain.
Pelvis	Gently palpate the pelvic bones for signs of instability, pain, crepitus and deformity
Perineal region	The prepuce, vulva and anus should be examined for signs of haemorrhage because signs of blood at these orifices may indicate that internal organs (e.g. the bladder) have been damaged. In cases of paralysis, it is useful to note the presence or absence of the anal ring reflex by watching for anal sphincter contraction when a thermometer is inserted into the anus
Tail	Observe the signs of voluntary movement, e.g. correct carriage of the tail, wagging, etc.
General body	Note any matting of the fur which may indicate an underlying wound. If in doubt as to the severity of the wound, assume the worst and treat accordingly. If foreign bodies are present, removal may be attempted unless they are embedded. Dislodging embedded foreign bodies may provoke more serious injury and must therefore be avoided.

Table 4.1 (Continued)

'A CRASH PLAN': EXAMINATION CHECK LIST	
Airway	Visualisation, palpation, ausolation, and examination of the oral cavity, the pharynx and the neck.
Cardiovascular	Visualisation, palpation and auscultation bilaterally.
Respiratory	Visualisation, palpation, auscultation and percussion bilaterally.
Abdomen	Visualisation, palpation, auscultation and percussion.
Spine	Visualisation, palpation
Head	Eyes, ears, nose, mouth (inc. teeth), gums, tongue, mucous membranes.
Pelvis	Perineum, perianal, rectal and external genitalia.
Limbs	Skin, muscle, tendons, bones and joints.
Arteries	All peripheral pulses.
Nerves	Motor and sensory output to limbs and tail.

General nursing care

The majority of accident victims and very ill patients needing emergency treatment are likely to be severely shocked. Many first aid measures are aimed at counteracting the effects of shock (a subject which is covered in Chapter 22, 'Fluid Therapy and Shock').

All veterinary nurses need to recognise the main signs of shock. These are:

- Pale mucous membranes.
- Decreased capillary refill time.
- Increased respiration rate.
- Rapid, weak pulse – sometimes not palpable.
- Cold extremities.
- Dull, depressed and lethargic.
- Convulsions and/or collapse if the patient is hypoxic due to hypovolaemic shock (severe haemorrhage) or asphyxia (obstructed airway).

Specific treatment varies depending on the primary cause of the shock, but the following principles apply to all cases:

(1) **Prevent any further haemorrhage.**
(2) **Do not apply direct heat or give alcohol or other peripheral vasodilator drugs** (e.g. acepromazine). Both cause dilatation of the cutaneous blood vessels, which are a non-essential part of the circulatory system as far as the shocked patient is concerned. The cutaneous blood vessels constrict in shock so that the circulating blood volume is directed towards maintaining sufficient blood supply to vital organs such as the brain, heart and lungs. This is why the extremities (paws and tail) feel cold to the touch and also why the mucosae are pale. If these non-essential blood vessels are encouraged to dilate, the blood pressure will fall as there is an increase of circulatory 'pipework' to be filled by the circulating blood. Vasodilatation in the skin is also more likely to restart haemorrhage from surface wounds.
(3) **Make the animal comfortable and prevent any further heat loss**. Lay the patient on an insulated surface such as thick blankets, vetbeds or polystyrene beanbags and cover the animal with further insulation to prevent heat loss from the body.
(4) **Set up an intravenous fluid drip** (the drip of choice is warmed Hartmann's solution but normal saline is adequate in an emergency). Intravenous fluids will help to

correct the metabolic acidosis of shock and expand the circulating blood volume quickly, therefore improving the supply of oxygen to all body tissues. It also allows the kidneys to function more normally again. If there has been extensive blood loss, a blood transfusion or a plasma expander may be required. In cases of brain damage, some veterinary surgeons use hypertonic solutions to decrease the oedema of the brain tissues (e.g. mannitol solution). These fluids may be warmed, ready for administration if the veterinary surgeon needs them.

(5) **Give fluids by mouth** (unless there are contraindications, e.g. vomiting, unconsciousness, severe mouth or throat injuries). Small volumes of oral electrolyte replacement fluids should be offered by mouth every 30 minutes (25–100 ml depending on size of the animal). Oral Hartmann's or an improvised solution of 1 litre of plain water with half a teaspoon of salt and half a teaspoon of bicarbonate soda dissolved in it is useful if no veterinary preparations are available.

(6) **Check dressings** every 10–15 minutes to ensure that they are comfortable, that the animal is not interfering with them and that any haemorrhage is being controlled.

(7) **Maintain constant observation**. The condition of the patient can deteriorate rapidly and the veterinary nurse must always remain on the alert. The state of consciousness, pupillary and palpebral reflexes, mucosal colour, capillary refill, and character and rate of pulse and respiration should be monitored every 10 minutes, or more frequently if the animal seems very distressed. **Make notes of the findings and time of each inspection and record them on the kennel chart**. This is essential in cases of brain injury, haemorrhage, dyspnoea and suspected poisoning.

(8) **TLC**. All the above measures are aimed at reversing the effects of shock and will therefore make the animal feel more comfortable. However, the emotional needs of the patient should not be overlooked. These animals are often in much pain; they are confused and disorientated because they are alone in a strange and hostile environment (few animals like the surgery!) and they need sensitive and sympathetic handling. It should also be remembered that brain-damaged patients may have lost some faculties (e.g. sight or hearing) in the accident and need even more careful handling.

The nurse can help patients greatly by keeping them in a quiet, warm, darkened room and moving quietly and calmly whilst talking in a soothing manner. It does not matter what is said, rather the tones used. When checks are made, the animal should not be rushed – a gentle approach is much less stressful. Contact with human hands is very important, especially to dogs, and a little fussing is a good idea if time permits, but attention should *never* be forced on the patient. If any apprehension is shown, the animal is best handled as little as possible and it may even be advisable to cover the front of the kennel or basket to allow the patient some privacy between regular check-ups.

As soon as possible, veterinary assistance should be obtained and comprehensive notes should be handed to the veterinary surgeon in charge of the case. Meanwhile, the veterinary nurse may prevent delays by preparing dressings, drips, transfusions, instruments, anaesthetic machines, the X-ray suite and the operating theatre in readiness for any further treatment that the veterinary surgeon may think necessary once the patient's condition is stabilised. The efficient nurse will save valuable time by being one step ahead and having equipment ready, drugs available, drips warmed, etc., for when the veterinary surgeon arrives.

Collapse, unconsciousness, death and resuscitation

The first thing a veterinary nurse needs to establish when presented with an immobile animal is whether the patient is alive, conscious/unconscious or dead.

- **Conscious** animals are aware of their surroundings, and able to respond to external stimuli. They respond normally to sound, sight and touch.
- **Unconsciousness** occurs when the brain has been affected and the animal is rendered unable to respond normally to external stimuli.

Conscious collapse and unconsciousness

Collapse is said to have occurred when a conscious animal is unable, or unwilling to stand up. It is the most common emergency reported by owners and it covers a multitude of situations ranging from an arthritic dog that is reluctant to go for a walk, to the deceased pet. The cause and severity of the collapse must be established before the correct first aid procedure may be carried out.

The difference between collapse and unconsciousness is whether the animal is conscious or not. Conscious animals are aware of their surroundings, and are able to respond normally to sound, sight and touch. They have normal eye reflexes and can focus on objects following movement with their eyes. Collapsed animals will respond to handling, either by becoming calm and affectionate, or aggressive. Caution should always be exercised, as the collapsed patient is able to bite, even if it is unable to get up.

A collapsed patient must be constantly observed and its reflexes regularly assessed to ensure the situation is not deteriorating. The patient should be treated with care because its condition may not be stable. In some instances the patient may lapse into unconsciousness, whilst in others there may be rapid improvements to normal health.

There are many different causes of collapse and unconsciousness, and sometimes there is not a clear line between the two. Table 4.2 outlines the common conditions that may result in a collapsed or unconscious animal. Some condi-

Body system	Collapse	Unconsciousness
Table 4.2 Cases of collapse and unconsciousness		
CNS	—	Epilepsy
	Brain trauma	Brain trauma
	Vestibular syndrome	—
	Disc protrusion	—
	Atlanto-axial subluxation	—
	Spinal fractures	—
Respiratory	Airway obstruction	Airway obstruction
	Fluid in the alveolar spaces	Fluid in the alveolar spaces
	Collapsed lungs	—
	Interference with respiratory movements	—
	Interference with oxygenation of the blood	—
Circulatory	Cardiac failure	Cardiac failure
	Hypovolaemic shock – acute haemorrhage	Hypovolaemic shock – acute haemorrhage
	Hypovolaemic shock – severe fluid loss	—
	Traumatic shock (e.g. road traffic accidents)	—
	Anaemia (long term blood loss)	—
	Thrombosis – brachial or iliac	—
Abdominal emergency	Gastric torsion, bowel rupture	—
	Bladder rupture	—
	Urethral obstruction	—
	Acute prostatitis	—
	Acute hepatitis	—
	Splenic torsion	—
	Acute pancreatitis	—
	Abdominal pain	—
Locomotor conditions	Dislocations and fractures of the limbs	—
	Arthritis, muscle wasting	—
Metabolic disturbances	Hyper/hypoglycaemia	Hyper-hypoglycaemia
	Hypocalcaemia	Hypocalcaemia
	Uraemic fits	Uraemic fits
	Toxaemia (e.g. pyometra)	—
Physical causes	—	Electrocution
	Hypothermia	Hypothermia
	Hyperthermia	Hyperthermia
Drugs and poisons	Any compound causing CNS depression	Any compound causing CNS depression

CNS = central nervous system (brain and spinal cord).

tions have been placed in both categories as all reasons for unconsciousness may cause the animal to collapse if the brain is only mildly depressed, and most causes of collapse may progress to unconsciousness if the situation deteriorates. Some conditions may be so severe or acute that the patient becomes unconscious almost immediately and the collapsed conscious state is scarcely noticeable. An example of a condition that can present in either scenario is hyperthermia (heat stroke). If an animal is confined and left in a car on a hot day for 20 minutes then it will probably arrive at the surgery collapsed but still conscious. If the same animal is left for a longer period of time then it is likely to be presented in an unconscious state.

Unconsciousness and death

There are two terms that can be used to describe the depth of unconsciousness in animals. Those in a **stupor** can be roused (with difficulty). Their pedal withdrawal reflex, pupil-

lary light reflex and palpebral reflexes are still present. Those in a **coma** cannot be roused. Their pedal reflexes are absent, and their eye reflexes indicate a surgical (or deeper) plane of anaesthesia. Pupils will dilate as the condition deteriorates, and death approaches.

Veterinary nurses should take every opportunity to practice monitoring vital signs in healthy unconscious animals undergoing routine surgery. Familiarity with technique leads to confidence in an emergency situation.

Comparisons between unconsciousness and death are outlined in Table 4.3.

Heartbeat   This can be listened to with a stethoscope or detected by palpation. If no heartbeat is immediately obvious, a stethoscope must be used to detect any cardiac activity.

The heartbeat may be felt by placing one hand either side of the chest wall so the fingertips rest on the costal cartilages of ribs 5–6 (bottom of the rib cage behind the elbow). If needed, gentle pressure can be applied with the fingertips

Table 4.3 Signs of unconscious collapse and death		
Sign	**Unconscious collapse**	**Death**
Heartbeat	Regular, though slowed	Absent for more than 3 minutes
Respiratory pattern	Varies according to depth of CNS depression. Mimics anaesthesia	Absent, although sometimes Cheyne–Stokes respiration is observed
Eyeball position	Turned down or central, according to depth of CNS depression. Mimics anaesthesia	Central
Cornea	Normally moist	Glazed
Corneal reflex	Present, unless eyelids paralysed	Absent
Pupil size	Varies in size, rarely fully dilated	Fully dilated
Pupillary light reflex	Usually present, unless iris is paralysed	Absent
Movement	May be roused in stupor, pedal reflexes present in mild cases. Varies according to depth of CNS depression	Absent except Cheyne–Stokes respiration
Body temperature	Remains constant	Begins to cool within 15 minutes

until the pulsations of the ventricles can be felt. In barrel-chested breeds (bulldogs), it may be impossible to feel an apex beat so a stethoscope must be used.

The head of the stethoscope should be placed over the area of intercostal space between ribs 7 and 8.

Respiratory pattern This can be observed through watching the chest wall rise and fall. Deep, regular breathing may quicken as the animal regains consciousness or it may progress to rapid, shallow gasps as the brain becomes more and more depressed. Fogging of a cold mirror or movement of a fine tuft of hair or a wisp of cotton wool held at the nostrils will detect the slightest expiration.

Cheyne–Stokes respiration (infrequent deep convulsive gasps for breath) heralds the onset of death.

Eyeball position In cases of flaccid unconsciousness, the eye position will often indicate the depth of CNS depression **unless the muscles of the eyeball are paralysed.** Evidence of **nystagmus** or **strabismus** should be noted. In cases of epileptiform convulsions, the eyeball may stay in its usual position but remains in a fixed, unfocused stare. The eyes do not follow movements, or turn towards the owner in recognition.

Cornea Glazing of the cornea is indicative of death. The surface of the cornea lacks its usual lustre.

Corneal reflex Because the cornea is easily damaged, its reflex should only be tested by touching it with a wisp of moist cotton wool. This should be sufficient to make the eyelids blink. The cornea is so sensitive that this is one of the last reflexes to be lost. However, in some cases of head trauma (where the motor nerves of the eyelid muscle are damaged) the corneal reflex may be absent.

Pupil size Compare the pupil size of each eye. **Anisocoria** can indicate unilateral brain damage.

Pupillary light reflex This reflex should be tested in a darkened room, using a torch or auroscope as a source

of bright light. As the light shines into the eye, both pupils should constrict equally. Failure to do so indicates brain damage. However, if the nerves to the pupil are damaged (prolapsed eyeball), this reflex may be absent as it is unable to work.

Body temperature and rigor mortis In the unconscious animal the body temperature remains constant. After death the body cools. This takes several hours and the speed is dependent on the room temperature.

In the dead animal the muscles totally relax, then they gradually stiffen due to chemical changes occurring in the muscle cells. Rigor mortis usually takes about 12 hours to set in throughout the body, but the rate is variable depending again on the room temperature, the cause of death and the physical condition of the animal.

Cardio-pulmonary resuscitation

If a veterinary nurse is presented with a dying patient then cardio-pulmonary resuscitation (CPR) needs to commence. Cardiac massage and artificial respiration need to be administered simultaneously as one is pointless without the other. The veterinary nurse should follow the **ABC** regime.

- **A**irway.
- **B**reathing.
- **C**irculation.

Airway

Check for a patent airway. Intubate, inflate cuff to avoid inhalation of fluids. If airway is obstructed:

(1) Remove collar, check mouth and throat for any obstruction, swab away fluid, remove foreign bodies.
(2) Give 5 or 6 abdominal thrusts.
(3) Check mouth, swab pharynx.

If this is not sufficient, then:

(4) Turn patient on its side and give several blows to its back.
(5) Repeat (only 2 or 3 times).
(6) Place a large-bore needle into the trachea and administer oxygen.
(7) Prepare to do a tracheostomy.
(8) Put patient in dorsal recumbency.
(9) Clip neck (distal to larynx).
(10) Make a 2–3 cm incision with a scalpel down the ventral midline through the skin and the subcutaneous tissue.
(11) Bluntly dissect the muscles with forceps/scissors until the tracheal rings are exposed.
(12) Incise between the tracheal rings ($\frac{1}{4} - \frac{1}{3}$ of the circumference).
(13) Separate the tracheal rings with a blunt object (forceps/scalpel blade handle).
(14) Insert a tracheostomy or endotracheal tube caudally and tie in place.
(15) Administer oxygen.

Breathing

If respiratory movements have ceased, respiratory stimulant drugs may be used (e.g. doxapram hydrochloride). Until the animal begins to breathe on its own again **the lungs must be mechanically inflated**. It is preferable to intubate these patients as an endotracheal tube ensures a patent airway, and if the cuff is inflated it eliminates the possibility of the animal inhaling any fluids. Artificial respiration via an endotracheal tube is much more hygienic than mouth-to-nose resuscitation.

Intubated patients should be connected to an oxygen supply from a closed circuit anaesthetic machine and the **reservoir/rebreathing bag used to inflate the lungs**. Two methods of respiration have been suggested.

(1) **Panting respiration** – gentle pressure given to mimic panting (i.e. 120 breaths per minute/2 breaths per second). Very useful if fractured ribs are suspected, as massive inflation of the lungs can drive the lungs against sharp fragments causing further damage.

   Panting respiration can be rested for 5 seconds every 15 seconds to see if breathing has restarted. If there are any signs of cyanosis the respiration must be maintained continuously.

(2) **Normal respiration** – the aim of this is to mimic the normal respiration pattern. Care must be taken **not to overinflate the lungs**, damaging the lung alveoli. Patients should be ventilated at the following rates:

   - > 15 kg: 20–25 breaths per minute.
   - < 15 kg: 25–30 breaths per minute.

Non-intubated patients should be placed in the recovery position (Fig. 4.2).

(1) Lay the patient on its right side.

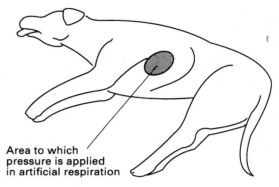

Area to which pressure is applied in artificial respiration

Fig. 4.2 The recovery position.

(2) Extend the head and neck.
(3) Pull the tongue forward to clear the airway.
(4) Pull front legs forward to relieve any pressure on the chest.

The palm of the hand can now be placed in the middle of the chest wall (just behind the mass of the triceps muscle of the foreleg). Firm, steady pressure should be applied then released allowing the rib cage to spring back, drawing air into the lungs. **Reapply pressure at 0.5–1 second intervals** depending on the size of the animal.

Do not use this method if there is suspected damage to the thoracic wall, as fractures can easily be displaced and puncture the lungs or heart during thoracic compression. In such cases **mouth-to-nose resuscitation** should be used if no intubation facilities are available. Always wear a face mask when attempting this procedure, and breathe in through your nose, and out through your mouth. Do not inhale the animals' saliva.

(1) Pull the tongue forward to clear the airway.
(2) Grasp the top of the patient's muzzle in the left hand (holding down the upper lip-folds).
(3) Put the right hand under the muzzle to support the weight of the head, and create an airtight seal (Fig. 4.3).
(4) Inflate the patient's lungs using gentle puffs directly up the nostrils. **Do not overinflate the lungs.**

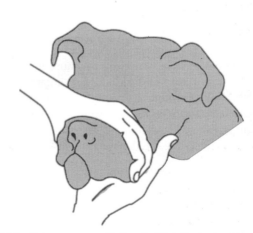

Fig. 4.3 Mouth-to-nose resuscitation: holding the nose.

Circulation

Cardiac massage must be started immediately if there is no pulse and no heartbeat can be felt or heard when using a stethoscope. The heart may be stimulated by rhythmical compression of the lower rib cage over ribs 3–6.

Patients such as cats, rabbits and rodents have small chests that are easily compressed by placing fingertips of both hands on either side of the thorax and applying gentle, firm pressure.

Patients with larger chests need to be laid on their side in the recovery position (Fig. 4.2) and punched with a closed fist to stimulate the heart effectively. A foam wedge or sandbag placed between the chest and table often provides useful support and balance, and stops the patient moving from the pressure of the chest compressions.

Chest compressions should mimic the patient's natural heart rate, ranging between 80–120 beats/compressions per minute.

Artificial respiration must be maintained at the same time as cardiac massage and therefore it is best if **two people** cooperate in resuscitating the patient. In optimum conditions the patient would receive one artificial respiration for every 2–3 chest compressions.

If resuscitation is being attempted alone then the veterinary nurse should administer 2 artificial respirations per 15 chest compressions (Plunkett, 2001).

Cardiovascular emergencies

Heart failure

Clinical signs

- Restlessness.
- Coughing.
- Haemoptysis (coughing blood).
- Dyspnoea/tachypnoea.
- Pallor.
- Decreased CRT.

Diagnostic aids

- Thoracic radiographs.
- ECG.

Treatment

- Oxygen therapy.
- Intravenous fluid therapy.
- Medical intervention, including:

  - Diuretics.
  - Bronchodilators.
  - Vasodilators.
  - ACE inhibitors.
  - Beta-blockers.

Cardiomyopathy

This is disease of the heart muscle, and has two forms:

- Dilated cardiomyopathy (DCM) – most commonly occurs in large-breed dogs.
- Hypertrophic cardiomyopathy (HCM) – most commonly occurs in cats.

Clinical signs

- Heart failure.
- Pallor/cyanosis.
- Dyspnoea.
- Lethargy.
- Anorexia
- Abdominal swelling (DCM).
- Thromboembolism (HCM).

Diagnostic aids

- Thoracic radiographs.
- Ultrasonography.
- ECG.

Treatment

- Oxygen therapy.
- Monitor core temperature.
- Intravenous fluid therapy.
- Medical intervention, including:
  - diuretics.
  - bronchodilators.
  - vasodilators.
  - ACE inhibitors.
  - beta-blockers.

Arterial thromboembolism

This is obstruction of an artery by a blood clot.

Causes

- Myocardial disease.
- Endocarditis.
- Hyperadrenocorticism.
- Coagulation disorder.
- Altered blood flow.
- Tumour.

Clinical signs (dependent on the site of the embolism)

- Pain (vocalising).
- Reduced blood flow.

- Absence of pulse.
- Cold to the touch.
- Pale/cyanosed skin.
- Paresis.

Diagnostic aids

- Haematology, biochemistry.
- Coagulation screening, thyroid function.
- Thoracic radiographs.
- Blood pressure.
- ECG.

Treatment

This is aimed at removing or dislodging and dissolving the clot.
- Oxygen therapy.
- Analgesia.
- Environmental warmth and comfort.

Medical intervention

- Intravenous fluid therapy.
- Antithrombotic agents.
- Thrombolytic agents.
- Vasodilators.
- Bronchodilators.

The clot can be removed surgically, but this is not first aid.

Respiratory emergencies

Laryngeal obstruction

Causes

- Obstruction (foreign body/tumour).
- Fight wounds.
- Laceration wound.
- Strangulation (caught by collar).

Clinical signs

- Dyspnoea (harsh and noisy).
- Asphyxia (swelling/foreign body).
- Swelling and pain (emphysema/bruising).
- Hissing (if wounds present).
- Frothy haemorrhage (if wounds are present).

Treatment

Sedation may be necessary.

- Remove animal's collar.
- Obtain/maintain an airway (tracheostomy may be necessary).
- Treat/remove primary problem:

  - Control haemorrhage.
  - Remove foreign body.

- Oxygen therapy.

Nursing care

When cleaning wounds, care should be taken not to introduce any fluid into the respiratory tract. Any dressings should be applied loosely to minimise pressure on the airway.

Laryngeal paralysis

This is paralysis of the muscles which move the vocal cords and the arytenoid cartilages outwards on inspiration. Most commonly seen in bull terriers.

Causes

- Congenital.
- Trauma.
- Inflammation.
- Idiopathic.

Clinical signs

- Dyspnoea.
- Increased breathing sounds.
- Exercise intolerance.
- Voice change.
- Hypersalivation.
- Coughing/gagging.
- Syncope.

Laryngoscopy under sedation can aid diagnosis.

Treatment

- Oxygen therapy.
- Intravenous fluid therapy.
- Surgical correction.

Nursing care

Before surgery, patients may be very stressed and inconsolable. Sedation may be required to keep them calm. It is also advisable to regularly check their temperature, as secondary hyperthermia may develop.

Following surgery, these animals should be monitored closely for any progression of dyspnoea. It is good practice to be ready and prepared in case laryngeal oedema becomes a complication and a tracheostomy is necessary.

Tracheal collapse

This is collapse of the tracheal rings. Most commonly seen in small toy breeds of dog.

Clinical signs

- Dyspnoea.
- Coughing.
- Exercise intolerance.
- Syncope.

Diagnostic aids

- Palpation.
- Radiographs.

Treatment

- Maintain/obtain a patent airway.
- Oxygen therapy.
- Intravenous fluid therapy.
- Strict rest.
- Medical intervention, including:

    – Bronchodilators.
    – Anti-inflammatories.

- Surgical intervention is possible for long-term management.

Pleural effusion and pneumothorax

This is fluid or air in the pleural cavity.

Causes

- Hydrothorax – fluid overload, heart failure.
- Pyothorax – bacterial/fungal/viral pleuritis.
- Chylothorax – neoplasia, thoracic duct dysfunction.
- Haemothorax – neoplasia, trauma, coagulopathies.
- Pneumothorax (closed) – trauma, diaphragmatic hernia.
- Pneumothorax (open) – trauma, penetrating foreign bodies.

Clinical signs

- Dyspnoea/tachypnoea.
- Abdominal breathing.

- Distress.
- Difficulty lying down.
- Coughing.
- Anorexia.
- Weight loss.
- Cyanosis/pallor.
- Hissing on inspiration (open pneumothorax).

Diagnostic aids

- Thoracic radiographs.
- Thoracic ultrasonography.
- Thoracocentisis/pleural tap.
- Pleural effusion analysis.

Treatment

Sedation with or without local nerve block may be required.

- Oxygen therapy.
- Bilateral thoracocentisis.
- Surgically place a thorocotomy tube.
- Apply a protective bandage (to prevent self-trauma/infection).
- Elizabethan collar (to prevent self-trauma).
- Treat primary cause.
- Antibiotics/analgesics.

Nursing care

- Ensure chest drain does not allow air in (creating a pneumothorax).
- Ensure chest drain entry site stays clean and non-infected.
- Ensure chest drain is removed when less than 2–4 mg/kg/day is drained.

Diaphragmatic rupture/hernia

This is a tear/hole in the diaphragm which results in abdominal viscera in the thoracic cavity:

- **Rupture** – the protrusion of viscera through a traumatic tear in the muscles or membrane bounding a cavity.
- **Hernia** – the protrusion of viscera through a natural opening in the muscles or membrane bounding a cavity.

Causes

- Trauma.
- Congenital.

Clinical signs

- Dyspnoea/tachypnoea.
- Abdominal breathing.

- Restlessness/weakness.
- Thin sunken abdomen.
- Shock.

Diagnostic aids

- Thoracic radiographs.
- Thoracic ultrasonography.

Treatment

- Oxygen.
- Intravenous fluid therapy.
- Surgical repair.
- Antibiotics/analgesics.

Nursing care

The severity of this condition depends on the extent of cardiac compression and lung collapse caused by the abdominal viscera in the thoracic cavity. Patients should be encouraged to lie on a slope with the head higher than the hindquarters to allow the abdominal viscera to return to their normal anatomical position.

Flail chest

This is where one or more ribs fracture in two places. Caused by trauma.

Clinical signs

- Pain.
- Dyspnoea.
- Free-floating segment of ribs.

Thoracic radiographs are an aid to diagnosis.

Treatment

- Place in lateral recumbence (flail-side down).
- Oxygen therapy.
- Prevent movement.
- Stabilise fracture (external/internal).

Nursing care

- It is important to remember not to stress these patients.
- When observing respiration the free-floating segment of ribs will move inwards on inspiration and outwards on expiration.

- External fixation methods (chest wraps, splints or external sutures) are usually adequate to stabilise a patient with flail chest.

PREVENTING HYPOXIA
- Encourage rest.
- Encourage to breathe oxygen.

100% oxygen can be administered via:

- Endotracheal tube (unconscious patients).
- Facemask (can cause distress).
- Oxygen tent (basket in a plastic bag).
- Nasal catheter (oxygen needs to be humidified).

Reproductive emergencies

Dystocia

This is abnormal labour or birth. It is a common problem for brachycephalic animals, and all breeds with large heads and wide shoulders. Causes are summarised in Table 4.4.

Clinical signs

- No foetus for 24 hours post onset of labour.
- > 30–60 minutes of unproductive active labour.
- > 3–4 hours rest between deliveries.
- > 24 hours (dogs) to 36 hours (cats) to deliver entire litter.

(Plunkett, 2001, p. 211.)

Productive labour should begin within 2 hours of **uteroverdin** (green vulval discharge). This discharge indicates that placental separation has taken place.

Diagnostic aids

- Abdominal radiographs.
- Ultrasonography.

Table 4.4 Causes of dystocia	
Material	**Foetal**
Uterine inertia	Oversized
Obesity	Badly positioned
Hypocalcaemia/hypoglycaemia	Foetal fatality
Septicaemia	
Exhaustion	
Stress/anxiety	

Treatment

There are three treatment options:

- Manual intervention – only useful in obstructive dystocia.
- Medical intervention – administration of ecbolic agents to stimulate uterine contractions.
- Surgical intervention – caesarean section.

Nursing care

If a caesarean section is indicated, the administration of a general anaesthetic will be necessary. It is important to minimise the anaesthetic time for the health of the pregnant animal and the survival of the neonates. It is good practice to be fully prepared before induction. In some cases it may even be possible to clip and prepare the surgical site before the anaesthetic is administered.

The neonate – revival and resuscitation

Once the neonates have been removed from the uterus resuscitation must commence:

(1) Remove the foetal membrane.
(2) Confirm heartbeat (using digital palpation).
(3) Clear the airway.
(4) Dislodge fluid by **gently** swinging the neonate (head down). The head and neck must always be supported.
(5) Stimulate and dry the neonate by rubbing it gently in a towel.

Doxapram hydrochloride drops may be used to stimulate respiration.

Continue stimulation until breathing is unassisted and regular and the neonate is moving.

Place the neonates in a prewarmed environment until the mother is fully awake from the anaesthetic.

The umbilicus must be clamped or tied off to prevent haemorrhage. A single ligature of suture material or the application of haemostatic forceps is usually sufficient to arrest bleeding.

Hand-rearing

It is sometimes necessary to hand-rear infants or to provide additional nutrition following a caesarean section. Nutritional support can be provided by the use of a commercial milk replacer. The milk replacer should be diluted and given according to the manufacturer's recommendation. If the neonate is capable of suckling then special hand-rearing bottles can be used. If this is not possible, then a 1ml syringe or dropper bottle can be utilised.

(1) Dilute milk replacer and warm to body temperature.
(2) Hold neonate in one hand with head held up and neck extended.

(3) Place feeder into its mouth.
(4) Allow the neonate to suckle at his/her own pace.
(5) Ensure that no milk bubbles enter the neonate's nose.

Following feeding it is important to stimulate the neonate to go to the toilet. This can be achieved by rubbing the underside of the caudal abdomen with a warm damp piece of cotton wool. This simulates the action their mother would create with her tongue, and encourages urination and defecation.

Fading neonatal syndrome

This is an illness that results in death within the first 2 weeks of life.

Clinical signs

- Persistent crying (> 20 minutes).
- Decreased feeding.
- Inactivity and weakness.
- Lack of growth and weight gain.
- Dry, rough coat.

Treatment

- Treat primary aetiology.
- Rehydration (intravenous or subcutaneous fluids).
- Dextrose or glucose.
- Warmth (monitor rectal temperature hourly).
- Provide nutritional support (if vomiting then a feeding tube may be placed).

Nursing care

Nursing care will include providing a warm, clean and quiet environment isolated from any risk of cross-contamination. Neonates should be barrier nursed for their own protection.

Pyometritis/pyometra

This is an infection in the uterus caused by hormonally induced changes. It most commonly occurs during dioestrus, 45 days after oestrus in entire middle- to old-age queens and bitches. It can also occur for up to 10 weeks following oestrogen therapy for accidental mating (Battaglia, 2001, p. 299).

Clinical signs

- Lethargy.
- Vomiting.
- Polydypsia/polyuria.
- Abdominal distension/pain.

- Purulent vaginal discharge (open pyometra).
- Dehydration.
- Collapse.

Diagnostic aids

- Haematology, biochemistry.
- Urinalysis.
- Vaginal cytology.
- Abdominal radiographs.
- Abdominal ultrasonography.

Surgical treatment

- Rehydration.
- Antibiotics/analgesics.
- Overiohysterectomy:

  - Immediately if closed pyometra.
  - As soon as possible if open pyometra.

Nursing care

Educate owners about the risk of pyometritis in intact female animals. Encourage preventative sterilisation of all non-breeding bitches and queens.

Paraphimosis

This is the inability to retract a protruding penis. This is more commonly seen in entire male dogs following copulation or sexual excitement. It can be congenital, due to muscle paralysis or a fracture of the penis. It may also occur in long-haired cats.

Clinical signs

- Engorged protruding penis (usually dry or necrotic).
- Haematuria/dysuria.
- Foreign material on penis (string or hair).
- Obsessive self-cleaning of the penis.

Treatment

- Gently rinse the penis with water or saline.
- Apply topical hyperosmotic agent (reduces swelling).
- Apply cold compresses.
- Lubricate.
- Manually replace.
- Gently pull the prepuce back into its normal position.
- Surgical intervention (if the situation recurs).
- Antibiotics/analgesics.

Eclampsia

This is hypocalcaemia due to pregnancy or lactation. It is more often seen in small-breed dogs, usually within the first two weeks post parturition, but may occur in pregnancy.

Causes

- Calcium losses during gestation or lactation.
- Poor appetite/bad diet.
- Excessive supplementing of calcium during gestation.
- Metabolic alkalosis.

Clinical signs

- Restlessness/anxiety.
- Irritability.
- Panting/hypersalivation.
- Tachycardia.
- Pyrexia.
- Stiffness.
- Ataxia.
- Collapse.
- Muscle spasms.
- Seizures.

Treatment

- Extremely slow intravenous infusion of 10% calcium gluconate.
- Constantly monitor heart rate and ECG.
- Stop infusion if brachycardia or arrhythmia develop.

Nursing care

Oral supplements of calcium (gluconate, lactate or carbonate) are advised. A good-quality complete growth diet should be given, and should be supplemented with a commercial milk replacer to minimise metabolic demands on the mother. If the condition re-occurs the puppies or kittens should be fully weaned.

Urological emergencies

Urinary obstruction

This produces an inability to urinate normally. It is most commonly seen in middle-aged, neutered overweight male cats, but can be seen in any animal of any age or sex.

Causes

- Physical obstruction.

- Urinary calculi.
- Urethral plug.

Clinical signs

- Depression (depending on duration and severity of obstruction).
- Stranguria (straining to urinate).
- Pollakiuria (small amounts frequently).
- Haematuria.
- Urination in unusual places.
- Obsessive cleaning of urethra.
- Distended, painful bladder.
- Dehydration.
- Vomiting.
- Uraemia (acute).
- Collapse.

Diagnostic aids

- Palpation of the bladder.
- Biochemistry, haematology, serum electrolytes.
- Urinalysis and urine culture (from a cystocentesis).
- ECG (cardiac arrythmia due to hyperkalaemia).
- Radiographs.
- Ultrasonography.

Treatment and nursing care

- Symptomatic treatment.
- Intravenous fluid therapy.
- Urinary catheterisation.
- Bladder decompression.
- Monitoring of urine output.
- Antibiotics/analgesics.

Ruptured bladder

This is a tear in the urinary bladder.

Clinical signs

- Shocked.
- Collapsed.
- Anuria.
- Uraemia.
- Peritonitis.

Diagnostic aids

- Pneumocystogram.
- Catheterisation (if there is a partial rupture urine may be collected from the bladder).

Treatment

- Intravenous fluid treatment.
- Surgical repair.
- Antibiotics/analgesics.

Acute renal disease

This is the failure or sudden inability to maintain renal function.

Causes

- Pre-renal: decreased blood flow to kidneys (haemorrhage, vomiting, diarrhoea, dehydration, heart disease etc.).
- Intrinsic renal parenchymal: damage to cellular structure (ischaemia or nephrotoxins).
- Post-renal: urinary obstruction.
- Glomerulonephritis.
- Hypercalcaemia.
- Bacterial/viral/fungal.

Clinical signs

- Depression.
- Dehydration.
- Vomiting/diarrhoea.
- Uraemia (uraemic breath/uraemic ulcers).
- Swollen painful kidneys.
- Polyuria/oliguria/anuria.

Diagnostic aids

- Biochemistry, haematology, blood gas.
- Urinalysis.
- Abdominal radiography.
- Abdominal ultrasonography.

Treatment

- Intravenous fluid therapy.
- Monitor urine output.
- Diuresis/peritoneal dialysis.
- Symptomatic treatment.
- Antibiotics/analgesics.

Nursing care

If diagnosed promptly and treated radically, acute renal failure is reversible.

Neurological emergencies

Seizures/fits/convulsions

This is acute disturbance of normal electrical activity and function within the brain:

- **Petit mal** (focal seizure) – affecting one part of the body.
- **Grand mal** (generalised seizure) – affecting the whole body.
- **Post-ictal period** – following a seizure the animal is confused, listless, restless, hungry, thirsty and sometimes sleepy.
- **Status epilepticus** – one seizure lasting more than 3–4 minutes, a cluster of more than 3 or 4 seizures in 30–40 minutes, a group of seizures over 12–24 hours.

Clinical signs – ictal phase

Focal seizure:

- Glazed non-focused stare.
- Lack of response to environmental stimulants.
- Face twitching.
- Vocalisation.
- Running.
- Circling.
- Self-trauma.
- Repetitive movements.

General seizure:

- Unconscious and recumbent.
- Frantic paddling of the limbs.
- Violent shaking.
- Mastication.
- Salivation.
- Rigidity.
- Hallucination.
- Involuntary defecation/urination.

Treatment

For patients in status epilepticus the primary concern is to arrest seizure activity immediately. This is highly important as prolonged seizure activity can cause permanent neurological damage, hyperthermia, disseminated intravascular coagulation and death (Battaglia, 2001, p. 310).

Not all animals respond in the same manner to the different medications or protocols that are aimed at controlling seizures.

Control of seizures is usually attainable by administering intravenous sedation (diazepam) or a general anaesthetic (pentobarbitol, propofol, thiopental) or by rapidly achieving therapeutic serum levels of anticonvulsant medications (phenobarbital, potassium bromide).

If intravenous routes are not accessible, then it is possible to administer medication rectally.

Nursing care

- Monitor vital signs.
- Monitor rectal temperature.
- Monitor for seizure activity.
- Maintain intravenous access.
- Turn patient (feet under) every 4 hours.
- Lubricate eyes.
- Consider urine output control (express bladder/place indwelling urine catheter).

TELEPHONE ADVICE
- Remain calm – don't panic.
- Contain the animal in a darkened room.
- Do not touch the animal.
- Move all objects out of the way to minimise any injury.
- Allow the animal to finish convulsing.
- Do not approach the animal in the post-ictal phase as this may trigger another fit.
- Only reassure the animal if it approaches you.

WARNING
If the patient shows signs of cyanosis, it must be observed carefully as the tongue may be obstructing the pharynx. **Do not attempt to move the tongue manually** – the animal will bite. The animal may be suspended by its hindlimbs in the hope that this will remove the obstruction, otherwise resuscitation will be necessary when the patient stops convulsing.

Head trauma

This results from a direct blow to the head (e.g. a kick from a horse, or a road traffic accident).

Clinical signs

Symptoms vary depending on the part of the brain injured, and the extent of the injury:

- Shock.
- Haemorrhage (from nose, mouth or ears).
- Fractures (cranium/hard palate).
- Anisocoria/nystagmus/strabismus.
- Absence of palpebral/corneal reflexes (severe case).
- Bradycardia.
- Uncoordination/vomiting.
- Circling, head tilt.
- Paralysis.
- Seizures.

- Cranial nerve deficits.
- Coma/death.

Diagnostic aids

Neurological examination repeated frequently (every 5–10 minutes), as deterioration can occur very suddenly.

Treatment

- Maintain airway.
- Maintain constant observation/monitor vital signs.
- Conserve heat.
- Treat shock.

Nursing care

These patients need to be kept under constant observation.

Spinal cord trauma

Causes

Intrinsic spinal cord trauma:

- Intervertebral disc disease.
- Pathological fractures.
- Dislocation of atlantoaxial joint (toy breeds).

Extrinsic spinal cord trauma:

- Direct trauma.

Clinical signs

These are dependent upon location and severity of injury.

Cervical injury:

- Intense pain.
- Reluctant to move (if able to stand).
- Uncoordinated.
- Vocalising if moved.
- Quadriplegia or tetraplegia.
- Pedal reflexes present.
- Reduced proprioception (due to nerve damage).

Thoracolumbar injury:

- Pain.
- Kyphosis (arched back) if able to stand.
- Vocalising if moved.
- Collapsed/uncoordinated.
- Rigid extended front legs.
- Tightly flexed hind legs.
- Paraplegia.
- Incontinence.
- Pedal reflexes present.
- Reduced proprioception.

Diagnostic aids

- Neurological examination.
- Radiographs.

Treatment and nursing care

There is no specific treatment for these cases but if spinal trauma is suspected it is vital to advise owners over the telephone:

- Not to move the animal unless it is absolutely necessary.
- To lift the animal as a unit, never twist the spine.

Transportation methods are described at the start of this chapter.

Once the patient has arrived at the surgery, treatment is aimed at stabilising the patient:

- Confine and limit movement.
- Physical and neurological examination.
- Stabilise respiratory and cardiovascular systems.
- Analgesia/sedation (do not compromise respiration).

Medical management

- Back/neck brace.
- Cage rest.

Surgical management

- Decompression of spinal cord.
- Stabilisation of vertebral column.

Vestibular disorders

- **Peripheral** vestibular disorders – affecting the vestibular portion of the vestibular cochlear cranial nerve. No brain stem disturbance.
- **Central** vestibular disorders – affecting the medulla, cerebellum and pons.

The causes of vestibular disorders are summarised in Table 4.5.

Table 4.5 Causes of vestibular disorders	
Central	**Peripheral**
Head trauma	Otitis interna/media
Metronidazole toxicity	Geriatric vestibular disorder
Thiamine deficiency	Idiopathic
Viral, bacterial or fungal	Aural neoplasia
Infarction	Head trauma
Neoplasia	Aminoglycoside toxicity

Clinical signs

- Head tilt.
- Leaning/falling/uncoordination.
- Circling.
- Nystagmus.

Physical and neurological examination aids diagnosis.

Treatment and nursing care

Treatment should be given for the primary aetiology. Animals with vestibular disorders should be contained and surrounded with extra padding to avoid any self-trauma from flailing and falling over.

Metabolic emergencies

Diabetic ketoacidosis

This is insulin deficiency which causes the breakdown of body fat and results in acidosis. It is more common in female dogs, but can occur in any dog aged from 4 to 18 years. It can also affect cats of any age.

Causes

- Increased glucose use (insulin overdose, insulin feeding tumour, renal glycosuria).
- Decreased glucose storage (glycogen storage deficit, starvation, malabsorption, hepatic disease).

Clinical signs

- Polyuria/polydipsia.
- History of polyphagia.
- Anorexia/weight loss.
- Vomiting.
- Muscle wastage/weakness.
- Dehydration.
- Ketotic breath.
- Panting.

Diagnostic aids

- Haematology, biochemistry, blood gases.
- Urinalysis.
- ECG.

Treatment

- Intravenous fluid therapy.
- Insulin.

- Treat symptoms.
- Nil by mouth if vomiting/high fibre diet if eating.
- Supplement potassium/phosphorus if necessary.
- Monitor blood glucose.
- Monitor urine for ketones.
- Antibiotics.

Hypoglycaemia

This is a low level of blood glucose.

Causes

- Increased glucose use (insulin overdose, insulin feeding tumour, renal glycosuria).
- Decreased glucose storage (glycogen storage deficit, starvation, malabsorption, hepatic disease).

Clinical signs

- Depression.
- Lethargy.
- Weakness/shaking.
- Seizures.
- Coma.

Diagnostic aids

- Biochemistry, haematology, blood glucose.
- Urinalysis.

Treatment and nursing care

- Rub glucose powder/glucose syrup/honey on the buccal mucosa.
- If able to eat, then a small meal may be given.
- Measured and monitored blood glucose.
- Intravenous dextrose bolus.
- Intravenous dextrose drip.

Hypoadrenocorticism

This is also called acute Addisonian crisis, a deficiency in the production of glucocorticoids and mineralocorticoids in the adrenal glands (mineralocorticoids help to regulate the electrolyte balance).

Clinical signs

- Anorexia.
- Vomiting/diarrhoea.
- Depression/lethargy.
- Weight loss.

- Weakness.
- Polyuria/polydipsia.
- Pale mucous membranes.
- Decreased CRT.
- Hyperkalemia.
- Cardiac arrhythmia.
- Shock.
- Collapse.
- Seizure/coma.

Diagnostic aids

- Haematology, biochemistry, electrolytes.
- Urinalysis.
- ACTH stimulation test, blood aldosterone concentration.
- Radiographs.
- ECG.

Treatment

- Intravenous fluid therapy.
- Balanced electrolytes.
- Hormone replacement therapy.
- Mineralcorticoid and glucocorticoid replacement therapy.

Gastrointestinal and abdominal emergencies

Foreign body in mouth

Examples are pieces of stick or bone, needles with or without thread, fishhooks.

Clinical signs

- Dysphagia.
- Difficulty swallowing.
- Pawing at face.
- Dyspnoea.
- Swelling.
- Hypersalivation, possibly with blood.

Treatment

- Removal of foreign body (general anaesthetic is sometimes needed).
- Oxygen (if dyspnoeic).

NB: No attempt should be made to pull out fishhooks or thread.

Fishhooks should be pushed further in until the barbed end comes through the skin. Once the barb is through, the hook can be cut in half and the two pieces removed separately. This is not an easy task to do and a local or general anaesthesia may be necessary.

Thread may be attached to a needle. If this is the case it is best to trace the thread to its source and see if the needle can be dislodged. If the needle cannot be dislodged and two ends of thread are present, then the ends should be tied together to avoid the needle becoming unthreaded.

Foreign body in oesophagus

Examples are balls, grass blades, needles with or without thread, fishhooks, pieces of stick or bone.

Clinical signs

- Gagging/wretching/gulping.
- Dyspnoea.
- Swelling/pain.
- Hypersalivation, possibly with blood.
- Dysphagia.
- Difficulty swallowing.
- Regurgitation if food is taken.

Treatment

- Removal of foreign body (general anaesthetic is often needed).
- Oxygen (if dyspnoeic).

Additional considerations

Asphyxia may occur as a complication. In this situation a patent airway will need to be created and maintained (see 'Cardio-pulmonary Resuscitation' – 'Airway' p. 109).

Vomiting (emesis)

This is the forceful expulsion of gastrointestinal contents, to be distinguished from **regurgitation**, the passive reproduction from the oesphagus of recently ingested food/water. The causes of vomiting are summarised in Table 4.6, and a guide to identification of expelled contents is given in Table 4.7.

Diagnostic aids

- Clinical history.
- Physical examination (ruling out ingestion of foreign material).
- Biochemistry, haematology, electrolytes, blood gases.
- Viral screening.
- Abdominal radiographs (contrast media).
- Endoscopy.

Table 4.6 Causes of vomiting	
Internal	**External**
Obstructory	Dietary
Neurological	Medication
Inflammatory	Toxins
Systemic	Foreign body
Endocrine	Infectious
Organ disorders	Motion

Treatment

- Treat the primary cause.
- Ensure patent airway.
- Intravenous fluid therapy.
- Nil by mouth.
- Antiemetics.

Nursing care

Grooming and TLC.

Diarrhoea

This is the passing of faeces of a liquid consistency.

- Small intestine – large volume of faeces usually passed at a normal frequency.
- Large intestine – small volumes of faeces passed at an increased frequency.

The causes of diarrhoea are summarised in Table 4.8.

Diagnostic aids

- Vaccination status?
- Faecal parasitology, culture and sensitivity, bacteriology and virology.
- Biochemistry, haematology, electrolytes.

Table 4.7 Identification of expelled contents by colour	
Colour	**Origin**
White	Gastric/oesophageal
Yellow	Gastric with bile (pancreatitis)
Green	Duodenal (bile) (pancreatitis)
Brown	Reflux of faeces
Red (haememesis)	Oesophageal/gastric/duodenal bleeding (ulcers)
Coffee grounds	Gastric duodenal with digested blood

Table 4.8 Causes of diarrhoea	
Internal	**External**
Obstructory	Dietary
Inflammatory	Medication
Systemic	Toxins
Organ disorders	Foreign body
Endocrine	Infectious (viral, bacterial, fungal)

Treatment

- Intravenous fluid therapy.
- Nil by mouth for 12–24 hours.
- Bland diet – feed little and often.
- Balance electrolytes.
- Anticholinergic, antispasmodic, intestinal absorbent/protectant.
- Treat underlying aetiology.

Nursing care

All diarrhoea should be managed as an infectious disease unless proven otherwise. Measures should be implicated to isolate and barrier-nurse individual cases. Vomiting and diarrhoea cases need lots of TLC. They need to be kept clean (baths, grooming, tail bandages, etc.).

Rectal prolapse

This is the protrusion of the rectum through the anal opening, caused by straining to pass faeces (**tenesmus**).

Clinical signs

Red/swollen protrusion from the anus.

Treatment

- Lubricate.
- Reduce/replace the prolapse.
- Local analgesia/anaesthesia.
- Elizabethan collar.

Nursing care

Even if the prolapse is easily reduced it very commonly re-occurs. It is advisable to surgically prevent this by the placement of a purse string suture around the anal ring.

Obstruction/intussusceptions

Causes

- Intralumen obstruction – foreign bodies.
- Extralumen obstruction – stricture, hernia, intussusception.

Clinical signs

- Anorexia.
- Depression.
- Vomiting.
- Constipation/diarrhoea/meleana.
- Dehydration.
- Weakness.
- Abdominal pain.

Diagnostic aids

- Abdominal palpation (gastric foreign bodies not palpable, intussusceptions feel like a sausage).
- Biochemistry, haematology, electrolytes, blood gases.
- Faecal examination.
- Urinalysis.
- Abdominocentisis.
- Abdominal radiographs.
- Abdominal ultrasonography.

Treatment

- Emetics (removal of gastric foreign bodies).
- Endoscopy.
- Surgical removal (only option for extralumen obstructions).

Nursing care

- Nil by mouth 24 hours post surgery.
- Then 8–12 hours on liquids.
- Follow with bland diet for 3–5 days.
- Reintroduce normal food after 5 days (gradually).

Abdominal rupture/hernia and evisceration

This is a tear/hole in the muscles bounding the abdominal cavity resulting in the protrusion of abdominal organs or intestines.

Causes

- Trauma.
- Surgical procedures.

Clinical signs

- Open/closed wounds.
- Swelling.
- Anatomical abnormalities.
- Pain/discomfort.
- Vomit/diarrhoea/constipation.
- Toxicity.
- Shock.
- Collapse.

Diagnostic aids

- Radiographs.
- Ultrasonography.
- Exploratory laparotomy.

Treatment

- Intravenous fluid therapy.
- Treatment for shock.
- Antibiotics/analgesics.
- Surgical repair.

Complications

- **Irreducible rupture/hernia** – Impaired venous return causes the organs to become blood engorged, swollen and painful. This also occurs if a distendable organ (such as the bladder) is involved. It is extremely difficult to replace these organs because of the increase to their size.
- **Strangulated rupture/hernia** – Impaired arterial flow creates tissue hypoxia which leads to necrosis (death of cells and tissue).

Nursing care

It is most often intestinal loops which protrude through ruptures/hernias. If evisceration occurs then it is necessary to protect the tissues from any attempt made by the patient to clean the wound. It is important to keep the tissue clean and moist to optimise viability. Warmed sterile saline should be used to thoroughly cleanse the wound and viscera, and sterile gauze swabs soaked in sterile saline can be placed and fixed over the wound with a bandage to increase/maintain tissue viability. If a temporary manual reduction is attempted, gravity can be used to assist replacement.

Gastric dilation and volvulus

This is twisting of the stomach, resulting in a one-way valve effect (at the gastro-oesophageal junction) which allows air to enter but not leave the stomach (Battaglia, 2001, p. 252).

Clinical signs (acute onset)

- Unproductive attempts to vomit.
- Restlessness.
- Hypersalivation.
- Abdominal distension.
- Tympanic resonance of bloated abdomen.
- Tachypnoea.
- Tachycardia.
- Splaying of legs.
- Collapse.
- Shock.

Diagnostic aids

- Radiography.
- Biochemistry, haematology, electrolytes and blood gases.
- ECG, plasma lactate level.

Treatment

- Intravenous fluid therapy.
- Analgesics and antibiotics.
- Stomach tube.
- Gastric lavage.
- Surgery.

If stomach tubing is not possible, tension may be alleviated by performing gastrocentesis through the lateral abdominal wall (caudal to the right 13th rib) using a 14–20 g /1–1.5 inch needle. This allows gas to escape. Stomach tubing may then be possible.

During surgery it is advisable to keep the stomach tube in place to decrease the risk of reflux oesophagitis and/or aspiration of stomach contents.

Surgical intervention

Surgical intervention is the ideal treatment for all cases of gastric dilation and volvulus (Battaglia, 2001, p. 253). The primary aim of surgery is to reposition the stomach. Partial gastrectomies may be necessary to remove any necrotic areas. Gastrotomies are performed to remove large quantities of stomach contents. After the stomach has been repositioned, a gastropexy can be performed to fix the stomach in place (see Chapter 19, Surgical Nursing).

Ruptured spleen

Causes

- Tumour.
- Trauma.
- Torsion.

Clinical signs

- Tachypnoea.
- Tachycardia.
- Weak pulse.
- Extreme pallor.
- Shock.
- Acute collapse.
- Abdominal pain.
- Abdominal distension.

Diagnostic aids

- Haematology, biochemistry.
- Abdominal radiographs.
- Abdominal ultrasonography.
- Exploratory laparotomy.

Treatment

- Intravenous fluid therapy.
- Shock treatment.
- Plasma expanders.
- Blood transfusion.
- Surgical intervention.

Nursing care

A pressure bandage around the abdomen may help to increase back pressure and reduce internal haemorrhage.

Hepatic damage/failure

Causes

- Disease.
- Tumour.
- Infection.
- Trauma.
- Poison.
- Inflammation.

Clinical signs

- Abdominal pain.
- Vomiting/diarrhoea.
- Anorexia.
- Jaundice.
- Polydypsia/polyuria.
- Abdominal distension.
- Coagulopathy.
- Neurological dysfunction.
- Seizures.
- Coma.

Diagnostic aids

- Biochemistry, haematology.
- Urinalysis.
- Coagulation panel.
- Abdominal radiographs.
- Abdominal ultrasonography.

Treatment

- Intravenous fluid therapy.
- Treat primary cause.

Nursing care

Remain aware of possible infectious or zoonotic diseases which can affect unvaccinated animals and be fatal in human beings (*Leptospira icterohaemorrhagia*). Isolate and barrier-nurse any suspected cases.

Acute pancreatitis

Causes

- Obesity/high-fat diet.
- Hyperadrenocorticism.
- Pancreatic duct obstruction.
- Infection.
- Trauma.
- Tumour.

Clinical signs

- Acute abdominal pain.
- Vomiting/diarrhoea.
- Dehydration.
- Jaundice.
- Shock.

Diagnostic aids

- Haematology, biochemistry, blood gas analysis.
- Urinalysis.
- Pancreatic screen (trypsin-like immunoreactivity).
- Abdominal radiographs.
- Abdominal ultrasonography.

Treatment

- Intravenous fluid therapy.
- Treat shock.
- Treat primary cause.
- Antibiotics/analgesics.
- Nil by mouth.

Nursing care

Certain pancreatic changes allow the release of trypsin (a proteolytic enzyme). This release sets off a chain reaction resulting in the pancreatic enzymes digesting the pancreatic tissue. This digestion stimulates more release of trypsin and therefore an increase in autodigestion. Pancreatitis rapidly escalates causing immense pain, shock, peritonitis and sometimes death.

Long-term maintenance of pancreatitis includes a low-fat, low-protein diet.

Peritonitis

This is inflammation of the peritoneum and peritoneal cavity.

Causes

Peritonitis can be due to a primary reason (feline infectious peritonitis) or a complication of another problem and therefore a secondary complaint.

Clinical signs

- Primary disease.
- Anorexic/vomiting.
- Depressed.
- Praying position/kyphosis (arched spine).
- Abdominal pain/distension.
- Hypo/hyperthermia.
- Dehydration.
- Weak peripheral pulse.
- Decreased CRT.
- Shock.

Diagnostic aids

- Biochemistry, haematology, electrolytes, blood gases, coagulation profile.
- Urinalysis.
- Abdominocentesis.
- Evaluation of peritoneal fluid (creatinine, bilirubin, PCV, TP).
- Peritoneal fluid cytology.
- Abdominal radiographs.
- Ultrasonography.

Treatment

- Treat primary cause.
- Oxygen therapy.
- Intravenal fluid therapy.
- Antibiotics/analgesics.
- Exploratory laparotomy.
- Peritoneal drainage.

- Nutritional support.
- Monitor blood parameters.

Nursing care

- Turn patient over every 4 hours.
- Ensure patient is comfortable (clean and dry padded bedding).
- Groom patient.
- TLC.

Emergencies involving the organs of special sense

Eye

Eyes are very sensitive organs and any discomfort will cause the animal to scratch and rub at the area repeatedly. Minor problems can occur that when left untreated can rapidly deteriorate. Most eye problems present to the owner in a very similar manner. Therefore, all problems relating to the eye can be considered potential emergencies and should be seen as soon as possible – if only to rule out severe ocular damage. Whatever the primary cause of the problem is, all patients will benefit from relief and analgesia, and this should decrease the likelihood of any further self-trauma.

> **WARNING**
> Antiseptics should never be used in or around the eye. For cleansing it is best to use isotonic sterile saline.

Acute ulcerative keratitis

Causes

- Physical trauma.
- Chemical.
- Bacterial/viral/fungal.
- Metabolic.
- Immune mediated (Plunkett, 2001, p. 265).

Clinical signs

- Squinting.
- Rubbing eyes/face.
- Discharge.
- Blephrospasm.
- Photophobia.
- Conjunctivitis.

- Uveitus.

Fluorescein stain aids diagnosis.

Treatment

- Treat primary cause if present.
- Topical with or without systematic anti-inflammatory.
- Topical mydriatic agent.

Nursing care

Warm compresses may be used on the eye to give comfort to the patient. It is also advisable to keep the animal out of bright lights.

Acute glaucoma

This is increased pressure in the eye (> 30 mmHg). It most often occurs in Cocker Spaniels, Basset Hounds, Poodles, St Bernards, Samoyed, Sharpei and Chow Chows.

Causes

- Primary glaucoma – structural or functional impairment of aqueous humour outflow.
- Secondary glaucoma – dysfunction of filtration due to other intraocular problem. (Wingfield, 1997, p. 124.)

Clinical signs

- Ocular pain.
- Blephrospasm.
- Translucent/opaque corneal clouding.
- Mydriasis (or myosis in some cases).
- Vision impairment/blindness.

Diagnosis

- Ophthalmic local anaesthetic.
- Measure intraocular pressure using

    - Indentation tonometry (Schick tonometer).
    - Applantation tonometry (electronic or pneumatic devices).

Treatment

- Anti-inflammatory agents.
- Hyptotonic/hyperosmotic agents (mannitol).
- Topical miotic agents (if indicated).
- Topical adrenergic agonists (epinephrine 1%).
- Referral to an ophthalmologist.
- Surgical intervention.

Nursing care

Acute glaucoma needs immediate emergency treatment. After only a few hours of increased ocular pressure, sight can be seriously compromised. The cellular damage that occurs during the period of increased pressure does not heal well, so permanent blindness becomes a likely complication if acute glaucoma is left untreated.

Proptosis/prolapse of the globe

This is abnormal protrusion of the eye, usually a result of trauma.

Treatment (general anaesthetic may be required)

- Lubricate eye – do not use steroids.
- Replace globe – slowly pull eyelids forward and gently push globe back into the socket using firm even pressure.
- Sometimes it is necessary to perform tarsorrhaphy (suture the eyelids closed).
- Antibiotics/analgesics.
- Elizabethan collar.

Ocular foreign body

Clinical signs

- Squinting.
- Rubbing eyes.
- Blephrospasm.
- Chemosis.
- Photophobia.

Visualisation of foreign body aids diagnosis (may require magnification or radiographs).

Treatment

- Ophthalmic local anaesthetic.
- Flush eye with saline.
- If foreign body moves then remove it (large objects, e.g. grass seeds, can be mechanically grasped, small objects can be flushed into the corner of the eye and lifted with a cotton bud/moistened lint/fine paintbrush).
- If foreign body does not move presume that it has penetrated the eye and do not attempt to pull it out.
- Possibly topical with or without systemic antibiotics.
- Possibly systemic anti-inflammatory.
- Elizabethan collar.

Removal of penetrating matter is best performed by an ophthalmologist who is specially equipped to perform limbal incisions and control intraocular haemorrhage (Plunkett, 2001, p. 267).

Uveitis

This is inflammation of the uvea (iris, ciliary body and choroid coat of the eyeball).

Causes

- Trauma.
- Inflammation.
- Infections (bacterial, viral, fungal).
- Tumour
- Metabolic.

Clinical signs

- Squinting.
- Blephrospasm.
- Photophobia.
- Ocular pain.
- Miotic pupil.
- Chemosis.
- Impaired vision.
- Uveitis may be unilateral or bilateral (bilateral uveitis suggests a primary systemic disease).

Treatment

- Treat underlying aetiology.
- Topical with or without systemic anti-inflammatory.
- Topical mydriatic.

Nursing care

Warm compresses may be used on the eye to increase the comfort of the patient. It is also advisable to keep the animal out of bright lights.

Ear

Aural haematoma

This is haematoma of the ear pinna.

Causes

- Self-trauma.
- Head shaking.

Clinical signs

- Shaking of the head.
- Scratching the ear.
- Swollen pinna (cool and soft).

Treatment

- Drainage of haematoma.
- Pressure whilst healing.
- Compressing/immobilising ear bandage.

Traumatic wounds

Wounds to the earflap should be treated by normal methods. Haemorrhage is very messy as the patient usually shakes their head repeatedly. Placement of an ear bandage (encircling the whole head) and a buster collar can prevent further self-trauma and blood spatters.

Aural foreign body

Clinical signs

- Pain.
- Irritation.
- Head tilt.
- Head shaking.
- Rubbing/scratching ear.

An auroscope aids diagnosis.

Treatment

- If visible mechanically remove.
- If not visible then sedation or a general anaesthetic may be necessary.

Nursing care

Warmed olive oil or liquid paraffin may be poured into the ear to alleviate discomfort.

Nose

Epistaxis

This is bleeding from the nose.

Causes

- Trauma.
- Tumour.
- Persistent sneezing.

Clinical signs

- Haemorrhage.
- Sneezing.
- Mouth breathing.
- Dyspnoea.
- Swelling.

Treatment

- Cold compress.
- Adrenalin swabs inside the nostrils.
- Close observation.

Nursing care

Animals suffering from epistaxis should not be muzzled. They should also be closely monitored for any signs of concussion.

Nasal foreign body

Examples are grass seeds, grass blades and splinters.

Clinical signs

- Sneezing.
- Head shaking.
- Rubbing.
- Nasal discharge.
- Epistaxis.

Treatment

Mechanical removal (may require sedation if not visible).

Nursing care

Infection is often a complication of nasal/nasopharyngeal foreign bodies. It cannot be controlled until the foreign body has been removed.

Environmental emergencies

Burns and scalds

Causes

Scalds are caused by moist heat. Burns can be caused by:

- Dry heat (fire, heat lamps, hot surfaces).
- Excessive cold (frostbite, cryosurgery).
- Corrosive chemicals (strong acids, petroleum products).
- Electrocution (electrical faults).
- Radiation (nuclear disaster).

Heat and electrical burns cause instant effects on the body. Radiation and cold burns may take several hours or days to manifest symptoms.

Clinical signs

All burns and scalds present (eventually) in a similar manner. Symptoms may include:

- Red, moist skin.
- Heat.
- Swelling.
- Pain (deep burns are less painful).
- Alopecia.

Diagnostic classification

Burns and scalds can be classified according to extent of the damage:

- **Percentage** of the total body surface affected by the burns should be estimated because it will give some idea to the extent of pain and dehydration suffered by the patient.
- **Superficial** penetrate no deeper than the skin surface (1st and 2nd degree burns).
- **Deep** penetrate through the skin thickness into the tissue beneath (3rd, 4th, 5th and 6th degree burns).

Treatment

Heat and electrical burns:

- Intravenous fluid therapy.
- Cool the damaged area.
- Monitor body temperature.
- Clean and dress the wound.
- Limit the animals movement (splint limbs if necessary).

For cleansing and dressing purposes sterile saline and sterile non-stick dressing with protective wound gel are advised. Minimal amounts of dressing material should be used to reduce absorption of fluid from the wound and keep the area as cool as possible. If no dressing materials are available clean cling film may be used to wrap around the burns (minimising fluid loss). Cold towels must be placed on top of the cling film to cool the area and prevent hyperthermia.

Chemical burns are rarely deep but may be extensive and irritating:

- Wear gloves when handling.
- Flush surface with copious amounts of water (hosepipe).
- Wash coat in a mild detergent.
- If the chemical is a known acid, then apply a concentrated solution of bicarbonate of soda/washing soda.
- If the chemical is a known alkali, then apply a weak acidic solution (vinegar and water).
- Give demulcents and absorptives.

- Observe for signs of toxicity.

Nursing care

Complications of heat burns can include dyspnoea, asphyxia, infection and scarring.

Smoke inhalation

Smoke inhalation can cause minimal to severe pulmonary damage, and is the leading cause of death following fires.

Clinical signs (evident 24–48 hours after incident)

- Smell of smoke.
- Singed whiskers/evidence of burns.
- Nasal discharge.
- Distress.
- Tachypnoea/bradypnoea/apnoea.
- Pale/brick red mucous membranes.

Diagnostic aids

- Thoracic radiographs (although not very reliable for detecting smoke damage).
- ECG.
- PCV, TP, blood gases.
- Carbon dioxide and oxygen levels.

Treatment

- Oxygen therapy.
- Ensure a patent airway.
- Intravenous fluid therapy.
- Treat for shock.
- Analgesics.

Nursing care

The major complication with smoke inhalation occurs when carbon dioxide and carbon monoxide molecules bind with the haemoglobin in the blood, replacing oxygen and causing severe hypoxaemia. Inhalation of smoke can also cause thermal and chemical injury to the respiratory tract.

Electrocution

Contact with a high-voltage source causes an electric current to flow through the body. If the path of electrical conduction passes through the heart the result is instantaneous cardiac arrest.

Clinical signs

- Collapse.
- Stiff and twitching.
- Spastic muscle contraction.
- Hair and ears standing on end.
- Sharp, short breaths.

Treatment

- **Switch off electricity supply.**
- Stand on **dry** insulated surface. Put on gloves.
- Remove animal from electrical source using a **dry** wooden pole.
- Airway.
- Breathing.
- Circulation.
- Treat burns.
- Observe for signs of meningeal oedema.

NB: Remember that water and metal are both very good conductors of electricity.

Hypothermia

This is subnormal body temperature.

Causes

- Disease.
- Anaesthesia/sedation.
- Overexposure to the cold.

Clinical signs

- Shivering.
- Depression/unconsciousness.
- Bradypnoea.
- Bradycardia.
- Cardiac arrhythmia.

Treatment (gradually rewarm the patient)

- Passive rewarming (increase ambient temperature).
- Active surface rewarming (heat pad/hot water bottle).
- Active central rewarming (warmed intravenous fluids).

Nursing care

- Monitor temperature every 10–15 minutes until it returns to normal.
- Turn collapsed/unconscious patients over every 2–4 hours.
- Conserve/maintain heat by laying patient on a thick bed (e.g. Vet Bed).

- Massaging with warm rough towels will help open up the cutaneous circulation and enable the body to pick up radiant heat.

Frostbite

This is exposure to extreme cold resulting in tissue necrosis.

Clinical signs

- Pain.
- Pale/cyanotic cold skin.
- Localised swelling.

Treatment

- Intravenous fluid therapy.
- Warm compresses/bathing.
- Monitor body temperature.
- Clean and dress the wound.
- Limit the animal's movement.
- Prevent self-trauma.
- Analgesics/antibiotics.

Hyperthermia/heatstroke

This is increased body temperature, most commonly seen in brachycephalic breeds, obese animals, or animals with thick coats.

Causes

- Overexposure to heat (hot cars, hot rooms, excessive sunlight).
- Overexertion.
- Obesity.
- Cardiac/pulmonary disease.

Clinical signs

- Restlessness.
- Excessive panting.
- Bright red/cyanotic mucous membranes.
- Hypersalivation.
- Vomiting.
- Ataxia.
- Collapse/unconsciousness.
- Seizures.

Treatment (gradually cool the patient)

- Oxygen therapy.
- Cold compresses/bathing.

- Cool ambient temperature (fan).
- Chilled intravenous fluids.
- Cold gastric/peritoneal lavage.
- Ice-water enema.

Nursing care

Monitor body temperature every 15 minutes whilst hyperthermic, every 30 minutes when core temperature returns to normal.

Toxicological emergencies

- Poison or toxin – substance which when enters the body in sufficient doses causes harmful effects.
- Poisoning – when the poison or toxin causes clinical effects.
- Antidote – substance which specifically counters the action of the poison.

Clinical signs

Directly dependent upon the type and amount of toxin exposure, can include:

- Vomiting.
- Diarrhoea.
- Trembling/shaking.
- Tachy-/brachycardia.
- Tachy-/brachypnoea.
- Dilated pupils (midriasis).
- Muscle weakness/stiffness.
- Coagulation problems.
- Convulsions/seizures.
- Coma.

Poisons can affect any body system and produce any variety/combination of clinical signs.

Diagnostic aids

- Haematology, biochemistry, electrolytes, blood gases.
- Urinalysis.
- Thoracic/abdominal radiographs.
- ECG.
- Blood pressure monitoring.
- Toxicology screening (stomach contents, urine, faeces, tissue/brain – do not freeze).

Treatment

Variable, depending on the poison or toxin (see Table 4.9). May include:

- Specific treatment for known poison (antidote if available).

- Treatment for clinical signs (control seizures etc.).
- Cease further absorption/exposure.
- Supportive therapy.
- Intravenous fluid therapy.
- Induce emesis (see Table 4.10) unless the patient:

  - Is unconscious.
  - Has CNS/respiratory depression.
  - Ingested acid/alkaline substances or petroleum products.
  - Ingested the toxin/poison > 4 hours ago.

- Gastric lavage.
- Give absorbent substances (see Table 4.11) orally to absorb toxins.
- Give laxative 30 minutes post charcoal (to clear out absorbed toxins).
- Give demulcents (see Table 4.12) – especially if corrosive poisoning.
- Bathe (see Table 4.13) if toxin or poison is topical.

Incidence of poisoning cases

Poisoning is not commonly seen in small animal practice but the veterinary nurse must always bear the possibility in mind when presented with an acutely ill patient. Sometimes the history offers a clue, e.g. a cat that has been dosed by the owner with paracetamol to ease the pain of an injured leg. At other times, careful questioning is necessary to establish the cause of the problem. Many humans are incurable hoarders and ancient bottles and boxes may be found in cupboards and garden sheds; strychnine has been banned from use in the UK for a long time but occasional poisonings still occur; some old houses still have linoleum, old lead pipes, lead paint, etc. Weedkiller, insecticides, rodenticides and human medication which has been eaten by pets are other common causes of poisoning cases.

History taking

Many poisons cause common symptoms. This means that, when asking routine questions over the telephone, it can be difficult to decide if an animal has actually been poisoned or has simply had severe gastroenteritis or an epileptic fit. The following points should be considered when trying to come to a conclusion.

What species is the patient?

Pups are indiscriminate chewers of everything from laburnum sticks to old lino, both of which are toxic, and many dogs will eat almost anything, including rat bait.

Cats are fastidious and cautious about what they consume, but they groom endlessly and are therefore most likely to ingest contact poisons on their coat. They also hunt more

Table 4.9 Effects of common poisons, and treatment

Category	Specific toxin	Effect of toxin	Treatment
Medicine	ACP (tablets)	Depression, collapse, hypotension	Induce vomiting, treat symptoms
	NSAID	Gastric ulceration, haematemesis, melaena, dehydration, kidney damage	Stop medication, induce vomiting, give absorptives and demulcents, IVFT
	Paracetamol (cats)	Cyanosis, hypoxia (haemoglobin transforms into methaemoglobin), incoordination, depression/excitement, facial swelling	Induce vomiting, give antidote (*N*-acetyl cysteine or methionine), oxygen therapy, give absorptives if no antidote is available
	Salbutamol	Stimulates sympathetic nervous system, peripheral vasodilation, tachycardia, panting, muscle weakness	General first aid, beta-blockers
	Calcipotriol (vit D derivative)	Hypercalaemia, hyperphosphataemia, nephritis, polyuria/polydypsia, gastrointestinal tract damage, haemorrhagic diarrhoea, collapse, seizures	Induce vomiting. Give absorbents, IVFT, diuretics Death may occur within 24 hours
Herbicide	Chlorates	Vomiting diarrhoea, abdominal pain, cyanosed to brown mucous membranes	Give antidote (4% methylene blue injection IV), general first aid
	Dinitro compounds	Depression, listlessness, muscle weakness, dyspnoea/tachypnoea, hyperthermia, fluorescent yellow/green urine	General first aid, monitor rectal temperature
	Paraquat	Inflamed mouth/tongue, vomiting/diarrhoea, abdominal pain, depression, progressive dyspnoea (lung oedema), cyanosis, death	Induce vomiting (even though it is irritant) as effects are so severe, administer fuller's earth (binding agent)
Insecticide	Borax (ant killer 'Nippon')	Vomiting/diarrhoea, collapse, seizures, paralysis, death	General first aid, avoid fatty food and drink for 1 week as it increases absorption
	Organophosphates	Vomiting/diarrhoea, salivation, constricted pupils, muscular twitching, excitement, weakness, incoordination, depression, seizures	General first aid, atropine sulphate
	Organochlorines	Muscle twitching (face and limbs), seizures, behavioural changes	Wash any topical contamination, give absorbents and/or liquid paraffin, treat symptoms, avoid fatty food/drink
Molluscicide	Carbamate	Vomiting/diarrhoea, salivation, constricted pupils, muscular twitching, excitement, weakness, incoordination, depression, seizures	General first aid, atropine sulphate
	Metaldehyde	Incoordination, hyperaesthesia, seizures, tachycardia, tachypnoea, cyanosis	General first aid, liquid paraffin (if no symptoms present) may delay absorption
Rodenticide	Alphachloralose	Hypothermia, progressive depression, incoordination, coma	General first aid (warmth is essential as this poison acts by lowering body temperature)
	Calciferol	Hypercalaemia, hyperphosphataemia, nephritis, polyuria/polydypsia, gastrointestinal tract damage, haemorrhagic diarrhoea, collapse, seizures	Induce vomiting. Give absorbents, IVFT, diuretics Death may occur within 24 hours
	Anticoagulant preparations	Depression, weakness, dyspnoea, haemorrhage (internal and external), haematemisis, epistaxis	General first aid, IVFT, blood transfusion/ fresh frozen plasma, vitamin K (orally with fatty food; best route if symptoms are present – IV can cause anaphylaxis, IM can cause internal haemorrhage, SC poor uptake if hypovolaemic)
Household commodities	Alcohol	Hyperaesthesia, incoordination, collapse, death	Induce vomiting, general first aid
	Chocolate	Nervous excitement, tachycardia, panting, seizures, coma	Induce vomiting, gastric lavage, absorbents, symptomatic treatment
Household chemicals	Phenol (cats)	Stomatitis, mouth ulcers, vomiting/diarrhoea, abdominal pain, seizures, coma, death	Do not induce vomiting, wash any topical contamination, general first aid
	Quaternary ammonium compound	Depression, anorexia, vomiting, salivation, stomatitis, mouth/tongue ulcers, skin ulcers	Do not induce vomiting, wash any topical contamination, general first aid
	Ethylene glycol	Incoordination, depression, tachypnoea, uraemia	General first aid, IV ethanol (antidote)
	Petroleum products	Depression, vomiting, collapse, inflammation (if topical exposure), aspiration pneumonia (if submersed), death	Do not induce vomiting, general first aid treatment

IVFT = intravenous fluid treatment. This table is included only to give the veterinary nurse an indication of the relative toxic effects and treatments of the most common poisons encountered in veterinary practice. It is not designed to ensure that the veterinary nurse can diagnose which poison has been consumed or absorbed. Accurate advice needs to be given immediately following ingestion or exposure to a toxin, and further information should be obtained from toxicology publications, or the Veterinary Poisons Information Service

Table 4.10 Inducing emesis

Substance	Dosage
Diluted hydrogen peroxide 1:3	1–2 tablespoons/10 kg, orally Can be repeated if no results in 20 mins
Washing soda	1–2 pea-sized crystals, orally On the back of the tongue
Apomorphine	0.1 mg/1 kg, subcutaneously At the direction of the veterinary surgeon
Xylazine	3 mg/1 kg, intramuscularly At the direction of the veterinary surgeon
Mustard	2 teaspoons in a cup of warm water, orally (If nothing else is available)

Table 4.11 Absorbent substances

Substance	Dosage (oral)
BCK granules	1–3 tablespoons (depending on size of patient) mixed to a slurry with water
Activated charcoal	1 g/1 kg bodyweight. Mix to a slurry with 5 ml of water per 1 g charcoal
Kaolin	Less effective than charcoal, but very effective in cases of paraquat poisoning

Table 4.12 Demulcents

Arrowroot
Glycerin
Bismuth subnitrate
Bismuth carbonate
Raw egg, milk, honey/sugar

Table 4.13 Cleaning solutions for topical contamination

Contaminant	Treatment
Non-oily compounds (disinfectants)	Copious amounts of water (detergents can increase absorption)
Liquid oily compounds (sump oil, creosote)	Swarfega (or liquid paraffin/cooking oil) wash coat clean with detergent and warm water until the smell of the contaminant has completely gone
Solid oily contaminants (tar)	Clip fur if possible, if not then apply liquid paraffin, vegetable oil or butter and bandage area to prevent grooming. After 15 minutes the combination of body heat and the action of the solvent may make it easier to remove. Once the solid contamination has been removed wash the area with soap and water

Always wear gloves when handling contaminated patients

and may eat their poisoned prey. The cat also has a poorly developed enzyme system in the liver, which means it is far less able to metabolise and excrete certain poisons. These chemicals therefore build up to toxic levels in the body tissues and poison the animal. The classic example here is paracetamol.

Birds are more susceptible to inhalation poisoning because of the structure of their respiratory system.

What could be the cause of any poisoning?

- **Accident**, e.g. cats falling into containers of old sump oil or dogs finding slug bait.
- **Overdosing**, e.g. owners who do not read and follow directions correctly.
- **Unusual reactions** to normally harmless substances.
- **Anaphylactic** reactions to wasp or bee stings, antibiotics or vaccines (some of these are not poisons but the reaction suggests it).
- **Carelessness** when an owner leaves medications where an inquisitive puppy can eat them.
- **Ignorance** of an owner who doses a pet with human preparations (ibuprofen/paracetamol).
- **Malicious poisoning** which in reality is extremely rare.

The questions the veterinary nurse should ask must therefore concern the species, age, whereabouts and movements of the patient prior to the onset of illness, and the actions of the owner.

Questions about the patient

(1) Has the animal been observed eating anything in the hours preceding the onset of illness? (A sample of the substance preferably with its packaging is very useful.)

(2) Is there any contaminating substance on the coat, e.g. a smell of creosote, sticky engine oil, grease or paraffin?

(3) What were the patient's movements prior to the illness? For example, was the cat out overnight, or had the dog been shut into a garden shed where slug bait was stored, or is there evidence of chewed tablet packets? Has the animal been anywhere unusual in the last 24 hours – has the dog perhaps been walked in a different area where it may have found something?

(4) How old is the patient? The young are curious and may eat anything. The very young and the elderly are more susceptible to being poisoned since the liver and kidneys may not be functioning efficiently and therefore the poison cannot be detoxified and excreted so quickly. These animals need more rapid treatment and more intensive nursing care.

(5) Are other animals in the household affected (if there is more than one animal)? Simultaneous illness is more likely to be caused by poisoning.

Questions about the home environment

(1) Have any medication (human or veterinary) been given in the last 24 hours?
(2) Have any toxic products been used by the owner recently in the house or garden, e.g. pesticides, rodenticides, wood preservative, paint?
(3) Have there been any recent upheavals in the house which may have exposed pesticides or toxic material previously inaccessible, e.g. moving to a renovated house, gutting a kitchen where rat bait has been laid, removing old (lead) pipework, stripping old paintwork where lead-based paints were originally used?
(4) Did any accidents occur recently in the home, e.g. overheating of fat or non-stick cooking utensils, accidental spillage of substances onto the animal's coat?

Nursing care

The role of the veterinary nurse in suspected poisoning cases is to:

(1) Be familiar with common poisons.
(2) Recognise whether a substance is likely to be toxic or harmless.
(3) Give appropriate first aid advice (induce emesis/do not reduce emesis, prevent animal from licking itself, etc.).
(4) Take a comprehensive case history and perform a thorough physical examination.
(5) Reserve any vomit, faeces or urine for possible toxicological screening (keep samples refrigerated not frozen, ensure samples are clearly labelled with the owner's or patient's name and address and the time and date of sample collection).
(6) Maintain a diplomatic silence about the cause of poisoning – do not suggest or agree with accusations of malicious poisoning – it is rare and very difficult to prove.
(7) Ensure that there is access to a poison information unit.

In the UK, The Veterinary Poisons and Information Unit (VPIS) provides a 24 hour information service supplying data on clinical effects, suggested treatments for specific poisons, and suggested antidote therapies (where advisable). VPIS is not a public access service and will only take calls from veterinary practices. Precise details need to be supplied to VPIS to ensure an accurate response. Information regarding the trade name of the toxin, the product constituents, the name of the manufacturer, the time and route of exposure and the amount exposed to needs to be supplied.

Treatment of oiled birds

The role of the veterinary practice is to admit the bird and decide if it is well enough to survive (many oiled birds are in too poor a condition or too badly poisoned, so euthanasia is often the kindest treatment). Further ingestion of the poison can be minimised by superficial cleansing whilst the appropriate organisation is contacted for continuing treatment.

WARNING
To thoroughly clean the plumage and maintain the patient while the bird's waterproofing oils are revived requires considerable experience. Special facilities and weeks of attention may follow – none of which can be easily provided by busy veterinary nurses in a routine small animal practice. There will also be the problem of returning a wild bird to its natural habitat, and this process of rehabilitation (which is vital to its survival) requires a great deal of knowledge and skill.

Snake bites

Most bites are seen on the head and paws of the animal.
There are two groups of venomous snakes:

- Viperidae (viper, rattlesnake and adder).
- Elapidae (cobra, mamba and coral snake).

The only indigenous venomous snake in the UK is the *Vipera berus* (adder). Other exotic reptiles are being kept as pets by ever-increasing numbers of people and if one of these animals escapes it is possible that it may bite.

The adder has a characteristic V or X marking on the head and zigzag markings along the body. It is usually found basking in the sun and may well strike and bite at chest level if disturbed by a dog.

Clinical signs

- Rapid painful swelling.
- Fang marks – may or may not be visible.
- Dull and depressed.
- Anaphylactic reactions are possible.

Treatment

Non-poisonous species:

- Wash with diluted hydrogen peroxide 1:4.
- Flush with saline.
- Give antibiotics (reptile oral flora is rich in Gram-negative bacteria).

Poisonous species:

- Identify the poison.

- Prevent further absorption.
- Restrict movement to slow circulation.
- Splint the bitten limb or bandage tightly.
- Do not use tourniquets (they prevent arterial blood from entering the area).
- Treat the symptoms – shock, collapse, unconsciousness.
- Give antidote/antivenom available from all major accident and emergency departments.
- Adder bite antivenom is called Zagreb.

Toad poisoning

The common toad secretes toxic venom onto its body surface. If the toad is picked up in the mouth of an animal this venom will cause notable clinical signs.

Clinical signs

- Hypersalivation.
- Pawing at the mouth.
- Distress.
- Nervous symptoms (if the toad or an excessive amount of venom have been ingested).

Treatment

- Flush mouth with sponge (or hosepipe if available).
- Symptomatic treatment if nervous signs develop.

Insect stings

Most stings in animals are seen on their paws or in the mouth. When the bee stings it detaches itself from the venom sac (which remains in the animal). Wasp stings do not detach from the wasp. The presence of a venom sack at the affected site confirms that a bee is responsible for the sting.

Bee and wasp stings cause similar side-effects but treatments vary, depending on the primary cause of the sting. Insect stings are classified according to Table 4.14. The clinical signs are summarised in Table 4.15.

Table 4.14 Classification for insect stings

Group	Type	Reaction
1	Toxic	Small location reaction – rarely needs veterinary treatment
2	Allergic	Large local reaction – sometimes needs veterinary attention (to reduce swelling)
3	Anaphylactic	Systemic allergic reaction – immediate veterinary treatment needed
4	Toxic	Systemic toxic reaction – (multiple stings) immediate veterinary attention needed

Source: Wingfield (1997, p. 376)

Treatment

Group 1 These can be treated at home if not too severe.

- **Bee**: Scrape the sting out (removes the sting without disturbing the poison sacs). Do not use tweezers as this empties the poison sacs into the animal. Bee stings should be bathed in bicarbonate solution (1 teaspoon in 250 ml of water), then apply ice pack.
- **Wasp**: Bathe in diluted vinegar (1:1 vinegar and water), then apply ice pack. If the swelling does not respond to these measures the sting should be classified as group 2.

Group 2 These can be treated at home or in the surgery.

- Treat as group 1.
- Give antihistamine with or without corticosteroids.

Group 3 The symptoms are usually observed within 15 minutes.

- Intravenous fluid therapy.
- Antihistamines.
- Intravenous glucocorticoids.
- Epinephrine.

Group 4 The symptoms have a chronic onset.

- Intravenous fluid therapy.

Table 4.15 Clinical signs for insect stings

Group 1	Group 2	Group 3	Group 4
Swelling	Swelling	Swelling	Chronic onset
Pawing at mouth	Pawing at mouth	Vomiting	Depression
Hypersalivation	Hypersalivation	Urination/defecation	Vomiting
Discomfort	Discomfort	Weakness/collapse	Melaena
Dyspnoea	Dyspnoea	Dyspnoea	Ataxia
		Ataxia	Seizures
		Seizures	Toxicity

- Symptomatic treatment.
- Intravenous glucocorticoids.

Traumatic emergencies

Haemorrhage

This is bleeding caused by trauma (or disease).

Clinical signs

Haemorrhage can be classified according to:

Type of blood vessel damaged   Arterial, venous or capillary?

Arterial haemorrhage (most serious form of haemorrhage):

- Bright red blood.
- Spurts forcefully.
- Spurts with the heart beat.
- Definite bleeding point.
- Issued from the side of the wound nearest the heart.

Venous haemorrhage (slightly less serious):

- Dark red blood.
- Steady stream.
- May pulsate slightly with heart beat.
- Definite bleeding point.
- Issued from the side of the wound furthest from the heart.

Capillary haemorrhage (occurs in all wounds):

- Bright red blood.
- Steady ooze.
- Little/no force.
- Multiple pinpoint sources.
- No definite bleeding point.

Mixed haemorrhage (most common in large wounds): characteristics of all of the above.

When the haemorrhage occurred   Primary, reactionary or secondary?

Primary haemorrhage (0–24 hours):

- Immediate result of damage to a blood vessel wall.
- Blood pressure falls.
- Blood clots (or a ligature is placed).
- Haemorrhage arrests.

Reactionary haemorrhage (24–48 hours):

- Blood pressure rises.
- Primary blood clot (or ligature) is displaced.
- Haemorrhage begins again.

Secondary haemorrhage (3–10 days):

- Primary blood clot (or ligature) remains in place.
- Blood clot (or ligature) is destroyed by infection in the wound.
- Haemorrhage begins again.

Where the blood escaped to   External body surface or internal tissues or body cavities?

External haemorrhage may originate from:

- Open wounds.
- Nose, ear or mouth.
- Stomach lining or intestines.
- Urinary tract or uterus.

Internal haemorrhage:

- Can be difficult to detect.
- May cause tissue swelling.
- May cause distension of a cavity.
- Will cause general signs of shock.
- May occur:
  - If there is severe mucosal bruising.
  - If an internal organ is damaged (lungs, liver or spleen).
  - If there is a disease which erodes blood vessel walls (tumour).
  - If there is a clotting deficiency (rat poison).

Natural arrest of haemorrhage

The body utilises **four factors** to naturally arrest haemorrhage:

(1) **Retraction of the cut ends** of arteries, arterioles and large veins is due to the elastic nature of their walls.

- Cut ends recoil.
- Elastic tissue contracts and bunches up.
- Reduces the hole through which blood is escaping.
- Decreased blood flow.
- Clot formation.

(If a vessel is stretched before it is torn then it recoils further. This causes less haemorrhage (but usually more tissue damage) than if a wound is cleanly incised.)

(2) **Drop in blood pressure** due to loss of blood:

- Less blood reaches affected vessel.
- Less pressure to force blood out of the cut end.

(3) **Back pressure**

- Internal haemorrhage fills a cavity or surrounding tissue.
- Low pressure in damaged vessel is equal to pressure of the cavity or surrounding tissue.
- No further blood can escape.

(4) **Blood clotting** (does not work if there is a clotting deficiency):

- Platelets adhere to the vessel wall.
- Fibrin and red blood cells adhere to the platelets.
- Platelets adhere to the fibrin and red blood cells.
- A solid plug is formed preventing further blood loss.

When haemorrhage has stopped, the body attempts to repair the damaged vessel. If the two ends have recoiled away from each other this is not possible. In such cases the blood will be redirected via other vessels (which enlarge to cope with the increased flow). New vessels will develop to re-establish natural circulation. If all the vessels supplying a part of the body are severed, the circulation cannot be re-established in time to prevent the tissue dying. This is often observed in crushing injuries to the tail and digits.

Treatment

Direct digital pressure controls haemorrhage by applying pressure to the wound with clean hands:

- Press fingers on the intact skin either side of the wound.
- Pinch wound edges together.
- If wound is too large, apply pressure directly on to the bleeding points within the wound.

Haemostatic forceps are useful if the cut ends of the vessel can be clearly seen:

- Occlude the end of the vessel with haemostatic forceps.
- Ligate the vessel with absorbable suture material.

Pad and pressure bandage controls haemorrhage by applying pressure to the wound:

- Pack wound with sterile gauze (if it is very large).
- Cover the wound with a pad of gauze swabs.
- Cover the swabs with a thick pad of cotton wool.
- Bandage firmly in place (if the wound is high up, include the whole limb to stop any tissue below the dressing swelling).
- If bleeding continues apply a second pad **over** the first.
- Do not remove the first dressing as this will disturb any clot formation.
- If internal bleeding is suspected a tight crepe bandage over the area will increase the back pressure in the affected tissue.

Pressure points are points in the body where it is possible to prevent arterial flow by pressing an artery against a bone. There are three points in the dog and cat but they are not of much practical use:

- **The brachial artery** – pressure here arrests haemorrhage from below the elbow. It runs down the medial shaft of the humerus and swings cranially behind the biceps muscle. The pulse can be felt in the distal third of the humerus.
- **The femoral artery** – pressure here arrests haemorrhage from below the stifle. It passes obliquely over the proximal third of the femur on the medial aspect of the thigh. It lies just in front of the small taut pectineus muscle.
- **The coccygeal artery** – pressure here arrests haemorrhage from the tail. It passes backwards along the underside of the tail.

Tourniquet stops bleeding by constricting all the arteries supplying blood to a wound on a limb or tail:

- Place tourniquet a few inches above the wound.
- Fix it firmly around the limb.
- Adjust until the pressure is just sufficient to stop haemorrhage.
- Do not leave an animal unattended with a tourniquet in place.
- As soon as bleeding is controlled, other methods of haemostasis should be attempted.

Tourniquets should only be used if haemorrhage is severe and cannot be controlled by any other means. If no custom-made tourniquet is available, one can be fashioned by using a thick elastic band, strong bandage, piece of material, rubber tubing, or narrow belt. If improvising a tourniquet, a half-hitch (stick/rod/ballpoint pen) can be tied against the skin and twisted if the tourniquet needs to be tightened.

Nursing care

Any haemorrhage should be regarded as serious, for a sudden or severe loss of blood may result in death. Even slight haemorrhage that continues over a period of time may result in sufficient blood loss to jeopardise life.

Open wounds

This is a visible break in the surface of the skin or mucous membranes. Open wounds can be classified as:

- **Incised** – clean cut with clearly defined edges.
- **Lacerated** – irregular in shape; jagged uneven edges.
- **Puncture** – small skin wound leading to a narrow penetrating track.
- **Abrasion** – graze wound not penetrating the entire skin thickness.
- **Avulsion** – skin flaps (still attached to the body) which have been torn away from the underneath tissue.

Treatment

- Arrest haemorrhage.

- Treat for shock.
- Clip hair from around the wound.
- Remove any contaminating foreign bodies (grit/dirt/hair).
- Remove the cause of the injury **unless it is**:

  - A deeply penetrating foreign body.
  - Penetrating the chest wall.
  - Penetrating the abdominal wall.

- Cleanse the wound (irrigate with isotonic sterile saline).
- Dress the wound (use a protective gel and sterile non-adhesive wound dressings).

Nursing care

Wounds with penetrating foreign bodies may be dressed using a ring bandage. If the foreign body protrudes it is advisable to cut it off close to the external body wall to avoid further trauma before placement of the ring dressing.

Never use cotton wool or gauze swabs directly on an open wound as they will stick and contaminate the wound. Do not use, or advise owners to use, antiseptic ointments unless they are soluble in water.

Wound healing (Table 4.16)

First intention healing can only take place in incised wounds where the edges remain close together. This may be achieved by stitching or bandaging while healing takes place.

Granulation tissue usually heals lacerated, avulsed and infected wounds and the repair process may take several weeks, as the wound edges are widely separated. Clusters of cells are produced on the exposed tissue of the wound and they multiply rapidly to form areas of granulation tissue. These areas gradually expand to cover the entire wound area, growing upward towards the skin surface level. When it is level with the surface, new epithelial cells can spread across the top to complete the healing process.

Factors delaying wound healing

- Movement.

- Infection.
- Disturbance in circulation.
- Self-trauma.

Fractures

This is a forcible break in the continuity of bony tissue, i.e. the bone is broken.

Fractures can be classified according to the damage done:

- **Incomplete fracture** – the bone cortex is broken on one side but not broken in two pieces.
- **Simple fracture** – bone broken cleanly into two pieces.
- **Compound fracture** – a wound is present between the fracture and the skin (or mucous membranes). Infection is often a complication of this type of fracture.
- **Complicated fracture** – important structures or organs surrounding the fracture site are damaged by the bone fragments (e.g. blood vessels, nerves, spinal cord, lungs or heart).
- **Comminuted fracture** – lots of bone fragments at the fracture site.
- **Multiple fracture** – one bone fracture in two or more pieces where there is an appreciable distance between fracture sites.

A fracture may be described by using several of the above terms. A fracture may be simple because the bone is broken in two pieces but also compound because the sharp proximal fragment has penetrated the skin. It may also be complicated if the sharp distal fragment damages local structures or blood vessels.

Clinical signs

- Pain at or near the fracture site.
- Swelling.
- Loss of function.
- Deformity.
- Unnatural mobility.
- Crepitus.

Radiographs aid diagnosis.

Table 4.16 Wound healing

First intention	Granulation
Incised wounds, simple puncture wounds	Lacerated and infected puncture wounds
Edges of wound stay close together	Wound edges are widely separated
Healing complete in 7–10 days	Healing can take weeks or months
No infection present	Wound often infected
Minimal scarring	Scarring is extensive

Table 4.17 Emergency support for limb fractures

Support	Materials	Method
Robert Jones dressing	Adhesive tape (2.5 cm) Cotton wool/orthopaedic wrap Conforming/WOW bandage Adhesive/cohesive bandage (7.5 cm)	Cut two strips of adhesive tape and fix longitudinally along the anterior and posterior aspects of the metacarpals/metatarsals Cover the entire leg with 4–5 layers of cotton wool, or 12–15 rolls of orthopaedic bandage Bandage cotton wool in place using conforming/WOW bandage Reflect the longitudinal strips of adhesive bandage upwards over the bandage to prevent the dressing from slipping Bandage strips in place using adhesive/cohesive roller bandage When flicked, a good Robert Jones dressing should sound like a ripe melon
Bandaging	A range of dressing material	Bandage affected part of the body firmly against unaffected parts of the body Useful for scapular, metacarpal, metatarsal or digital fractures
Splinting Can only be used for fractures below the elbow or stifle. Time consuming and painful to fit	Wooden splint Cotton wool/orthopaedic wrap Conforming/WOW bandage Adhesive tape	Needs to be long (to immobilise joints either side of the fracture), rigid (minimising movement), smooth and conforming Cover leg with two layers of orthopaedic bandage (unless splint is padded) Fix in place using 2.5 cm adhesive tape (do not encircle limb at fracture site) Bandage entire limb with cotton wool wrap, or orthopaedic wrap Fix in place with conforming or WOW bandage
	Preformed metal splint (tin/aluminium) Cotton wool/orthopaedic wrap Conforming/WOW bandage Adhesive tape	Zimmer splints (malleable aluminium) useful as they can be manipulated to conform to the shape of the leg Cover leg with two layers of orthopaedic bandage (unless splint is padded) Fix in place using 2.5 cm adhesive tape (do not encircle limb at fracture site) Bandage entire limb with cotton wool wrap, or orthopaedic wrap Fix in place with conforming or WOW bandage
	Plastic gutter splint Cotton wool/orthopaedic wrap Conforming/WOW bandage Adhesive tape	Lined with foam. May be cut to size Cover leg with two layers of orthopaedic bandage (unless splint is padded) Fix in place using 2.5 cm adhesive tape (do not encircle limb at fracture site) Bandage entire limb with cotton wool wrap, or orthopaedic wrap Fix in place with conforming or WOW bandage
	Plaster cast or resin Cotton wool/orthopaedic wrap Conforming/crepe bandage	Wrap 1–2 layers of orthopaedic bandage around limb Cut a suitable length of cast material from a roll and soften as appropriate or soak plaster of Paris in water, wring out, unroll out and fold 3–4 times to form a slab Mould it onto the affected limb Secure in position with conforming bandage/crepe bandage Do not use to encase the limb (this is beyond the scope of first aid)
	Inflatable airbag	Human first aid appliance Inflated around the limb to immobilise fracture

In all cases where a support dressing is used the toes should be left out so they can be frequently examined to ensure that the circulation is not hindered. Overtight bandages obstruct venous return up the leg, causing the toes to swell. Patients should be constantly monitored for signs of discomfort (biting at the dressing) or distress. WOW = white open weave

Treatment

- Clean wounds – flush with sterile saline.
- Minimise movement – confine patient.
- Control haemorrhage – pressure/ring pad dressings.
- Support limb fracture – (see Table 4.17).
- Analgesia.
- Antibiotics.

Nursing care

It is really only practical to support limb fractures. Support for the fracture should be applied as soon as possible to limit movement and prevent further damage. However, splinting should be abandoned if it is impossible without a struggle – provoking the animal to thrash around will do it more harm than the splint will do good. Such animals are best kept still, warm and comfortable until professional help is available or until the animal has calmed down and will allow a splint to be applied without a struggle.

Dislocation/luxation

This is a persistent displacement of the articular surfaces of the bones which form a joint. A partial displacement of the articular surfaces at the bones which form a joint is called **subluxation**.

Clinical signs

- Pain on manipulation.
- Swelling.
- Loss of function.
- Deformity.
- Usually affects carpus, tarsus, hip joint or patella.

Treatment

- Do not attempt to reduce.
- Cold compress.
- Apply support bandage.
- Analgesia.

Sprain

This is a joint damaged by overstretching the synovial membrane. Ligaments and soft tissue may be damaged in the process but the joint is anatomically correct.

Clinical signs

- Pain.
- Swelling.
- Loss of function.
- No gross deformity.
- Usually affects shoulder, stifle, carpus or tarsus.

Treatment

- Rest.
- Cold compress.
- Support bandage.

Strain

This is stretching or tearing of muscle or tendon.

Clinical signs

- Sudden loss of use.
- Tenderness and swelling.
- No deformity.
- Usually affects muscles of the legs.

Treatment

- Enforced rest (splint if necessary).
- Cold compress.
- Support bandage.
- Warm compress (longer-term use).

Ruptured tendon

This is partial or complete tear of a tendon as a result of direct or indirect trauma.

Clinical signs

- Lameness, due to loss of support.
- Unusual foot/leg conformation.
- Flexor tendon injuries – claws of the affected toes stick upwards (knocked-up toe).
- Gastrocnemius tendon – hock sinks downwards and animal walks with the metatarsus on the ground (kangaroo foot).
- Torn ends of tendons may be palpable through the skin or visible through a wound.

Treatment

- Flush wounds with saline and dress with sterile dressings.
- Support bandage (try to position the leg so the cut ends of the tendon stay together).
- Flexor tendon injuries – keep toes flexed.
- Extensor tendon injuries – keep foot in normal position.
- Gastrocnemius tendon injuries – keep hock extended.
- Surgical intervention to repair rupture.

KEYPOINTS
- Remember the aims of first aid are to preserve life, prevent suffering and prevent the situation deteriorating.
- Be aware that owners faced with emergencies involving their pets are often in a state of panic. Always remain calm, sympathetic and patient, whilst being specific, clear and concise.
- Remember that injured animals are usually frightened and shocked and need to be handled and restrained in a way suitable for their condition.
- Always try to be ready and prepared for an emergency before it arrives at the surgery.
- Triage should be used to prioritise treatments. This applies when faced with multiple emergencies or when an individual patient has multiple problems.
- During the primary examination remember to record all information accurately.
- The assistance of a veterinary surgeon must be sought as soon as it is reasonably possible.

Further reading

Battaglia, A. M. (2001) *Small Animal Emergency and Critical Care*, W. B. Saunders Company, Philadelphia, Pennsylvania.

Plunkett, S. J. (2001) *Emergency Procedures for the Small Animal Veterinarian*, Harcourt Publishers, London.

Wingfield, W. E. (1997) *Veterinary Emergency Medicine Secrets*, Hanley & Belfus, Philadelphia, Pennsylvania.

5

Occupational hazards

R. Butcher and *S Bowden*

Learning objectives

After studying this chapter, students should be able to:

- Identify the legislation that pertains to veterinary practice.
- Describe the key features of Health and Safety management.
- Discuss the procedure for dealing with first aid and accident reporting.
- Describe how to carry out a risk assessment.
- List the categories of hazards in a veterinary practice.

The laws relating to occupational health

The very nature of veterinary practice means that staff, clients and visitors can be exposed to potential hazards such that accidents are possible. The Health and Safety legislation attempts to make the workplace as safe an environment as possible, by ensuring that practices examine their working procedures and adapt them to reduce to a minimum the risk of exposure to hazardous materials or circumstances in which accidents can occur. Even so, accidents will happen and practices should draw up contingency plans to deal with them. The legislation also makes provision for the recording and reporting of diseases and injuries that occur in the workplace (Reporting of Diseases and Dangerous Occurrence Regulations (1995) (RIDDOR)).

It is important that veterinary nurses are familiar with Health and Safety legislation, not only because they have specific obligations as employees but also because they may become involved in formulating the practice policy or ensuring that other staff adhere to it. The two most important general pieces of legislation are the **Health and Safety at Work Act (1974) (HSW Act)** and the **Management of Health and Safety at Work Regulations (1999) (MHSW Regulations).**

The Health and Safety at Work Act (1974)

This Act applies to all businesses, however small, and relates to all persons in the workplace, whether employers, employees or visitors. It sets out the specific duties of both employers and employees, and indicates that the ultimate responsibility rests with the senior partner of the practice.

The general provisions of the Act dictate that every *employer* should ensure that:

(1) Proper provision is made to establish safe systems of work. These should be written down as '**Local Rules**' and be displayed on Health and Safety notice boards at the appropriate work stations.
(2) All equipment is adequately maintained to the manufacturer's specification.
(3) The premises (including vehicles) should be kept in a good state of repair and adequate attention given to providing safe access or exit in times of emergency.
(4) All articles and substances used within the practice should be handled, stored and transported in a safe manner.
(5) Information, instruction and supervision of employees should be carried out regularly.
(6) All appropriate protective clothing is provided free of charge.
(7) A satisfactory working environment is maintained with adequate facilities and arrangements for employees' welfare at work. This should include adequate washing and toilet facilities as well as a separate hygienic area for rest and refreshment.
(8) Appropriate first aid facilities are available. All accidents should be recorded, and the more serious ones reported to the Health and Safety Executive (HSE).

An employer with five or more employees must prepare, and when necessary revise, a written **Health and Safety Policy Statement**. This must outline the general policy of the practice, as well as listing the general duties of all members of the practice. It is necessary to appoint (in writing) individual members of staff to jobs with special responsibilities (e.g. practice safety officer, fire officer, first aid officer, etc.), providing written job specifications for these posts. It is essential that this statement, and any revision, is brought to the attention of all employees. The HSE document *Stating Your Business – Guidance on Preparing a Health and Safety Policy Document for Small Firms* provides a useful template with blanks that can be completed by the individual practice to ensure they are complying with the law.

The Act highlights the responsibilities of all *employees*, who must:

(1) Take reasonable care for the health and safety of themselves and of other persons who may be affected by their acts or omissions.

(2) Cooperate with the employer so far as it is necessary to enable any duty or requirement under the Act to be performed or complied with.

(3) Not interfere, recklessly or intentionally, with anything provided in the interests of health, safety and welfare.

These broad guidelines to the Act are highlighted on a poster and leaflet produced by the Health and Safety Executive (HSE) entitled *Health and Safety Law – What You Should Know*. The poster should be displayed on the practice notice board and the leaflets should be provided to all staff.

Management of Health and Safety at Work Regulations (amended 1999)

These regulations build on the HSW Act and include duties to assess risks and ensure that the arrangements for Health and Safety are effective. It requires the following steps:

* Planning.
* Organisation.
* Control.
* Monitoring.
* Review.

These regulations stress the requirements for health surveillance. The essential element of the effective management of Health and Safety is a thorough Risk Assessment (see below).

Additional legal requirements for specific health risks at work

Although the HSW Act and the MHSW Regulations provide the overall framework, there are some specific laws that relate to particular risks and the Special Waste regulations 1996 (as amended). The requirements of these laws must be incorporated in the overall Health and Safety management plan for the practice.

In addition to these major regulations, a number of others have relevance to the practice of Health and Safety and some of these are considered in Chapter 8 (The Law and Ethics of Veterinary Nursing). The following paragraphs highlight some of the particular provisions of these specific regulations.

Ionising Radiation Regulations (1985)

These apply specifically to the hazards associated with radiography and are dealt with in Chapter 24 (Radiography).

SPECIFIC HEALTH AND SAFETY LEGISLATION OF RELEVANCE TO VETERINARY PRACTICE

* Special Waste Regulations (as amended) (1996)
* The Fire Precautions Act (1971).
* The Control of Pollution Act (1974).
* The First Aid at Work Regulations (1981).
* The Ionising Radiation Regulations (1985).
* The Electricity at Work Regulations (1989).
* The Environmental Protection Act (1990).
* The Manual Handling Operations Regulations (1992).
* The Health and Safety (Display Screen Equipment) Regulations (1992).
* The Reporting of Diseases and Dangerous Occurrences Regulations (RIDDOR) (1995).
* Chemicals (Hazard Information and Packaging for Supply) Amendment Regulations (2002) (CHIP 96).
* The Control of Substances Hazardous to Health (COSHH) Regulations (1999).
* The Fire Precautions (Workplace) (Amendment) Regulations (1999).
* Personal Protective Equipment (PPE) regulation (1992).

The Control of Substances Hazardous to Health (COSHH) Regulations (1999)

These Regulations were introduced to specifically cover the management of risks associated with hazardous substances and relate to all pharmaceutical products and chemicals used in veterinary practice. Manufacturers should supply **COSHH Hazard Data Sheets** with all such products to help the practice formulate their **COSHH Assessment**. This is simply part of the Risk Assessment demanded by the MHSW Regulations and will be dealt with below.

Clinical Waste Regulations

The principal regulations relating to this subject are the **Control of Pollution (Amendment) Act (1974).** Together they regulate the correct segregation, storage, transfer and eventual destruction of waste products produced at the surgery. The waste produced at veterinary practices must be classified (clinical waste, 'sharps', special waste, cadavers and industrial waste), labelled and disposed of correctly.

Clinical waste includes all waste that consists wholly or partly of animal tissues, blood or other body fluids, excretions, drugs or pharmaceutical products likely to be hazardous to health. It should be collected and stored in approved colour-coded plastic sacks (yellow with the words 'Clinical waste' and the name of the practice clearly printed on the outside).

'Sharps' is a special category of clinical waste that includes used needles, scalpel blades or other sharp instruments. These should be discarded *immediately* after use, into special yellow plastic tubs that can be sealed once full.

Special waste, a further category of clinical waste, includes bottles and vials contaminated with pharmaceutical products. These too are stored in specific yellow plastic bins.

Cadavers are technically clinical waste. Strict interpretation of the law would cause problems for owners who wish to bury their pets in their garden. The Department of Environment Management Paper No. 25 states:

> Pets deceased at a veterinary practice remain the property of the owner and may be disposed of by the owner within the curtilage of their dwelling in their capacity as a private individual without breach of duty of care. Where the pet suffered from an infectious disease or for other reasons may be significantly hazardous, then it should be dealt with by the veterinary surgeon as clinical waste. Low hazard deceased pets should be classed as non-clinical commercial waste where the owner requests disposal by the veterinary surgeon, who will be subject to the duty of care.

This is of importance to the owner who wishes to bury their own pet in their garden.

The remainder of the practice waste is regarded as **non-clinical commercial waste**. This is non-hazardous and can be removed by the local authority or other registered carrier (an appropriate charge may be levied for the service).

Segregation and storage within the practice

The practice must have a strict policy on the segregation of waste. To be practical this must allow for the immediate disposal of material after use and hence there must be sufficient receptacles to allow for segregation at each work station. This should also apply to practice vehicles. Prior to collection, clinical waste should be stored in a secure place within the practice.

Transport and disposal

Clinical waste is collected by a registered carrier in a 'dedicated' vehicle, licensed specifically for the transport of clinical waste. It is transferred to a licensed plant where final disposal is achieved, preferably by high-temperature incineration. Each collection (or batch of collections) should be accompanied by the appropriate certification and copies of which should be kept by the practice.

The regulations place a **duty of care** on the producers of clinical waste to ensure that, from production to ultimate disposal, the waste is dealt with according to the law. The practice itself is responsible for checking that both the carrier and incineration plant have the appropriate licences (ideally keeping photocopies for its own records).

General maintenance of buildings and equipment

It is important that all buildings are kept in a good state of repair, especially with regard to electrical or gas installations and fittings. All equipment (X-ray machines, anaesthetic machines, autoclaves, etc.) should be regularly serviced according to the manufacturer's recommendations and service records should be kept.

The Electricity at Work Regulations (1989) state that all systems should be maintained so as to prevent, as far as is reasonably practicable, all dangers. HSE guidelines on maintaining portable electrical equipment in offices and other low-risk environments recommend a regular visual inspection and recording system. The frequency of inspection is dependent on the type of equipment, the suggestions ranging from every 6 months for hand-held equipment to every 2 years for static equipment (e.g. photocopiers).

Fire precautions

Adequate precautions should be taken to avoid or combat fires. This is covered by the **Fire Precautions Act 1971** and involves:

(1) The provision of adequate fire-fighting equipment (advice needs to be taken on the correct extinguishers for different work stations, and these should be checked regularly).
(2) An alarm system, regularly maintained.
(3) Well-signposted emergency exits.
(4) Emergency lighting.
(5) Clear local rules stating what to do in case of fire. These should be posted in strategic places, and reinforced by regular fire practices.
(6) Care in the storage of inflammable and explosive material.
(7) The provision of fire doors where appropriate.

Further to this the **Fire Precautions (Workplace) (Amendment) Regulations (1999)** specify a requirement:

(1) For competent assistance to deal with general fire safety risks.
(2) To provide employees with information on fire provisions.
(3) On employers and self-employed people in a shared workplace to cooperate and coordinate with others on fire provisions and to provide outside employers with comprehensive information on fire provisions.

The practice should appoint a fire officer to oversee these provisions. Very valuable advice can be obtained from the local Fire Prevention Officer.

Oxygen cylinders and other flammable substances

The HSE document *Safe Working with Flammable Substances* (1997) highlights five principles when considering working safely with flammable substances ('VICES'):

- Ventilation.
- Ignition.
- Containment.
- Exchange.
- Separation.

Special consideration should be given to the transport and storage of oxygen cylinders – ideally they should be stored in a locked construction away from the main building.

Protection of the person against physical attack

Unfortunately, veterinary practices are not immune from the attentions of criminals. Nurses or veterinary surgeons 'on call' at night and weekends are especially vulnerable and it might be worth incorporating personal 'panic buttons' into the practice alarm system. The local Crime Prevention Officer may give useful advice on this matter.

It is wise to have a practice policy of noting names, addresses, phone numbers of clients being visited. Staff members should *never* go out on a visit without informing other staff of their whereabouts.

First aid and reporting accidents

First aid

Despite every precaution, accidents will occur. The **First Aid at Work: Approved Code of Practice and Guidelines (1997)** states the requirement for a suitably stocked accessible first aid box and the appointment of a nominated first aider. There are no hard and fast rules about the contents of the first aid box, but it must reflect the number of staff and the type of hazards encountered.

The personnel responsible for first aid include:

(1) A First Aid Appointed Person – responsible to take charge when someone is injured or falls ill, including calling an ambulance if required. They are also responsible for maintaining and stocking the first aid box and ensuring that records of accidents are recorded in the accident book. They should not attempt to administer first aid.
(2) A qualified first aider – this person must have attended an HSE approved training course and hold a current First Aid at Work Certificate.

The recommended numbers of first aid personnel for a 'medium risk' business is given in Table 5.1. Clearly, in veterinary practice, availability of staff during different shifts should be taken into account, as well as the fact that

Table 5.1 Recommendations for numbers of first aid staff	
Number of employees	**Suggested first aid staff**
< 20	At least one appointed first aid person
20–100	At least one qualified first-aider for every 50 employees (or part thereof)
>100	One additional qualified first-aider for every additional 100 persons

clients attending the clinic may significantly increase the number of people at risk at any one time.

Recording accidents

It is the duty of the practice to record all accidents and injuries that occur. An accident book approved by HSE (Form B1 510) is available from HMSO. The information that is to be recorded includes:

(1) The full name, address and occupation of the person who had the accident.
(2) The signature (with date) of the person filling in the book. This must also include the address and occupation if the person is different from (1).
(3) When and where the accident happened.
(4) Details about the cause of the accident. Record details of any personal injury.
(5) Indicate whether the injury needs to be reported under RIDDOR.

Reporting accidents

Under the provisions of **RIDDOR (1995)**, the practice is obliged to report certain serious events direct to the HSE. These can be broadly divided into three categories:

(1) Major or fatal accidents.
(2) 'Three-day' accidents.
(3) Dangerous occurrences and near misses.

Major or fatal accidents must be reported as soon as possible by telephone, followed by written confirmation within 7 days on **Form 2508**. Major accidents are defined as:

(1) A fracture of the skull, spine or pelvis.
(2) A fracture of a long bone of the limb.
(3) Amputation of a hand or foot.
(4) Loss of sight of an eye.
(5) Any other accident which results in an injured person being admitted into hospital as an inpatient for more than 24 hours, unless only detained for observation.

Fatal accidents include those instances where a fatality occurs within 1 year as a result of an original accident at work.

'Three-day' accidents relate to absences from work for a minimum of 3 days as a result of an accident at work. The DHSS will notify the HSE, who in turn will require a written report from the practice.

There is a list of **dangerous occurrences** that should be reported to the HSE (Form F2508) whether or not an injury occurs. These include:

(1) Explosion from a gas cylinder or steriliser.
(2) Uncontrolled release of substance (including gases, vapours and X-rays) liable to be hazardous to health.
(3) Any escape of substances that might result in problems due to inhalation or lack of oxygen.
(4) Any cases of acute ill-health that could have resulted from exposure to pathogens in infected material.
(5) Any unintentional ignition or explosion.

(See also Chapter 13.)

Manual handling procedures

More than a quarter of the accidents reported each year to the enforcing authorities are associated with manual handling, i.e. the transporting or supporting of loads by hand or body force. Indeed, statistics published by the HSE indicate that this may be as high as 55% for those working in medical, veterinary and other health services. Sprains and strains arise from the incorrect application and/or prolongation of bodily force. Poor posture and excessive repetition of movement can be important factors in their onset. Many manual handling injuries are cumulative rather than being truly attributable to any single handling incident.

The Manual Handling Operations Regulations (1992) expand on the general provisions of the HSW Act (1974) in this regard. The HSE booklet *Manual Handling – Guidance on Regulations* clearly outlines the requirements and application of these regulations. The general provisions highlight a hierarchy of measures:

(1) Avoid hazardous manual handling operations so far as is reasonably practicable.
(2) Assess any hazardous manual handling operations that cannot be avoided.
(3) Reduce the risk of injury so far as is reasonably practical.

Assessment of manual handling procedures

Though the HSE Guidelines give some practical help, the regulations set no specific requirements such as weight limits. The importance of an ergonomic approach to the assessment of each procedure is stressed – giving consideration to the **task**, the **load**, the **working environment**, the **individual's capability** and the relationship between them. The intention is to fit the operation to the individual rather than the other way around.

Factors to be considered in making an assessment are fully explained in the HSE Guidelines and specific references to some problems in veterinary practice are made. When carrying animals, for example, the load lacks rigidity, there is a concern on the part of the handler to avoid damaging the load and sudden movements of the load add an element of unpredictability. All these factors serve to increase the likelihood of injury compared to handling an inanimate load of similar weight and shape.

It should be realised that an individual's physical capability varies with age, the risk of injury being higher in the teens or above the age of 50 years. Pregnancy also has significant implications for the risk of manual handling injuries. Hormonal changes can affect the ligaments, increasing the susceptibility to injury; and postural problems may increase as pregnancy progresses. Particular care should also be taken for women who may handle loads during the 3 months following a return to work after childbirth.

Display screen equipment

Possible hazards associated with the use of display screens are those leading to musculoskeletal problems, visual fatigue and stress. The likelihood of experiencing these is related mainly to the frequency, duration, intensity and pace of spells of continuous use on the display screen equipment.

The HSE booklet entitled *Display Screen Equipment Work – Guidance on Regulations* clearly outlines the provisions and requirements of the regulations (e.g. the provision of appropriate eye and eyesight tests for designated '*operators*' and '*users*').

In general it is very unlikely that many staff working in a veterinary practice would be classified as 'operators' or 'users' under the provisions of the regulations, since most of the display screen work is intermittent. However, the guidelines do give some useful points to consider in relation to the physical layout of the work station (e.g. lighting, correct posture, layout of screen and keyboard, etc.). Such considerations would be part of the normal Health and Safety assessment irrespective of whether the specific Display Screen Equipment Regulations apply.

Risk assessments

The MHSW Regulations require that all employers and self-employed people assess the risks to workers and any others who may be affected by their work or business. Moreover, those who employ five or more employees should record the significant findings of that risk assessment. The five basic stages that are required are outlined:

(1) Identify what the hazards are.
(2) Identify who might be harmed and how.
(3) Evaluate the risks from the identified hazards.
(4) Record.
(5) Review and revise.

Hazards and risks

- **Hazard** – anything with the potential to cause harm.
- **Risk** – the likelihood of the hazard's potential being realised.

The essence of Health and Safety management is to identify all the hazards to which the staff are exposed and then to develop work protocols that reduce the risks from these hazards to a minimum.

The HSE Health Risk Management Guide identifies the broad categories of hazard as:

(1) Hazardous chemicals.
(2) Sprains, strains and pains.
(3) Noise.
(4) Vibration.
(5) Ionising radiation.
(6) Extremes of temperature, pressure and humidity.
(7) Hazardous micro-organisms.
(8) Stress.

The range of potential hazards within a veterinary practice is vast, and the authors have found the accompanying classification (see box) of practical use in making their own risk assessment.

> *SUGGESTED CATEGORIES OF HAZARD IN*
> *VETERINARY PRACTICE*
> Chemical agents:
> - Dispensed drugs.
> - Laboratory chemical reagents.
> - Cleaning materials.
> - Inhalation of dust and fumes.
> - Explosive/flammable agents.
> - Miscellaneous non-laboratory solvents.
> Biological agents:
> - Non-specific organisms.
> - Specific zoonotic infectious agents.
> - Non-zoonotic infectious agents.
> - Animal tissues – allergens.
> - Unidentified allergens.
> Traumatic injuries:
> - Sharps:
> - Manual lifting.
> - Direct injury inflicted by animals.
> - Burns and scalds.
> - Accidental falls.
> - Accidents in the car park and entrance.
> Hazards from using equipment:
> - Electrocution.
> - Burns and scalds.
> - Eye strain from visual display screens.
> - Repetitive strain injuries.
> - Back injuries from poorly adjusted seating.
> Hazards from poor environmental control:
> - Heating/air conditioning.

> - Humidity.
> - Ventilation.
> - Contamination of water supply.
> - Noise.
> Radiation.

Warning label (Fig. 5.1)

All hazardous chemicals have clear warnings on the bottle and are classified as either toxic, highly flammable, corrosive, harmful or irritant. A more complex numerical code system employed for the purposes of the classification and labelling of hazardous chemicals was introduced as a result of the **Chemicals (Hazard Information and Packaging for Supply) Amendment Regulations (1996) (CHIP 96)**. This classification includes data relating to the potential risks and safety precautions required for these chemicals. Although much is of little relevance to veterinary practice, the veterinary nurse should be aware of its existence. The HSE have produced an explanatory booklet called *The Complete Idiot's Guide to CHIP*.

The risk assessment and the development of a management plan

In making the risk assessment, the first three steps involve identifying the hazards, identifying who might be at the greatest risk and assessing the nature of the risk. In the case of hazardous substances, some may have specific Maximum exposure limits (MEL) while others may have Occupational exposure standards (OES).

The MEL of a hazardous substance is assessed in relation to a specific reference period when calculated by a method approved by the Health and Safety Commission. Exposure should not exceed this level. Where an OES has been approved for an inhalation agent, control can still be regarded as adequate if the level is exceeded and yet the employer identifies the reasons and takes the appropriate action to remedy the situation as soon as is reasonably practical.

Thus when considering a particular hazard, consideration should be given to:

- **The nature of the hazard**. What symptoms are seen if exposure occurs? Is there a published MEL or OES? Is there an available COSHH Hazard data sheet, or does the material carry a specific warning label?
- **Route of exposure**. Remember that there may be more than one for each substance, and that accidents may result in unexpected routes of exposure (e.g. injectable drugs could enter the body by accidental self-injection, but also via the skin or eyes if the bottle is broken).
- **First aid**. Are there any specific first aid measures if accidental exposure occurs? Such information should be included in the COSHH Hazard data sheet.

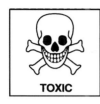 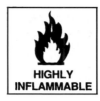 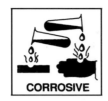

Fig. 5.1 Hazard warning labels.

- **Preventative measures**. Does this particular substance need to be used or is a safer alternative available? Will strict Standard Operating Procedures (SOPs), possibly involving the use of protective clothing, greatly reduce the risk?
- **High-risk staff**. Are there any members of staff who may be at a greater risk (e.g. those with known allergies or at risk during pregnancy)? In this regard it is important that staff feel able to notify the practice safety officer or senior partner in confidence if they consider there is any chance of being pregnant, or if they have any disease or condition that might increase the risks when working in a particular environment.
- **Recording of exposure**. Are there any monitoring schemes available to record exposure? This would include dosimetry for X-ray radiation exposure and any monitoring for halothane and nitrous oxide.

Many of the individual hazardous substances can be grouped together since the hazards are similar.

Standard Operating Procedures (SOPs).

Having identified the types of hazard, those at particular risk and the nature of the hazard, the Health and Safety management system should develop working protocols to make the hazards as low risk as possible. This generally requires the production of written SOPs that cover the full range of all work performed at the surgery. They must above all be clear and concise, and be tailored to the work protocols of each individual practice. Copies should be posted at the appropriate work stations, so that the group of SOPs in that area forms the basis of the Local Rules as required by the general Health and Safety legislation. A pictorial component would give more impact to SOPs posted on notice boards. Specimen SOPs are available as part of the BSAVA Members' Information Service.

The actual SOPs required by each practice may vary, but suggested topics (some of which are discussed in greater detail in relevant chapters of this book) are given in the accompanying list.

Practical risk assessment at each work station

This builds on the information collated above and is basically a critical look at the safety of each work station within the practice. The format discussed below is that suggested in

SUGGESTED LIST OF STANDARD OPERATING PROCEDURES (SOPs)
- Radiation protection.
- Accidents and first aid.
- Health surveillance.
- Laboratory procedures.
- Postage of laboratory specimens.
- Safe prescribing and handling of medicines.
- Injections.
- Restraint of animals.
- Spillages.
- The dental scaler.
- Waste disposal.
- Disinfectants and floor cleaning.
- Kennel management.
- Bathing animals.
- Anaesthetic gases – scavenging and monitoring.
- Fire precautions.
- The mortuary/post-mortems.
- X-ray processing.
- Sterilisers.
- Visits/the practice vehicle/on the farm or stable.
- Manual handling/lifting.
- Display screens.
- Refreshments/the staff kitchen.
- Staff children

COSHH: BVA Guide to the Initial Assessment in Veterinary Practices. At each work station (or room or department) the assessment involves the methodical listing of:

(1) Hazards that may be encountered in that area. For each one the practice must assess the degree of risk and allot a hazard code (H = high; M = moderate; L = low; N = negligible).
(2) If the substance has a known MEL or OES, this too should be recorded.
(3) All the members of staff present in this area. This should include their gender, official job title and a brief summary of their involvement in this area. A note should be made if the member of staff is of particular risk (e.g. pregnant, under 18 years of age, etc.).
(4) All the practice SOPs that may be of relevance in this area.

(5)   The control measures in use in the area. This may simply require reference to specific SOPs.
(6)   Safety clothing provided and used.

Having completed this stage of the assessment, it is important to record a comment that represents an overview of the exposure and actual risks in that area. It is possible that various deficiencies are highlighted. These should be listed and a note made when they have been corrected.

An important part of the assessment is to ascertain where further staff training or instruction is required. This too should be planned and a note made when completed. Finally, the date of the next assessment should be set (at least annually). The risk assessment is therefore an ongoing process promoting continual improvements to the practice's safety standards.

General points

Many items covered by the SOPs will be common to all parts of the practice (e.g. first aid, fire precautions, floor cleaning and disinfectants, etc.) and will not be mentioned below. In all work areas where hands are likely to become contaminated, it is worth considering the use of elbow taps on sinks and disposable towels.

Waiting room/reception

Probably the major potential hazard in this area is injury from unrestrained animals. The practice is liable for injuries sustained by any person on their premises, so it is important that clients are made aware (ideally by a sign outside the building) that all animals must be suitably restrained. Leads and cat baskets should be available in reception for clients who arrive without them and reception staff should give a verbal reminder to clients arriving with unrestrained animals.

Recently washed floors must be dried well or 'wet floor' warning notices displayed.

Should an accident occur, whether it involves a member of staff or a client, it is important that it is recorded in the accident book.

The consulting room

A special consideration here is the potential hazard of children becoming injured by contact with sharps or pharmaceutical products. Ideally drugs should be stored outside the consulting room. Where this is not practical, they must be kept well out of reach of children.

Clinical waste, including sharps, should be disposed of in the appropriate manner immediately after use.

The dispensary

The correct storage and dispensing of drugs (as recommended by the RCVS), including special provisions for controlled drugs, is an important factor and is discussed fully in Chapter 12 (Medicines, Pharmacology, Therapeutics and Dispensing).

Care must be taken when dispensing drugs that can be absorbed through the skin (e.g. cytotoxic drugs). Some individuals show skin hypersensitivity to antibiotics and so disposable gloves should be considered when handling tablets. The use of automatic tablet counters avoids direct handling altogether. Care must also be taken when dispensing small quantities of powdered material that could be a hazard if inhaled. Face masks should be worn. Similarly, precautions may be needed if dispensing small volumes of liquid from a larger stock solution.

Stores

In most practices, space is at a premium and so storage often involves high shelving. Full consideration of the provisions of the Manual Handling Regulations should be made. Avoid putting heavy material on the highest shelf and provide non-slip stools in each storeroom where they may be required. Where heavy items need to be transported within the practice (e.g. trays of petfood or anaesthetised dogs), a trolley should be available to avoid back injury. It is important to keep corridors free from stored material as this could impede rapid exit in the case of fire.

The practice laboratory

There are many potential hazards in the practice laboratory and strict attention to SOPs is required. This is considered in more detail in Chapter 13 (on diagnostic aids). In practices without a laboratory, it is important to adhere to the regulations for the postage of pathological specimens.

The X-ray room

The problems associated with radiation hazards are discussed fully in Chapter 24 (Radiography). It is worth considering here the problems of disposing of spent developer and fixer solutions. The appropriate protective clothing should be worn when dealing with these chemicals and good ventilation is essential to avoid inhalation of fumes. Spent developer and fixer should not be discharged into the normal waste water supply, but stored in appropriate containers and removed by a licensed agent.

The preparation area

The problems related to anaesthetic gas scavenging and monitoring are of significance in this area. In addition, the amount of animal hair should be reduced to a minimum, not only to improve general hygiene but also to reduce the risk of hypersensitivity reactions in some individuals.

Dental scalers are often used in this area, and a SOP should be formulated to cover the use of masks and eye protection. In practices using oscillating saws to remove plaster casts, thought should be given to the control of the amount of dust, which could be hazardous if inhaled.

The operating area

There are no specific problems here not already dealt with elsewhere but it is worth considering the transport of animals to and from the theatre using trolleys and providing hydraulic tables to avoid excessive heavy lifting of animals.

The level of waste anaesthetic gases in the recovery area may be high as the animals exhale it on recovery. To keep this problem to a minimum it is desirable to keep the animal connected to the anaesthetic circuit for as long as possible to make use of the scavenging system (ideally until extubation). Nevertheless, good ventilation is still essential in this area.

Hospital kennels and catteries

Thought should be given to hygienic kennel protocols that reduce the risk of infection from zoonotic agents. The practice might consider the provision of isolation facilities (see Chapter 6) in cases where there is a known risk of zoonoses.

There should also be clear instructions to staff relating to the handling of animals and their transport within the building to avoid physical injury from bites and scratches, as well as from manual lifting procedures.

Mortuary

Correct protective clothing and disinfection regimes are essential in this area. Special thought should also be given to precautions taken if post-mortems are performed on parrots, since there is the additional risk of the inhalation of the agent causing psittacosis from feather debris.

Staff rest room

Adequate rest room facilities should be provided to allow refreshments to be enjoyed away from the working areas. A sink should be provided specifically for the supply of drinking water and for washing up crockery.

Office

This is an area of the practice that is often ignored from the Health and Safety point of view. Hazards do occur, and further information can be obtained from the HSE booklet *Officewise*. There are guidelines relating to the minimum temperatures and lighting conditions for the workplace. The use of display screen equipment is referred to earlier.

Car park/entrance

The Health and Safety legislation extends to the limit of the practice boundaries. Ensure adequate lighting at night and consider providing bins for the disposal of dog faeces.

Practice vehicles

Within vehicles, ensure that all drugs are stored safely and securely. Also make provision for the immediate disposal of clinical waste and sharps. The habit of bringing trays of used syringes and needles back to the surgery for others to dispose of greatly increases the risk of accidental self-injection (especially important in relation to drugs like prostaglandins).

On the farm

The same principles of Health and Safety apply when working on the farm. Many potential hazards relate to zoonotic infections and the BVA guidelines are very useful in this regard. Farmers also have responsibilities under the Health and Safety at Work Act and the COSHH Regulations, and the veterinary surgeon's advice is very important in helping farmers to formulate their own SOPs with regard to zoonotic infections.

BE SAFE: KEY POINTS
Be aware of the following in your practice:
- How to lift correctly.
- Personal hygiene when working with animals.
- How to handle animals.
- What to do if a chemical spill onto your skin or clothes occurs.
- The fire drill procedure.
- The first aid arrangements.
- How to operate machines properly.
- How to use electrical equipment safely.
- The correct protective clothing for the task in hand.

Further reading

The HSE's website address is www.hse.gov.uk

BSAVA Members' Information Service (1993) *Guides to Local Health and Safety Rules.*

BVA (revised 1989) *Health and Safety at Work Act – A Guide for Veterinary Practices.*

BVA (1991) *COSHH: BVA Guide to the Initial Assessment in Veterinary Practices.*

HSE (1997) *First Aid at Work – Approved Code of Practice and Guidance,* ISBN 0 7176 1050 0.

HSE (1998) *Five Steps to Risk Assessment,* ISBN 0 7176 1565 0.

HSE (1998) *Manual Handling Regulations 1992 – Guidance on Regulations,* ISBN 0 7176 24153.

HSE (1999) *Essentials of Health and Safety at Work,* ISBN 0 7176 0716 X.

HSE (1999) *COSHH – A Brief Guide to the Regulations,* ISBN 0 7176 2444 7.

HSE (1999) *RIDDOR Explained,* ISBN 0 7176 2441 2.

HSE (2000) *Management of Health and Safety at Work Regulations 1999 – Approved Code of Practice and Guidance,* ISBN 0 7176 2488 9.

HSE (2000) *First Aid at Work – Your Questions Answered,* INDG214 11/00 C1500.

NOAH (1990) *The Safe Storage and Handling of Animal Medicines.*

RCVS Guidelines (1988) *Dispatch of Pathological Specimens by Post* (reprinted by BSAVA Members' Information Service).

6

Basic animal management

C. A. van der Heiden and *Jean Turner*

Learning objectives

After studying this chapter students should be able to:

- Describe the legal requirements for animals regarding boarding establishments.
- Discuss the sizes and materials required for animal accommodation.
- Describe appropriate accommodation for different categories of animal.
- Discuss suitable situations for kennel siting.
- Apply appropriate environmental conditions in animal accommodation by monitoring and controlling ventilation to suit animals' requirements.
- Explain how extra heat may be supplied to a unit and the normal ambient temperature for housing various categories of dog.
- Discuss methods and safety measures for lighting a unit.
- Discuss types of bed/bedding materials, their advantages/disadvantages and how to clean them.
- Describe the appropriate disposal of waste materials (including clinical).
- Explain the principles of cleaning and disinfection and apply safely to animal accommodation and equipment in various situations.
- Discuss hygiene procedures for a hospitalised pet.
- Recognise and describe the use of various items to groom an animal.
- Explain the grooming of an animal, describing the areas requiring particular attention.
- Describe the equipment and procedure required to bath an animal.
- Describe the equipment and procedure to clip claws.
- Describe the appropriate measures for quarantine and isolation.
- Discuss the requirements for the PETS travel scheme.
- Discuss the action taken if a rabies case is suspected.
- Identify the different groups of pedigree dogs as recognised by the Kennel Club and the main groups of pedigree cats as recognised by the Governing Council of the Cat Fancy.

It is essential that those persons who are responsible for animals should have a good basic knowledge of the needs, care and welfare of the normal healthy domestic animal, whether it is in a one-pet household or in a large kennel or cattery. This knowledge can then be built upon so that the many and varied requirements of patients that are entrusted to the care of the veterinary nurse can be taken into account.

Although this chapter is relevant to accommodation for pets and is therefore likely to assist the nurse in advising pet owners, it deals mainly with the care of groups of dogs and cats in kennels or catteries. Veterinary nurses are often responsible for running the hospital kennels, and it is important to understand fully the construction and efficient management of such establishments and their effects on the health and well-being of the animals.

Basic requirements for a kennel or cattery

The design and construction of a kennel or cattery will depend upon its main use. Kennels and catteries range from those owned by private individuals (for housing their pets, breeding and show animals or working dogs) to large boarding, quarantine or dog training establishments, as well as the specialist hospital accommodation provided within veterinary practices. The requirements for the housing of all dogs and cats are basically the same, with some variations for different use of accommodation.

Construction requirements

Essential requirements

Above all, kennels should be designed and managed to meet the needs of the animal to be housed in comfort. This first and most important consideration for the housing of any animal should not be prejudiced by other requirements such as ease of management, as this could result in housing to suit the human operators rather than the animals.

BASIC NEEDS
The animals' basic needs are:
- Warmth, comfort and security.
- Companionship, mental stimulation and opportunities for expression of normal behaviour.
- Exercise as appropriate to the animal.
- Protection as appropriate to the animal.
- Protection from disease and injury.
- Protection from fear and distress.
- Provision for appropriate feeding.
- Opportunities for defecation and urination away from the sleeping area.

Warmth, comfort and security

For the normal healthy dog, a relatively cool environmental temperature is quite acceptable (though it should not drop below 7°C (44°F)) as long as the accommodation is dry and draught free and with suitable and sufficient bedding material. The working party report 'Model Licence Conditions and Guidance for Dog Boarding Establishments' recommends that there must be some part of the dog's sleeping area where the dog is able to enjoy a temperature of at least 10°C (50°F). A higher temperature is required by very young, elderly or ill animals and by some specialist breeds. Under normal circumstances a maximum temperature of 26°C (80°F) should not be exceeded as this becomes uncomfortable for dogs (see Table 6.6, p. 163).

Dogs are generally more relaxed when they feel comfortable and secure. The design of the sleeping area will aid this: they tend to seek out darker areas where they can lie behind or underneath something, or in a corner. All dogs should be given the opportunity to sleep in a conventional sleeping area, which they will usually prefer once settled into kennel life, but they often initially have the desire to create their own sleeping area by moving the bedding material. Some individuals pull the bedding out to the centre of the kennel or into the run if they can. This is a form of nesting behaviour and the dog will often be much more relaxed if it has been able to achieve this, though at times there seems to be quite a frantic period of activity before the dog finally settles.

Cats require a comfortable ambient air temperature of at least 10°C (50°F) in the sleeping area (recommended maximum temperatures as for dogs). The sleeping area should be sited and designed to encourage cats to feel secure and comfortable. A bed should be provided with adequate protective sides. Many shy cats take to the 'igloo' style of bed, which has its own roof. Even a simple upturned cardboard box can give a greater feeling of security in an unfamiliar environment.

Companionship, mental stimulation and opportunities for expression of normal behaviour

Dogs are pack animals by nature and prefer companionship. Domesticated dogs need the attention and physical presence of humans as well as other dogs. Association with the latter can (or, in quarantine, must) be achieved without actual physical contact (see 'Quarantine and Isolation', p. 184).

Kennelled dogs and cats need stimulation – by sight, sound, smell and touch, as found in their normal environment – to avoid boredom and, ultimately, the stereotyped behaviour patterns that boredom would produce. This can be a particular problem in long-stay establishments and in institutional or 'rescue' kennels. Opportunities to look out at distant views may be preferable to face-to-face kennels that encourage dogs to bark at each other.

Exercise

To understand the dog's natural exercise behaviour, it is necessary to look at the domestic animal's wild cousins. These dogs would exercise at a trot over many miles per day, with short bursts at full speed when hunting or at play, interspersed with rest periods (particularly after feeding). This behaviour is modified in the domestic dog, though it is still seen in some working dogs.

Age and health affect exercise requirements, e.g. young adult dogs require more than the middle-aged, elderly or very young. The breed of dog also has an enormous influence on the amount of exercise required. All dogs require daily exercise, though the requirement of gun dogs, herding dogs and sight hounds, for example, is much higher than for toy breeds. Dogs are more contented and relaxed when exercised on a regular daily basis, and so kennel design and practices must take the need for exercise into account.

Cats in a domestic environment exercise themselves by playing hunting games where stalking, pouncing and killing are practised on small inanimate objects. Cats at liberty act in contrast to dogs: they usually walk and then stalk, with jumping and running over short distances only. They jump much higher than dogs and they have the ability to climb. Cats that have outdoor access sometimes range a considerable distance when hunting. They are territorial and identify their territory by scent marking, guarding the area against intruding cats. Intruders have the choice of standing and fighting or running away when challenged.

The normal exercise requirements for cats differ from those of dogs and this should be borne in mind when keeping cats indoors or in a cattery. The cat should be provided with suitable 'toys' to stalk and chase, some of which can be suspended to simulate airborne prey. Opportunity should be provided for cats to climb and jump by providing ledges or similar at different heights. In a cattery, window-sills or similar vantage points are provided within the run.

Protection from disease and injury

This is one of the major contributions made by humans to the well-being of the domestic dog and cat. Many factors contribute to this and in a kennel or cattery environment they are as follows:

- Safe housing: no sharp edges; escape-proof accommodation and secure run fencing; no areas to get caught or fall into; use of non-toxic and non-combustible materials; prevention of access to dangerous areas or materials.
- Hygiene and cleanliness of the living areas, and surrounding environment: specialist kennels for sick dogs (e.g. hospital for non-infectious, isolation for infectious cases).
- Health care: vaccination and antiparasitic control programmes; grooming and checking for abnormalities; prompt recognition of any signs of ill-health, presentation to the veterinarian and subsequent application of prescribed treatments.

Protection from fear and distress

It is important to take into account that if kennelled animals have been parted from their owners and are accustomed to living in a domestic situation, when put into kennels or a cattery for the first time they may be distressed until they become accustomed to the new routine. They should be handled with consideration and care, taking into account their temperament and mental state (recognised by body posture and behaviour). Time should be taken to reassure distressed animals, particularly recent admissions.

Provision of appropriate feeding

Dogs and cats must receive adequate nutrition appropriate to their specific requirements and must have access to clean, fresh drinking-water at all times (unless contraindicated by a specific condition). Automatic drinking-water systems can be incorporated into the design of the kennel. Nutrition requirements are dealt with in Chapter 9.

Opportunities for defecation and urination

Dogs are instinctively reluctant to foul their sleeping area. During early training this instinct is extended to human living areas via house-training. It is therefore necessary to provide frequent opportunities for urination or defecation in designated areas to avoid the breakdown of this training.

Dogs prefer to relieve themselves on a similar surface to the area they used as puppies, which is often grass. This behaviour will probably have to be modified during a stay in the kennels, as grass is not practical for kennel 'relief areas' due to reasons of hygiene. However, the preference should be borne in mind if a particular dog is very reluctant to relieve itself in the designated concrete area.

Exercise is the time used by many owners to give their dogs the opportunities for urination and defecation, but elimination behaviour should be separated from free exercise where possible. Many local authorities have laws on the fouling of public areas by dogs and so owners are encouraged to 'relieve' their dogs on command in their own gardens before exercising. Alternatively they should clean up after their dogs; this is easier if the command is given just before exercise so that the faeces are easily found and removed.

When dogs are in kennels, therefore, it is important that opportunities for urination and defecation are regular and are separate from exercise periods, so that training habits are not disrupted.

Cats are also instinctively reluctant to foul their sleeping area and they usually have the desire to bury their excreta. This assists greatly in normal domestic house-training as loose, readily dug materials considered suitable by the cat can be provided by the owner in a 'litter' tray. Sometimes cats will deposit faeces that remain uncovered for marking their territory.

Cats which do not have free access to areas that they would naturally find suitable (e.g. loose soil) should be provided with litter trays containing material that they find acceptable. The trays should be regularly cleaned and replenished.

Design factors for kennels and catteries

They should be built for the purpose for which the animals are housed (Table 6.1).

They should meet all local authority licensing, building, planning requirements and regulations.

They should be designed with reference to the factors set out in Table 6.2 together with the frequently incorporated facilities as set out in Table 6.3.

The sizes and construction materials depend upon the proposed use of the kennels. Many kennel owners refer to recommended boarding kennel sizes and construction details when building private kennelling, and this is increas-

Table 6.1 Examples of kennels and uses
Private owner unlicensed: pet dogs   gun dogs/herding dogs   small-scale breeding (one or two bitches)   show dogs
Private owner licensed breeding (two breeding bitches or more)[*]
Boarding kennels/cattery[a]
Training kennels: Police, customs, security, defence   Guide dogs for the blind, hearing dogs for the deaf, dogs for the disabled, etc.
Charity rescue kennels   e.g. Blue Cross, NCDL, RSPCA, Wood Green Animal Shelters, etc.
Quarantine kennels
Veterinary practices with hospital kennels

[a] *Need to be licensed. Requirements are available from the licensing body as regards building materials and accommodation sizes*

Table 6.2 Factors in kennel and cattery design
Adequate accessibility for safe handling, cleaning maintenance and emergency
Maximum efficiency, e.g. easy to clean, positioning of fixtures and fittings
Adequate care facilities such as grooming, food preparation and treatment areas
To meet all current health, safety and fire prevention regulations
Designed for the purpose, e.g. quarantine kennels – high security and no contact between animals
To meet all licensing and planning and building regulations
Proposed kennel site has suitable: Ground for building   Size of plot   Water drainage   Access and availability of local services

Table 6.3 Frequently incorporated facilities in a kennel or cattery	
Kitchen with food stores	It is advisable to have the kitchen separate from the kennel blocks, particularly if it is to service more than one block. Where it is separate, each kennel block should have a small utility area with worktops and sink, for final mixing of feeds, washing of dishes, etc. The main dog and cat kitchen should be easy to clean and disinfect
Stores for equipment, disinfectants, cat litter, bedding, etc.	The size of the stores will depend upon the size of the kennels and the types of material used. Relatively large storage areas may be required if it is possible to bulk-buy items
Grooming and bathing room	The size of the grooming area, type of bath and equipment held depend on the use. Some kennels run animal grooming services where owners bring the animals in for the day; they therefore require a large fully kitted grooming and bathing room with small holding kennels. Where the grooming facilities are for boarding/hospitalised animals a small area in each kennel block may be used for grooming individuals. A small central bath room/area can then be used if bathing of animals is fairly infrequent
Surgery or veterinary consulting room	This room, built as a separate facility for non-veterinary practice kennels, is usually only necessary for large establishments. Separate facilities are particularly useful where the animals are long-stay and the population is relatively static. It is more usual for the animal to be examined and treated either in its own housing or in a hospital ward where suitable examination facilities are made available.

ingly made easier by the availability of ready-made sectional kennelling. Medium-sized to large establishments tend to build traditional permanent buildings, built to a specific design using suitable permanent materials such as brick or breeze-block structures.

The walls have impervious coverings and are built on foundations. Internal concrete flooring is laid with a minimum fall of 1 in 80 running towards built-in drains, or guttering and drains. The floor is then either painted, tiled, or covered with asphalt, vinyl or similar internal flooring material in such a way as to prevent pooling of liquids. Materials that can be moulded up at the edges and secured to create a watertight seal with the walls are particularly useful. Any material for kennel or cattery flooring must be impervious and capable of being regularly hosed and disinfected, in addition to being non-slip (even when wet) for the safety of both animals and kennel personnel.

Sound-proofing

All kennels have a potential noise problem caused by the barking of the dogs and every effort should be made to prevent barking becoming a problem. The effective handling and control of the dogs is of great importance. All staff should be aware of dog behaviour, including why dogs bark and how to reduce the noise. Where a dog is barking from excitement, it should be handled calmly and firmly – and without shouting, as this can in itself contribute to further excitement and noise.

Staff cannot be in the kennel 24 hours a day and spontaneous barking will usually occur if the dogs are disturbed by external noises. Efficient sound-proofing will reduce the likelihood of such disturbance as well as assist in reducing the noise of barking reaching outside the kennels. Sound-proofing is achieved by either absorbing the sound, deadening it with suitable materials rather than reflecting it from hard surfaces, or preventing the free passage and escape of the sound from the buildings and perimeters (Table 6.4).

Purpose-built kennel blocks

Individual kennels designed and arranged together in a group under one roof are generally referred to as a kennel block. There are many different designs for differing requirements, each with certain advantages and disadvantages. The main features of the more common designs (run-access, corridor kennels, circular 'parasol' and 'H'-block kennels) are illustrated in Fig. 6.1.

Surfaces and materials used in modern kennelling

(1) Wood – traditionally used for animal housing:

- Inexpensive.
- Warm.
- Easy to erect.
- Has a relatively short life.
- Requires constant maintenance.
- Easily damaged by animals.
- Difficult to clean and disinfect.
- As more modern materials become available it is being used less.

(2) Stainless steel:

- Durable.
- Easy to clean and disinfect.
- Easy to maintain.
- Can be cold and hard, so good bedding required.
- Can be noisy when animals bang or move about.

Table 6.4 Sound-proofing	
Absorbing the sound	Use of acoustic tiles or materials with similar properties on upper walls and ceiling (hard surfaces are preferable for hygienic reasons lower down)
	Tiles must be out of dogs' reach (easily damaged if chewed or scratched)
	Some acoustic tiles cannot be cleaned/disinfected easily – careful use of spray disinfectant for those that should not be wetted may be possible (check with tile manufacturer). Washable tiles are now available but can be damaged with rough use
Preventing the free passage and escape of sound	Construct the building to prevent free passage of sound down corridors: use double doors offset to one another
	Double glazing throughout the kennels
	Perimeter structures such as earth mounds or 'bunds' surrounding the kennels – require additional space and are expensive but can be very effective
	To be fully effective they must be at least as high as the kennel roof
	There must be no near neighbours with buildings higher than the mounds
	Other structures that take up less space:
	'Green' or 'willow' walls of woven willow fencing and earth. Shrubs are planted in these 'walls' to stabilise and create an attractive appearance
	Tree belts require a large area for maximum effect with bushy non-deciduous trees/shrubs

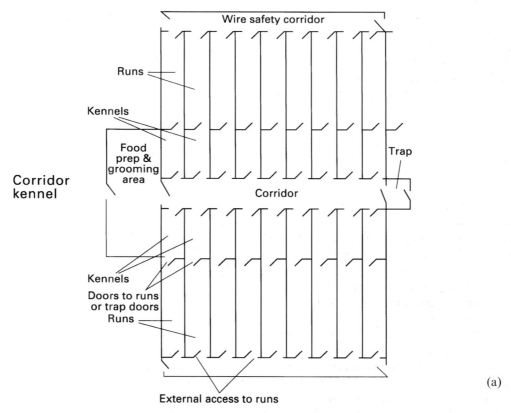

(a)

Fig. 6.1 Main kennel types. (The design of the 'H'-block kennel is credited to the Guide Dogs for the Blind Association and architects Abbey Hanson Rowe Partnership. The circular kennel plan is courtesy of the Animal Inn, Deal, Kent.)

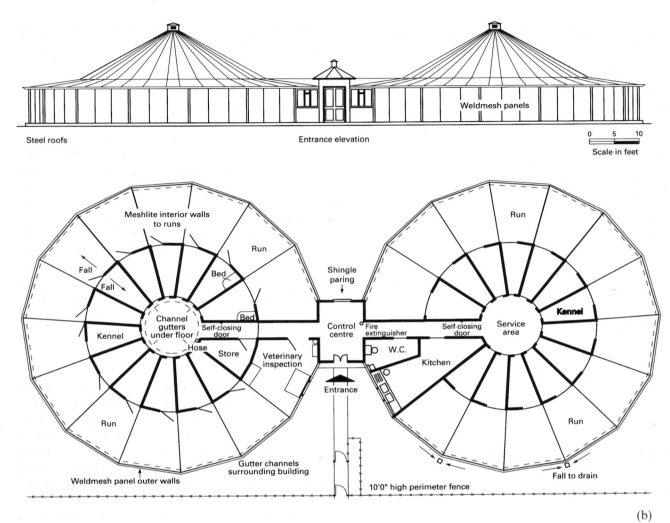

Steel roofs   Entrance elevation

Weldmesh panels

Scale in feet
0   5   10

Meshlite interior walls
to runs

Run

Fall

Fall

Bed

Bed

Channel
gutters
under floor

Self-closing
door

Kennel

Hose

Store

Run

Veterinary
inspection

Shingle
paring

Control
centre

Fire
extinguisher

Self-closing
door

W.C.

Kitchen

Service
area

Kennel

Run

Run

Entrance

Gutter channels
surrounding building

Weldmesh panel outer walls

Fall to drain

10'0" high perimeter fence

(b)

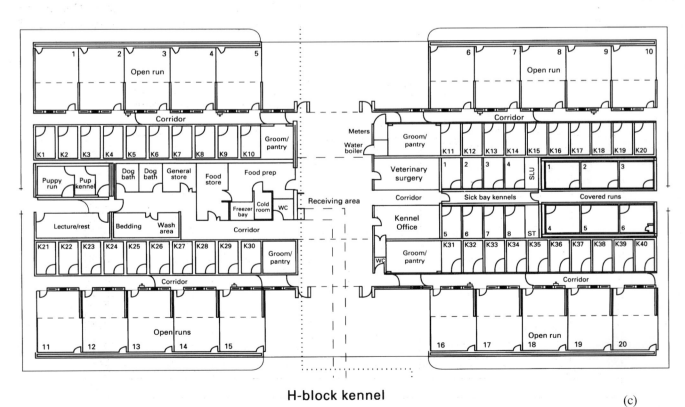

H-block kennel

(c)

Fig. 6.1 (*continued*)

(3) Metal – used for doors, frames, supports and run panels:

- Durable if correctly maintained.
- Maintenance is considerably less if galvanised metal is used.

(4) Tiles – often used for floors and lower walls:

- Easy to clean and disinfect.
- Attractive appearance.
- Can be expensive to install.

(5) Plastic – modern forms of plastic are evolving and used more frequently within animal accommodation as beds.
- Inexpensive and lightweight.
- Care should be taken regarding cleaning and disinfection as some plastic is susceptible to damage.

Ease of cleaning, low maintenance costs and noise reduction will influence the choice of construction.

Check with manufacturers that materials are suitable for use in animal housing both for construction and cleaning.

Cattery design and construction

The essential requirements in cattery design are similar to those for housing dogs, but two further factors must be taken into account:

- The cat's agility in climbing to escape.

- The greater risk of infectious respiratory disease among cats, which means that segregation is more important.

Outdoor catteries

These are similar to the run-access kennels for dogs, with entrance to the cat accommodation through the outdoor run. Major differences are that the run is totally roofed (part of which must be translucent) and that the run access is via a safety passage covered with mesh to prevent any likelihood of escape. The cat accommodation units are side by side, with full height 'sneeze barriers' and/or gaps of 0.6–1.2 m (2–4 ft) minimum between the runs (Fig. 6.2). Correctly positioned and managed, outdoor catteries provide the least risk for cross-infection between cats. This advantage can be lost if two of the blocks are positioned with their runs facing into the same safety passage from opposite sides.

Indoor catteries

Indoor catteries are similar in layout to corridor kennels for dogs, with access to each cat housing unit via a central passage. The major disadvantage is the risk of cross-infection due to air exchange between the units via the central passage. The exterior doors from the units on both sides of the block open into totally enclosed runs. Each unit is completely enclosed, to prevent escape, with roofing of runs as for outdoor catteries. Within the cattery building, the doors and internal partitions should be solidly constructed to prevent air circulation between the units. Due to the increased risk of cross-infection, good ventilation is of

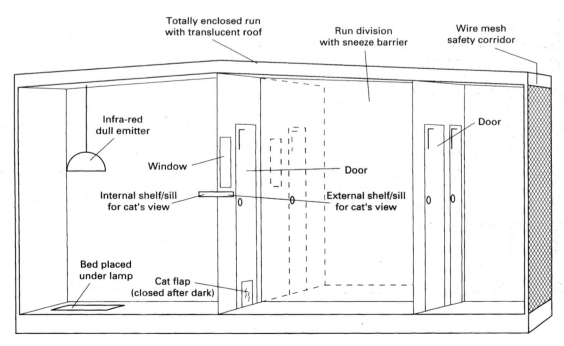

Fig. 6.2 Outdoor cattery design.

major importance in an indoor cattery. (Ventilation is discussed later in this chapter.) The solid doors between the units and central corridor must have viewing panels incorporated in all new catteries to allow the inspection of the whole area.

Cattery windows

It is recommended in the 'Model Licence Conditions and Guidance for Cat Boarding Establishments' that each sleeping compartment should have its own window, with a shelf beneath it to allow natural daylight into the unit and to permit the cat to look out. Due to the agility of cats, windows may pose a security risk and therefore must be escape-proof at all times. It is therefore recommended that windows are either protected by welded mesh, or be made of reinforced glass, polycarbonate or other impact-resistant material.

CATTERY UNIT SIZES
Recommended in 'Model Licence Conditions and Guidance for Cat Boarding Establishments'. Sleeping areas can be at ground level or raised (penthouses).

No. of cats	Sleeping area size (min) sq m (sq ft)	Exercise area size (min) sq m (sq ft)
1 cat	0.85 (9)	1.70 (18)
2 cats	1.50 (16)	2.23 (24)
4 cats (max)	1.85 (20)	2.79 (30)

Height of sleeping area at least 91 cm (3ft).

Raised sleeping areas must be a minimum of 91 cm (3 ft) above floor level with a maximum depth of 106 cm (3 ft 6 inches).

Minimum internal height of unit 1.8 m (6 ft).

Specialised animal housing

Specialised housing is used for animals that have specific needs regarding their environment and care. Specialised housing includes:

- Hospital kennelling.
- Whelping kennelling.
- Puppy kennelling.
- Isolation kennelling (covered later in this chapter).
- Dangerous and stray dog kennelling.

Hospital kennelling

Hospital kennels or cages are designed and constructed for animals that are undergoing treatment or for post-operative convalescence. These short-stay animals require a high degree of supervision and the kennelling is deliberately restrictive in size (Table 6.5). In many cases strict rest is required, particularly for post-operative animals that may dislodge sutures, etc.

It should be remembered that these units are designed for a short stay. Where animals do not specifically require confinement and their stay is likely to be medium to long term, they should be housed in a larger kennel.

Hospital kennelling can be either of the 'walk-in' type or the more restricting 'locker' type. It is usual to have a choice of both types in a hospital ward to allow selection of the most suitable housing for each animal, depending upon the animal's size and temperament and the degree of confinement required.

Metabolic kennels

Metabolic monitoring kennels, available in some veterinary hospitals, are usually smaller and therefore even more confining than standard hospital kennels. Animals are only housed in them for the short duration of any tests before

---

Table 6.5 Hospital kennel sizes (locker type): some size ranges in common use

Type/size of animal	Width cm	(inches)	Height cm	(inches)	Depth cm	(inches)
Cats	45.72	(18)	45.72–60.96	(18–24)	72.39	(28.25 or slightly less)
Dogs Small breeds	60.96–76.20	(24–30)	45.72–76.20	(18–30)	72.39	(28.25 or slightly less)
Medium breeds	76.20–91.44	(30–36)	76.20–91.44	(30–36)	72.39	(28.25 or slightly more)
Large breeds	121.92	(48)	(76.20–91.44)	(30–36)	72.39–100	(28.25)–(39.4)
Giant breeds	152.40–182.88	(60–70)	91.44	(36)	72.39–100	(28.25)–(39.4)
Walk-in kennels	approx 140 cm	55	180	70	100	(28.25)–(39.4)

With the smaller sized kennels where space is limited and for top rows the depth can be reduced from 72.39 cm (28.25 inches) to 60.96 cm (24 inches) or a minimum of 45.72 cm (18 inches)

being rehoused in standard hospital kennelling. Facilities to collect urine may be required which can be achieved by installing suitable flooring.

Intensive care kennels

Some form of intensive care kennelling is available in many hospitals. It is usually in the form of an airtight kennel with the supply of oxygen to the interior. The front of the kennel is transparent to allow constant observation of critically ill animals.

Specialist requirements

Due to the diversity of animal sizes and their conditions it is necessary to provide some kennels that enable specialist care to be given both for the comfort of the animal and procedures to be carried out. One example of a specialist requirement is for a paraplegic animal. The access for staff for safe and appropriate lifting and handling operations in addition to the comfort of the animal is most important.

Whelping kennelling

A whelping kennel and its run should be large enough to accommodate a whelping bitch and her litter up to at least 6 weeks of age. The whelping box should be designed to allow the use of an additional heating unit (such as an infrared dull emitter) and to give the bitch privacy, with an observation panel that enables staff to observe her unnoticed. Kennelling must be escape-proof; a bitch should never leave the confines of the whelping area, because of the high risk of introducing disease to her pups from contact with other dogs. The whelping kennels should be situated away from other dog housing and be managed in a similar manner to the isolation unit detailed later in this chapter, to achieve 'protective isolation' for the vulnerable pups.

In a hospital, it is highly unlikely that the bitch and pups will be housed longer than the duration of the whelping itself. It is therefore only necessary to have a kennel large enough to hold the whelping bed but it should be in the quietest site available. The bitch and pups should still be subject to protective isolation procedures within the hospital environment.

Puppy kennelling

Breeding kennels and others that commonly house very young animals for a short time usually require safe housing for these vulnerable animals. Puppy kennels should be situated away from adult dogs and managed so as to reduce the risk of unvaccinated youngsters coming into contact with disease. A puppy kennel should be able to house an additional heating unit, with any possible contact with electric wiring totally eliminated.

There must be no gaps between the dividing partitions and the floor of kennelling and runs as puppies can squeeze through very small spaces, including those used for drainage in the kennels of adult dogs.

Where litters of puppies are to be housed, a divided 'stable door' is invaluable: when its top half is opened, attending staff can step over the closed bottom half which confines the pups. When a standard kennel door is opened, it can be very difficult to stop a number of pups escaping or, worse, getting trapped by the door.

Dangerous and stray dogs

Any dog, irrespective of breeding or size, can be difficult or dangerous under certain circumstances. This does not refer to the types specifically referred to in the Dangerous Dogs' Act of 1991 (amended 1997). Stray dogs of unknown origin can be unpredictable often due to stress rather than inherent aggression. Any considered even potentially dangerous should be treated with care. Security is paramount. Ideally, access to both the kennel and the run should be via separate secure service passages with separate doors into the kennel and run. When accessing the kennel or run, care should be taken to ensure that security doors/ gates to the service passages and to the dog's accommodation area are securely closed. For particularly nervous and potentially unpredictable dogs, a well-adjusted collar and trailing lead is beneficial both for handlers and inmates initially. However, this should be removed as soon as the dog's confidence is gained. Communication is essential. Initially, staff levels permitting, approach by two people is useful, particularly if housing conditions are not ideal, i.e. no access from run to exterior. It is not unknown for personnel to be trapped in a kennel with a difficult dog and unable to summon help because of the noise surrounding the inmates. Many kennels specialise in accommodating dogs known to be difficult. They provide means of personal communication to all members of staff, e.g. mobile phone, walkie-talkies, etc. Consider also communication in the form of meticulous labelling with any notes regarding particular idiosyncrasies such as not attempting to groom without muzzling. Conventional red lettering alerts personnel. A quick release grasper should be readily available but remember a nervous/ difficult aggressive dog, once secured on a grasper, is likely to be more difficult next time!

Kennel services

Ventilation

Ventilation must be provided in kennels and catteries to:

- Provide transmission of clean air for the animals and staff by removing any foul air containing fumes, obnoxious gases and smells, e.g. stale air (CO_2 from exhalation), ammonia, methane and unpleasant odours from animal soiling.

- Reduce to a minimum the concentration of possible airborne infective agents that may cause disease.

The two types of ventilation commonly used in kennels are known as active and passive.

Active ventilation

Active ventilation mechanically pulls air into or out of the kennels, usually by means of extractor fans or an air-conditioning system. In the case of air-conditioning, a heat exchange system to prevent loss of heat from the unit can be incorporated with a heating system, providing a dual-purpose ventilation and heating system.

In some specialised kennels much thought is given to the ventilation system and attempts are made to reduce the potential transmission of airborne infection. The aim is to introduce clean air into each kennel, and extract the 'used' air from the kennel, in such a way as to reduce the likelihood that the air exhaled by one animal is inhaled by another. There are two common systems: either air-conditioning with induction vent or extractor fan with vent.

Air-conditioning system with induction vent

In this system there is an induction vent in each kennel unit, actively pushing air into the kennel from an external 'clean' source such as the central area of the kennel roof. The air is actively extracted by another vent immediately outside the individual kennel in the corridor (Fig. 6.3).

Air-conditioning units are usually installed to suit the conditions within the unit when closed, which means that leaving doors and windows open can affect their efficiency. Always seek advice from the manufacturers or installation engineers to ensure effective management and operation.

Active ventilation enables control over the number of air changes per hour, usually set at 6 for kennels, with the ability to increase up to 12 changes (or to decrease the rate in some circumstances), depending on weather conditions, number of kennel occupants, etc.

Extractor fan and vent
Vents to introduce air are placed in the kennels and are themselves passive, the air being drawn through them by the activity of the extractor fan. The success of the system depends upon the correct placing of the vents in relation to the extractor fan. Figure 6.4 demonstrates the system in use in a circular 'parasol' kennel. The system is also suitable for the smaller indoor catteries and small-scale hospital accommodation.

This system can be used in reverse, with air drawn in through the central fan rather than being extracted by it. This creates positive pressure so that the air is forced out through the passive vents.

Even though a ventilation system is designed to reduce airborne infection in a working kennel, it should be remembered that it is not infallible. There is a strong possibility of the transmission of airborne infection if the dogs are passing along the corridor to grooming, relief areas or for exercise, also if they are allowed to exercise in adjoining runs with free airflow between them. For disease control, in addition to a scientific ventilation system:

- The kennels should be managed in such a way as to reduce likely contact, particularly at high-risk times (e.g. when kennel cough is known to be affecting dogs in the area, or the kennels are full). All staff should be aware of the risk of airborne disease and be able to quickly identify suspect cases.
- Animals infected or suspected of being infected should be placed in an isolation unit immediately and their living area promptly and thoroughly disinfected.

Passive ventilation

Passive ventilation is achieved by opening and closing vents, windows and doors. Although widely used in many kennels

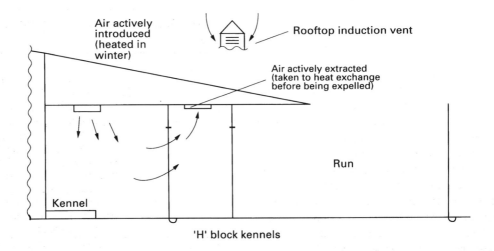

Fig. 6.3 Active ventilation: air-conditioning system with vents.

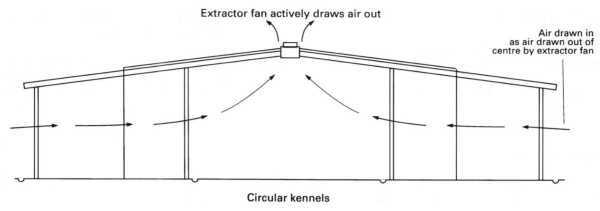

Fig. 6.4 Active ventilation: extraction fan and vents.

and found to be satisfactory for situations where only a few animals are kept, there are some disadvantages:

- No control over air changes.
- Draughts may be caused.
- Loss of heat may be a problem.
- Open windows and doors increase noise risks.

Insulation and heating

Insulation and heating are provided for several reasons:

- For the warmth and comfort of the dogs.
- To enable rapid drying of kennels and service areas after cleaning and disinfection (heating combined with through airflow provides the most rapid drying).
- For the maintenance of buildings and contents (without heating, some deterioration or damage may occur – such as the freezing and fracturing of insufficiently insulated water pipes). A good heating system, combined with proper ventilation, also controls condensation, the dampness of which leads to mould and other problems.
- To a lesser extent, for the comfort and health of staff working in the kennel area: they will also benefit from dry, well-ventilated and warm environments.

Temperature control

It is advisable to check the temperature at different sites within the kennel building, particularly within the kennels themselves. The use of a 'maximum/minimum' environmental thermometer can be helpful in assessing the variations in temperatures throughout the day and night. The range may be significant enough to warrant changes to the system. During the day the general opening and closing of doors associated with the normal running of kennels may have a noticeable effect. During the night, when there is no movement, the temperature range and air quality may be significantly different from that in the daytime. Table 6.6 gives recommended environmental temperatures for housing dogs.

Types of heating

Heating for kennelling and catteries should be:

- Economical to install and run.
- Easy to control, operate and maintain.
- Safe, i.e. not easily knocked over, with no naked flames and free from fumes.

Various options are available for heating kennels but they generally fall into two groups: environmental or 'central' heating of the whole kennel space and local heating for individual animals.

Central heating is controlled by a thermostat. Local heating is more economical to run: it provides additional heat for individuals with special needs, enabling the overall environmental temperature of the block to be lower so that it is more comfortable for individuals not requiring such a high degree of warmth. This allows animals with different needs to be housed in the same block. Table 6.7 sets out the advantages and disadvantages of typical systems used for both central and local heating.

Table 6.6 Environmental temperatures for housing dogs	
Adult dogs	Should not drop below 7°C (44°F). Boarding/private kennels in sleeping area at least 10°C (50°F)
Whelping and puppy accommodation	18–21°C (65–70°F), with the temperature in the whelping bed for pups in the nest at 26–29°C (80–85°F) during their first week, 21–26°C (70–80°F) in their second week, then 20°C (68°F) thereafter until weaning The pups require a higher temperature than the bitch. The bitch can leave the bed if she becomes too hot without the pups becoming chilled
Hospital and isolation kennels	Usually 18–21°C (65–70°F) Should not fall below 15.5°C (60°F)

Table 6.7 Types of heating: advantages and disadvantages

Type	Advantages	Disadvantages
Central heating:		
Gas, oil or electrical boilers	Easy to operate and maintain Commonly available	The corridor can be often warmer than the kennels if a thermostat or thermometer is not correctly positioned
Electrical underfloor heating	Floors dry very quickly Animals have local heating	Floors can become uncomfortably hot if the unit is poorly insulated Animal faeces dry hard to the floor making removal difficult. Repair costs can be expensive
Electric fan-assisted warm air heating	Provides rapid heat by circulating heated air	Placing a heater too close to a patient's kennel could be dangerous and overheating of the patient could occur Can be noisy and expensive to run with prolonged use
Total air conditioning/heating system	Heat and clean air can be fed directly into individual kennels and extracted in the corridor, ensuring the kennels themselves are the correct temperature and air extraction reduces the air flow from kennel to kennel, which is advantageous in reducing the distribution of airborne infections	Expensive to install and not suitable for many types of kennel design with low roofs Running costs may be higher in winter
Local heating		
Infra-red dull emitter	Easy to install Produces direct heat without light, aiding restfulness The height of the unit can be adjusted	Requires a power point either in each kennel or the means to direct an electric lead safely into the kennel, with lead and unit well out of reach of the animal Unless correctly positioned or is thermostatically controlled the animal may be either too hot or cold Fires can occur if hung too low or not firmly fixed If water is splashed onto the bulb this may cause it to burst
Heated bed/pad	The animal can be directly heated by contact with a low constant heat being emitted from directly below	Frequently damaged by chewing (even when metal casing is used for wires) leading to a risk of electrocution of animal. These should be used with a circuit breaker to minimise the risk There is an increased risk of contamination as they are in direct contact with an animal and may prove difficult to disinfect thoroughly Some users feel that continual contact with a heated surface can lead to hair loss
Hot-water bottles	Inexpensive, rapid, direct warmth They are suitable for sending home with tiny puppies or kittens after a caesarean operation (with the water at normal body temperature)	There is a danger of the water being too hot and burning the animal Risk of bursting/wetting and/or scalding the animal, if it bites or claws the hot water bottle. Water cools rapidly and therefore should only be used for short-term emergency use where an animal can be supervised
Electrically heated oil-filled radiators	Mobile and relatively safe as there is no single concentrated heat source	Can take some time to heat up and may not benefit the animals for some time after switching on

Important note. For all types of heating the manufacturer should be consulted as to its suitability for the use intended. It should always be maintained and used as recommended by the manufacturer

Insulation and draught-proofing

Whatever type of heating is installed, it will not be efficient or economical if heat can easily be dissipated due to poor insulation or draughts.

Automatic door closers may be found helpful. If doors and windows are unnecessarily left open when the heating is operating, this will obviously also reduce the effectiveness of the heating systems.

In cat accommodation, cat flaps are required in the door from the sleeping area to permit access for the cat to the run. As this is a potential source of draughts, positioning and design of the flaps should be taken into account when constructing catteries.

Lighting

It is necessary for the kennels to be well lit so that all procedures can be carried out effectively and safely, from cleaning the kennels to safe handling and effective observation of the boarders.

Lighting and its effects on dogs

Dogs require mental stimulation for their general wellbeing, and in this the use of sight plays its part. It is therefore important for the welfare of the dog that adequate lighting is provided during the active hours of daylight. This may seem obvious but, in kennels that have no natural light through windows, the dogs can be left in total darkness when staff switch off the lights. The dog should be able to observe other dogs and staff, creating an interesting environment, preventing boredom.

It is preferable to allow as much natural light as possible but to bear in mind the likelihood of overheating the kennels in mid-summer.

Lighting and restfulness

While it is necessary to have good lighting to create an interesting environment during the active daylight hours, it is also necessary to have reduced lighting in sleeping areas to encourage rest.

During daylight periods of inactivity, dogs take short periods of rest. To sleep, they often seek out darker areas. This should be taken into account when designing kennel sleeping areas, e.g. a 'skylight' over the sleeping bench should be avoided. Where a great deal of natural light is provided (via windows and glass doors) it is useful to be able to reduce this overnight so that the dogs are more restful and less likely to bark. In winter, the long hours of darkness achieve this naturally, but in summer months the dogs become restless at dawn and start to bark, which can cause problems with neighbours.

Artificial lighting

It is usually necessary to supplement natural light with some form of artificial lighting in a kennel block. The most commonly used is fluorescent strip lighting with a diffuser, which provides few shadows and is therefore helpful when cleaning.

The lighting is usually situated in the corridor, or in the central area of circular kennel blocks. If this does not provide sufficient visibility for cleaning, bulkhead lights can be positioned in the kennels. These are securely attached, to either the ceiling or the upper wall, and are completely covered. Hanging light-bulbs are not recommended: some dogs may try to grab them if they dangle low, and there is also a danger of kennel staff knocking the bulbs while scrubbing out the kennels.

All wiring and switches should be inaccessible to the dogs and all electrical fittings should be protected from contact with water. One method is to use waterproof switch units and screw-on covers for power points when not in use.

Beds and bedding

Beds are used to contain the animal while resting or sleeping. They should provide a sanctuary where the animal may retire to feel safe and secure. The bed will represent its own territory in the kennels.

For these reasons all dogs and cats, whether housed in human accommodation or in any type of kennelling, should have a bed. The basic requirements for most types of bed are that they should:

- Be raised to some extent from the floor.
- Give easy access for the animal (particularly the old and very young).
- Have sides and back (and front where used) high enough to prevent draughts, to promote the animal's feeling of security and to contain the bedding material.

Types of bed

Many types of bed are available for purchase (Table 6.8). The majority are designed with the domestic pet owner in mind, rather than for kennel use, although some are suitable for both. Most require the addition of bedding material but some have this incorporated in the bed.

Bedding

Bedding is used:

- To provide warmth by insulation of the animal's body heat.
- To provide comfort, by allowing padding between the animal and hard surfaces.
- To avoid injury from constant contact between skin over bony areas and hard surfaces that cause pressure or 'bed' sores.

Table 6.8 Types of bed for domestic animals

Type of bed	Use	Advantages	Disadvantages
Wicker basket (with blanket or similar)	Domestic	Popular with owners, flexible, attractive, traditional	Chewed by some dogs, difficult to clean/disinfect, may harbour flea eggs
Bean bag (with outer cover)	Domestic	Polystyrene beads insulate and mould to body shape assisting comfort can be arranged by dog Outer cover is washed/disinfected	Bean bag difficult to wash. Not suitable for chewers as small holes allow the polystyrene beads to escape
Foam and fabric (traditionally shaped) Used with own foam pad, additional blankets can be used	Domestic	Flexible, beds are machine washable Light and easy to transport	Easily destroyed by chewing
Metal frame bed	Domestic	Raises animal well off floor, removable covers or blankets used to allow washing, folds up for transport	Some elderly animals may have difficulty getting in
Radiator cat beds Fixed, radiator used with own cover, additional blankets can be used	Domestic	Removable washable cover	Cannot always be conveniently placed as it protrudes from the top of a radiator. Elderly/very young or infirm cats may not be able to get in. Warm while radiator is on, but will be less comfortable when the heating is off, e.g. at night
Plastic moulded Used with foam pad/blankets	Domestic or kennels	Widely available in many sizes They can be washed and adequately disinfected	May be chewed by some dogs, resulting in quite sharp edges being formed Occasionally animals have allergic reactions to prolonged contact with some types of plastic, especially if the dog's nose rests on the plastic
Sleeping benches *Fixed (built-in plinth):* Benches are either a slightly raised floor in one area, or projecting from a wall with supports. Bedding material must be used	Kennels	Permanent and not easily damaged	They may have difficult corners to clean/disinfect depending on design
Removable: Slide/lift out. Fold down Wood laminated (aluminium reinforced edges) Bedding material must be used		Are removable for cleaning etc	Some benches may be chewed by some dogs if any unreinforced edges are accessible

Properties of suitable bedding material:

- It should be a good insulator.
- It should be soft and flat with some give, and large enough to accommodate a stretched-out animal (it is important that older animals should not be forced to sleep curled up), but it can be arranged by the animal when curling up to sleep.
- It should permit drainage of body fluids. This is essential in keeping ill or incontinent animals dry.
- It should not contain anything that is harmful if ingested or is irritant, for example, to skin or eyes.
- It should be easy to physically manage.
- It should be easily cleaned, disinfected or disposed of.
- It should be easy to store.

- It should not soil or damage the animal's coat.
- It should be economical to use – inexpensive if disposable – durable, long-lasting and not easily chewed or destroyed if reusable.

The materials that are commonly used for bedding are either disposable or non-disposable (Table 6.9).

Non-disposable bedding   Non-disposable materials are laundered, disinfected and re-used; they are used mainly in longer-stay kennels. They can be expensive to purchase and require suitable facilities for laundering and disinfection. The size of storage area for this type of bedding is far less than for the disposable type as less stock is required. Non-disposable bedding includes blankets, acrylic bedding and covered foam pads.

Table 6.9 Types of bedding	
Non-disposable	**Disposable**
Blankets Expensive unless donated or old blankets used, may be chewed and torn up by some destructive dogs. Not suitable for dogs with allergies due to dust mites unless laundered regularly using very hot washing water Blankets are traditional, warm and are often used in domestic circumstances. Owners like to see them in kennels and many dogs benefit from being able to make their own 'nest' and therefore reduce kennel stress Not suitable for hospital kennels or for animals with infectious illness as they are difficult to sterilise	**Newspaper** Widely used by kennels and hospitals It is freely available and absorbent Used to line the bed area with a blanket or similar on top It is not warm or comfortable by itself (unless shredded) Newsprint may stain light coloured coats and kennelling, particularly when wet
Deep pile 'veterinary' bedding Widely used both domestically and in kennels Expensive to purchase but more resistant to chewing than blankets Easier to launder than blankets as resorbent to organic material/dried-on debris usually removed by soaking Suitable for hospital use as it allows body fluids through, keeping animals relatively comfortable and dry Helps to reduce the occurrence of pressure sores in elderly and recumbent animals	**Shredded paper** Warmer than newspaper due to bulk If shredded newspaper is used staining as mentioned may occur Can be messy to deal with in kennels, unless properly retained It may stick to wounds (particularly if weeping) and to animal's coat, if damp Healthy dogs appear to enjoy arranging it and burying their toys in it. Some dogs may eat small quantities usually causing them little harm
Covered foam pads Used with a traditionally shaped foam-and-fabric or plastic-moulded bed. They can be badly damaged or destroyed by destructive dogs Easily laundered, warm and comfortable. Helps to reduce the occurrence of pressure sores Thick foam pads covered with waterproof material are useful in a hospital where very large breeds are recumbent Due to the thickness and size they are very difficult to launder. The waterproof covering can be cleaned/disinfected by using chemical disinfectant	

Disposable bedding   Disposable materials are relatively inexpensive and are discarded once soiled. A large stock of materials will be required and needs a suitable storage area situated as near to the kennel accommodation as possible.

Provision must also be made for disposal according to current regulations. Commonly used disposable materials include newspaper, shredded paper and woodwool. Less frequently used (and not advised for regular use) are straw, straw bags, peat, woodshavings and sawdust.

General principles of kennel and cattery management

Kennel and cattery management consists of ensuring a planned and methodical approach, by designing and executing efficient routines and procedures for the care and welfare of the animals. Such management will ensure that:

- All tasks are carried out in a logical order, with the needs of the animals high in priority.
- The best possible use is made of labour and materials.

- All staff are fully instructed about how to carry out their tasks.
- All staff are aware of set standards and can recognise when they have been achieved.
- Health and safety regulations observed.
- Consistency of standards is maintained by supervision and by checking procedures.
- Morale of staff is kept high by making them fully aware of what is expected and the reasons for carrying out their tasks.
- Confidence generated by the staff and management conveys to clients that their animals are being well cared for.

Kennel management procedures

The kennel manager should design and introduce set procedures within the kennel to ensure smooth running and minimise error. These should be supported by some form of documentation for records and checking purposes. Set procedures should include admission (intake of animals), discharge (animals leaving the kennels) and others as appropriate to the type of kennels.

Documentation

All documentation must be:

- Legible and accurate.
- Up-to-date and relevant.
- Able to record action taken.
- In the correct terminology.

Kennel cleaning and disinfection

All animals require a hygienic environment in order to remain healthy. Where animals are housed in large numbers or the population is constantly changing, an effective cleaning and disinfecting routine should be in place and strictly followed.

Daily cleaning

Whilst animals are resident, one thorough daily cleansing (and disinfection where conditions dictate) using the method described later should be sufficient and is better than, say, three half-hearted floor wipes with a cloth or mop and bucket. When animals accidentally soil their accommodation, this should be dealt with on a local area basis and must be attended to at once.

Tidying kennels

For removal of dust and hair from the kennel during the day, consider the use of a vacuum cleaner. It is more effective and less time consuming than a broom or dustpan and brush and it reduces the amount of water used in kennels. (Take care to use a quiet machine and be aware that some animals may object to the noise). At this point the bedding is usually tidied and shaken out.

Cleaning and disinfection on departure

On an animal's departure from the kennels, its accommodation and fittings must be thoroughly cleaned and disinfected, and preferably left empty for a few days. All bedding is removed and either disposed of or disinfected. If disinfecting bedding, some types of detergent/disinfectant may be used in washing machines, e.g. halogenated tertiary amines (that are a mix of special detergents and disinfecting agents). However, strongly acidic oxidising or bleaching agents should not be used (always check the manufacturers' recommendations before use).

All toys belonging to the kennels (rather than to the individual) should be disinfected, or discarded if this is not possible.

Post-operative kennelling

The highest possible standards of disinfection are essential in veterinary hospital kennels, especially where a risk of infection is likely, as in post-operative kennelling.

Principles and methods of cleaning and disinfecting kennels

The cleaning and disinfection of kennels is achieved by physical and chemical actions. The action of all chemical disinfectants is dependent upon being in direct contact with the target micro-organisms. This means that all traces of organic material such as dirt, grease, faeces, urine, blood and vomit must be physically removed from the surface prior to disinfection, as it will prevent such contact. Begin by removing the bulk of the material with a shovel and scraper (or similar). Tackle the remainder by hosing out the kennel liberally with water; then use a detergent and energetically scrub with a suitable brush.

Precautions and use of chemical disinfectants

When using any chemicals, including disinfectants and cleaning materials, care should be taken to ensure their correct handling:

- Store in the original containers with the lids fully secured.
- Keep away from animals and children.
- Wear protective clothing when recommended and take care to avoid contact with skin.
- Wash hands thoroughly after use, particularly before eating and drinking.
- Only use disinfectants for the purpose recommended by the manufacturer.
- Use the correct concentration.
- Wear gloves.

Manufacturers of disinfectants give recommended dilution rates. There is usually more than one rate, depending upon where the chemical will be used and the type of organisms to be killed or inactivated. To simplify use, most manufacturers do not provide a list of micro-organisms and a recommended strength for each, but they give a recommended strength for routine or general use and (usually) a stronger solution for certain specific disease-causing organisms.

In some kennels the recommended 'routine' strength is used for the normal daily cleaning and disinfection of kennels where no specific problems exist. A recommended higher concentration is often used in disinfecting a kennel after its occupant has been discharged and before admitting another animal into it. Some general rules can be applied to the use of disinfectants:

- Too weak a solution will be ineffective, whereas a solution that is stronger than the recommendation is not only wasteful but also may, with some types of disinfectant, lead to problems with the animals' feet, eyes and other sensitive areas. Inadequate rinsing may lead to similar problems.

- A disinfectant should have no substances other than water added to it. It is potentially dangerous to mix disinfectants together or disinfectants with detergents, unless recommended by the manufacturer, as combinations of chemicals can negate the effect of the active ingredient in both products as well as producing noxious gases or cause corrosive action. This problem can occur accidentally if adequate safeguards are not in place – always be cautious of the chemicals and always use and store as recommended.
- Use at the chemicals' optimum temperature for action. Many disinfectants are more effective when used with hot water than with cold, although with others there is no advantage. It is advisable to check this feature.
- Using very hot water can be hazardous. If it spills on the operator or the animal, injury will occur. Safety should be of paramount importance, as with all actions in kennels.
- The contact time should be taken into account when planning a disinfection routine. All disinfectants require time to kill or inactivate micro-organisms and are ineffective if rinsed off immediately after application. The required contact time varies considerably, depending on the type of disinfectant and the organisms to be killed. Take note of the manufacturers' recommended contact times when selecting a disinfectant: it may be able to kill certain organisms but may take up to 24 hours' contact time to do its work.
- Use freshly made-up solutions to ensure effectiveness. Some disinfectants begin to deteriorate when made into solution with water.
- Equipment and receptacles used with disinfectants should be thoroughly cleaned and rinsed before use. Any organic material present may reduce the effectiveness of the disinfectant.
- It should also be noted that the efficiency of some disinfectants may be hindered by 'hard' water, some plastics and certain other materials. Read all the literature relating to the chemicals before use.
- All disinfectants should be thoroughly rinsed off once the contact time is completed, unless otherwise recommended.
- Always adhere to recommendations on product COSHH sheets. Specific use and precautions to be taken when using chemical disinfectants are stated on the COSHH sheet provided by the manufacturer (see Chapter 5).

Cleaning and disinfection of kennel equipment

Equipment such as shovels, buckets, mops, dustpans and brushes, kitchen utensils, feed bowls, beds and bedding must all be cleaned and disinfected regularly. Wash them first in detergent and water to remove any organic material. To disinfect, soak the equipment in a solution of disinfectant appropriate to the material at the manufacturer's recommended strength and for the recommended contact time, then thoroughly rinse and dry the equipment before storing it.

Special care must be taken that the disinfectant is in fact 'appropriate to the material' as some items can be corroded by certain chemicals. Particular care should be taken with the disinfection of items made of plastic (including thermoplastic floor tiles), rubber and mild steel; the soaking of these materials in an oxidising disinfectant should be avoided unless the manufacturer states otherwise (if so, the stated contact times should not be exceeded, with items being thoroughly rinsed and dried). If bedding

---

SUMMARY OF ROUTINE PROCEDURE FOR CLEANING AND DISINFECTION OF KENNELS

(1) Remove animal from kennel into a run or other secure holding area (not another dog's kennel).
(2) Remove bed, bedding, toys and any other portable objects.
(3) Remove any gross soiling with shovel and scraper or similar equipment.
(4) Hose out hair and any debris. Pressure hoses or steam cleaners are used in some establishments.
(5) Scrub out with detergent.*
(6) Rinse with water.*
(7) Apply disinfectant* (or scrub out with detergent/disinfectant).
(8) Time contact.
(9) Rinse thoroughly.
(10) Dry (remove excess water with a 'squeegee' drier).
(11) Leave to air dry.
(12) Return/replace bedding as necessary.
(13) Return animal to kennel.

*Many of the more recently developed kennel disinfectants are a combination of specialist detergents and disinfectant agents. These specialist detergent/disinfectants are mixed by manufacturers as part of the active ingredient formulation. This principle potentiates the activity of the disinfectant and accelerates the microbiocidal process.

When using these products follow actions 1–4 (using the correct dilution), cut out steps 5 and 6 and proceed with step 7, second option.

These products are often used in low-risk areas for routine cleaning/disinfection where no disease problems exist.

is disinfected by soaking it can be laundered in the normal way afterwards.

Antiseptics and disinfectants

The terms 'antiseptic' and 'disinfectant' are often used loosely when referring to chemical agents but they actually describe the chemicals' action against micro-organisms.

DEFINITIONS

- **Antiseptics** are chemicals that cause the destruction or inhibition of micro-organisms, preventing their growth or multiplication, without damaging an animal's cells. Antiseptics applied topically have many uses, such as the cleansing of wounds or the skin.
- **Disinfection**. This term describes a process that is used to reduce the number of micro-organisms (but not all bacterial spores) to a level which is not harmful to health. This term applies to the treatment of inanimate objects and materials and may be also applied to the treatment of skin, mucous membranes and other body tissues and cavities. Methods of achieving disinfection include the use of chemicals and some physical processes such as boiling.
- **Skin disinfectants** are antiseptic preparations designed either for pre-operative skin cleansing or for use on inanimate objects.
- **Environmental disinfectants** are designed for use on inanimate objects only; many of them require the user to wear protective clothing and they should *never* be used on the skin.
- **Sterilant** is a term used to describe some types of chemical disinfectant which can under certain conditions destroy bacterial spores, viruses and vegetative organisms. Physical methods of sterilisation are superior to chemical sterilants in their effectiveness, e.g. steam sterilisation.
- **Sterilisation** is the term applied when an inanimate object is rendered free from all micro-organisms, including bacterial spores, by their removal or destruction. This procedure must be used when the efficient destruction of all micro-organisms is vital, such as in the preparation of instruments for surgery. When selecting methods for destroying micro-organisms on inanimate objects, it is important to remember that a method producing sterilisation is far more satisfactory than one that produces disinfection.
- **Decontamination** refers to rendering an item safe by the destruction or removal of microbial contamination. This is usually achieved by cleaning, disinfection or sterilisation.

SUFFICES

- **-cide** indicates that a chemical kills a particular type of micro-organism. For example, a bactericide kills bacteria; a fungicide kills fungi.
- **-stat** describes the action of a chemical that prevents or inhibits the growth of a particular type of micro-organism, for example, a bacteriostat inhibits the growth of bacteria. Some antiseptics have this characteristic, although it is preferable to select a chemical with the ability to kill the micro-organism rather than one that merely prevents or inhibits its growth.

Selecting disinfectants and antiseptics

The choice of product depends upon many factors but some of the main considerations are:

- The intended use of the product:

    - environmental (kennels, runs, equipment)
    - on living tissue (skin, wounds, body cavities, etc).

- The product's activity against specific micro-organisms.
- The contact time required.
- Known local conditions (e.g. water hardness).
- Safety of staff and animals – ideally the product should be non-irritant, non-toxic and non-corrosive – check manufacturer's COSHH sheets for details of any hazards and for recommended suitable protective clothing for the user.
- Stability of the product in storage.
- Odour of product. Ideally products should be either odourless or have a pleasant aroma that is acceptable to staff and animals.
- Ease of use – it should disperse easily in water if dilution is required.
- Economy of use, assessed by cost per litre of ready-to-use solution.

It should be noted, for example, that:

- Some products which are very effective for kennel disinfection will stain bedding and other porous materials.
- The presence of even relatively small amounts of organic material in water may affect some products.
- Some animal species are sensitive to some types of disinfectant (e.g. cats are sensitive to phenol; and vapours given off by some chemicals such as glutaraldehyde will cause irritation to the eyes of many animals).
- Strong odours or perfumes are offensive to some animals, promoting sneezing and irritation to the ocular mucous membranes.

Effectiveness   The product should have been tested for action against specific significant organisms, for example, parvovirus. The results of these tests should be available so that the user knows what strength/dilution and contact time are effective. Early tests, such as the Rideal–Walker and Chick–Martin tests, only give accurate results for phenolic-based disinfectants; more modern techniques such as the Kelsey–Sykes test are suitable for the assessment of most disinfectants.

The bacteria-killing capability of a disinfectant varies as some forms of bacteria are more resistant than others. The Gram-positive group are the most easily destroyed; the Gram-negative group, acid-fast group and bacterial spores are progressively more difficult to destroy. The literature for many disinfectants now available for use in kennels and catteries states that they are effective against specific important viral diseases of the dog and cat.

Types of disinfectants and antiseptics

There are a number of different products available on the market, with new products appearing frequently. Most chemical disinfectants available will fit broadly into the main groups, some of the recognised general characteristics of these chemicals being listed below. However, it should be recognised that advances in manufacturing and blending of chemicals may mean that certain disinfectants may perform slightly differently. It is therefore advisable when selecting products to refer to the manufacturers' performance data.

The main groups of disinfectants

Phenolics

The phenolic disinfectants have a wide range of bactericidal activity but variable activity against viruses (usually poor against non-enveloped viruses such as parvovirus). The activity against bacterial spores is poor. All are toxic to cats, and care in use must be taken.

Black, white and clear phenolics These disinfectants are inexpensive and not as susceptible to inactivation by organic materials as some other chemicals. They are toxic and irritant to varying degrees and should not come into contact with the skin. These types of disinfectant can be absorbed by rubber and plastics. They are also strong smelling, and black fluids can leave sticky residue on some materials.

Chloroxylenols (synthetic phenol/chlorinated phenol) Chloroxylenol is less irritant than other types of phenolic but can be inactivated by hard water and organic material. It is active against Gram-positive bacteria, but has poor activity against Gram-negative bacteria (though improved by the addition of EDTA in some products).

Hexachlorophane This type of chemical is more active against Gram-positive than Gram-negative bacteria, but has little other activity. Hexachlorophane has been used in soap and detergent preparations, for skin disinfection, as it has a good residual effect. Recently there have been

concerns regarding its possible cumulative toxicity (with human neonates). This has restricted its use in some areas.

Triclosan (cloxifenol) Has similar characteristics to hexachlorophane but no concerns regarding toxicity. It is now used in a similar manner to a skin disinfectant.

Halogens

Hypochlorites (bleach) These disinfectants are generally inexpensive and are effective against bacteria, fungi, viruses and spores when used correctly. However, there are some disadvantages: chlorine is a strong oxidising agent which is corrosive to metals, and bleaching of some materials occurs. Chlorine gas may be liberated if in contact with acids, therefore, it should not be used in the presence of urine. It should be noted that these chemicals can gradually lose strength in storage and that the presence of organic matter can affect the disinfectant activity.

Halogenated tertiary amines (HTA) This is a group of compounds developed in the UK. The term 'halogenated' provides association with the chlorine derivative which is reacted in combination with other complex chemistries. Generally these new compounds contain one or more highly sophisticated **quaternary ammonium compounds** (QACs) which work with very specific amine salts. These products with their specialist detergents have wide-ranging activities. These include action against Gram-negative and Gram-positive bacteria. There is also good action against viruses, including enveloped and non-enveloped types. These disinfectants also act against spores and fungi. These compounds are more resistant to inactivation by organic materials than some other types of disinfectant. Although they are thought to be irritant at concentrate level (the use of gloves is recommended), they are generally of low toxicity and low corrosion potential.

Dichloroisocyanurates Sodium dichloroisocyanurate is a chlorine-releasing agent available in tablet/powder or granule form. Advantages are that they have similar disinfectant activities to hypochlorite but less of a corrosive tendency. They are also generally more resistant to inactivation by organic materials and although unstable when made up into solution they are very stable when stored correctly as powder, granules or tablets.

Iodine/iodophors This group of disinfectants has a wide range of activity including some activity against bacterial spores. Iodine has been used for well over one hundred years in the treatment of wounds. The properties of iodine and iodophors ('iodine carriers') are similar in many ways to the hypochlorites but are most often used on the skin rather than environmentally. It should be noted, however, that some people may be allergic to iodine. Staining can also be a problem with iodine products. Iodophors have an added substance (often a non-ionic surfactant). These products are less irritant and do not stain in the same way as iodine. Povidone–iodine products (water-soluble complex of iodine and polyvinylpyrrolidone) are used in veterinary practice.

Others

Peroxides
Peroxygen compounds (peracetic acid, hydrogen peroxide, potassium monopersulphate, peroxygenated chlorine compounds). Hydrogen peroxide and peracetic acid are oxidising agents that have a wide range of bactericidal, virucidal and fungicidal activity when used appropriately. There is, however, variable sporicidal activity with hydrogen peroxide, but good activity for peracetic acid. The activity is greatly reduced in the presence of organic matter and there can be corrosion of some metals. Hydrogen peroxide has low irritancy and toxicity but peracetic acid is highly toxic and irritant. The characteristics of other peroxygen compounds are similar to those of peracetic acid and hydrogen peroxide but some can be highly corrosive to many metals and break down plasticisers in rubber and plastic products. Manufacturers' approval must be obtained for use of their products with equipment that may be prone to corrosion or degradation.

Biguanides
This group contains chlorhexidine preparations which have low toxicity and irritancy, and are therefore frequently used in skin cleansing agents and surgical scrubs. Biguanides are more active against Gram-positive than Gram-negative bacteria but have no activity against bacterial spores. There is good fungicidal activity but limited activity against viruses. They can be inactivated by organic matter, soap and other anionic detergents.

Alcohols
Alcohols are very effective against many organisms with the notable exception of spores and some viruses (but only if organic material has first been removed). Ethanol (70%) and isopropanol (70%) are used for clean areas such as trolley tops. Hand rubs containing alcohol and other chemicals such as chlorhexidine and glycerine are often used for disinfection of hands between clean tasks. Alcohols are flammable and care should be taken when using and with storage.

Aldehydes
Glutaraldehyde This chemical has a wide range of bactericidal activity and is known to be active against many bacterial spores and some viruses. Glutaraldehyde is relatively slow acting but organic matter has less effect on its activity than some other disinfectants. Some products containing glutaraldehyde may also have QAC combined. This type of disinfectant is useful for disinfecting some types of equipment that cannot be heat sterilised. Disadvantages include high irritancy and toxicity; it is irritant to the skin, eyes and respiratory mucosa. Glutaraldehyde can also cause sensitisation, leading to further health problems with continued exposure. It is therefore only used where the recommended necessary precautions for user protection can be applied. The Health Service Safety Council recommends that disinfectants employing this substance should not be used as general 'wash down' disinfectants.

Formaldehyde Formaldehyde is active against many microbes but is considered too irritant to be used as a disinfectant.

Surfactants
These are chemical compounds that lower the surface tension of an aqueous solution. Commonly used as wetting agents, detergents and emulsifiers.

The types of surfactant are:

- Anionic.
- Cationic.
- Amphoteric (ampholytic).
- Non-ionic.

Anionic surfactants These types are generally referred to as soaps. The most important action is the physical emulsification of lipoidal secretions of the skin which contain bacteria; the bacteria are thus suspended in the lather and are rinsed away. The inclusion of certain antiseptics has increased the antibacterial action of anionic surfactants.

Cationic surfactants The most important example of this type of surfactant is the QACs. QACs have low toxicity and some detergent properties. These disinfectants are more active against Gram-positive than Gram-negative bacteria, have good fungicidal activity, but have variable activity against viruses. They are not active against bacterial spores. They are widely used in the cleansing of food preparation areas. They can be inactivated by many materials including soaps and organic matter. These surfactants are frequently used in products in combination with other chemicals to increase the disinfectant activity. Benzalkonium chloride is one type of QAC used in veterinary practice.

Amphoteric (ampholytic) surfactants These agents have similar characteristics to the anionic and cationic surfactants in that they have good detergent and bactericidal properties. The food industry uses compounds based on dodecyl-di(aminoethyl)glycine.

Non-ionic The non-ionic surfactants are considered to have no antimicrobial properties; however, polysorbates are believed to weaken some bacteria, making them more sensitive to other agents. For example, they are frequently used in iodophor preparations.

Table 6.10 lists some disinfectants that are available, their main active ingredients and recommended uses (for detailed information regarding each product's suitability in veterinary practice, the manufacturer's data sheets should be read).

Disposal of waste

All establishments, whether domestic or industrial, have to dispose of waste materials. Veterinary practices and commercial kennels are classed as industrial users for this purpose.

Table 6.10 Antiseptics and disinfectants – some examples of types available

Active ingredient	Examples of products	Presentation and recommended use
Phenol compound (black fluids) (white fluids) (clear soluble)	Jeyes fluid Izal Clearsol	Liquid concentrate – environmental use Liquid concentrate – environmental use Liquid concentrate – environmental use
Chloroxylenol (chlorinated phenol)	Dettol Ibcol	Liquid concentrate – environmental use and skin disinfectant Liquid concentrate – environmental use and skin disinfectant
Hypochlorites (bleaches)	Chloros Domestos	Liquid concentrate – environmental use Liquid concentrate – environmental use
Halogenated tertiary amine	Trigene	Liquid concentrate – disinfectant cleaner Environmental use
Sodium tosychloramide	Halamid	Powder concentrate – environmental use
Sodium dichlorisocyanurate	Vetaclean Parvo	Tablet – environmental use
Povidone–iodine	Pevidine Antiseptic Soln	Solution – topical application – burns, wounds, etc.
Peroxyacetic acid	Vetcide 2000	Liquid concentrate
Acetic acid		Environmental use
Hydrogen peroxide surfactants Peroxygen compound Inorganic salts, organic acid, anionic detergent	Vircon (concentrate)	Powder Environmental use
Chlorhexidine gluconate 4% Chlorhexidine gluconate	Dinex Scrub Hibiscrub Vet	Liquid concentrate – pre-op. skin disinfectant Rapid bactericidal skin cleanser/surgical scrub
Chlorhexidine acetate 0.1% Chlorhexidine acetate	Nolvadent Nolvasan Surgical Scrub	Solution and spray – oral cleanser Solution – skin and wound cleanser
Chlorhexidine gluconate cetrimide	Savlon Vet Concentrate	Solution – wounds (dilute). Pre-op. instruments
Glutaraldehyde	Cidex Formula H routine spray Formula H concentrated disinfectant	Liquid concentrate – environmental use Spray – environmental use Liquid concentrate – environmental use
Cetrimide (quaternary ammonium compounds)	Cetavlon	Liquid concentrate – environmental use and skin disinfectant
Ampholytic surfactants	Tego	Liquid concentrate – environmental use
Quaternary ammonium compound Non-ionic surfactant	Vetaclean	Liquid concentrate – surface disinfectant, sanitising feeding utensils, etc.
Octyl decyl dimethyl ammonium chloride	Quinticare	Liquid concentrate
Dioctyle dimethyl ammonium Alkyl dimethyl benzyl ammonium chloride	(Quinticide)	Environmental use – especially stainless steel
Benzalkonium chloride	Roccal	Liquid concentrate – environmental use and skin disinfectant
Benzalkonium chloride	Marinol Blue	10 or 50% solution. Pre-op. Topical (diluted) or environmental

The Environmental Protection Act 1990 imposed a 'duty of care' on the disposal of waste classed as Controlled Waste, of which there are three types; household, industrial and commercial. Of particular importance to the veterinary practice is the fact that some of the items in the Industrial class are further classified as Clinical Waste and it is essential that the veterinary nurse should be aware of items in this category, with particular regard to methods of disposal and how they should be handled and stored prior to disposal (see Chapter 5). Table 6.11 identifies items classed as clinical waste and their ultimate disposal.

Table 6.11 Clinical waste and its disposal		
Sharps Needles, syringes, broken glass, scalpel blades, etc. Unless rendered safe is clinical waste	Waste containing blood, body fluids, excretion, drugs Swabs and dressings, blood/body fluids	Non-agricultural animal carcasses and animal tissue Non-domestic kennel excreta and bedding
Pre-disposal handling Sharps Approved sharps container (sealed)	Swabs and soiled disposable bedding Kennel excrement Approved yellow containers or bags identifiable (with name and source of waste) prior to collection	Cadavers May be deep frozen for storage prior to collection
Collection by local authority or licensed contractors All clinical waste is destroyed by high temperature incinerator, licensed for this use		

Handling clinical waste

For the health and safety of staff and to comply with the regulations, clinical waste must be handled, segregated and disposed of with great care. See 'Clinical Waste', p. 144.

Disposal of clinical waste

All items classed as clinical waste must be disposed of by incineration in a licensed high-temperature incinerator. These incinerators must conform to the regulations regarding clean discharge into the atmosphere (see Chapter 5).

Non-clinical practice waste

Non-clinical waste is classed as domestic waste. This includes empty food cans, outer packaging and office waste. (All confidential records should be shredded prior to disposal.) Domestic waste continues to be collected regularly by the local authority. Normal 'day-to-day' deposits of pet owners' dog faeces are also classed as refuse rather than clinical waste. Black plastic bags are commonly used for the refuse that is not classified as clinical waste.

Small animal care

Daily care of hospitalised animals

The specific requirements in the care of hospitalised animals depend to some degree on the conditions under treatment. Table 6.12 suggests a care routine.

Defecation and urination

Dogs   The opportunity to defecate and urinate is sometimes referred to as 'relief' and sometimes as 'exercise'. Most hospitalised dogs require restricted exercise but frequent opportunities to relieve themselves. It is therefore less confusing to refer to 'opportunity for relief' rather than 'exercise' in this context.

All dogs should be taken to a run and given frequent opportunities for relief, unless they are not mobile or movement is contraindicated by their condition. It is important

Table 6.12 Care routine for hospitalised animals	
Check	**Care routine**
General check	All animals are inspected briefly by touring the kennels/cages. This is to establish that there are no urgent problems that require immediate attention
Individual check	Each individual should be looked at for some time, noting the behaviour of the animal compared with its normal, e.g. whether it is lively, aggressive, unresponsive. Its posture should be noted – whether it is standing, lying down or in an abnormal position
Observe respiration	This should be done before the animal is disturbed
Pulse and temperature	The animal's pulse and temperature may be taken (before exercise)
Soiling, etc.	Check for soiling of kennel, and record details of quantity and type of eliminations. If the animal has urinated or defecated, note if it is normal. If the animal has vomited, note the appearance or amount, assess what has been eaten and record the observation before removing it. It is not usual practice to leave food in with dogs overnight except in the case of difficult or shy feeders. It is more frequently necessary to leave food in with cats, as overnight is often the only time that some hospitalised cats will eat
Check the water bowl	Note how much has been taken and if any spilling has occurred (if there is spilling the assessment of intake will be inaccurate)
Physical check on patient	Any abnormalities should be noted and recorded. Wounds may be inspected. Any discharges should be gently removed

not to leave a dog so long that it is forced to urinate or defecate in its kennel, which would cause considerable distress to normally clean house-trained dogs.

When the dog is taken to a run, its gait and general body stance should be noted. When it passes urine and faeces, any difficulty should be noted along with the appearance and the amount passed.

Reluctance to urinate or defecate in kennel runs A reluctant dog should not be returned to its kennel until every effort has been made to encourage it to urinate and defecate. This is particularly important if the dog has been confined for a long period (such as overnight) and has not soiled its kennel.

Some dogs are reluctant to relieve themselves with the handler in close proximity. If so, retire a suitable distance to observe. If the dog is still reluctant, it may be unused to defecating on a hard surface such as concrete or slabs (as described in the discussion on kennel design earlier in this chapter). These dogs may be used to relieving on grass or soil surfaces, and it may need a little ingenuity to encourage them. Initial effort will ensure less stress to the dog and will save time for the handler on future occasions as the dog should relieve itself without delay once it understands the routine.

Put some sawdust or peat on a small area at the end of a run and then praise the dog when it urinates or defecates there, so that it understands that this is the right place. The sawdust or peat can be lifted along with any urine or faeces and the run cleaned as normal.

If this ploy fails, it may be necessary to walk the dog for some distance and then 'leash relieve' it on grass. However, this is not generally recommended as it is unhygienic: grass cannot be disinfected. (Dogs with suspected infectious disease should never be relieved on an area that cannot be adequately disinfected.)

Cats All hospitalised cats should be provided with a litter tray unless their condition contraindicates. Clean the tray regularly and record the presence and characteristics of the faeces and urine produced. If the tray is not cleaned frequently enough, some cats are so fastidious that they will not re-use the tray but will soil elsewhere in the kennel.

Some cats prefer privacy, which can be provided by covering the litter tray with an upturned box with an entrance hole cut into it.

Feeding

All animals should be observed when feeding to check that they are eating normally and without difficulty.

Each animal should have the same feed and water bowls throughout its stay to reduce the possibility of cross-infection. The bowls can be labelled or numbered to identify them with the kennel or animal.

Medication

Adhere strictly to any specific medication times, as instructed by the veterinary surgeon. Keep up-to-date records of all medications given.

Where medication has been given with food, check that the food has been consumed.

Weighing

All dogs should be weighed on entry to the hospital and weekly thereafter. This is important with long-stay animals to ensure that the feeding and exercise regime maintains the dog's condition and that any loss of weight due to illness is monitored and reported.

Grooming of hospitalised animals

Every effort should be made to keep hospitalised animals in a hygienic and comfortable condition. The grooming of hospitalised dogs should be carried out as part of their general nursing care, unless their condition contraindicates it (e.g. an animal admitted for warfarin poisoning should not be handled vigorously – see Chapter 4).

Grooming as part of normal animal care

There are various reasons why grooming is beneficial and all of them can be placed broadly under five headings:

- **C**leanliness.
- **H**ealth.
- **A**ppearance.
- **I**nspection.
- **R**elationship.

The initial letters of these headings form a useful memory aid: CHAIR.

Cleanliness

Keeping the animal clean by the removal of dirt and discharge and assisting in the casting of hair contributes towards the animal's health and well-being. At home, the regular grooming of dogs and cats reduces the amount of hair deposited on furniture and carpets.

It is important that animals with dense or long coats are groomed regularly, as their coats rapidly become tangled, matted and soiled.

Health

By keeping the animal's coat clean, grooming assists the condition of the skin and hair and thus contributes to the animal's health:

- Grooming stimulates anagen (the hair growth stage) by the removal of dead, shedding hairs.
- The removal of discharge and prevention of matting prevents skin irritation.
- The close inspection of the animal during grooming assists in early problem recognition.
- During grooming, daily care and attention to any bony prominences, skin folds, feet and claws, eyes and ears, mouth and teeth, anus, vulva and prepuce contribute to the health of the animal.

Appearance

Owners usually give this as the first reason for grooming, though it is the least important for the animal itself. Many owners take a pride in the appearance of their animals – and this becomes very apparent when a post-operative animal with large areas of denuded skin is returned to an owner who was not forewarned. Owners of pedigree dogs often want their pets to look like the breed as seen at championship dog shows and this means that many dogs are trimmed and clipped by professional groomers, a practice that also assists the owner's daily grooming of the dog. The appearance of the true show dog is of major concern to its owner and show preparation often involves hours of careful grooming and trimming or clipping. Nurses should be careful not to remove hair from show dogs without the owner's consent.

The veterinary nurse needs to appreciate this emphasis on appearance: many owners, rightly or wrongly, judge the standard of care at the practice or kennels by the appearance of the animal when it is returned to them.

Inspection

The daily inspection of an animal during the grooming routine contributes to its health by giving an opportunity for early recognition of problems. For example, flea excreta will only be discovered on close examination of the coat. It is recommended that inspection is carried out in a logical daily sequence so that any problems found can be attended to before further damage or discomfort is caused to the animal during the actual grooming.

Relationship and human contact

This is an important reason for grooming; for the dog in the wild state, mutual grooming is part of pack socialisation activities. Dogs lower in the pack order submit to grooming by a more dominant member, while dominant dogs make it clear whether or not they consent to being groomed by other members of the pack. When dogs are groomed by their handlers, the activity strengthens the bond between them and confirms to the dog its place in the hierarchy: the handler is the 'pack leader'. The act of grooming, therefore, should assist in the handling and training of the dog.

Grooming can also assist in teaching a dog to sit or stand still whilst the procedure is carried out, which will be of great assistance for veterinary examinations. If a dog resents grooming for no physical reason, it is likely to prove generally difficult to handle.

Introducing an animal to grooming

Ideally the process of grooming should be introduced (to all domesticated species) at a very young age as part of socialisation and habituation. Even short-haired puppies and kittens should be handled each day and introduced gently to brushes and combs. The experience should be made pleasant for the animal, with praise given for good behaviour but a firm tone if the animal struggles.

As with all training, grooming should be carried out for a few minutes at a time at first and gradually built up as the animal becomes accustomed to it. Each session should end on a successful note with the animal being praised for compliance.

Owners of long-haired animals should in particular be advised that time spent in the early stages of ownership will ensure that the animal is easier to groom in later years and is less likely to be presented at the practice for de-matting when an owner is unable to groom the pet because it objects, struggles or even attempts to bite.

Routine grooming

Routine grooming is part of the daily care of a normal healthy animal, but the veterinary nurse can be faced with quite a problem as there are so many different types of coat. In addition, various factors have a direct effect on the coat and it is necessary to have a broad understanding of them so that the coat can be correctly maintained while the animal is in the nurse's care and so that owners' queries regarding grooming at home can be answered. It can be seen from Table 6.13 that the major factors affecting hair growth include:

- Environmental temperature and time of year.
- Health.
- Endocrine and reproductive status.
- Feeding and nutrition.

The type of coat is governed by combinations of individual hair types that make up the coat. These are the rigid primary or 'guard' hairs and the soft, thinner secondary or 'lanugo' hairs. The various proportions, lengths and weights of these hair types account for the many and varied types of coat seen in dogs and cats (Table 6.14).

Grooming equipment and methods

A fairly wide range of attention and equipment is required to deal with the various types of coat. For the routine main-

Table 6.13 Factors affecting hair growth and type

Factors	The average rate of hair growth in the dog is 0.5 mm per day An average smooth-coat type takes about 6 months to regrow completely. Fine, silky long-haired coats take up to 18 months; a similar growth rate can be expected in cats

Environmental temperature and time of year	Dogs kept in housing with constantly high environmental temperature (usually centrally heated) will often shed hair almost continuously throughout the year but with noticeable increases in spring and autumn. Shedding in dogs kennelled out of doors or with less environmental heating tends to be more obviously seasonal – shedding is very noticeable in spring and autumn. This seasonal coat change is a natural process triggered by increasing day length in spring and decreasing day length in autumn
	
	Spring = increasing day length
	      Production of summer coat triggered
	      Increased hair shedding (of winter coat)
	      Coarser coat with reduced density
	   plus
	Increased sebaceous gland activity = Summer coat
	Allowing increased air circulation through coat
	Autumn = decreasing day length
	      Production of winter coat triggered
	      Increased hair shedding (of summer coat)
	   plus
	      New coat growth and reduced sebaceous gland activity = Winter coat
	Increased coat density = insulation against the cold

Health and reproductive status	Condition can often be assessed by observing the coat and noting any unseasonal loss or thinning of hair Thinning during periods of ill-health is due to interruption of the growth cycle: fewer individual hairs are in the growth stage An animal suffering from ill-health may also have a dull and harsh coat. The reproductive status of an animal can have an effect on the coat growth and this can be quite obvious during pregnancy and lactation and occasionally after neutering These and other so-called hormonal alopecias usually involve thinning of hair on certain areas of the body
Feeding and nutrition	Diet affects hair growth, as it does all other functions Nutrients essential for good health of skin and hair include amino acids, essential fatty acids, zinc, iodine, etc. (see Chapter 9)

Table 6.14 Coat types

Coat	Type	Example
Most coat types can be divided into five broad groups for the purpose of grooming:		
1. Smooth coat	Short	Boxer, Dachshund, Chihuahua
	Intermediate or coarse	German Shepherd dog, Pembroke Corgi. Wild dogs and
	Dense	wolves have this type and it is therefore sometimes referred to as a normal coat
2. Wire coat		Wire-Haired Terriers
3. Double coat		Rough Collie, Long-Haired German Shepherd dog
4. Silky coat	Medium	Most spaniels, setters and some retrievers
	Long fine	Afghan Hounds, Bearded Collies
5. Woolly coat		Poodle, Bedlington Terrier, Curly-Coated Retriever, Irish Water Spaniel

There are some more unusual or specialised coat types, such as corded coats. Where animals with such coats are under the nurses' care, a professional groomer or the individual breed society should be contacted for specific advice if the owner is unable to provide details on coat maintenance

tenance grooming of patients and boarders, it is advisable to stock a range of basic grooming equipment (Table 6.15).

Although different coats require different attention, a logical general sequence can be adopted for all common breeds to ensure that nothing is missed out during the grooming session:

- Assess the animal's temperament.
- Carry out a physical inspection of the animal (Table 6.16).
- Remove loose hair.
- Comb, brush and finish (Table 6.17).

Table 6.15 Grooming and trimming equipment		
	Types	**Features and use**
Brushes	Double-sided grooming brush (pins and bristles) 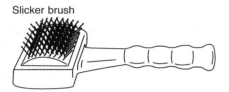	Metal pins with rounded ends. The straight pins more effectively than bristle with silky coats. Used for silky, double coats and feathering to separate hairs and smooth and lay the coat. Not so useful for tangled coats Natural or synthetic bristles. Denser than pin brushes and less able to brush through thick coats for hair separation. The bristles are flexible for removal of dirt deep in the coat this brush is most commonly used for routine grooming of short-coated breeds
	Slicker brush 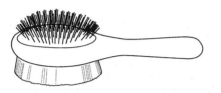	One-way hooked pins. The hooks assist in pulling out loose hair. Pressure should not be used as the hooks easily damage the dog's skin. Used for removing loose hair from thick coats, grooming silky coats (especially feathering), wire, woolly and double coats
	Hound glove 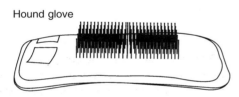	Flexible, with bristles, small plastic projections or a velvet type surface, often double sided. Used to assist moulting and for the routine grooming of short-coated breeds. Pressure and vigorous use should be avoided with wire bristles
Combs	Metal combs 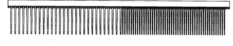	Handle and non-handle combs. Both are available in various tooth widths. Used for grooming of longer hair behind ears in silky coats etc. Also used for detangling and breaking up small mats
	Rake 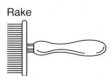	Designed for greater pull through dense coats. Used for removal of loose undercoat and breaking up some small mats (with great care as damage can easily be inflicted on the dog's skin)
	De-matting comb with specialised teeth 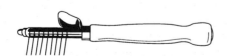	Only used to cut out mats; it is a much safer way to remove mats than by the use of scissors, allowing the maximum amount of coat to be preserved once the mat is removed
Scissors	Trimming scissors 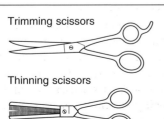	Long very sharp blades tapering to a point. Different sizes available. Used to trim neatly around the edges of ears, etc.
	Thinning scissors	Specialised blades for thinning without leaving 'steps' in the coat Used to enhance features, e.g. the shoulders, sides of chest

Table 6.16 Physical inspection routine before grooming

Aims	Method
Assess the state of the animal's coat and therefore the need for the use of non-routine equipment such as the de-matting comb	The inspection should be carried out in a logical sequence, checking the dog from head to tail, checking closely both visually and by running the hands carefully over the animal. Areas requiring special attention, particularly with elderly or hospitalised animals, include:
Assess the state of the animal's health. This is very important as it ensures close observation of the animal so that lesions normally obscured by the coat are found prior to the use of any equipment that may cause injury to the animal. (It is too late to find a wart once you have stuck the comb in it causing it to bleed!)	Mouth, teeth, gums, and lip folds Eyes and ears – discharges wiped away with clean damp cotton wool. In some breeds the long hair on the ears (and face) may gather food whilst the animal is eating. This should be removed by washing. Either trim the hair carefully to prevent recurrence, or, for a pedigree breed where this long hair is a feature, make a note to use a 'snood' when feeding the dog (these hold the long hair and ears back during feeding and are often used for Afghan Hounds) or a narrow deep feeding bowl that allows the long hair and ears to fall on each side of the bowl and not in the food Hocks and elbows – any pressure sores noted and attended to (improve bedding and apply white petroleum jelly if there is hard skin but no sign of breaks in the skin) Foot pads – may be cracking, or in dogs that pace about continually in hard surfaced runs they may be reddened and thin due to the abrasive action Claws – these should be checked for injury and condition (e.g. they may be overgrown when a dog has restricted exercise or is walked on grass). Some dogs that have a long term abnormal gait may wear their claws unevenly, resulting in the need to trim some of the claws on a regular basis Body orifices – anus, vulva and prepuce may require the regular removal of discharges/soiling. With long-haired animals it may be necessary to trim or clip away some of the surrounding hair to allow easier cleaning of these areas. Any treatment or attention to any abnormalities found should be dealt with at this stage

De-matting

Sometimes the coat of a long-haired animal has been so grossly neglected and become so matted that it would be unkind to try to de-mat it while the animal is conscious. The neglect may have arisen because the animal has been so difficult to groom when conscious anyway.

In such cases the veterinary surgeon might sedate or anaesthetise the animal and request the veterinary nurse to 'de-mat' it. This should be carried out with great care: it is very easy to cut the skin, and scissors should not be used by unskilled nurses. Cats are especially at risk when hair lumps are cut away.

Clipping and trimming

Under normal circumstances a nurse is unlikely to be involved in the long-term maintenance of a coat that requires clipping or trimming. However, it is essential that all those who care for hospitalised animals should know how to look after a variety of coat types.

The routine clipping or trimming of some areas in long-haired dogs will assist in maintaining cleanliness but care should be taken. **Do not trim or clip an animal without its owner's consent** – it may be a pedigree show dog which should either not be trimmed or needs specialised clipping and trimming.

The clipping, hand stripping and trimming of specific breeds is generally within the realms of the professional dog groomer and showing kennel. Interested veterinary nurses can attend special courses on this art, but in general practice it is more usual for a nurse to clip or trim a pet dog at its owner's request because the animal is difficult or impossible to groom. This may be due to the animal's temperament, or because the dog is elderly or infirm with perhaps an elderly owner. In the latter case, trimming and clipping may be carried out as part of a geriatric care policy (for the dog, that is). Where temperament is the problem, it is usually necessary to sedate the dog or, in extreme cases, to anaesthetise it as already discussed for de-matting.

In general practice, the veterinary nurse needs to know how to use common equipment for trimming or clipping a dog neatly and tidily. The regular trimming of some types of coat assists grooming and general hygiene, while clipping can assist in grooming by keeping the coat short enough to be managed easily.

Trimming is carried out with special scissors. Areas that are commonly trimmed to assist in grooming are those prone to matting or collection of soiling in breeds such as some spaniels and setters. This includes the ears, to avoid the collection of food when eating, and the matting of the long silky hair just behind the ears. Feet are trimmed particularly between the toes, where mud can collect and dry on the hair so that it causes discomfort by rubbing and by pushing the toes apart. In bitches, it may be necessary to

Table 6.17 Grooming procedures	
Procedure	**Aim**
Loosening the dead hair	Most coats will benefit from the groomer pulling the fingertips along the skin through the coat against the lay of the hair. This will help to remove the loose hair and therefore stimulate normal hair growth. Dogs tend to find this procedure pleasant and some will get excited and see it as a game, so firm but friendly handling is required to insist that the dog stays fairly still
Combing	Using a traditional comb, any tangles can be eased out gently and any loose hair removed from the coat at this stage. The comb is used with the lay of the hair at an angle usually about 45°. Particular attention should be paid to areas on the longer haired breeds that have a tendency to tangle and mat such as behind the ears and feathering between and on the backs of the hindlegs. As the comb is more accurate than a brush and is usually smaller it can be used with care on areas that are difficult to assess, ensuring that no areas are missed or tangles remain underneath a superficially groomed coat. If mats are found during combing and they are not able to be removed or teased out gently during a traditional comb, then a specialised de-matting comb can be used where appropriate to remove the mat, followed by a combing out of the remaining hair gently with the traditional comb. Where a mat has been removed it is important to check the skin underneath it for damage as the area may be reddened or even suppurating. If the mat has caused irritation to the skin, this should be dealt with, depending on the severity
Brushing	This is carried out with a brush type depending upon the coat; the action of brushing depends on the brush. Exercise great care when grooming with pin or slicker brushes, as it is possible to damage the skin with some types if used too vigorously. It is not generally advisable to use this type of brush against the lay of the hair. For a smooth coat of the intermediate type the following brushing technique could be adopted. Once the combing is complete a bristle brush can be used. Firstly it is used on the hair covering the trunk. The brush is used against the lay of the hair in short straight strokes. This is begun at the base of the tail and thighs and moves gradually forward as each area is brushed. The brushing against the lay stops at the back of the head and at the base of the skull, leaving the head untouched at this stage. The brush is then used gently on the head with the lay of the hair and thereafter working downwards and backwards with short straight strokes, until the entire body and legs have been brushed. Taking hold of the tail, gently but firmly brush carefully from base to tip. Care is required when grooming tails as many dogs are quite sensitive about their tails being groomed and some may react sharply to all but the most gentle brushing. During the brushing phase the brush should be periodically cleaned to remove any build-up of hair. This can be done by drawing a traditional comb through the bristles
Finishing	After combing and brushing, a smooth or silky medium type of coat can be finished off by using a damp cloth or smooth hound glove (or a piece of velvet or damp synthetic chamois cloth). The face is gently wiped over followed by the remainder of the body, working from front to back. This action smooths down the coat and removes stray hair and dust from the coat surface, giving a sleek shine to a healthy coat. This is not done generally with coats that are the woolly or wire coat type, as these are usually required to stand up and are brushed into shape and left

trim soiled areas post-whelping if soiling and staining from whelping fluid cannot be removed easily any other way.

If a dog soils itself or mats easily, grooming will be simplified if hair is judiciously trimmed from the anal area and hindleg feathering – but do not be scissor-happy. Strike a balance between the need to keep the dog hygienic and the owner's need for the dog's appearance to be acceptable.

Clipping is by means of special clippers. There are set styles of clip designed to enhance breed features, e.g. some of the hair of terrier breeds is removed or thinned out by professional hand-stripping. Non-showing owners of breeds with long, heavy coats such as the Old English sheep dog may have their animals clipped out for the summer. Dogs such as poodles do not moult normally and it is essential to clip the coat regularly, otherwise it would become unmanageable for the owner and would cause discomfort and distress to the dog.

Clippers should only be used according to the manufacturer's instructions as they are easily damaged by misuse. For example, the hair must be completely dry, as wet hair quickly blunts the blades. The blades should not be forced through a thick coat or matting as they may be clogged by the hair and stop the machine, possibly causing damage to the equipment. If the clippers become hot during use, they should be allowed to cool down before continuing.

Clipping machines should be regularly serviced and maintained. They need to be thoroughly cleaned and oiled after each use and then stored in a dry environment. A variety of blades should be available, with spares of those used most commonly to enable a rotation for regular sharpening.

Bathing

Bathing is carried out for three main reasons:

- To eradicate and control ectoparasites.
- To treat skin conditions and apply topical medication.
- To cleanse and condition the coat.

Cleansing may be required for various reasons, such as:

to disease are generally more common in a hospital situation (e.g. post-operative cases are more susceptible than the average healthy adult animal) and hospital accommodation is therefore designed and managed to reduce this risk by means of high standards of hygiene. Unfortunately, even with the best standards of kennel design and hygiene, risks can never be totally removed, particularly where there is a potential mechanism by which micro-organisms can be transferred.

Thus it becomes apparent that three out of the four factors in the above list can never be wholly removed. It is therefore important to concentrate on the other factor – the essential link of the transfer mechanism by which a micro-organism is transferred from one animal to another. The prevention of this mechanism is achieved by barrier nursing or isolation nursing of the infected animal.

To achieve effective isolation of an infected animal, the particular transfer mechanism of the specific disease must first be understood (see Chapter 17).

Admission of infected animals

As general kennel or practice policy, ideally no animal should be admitted that has (or is suspected of having) an infectious disease which poses a potential risk to other animals housed. An infected animal should never be admitted into a hospital or kennels where no separate, specific isolation facilities exist.

The usual reason for providing isolation facilities in kennels and catteries is to enable the isolation of animals that have developed suspicious symptoms after they have been admitted. By then, this will be the only course of action to protect the other animals housed. Where this occurs, the correct care and housing depends upon the nature of the disease and the type of infection risk.

Isolation kennelling

The size of isolation facilities is dependent on the numbers of animals housed. The recommended rate for dog isolation is at least one isolation kennel for up to 50 kennels (licensed for 50 dogs) and pro rata above that number.

The recommended rate for cat isolation is at least one isolation unit for up to 30 units (licensed for 30 cats).

When isolation kennelling is being designed, all possible disease transmission factors should be taken into account. The kennelling should comprise a totally self-contained unit so that all procedures can be carried out within the unit itself.

If space does not permit the recommended distance for the isolation units, care must be taken to ensure there is no possibility of cross-infection, e.g. windows and doors must not open towards non-isolation units. Personnel should be allocated separately to handle these cases. If this is not possible, all 'clean' animals should be attended to first and then those in isolation, with strict attention being paid to protec-

tive clothing, changes of footwear, etc. An alternative is for a member of staff who is not on kennel or ward duties to be allocated to the isolation unit.

Isolation kennels must be separate from the main kennels and are usually physically separated by at least 5 m (15 ft) (this distance is based upon the distance that a dog sneeze travels). In existing catteries there must be a minimum of 3 m (10 ft) physical separation from the main cat accommodation units.

Where new kennels or catteries are being built it is recommended that isolation facilities are built 10 m (30 ft) from the main accommodation units. However, intervening buildings and other constructional details such as the positioning of doors, windows and exercise runs, when taken into account, may allow for variation of the distance.

All equipment should be kept and used in the isolation unit only and the unit should be equipped to enable the intensive care of acutely ill patients.

Isolation and infectious disease

Certain disease management methods are used routinely when managing a case in isolation:

- If possible, one or two staff members should be allocated to deal only with the infected animal and they should not handle any other animals. If this is not practical, they should be restricted to handling animals that have a low risk of contracting the disease. On no account should they also care for high-risk animals such as the very young.
- A foot-bath should be used at the entrance of the isolation unit and should contain a freshly prepared disinfectant solution. The disinfectant type depends upon the disease.
- All hygiene procedures should be carried out using disinfectants known to be effective against the disease concerned.
- A change of protective clothing should be available in a suitable area at the entrance to the isolation unit. The type of clothing depends upon the disease but may be:

  - a boiler suit or other coverall;
  - wellington boots;
  - disposable gloves and apron;
  - surgical mask;
  - hat (particularly for staff with long hair).

- There should be facilities for washing and disinfection and for safely discarding disposable items at the exit from the isolation unit.
- The infected animal should be nursed and treated as is appropriate to the disease.

Where purpose-built isolation facilities are not available, a measure of isolation can be achieved in less than ideal situations by strict nursing techniques (see Chapter 17).

Quarantine in the UK

The British Isles are fortunate in being separated by sea from mainland Europe. This separation has provided a natural barrier to diseases that spread through wild or domestic animals where free passage across borders is otherwise difficult to prevent. Pet animals require human assistance to cross the sea and it is therefore relatively easy to control and restrict the entry of animals, despite the constant movement of humans.

Britain has been free from the disease of rabies for many years and the continued prevention of its entry is of major concern. The principal control measure has been the quarantine of all animals susceptible to transmitting the disease, i.e. dogs, cats, etc., entering the country, but in recent years there has been much debate with the other European Community member states regarding the freer movement of animals. The argument put forward is that effective vaccination is now possible and so is thought to reduce the likelihood of rabies entering the UK. Although the use of quarantine still stands as the principal method of preventing the entry of rabies, Britain has now agreed to certain new arrangements regarding the movement of animals, but only in cases where the conditions provide controls at least as stringent as quarantine. The Ministry of Agriculture, Fisheries and Food (now DEFRA) announced changes relating solely to commercially traded breeding animals in July 1994. These arrangements were known as the 'Balai' arrangements. In February 2000 the PETS Scheme (Pet Travel Scheme) came into operation allowing animals from Europe and other authorised countries to enter the UK without undergoing the statutory 6 months quarantine period provided they satisfy all the regulations.

PETS – Pet Travel Scheme

Since February 2000 the system allows pet animals from certain countries to enter the UK, without going into quarantine. This is known as The Pet Travel Scheme (PETS).

The scheme was introduced for dogs and cats travelling from certain European countries and additional countries have been added since its commencement. Since qualifying countries are being added from time to time, particularly rabies-free islands, it is advisable for clients to check before making their arrangements.

The Pet Travel Scheme applies to England, Wales and Scotland only. Pets entering the Republic of Ireland from all countries other than the UK, Channel Islands and Isle of Man will still be required to undertake quarantine.

Guide dogs and registered assistance dogs must fulfil the same criteria but individual carriers may permit different travelling conditions.

Booster vaccinations against rabies must be administered at the intervals specified by the manufacturer of the vaccine. It is essential that owners keep these up to date to avoid having to have the animal revaccinated and blood tested and the 6 months rule being imposed again.

Treatment against tapeworm and ticks must be administered in the 24–48 hours period before the animal re-enters the UK. This has to be carried out every time. If the animal is leaving the UK on a day trip, this treatment should be carried out in the UK, again 24–48 hours before the re-entry.

The animal must be treated with praziquantel for the tapeworm and for those treated in rabies-free islands, the tick treatment must contain fipronil.

The veterinary nurse should be aware that there are diseases prevalent in other countries which do not occur in the UK. These include parasites such as heartworm, tapeworm and diseases transmitted by ticks and other insects such as sand flies. Preventative treatment is available for some conditions.

Clients should also be counselled on whether the animal would be happy travelling abroad and whether kennelling or home sitters might be preferable to travel stresses.

PETS only applies to pet cats and dogs (excluding those banned under the Dangerous Dogs' Act of 1991): it is limited to pets coming into the UK from certain countries and territories and it only operates on certain sea, air and rail routes to England.

The basic requirements are that the pet must be:

(1)   Microchipped (tattooing is not acceptable).
(2)   Vaccinated against rabies.
(3)   Blood tested and the result must show the vaccine has given satisfactory protection against rabies.
(4)   Issued with an official PETS certificate.
(5)   Treated against tapeworm and ticks.

The procedures must be undertaken in the order shown.

Additionally, when returning with the pet into the UK, owners are required to have an official PETS certificate which shows the animal has been microchipped, vaccinated and blood tested. The animal must have an official certificate showing it has been treated against tapeworm and ticks and have an official declaration that the animal has not been outside the PETS countries.

Veterinary advisers must strongly recommend owners to obtain all the necessary certification before travelling, including any certificates required for entry into other countries.

A further essential requirement is that the animal cannot enter the UK until at least 6 calendar months after the blood sample taken giving a successful test result. The reason for this is that should the animal have been infected before or at the time of vaccination it would not be protected against rabies. Most infected animals will display any clinical signs of rabies by this time. This is equivalent to the period of quarantine required.

Entry to the UK must be by specified air, sea and rail routes to specified entry ports. These are subject to alteration and students should advise clients to ring the PETS helpline or visit the PETS website.

Should the pet not meet all the requirements of the PETS scheme, it must go into quarantine. An import licence must be obtained before travelling. Should the animal subsequently fulfil the requirements of the PETS, it can become eligible for early release from quarantine.

To apply for an import licence, owners must contact the Quarantine Section of DEFRA, Area 211, 1a Page Street, London SW1P 4PQ.

Other considerations in some countries (e.g. France and Germany) require that dogs such as Staffordshire Bull Terriers and Rottweilers are to be kept on a lead and muzzled in public. Advice on whether a pet is allowed into a country should first be obtained from the Embassy of the country clients intend to visit.

Other requirements

Some qualifying countries require a veterinary health certificate before entry. These requirements are totally separate from the Pet Travel Scheme. Some countries also require a separate rabies vaccination certificate.

Other categories of captive bred rabies susceptible animals present no real risk of bringing rabies into the British Isles, e.g. rabbits, rats and guinea pigs. From 1 January 1994 there was no requirement to quarantine such animals, provided that they have been born and reared on the holding of origin without coming into contact with any other rabies susceptible animal. (Domestic farm livestock and horses have never been included in the rabies quarantine arrangements as they are not considered a risk on import.)

Animals still subject to quarantine are:

- Primates.
- Carnivores.
- Wild mammals not born and kept in captivity.

In view of further changes to the rules, it is strongly recommended that those who wish to import or export dogs and cats into or from the UK should contact DEFRA for the most recent information regarding relevant regulations and the specific requirements for each country of destination. At present the quarantine period for dogs and cats entering the UK is 6 calendar months, the only exceptions being those previously mentioned.

The requirements of quarantine kennelling

The principles of quarantine kennelling for the prevention of rabies entering Britain are that the animal should be confined humanely for a period of 6 months in a secure establishment. The animal must have no possibility of contact with other animals (either internally or external to the kennels) that may risk being infected by rabies. To meet these principles:

- No physical contact of any kind is allowed between animals.
- No animal may have contact with the body fluids of another animal (e.g. urine must not seep through or be directed from one run to another through fences, and screens must protect cats from spitting at one another).

No animal may have contact with any item used by another animal prior to disinfection (e.g. dog beds and non-disposable bedding materials).

- There must be no possibility of escape from the kennel or compound.
- The only exception to the above is where animals from the same household share a kennel, in which case both animals are isolated from others as if they were one animal.

The standard sizes and other factors regarding quarantine accommodation for dogs and cats are set out in Table 6.18.

Licensing of quarantine kennels

Kennels and catteries used for the quarantine of animals in the UK are authorised by DEFRA. The primary concern is that the kennels should be secure and meet standard requirements necessary to achieve all the principles previously mentioned in relation to the design, construction, operation and management.

If a lay person owns the kennels they must employ a veterinary surgeon who is appointed as veterinary superintendent and who must visit the premises daily from Monday to Saturday, and on Sunday when necessary.

General safety procedures in quarantine establishments

- All staff must be instructed on the dangers of rabies.
- Quarantine kennels must be run separately from all other units on the same site.
- Security and fire precautions and procedures must comply with current regulations.
- All animals must be transported to the kennels by an authorised carrying agent from the airport or ship's dock, and in a special vehicle and container.
- A high-security area must be used for the transfer of animals from the transporting vehicle to the kennel accommodation units.
- Rabies vaccination should be carried out on arrival or within 24 hours (regardless of current vaccination status).
- An animal must be kept in one accommodation unit for the duration of its stay.
- Animals housed in each accommodation unit should be clearly identified.
- Strict hygiene procedures should be observed at all times, using approved disinfectants.
- Animals in quarantine have restricted access by owners or any other person. Special authorisation is required if owners visit within 14 days of the arrival in quarantine.
- Strict recording procedures must be carried out regarding any movements of the animal, visits by the owner and all health records.

See 'Rabies', Chapter 17.

Table 6.18 Quarantine facilities

	Sleeping area (not less than)	Adjoining exercise area (run) (not less than)	Other comments
Small dogs (less than 12 kg (26 lb))	1.1 m² (12 sq ft) Width and length 0.9 m (3 ft)	3.7 m² (40 sq ft) Width: 0.9 m (3 ft)	*Height of dog compartment*: not to be less than 1.8 m (6 ft). Walls of sleeping area must be floor to roof or with all walls measuring at least 1.8 m (6 ft) and any gap above partitioned with escape-proof weld mesh. Wire diameter must not be less than 2 mm (14 swg), with mesh size not exceeding 50 mm (2 inches)
Medium-sized dogs (12–30 kg (26–66 lb)	1.4 m² (16 sq ft) Width and length 1.2 m (4 ft)	5.5 m² (60 sq ft) Width: 1.2 m (4 ft)	
Large dogs (more than 30 kg (66 lb))	1.4 m² (16 sq ft) Width and length 1.2 m (4 ft)	7.4 m² (80 sq ft) Width: 1.2 m (4 ft)	Runs should be constructed to allow dogs to see beyond the confines of the unit wherever possible They must be constructed to allow no nose or paw contact and no passage of urine from one to another
			Dividing partitions between runs: At least 1.8 m (6 ft) high An impervious material with a smooth hard finish is used for the first part of the dividing partition, to a height of 0.4 m (18 inches) for small to medium-sized dogs and 0.6 m (2 ft) for large dogs The upper part of the dividing partition must be constructed of a see-through material that is nose and paw proof
			Run fencing: Minimum height of 0.3 m (10 ft) with a weld mesh guard of 0.6 m (2 ft) set at an inward 45° angle; or runs roofed over completely
Cats	Total floor area (sleeping compartment and run) not less than 1.4 m² (15 sq ft) Width and length: 0.9 m (3 ft) Height not less than 1.8 m (6 ft)		Quarantine accommodation for cats should be of the 'walk-in' type. It must be securely roofed with all partitions solid to prevent cats spitting at one another

The welfare of dogs and cats in quarantine premises

A voluntary code of practice regarding the welfare of dogs and cats held in quarantine premises has been produced. These standards were compiled by DEFRA in consultation with the owners of quarantine premises and animal welfare organisations.

The standards include:

- Identification of who is responsible for the welfare of the animals.
- Transport to and moves within the premises.
- Minimum standards for sizes of units housing dogs and cats.
- General standards including hygiene, non-slip and other construction hazards, visual stimulation and ventilation, sleeping compartment, and heating recommendations.
- Feeding and management standards include weighing, feeding and supervision, provision of water, diet, and condition and frequency of feeds.
- Recommended animal checking intervals.

- General conduct including reporting structure, supervision and training of staff.

Copies of the booklet are available on request.

Procedure if a rabies case is suspected

Where the suspected case is held in quarantine

If an animal in quarantine displays unexplained nervous signs, it should immediately be confined and the DEFRA should be informed that a case of rabies is suspected.

If the suspect case dies or is euthanased, the animal is removed by the Ministry veterinary officer. Its head will be removed and taken to the DEFRA diagnostic laboratory where the brain is removed under very strict conditions for tests to determine if the animal was infected by rabies.

It is possible that an animal brought into the practice for consultation with a veterinary surgeon displays clinical signs and a case history which raise the suspicion that it may be a case of rabies. Even a sick bat brought in might have to be viewed with suspicion. The veterinary surgeon will take into account all the symptoms and the history in making a decision to report the case as suspected rabies.

Where an animal is a suspected case but with insufficient grounds to report

In these circumstances a second opinion may be requested. The DEFRA Duty veterinary officer at the local Animal Health Divisional Office (AHDO) should be contacted to arrange for a veterinary officer to visit and examine the animal in consultation with the veterinary surgeon. The animal will be isolated and the veterinary surgeon will remain with the suspect animal until the veterinary officer arrives.

Where the veterinary surgeon makes a decision to report a suspected case

There is a statutory requirement that any suspicion of a case of rabies must be reported to:

- A DEFRA inspector (veterinary officer).
- The local authority animal health inspector.
- A police constable.

Where a case is suspected in general practice, it is likely that the first contact will be with the Duty veterinary officer at the AHDO, by telephone.

The owner or person in charge of the animal should be advised by the veterinary surgeon:

- That rabies is suspected.
- That the animal must be detained and isolated.
- That it will be necessary for an official inquiry to be carried out by the Department's veterinary officer who is being called to attend the case.

Isolation of the suspected case

The suspect animal must be isolated in escape-proof accommodation in order to prevent any further contact with animals or humans. It must remain on the premises on which it has been examined by the veterinary surgeon until the Department's veterinary officer's enquiries are completed.

Where a suspected case occurs in general practice

The veterinary nurse should always have emergency plans prepared for various events, including natural disasters such as fire and flood. Rabies should be considered as a potential 'disaster' and requires a plan of action by the head nurse to keep the veterinary practice prepared.

Identification of all contact animals

The names and addresses of the owners or person in charge of all animals that may have come into direct contact with the suspect case, along with descriptions of those animals, should be recorded. Reception records for the day will be needed for verification.

Any animal that has been bitten, scratched or come into contact with the saliva of the suspect animal should be detained at the premises until the Department's veterinary officer's enquiries are completed.

The officer will advise if any further action is necessary with regard to contact animals.

Human contacts

Once the animal has been detained and isolated, all persons who have handled it should carry out a thorough personal disinfection:

- Hands should first be washed with soap or detergent and hot water.
- Clothing or overalls, if contaminated with discharges from the suspected animal, should be removed and sterilised before re-use.
- Equipment used on the animal should be removed and sterilised before re-use.

All cases of human contact with the suspected animal must be referred to the medical officer or the Environmental Health Office for further action and advice immediately.

WARNING

It is of paramount importance that anyone bitten or scratched by the suspected animal should have the wound treated immediately.

(1) Wash and flush the wound with soap or detergent and water.

(2) Flush repeatedly with running water alone – this is imperative.

(3) Apply either:
  - 40–70% alcohol; or
  - tincture of aqueous solutions of iodine; or
  - 0.1% quaternary ammonium compounds (NB: soap neutralises quaternary ammonium compounds, therefore all traces of soap must be removed before application).

General routine of admission of dogs and cats into the UK

The routine of admission at the time of writing is as follows. For information on imports, contact the Department of the Environment Food and Rural Affairs (DEFRA).

The Dangerous Dogs Act 1991

The Government has, under the Dangerous Dogs Act 1991 (as amended 1997) placed a ban on the ownership of certain breeds of dog. The dogs affected by the ban are certain breeds bred for fighting and cross-breeds of these types.

The following are affected by the ban:

- Pit Bull Terrier.
- Japanese Tosa.

- Dogo Argentino.
- Fila Braziliero.

The UK police and local authorities may seize any dog that **appears** to belong to one of these breeds. The owner will then be prosecuted.

If convicted the owner will face a fine or imprisonment and the dog may be destroyed on the order of the court.

An amendment was made to the Dangerous Dogs Act in 1997 which gives the Courts some discretion in that a destruction order may not be imposed if certain conditions are met, such as muzzling when in a public place, neutering, etc.

Import licence

No pet dog or cat may be imported unless an import licence has been granted by or on behalf of DEFRA (or the Secretary of State for Scotland, Northern Ireland or Jersey or the Welsh Office Agriculture Department if appropriate). Commercial trade in dogs or cats may be allowed under the 'Balai' arrangements, provided that all of the conditions can be met. A condition of the licence is that the animal will be held in quarantine for 6 calendar months from the date of its landing in the UK.

Application for import licences must be made in good time. As it is essential that the licence is issued on time, it is necessary for applications to be made at least 8 weeks in advance of the proposed date of importation.

Licences will not be granted unless the DEFRA is satisfied that the necessary arrangements have been made, i.e. that the quarantine kennels and carrying agent have given notice of the booking.

Quarantine kennels
Accommodation must be reserved at approved quarantine premises well in advance of the proposed date of importation. A list of approved premises is available from DEFRA.

Authorised carrying agent
The services of an authorised carrying agent must be reserved to meet the animal at the port or airport and be responsible for its safe custody to the quarantine premises (some quarantine premises are also authorised carrying agents).

The port of entry
Animals may only be landed at certain ports and airports. A list is available from DEFRA.

If arriving by air, animals going directly into quarantine may only be landed at the following UK airports:

- Birmingham.
- Leeds.
- Edinburgh.
- Manchester.
- London Gatwick.
- Prestwick.
- Glasgow.
- Belfast.
- London Heathrow.

DEFRA will forward to the owner or representative a red label which has to be completed and attached to the travelling crate. This ensures the crate is identifiable as one containing an animal subject to quarantine.

Crates must meet International Air Transport Association (IATA) standards. Airlines will advise owners of the correct size. Pets are not allowed to travel with owners in the passenger cabin under any circumstances.

If arriving by sea route, there are specific ports of entry where animals going directly into quarantine may be landed. At the time of writing (July 2001) these are:

- Dover Eastern Docks.
- Harwich, Parkeston Quay.
- Hull.
- Portsmouth.
- Southampton.

Before leaving the vessel, the pet must be crated and the red label attached. At most ports of entry the carrying agent will board the vessel to collect the animal. At all times, owners must be advised by the veterinary nurse to contact DEFRA to obtain current information since this may be subject to change.

Rabies vaccination should be carried out on arrival or within **48 hours** of landing.

Granting of the licence
DEFRA will confirm the booking with the quarantine premises and carrying agent. They will then:

- Send the import licence to the carrying agent. (The carrying agent is responsible for clearing the animal through customs.)
- Send a boarding document to the applicant (usually owner of the animal) or a named representative. (The boarding document will confirm the licence number and act as written evidence that a licence has been granted. This document will be shown to the shipper or airline before the animal will be allowed to leave for the UK.)
- Send a red label to the applicant or named representative if the animal is to be transported by air. The red label is to be completed and affixed to the crate prior to embarkation.

Container or crate
If the animal is to travel by air, the container or crate must conform to IATA standards, i.e. it must be large enough for the animal to stand and lie in a natural position and turn around (Fig. 6.7).

The animal will travel to the UK as manifest cargo in the freight compartment.

Procedure for exporting dogs and cats from the UK

The factors governing the requirements for the export of dogs and cats from the UK are determined by the country to which the animal is being exported. No British laws are in

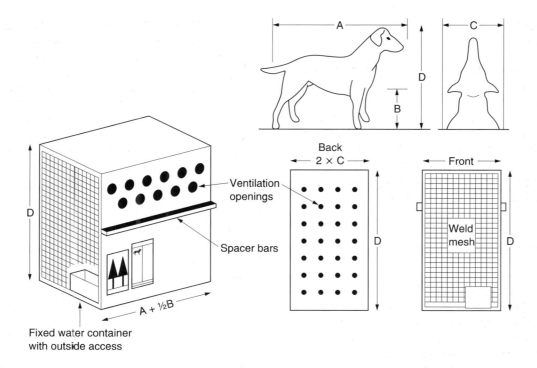

Fig. 6.7 IATA container requirements for cats and dogs. (Reproduced by kind permission of the IATA.)

force which govern the export of animals – the only laws presently in force govern imports.

The regulations relating to the export of dogs and cats to other countries vary considerably and may change depending upon the circumstances within the individual country at the time.

It is recommended that the export section of DEFRA be contacted for the up-to-date requirements for each country.

Breeds: the recognised groups of dogs and cats

Pedigree dog breeds: The Kennel Club

The Kennel Club has been in existence since 1873 and its main aim is 'To promote in every way the general improvement of dogs'. The Kennel Club is the governing body for all official shows, trials and competitions held in the UK. All dogs exhibited in the UK at breed shows must be recognised and registered by the Kennel Club through their formal registration system. Change of ownership is also registered with the Kennel Club. The breeds recognised by the Kennel Club are broadly classified as 'sporting' and 'non-sporting', subdivided into 'groups'. The following includes three examples of breeds within each group:

- **Sporting**

  - Hound group (e.g. Beagle, Dachshund, Whippet).
  - Gundog group (e.g. English Setter, Labrador Retriever, Cocker Spaniel).

  - Terrier group (e.g. Cairn Terrier, Lakeland Terrier, Staffordshire Bull Terrier).

- **Non-sporting**

  - Utility group (e.g. Dalmatian, Keeshond, Lhasa Apso).
  - Pastoral group (e.g. Bearded Collie, German Shepherd Dog, Samoyed).
  - Working group (e.g. Dobermann, Great Dane, St Bernard).
  - Toy group (e.g. Chihuahua, Italian Greyhound, Yorkshire Terrier).

Within these groups there are many different breeds eligible for registration; each of these breeds has a breed standard. The breed standard describes the ideal of each breed's appearance, behaviour and movement. The breed names are not necessarily a guide to the breed's group. For example, not all dogs with the word 'terrier' in their name are classed as terriers. The Australian Silky Terrier, English Toy Terrier and Yorkshire Terrier are in the Toy group, while the Boston and Tibetan Terriers are in the Utility group. Most but not all spaniels are in the Gundog group but the Tibetan Spaniel is in the Utility group and the King Charles and Cavalier King Charles Spaniels are in the Toy group.

Cats

There are more than 5 million non-pedigree cats in Britain and the numbers are increasing. All types are seen due to the free-range nature of the breeding of cats in this country and resulting mix of genes. Both long- and short-hair types occur naturally in the present population. All colours are found but the most common is tabby, of which there are two types: those with 'mackerel' stripes (narrow bands of colour similar to the coat of the Scottish wildcat) and those with the more common blotched tabby markings. The tabby colouring is followed in frequency by black and white colouring. More unusual colours like chocolate, colour point and chinchilla suggest that a pedigree cat has been involved in an individual ancestry.

Pedigree cat breeds are recognized and classified in the UK by the Governing Council of the Cat Fancy (GCCF), which is similar to the Kennel Club in that it:

- Classifies breeds and issues breed standards by which cats may be judged.
- Licenses cat shows and appoints judges.
- Prepares and publishes the rules to control these functions.
- Protects the welfare of cats and improves cat breeding.
- Protects the interests of cat owners.
- Exercises disciplinary powers.

In 1992 there was a major change in the GCCF's classification and grouping of cats with the introduction of a new section, the 'semi-long-hairs'. The major groups are now:

- Long-hairs.
- Semi-long-hairs.
- British short-hairs.
- Foreign.
- Burmese.
- Orientals.
- Siamese and Balinese.

The GCCF has a breed numbering system first adopted in 1910, which has evolved into a master series of numbers and letters. Each cat breed is individually numbered according to the major group, breed type, coat pattern and colour.

KEY POINTS
- The basic needs and category of the animal should always be taken into account when housing.
- Kennels and catteries should always be managed using a planned and methodical approach.
- Cleaning and disinfection routines must be followed in a strict protocol according to the situation.
- Basic care of hospitalised animals should always take into account their underlying condition.
- Isolation procedures are in place to prevent the spread of disease.
- Quarantine in the UK is in place as a principal control measure to prevent the ingress of disease not normally occurring.
- The manufacturers' recommendations regarding all equipment, materials and products should always be consulted and adhered to.

References and further reading

Kennel and cattery construction

Hamilton-Moore, S. and Cruickshank, C. (1988) *Boarding Cattery Construction and Management*, Feline Advisory Bureau Boarding Cattery Information Service.

Heginbotham, G. and S. (1984) *Boarding Kennels and Catteries (Their Design and Management)*, 2nd edn, The Kennels Agency and Hurst Publications, Reading.

Key, D. (2000) *Essential Kennel Design 'The Owners Complete Guide to Design and Specialisation'*, Uniskill, Witney.

Working Party Report (1995) *Model Licence Conditions and Guidance for Dog Boarding Establishments*, Chartered Institute of Environmental Health, London.

Working Party Report (1995) *Model Licence Conditions and Guidance for Cat Boarding Establishments*, Chartered Institute of Environmental Health, London.

Zabawa, S. (1988) *Running Your Own Boarding Kennels*, Kogan Page, London.

Antiseptics and disinfectants

Ayliffe, G. A. J., Coates, D. and Hoffman, P. N. (1993) *Chemical Disinfection in Hospitals*, 2nd edn, PHLS, London.

Rutala, W. A. (1990) APIC guideline for selection and use of disinfectants. *American Journal of Infection Control*, vol. 18, no. 2, pp. 99–117.

Smith, J. (1998) A guide to disinfectant. *Veterinary Nursing*, vol. 13, no. 6, pp. 207–212.

Stucke, V. A. (1993) *Microbiology for Nurses*, 7th edn, Baillière Tindall, London.

Management and hygiene

Officers of the BVA (1993) The veterinary surgeon's duty of care in handling and disposing of clinical waste. *The Veterinary Record*, January 9, pp. 25, 43, 44, 45.

Price, C. J. (1991) *Practical Veterinary Nursing (Nursing of Inpatients)*, 2nd edn, BSAVA, Cheltenham.

Taylor, R. (1992) An introduction to dog grooming (parts 1 and 2). *BVNA Journal*, vol. 7, nos 5/6, pp. 158–164.

Watson, D. (1992) The skin, mother nature's barometer of health. *Veterinary Practice Nurse*, vol. 4, no. 2, pp. 9–11.

Quarantine, isolation and quarantine kennels

Chandler, S. (1994) Isolation. In Simpson, G. (ed.), *Practical Veterinary Nursing*, 3rd edn, pp. 182–183, BSAVA, Cheltenham.

DEFRA Rabies information literature, including *Rabies – Guidance Notes for Practising Veterinary Surgeons*, provided by MAFF Tolworth, Surbiton.

DEFRA website: www.defra.gov.uk.

Evans, J. (ed.) (1989/90), *Rabies – Guidance Notes, Henston Vade mecum (small animal)*.

MAFF (1995) *The Welfare of Dogs and Cats in Quarantine Premises, Voluntary Code of Practice*, DEFRA Publications, London.

Dog and cat breeds

Governing Council of the Cat Fancy (March 1998) *List of Breeds to be Catered for at GCCF Championship Shows*, GCCF.

Spall, J. (ed.) *Showing Cats (the GCCF Guide to Shows and Show Cats)*, GCCF/Pedigree Petfoods.

The Kennel Club (1998) *The Kennel Club's Illustrated Breed Standards*, Ebury Press, London.

7

Basic organisation and management

Sue Morrissey

Learning objectives

After studying this chapter, students should be able to:

- State the basic principles of practice management.
- Identify the interpersonal skills required by veterinary nurses.
- Describe the methods used for record keeping.
- List the methods of payment.
- Describe the principles of ensuring security of the practice premises and property.
- Describe how personal safety can be maintained at work.

Why profit?

A veterinary practice is an expensive business to run; the cost of drugs, salaries of staff and all the other overheads associated have to be met by the fees paid by clients. It is imperative that a fee structure is in place which will not only cover these costs but also generate a surplus (profit) which can be used both to continue to develop the practice and also reward the owners for their investment.

Planning for success

A successful practice is one which achieves its objectives. Objectives should always include profitability. Success does not just happen – plans must be made, systems set up and monitored, and changes made to meet changing circumstances.

It is of fundamental importance that the aims and objectives of the practice are defined and known, understood and accepted by all members of the practice. These aims are most usually set out in the following two documents.

The **Mission Statement**. This is a written statement of the practice's purpose and ethos. It is usually brief and may cover such items as

- The geographical area served by the practice, e.g. '10 mile radius of Anytown'.
- The type of work undertaken by the practice, e.g. 'companion and farm animal work'.
- Whether the practice is first opinion or referral or both.
- The standard of patient care to which the practice aspires.
- How clients may expect to be treated when they visit the practice.
- Pricing policy.

The Mission Statement is normally displayed in a public area for clients to see and may even be incorporated into literature produced by the practice such as the practice brochure, or website.

The **Business Plan**. This is a written statement, which sets out in precise terms what the practice aims to achieve over a given period (3–5 years), and how it will achieve those objectives. It is a living document which is constantly being updated to take account of changes in circumstances.

Before formulating its Mission Statement or Business Plan, the practice must first analyse its current position, performing what has come to be known as a 'SWOT' analysis.

- **S** – *Strengths*. What are the strengths of the practice? (Excellent location? Longstanding reputation for good service? Highly trained and committed staff?)
- **W** – *Weaknesses*. What are the weaknesses of the practice? (Poor premises? Lack of equipment? Inadequately trained staff?)
- **O** – *Opportunities*. What opportunities are open to the practice? (Neighbouring practice closing down? Growth in local population bringing potential new clients?)
- **T** – *Threats*. What is the potential threat to the practice? (A new competitor opening locally? Declining population?)

The whole practice should be involved in the SWOT analysis, initially often most successfully undertaken as a 'brainstorming' session. The SWOT analysis should be performed on an annual basis and changes reflected in the Business Plan.

Armed with the self-knowledge derived from the SWOT analysis and Mission Statement, the practice can then set about the task of writing a Business Plan.

To be successful it is essential that the Business Plan is:

- *Achievable*. Planning to have 100% of the cat-owning population of an area as clients within 12 months is unrealistic, as is seeking to convert an inner city small animal practice into a profitable farm business.
- *Resourced*. The Business Plan must take account of financial and human resources required and available.
- *Targeted*. The Business Plan should set very specific goals.
- *Measurable*. To assess whether a target has been achieved, that target must be measurable and the method of measurement laid down.

Either as part of the Business Plan, or as a series of associated documents, detailed Action Plans for all the tasks necessary for achievement of the plan will be made.

An example

To illustrate this process, let us follow through a simple example. The Anywhere Veterinary Practice conducted a SWOT analysis. Amongst the results of this were:

- Strengths – a highly trained nursing team.
- Weaknesses – included the lack of any programmes designed to encourage client loyalty and market practice services, and poor morale in the practice.
- Opportunities – included an increased number of potential clients from a newly completed housing estate.
- Threats – thought to exist from the planning consent which had been granted to another competitor to open a new practice in the same locality.

The practice discussed these SWOT results at some length and decided that considerable improvements were required, wishing instead to be perceived as a practice which was interested in maintaining the health of pets rather than one where the only contact between client and surgery was when an animal was sick. In addition, it was concluded that practice members would be happier and more fulfilled if they had the opportunity to use more of their skills. When the Mission Statement was written, it included 'This practice seeks to work with clients to keep pets as happy and healthy family members'.

Through a series of meetings, practice members were encouraged to put forward ideas for ways in which the aspirations expressed in the Mission Statement could be fulfilled and the positive and negative points arising from the SWOT analysis tackled. Amongst other ideas, the nurses said that they would like to set up puppy parties, as this was a service requested by clients and an area in which they felt they could use skills which were currently redundant. It was agreed that puppy parties would be a positive development of practice services and that they should be incorporated in the Business Plan.

The entry in the Business Plan read 'Puppy parties will commence on 1st March 1999. The programme of material to be included at the parties, and a suggested marketing plan for them, will be drawn up by the Head Nurse and submitted for Partners' approval by e.g. 1st November 1998. Initially the parties will be held once a month. No charge will be made for the parties. Annual costs, including promotional material and overtime payments, are estimated to be c£1000 per annum'.

No practice will achieve the goals set out in the Mission Statement and Business Plan unless practice members accept responsibility for and understand their personal role in fulfilling those goals. Plans which are formulated by practice owners without the involvement of the rest of the practice and issued simply as sets of instructions are less likely to succeed than those which have involved staff and sought input from everyone in the practice from their inception.

The purpose of management is to achieve the objectives of the practice, using resources effectively and efficiently. It is the responsibility of every member of the practice to contribute to this, often outside what may be considered the narrow confines of their professional discipline. **This is probably more true for veterinary nurses than for any other group of staff.**

We will now consider in more detail those areas of practice activity, outside clinical work, where the veterinary nurse can, quite literally, 'make or break' a practice.

Client contact: interpersonal skills

A veterinary nurse, whether officially designated 'receptionist' by the practice or not, will often be the first point of contact between the client and the practice. Poor interpersonal skills at this stage may lead to clients taking their pets elsewhere with consequential loss of fee-earning potential to the practice. Brusque treatment of a client who has come to purchase wormers for their puppy does not result simply in the loss of that £5 sale for the practice, it means that the practice has lost the capacity to earn hundreds of pounds over the lifetime of the dog in vaccination and neutering fees alone, without even considering any fees resulting from treatment for illness. **An even more damaging consequence of poor client service is that the client concerned will undoubtedly tell friends and family of their dissatisfaction, harming the reputation of the practice and possibly causing other existing or potential clients to go elsewhere.**

The receptionist is usually the first person with whom a client or the general public have contact when they telephone or come into the practice. The image that the receptionist portrays at that point of contact will be what the person remembers and perceives as the image of the practice as a whole. It is essential that this first impression, be it by telephone, direct contact or letter, is the one the practice wishes to portray. Reception is often the hub of internal and external communication within the practice.

Those working in reception must understand and deliver the policies and procedures of the practice for greeting visitors and clients and for security, safety and emergencies, as well as policy relating to routine work such as neutering, vaccination, worming and dealing with second opinion or referral cases. All these protocols should be incorporated into a staff handbook which forms the basis for induction training.

The reception area must be kept clean and tidy. With the use of plants, attractive and well-maintained posters or pictures, up-to-date reading material and comfortable seats, the area can project a warm, pleasant feeling which will encourage client confidence.

The personal appearance and hygiene of all members of staff are often perceived as representing the cleanliness and quality of the entire practice. Therefore it is important that a professional image is given. Clients like to know to whom they are talking and many practices now provide name badges, detailing job roles.

Clients are paying guests and they should be greeted as soon as they arrive. Ascertain the purpose of the visit and obtain all relevant details. Listen carefully and interpret the information that is given. Also look at the person who is communicating with you: non-verbal communication (body language) may tell you more than you are hearing.

Client contact

Interpersonal skills

Answering the telephone

The telephone should be answered promptly, confidently and efficiently, saying 'Good morning' (or afternoon or evening) and giving the name of the practice. Speak clearly and remember that your greeting will create a favourable or unfavourable impression of the practice as a whole.

Some practices may require that you then state your name and ask, 'How may I help you?' However, this will vary. Always ask who is calling. If you are unable to deal with the enquiry yourself, obtain as much information as possible and notify the caller that you are placing them 'on-hold' while you see if someone else is able to assist.

Pre-empt any queries or lapses of memory by surgery staff about the waiting caller by giving them the relevant information before putting the call through. This will also create a favourable impression with the client. In the meantime, keep going back to the caller 'on-hold' to apologise for any delay. They may be required to call back at a more appropriate time or you may need to obtain details from them so that the call can be returned. All telephone messages should be recorded in writing.

The practice should have a clear policy about the information that may be given over the telephone to clients and non-clients. All staff must be aware of these policies and then the relevant information can be given out in a clear and informed manner. If there is any doubt, the veterinary surgeon should be consulted and the client asked to bring the animal into the practice for examination.

A client may require telephone advice on animal first aid procedures. This should be given in a clear, calm manner by someone who has received training or instruction in the aims and procedures of animal first aid. You may need to advise the owner on how best to transport the animal to the practice or alternatively arrange a visit depending on the situation.

Rules for good communication

A few basic rules should ensure an accurate and effective system of internal and external communication:

- All forms of communication must be polite, clear and unambiguous.
- Information must be easily understood by both parties. Do not forget that the style and tone of a message or conversation can affect the response given.
- One of the most important aspects of communication is to be able to listen to others, to understand their view-point or requirements and to take action to fulfil their expectations.

There will be occasions when communication fails, leading to a complaint from the client. In the case of complaints made at the reception desk, try to take the client to a private area where the problem can be discussed, and hopefully resolved, without interruption. At all times the client must be treated with courtesy and respect.

Accuracy and efficiency

Appointments for consultation
Ensure that all those booking appointments know who is consulting and what length of consultation they require for certain procedures. Primary kitten vaccination consultations are sure to take longer than a post-operative check on a dog castration.

Nothing annoys clients more than surgeries that always run late. Try to ensure that surgeries start on time and that time is allotted for possible unexpected cases or emergencies.

Appointments for surgery
Ensure that all those clients booking animals in for operative or medical procedures are aware of the practice protocol for such cases. All animals should have been examined recently by the veterinary surgeon or be booked in for an appointment on the day of admission. Full details about the animal in question should be obtained from the owner plus a detailed list of procedures required to be undertaken whilst admitted into the practice.

Clients should be given accurate and detailed instructions on the preparation of the animal prior to admission.

Appointments for second opinions
When clients indicate to a veterinary surgeon that they are seeking referral for a second opinion from another veterinary surgeon, the original veterinary surgeon should make all the arrangements for such a consultation, including providing a full case history to the second veterinary surgeon.

Clients often telephone the practice themselves to arrange for a second opinion and it is essential that all staff dealing with such calls know what procedures should be followed to avoid the unethical situation of supersession. The original veterinary surgeon should be contacted by the practice and notified of the client's wish, so that both veterinary surgeons can discuss the case.

If the owner subsequently decides not to use the services of the original veterinary surgeon, the latter should be notified as soon as possible.

The following relevant definitions are given in the RCVS's *Guide to Professional Conduct*:

- **Second opinion** – when the original veterinarian or the client requests a second opinion from another veterinarian on diagnosis or on treatment, the intention being that the continued responsibility for treatment of the case should remain with the original veterinarian.

- **Referral** – when at the request of a veterinarian or client a case is referred to a second veterinarian or to another therapist for further diagnosis and treatment with the objective of return to the responsibility of the referring veterinarian at a mutually agreed time.
- **Supersession** – when a second veterinary surgeon assumes responsibility for diagnosis and treatment of the case without reference to the first veterinary surgeon or against the latter's wishes.

House calls Ensure that the client's full name, address and telephone number are obtained when arranging a house call. It is helpful if the client gives suitable directions on how to reach the house. It is essential to obtain as full a description of the animal's condition as soon as possible to ensure that the veterinary surgeon takes not only the correct equipment and drugs but also support staff if necessary. Staff should be aware that the personal security of a veterinary surgeon going out on a visit may require that a nurse is taken along for safety in numbers. The time of the visit should therefore be arranged according to the urgency of the visit and the availability of staff.

Admission of animals for surgery The admission of animals for surgery is best carried out by appointment in a separate room, allowing the owner time to discuss the case with the veterinary surgeon or nurse. This is usually done the evening prior to surgery, or at least 2 hours prior to surgery, thus giving time for the animal to settle and any preoperative procedures to take place.

Owners are frequently concerned about leaving a pet and often need the reassurance of a talk with a neatly dressed, friendly and knowledgeable person. There should be clear practice policies on who admits animals (if not the veterinary surgeon) and when an animal's preoperative check should take place. Owners often wish to see the premises where their animal will be hospitalised and there should be a clear practice policy and procedure to deal with such requests.

On admitting an animal, the nurse should write down routine details and ask relevant questions about the condition of the animal. These should include checking the owner's details and contact telephone number, the animal's details and the animal's weight recorded. Ask the following questions:

- Have there been any changes since the veterinary surgeon last saw the animal?
- When did the animal last eat any food?
- When did the animal last take fluids?
- When did the animal last have any medication, particularly if on a current course prescribed by the veterinary surgeon?
- To the owner's knowledge, does the animal have any allergies or adverse reactions to particular foods or drugs?
- When was the last bowel movement/urine passed?
- If the animal is female and entire, when was she last 'in season'?

- Vaccination status?
- Temperament?
- Have any abnormalities been noticed?

Also take the following action:

- Make a note of all objects brought in with the animal, to ensure that they are returned with the animal when it is discharged.
- All cats should be brought into the surgery in some form of carrier – if not they should be placed in one immediately. For security, cats should always be carried in a carrier, even from one room to another.
- To ensure that dogs do not escape by slipping collars and leads provided by the owner, place practice slip-leads on all dogs when transferring them to and from the kennels.
- It will depend on practice policy whether owners accompany their pets to the kennels. If not, it is best to ask the owner to leave the room before the dog is taken through.
- Any animal booked in for a procedure requiring the administration of a general or local anaesthetic should normally be admitted only after the owner or agent has read, understood and signed a fully completed anaesthetic consent form. Only someone over the age of 18 years may sign this form.
- It is often practice policy that all operative and investigative procedures are paid for on collection of the animal. The veterinary surgeon admitting the animal should be able to give the owner some idea of the cost, but this can always be confirmed when the owner arranges an appointment on the date of collection.

Kennels Kennels and cages must be labelled clearly and a system used to ensure that animals are not mixed up. It is possible to obtain identification collars for dogs and cats similar to the wrist bands placed on people when in hospital.

There must also be some method of correctly linking an animal in a kennel or cage with its full records, wherever these are kept. They might be on the front of the cage, or on clipboards kept in a place corresponding to the appropriate kennel. If a computerised system is used, there must be a proper reference on the kennel which can be used to access with certainty the right patient's data on the computer.

The allocation of cages according to the species and the disease is important:

- Cats are best separated from dogs.
- Small animals need to be put in an appropriate place and type of cage.
- Birds and nocturnal animals prefer a secluded, dimmed area.
- Infectious animals must be isolated and their cages labelled with relevant information so that staff may handle and care for them accordingly.

The stress for a hospitalised animal can be reduced to a minimum with gentle, caring nursing and a little thought. Animals often settle very well if regularly visited by the owner, who may bring in a well-loved blanket or toy (as long as the animal is unlikely to eat it). Feeding an animal from its own bowls may also reduce stress. If this does not work, early discharge may need to be considered in the interest of the animal's well-being.

Discharging of animals This process must be undertaken by someone who will be able to answer the owner's routine questions about the case.

No animal should be allowed to go home if the owner feels unable to care for it properly, be it wound management, stabilisation of an animal's fluid balance, digitalisation or diabetic stabilisation. Some animals are bright and well enough to go home but it is more convenient if the practice keeps the animal hospitalised, e.g. when a dog has a discharging Penrose drain in a wound that needs flushing four times daily. A sleepy Pomeranian is easy enough to care for post-operatively, but this may not be the case with a Great Dane. Each case should be considered individually and discharged at an appropriate time that is convenient for the owner, but in the best interest of the animal.

Before discharging the animal:

- The owner should be given full details on the procedures undertaken and any results of investigative procedures carried out on the animal.
- Detailed information on immediate post-operative/investigative care with regard to wound care, diet, exercise and medication should be given.
- If the animal is present whilst this information is being given, the owner is likely to take in very little – it is better to give the information before the animal is brought through. Many owners benefit from being given these instructions in writing as well. They should always be reassured that they can contact the surgery if they have any queries.
- If any medication is being dispensed, owners are often very glad to be given a practical demonstration on how best to administer it, particularly if they have no previous experience.
- All drugs should be suitably packaged and labelled.
- Remember to return the animal's belongings and always ensure that the animal is clean before being discharged. Regardless of the animal's state on arrival for admission, every effort should be made to ensure that it goes out clean and well groomed. Frequently the animal's coat is in such a bad state on admission that it would require more than a good brush to remove the dirt and mats. Permission from the client must be sought to go ahead with such a procedure.
- Finally, make an appointment for a return visit if required and deal with payment of the account according to the practice policy.

Record keeping

Computers

The use of computers is growing rapidly and they are playing an increasingly important role in the day-to-day running of veterinary practices. They can be extremely useful in a number of areas, including:

- Client record keeping.
- Sales and purchase controls.
- Stock control.
- Practice activity reporting.
- Costing and budgetary control.
- Personnel records.
- Wages/salary systems.
- Market research.
- Cash-flow analysis.
- Word processing.
- Desktop publishing.

All users of computers must be aware of the Data Protection Act 1984, which is supervised by the Data Protection Registrar. All employers holding computerised data including personnel records need to decide whether or not they need to register as 'data users'. The following points are relevant to the decision:

- The types of data held.
- Why the data is held.
- From whom and how the information is obtained.
- To whom the information will be disclosed.

Employees and clients have a statutory right to access all computerised and manual information held about themselves.

Eight principles within the Act govern the processing of computerised personal data:

- Data must be obtained fairly and lawfully.
- Users are required to register the personal data held with the Data Protection Registrar and it must be held only for specified and lawful purposes.
- Data must only be disclosed and used for the purpose registered.
- Data must be relevant, adequate but not excessive for its requirement.
- Data must be accurate and up to date.
- Data must not be held any longer than necessary.
- Individuals have a right to be granted access to their own personal data at reasonable intervals without undue expense and must be provided with a copy of it, in an understandable form. Data must be amended or removed where appropriate.
- Necessary precautions must be taken by data users to ensure security in order to prevent unauthorised access, disclosure, alteration or removal of personal data and accidental loss of data.

Computer systems

There are two main types:

- **Single-user** systems – computers that are not connected to other computers via a network.
- **Network** systems – groups of single-user personal computers (PCs) linked (by cable) to a central main computer – the file-server. Data is stored on the file-server but can be accessed by any of the PCs (called workstations) on the system. Networks allowing the sharing of resources such as printers are commonly used in veterinary practice.

Computer hardware

The physical parts of a computer are described as hardware:

- **Peripheral device** – any input or output device that is used to communicate with the computer; a typical set includes keyboard, mouse, visual display and printer.
- **Central processing unit (CPU)** – controls the operation of the computer.
- **Keyboard**, through which the operator enters data into the computer.
- **Visual display unit (VDU)** – displays data on a screen.
- **Mouse** – portable input device on a rolling ball; it is used to move a pointer on the screen, the position of which is activated when the mouse button is 'clicked'.
- **Printer** – data printed out on paper by the printer is described as **hard copy**. The wide choice of printers fall into two main categories: inkjet and laser.

Computer data storage

Hard disks are fixed within the computer and used for permanent storage of large quantities of data.

Floppy disks are of thin, flexible plastic protected by a hard or soft plastic cover, usually 3.5 inches in size (though some 5.25 inch disks are still available for old machines). The size and the density of the disk determines the volume of data that can be stored on it. A 3.5 inch disk holds more information than a 5.25 inch disk; high-density (HD) disks hold more than single-density (SD) or double-density (DD) disks. The choice of size and density is dictated to some degree by the central processor unit (CPU).

Floppy disks are placed into the appropriate **disk drive** mounted on the computer. They can be used as a method of storing small volumes of data (usually up to 1.44 Mb) and are useful as a means of back-up and transferring data from one computer to another. It is important that floppy disks are correctly labelled to show contents and date.

Tapes are used for back-up storage where fast access is not required and are used for backing-up (copying) data from the hard disk.

Optical disks include compact disk (CD) read-only memory (ROM) disks that look like audio CDs and are designed as bulk storage systems for information that does not require changing. They are usually produced commercially and hold data such as textbook information – they have an important role in teaching. CDs onto which information can be written are also available: these are known as 'CD recordable' (CDR) disks, which can be written to once only, and hold data permanently, and 'CD rewritable' (CDRW) disks, which can be erased, and so used like floppy disks.

Software

The program that dictates what the hardware does is described as the **software**. The process of switching on the computer and loading the software into its memory is described as **booting up**.

Software application packages are written for particular functions. For example:

- Games.
- Drawing or painting.
- Design drawings.
- Management information systems (appointment system/ meetings).
- Database (sales/purchases/wages systems).
- Word processing.
- Spreadsheets (calculations and accounts).

Database programs are designed to manage and store large quantities of data. They are often custom-written and a veterinary practice's database program might include information on vaccinations, species, coat colours, etc. The program allows the creation, amendment and deletion of records so that client and animal information is kept up to date.

Spreadsheets are powerful calculating tools used in managing numerical information quickly and efficiently. For example:

- Plotting graphically the values of monthly vaccination sales.
- Calculating the costs of an operation by inputting figures, e.g. if you enter the number of hours an animal is under an anaesthetic, the flow rate of the gases and the unit cost of the gases, the computer will calculate how much it costs to provide the gases for that particular operation.
- Calculating averages and standard deviations, e.g. calculating the average transaction fee. If the practice price list is stored on a spreadsheet it is very simple and quick to increase prices by the rate of inflation without having to calculate and change each price individually.
- Accounts and VAT records can also be kept.

Word processing programs can be used to create a variety of documents. The screen displays typed input or text, either with codes that control its design and layout or as straight text on the basis of WYSIWYG ('what you see is what you get'). There are many word-processing applications:

- Processing articles, letters, reports, minutes, etc.
- Amending and updating documents without retyping all of the information (e.g. drug lists, mailing lists, price lists, telephone numbers).
- 'Merge-printing' standard letters with a mailing list so that each letter is individually addressed and detailed (e.g. booster reminders).

Desktop publishing is a more advanced facility for preparing documents containing both text and graphics of a quality adequate for use in publications – incorporating pictures with the text, laying out pages with multiple columns, etc., as required for a practice newsletter.

Computer communication It is possible to create high-speed links between computer systems at different locations and these are increasingly being used both by practices with more than one site as a means of transferring or viewing information and also by practices as a means of placing orders with drug wholesalers. The most common types of linkages are made using telephone lines, and include modem, ISDN and kilostream. All have significant costs for installation and usage but can repay these costs to the practice through increased efficiency.

The internet The internet is playing an increasingly important role in veterinary practice. Many practices now have a website to advertise their services and there are an increasing number of websites offering veterinary advice and information. There is no jurisdiction over what is published on 'the web' and so care most always be taken to ensure that information is accurate.

Data safety Floppy disks are prone to damage which can corrupt the information stored on them unless they are handled and stored correctly:

- Do not handle the exposed parts of a floppy disk.
- File disks in a dust-free box when not in use.
- Do not drop them.
- Keep coffee and other liquids well away from disks (and keyboards).

Information held on the computer in a veterinary practice is irreplaceable. It is essential to have a **back-up routine** that will minimise the loss of information in most eventualities. Each practice should devise a regular back-up routine and should ensure that the routine is followed rigorously. The essence of backing up is to copy data on to a separate disk or tape, stored separately from the originals.

Back-up daily (or more frequently in a very busy practice). Daily back-ups are often scheduled to perform automatically overnight.

In addition, back-up weekly to ensure that data is saved in case corruption of information goes unnoticed for a number of days.

For added insurance, back-up on a monthly basis as well. (This is a 'belt-and-braces' system – many practices follow only a daily back-up routine.)

Intelligent tills Intelligent tills incorporate some of the elements of a computer. They may be able to read item prices, using a bar-code reader or have dedicated buttons for items and services sold. Some also have the capacity to check stock levels and create automatic orders. Certain intelligent tills can be used to update vaccination reminder information. If a practice uses a manual medical record-card system, an intelligent till provides a cheap and effective way of automating certain routines such as stock control and vaccination reminders.

The future of electronic technology Increasingly, computers are replacing manual filing systems. Digital data may be stored (filed) 'on-line' in a computer, or 'off-line' on disks or other magnetic media. Advances in technology have resulted in significant changes in the way that data is generated, stored and utilised, particularly in the fast-moving world of veterinary medicine. It is now possible to use the following in the day-to-day running of many practices:

- Storage of ECGs on computer.
- Interpretation of ECGs by computer.
- Storage of radiographs on computer.
- Scanning of radiographs by computer.
- Digital cameras linked to the computer to take and store information such as skin conditions.
- Electronic drug-ordering – the order to the wholesaler is transmitted direct from the computer.
- Laboratory reports transmitted electronically from the laboratory directly to the practice computer.

The management of information may be in the form of one or a combination of the following increasingly sophisticated systems:

- Card system and an ordinary till.
- Card system and an intelligent till capable of stock control.
- Card system and an intelligent till capable of stock control and producing vaccination reminders.
- Word processor and intelligent till holding clinical data as well as controlling stock and producing vaccination reminders.
- Multi-user system.
- Computer system at the main surgery linked to the branch surgeries by dedicated lines, ensuring immediate access of information gathered at all sites.

Clinical information held on a card system at a practice that runs more than one site can be difficult to access when, say, an animal normally seen at a branch is brought into the main surgery out of normal working hours. Practices that encounter this problem will probably favour the computer-link system described above.

Filing systems

Filing is often an unpopular job but it is a vital one. A poorly managed system will produce hours of extra work spent looking for misfiled or lost material. If the filing of records is carried out regularly and accurately, a fast efficient system for the retrieval of information can be developed.

The storage system must be suitable for the information being stored and accessibility required. The storage of radiographs in labelled envelopes or cardboard sleeves placed in suspension filing cabinets is more appropriate than stacking them all on top of one another in a box.

The ideal filing system should incorporate the following features:

- Guaranteed fast retrieval of information.
- Easy identification of misfiled material.

- Easy identification of active material and archive material.
- Allowance for expansion of the system.
- Determination of the period of retention of documents.
- Consideration of security and safety.
- Identification of file users by a system of tracer cards or 'out' guides showing users' names and date borrowed, placed in position of file removed.
- Suitable system of indexing.
- Index and cross-references if necessary.
- Colour coding for awareness of misfiling and for ease of identification.

Commonly used indexing systems include:

- Alphabetical.
- Numerical.
- Alpha-numerical.
- By subject.
- Geographical.

The alphabetical system is most commonly used in practice for client files.

Storage of documents   Due to the nature of the work carried out in a veterinary practice, a variety and large volume of documents and correspondence need to be stored. Each practice should draw up an appropriate retention and disposal policy to ensure that essential, irreplaceable information is protected and non-essential documents and records are disposed of at appropriate intervals. Depending on the subject matter and legal obligations, certain correspondence and documents must be kept for certain periods:

- Accident records: 3 years.
- VAT records: 6 years.
- PAYE records: at least 3 years after the income tax year to which the earnings relate.

There is no statutory obligation to keep the following records but the Veterinary Defence Society recommends that they are kept for a minimum of 2 years; if there is any possibility of dispute about a case, keep them for longer:

- Anaesthetic consent forms.
- Medical/hospital records.
- Laboratory reports.
- Radiographs.
- ECG/EEC traces.

The Royal College of Veterinary Surgeons recommends that records are kept for a minimum of 6 years. In disputed cases that are taken to the Veterinary Defence Society, the Society is advised to keep papers and documents with reference to the case, for court purposes, for 6 years and 364 days.

Many practices keep documents and records for longer than is legally required. These are termed 'dead files' and it is important to ensure that the storage system is both cost-effective and easily accessible.

Financial control

Every successful practice has a written budget which includes targets for fees earned and estimates of overheads, etc. It is formulated annually, based on the Business Plan. During the year, financial management reports are produced regularly for the practice owners so that they can assess progress against budgets, identify problems quickly, and implement appropriate corrective action where required.

Methods of payment

Strict procedures must be in place for the handling of payments made by clients, and accuracy of recording is vital.

Each method of payment has advantages and disadvantages:

- **Cash**. This has the benefit of being instant but it is easy to make mistakes, e.g. in counting change, when working under pressure. The security of cash in the practice and when being taken to the bank also has to be considered, as well as the possibility of theft within the practice.
- **Cheques**. A more secure form of payment in that it is less subject to dishonesty or mistakes than cash, but it has disadvantages in that there is a delay in the cheque clearing through the banking system. Banks usually charge the practice for processing cheques and unless the cheque is covered by a guarantee card, a bank may refuse to honour it.
- **Credit/debit cards**. These are increasingly being used by clients and should be accepted by all practices. Electronic terminals give instant authorisation and same-day credit of the amount paid directly into the practice account. The practice is charged a percentage of each transaction by their service provider for credit card transactions and a flat fee for debit card transactions.

All monies received from clients must immediately be accounted for, either through the computerised or manual cash book.

At the end of each day, or when a change of shift occurs, cash/cheques/credit and debit card slips in the till must be reconciled against the cash book and any discrepancies immediately investigated. It is just as serious to be 'over' in the till as 'under', as it means that payments have not been attributed to a client's records and the potential for a non-existent debt to be chased in the future by the practice, to the considerable annoyance of the client concerned.

Debt control

Constant vigilance is required to ensure that all fees earned by the practice are collected. All practices have a policy for collection of fees and this procedure must be followed at all times. Small animal practices usually operate on the basis of payment at the time work is done (though there may be a few exceptions, e.g. breeders may be allowed account facilities with settlement on a monthly basis), whereas large animal practices usually bill their clients at regular intervals. The practice's terms of business must be made known to clients before the provision of services, though care must be taken with the tone of any communication to avoid the impression that the practice's primary concern is financial rather than clinical.

Debt must be dealt with assertively and promptly. Many practices use the services of solicitors, debt collecting agencies or the County Court to collect outstanding debts.

Security

Security in a veterinary practice covers many areas and all members of staff should be aware of the implications of a lax system with reference to theft, damage and personal safety of staff and clients alike.

Premises

Burglaries are not uncommon and it is wise to ask the local Crime Prevention Officer for advice on how best to secure the premises. All doors, windows, skylights and shutters should be locked and checked before the building is left unattended.

Personal safety

It is unwise for anyone on their own at the practice to open the surgery door to a caller who may appear to be the owner of an animal in distress. A telephone intercom may be fitted so that you may speak directly to the person without opening the door. Then contact the veterinary surgeon on call before proceeding any further. A good source of light should make it easier to see and identify the caller and their vehicle (write down its colour, make and number).

To minimise the risk of personal danger to staff, arrangements can be made with known clients to call at the surgery at a specified time. They should have given a description of themselves, their vehicle and the animal. Ensure that all staff are aware of practice policy on this matter and that they all **think** before putting themselves in potentially dangerous situations. The fitting of 'panic buttons' in strategic places within the practice can make staff feel more secure.

Tills

Never leave an open, unlocked till unattended, even if you are staying in the same room. Never place the money tendered by the client into the till until you have counted out and given them their change and receipt.

It is very easy to accept into the till a £10 note for a small transaction only to be told, on giving the person their change, that they had given you a £20 note. Unless there is a detailed list of what was in the till, it is very difficult to prove that they did not in fact pass over £20.

Dangerous drugs cupboard

Only veterinary surgeons and nominated staff should hold keys to the dangerous drugs cupboard and these should never be left lying around or lent to unauthorised staff. Nor should the cupboard be left unlocked.

Staff-only areas should be well signposted and clients should never be left unattended in areas that contain anything other than GSL drugs.

Prescription pads and headed paper should not be left lying around. Stolen pads have sometimes been used by drug users trying to obtain prescription-only medicines or controlled drugs.

Animals

Always ensure the security of the animals in your charge and lock cages if necessary to prevent escape.

Measuring practice success

In order to assess progress in achievement both of the specific objectives of the practice as set out in the Business Plan and also its general health as a profit-making organisation, regular measurements must be taken. Most practices use broadly similar measurements, adding parameters to suit their particular circumstances. All practices produce annual Profit and Loss Accounts. Additional commonly used methods of assessing practice performance are:

- **Average transaction value (ATV)**. The total value of turnover in a period, divided by the number of invoices raised in that period. For example, if in a month the practice has achieved a turnover of £60 000 and during that time 3000 invoices have been raised, then the average transaction value would be £20. ATV should be regularly monitored and changes investigated.
- **Annual health check and booster appointments**. Responses to reminder letters should be monitored each month and compared with previous months. The practice should aim to achieve as near 100% compliance from clients as possible.
- **Active and bonded clients**. An active client is one who has used the practice within a given period – often taken as the preceding 2 years. Definitions of 'bonded' vary but commonly a bonded client is said to be one whose pets' vaccinations are kept up to date. Practices seek both to increase the number of active clients and ensure that these clients are bonded. The practice should target these clients for marketing of services available.

- **Practice activity**. The number of procedures and appointments in a given period, compared with past months or years.
- **Team member's activity**. The income achieved by each member of the practice. Care should be taken in interpreting the results of this analysis as almost inevitably not all individuals will have the same opportunities or job roles to contribute directly to the income of the practice.
- **Overheads.** These are the costs associated with running the practice and must be constantly monitored, with any variations against budget investigated promptly.

Particular care should be taken following any increase in the price of services. Some areas of practice activity are likely to be more 'sensitive' to an increase in prices than others. These 'sensitive' areas are generally those where the service is elective and it is apparently straightforward to the client to compare prices between practices, e.g. neutering and vaccination.

Further reading

Corsan, J. (2002) *Veterinary Receptionist*, Butterworth-Heinemann, Oxford.

LeGood, G. (1999) *Veterinary Ethics: A Principled Approach*, Macmillan, Oxford.

Shlock, N. (2002) *Veterinary Practice Management*, Butterworth-Heinemann, Oxford.

www.hse.gov.uk

8

Legal and ethical aspects of veterinary nursing practice

Elizabeth Earle

Learning objectives

After studying this chapter, students should be able to:

- Outline the legal accountability of the veterinary nurse.
- Describe the differences between civil and criminal law.
- Outline the concept of informed consent.
- Describe the legal and ethical requirements for record keeping.
- Describe the legal scope of veterinary nursing practice.

Introduction

Veterinary practice, like other professions and businesses, operates within the framework of the law. The role of the veterinary nurse has expanded with the provisions laid down within Schedule 3 of the Veterinary Surgeons Act[1] and continues to evolve. This module provides a background to the legal obligations of the veterinary nurse. Ethical issues often arise in relation to the law; these are highlighted where they are important.

Basics of the legal system

The legal system comprises two main branches, criminal and civil law. **Criminal law** is concerned with the punishment of offences by the State. It exists in order to protect the individual and prevent harm to others. Generally speaking, criminal law intervenes only where there is a real justification for interfering with the liberty of others; for example the law avoids areas of private morality where there is no clear consequence of harm to others.[2] Criminal prosecutions are usually brought by the police through the Crown Prosecution Service. Criminal offences are classified as indictable or summary.

A summary offence is a relatively minor offence, such as breaking the speed limit, minor assault or some animal cruelty cases. It is tried in the Magistrates Court. This is a local court where evidence is heard and judged by magistrates. These may be specially trained members of the public (lay magistrates) or stipendiary magistrates who are quali-

fied lawyers. An indictable offence is a more serious matter such as murder, rape, serious drugs offences or fraud. It is heard in the Crown Court before a judge and jury.

A criminal case is referred to as *Regina* versus *Brown*, meaning the Crown against Brown. It is usually written as *R* v *Brown*.

Civil law is concerned with addressing harm or loss to an individual brought about by another person or organisation. The types of civil action most likely to affect a veterinary practice are breach of contract and actions in tort. A tort is a civil, rather than a criminal, wrong. The law of tort provides protection for a person's personal security, property and reputation. Thus they may bring an action for negligence if they suffer injury as a result of poor medical practice, or an action for defamation if someone publishes information which damages their reputation.

Civil law cases are heard in the County Court or, for major cases involving potentially large sums of compensation, the High Court. The person bringing the action is called the *claimant* and the person or organisation alleged to have caused the harm or loss the *defendant*. A civil case is usually referred to as *Jones* v *Smith*. Remedies in tort may involve the payment of compensation for injury and/or the award of an injunction to prevent the defendant from causing further harm.

Public law and judicial review

Government organisations and other public bodies exercise their own internal regulations granted by statute. Examples are Government departments, such as the Department for Work and Pensions, universities and professional regulatory bodies such as the Royal College of Veterinary Surgeons. An individual wishing to challenge a decision made by such a body may request a procedure known as judicial review. In judicial review cases the court must decide whether or not the public body has acted legally within its powers.

Sources of law

Law originates from Statutes, or Acts of Parliament and from the Common Law, based on case law decided in the courts. Britain is part of the European Union and, as such, is also governed by European law.

The Common Law results from case law arising from previous decisions taken by the courts. Decisions taken by the higher courts are binding on all lower courts. Thus, a

[1]Veterinary Surgeons Act 1966.
[2]Report on the Committee on Homosexual Offences and Prostitution (1957 Cmnd 247), HMSO, London.

case decided in the House of Lords will bind all courts whereas a decision taken by the High Court, whilst binding lower courts, may be overturned by the Court of Appeal or the House of Lords. This system is known as precedent. Some Common Law precedents are very long-established, for example the case of *Tuberville* v *Savage*,[3] which still helps to define the law on assault, dates from the seventeenth century.

Statutes are Acts of Parliament. These are developed from Bills presented to both Houses of Parliament. Bills may be Government sponsored or may be Private Member's Bills presented by an individual MP. Government-sponsored Bills are allotted more parliamentary time than Private Member's Bills and, as a consequence, have less chance of becoming law unless they also have Government support. Private Member's Bills are often concerned with social and ethical issues such as abolition of the death penalty,[4] abortion[5] and animal welfare.[6] In order to become law, a Bill must proceed through three readings in the House of Commons and House of Lords. It must then receive the Royal Assent. Statutes may be general, such as the Sale of Goods Act 1979 or specific and aimed at a small sector of the population, such as the Veterinary Surgeons Act 1966.

More recent statutes are often what is termed an 'enabling Act'. These statutes provide a broad legislative framework and allow powers for ministers to produce detailed regulations for the operation of the law. These regulations are known as **statutory instruments.** This sort of legislation is more flexible in that it allows ministers to make effective changes in the law without the time-consuming need for a new statute. Some 2000 statutory instruments are produced from Government departments each year.

When the Veterinary Surgeons Act is eventually redrafted it is likely to become an enabling Act. This will, for example, allow much greater flexibility than does the present Act in regulating the work of professionals allied to veterinary science such as equine dentists and veterinary nurses.

As a result of joining the European Community, Britain is subject to **European law.** The European Community Act[7] provides that rights arising out of Community Treaties shall have effect in UK law. In effect, the member states 'pooled' their national sovereignty and, as a result, formed a superior legal order which has precedence over their individual domestic systems. This is why cases decided in British courts may be overturned in the European Court. In addition, EC member states are subject to EU regulations and directives. Many of these have a major impact on veterinary practice.[8]

Legal and ethical accountability of the veterinary nurse

Veterinary nurses are accountable in law in four key areas. These cross both civil and criminal law as outlined above. Nurses are also accountable to themselves morally for their actions. In most cases moral and legal accountability are closely linked; however, there are some instances where a veterinary nurse may have a moral obligation but no legal liability. An example of this would be a nurse who declines to offer first aid to an injured animal outside of her practice environment. The law does not require that help must be offered and any legal action brought against the nurse would fail. In many instances several different fields of accountability will be involved in a single case. For example:

> Mrs Jane Jones' pedigree brood bitch died under anaesthetic during a caesarean section. Consequently the five puppies required hand-rearing and only two survived. It transpired that the anaesthetic was induced and administered by a veterinary nurse. She had qualified in 1999 but had not remained on the RCVS List.

Public accountability

As citizens, veterinary nurses are expected to conduct themselves within the law. Nurses may be prosecuted for a breach of the law, either within the context of their work (e.g. drug offences, theft) or private lives. Veterinary nurses may also be called as witnesses in criminal prosecutions brought against animal owners, for example cruelty cases. In the example given, a lay person may not perform any veterinary procedure, such as the administration of an anaesthetic agent, on an animal. An unlisted veterinary nurse is classed as a lay person and may accordingly be prosecuted in the criminal courts under the provisions of the Veterinary Surgeons Act.

Figure 8.1 shows various elements of accountability arising out of this case. The veterinary nurse was not on the RCVS list and therefore not eligible to perform a Schedule 3 procedure.

[3]*Tuberville* v *Savage* (1669) 1 Mod R 3.
[4]Murder (abolition of the Death Penalty) Act 1965.
[5]Termination of Pregnancy Act 1968.
[6]Welfare of Animals at Slaughter Act 1991.
[7]European Community Act 1972.
[8]Control of Substances Hazardous to Health Regulations (COSHH) 1988.
Manual Handling Regulations 1992.

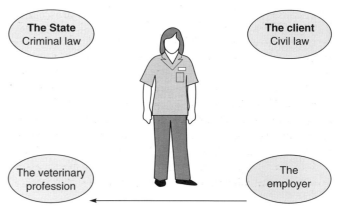

Fig. 8.1 The accountability of the veterinary nurse.

Accountability to the client

Clients may bring an action in the civil courts if they have suffered loss or injury as a result of negligence or a breach of contract. This action may be brought against one or more individuals personally or against an organisation. An organisation, such as a veterinary hospital, may be directly responsible for the loss of an animal because its policies and procedures are at fault. Alternatively it may be indirectly (or vicariously) liable for the negligent actions of its employees. In the example given, it is likely that the client would sue the veterinary practice for the loss of a valuable dog and puppies. If the client is successful and is awarded damages for her loss, the practice may decide to take action against the negligent employees.

Duty to the employer

As employees, veterinary nurses have a duty to obey all reasonable instructions given by their employers and to carry out their work with due care and diligence. This expectation is an implied term of any contract of employment, meaning that it does not have to be expressly written down. Employees may not be required to break the law or to act negligently as part of a 'reasonable instruction'. In the example, if it were found that the nurse and the veterinary surgeon were acting outside of the normal policy and procedures of the practice, they could be subjected to a disciplinary hearing and could be dismissed from their posts. Additionally, the practice may sue the employees personally for any loss incurred by the practice as a result of their action.

Professional accountability

A veterinary nurse's professional accountability is channelled through the employing veterinary surgeon. Veterinary Surgeons are accountable to the Royal College of Veterinary Surgeons which regulates the practice of veterinary surgery, in accordance with the Veterinary Surgeons Act 1966, in the United Kingdom. The client, in the example given, may make a complaint to the RCVS against the veterinary surgeon involved in the care of her dog. The RCVS would investigate the conduct of the vet, an issue of which would be his apparent delegation of an act of veterinary surgery to a lay person (the unlisted veterinary nurse). At present veterinary nurses have no direct professional accountability for their actions. It is for this reason that Schedule 3[9] of the Veterinary Surgeons Act permits veterinary nurses to undertake specified delegated acts of veterinary surgery only under the direction of an employing veterinary surgeon. The RCVS List of Veterinary Nurses is thus a list only of those who have reached the necessary standard of qualification and continue to pay the required annual retention fee. No nurse may be removed from the List for misconduct; the primary safeguard against 'unfit' veterinary nurses being through the diligence of their veterinary employers.

Moral accountability and codes of professional conduct

The law provides a broad and fairly blunt framework within which veterinary nurses must practice. However, it does not provide answers for the many occasions on which nurses may wonder what is the 'right' thing to do. Modern veterinary medicine and surgery has pushed back the boundaries of treatment for animals, and owners have access to more information and are consequently more demanding of veterinary professionals.

Codes of professional conduct set out the expected standards of practice within a profession and provide valuable guidance to the courts and professional conduct tribunals of regulatory bodies (such as the RCVS) when they are called to judge the conduct of a defendant. The RCVS *Guide to Professional Conduct*[10] provides guidance on ethical issues which has been agreed by the veterinary profession. The Guide provides ten 'guiding principles' which are relevant to all those, including veterinary nurses, working in veterinary practice. The RCVS also provides some additional specific guidance for veterinary nurses.

As with any code of professional conduct, the RCVS Guide represents a broad agreement of the veterinary profession on ethical standards of conduct. It is designed to provide a basis for ethical practice but cannot provide easy answers to the many specific moral dilemmas which may arise in veterinary practice. Those working in veterinary practice must, in addition to heeding the *Guide to Professional Conduct*, also be able to recognise moral problems and arrive at considered solutions which meet the best interests of all concerned.

Negligence

Veterinary nurses have a duty in law not to cause harm or loss to clients. Animals count as property and any harm to them must, for an action in negligence to be successful, result in loss to the owner. An example would be damage to a pedigree cat which prevented the owner from showing and/or breeding from it.

In order for negligence to be established, four questions must be addressed:

- Is there a 'duty of care'; when does the veterinary nurse owe a duty of care and to whom?

---

[9]Veterinary Surgeons Act (1966) Schedule 3 Amendment Order 1991.

[10]*Guide to Professional Conduct for Veterinary Nurses* (2000) Royal College of Veterinary Surgeons, London. (See Appendix to this book.)

- What is the appropriate standard of care expected and how will the courts decide if that has been breached?
- Was the injury or loss foreseeable and how must the claimant prove this?
- What type of harm or loss can be compensated?

The duty of care

Veterinary nurses owe a duty of care to clients of the practice, their colleagues and employer, and certain other individuals. It is important to recognise that, whatever the moral obligation, there is no legal duty of care owed to an animal patient. The duty of care concerning an animal is owed to its owner.

In order to establish a duty of care, there must be a recognisable relationship of dependence between the nurse and the injured party. In the context of medical (or veterinary) practice this is not usually difficult. It is accepted that the staff of a practice have a duty of care to clients and colleagues; the question is more likely to be whether there has been a breach of that duty and whether this caused damage.[11]

A difficulty may arise where a nurse acts as a 'Good Samaritan' and causes further injury by administering negligent first aid treatment outside the practice environment. However morally obliged a veterinary nurse may feel, there is no legal obligation to provide care and treatment for a stranger. A nurse may walk past an accident with legal impunity.[12] The reason for this may, at first, seem obscure. However, the law must respect an individual's right to judge whether or not they are competent to deal with a situation and to 'opt out' if they are not. In contrast, professional regulatory bodies often require a different approach in their codes of professional conduct. The RCVS would expect a veterinary surgeon to provide 24-hour emergency cover to all species, to include first aid and pain relief and not to allow any animal to suffer through neglect.[13] The UKCC, in its Guidelines for Professional Practice for nurses makes specific recognition of the difference between legal and professional duty in circumstances such as these. Regulatory bodies thus sometimes place additional moral duties upon their registrants which are over and above the legal definition of a duty of care.

Standards of care and breach of duty

Once it has been established that a duty of care is owed, the injured party (the claimant) must be able to establish negligence. In order to do this, he must be able to show that the veterinary nurse concerned fell below a reasonable standard of practice. The courts will decide what is a reasonable standard of practice by determining what the 'ordinary skilled veterinary nurse' would have done in the circumstances of the case.

A person who claims to have a special skill is judged according to the standard of the reasonable person who has the skill or qualification he or she professes to possess. Factors which would assist the case would be documentary evidence of the standard of competence required for registration as a veterinary nurse, for example the Veterinary Nursing Occupational Standards, and advice from expert witnesses qualified to comment on standards of veterinary nursing competence. The legal precedent for this comes from a medical case in which a doctor was held to have given an inappropriate treatment to a psychiatric patient which led to injury.[14] In the case, the Judge stated:

> The test is the standard of the ordinary skilled man exercising and professing to have that special skill ... he is not guilty of negligence if he has acted in accordance with a practice accepted as proper by a responsible body of medical men skilled in that particular art.

This became known as the Bolam Test and is the starting point in judging all cases of professional negligence.

It is important to recognise that a person acting as a veterinary nurse, regardless of experience and whether qualified or not, is expected to demonstrate a level of care and skill in accordance with the Bolam Test. Clients cannot be expected to distinguish between veterinary nurses and students or unqualified staff for themselves. In *Wilsher* v *Essex AHA* (a case concerning the negligence of a junior doctor), Glidewell L.J. said:

> ... the law requires the trainee or learner to be judged by the same standard as his more experienced colleagues. If it did not, inexperience would frequently be urged as a defence to and action for professional negligence.[15]

Name badges, uniforms, etc. should therefore identify and describe staff clearly and accurately and personnel should not be permitted to act outside their remit or without adequate supervision, i.e. an unqualified nursing assistant should not perform the work of a listed veterinary nurse.

It can also be seen that maintaining competence and skill after qualification is important. Veterinary nurses must be able to offer care and treatment in accordance with current practice and need to ensure that they remain abreast of changes in approach and new skills through effective continuing professional development (CPD).

[11]Jones, M. A. (1992) Medical negligence. In Dyer, C. (ed.), *Doctors, Patients and the Law*, Blackwell, Oxford.

[12]Tingle, J. (1998) Nursing negligence: general issues. In McHale, J., Tingle, J. and Peysner, J. (eds), *Law and Nursing*, Butterworth–Heinemann, Oxford.

[13]*Guide to Professional Conduct for Veterinary Nurses* (2000) Royal College of Veterinary Surgeons, London.

[14]*Bolam* v *Freirn Hospital Management Committee* (1957) 1 WLR 582.

[15]*Wilsher* v *Essex AHA* (1986) All E R 801.

Forseeability and remoteness

The consequences of a negligent act must be foreseeable by a reasonable person in the circumstances. Thus if a veterinary nurse fails to dispose of sharps in a bin made for the purpose, it is foreseeable that a colleague may suffer injury as a result. The courts must decide how likely it would be that an action might cause harm. For example, in *Bolton* v *Stone*[16] a woman was hit by a cricket ball whilst standing in the road outside her home. The cricket ball had been 'hit for six' and had travelled some 100 yards, up a slope and over the boundary fence which was 7 ft high. Cricket balls had been hit out of the ground before but only about six times in 30 years. The defendants were found not to be negligent as it would be 'intolerable if the ordinary careful man were to attempt to take precautions against every risk which he can foresee'. However, had the defendants been playing cricket on an unfenced pitch next to a major road, the situation would clearly have been different.

It is important to recognise that, provided damage to a person is foreseeable, it does not matter that the consequences to the person are unforeseeable. The case of *Bradford* v *Robinson Rentals*[17] illustrates the point. In this case a van driver's employers required him to drive from Bedford to Exeter on an exceptionally cold day in winter. There was no heater in the van. As a result of the cold, he suffered frostbite, a very rare condition in England. His employers were held liable, no matter that frostbite is rare or that the driver may have been unusually susceptible to it.

Res ipsa loquiter

This phrase means 'the thing speaks for itself'. This principle is applied where the court is prepared to infer that the defendant was negligent purely from the effect on the claimant. An example of *res ipsa loquiter* would occur if a swab were inadvertently left inside a patient at operation. It does not matter how this happened, the fact that it should never happen if reasonable care is taken is sufficient. In order for *res ipsa loquiter* to apply, three conditions must be satisfied. First, the defendant must be in control of the thing which caused injury to the claimant. Second, the accident must be of such a nature that it would not have occurred but for negligence. Lastly, there must be no explanation for the incident.

Establishing loss – causation

A claimant must establish that the harm or loss they have suffered has been caused by the negligence of the defendant. In other words, if a client slips on the surgery floor, she must prove that, but for the negligence of the practice, she would not have suffered injury. However, the courts must take care to establish that the injury is not due to a pre-existing condition. For example, the veterinary surgeon whose car backs into that of a client, is only liable for the resulting dent, not the damage caused previously when the client hit a lamp post! Sometimes it can be extremely difficult to establish the cause of an injury. In this case, the courts will decide liability on the balance of probabilities.[18]

Compensation – what can be claimed?

In the UK, the principle which underpins the payment of damages is that the injured party should be put in the position he would have been in had the negligent act not have occurred. This should not be confused with the situation in the USA where courts will often award punitive damages (to punish negligent action) which often amount to very large sums.

The courts will compensate loss of earnings, medical expenses and loss of property and will also allow damages for loss of future earnings and pension (in serious/long lasting injury), pain, suffering and loss of amenity (reduced ability to lead a normal life).

If an animal has been damaged or lost owing to negligence, the owner may sue for the reduction in value or the loss of the animal. As most pets are of limited financial value, it is often not practical to litigate.

Negligence and animals

An individual may be liable for the damage caused by an animal both in tort and under statute law. The most significant legislation in this area is the Animals Act 1971. This area of law is of special importance to veterinary practices which may have a number of animals under their control and which may cause damage to another person or property.

An individual may be liable in tort for the actions of an animal which he owns or has control of. The range of torts is wide and includes not just negligence (e.g. a dog escapes and causes a road accident) but battery (setting the dog on someone), nuisance (noise or smell from kennels), trespass (allowing animals to enter someone else's land) and, not least, defamation (teaching a parrot to utter slanderous statements).

The Animals Act 1971 provides a framework under which individuals may be liable for damage caused by dangerous species (Section 2(1)) and non-dangerous species (Section 2(2)).

Section 2(1) states:

> where any damage is caused by an animal which belongs to a dangerous species, any person who is a keeper of the animal is liable for the damage, except as otherwise provided by this Act.

---

[16]*Bolton* v *Stone* (1951) AC 850.
[17]*Bradford* v *Robinson Rentals* (1967) 1 WLR 337.

[18]*Wilsher* v *Essex AHA* (1988) AC 1074.

There are two crucial definitions to note. The first is the meaning of the word 'Keeper'. Section 6(3) states that a person is the keeper of an animal if:

a. he owns the animal or has it in his possession; or

b. he is the head of a household of which a member under the age of sixteen owns the animal or has it in his possession.

Section 6(3) also provides that the keeper only ceases to be so once another person has taken ownership or possession of the animal. In other words, he cannot abandon responsibility. Section 6(4) permits a person to deal with a dangerous species in an emergency (to prevent it from causing harm or to restore it to its owner) without being deemed a keeper. A veterinary surgeon who has temporarily taken responsibility for the care of an animal from its owner thus becomes its keeper and is accountable in law for any damage it may cause to other people or property.

The second definition is of a 'Dangerous species'. S6(4) defines this as a species:

a. which is not commonly domesticated in the British Isles; and

b. whose fully grown animals normally have such characteristics that they are likely, unless restrained, to cause severe damage or that any damage that they cause is likely to be severe.

It is important to note that the Act refers to the species which is dangerous, not to a particular animal. It is therefore no defence to say that a particular animal was tame. It should also be noted that the definition depends upon the characteristics of a fully grown animal. Again, it would be no defence to say the animal was only a baby.

The increasing number of exotic pets which find their way into veterinary practices, in particular reptiles, means that veterinary nurses must be particularly mindful of their duty of care.

Section 2(2) provides for non-dangerous species:

Where damage is caused by an animal which does not belong to a dangerous species, a keeper of the animal is liable for damage . . . if:

a. the damage is of a kind which the animal, unless restrained, was likely to cause or which, if caused by the animal, was likely to be severe; and

b. the likelihood of the damage or of its being severe was due to characteristics of the animal which are not normally found in animals of the same species or are not normally found except at particular times or in particular circumstances; and

c. those characteristics were known to that keeper or were at any time known to a person who at that time had charge of the animal as that keeper's servant or, where that keeper is the head of a household, were known to another keeper of the animal who is a member of the household and under the age of sixteen.

This section of the Animals Act means that it is important to take all reasonable precautions against any animal in the care and control of the veterinary practice from causing injury or damage. However, Section 5(2) provides that a keeper is not liable where the person suffering damage accepted the risk of such damage. In other words, they volunteered. This does not extend to veterinary practice staff who, as employees of a (temporary) keeper, are provided for by s6(5).

The Dangerous Dogs Act (1991) makes specific provision for types of dog which are bred for fighting. The principle of deciding who is the keeper of such a dog (and thus responsible for ensuring that the requirements of this Act are complied with) is similar to that described above. Practices need to take special care when dealing with an animal which, although the owner might not treat it as such, might be legally construed as a dangerous dog.

Consent to treatment

Consent to treatment is an area where veterinary nurses must demonstrate an understanding of both legal and ethical issues. In legal terms, written, verbal or tacit consent to treatment constitutes evidence of the contract which exists between the veterinary practice and the client. This one area gives rise to more disputes and complaints than any other single issue. It is thus of paramount importance that the veterinary practice should ensure that clients, wherever possible, are able to give fully informed consent to treatment.

Informed consent

As a general rule, an individual is legally bound by his signature to a document, whether or not he has read it or fully understood it. A consent to treatment form is often a key document providing evidence of the contract which exists between the veterinary surgeon and the client. Problems can, and do, arise when clients sign such a form without fully appreciating the implications of treatment.

Misunderstandings occur for a number of reasons, commonly because the outcomes of treatment do not meet the expectations of the client or/and the cost is greater than the client envisaged. Consent forms should therefore be signed by the client only when he/she understands as fully as possible the implications of treatment. Informed consent must always be judged from the perspective of the client and is therefore difficult to define precisely. In general terms it means that the owner of an animal should be given all the relevant information he/she needs in order to decide on the best course of action. Where relevant and appropriate, this should include the option of euthanasia. In ethical terms it is important that a client is enabled to make a decision about treatment which gives the best possible outcome for the animal in the circumstances. Where a client does not have the means to fund complex surgery or follow-up treatment, a palliative alternative or euthanasia may need to be offered.

The experience and intellectual ability of clients varies widely, as do their financial means. Many people have little knowledge of medical or veterinary issues and may not appreciate the implications of even quite routine procedures. Some will worry about meeting the cost of treatment. Coupled with these factors, the illness of an animal and associated visits to the veterinary surgery may be stressful. The existence of stress always interferes with an individual's ability to process and retain information to some degree and must always be allowed for. There are a number of simple measures which can be taken to assist clients to relax and be able to take part in rational decisions about treatment. These include the availability of attractive and clearly written advice leaflets for common procedures and adequate consulting time in which to assess both the animal and its owner before discussing and deciding upon treatment options. More time will be needed where an owner faces difficult decisions about the treatment (and associated cost) of serious illness. The communication skills and approach of the veterinary surgeon and practice staff are crucial factors in achieving informed consent to treatment and thus avoiding unnecessary distress and the possibility of disputes.

Veterinary nurses are often in a position to support clients during the decision-making process; clients may approach a nurse with their concerns, often expressed obliquely because of embarrassment. It is important to be aware of possible anxieties and always be prepared to explore them. Where a client appears to have serious doubts or misconceptions it is important that these are reported to the veterinary surgeon.

Confidentiality and clinical records

A successful relationship between client and veterinary surgeon is built upon trust. The confidentiality of information about clients or their animals, and the way in which such information is handled within the practice is central to this relationship. Clients do not expect any information concerning themselves or their animals to be made available to a third party without their consent. They also expect that records kept by the practice are accurate and do not contain prejudicial or defamatory statements or implications.

Standards of record keeping

Record keeping is a fundamental part of veterinary practice; records are an essential tool of clinical practice and, as such, must be kept diligently and accurately by everyone involved in veterinary care. Good record keeping helps to protect the welfare of animals and clients by promoting high standards of care, continuity, and communication between members of the veterinary team. It also ensures a comprehensive record of treatment, care and the decision-making processes involved.

Each veterinary practice will have a different policy and practice concerning the keeping of records; using electronic or manual systems or a combination of both. No matter what the system in place, certain principles apply to all record keeping.

Records should:

- Be written as soon as possible after an event has occurred.
- Be factual, concise and accurate.
- Be written legibly and in a manner which cannot be erased.
- Contain clear indications of alterations (dated, timed and signed) should never employ the use of correction fluid. Original entries must remain legible.
- Be accurately dated and signed by the author.
- Be devoid of abbreviations, jargon, speculation and subjective statements.

It is important to recognise that, in addition to their primary purpose of supporting patient care, clinical records may also be used in evidence where a complaint is made against a veterinary surgeon or practice. This may either be in a Court of Law or before the Disciplinary Committee of the Royal College of Veterinary Surgeons.

Who may see clinical records

The Data Protection Act 1984 gives individuals rights of access to their computer-held records. Although clients do not have legal access to manual records, it is good practice to write such records as if they were able to read them. In other words, both computerised and manual records should contain nothing which might be offensive, defamatory or prejudicial to them.

Other members of the veterinary team will, of course, have access to client records. However, should a client ask that access to their record is restricted, for example if a member of the practice team is a personal friend, this should be respected. In a referral practice clinical records may be used for research. This should always be subject to the client's consent and also any conditions imposed by the university research ethics committee concerned.

Security

Practices must ensure that records, whether kept electronically or manually, are secure. This especially includes the use of email attachments and fax, both of which are difficult to control once they leave the practice. Practices must have clear protocols for access to records and for their safekeeping at all times.

Confidentiality

Client confidentiality may only be broken in exceptional circumstances and only then when this can be fully justified in the public interest or by law, or on overwhelming grounds of animal welfare. Some of these instances are straightforward, for instance where a criminal offence is known to have been committed or the animal has a notifiable disease. Other issues are less simple and will involve reasoned ethical decision making. For example, it could be argued that all cases of apparent animal cruelty should be reported. However, would it be the right thing to report the elderly man who refuses euthanasia for his dog, although it is cachexic and clearly suffering, because he cannot bear to be parted from his only companion? Abuse of an animal is not always easy to identify but may also indicate that the abuser has other targets such as elder or child abuse. A veterinary surgeon must weigh the potentially serious consequences of overlooking the situation against the trauma to a family of investigation should he be mistaken.

Wherever a veterinary surgeon, or nurse, is in doubt concerning the disclosure of client information, the RCVS or a representative body should be consulted for support and advice.

Conflicts between confidentiality and upholding standards of care

Veterinary nurses have an ethical duty to uphold standards of care for clients and their animals. This may sometimes lead to conflicts between the duty of loyalty of nurses to their employers and the requirement to maintain client confidentiality on the one hand and the need to address poor standards of care on the other. A significant number of nurses experience these conflicts and yet feel powerless to do anything about them. As employees in a small workplace they understandably feel vulnerable to a breakdown in working relationships or to losing their job.

Concerns about standards of care should first be reported to a nurse's employer wherever possible, even if it seems likely that no action can or will be taken. Such reporting should be well thought out and prepared; it is almost never constructive to raise such issues in the heat of the moment. Advice from a professional association or the RCVS should be sought beforehand. When raising issues of concern, examples of the practice in question should be given, along with reasons for the nurse's concern. Workable suggestions for improvements and change should be offered wherever possible so that the discussion may be seen to be constructive. If issues are raised verbally, it is prudent to keep a written note of the date, issues discussed and the outcome for future reference. This record may be of importance should the matter need to be reported to the RCVS.

Whistle-blowing

Sometimes, despite discussing concerns with an employer, a veterinary nurse may feel that little or no action has been taken to address the issues raised. In this situation the nurse may consider disclosing their concerns publicly. This is known as whistle-blowing. One of the first and widely publicised incidents of whistle-blowing concerned Graham Pink, a charge nurse working on night duty in a NHS care of the elderly ward. He expressed concerns about low staffing levels and consequent poor standards of care to his employer, and subsequently at every level including the Department of Health. When nothing was done, in desperation he wrote to the local paper and made the matter public. He was sacked by his employers on the grounds that he had breached patient confidentiality but later reinstated by an industrial tribunal.

Mr Pink's case illustrates three essential elements[19] of whistle-blowing:

- The perception of someone within an organisation that something is morally amiss.
- The communication of those concerns to outside parties.
- The perception by those in authority in the organisation that such a communication ought not to have been made.

Unauthorised public disclosure of concerns about standards of care is a serious step to take and the consequences for an employee may be far-reaching. Such a move may well alienate a nurse within the practice team and could lead to disciplinary action. It is therefore essential to consider the justifiability of 'going public'.

Whistle-blowing should only be considered when:

- It will do more good than harm.
- It serves some purpose in correcting or preventing poor practice.
- It will be done in a responsible manner.
- All other internal channels of complaint and redress have been exhausted.

Making an unauthorised public disclosure should always be the last resort when trying to address a major problem within veterinary practice. It should only be considered where it holds a real prospect of change and the possible harms that may result (loss of public confidence in veterinary medicine, individual distress for clients of the practice, etc.) must be balanced against the good.

The scope of veterinary nursing

The Veterinary Surgeons Act 1966

The Veterinary Surgeons Act, in common with other animal protection legislation, sets out to prevent unnecessary suffer-

[19]Hunt, G. (1997) *Encyclopaedia of Applied Ethics*, Academic Press.

ing to animals. This is achieved through regulating who may provide veterinary care and treatment. The Act provides for the regulation of veterinary training, the provision of a register for veterinarians who practice in the UK and for the regulation of their professional conduct whilst entered on the register. The title of **veterinary surgeon** is reserved by law to those whose names appear in the Register of Veterinary Surgeons maintained by the RCVS. Individuals so registered are members of the RCVS and use the letters MRCVS or FRCVS if they are qualified as Fellows. Veterinary surgeons may also be colloquially referred to as **veterinarians**, a title that was one of the earliest names used and it is one widely recognised in North America and continental Europe. **Veterinary practitioner** is a title which the members of the Supplementary Veterinary Register may use. This small group of persons do not have formal qualifications in veterinary medicine and no further names may be added to this Register.

Veterinary surgery is defined in the Act as meaning:

> . . . the art and science of veterinary surgery and medicine and without prejudice to the generality of the foregoing, shall be taken to include:
>
> a. the diagnosis of diseases in, and injuries to animals, including tests performed on animals for diagnostic purposes;
> b. the giving of advice based on such diagnosis;
> c. the medical or surgical treatment of animals; and
> d. the performance of surgical operations upon animals.

As the range of veterinary work becomes more specialised and sophisticated, some of this work has been taken up by **para-veterinarians**. These are individuals who have a degree of specialised knowledge, training and experience in a specialised aspect of veterinary work, for example bovine blood samplers. Their work is regulated by a specific exemption to the normal provisions of the Veterinary Surgeons Act. Exemption Orders are a useful way of enabling well-defined areas of veterinary work to be undertaken by suitably trained lay specialists. However, Exemption Orders are very narrow in their scope and must usually be redrafted where advances in practice lead to a change in the way para-professionals covered by these orders work. This process is lengthy and could be said to impede the implementation of clinical advancements.

Schedule 3

This schedule of the Veterinary Surgeons Act sets down what the owners of farm and companion animals may provide by way of care and treatment. It also provides for the work of veterinary nurses.

In June 2002 an amendment to Schedule 3 became law. This widens the scope of veterinary nursing work, previously restricted to the provision of treatment to companion animals, i.e. not farm animals, horses, wild animals or animals kept other than as pets.

The amendment order permits:

6. Any medical treatment or any minor surgery (not involving entry into a body cavity) to any animal by a veterinary nurse if the following conditions are complied with, that is to say –

   a. the animal is, for the time being, under the care of a registered veterinary surgeon or veterinary practitioner and the medical treatment or minor surgery is carried out by the veterinary nurse at his direction; and
   b. the registered veterinary surgeon or veterinary practitioner is the employer or is acting on behalf of the employer of the veterinary nurse;
   c. the registered veterinary surgeon or veterinary practitioner directing the medical treatment or minor surgery is satisfied that the veterinary nurse is qualified to carry out the treatment or surgery.

7. Any medical treatment or any minor surgery (not involving entry into a body cavity) to any animal by a student veterinary nurse if the following conditions are complied with, that is to say –

   a. the companion animal is, for the time being, under the care of a registered veterinary surgeon or veterinary practitioner and the medical treatment or minor surgery is carried out by the student veterinary nurse at his direction and in the course of the student nurse's training;
   b. the treatment or surgery is supervised by a registered veterinary surgeon, veterinary practitioner or veterinary nurse and, in the case of surgery, the supervision is direct, continuous and personal; and
   c. the registered veterinary surgeon or veterinary practitioner is the employer or is acting on behalf of the employer of the student veterinary nurse.

In the above paragraphs:

- 'Veterinary nurse' means a nurse whose name is entered in the list of veterinary nurses maintained by the College.
- 'Student veterinary nurse' means a person enrolled under bye-laws made by the Council for the purpose of undergoing training as a veterinary nurse at an approved training and assessment centre or a veterinary practice approved by such a centre.
- 'Approved training and assessment centre' means a centre approved by the Council for the purpose of training and assessing student veterinary nurses.

There are several important points which must be recognised concerning the provisions of Schedule 3:

- It does not provide a definitive list of care and treatment which may be provided by a veterinary nurse. The intention is that a veterinary surgeon may delegate, provided that he is satisfied that a nurse is qualified and competent, any procedure or aspect of care which is not **excluded** (such as surgery which entails entry into a body cavity). Schedule 3 thus provides for advances in veterinary treatment over time and the individual qualifications, skills and competence of veterinary nurses.

- The broad scope of Schedule 3 means that it covers virtually all clinical work undertaken by veterinary nurses, from the administration of simple medications to minor surgery. The amendment order also permits animal owners or their employees to provide minor medical treatments.
- The competence of a newly qualified veterinary nurse is defined by the national Occupational Standards for veterinary nursing. However, most veterinary nurses will improve and increase the range of their knowledge and skills after qualification. They may therefore become competent to undertake more complex or specialised care and treatment. Once again, the employing veterinarian must actively ascertain this competence before delegating such work. Conversely, veterinarians must be aware that some nurses do not achieve this progression and must not be expected to undertake work for which they do not possess the necessary expertise.
- The provisions of Schedule 3 apply **only** to veterinary nurses listed by the RCVS, and to enrolled student veterinary nurses (see below). It is therefore important for employing veterinarians to check a nurse's Listed status annually and especially when employing locum staff. Clinical work, which falls within the definitions set out in Schedule 3, undertaken by a qualified but unlisted nurse is outside the law, as is such work undertaken by any unqualified nursing assistant.
- Student veterinary nurses may undertake medical treatments or minor surgery **only** as necessary to further their training. Student nurses must always conduct such work under supervision. In the case of a student undertaking minor surgical procedures, that supervision must be direct, continuous and personal. This means that the supervisor must be present, in control of the situation and able to intervene if necessary throughout the procedure.

Further guidance may be obtained from the RCVS (website address www.rcvs.org.uk).

KEY POINTS

- Remember that, as a student or qualified veterinary nurse, you are accountable in law (civil and criminal) for what you do in practice.
- As an employee, you have legal duties towards your employer, as your employer has to you.
- If you are negligent at work, a claim for compensation may be made against your employer rather than you as an individual. This is called vicarious liability.
- Your work as a student or qualified veterinary nurse is subject to the provisions of the Veterinary Surgeons Act 1966 Schedule 3.
- Your employing veterinary surgeon is professionally accountable to the Royal College of Veterinary Surgeons. This professional accountability includes his/her direction and supervision of veterinary nurses.
- Your work as a veterinary nurse may lead to moral conflicts which need careful resolution, taking into account both legal and ethical considerations.

Further reading

Bloy, D. and Parry, P. (1997) *Principles of Criminal Law*, Cavendish, London.

Dimond, B. (2001) *Legal Aspects of Nursing*, 3rd edn, Prentice Hall, London.

Dunstan, G. R. D. and Seller, M. J. (eds) (1983) *Consent in Medicine*, King Edward's Hospital Fund for London.

Legood, G. (2000) *Veterinary Ethics*, Continuum, London.

Mackay, L. (1993) *Conflicts in Care: Medicine and Nursing*, Chapman & Hall, London.

Mason, J. K. and McCall-Smith, R. A. (1999) *Law and Medical Ethics*, 5th edn, Butterworths, London.

McHale, J., Tingle, J. and Peysner, J. (1998) *Law and Nursing*, Butterworth-Heinemann, London.

Rollin, B. (1999) *An Introduction to Veterinary Medical Ethics*, Iowa State University Press.

Royal College of Veterinary Surgeons (2000) *Guide to Professional Conduct for Veterinary Nurses*, RCVS, London.

Suff, M. (1997) *Essential Contract Law*, Cavendish Publishing, London.

Lord Templeman, and Pitchfork, E. D. (eds) (1997) *Obligations: The Law of Tort*, Old Bailey Press, London.

9

Nutrition

S. McCune

Learning objectives

After studying this chapter, students should be able to:

- Describe the nutritional needs of dogs and cats in a variety of settings and life stages.
- Describe the organs and their role in digestion, absorption and excretion.
- Discuss the dietary requirements of a range of small mammals including rabbits, guinea pigs, rats, mice, hamsters, chinchillas, gerbils, ferrets, reptiles, cage birds, amphibians and ornamental fish.

Introduction

Proper nutrition is essential for the maintenance of optimum health and activity in all living creatures. Wild animals can obtain all the nutrients they need through a combination of hunting, scavenging and foraging but the opportunity for companion animals to access their natural diet has been limited by the process of domestication. It is the responsibility of the owner, therefore, to ensure that the diet they provide meets all the nutritional and behavioural needs of their pet and professional advice in this area is frequently sought.

Failure to provide a nutritionally adequate diet can result in disease or suboptimal performance, but nutritional factors may impact on the health of animals in a number of other ways. Many medical conditions will respond to modification of some aspect of the diet, and nutritional support is particularly important at times of illness or other forms of stress.

Research into the nutritional needs of pets has advanced significantly over the past few decades. Compared to where we were 40 years ago, we have a vastly improved understanding of what is necessary to feed in a balanced diet to prevent certain deficiencies, as well as throughout the various life stages and lifestyles of our pets as they grow, mature and age. As in human nutrition, attention is now turning towards achieving optimal health through functional foods, i.e. those nutrients which have a health benefit beyond preventing a deficiency, such as antioxidants to boost the function of the immune system, improve cognitive health, decreased cellular damage to DNA, and help slow the progression of ageing. Nutrition plays an essential role in the lifelong health and well-being of both humans and pets and should be an important consideration to discuss with owners at every health check (Fig. 9.1).

Nutrients and nutrient requirements

Food may be defined as any solid or liquid which, when ingested, can supply any or all of the following:

- Energy-giving materials from which the body can produce movement, heat or other forms of energy.
- Materials for growth, repair or reproduction.
- Substances necessary to initiate or regulate the processes involved in the first two categories.

The components of food which have these functions are called **nutrients** and the foods or food mixtures which are actually eaten are referred to as the **diet**. Any nutrient which is required by the animal and cannot be synthesised in the body is called an **essential nutrient** and a dietary source must be provided. If any essential nutrient is lacking or present in insufficient quantity in the diet, then the diet, as a whole, must be considered inadequate.

Energy

In addition to providing specific nutrients, food also supplies energy. Energy is a fundamental requirement of all living species and provides the power for cells to function. The energy content of the diet is derived from carbohydrates, fats and protein, and the amounts of each of these nutrients in a food will determine its energy content. Dietary fat supplies just over twice as much energy as protein or carbohydrate per gram and is therefore a more efficient fuel for metabolism. Water has no energy value so the energy density of food varies inversely with its moisture content.

Energy intake must be carefully regulated and maintained at a level close to requirements. When maintained over long

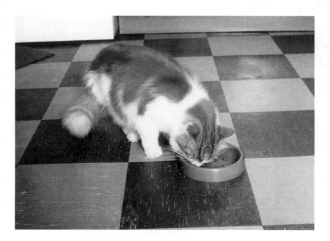

Fig. 9.1 Cat feeding.

periods, energy intake in excess of energy expenditure can be detrimental and leads to obesity or, in some young dogs, growth abnormalities. An inadequate energy intake results in poor growth in young animals and weight loss in adults. Although most animals are efficient self-regulators of their energy intake, this ability may be overridden by a number of factors, particularly in dogs.

No animal is able to utilise all the energy from its food. Energy intake is therefore considered at three different levels: gross energy (GE), digestible energy (DE) and metabolisable energy (ME).

- **Gross energy** of ingested food is the maximum amount of energy that can be released by a food and is assessed by bomb calorimetry. Although a substance may have a high GE content, it is of no use unless the animal is able to digest and absorb it.
- **Digestible energy** is the energy available from a food when it has been absorbed into the body after digestion in the digestive tract and is calculated as GE minus faecal losses.
- **Metabolisable energy** is the energy which is ultimately utilised by the tissues and is calculated as DE minus urinary losses.

The DE and ME contents of foods depend both upon their composition and upon the species which consumes them. The digestive systems of animals differ markedly between species, and even two fairly similar animals, such as the dog and the cat, show differences in digestibility values when fed the same food. In addition to these species differences there will be variations between individual animals in their own metabolic efficiency.

Simple formulae have been developed which give reasonable approximations of the ME in a food from its carbohydrate, fat and protein contents, allowing for the losses in absorption and efficiency (Table 9.1).

Within the body, energy is used to perform muscular work, basic processes such as breathing and physical activity to maintain body temperature. There are two components of energy expenditure, basal metabolic rate and thermogenesis:

- **Basal metabolic rate (BMR)** is the amount of energy required to keep the body 'ticking over' and includes processes such as respiration, circulation and kidney function. It may be affected by many factors including bodyweight and composition, age and hormonal status.
- **Thermogenesis** is simply an increase in metabolic rate over the basal level and includes the cost of digesting, absorbing and utilising nutrients (the 'thermic effect of food'); of muscular work or exercise; of stress; or of maintenance of body temperature in a cold environment. Unlike BMR, the degree of thermogenesis can vary widely and may cause large variations in daily output.

Energy requirements of individual animals are based on the weight of actively metabolising tissue and may be influenced by bodyweight, body surface area, body composition and hair type. Dogs are a unique species in that there is such a wide variation in normal adult bodyweights, and estimations of energy needs are calculated from an allometric equation which relates energy requirements to the animal's metabolic bodyweight, BW $(kg)^{0.75}$ (see later). For other species, including cats, with a relatively narrow range of bodyweights, a linear equation which links energy requirements directly to bodyweight is appropriate in most situations (see later). These basic energy requirements may then be modified according to the animal's physiological status (including life stage and state of health or disease), level of activity and environmental conditions (Tables 9.2 and 9.3).

The energy density of the diet must be high enough to enable the dog or cat to obtain sufficient calories to maintain energy balance. An animal is said to be in energy balance when its expenditure of energy is equal to its intake, with the result that the level of energy stored in the body does not change. Energy density is the principal factor determining the quantity of food eaten each day and thus the amount of each nutrient ingested by the animal. Nutrient requirements

---

Table 9.1 Calculation of metabolisable energy in cat and dog foods (kcal/100 g food[a]) (after Wills, 1996)

Species	Food type and ME equation
Cat	Canned $(P \times 3.9 + F \times 7.7 + C \times 3.0) - 5$
	Dry $(P \times 5.65 + F \times 9.4 + C \times 4.15)\,0.99 - 126$
	Semi-moist $(P \times 3.7 + F \times 8.8 + C \times 3.3)$
Dog	All $(P \times 3.5 + F \times 8.5 + C \times 3.5)$

P = protein g/100 g of food, F = fat (acid ether extract) g/100 g of food
C = carbohydrate (calculated by difference) g/100 g of food
[a] *For result in kJ/100 g food, multiply by 4.18*

Table 9.2 Estimated energy requirements of healthy dogs in various physiological states

Physiological state	Energy requirement
Work 1 hour light work	MER × 1.1
1 full day light work	MER × 1.5
1 full day heavy work (sledge dog)	MER × 2–4
Gestation (< 42 days)	MER × 1
(> 42 days)	MER × 1.1–1.3
Peak lactation (21–42 days)	MER × (1 + (0.25 × no. in litter))
Growth birth to 3 months	MER × 2
3 months to 6 months	MER × 1.6
6 months to 12 months	MER × 1.2
Cold wind chill factor of 8.5° C	MER × 1.25
wind chill factor of < 0°C	MER × 1.75
Heat – tropical climates	MER × 2.5
Inactivity	RER × 1.3

RER = resting energy requirement (kcal) = 70 × BW$^{0.75}$ (kg)
RER (kJ) = 4.184 × 70 × BW$^{0.75}$ (kg)
MER = maintenance energy requirement = RER × 2

Table 9.3 Estimated energy requirements for healthy cats in various physiological states		
Age	**Physiological state**	**MER^a (kcal [kJ]/kg BW)**
10 weeks	Growth	250 [1046]
20 weeks	Growth	130 [544]
30 weeks	Growth	100 [418]
40 weeks	Growth	80 [355]
Adult	Inactive	70 [293]
Adult	Active	80 [335]
Adult	Gestation	80 [335] × 1.1–1.3
Adult	Lactation	80 [335] × (1 + (0.25 × no. in litter))

^{a} *Maintenance energy requirement*

Table 9.4 Essential amino acids for dogs and cats		
Amino acid	**Dog**	**Cat**
Arginine	✓	✓
Histidine	✓	✓
Isoleucine	✓	✓
Lysine	✓	✓
Methionine	✓	✓
Cystine	✓	✓
Phenylalanine	✓	✓
Tyrosine	✓	✓
Threonine	✓	✓
Tryptophan	✓	✓
Valine	✓	✓
Taurine	✗	✓

✓ = essential; ✗ = non-essential

are usually expressed in terms of the ME concentration so that the values are applicable to any type of food or diet regardless of its water content, nutrient content or overall energy value.

Macronutrients

Protein

Proteins are large complex molecules which are composed of long chains of amino acids linked together by peptide bonds. There are only about 20 amino acids commonly found as protein components but these may be arranged in any combination to give an almost infinite variety of naturally occurring proteins, each with its own characteristic properties. Proteins are essential components of all living cells where they have several important functions including regulation of metabolism (as enzymes and some hormones) and a structural role in cell walls and muscle fibre. They are thus an important requirement for tissue growth and repair. Proteins are also a source of energy in the diet.

Animals need a dietary source of protein to provide the specific amino acids that their tissues cannot synthesise at a rate sufficient for optimum performance. Amino acids may be classified as either **essential (indispensable)** or **non-essential (dispensable)**. *Essential* amino acids cannot be synthesised by the body in sufficient amounts and must, therefore, be provided in the diet (Table 9.4). *Non-essential* amino acids are equally important as components of body proteins, but they can be synthesised from excesses of certain other dietary amino acids or other sources of dietary nitrogen.

Protein is required during normal maintenance to replace protein lost during the natural turnover of epithelial surfaces, hair and other body tissues, and in secretions. Additional protein is needed during periods of growth, pregnancy, lactation and for repair of damaged tissue. It is during these critical stages that protein quality (the amino acid composition of the protein) and digestibility are most important. Animal proteins generally have a more balanced amino acid profile, with a greater proportion of essential amino acids, and better digestibility than plant proteins.

The biological value of a food protein is the proportion which can be utilised for synthesising body tissues and compounds and is not excreted in urine or faeces. Good-quality animal proteins have a higher biological value than plant-based proteins.

Protein deficiency can result from either insufficient dietary protein or from a shortage of particular amino acids. Signs of protein deficiency include poor growth or weight loss, rough and dull hair coat, anorexia, increased susceptibility to disease, muscle wasting and emaciation, oedema and finally death. Deficiency of a single essential amino acid results in anorexia and subsequent negative nitrogen balance.

Cats exhibit a number of nutritional peculiarities, many of which are reflected in their protein and amino acid requirements. Not only do they have a higher maintenance protein requirement than many other mammals, but they are also particularly sensitive to an arginine-deficient diet and they have a specific dietary need for the amino-sulphonic acid, taurine. **Taurine** is vital to the functioning of a wide range of mammalian organ systems, but unlike other animals, cats are unable to synthesise sufficient quantities to meet their exceptionally high requirements. A deficiency of taurine in cats results in **feline central retinal degeneration** and has also been linked to **dilated cardiomyopathy**, reproductive failure in queens, developmental abnormalities in kittens, and impaired immune function.

Dietary protein in excess of the body's requirements is not laid down as muscle but is, instead, converted to fat and stored as adipose tissue.

Fat

Dietary fats consist mainly of mixtures of triglycerides, where each triglyceride is a combination of three fatty acids joined by a unit of glycerol. The character of each fat is determined largely by the different fatty acids in each. Fatty acids may be described as *saturated*, where there are no double bonds between carbon atoms, or *unsaturated*, where one or more double bonds are present. Those containing only one double bond are referred to as *monounsaturated*, while those containing more than one double bond are referred to as *polyunsaturated*. Most fats contain all of these types but in widely varying proportions.

Dietary fat has several roles. It serves as the most concentrated source of energy in the diet and it lends palatability and an acceptable texture to food. However, its most important functions are as a provider of essential fatty acids (EFA) and as a carrier for the fat-soluble vitamins A, D, E and K. There are currently three recognised EFA, all of which are polyunsaturated; linoleic, α-linolenic and arachidonic acids. Linoleic and α-linolenic acids are the parent compounds from which the more complex, longer chain compounds (derived EFA) can be made. The cat is unusual in that it is unable to convert the parent EFA into longer chain derivatives and therefore requires a dietary source of arachidonic acid, which in practical terms means a requirement for EFA of *animal* origin.

The EFA are involved in many aspects of health, including kidney function and reproduction. They are essential components of cell membranes and they are necessary for the synthesis of prostaglandins. Signs associated with EFA deficiency in dogs and cats include dull, scurfy coat, hair loss, fatty liver, anaemia and impaired fertility. It should be noted that diets high in polyunsaturated fatty acids may become rancid through oxidation, which can lead to the destruction of other nutrients, particularly vitamin E.

There are several families of fatty acid, named according to the position of the first double bond. Fatty acids with the first double bond between the 3rd and 4th carbon are in the n-3 family (e.g. α-linolenic acid, eicosapentaenoic and docosahexaenoic acids), 6th and 7th carbon the n-6 family (e.g. linoleic acid, α-linolenic acid and arachidonic acid) and 9th and 10th the n-9 family (e.g. oleic acid).The n-3 and n-6 families are EFA because they cannot be synthesised *de novo* in mammals, whereas saturated fatty acids and fatty acids of the n-9 series up to 18 carbons can be synthesised *de novo*.

Carbohydrate

Carbohydrates provide the body with energy and may be converted to body fat. This group includes the simple sugars (such as glucose) and the complex sugars (such as starch) which consist of chains of the simpler sugars. All animals have a metabolic requirement for glucose, but provided the diet contains sufficient glucose precursors (amino acids and glycerol), most animals can synthesise enough to meet their metabolic needs without a dietary source of carbohydrate.

Sugars and *cooked* starches are economical and easily digested sources of energy, whereas uncooked starches are less readily digested. Some species (some dogs for example) may find starch palatable, but others, such as the cat do not respond to the taste of sugar. The value of **disaccharides**, such as sucrose or lactose is limited in most animals by the activity of the intestinal disaccharides, such as sucrase and lactase. In particular, the activity of lactase declines with age and an excessive consumption of lactose-containing (dairy) products can lead to the production of diarrhoea.

Dietary fibre

Dietary fibre, or roughage, is the term applied to the group of indigestible polysaccharides such as cellulose, pectin and lignin. They are usually associated with plant material and typically constitute the cell walls of plants. These materials generally escape digestion and pass through the digestive tract relatively unchanged. The role of dietary fibre in the animal depends to a large extent on the physiology of the animal's digestive tract, but in most species, a limited amount of dietary fibre may provide bulk to the faeces, regularising bowel movements and thus helping to prevent constipation or diarrhoea. Soluble and insoluble sources of dietary fibre are used to improve glycaemic control in dogs with diabetes mellitus and in the dietary management of a number of other 'fibre-responsive' diseases.

Micronutrients

Minerals

Minerals are inorganic nutrients, which are sometimes referred to collectively as 'ash'. They may be divided into **macrominerals** (which are required in relatively large amounts) and trace elements or **microminerals** (which are required in relatively small or trace amounts). Electrolytes are minerals in their salt form as found in the body tissues and fluids. Table 9.5 lists the function of the main minerals and Table 9.6 the dietary requirements.

Macrominerals

Calcium (Ca) and Phosphorus (P)   Calcium and phosphorus are closely interrelated nutritionally and will therefore be discussed together. They are the major minerals involved in maintaining the structural rigidity of bones and teeth and approximately 99% of body calcium and 80% of body phosphorus are stored in the skeletal tissues. Calcium and phosphorus requirements are increased during growth, late pregnancy and lactation. The metabolism of calcium and phosphorus is closely linked with vitamin D.

Calcium is also essential for normal blood clotting and for nerve and muscle function. The level of calcium in the blood plasma is crucial to these functions and is very carefully regulated.

Phosphorus also has many other functions (more than any other mineral) and a complete discussion would require coverage of nearly all the metabolic processes of the body. Phosphorus is involved in many enzyme systems and is also a component of the so-called 'high-energy' organic phosphate compounds. These are mainly responsible for the storage and transfer of energy in the body.

Table 9.5 Established functions of minerals in the dog and cat

Element	Function
Macrominerals	
Calcium	Bone and teeth development. Required for blood clotting, nerve and muscle function
Chloride	Maintains osmotic pressure, acid–base and water balance
Magnesium	Bone and teeth development. Energy metabolism
Phosphorus	Bone and teeth development. Required for energy utilisation and various enzyme systems
Potassium & Sodium	Maintain osmotic pressure, acid–base and water balance. Required for nerve and muscle function
Microminerals	
Arsenic	Required for growth and red blood cell formation
Chromium	Required for carbohydrate metabolism
Cobalt	Component of vitamin B_{12}
Copper	Required for haemoglobin synthesis, structure of bones and blood vessels, melanin production and various enzyme systems
Fluoride	Bone and teeth development
Iodine	Thyroid hormone production
Iron	Component of haemoglobin and myoglobin. Needed for the utilisation of oxygen
Manganese	Required for chondroitin sulphate and cholesterol synthesis. Various enzyme systems associated with carbohydrate and fat metabolism
Molybdenum	Various enzyme systems
Nickel	Function of membranes and nucleic acid metabolism
Selenium	Component of glutathione peroxidase
Silicon	Bone and connective tissue development
Vanadium	Growth, reproduction and fat metabolism
Zinc	Various enzyme systems including alkaline phosphatase, carbonic anhydrase and digestive enzymes. Maintenance of epidermal integrity and immunological homeostasis

Although the absolute concentrations of these minerals in the diet are of paramount importance, the ratio of calcium to phosphorus is also of great significance.

> The minimum calcium : phosphorus ratio for growth is generally considered to be about 1 : 1.

For adult animals it is somewhat less critical. Imbalance in this ratio, where calcium is much less than phosphorus, leads to a marked deficiency of calcium in relation to bone formation.

Calcium deficiency (absolute or relative) results in **nutritional secondary hyperparathyroidism** in which there is increased bone resorption to restore circulating calcium levels. This results in skeletal deformities and lameness in the growing animal. Calcium–phosphorus imbalance may also occur in association with deficiency of vitamin D. This gives rise to **rickets** in the growing animal or **osteomalacia** in the adult. Hypocalcaemia in lactating bitches (particularly of the toy breeds) causes **eclampsia**, with nervous disturbances. This occurs where there is an inability of the calcium regulatory mechanism to compensate for the loss of calcium in milk.

There is evidence that very high levels of calcium and phosphorus or a very high ratio are also harmful.

> Conditions such as **hip dysplasia, osteochondrosis syndrome, enostosis** and **wobbler syndrome** have been related to excessive calcium intake in the growing dog.

Magnesium (Mg) In association with calcium and phosphorus, magnesium is required for healthy bones and teeth. About 60% of body magnesium is found in skeletal tissue, but it is also to be found in the soft tissues of the body. Heart and skeletal muscle and nervous tissue depend on a proper balance between calcium and magnesium for normal function.

Magnesium is also important in sodium and potassium metabolism and plays a key role in many essential enzyme reactions, particularly those concerned with energy metabolism.

A deficiency of magnesium is characterised by muscular weakness and in severe cases, convulsions. Nevertheless, a dietary deficiency of magnesium is very unlikely. In contrast, very high intakes of magnesium have been associated with an increased incidence of **feline lower urinary tract disease**.

Potassium (K) Potassium is found in high concentrations within cells and is required for acid–base balance and osmoregulation of the body fluids. It is also important for nerve and muscle function and energy metabolism. Potassium is widely distributed in foods and naturally occurring deficiencies are rare; however, its requirement is linked to protein intake, so care may be needed in ensuring that high-protein diets contain adequate potassium.

A potassium deficiency causes muscular weakness, poor growth and lesions of the heart and kidney. In cats, the use of diets containing urinary acidifiers with a marginal potassium content has recently been associated with hypokalaemia. Potassium excess is rare but results in paresis and bradycardia.

Sodium (Na) and Chloride (Cl) Together, sodium and chloride represent the major electrolytes of the body water and are required for acid–base balance and osmoregulation of the body fluids. Chloride is also an essential com-

Table 9.6 Dietary requirements: minerals

Mineral	Cat		Dog	
Calcium	Growth:	110–173 mg/kg BW/day or approximately 160–250 mg/100 kcal (418 kJ) ME	Growth:	320 mg/kg BW/day or approximately 275 mg/100 kcal (418 kJ) ME
	Maintenance:	87–156 mg/kg BW/day or approximately 125–200 mg/100 kcal (418 kJ) ME	Maintenance:	119 mg/kg BW/day or approximately 130–160 mg/100 kcal (418 kJ) ME
Phosphorus	Growth:	90–150 mg/kg BW/day or approximately 120–200 mg/100 kcal (418 kJ) ME	Growth:	240 mg/kg BW/day or approximately 200–225 mg/100 kcal (418 kJ) ME
	Maintenance:	90 mg/kg BW/day or approximately 120 mg/100 kcal (418 kJ) ME	Maintenance:	89 mg/kg BW/day or approximately 120–160 mg/100 kcal (418 kJ) ME
Copper	Growth:	100–160 µg/kg BW/day or approximately 300–460 µg/100 kcal (418 kJ) ME	Growth:	160–500 µg/kg BW/day or approximately 150–440 µg/100 kcal (418 kJ) ME
	Maintenance:	75 µg/kg BW/day or approximately 100 µg/100 kcal (418 kJ) ME	Maintenance:	80 µ/kg BW/day or approximately 150 µg/100 kcal (418 kJ) ME
Iodine	Growth:	20–309 µg/kg BW/day or approximately 27–33 µg/100 kcal (418 kJ) ME	Growth:	30–50 µg/kg BW/day or approximately 16–25 µg/100 kcal (418 kJ) ME
	Maintenance:	7–15 µ/kg BW/day or approximately 10–20 µ/g /100 kcal (418 kJ) ME	Maintenance:	12 µg/kg BW/day or approximately 16–24 µg/100 kcal (418 kJ) ME
Iron	Growth:	4–4.5 mg/kg BW/day or approximately 12–18 mg/100 kcal (418 kJ) ME	Growth:	1.74–2.3 mg/kg BW/day or approximately 1–2 mg/100 kcal (418 kJ) ME
	Maintenance:	1.2 mg/kg BW/day or approximately 1.6 mg/100 kcal (418 kJ) ME	Maintenance:	0.65 mg/kg BW/day or approximately 100–130 mg/100 kcal (418 kJ) ME
Magnesium	Growth:	7.5–9.4 mg/kg BW/day or approximately 10–12.5 mg/100 kcal (418 kJ) ME	Growth:	22 mg/kg BW/day or approximately 25 mg/100 kcal (418 kJ) ME
	Maintenance:	6 mg/kg BW/day or approximately 8 mg/100 kcal (418 kJ) ME	Maintenance:	5.5–8.2 mg/kg BW/day or approximately 11 mg/100 kcal (418 kJ) ME
Manganese	Growth and Maintenance:	80–250 µg/kg BW/day or approximately 100–250 µg/100 kcal (418 kJ) ME	Growth:	280–1000 µg/kg BW/day or approximately 200–600 µg/100 kcal (418 kJ) ME
			Maintenance:	100 µg/kg BW/day or approximately 140–200 µg/100 kcal (418 kJ) ME
Selenium	Growth:	5–13 µg/kg BW/day or approximately 2–5 µg/100 kcal (418 kJ) ME	Growth:	6–13 µg/kg BW/day or approximately 3–8 µg/100 kcal (418 kJ) ME
	Maintenance:	5 µg/kg BW/day or approximately 6 µg/100 kcal (418 kJ) ME	Maintenance:	6 µg/kg BW/day or approximately 7 µg/100 kcal (418 kJ) ME
Sodium	Growth:	15–30 mg/kg BW/day or approximately 20–40 mg/100 kcal (418 kJ) ME	Growth:	30 mg/kg BW/day or approximately 20–25 mg/100 kcal (418 kJ) ME
	Maintenance:	14 mg/kg BW/day or approximately 18 mg/100 kcal (418 kJ) ME	Maintenance:	14 mg/kg BW/day or approximately 18 mg/100 kcal (418 kJ) ME
Chloride	Growth and Maintenance:	29 mg/kg BW/day or approximately 38 mg/100 kcal (418 kJ) ME	Growth:	46 mg/kg BW/day or approximately 40 mg/100 kcal (418 kJ) ME
			Maintenance:	17 mg/kg BW/day or approximately 21–30 mg/100 kcal (418 kJ) ME
Potassium	Growth and Maintenance:	100–125 mg/100 kcal (418 kJ) ME	Growth and Maintenance:	100–125 mg/100 kcal (418 kJ) ME
Zinc	Growth and Maintenance:	2.5–3.9 mg/kg BW/day or approximately 1–2 mg/100 kcal (418 kJ) ME	Growth:	1.9–3.3 mg/kg BW/day or approximately 0.97–2 mg/100 kcal (418 kJ) ME
			Maintenance:	0.72 mg/kg BW/day or approximately 0.92–1.200 mg/100 kcal (418 kJ) ME

ponent of bile and hydrochloric acid (which is present in gastric juice).

Common salt (NaCl) is the most usual form in which these two minerals are added to food, so the dietary recommendation is often expressed in terms of sodium chloride. As with potassium, salt is widely distributed in normal diets so deficiencies are rare.

Signs of deficiency may include fatigue, exhaustion, inability to maintain water balance, decreased water intake, retarded growth, dry skin and hair loss. Excess will cause greater than normal fluid intake and it has been suggested that some dogs with hypertension may benefit from a lower sodium diet.

Microminerals

Iron (Fe) Iron is an essential component of the oxygen-carrying pigments, haemoglobin (in blood) and myoglobin (in muscle). It is also an essential part of many enzymes (haem enzymes) which are involved in respiration at the cellular level.

A deficiency causes anaemia with the typical clinical picture of weakness and fatigue. Conversely iron, like most trace elements, is toxic if ingested in excessive amounts and is associated with anorexia and weight loss.

Copper (Cu) Copper is required for the formation and activity of red blood cells, as a cofactor in many enzyme systems, and for the normal pigmentation of skin and hair. Copper deficiency impairs the absorption and transport of iron and decreases haemoglobin synthesis. Thus a lack of copper in the diet can cause anaemia even when the intake of iron is normal. Bone disorders can also occur as a result of copper deficiency, and in this case the cause is thought to be a reduction in the activity of a copper-containing enzyme, leading to diminished stability and strength of bone collagen. Other signs of deficiency include hair depigmentation, decreased growth, neuromuscular disorders and reproductive failure.

Ironically, *excess* dietary copper may also cause anaemia, which is thought to result from competition between copper and iron for absorption sites in the intestine. Bedlington Terriers are known to display an unusual defect which results in hepatitis and cirrhosis and appears to be inherited. It has also been identified in other breeds including West Highland White Terriers and Dobermann Pinschers. For these particular breeds, foods with a high copper content and copper-containing mineral supplements should be avoided.

Zinc (Zn) Zinc is an essential component of many enzyme systems, including those related to protein and carbohydrate metabolism, and is essential for maintaining healthy coat and skin. Zinc is required by all animals, but the zinc requirement is particularly affected by the other components of the diet. For example, a high dietary calcium content or a vegetable protein-based diet can dramatically increase the zinc requirement and this latter effect may be related to that reported for iron absorption.

Zinc deficiency is characterised by poor growth, anorexia, testicular atrophy, emaciation and skin lesions. Although all nutrients are important, the link between zinc and skin and coat condition makes this trace element particularly crucial for the companion animal. This is because a marginal deficiency may occur where an animal is not obviously unwell but its skin or coat condition is suboptimal and significantly detracts from its appearance.

Zinc is relatively non-toxic, but high levels may interfere with the absorption and utilisation of iron and copper.

Iodine (I) Iodine an essential component of thyroid hormones, which regulate basal metabolism in the body, and this is its only recognised function. **Goitre** (enlargement of the thyroid gland) is the principal sign of iodine deficiency but other factors may also produce goitre.

Hypothyroidism has been reported in dogs and iodine deficiency has also been observed in zoo felids, domestic cats, birds and horses. Clinical signs include skin and hair abnormalities, dullness, apathy and drowsiness. There can also be abnormal calcium metabolism and reproductive failure with fetal resorption.

Excessive iodine intakes can be toxic producing acute effects similar to those of a deficiency. The high doses in some way impair thyroid hormone synthesis and can produce so-called iodine myxoedema or toxic goitre. Anorexia, fever and weight loss may occur in cats.

Selenium (Se) Selenium is closely interrelated with vitamin E, such that the presence of one nutrient can 'spare' a deficiency of the other and together, they protect against damage to cell membranes. Nevertheless, it has been shown that selenium cannot be completely replaced by vitamin E and has a discrete, unique function. Selenium is an obligatory component of glutathione peroxidase, the enzyme which protects cell membranes against damage by oxidising substances. Selenium may also have other roles including protection against lead, cadmium and mercury poisoning and has been implicated as an anticancer agent.

Selenium deficiency has many effects, but one described in dogs is degeneration of skeletal and cardiac muscles. Effects of deficiency in other species include reproductive disorders and oedema.

Selenium is highly toxic in large doses and the difference between the recommended allowance and the toxic dose may be quite small. Effects of excess include vomiting, spasms, staggered gait, salivation and decreased appetite. Injudicious supplementation of foods is therefore particularly dangerous in this respect.

Manganese (Mn) Manganese is involved in many enzyme-catalysed reactions and is required for carbohydrate and lipid metabolism, cartilage formation, reproduction and cell membrane integrity. A deficiency is characterised by defective growth, reproduction and disturbances in lipid metabolism. Manganese is relatively nontoxic.

Cobalt (Co) Cobalt is an integral part of the vitamin B_{12} molecule and a deficiency is unlikely to occur if adequate vitamin B_{12} is present in the diet.

Other trace elements A number of trace elements have been demonstrated as necessary for normal health in mammals, although specific requirements have not been established for companion animals. These elements are listed in Table 9.7 with a brief summary of their functions. It appears that the amounts required in the diet are very low and the likelihood of a deficiency of any of these nutrients in a normal diet is consequently almost non-existent.

Conversely, as with the majority of the trace elements, these substances are all toxic if fed in large quantities, although the amounts which can be tolerated vary from one element to another. Arsenic, vanadium, fluorine and molybdenum are the most toxic, whereas relatively large amounts of nickel and chromium can be ingested without adverse effects.

Table 9.7 Functions of additional trace elements (after Wills, 1996)	
Element	**Function**
Chromium	Carbohydrate metabolism, closely linked with insulin function
Fluoride	Teeth and bone development, possibly some involvement in reproduction
Nickel	Membrane function, possibly involved in metabolism of the nucleic acid RNA
Molybdenum	Constituent of several enzymes, one of which is involved in uric acid metabolism
Silicon	Skeletal development, growth and maintenance of connective tissue
Vanadium	Growth, reproduction and fat metabolism
Arsenic	Growth, also some effect on blood formation, possibly haemoglobin production

Mineral interactions   A large number of mineral–mineral interactions exist. These interactions tend to be of two types:

- **Antagonistic** – the presence of one mineral reduces the transport or biological efficiency of the other.
- **Synergistic** – the two minerals act in a complementary way, either by sparing or substituting for the other mineral, or the two together enhance a biological function.

Most mineral interactions are antagonistic and can occur via a number of different mechanisms. Interactions may be:

- In the diet during processing and therefore before consumption.
- In the digestive tract where there is competition for uptake sites or other cellular mechanisms.
- At the tissue level either at storage sites or by inhibition of enzyme activity.
- At the time of transport.
- In the excretory pathway.

Vitamins

Vitamins are organic compounds which help to regulate the body processes. Most vitamins cannot be synthesised in the body and must, therefore, be present in the diet. They may be classified as **fat-soluble** (vitamins A, D, E and K) or **water-soluble** (B-complex vitamins and vitamin C). A frequent intake of water-soluble vitamins is necessary since they are poorly stored in the body, with excesses being lost via the urine. The fat-soluble vitamins are stored to a much greater extent and consequently, a daily intake is less critical. However, because they are stored, the risk of toxicity arising through excessive intake is far greater with the fat-soluble vitamins. Tables 9.8 and 9.9 list the essential features of vitamins and the cat's and dog's dietary requirement.

Table 9.8 Essential features of the major vitamins	
Vitamin	**Features**
A	Fat soluble. Essential in diet. Found in liver, fats, oils, egg yolks and cereal grain germ. Exists as a pro-vitamin in vegetable sources. Stored in the body. Deficiencies affect vision, hearing, respiratory tract lining, skin and bones. Excesses are toxic
B group	Comprises thiamine (B_1), riboflavin (B_2), niacin, pyridoxine (B_6), pantothenic acid, folic acid, biotin and cobalamin (B_{12}). Water soluble. Many are produced by intestinal bacteria. Found in liver, egg yolks, yeast and whole cereal grains. Exists as the active form in vegetables. Not stored in the body, except vitamin B_{12}. Deficiencies affect appetite and metabolism. Excesses are not usually toxic
C	Water soluble. No dietary requirement in healthy dogs and cats. Found in fresh fruit and vegetables. Found as the active form in vegetables. Not stored in the body. Deficiencies affect wound healing and capillary integrity. Excesses are not toxic
D	Fat soluble. Essential in diet. Found in liver, fats, oils, egg yolks and cereal grain germ. Exists as a pro-vitamin in vegetable sources. Stored in the body. Deficiencies affect bone, teeth and calcium-phosphorus absorption/utilisation. Excesses are toxic
E	Fat soluble. Essential in diet. Found in liver, fats, oils, egg yolks and cereal grain germ. Found as active form in vegetables. Stored in the body. Deficiencies affect muscle, fat and reproductive ability
K	Fat soluble. Minimal requirement in diet as it is manufactured by intestinal bacteria. Found in liver, fats, oils, egg yolks and cereal grain germ. Exists as a pro-vitamin in vegetable sources. Not stored in the body. Deficiencies cause a coagulopathy

Fat-soluble vitamins

Vitamin A   In nature, vitamin A (retinol) is found to a large extent in the form of its precursors, the carotenoids, which are the yellow and orange pigments of most fruits and vegetables. Of these, β-carotene is the most important. Vitamin A is a component of the visual pigments (which transmit light) in the eye and is important for proper vision. It is also concerned with cell differentiation and maintenance of normal cell structure, so is important for sustaining healthy skin, coat, all mucous membranes and for normal bone and teeth development.

A deficiency of vitamin A may be associated with anorexia, weakness, ataxia, weight loss and abnormalities of the squamous epithelium which are usually manifest as seborrhoeic coat conditions; xerophthalmia, which will ultimately lead to corneal opacity and ulceration; increased susceptibility to microbial infections; crusting lesions of the external nares and accompanying nasal discharge; and epithelial degeneration of the seminiferous tubules and endometrium, leading to infertility.

Deficiencies of vitamin A are not common and dogs are able to synthesise vitamin A from plant-derived β-carotene.

Table 9.9 Dietary requirements: vitamins

Vitamins		Cat per kg BW/day	Cat per 100 kcal (418 kJ)		Dog per kg BW/day	Dog per 100 kcal (418 kJ)
Vitamin B						
Choline	Growth:	120–130 mg	48 mg	Growth:	50 mg	34 mg
	Maintenance:	120–130 mg	48 mg	Maintenance:	25 mg	34 mg
Biotin	Growth:	1.5–3 µg	1.4–3.2 µg	Growth:	20 µg	12.5 µg
	Maintenance:	1.5 µg	1.4 µg	Maintenance:	20 µg	12.5 µg
Cobalamin	Growth:	1 µg	0.4–1.25 µg	Growth:	1 µg	0.7 µg
	Maintenance:	0.32 µg	0.4–0.5 µg	Maintenance:	0.5 µg	0.7 µg
Folate	Growth:	25–40 µg	16–25 µg	Growth:	8 µg	5.4 µg
	Maintenance:	16–20 µg	27 µg	Maintenance:	4 µg	5.4 µg
Niacin	Growth:	1.8 mg	1.8–2.4 mg	Growth:	0.45 mg	0.3 mg
	Maintenance:	0.9 mg	1.8 mg	Maintenance:	0.225 mg	0.3–0.45 mg
Pantothenic acid	Growth:	75–180 µg	100–250 µg	Growth:	400 µg	270–330 µg
	Maintenance:	75–180 µg	100–250 µg	Maintenance:	200 µg	270–400 µg
Pyridoxine	Growth:	0.128–0.2 mg	0.08–0.16 mg	Growth:	0.06 mg	0.03 mg
	Maintenance:	0.07 mg	0.08–0.1 mg	Maintenance:	0.022 mg	0.03 mg
Riboflavin	Growth:	150–320 µg	130–280 µg	Growth:	100 µg	68–80 µg
	Maintenance:	90 µg	120 µg	Maintenance:	50 µg	68 µg
Thiamine	Growth:	100–250 µg	0.125–0.16 mg	Growth:	54 µg	27–40 µg
	Maintenance:	80 µg	0.1 mg	Maintenance:	20 µg	27 µg
Vitamin A	Growth:	64–75 U	80–100 U/kg	Growth:	202 U	100–170 U
	Maintenance:	64–75 U	80–100 U/kg	Maintenance:	75 U	100–150 U
	Reproduction:	90–100 U	120–140 U/kg			
Vitamin D	Growth:	18–22 U	15–25 U	Growth:	22 U	11–18 U
	Maintenance:	8 U	10 U	Maintenance:	8 U	11–15 U
Vitamin E	Growth:	1–1.5 U	0.9–1 U	Growth:	1.4 U	1.25 U
	Maintenance:	0.45 U	0.6 U	Maintenance:	0.5 U	0.6–1 U
Vitamin K	Growth:	16–60 µg	2–20 µg	Growth:	16–60 µg	2–20 µg
	Maintenance:	16–60 µg	2–20 µg	Maintenance:	16–60 µg	2–20 µg

One international unit (1 U) of Vitamin D is equivalent to 0.025 mg
One international unit (1 U) of α-tocopherol is equivalent to 1 mg

Cats, however, are unable to perform this conversion and their diet must therefore include a source of preformed vitamin A, which may only be found in animal fat.

Excesses of vitamin A are stored in the liver and a toxicity can lead to liver damage. Clinically, the most recognisable signs of **hypervitaminosis A** are those of a crippling bone disease which results in the formation of bony exostoses and ankylosis of joints, particularly in the cervical vertebrae and the long bones of the forelimb. Cats are particularly susceptible to hypervitaminosis A and the problem usually arises following prolonged oversupplementation of the diet with vitamin A (in cod liver oil, for example) or by feeding large quantities of liver.

Vitamin D Metabolites of vitamin D stimulate calcium absorption in the intestine and, in conjunction with parathyroid hormone, stimulate resorption of calcium from bone. The requirements for vitamin D are closely linked to the dietary concentrations of calcium and phosphorus. Most mammals are able to synthesise vitamin D_3 from lipid compounds in the skin provided they have exposure to sunlight and are otherwise well nourished.

There are several compounds which have vitamin D activity but the most important are ergocalciferol (vitamin D_2) and cholecalciferol (vitamin D_3). Both of these forms are effective as sources of vitamin D activity.

A deficiency of vitamin D is extremely rare but is frequently confounded by a simultaneous calcium and phosphorus imbalance, which causes **rickets** in the young animal and **osteomalacia** in the adult, characterised by a failure of mineralisation of newly-formed osteoid. In the young animal, **endochondral ossification** of the growth plates is disturbed, giving rise to the typically enlarged metaphyses, particularly of the radius-ulna and ribs.

Adverse effects of excess vitamin D are generally related to hypercalcaemia which, if prolonged, results in extensive calcification of the soft tissues, lungs, kidneys, and stomach. Deformations of the teeth and jaws can also occur and death can result if the intake is particularly high.

Vitamin E Acting with selenium, vitamin E protects cell membranes against oxidative damage. The requirement for vitamin E is increased when dietary levels of polyunsaturated fatty acids (PUFA), which are easily oxidised, are high. Recent studies of healthy animals have demonstrated an increased immune response to vaccination when fed diets high in vitamin E and other antioxidants. Given the low potential for toxicity, this work indicates that there are likely added benefits to feeding higher quantities of vitamin E than that required to prevent a deficiency.

In cats, vitamin E deficiency can be induced by feeding diets of oily fish (especially red tuna) which are rich in polyunsaturated fatty acids or feeding rancid, oxidised fat. This causes a painful inflammatory condition of body fat (especially subcutaneous fat) known as *pansteatitis (yellow fat disease)*. Vitamin E deficiency in dogs has been associated with skeletal muscle dystrophy, reproductive failure and impairment of the immune response.

In practice, vitamin E toxicity is unlikely to occur. Vitamin E is one of the least toxic vitamins and relatively high doses may be tolerated.

Vitamin K   Vitamin K regulates the formation of several blood-clotting factors (factors VII, IX, X and XII). In normal, healthy animals the requirement for vitamin K is met by bacterial synthesis in the intestine and a simple deficiency is unlikely to occur. **Hypoprothombinaemia** and **haemorrhage** may occur in some animals when bacterial synthesis is suppressed, or there are vitamin K antagonists (such as warfarin or other coumarin compounds) in the diet.

Excess vitamin K has low toxicity but very large intakes may produce anaemia and other blood abnormalities in young animals.

Water-soluble vitamins

B-complex   The B-complex vitamins are used to form coenzymes (cofactors) which are involved with normal metabolic function, especially energy metabolism and synthetic pathways.

> Water-soluble vitamins are now usually referred to by their chemical names rather than by a letter/number combination.

Thiamin (aneurin, vitamin B$_1$)   Thiamin is involved in carbohydrate metabolism and the requirement for this vitamin is dependent on the carbohydrate content of the diet. Thiamin deficiency can occur in cats as a result of feeding large amounts of certain types of *raw* fish which contain the enzyme thiaminase. In addition, the vitamin is progressively destroyed by high temperatures and under certain conditions of processing. Most pet food manufacturers supplement their products to compensate for possible losses, but some home-prepared diets may require additional thiamin.

Thiamin deficiency is expressed clinically as anorexia, neurological disorders (especially of the postural mechan-

isms) followed ultimately by weakness, heart failure and death. Like other water-soluble vitamins, thiamin is of low toxicity when ingested at high levels.

Riboflavin (B$_2$)   Riboflavin is a constituent of two coenzymes which are essential in a number of oxidative enzyme systems. Cellular growth cannot take place in the absence of riboflavin.

Riboflavin deficiency is associated with eye lesions, skin disorders and testicular hypoplasia. Toxicity of this vitamin has not been reported in dogs and cats.

Pantothenic acid   Pantothenic acid is a constituent of coenzyme A which is essential for carbohydrate, fat and amino acid metabolism. This vitamin is widespread in animal and plant tissues and a deficiency is unlikely to occur in normal circumstances.

Signs of experimentally induced deficiency include depressed growth, fatty liver, gastrointestinal disturbances (including ulcers), convulsions, coma and death. Toxicity has not been reported in any species following ingestion of large doses.

Niacin (nicotinamide and nicotinic acid)   Niacin is a component of two important coenzymes, the nicotinamide adenine dinucleotides, which are required for oxidation–reduction reactions necessary for the utilisation of all the major nutrients. In mammalian species, the requirement for niacin is influenced by the dietary level of the amino acid tryptophan, which can be converted to the vitamin. In cats, however, this conversion does not occur because an alternative pathway in the metabolism of tryptophan is favoured, so the dietary requirement for niacin is greater.

A deficiency of niacin causes a condition known as pellagra in humans and blacktongue in dogs and cats, which is characterised by inflammation and ulceration of the oral cavity with thick, blood-stained saliva and foul breath. Both forms of niacin are considered to be of low toxicity.

Pyridoxine (vitamin B$_6$)   This vitamin is involved in a wide range of enzyme systems associated with nitrogen and amino acid metabolism and consequently, increased levels are required as the protein content of the diet increases.

A deficiency of pyridoxine results in anorexia, weight loss and anaemia. In cats, irreversible kidney damage can occur. Pyridoxine and its derivatives are not considered toxic. Prevalence of pyridoxine toxicity appears to be low. Earliest detectable signs include ataxia and loss of small motor control. Many of the signs of toxicity resemble those of B$_6$ deficiency.

Biotin   Biotin is required for a variety of reactions involving the metabolism of fats and amino acids. The vitamin is important in maintaining the integrity of keratinised structures, such as the skin and hair.

Deficiencies of biotin are unlikely to occur since the daily requirement is normally met by intestinal bacterial synthesis. However, a deficiency may develop following the prolonged use of oral antibiotics which suppress microbial synthesis or the feeding of large amounts of raw egg-white, which contains avidin, a protein which binds biotin. **Eggs should, therefore, be cooked** if they are to form a significant proportion of the diet.

Signs of biotin deficiency include dry, scaly skin with dull, brittle hair, hyperkeratosis, pruritus and skin ulcers. No toxicity has been reported in dogs and cats.

Folic acid (pteroylglutamic acid, folacin) The folates are important for a number of reactions including the synthesis of thymidine, an essential component of DNA. It is essential for normal maturation of red blood cells in bone marrow and the typical signs of folic acid deficiency are anaemia and leucopenia. However, deficiencies are unlikely to occur since it is likely that most, if not all of the daily requirement can be met by intestinal bacterial synthesis. Folic acid is considered to be non-toxic.

Vitamin B$_{12}$ (cyanocobalamin) The function of vitamin B$_{12}$ is closely linked to that of folic acid. It is also involved in fat and carbohydrate metabolism and in the synthesis of myelin. A deficiency results in pernicious anaemia and neurological signs.

Choline Choline is a constituent of phospholipids which are essential components of cell membranes and it is also the precursor of acetyl-choline, a neurotransmitter chemical. A dietary deficiency of choline is unlikely to occur, but experimentally it causes fatty infiltration of the liver. No toxicity has been described for dogs and cats.

Ascorbic acid (vitamin C) Vitamin C is required for many intracellular reactions and protein synthesis, but most mammals are able to synthesise it from glucose. The main exceptions are man, other primates and the guinea pig. Although there is no dietary requirement for vitamin C in normal, healthy companion animals, some researchers believe that a dietary source may be beneficial under certain circumstances (such as stress or high activity levels) or in certain individuals. No signs of either deficiency or excess have been reported in normal cats or dogs.

VITAMIN-LIKE COMPOUNDS
There are substances that exhibit properties similar to those of vitamins, but do not fit the strict definition of a vitamin. These compounds have physiological functionality but can be 'conditionally essential' depending upon the metabolic capacity of the animal. Examples include carnitine, carotenoids, bioflavenoids, ubiquinones and para-aminobenzoic acid (PABA). Research into these nutrients and their functions continues.

Water

An animal's requirement for water is at least as important as that for any other nutrient; life may continue for weeks in the absence of food but only for a few days, or even hours, when water is not available. Water performs many vital functions within the body and the body water content is regulated within quite narrow limits. A daily intake is necessary to replace obligatory water losses from the body which occur mainly via the urine, faeces, skin and lungs and in productive secretions such as milk.

Water is taken into the body in several forms: as fluid drunk, as a component of food or as metabolic water (that released during the breakdown of protein, fat and carbohydrate). The daily water intake of any individual will depend on a number of factors including the moisture content of the food, environmental temperature, level of activity and physiological state. A plentiful supply of fresh drinking water should, therefore, always be available.

A balanced diet

In the last several decades much has been learned about the nutritional needs of pets, in particular dogs and cats. With the advent of feeding balanced, prepared diets, nutritional deficiencies are a rare occurrence. A diet which is balanced will supply all the key nutrients and energy needed to meet the daily needs of the animal at its particular life stage. Nutrient and energy content are therefore important considerations but other related factors include digestibility and palatability of the food. Animals eat to satisfy their requirement for energy, so if all key nutrients are balanced to the energy content of the diet, then providing the correct quantity of energy also ensures an appropriate intake of essential nutrients. The need of animals requiring a higher plane of nutrition (as in gestation or lactation) will inevitably receive a higher intake of all key nutrients when they increase the amount of food consumed to meet their energy demands.

Nutrient balance

Nutrient requirements are bounded by a minimum and, in some cases, a maximum value. In other words, the amount of nutrient needed in the diet must lie on a 'plateau' between deficiency on the one hand and toxicity on the other (Fig. 9.2).

Nutrient interactions

Deficiencies of a specific nutrient may occur as a result of interactions with other components of the diet, which reduce

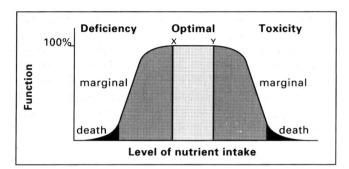

Fig. 9.2 Relationship of nutrient intake to health.

The main criteria for what constitutes a complete diet can be summarised as:
- The content of each nutrient must be on the plateau.
- Each nutrient must be present in the correct ratio to the energy content of the diet.
- Each nutrient must be at the correct ratio to other nutrients (where appropriate).
- Each nutrient must be in a form that is usable by the animal for which the diet is made.

---

their bioavailability. For example, excessive amounts of phytate (as is found in cereal-based diets) will interfere with the intestinal absorption of zinc and high levels of calcium will reduce the absorption of both copper and zinc. The absorption of iron is known to be influenced by a number of factors. Ferrous iron is better absorbed than ferric iron and iron contained in foods of animal origin tends to be better absorbed than that from vegetable sources.

Digestibility

The **digestibility** of a food is a measure of the **biological availability** of its constituent nutrients to the animal. Although analysis of a particular food may give an indication of its total nutrient content, it is only the portion of nutrients which are actually absorbed from the gut that have any true nutritional value.

Factors which affect the digestibility of a substance include chemical composition of the food, its state of subdivision and its method of preparation or processing.

Palatability

The palatability of food is a complex subject including a knowledge of the factors affecting appetite and behaviour, as well as an understanding of taste, smell and texture of food and their interrelationships. The importance of palatability cannot be overemphasised, since a food which is left uneaten, whatever its nutrient content, is of no nutritive value to the animal.

First impressions of a food are always important and food must always be presented in a manner which is appropriate to the size of the animal. Cats and small dogs prefer food in small pieces which are not too sticky, whereas larger dogs are able to eat foods with a much broader spectrum of shape and size.

Smell and taste are necessary sensory components of any meal and animals with poor appetites can often be tempted to eat by providing strong-smelling foods, particularly if the food is warmed to about 35°C. Cats can distinguish between sweet and bitter tastes but do not respond to the addition of glucose in their food. In general, meat is very palatable to dogs and cats and its acceptance can often be further enhanced by the addition of fat, especially animal fat.

Most animals enjoy variety in their diet, although they may be initially suspicious of a food which differs markedly from their previous diet. Above all it is important to recognise that, like humans, all animals are individuals with their own dietary likes and dislikes.

Foods and food types

Prepared pet foods

In the developed countries, the vast majority of dogs and cats are fed commercially prepared pet foods. The enormous range of manufactured pet foods available offer the pet owner a convenient method of feeding their pet; the preparation time involved is minimised and the animal can be provided with a variety of flavours and textures in its diet. All these diets are nutritionally balanced when fed according to the instructions on the label, and are all prepared to the same exacting standards.

Prepared diets for pets may be categorised on their nutrient content as either complete or complementary and this information should be stated on the product label. A **complete** diet will provide a balanced diet when fed alone, although the specific life stage (such as growth, reproduction or adult maintenance) for which it is designed must be specified. They require no supplementation except that clean fresh water should always be available. A **complementary diet** is designed to be fed in combination with an additional, specified food source, such as canned meat and biscuit mixer.

There are three main forms in which prepared pet foods are usually presented:

- **Dry foods**, which have a moisture content of 10–14%, include both complete diets and biscuits. The complete diets are usually a mixture of dry, flaked or crushed cereals and vegetables, and many include a meat-based dry protein concentrate. They may be fed dry or the owner may add gravy or water before feeding. Biscuits are generally made from wheaten flour and may be fed whole or broken and used as a mixer with moist foods.
- **Moist foods** are the most popular means of feeding pet dogs and cats. Their moisture content is 60–85% and they may be packed in cans, plastic or semirigid aluminium. They tend to have a higher meat content and are filled with gravy or set in jelly, both of which provide important vitamins and minerals and improve the palatability of the product. Canned meat products tend to be the most palatable.
- **Semimoist foods** have a moisture content of 25–40% and are composed of a meat and cereal mixture which is cooked to a paste and extruded into small, shaped pieces. The main advantage of this type of diet is its convenience.

The product packaging provides useful data, some of which is legally required, that should help the pet owner to make important decisions about how to feed the product. In addition to information which identifies the product and the species for which the food is intended, the pet food label should state:

- The ingredients in descending order of predominance by weight (Table 9.10).
- The typical (or guaranteed) analysis giving the concentrations of protein, oil, fibre, ash and moisture (if over 14%) in the product.
- Whether the food is complete or complementary in respect of the particular life stage for which it is designed.
- The manufacturer's directions for use including feeding recommendations or guidelines.

EC regulations do not currently permit the declaration of energy content on pet food labels, but this may be roughly estimated from its carbohydrate, fat and protein contents (Table 9.1). This reinforces the importance of reliable feeding recommendations, but these should always be regarded as guidelines only. Observation of the health, condition and bodyweight of the animal will help to determine whether adjustments are necessary in the amounts fed. Where supplementary foods are provided, as snacks, treats or table scraps, their nutritive value must be taken into account when determining the daily food allowance.

Home-prepared diets

For a variety of reasons, many dog and cat owners prefer to feed their pets on fresh foods prepared at home. However, formulation of a balanced diet for any animal requires a detailed knowledge of its specific nutritional needs; of the nutritive value of different foodstuffs from which the diet is to be prepared; of dietary interactions; and of methods of preparation and storage which may affect the availability of individual nutrients (Tables 9.11 and 9.12). Considerable time, effort and expertise are therefore required to be able to offer the animal a consistent and nutritionally adequate diet.

The following foods are common ingredients of home-prepared diets for dogs and cats:

- **Meat**. Lean muscle meat is a poor source of calcium and the feeding of an 'all-meat' diet is the most common cause of **nutritional secondary hyperparathyroidism**.
- **Offals**. These do not constitute a balanced diet and should not be fed exclusively. In particular, cats may become 'addicted' to liver and risk the development of **hypervitaminosis A**.
- **Fish**. Care should be taken when feeding raw fish as some types contain thiaminase, leading to **thiamine deficiency** with prolonged feeding. Large amounts of oily fish, especially red tuna, can precipitate **pansteatitis** (yellow fat disease) due to vitamin E deficiency.
- **Eggs**. These are a valuable source of good quality protein but should be fed cooked to destroy avidin (which binds biotin).

Table 9.10 Some ingredients used in commercial pet foods		
Dry foods	**Canned foods**	**Semi-moist**
Ground cereals (corn, oats, wheat, sorghum)	Ground cereals (corn, oats, wheat, sorghum)	Ground cereals (corn, oats, wheat, sorghum)
Meat and bone meal	Meat and bone meal	Sucrose
Whey	Meat	Meat and bone meal
Soyabean meal	Meat by-products	Wheat bran
Animal fat	Liver	Meat
Iodised salt	Lung	Meat by-products
Vitamin/mineral mix	Corn flour	Tallow
	Heart	Milk
	Lard	Soy flour
	Blood	Propylene glycol
	Vitamin/mineral mix	Iodised salt
		Vitamin/mineral mix

Table 9.11 Selected common protein sources and quantities required to supply 10 g of protein in home-made diets

Type of food	Approximate amount (g) required to supply 10 g protein[a]	Ca	P	Na	Cu	Fi	Fa	BV
Chicken meat	50	L	M	L	L	L	L	H
Chicken skin	62	L	M	L	M	L	H	M
Giblets	47	L	M	L	M	L	L	H
Cod	57	L	M	L	M	L	L	H
Haddock	53	L	M	L	L	L	L	H
Halibut	48	L	M	L	M	L	L	H
Shrimp	55	L	M	H	M	L	L	H
Tuna canned in oil	41	L	M	H	M	L	H	H
Tuna canned in water	36	L	M	L	M	L	L	H
Beef lean meat	48	L	M	L	H	L	M	M
Beef normal meat	56	L	M	L	H	L	H	M
Beef heart	59	L	M	M	–	L	L	M
Beef kidney	65	L	M	H	–	L	M	M
Beef liver	50	L	M	H	–	L	L	M
Lamb meat	65	L	M	M	–	L	H	M
Cottage cheese creamed	74	L	M	H	L	L	L	M
Cottage cheese non-creamed	59	L	M	H	L	L	L	M
Cheddar cheese	40	M	M	H	L	L	H	M
Egg whole	78	L	L	M	L	L	L	H
Egg white	92	L	L	M	L	L	L	H
Egg yolk	63	L	L	L	L	L	L	H

[a] The amounts required will vary between products. The amount required to supply 10 g protein can be calculated in the following way: amount required in g = (100 + protein content per 100 g of the food) × 10

Ca, calcium; P, phosphorus; Na, sodium; Cu, copper; Fi, fibre; Fa, fat; BV, protein biological value.

L = low levels (provides <50% of daily requirements on an ME basis)

M = medium levels (provides <50–150% of daily requirements on an ME basis)

H = high levels (provides >150% of daily requirements on an ME basis)

– = unknown or variable levels

The sodium levels are assuming food is cooked in unsalted water

- **Milk, cheese and other dairy products**. These are a good source of protein, fat, calcium and phosphorus but some individuals may be intolerant of lactose.
- **Cereals and vegetables.** These should be cooked to improve digestibility. High levels of phytate in cereals may reduce the availability of some minerals, especially zinc. Palatability may be low for some dogs and cats and being obligate carnivores, cats cannot be maintained on an exclusively plant-based diet.

Cooking is advisable for most foods, especially meats, since this will kill most bacteria and parasites and will improve the digestibility of some materials. Overcooking should be avoided, however, since this will destroy vitamins and reduce the food value of proteins. A minimal amount of cooking water should be used and, if possible, fed with the meal in order to conserve vitamins and minerals. Home-prepared diets will almost certainly require careful vitamin and mineral supplementation.

Dietary supplementation

Contrary to many advertisements and popular beliefs, young animals and lactating females do not require large quantities of minerals and vitamins. Provided they are fed a balanced diet appropriate to their life stage, their needs will be met as their food intake increases to meet their energy requirements. However, as our knowledge of nutraceuticals and functional foods increases, we are understanding the potential benefits of increasing certain types of nutrients which are safe and relatively non-toxic at high levels, e.g. vitamin E and other antioxidants to help slow the ageing process, and green-lipped mussel powder to alleviate arthritic symptoms.

Non-specific supplementation should be undertaken with care as this may unbalance an otherwise balanced diet, and many nutrient interactions can result in a reduced availability of specific nutrients. This can lead to the possibility of

Table 9.12 Selected common protein sources and quantities required to supply 100 kcal (418 kJ) in home-made diets

Food	Approximate amount (g) required to supply 100 kcal (418 kJ) energy[a]	Ca	P	Na	Cu	Fi	Fa	BV
Bread white	37	L	L	H	M	H	L	L
Bread whole wheat	41	L	L	H	M	H	L	L
Corn flour	27	L	L	L	–	M	L	L
Corn meal	27	L	L	L	–	M	L	L
Corn flakes (breakfast cereal)	26	L	L	H	M	M	L	L
Macaroni, cooked	75	L	L	L	L	M	L	L
Oatmeal, cooked	181	L	L	L	–	M	L	L
Potato, cooked	133	L	L	L	–	M	L	L
Rice long grain, cooked	80	L	L	L	L	M	L	L
Soybean flour high fat	26	L	M	L	–	–	L	L
Soybean flour low fat	28	L	M	L	–	–	L	L
Spaghetti (quick cook), cooked	77	L	L	L	L	M	L	L
Spaghetti (ordinary), cooked	91	L	L	L	L	M	L	L
Wheat dry	27	L	L	L	–	M	L	L
Wheat cooked	240	L	L	L	–	M	L	L
Wheat flour	30	L	L	L	–	M	L	L
Fat, trimmed from beef	14	L	L	L	L	L	H	0
Lard	11	L	L	L	L	L	H	0
Margarine	14	L	L	H	L	L	H	L
Oils – salad/cooking	12	L	L	L	L	L	H	0

[a] The amounts required will vary between products. The amount required to supply 100 kcal can be calculated in the following way: amount required in g to supply 100 kcal = 100 ÷ energy density kcal/g; amount required to supply 418 kJ = 418 ÷ energy density kJ/g

Ca, calcium; P, phosphorus; Na, sodium; Cu, copper; Fi, fibre; Fa, fat; BV, protein biological value
L = low levels (provides <50% of daily requirements on an ME basis)
M = medium levels (provides >50–150% of daily requirements on an ME basis)
H = high levels (provides >150% of daily requirements on an ME basis)
– = unknown or variable levels
0 = does not apply to these ingredients
The sodium levels are assuming food is cooked in unsalted water

toxicities occurring, as may readily occur with vitamins A and D, for example. Dietary supplementation can be expensive and is unlikely to be of benefit in non-deficient animals. Table 9.13 lists the deficiencies of foods commonly used in home-prepared diets.

The value of vitamin/mineral supplements used in moderate amounts should not be dismissed. They can act as an insurance for those individual animals who may experience difficulties in either absorption or utilisation of specific nutrients. Although they are unnecessary when a commercially prepared pet food is fed, supplements are likely to be required in order to produce nutritional balance in home-prepared diets. In addition, they have a psychological benefit for people who need to give what they see as extra care. Nevertheless, in cases of diet-related nutrient deficiencies, it is considered preferable to correct the deficient diet itself rather than to rely on blanket supplementation.

Feeding healthy dogs and cats

Pet owners tend to treat their dogs and cats as individuals and will develop their own feeding practices which must take account of the particular circumstances, likes and dislikes of the animal and their own view of convenience, cost, variety and suitability of foods. They must identify the particular needs of their animal and find a combination of foods to meet them.

The feeding recommendations in the following sections are intended only as *guides* for the average dog or cat in the usual range of environments found in European households. These guides can be used as a starting point to obtain an approximate estimate of a pet's needs, then by observation of the animal to decide whether to feed more or less, and by substitution of one food for another, the owner will arrive at a suitable regimen.

Table 9.13 Nutrient imbalances of selected foods		
Food	**Deficiencies**	**Excesses**
Meat	Calcium, phosphorus, sodium, iron, copper, iodine, vitamins A, D, E	Protein
Fish (bones removed)	Calcium, phosphorus, iodine, vitamins A, D, E	
Fish (including bones)[a]	Iron, vitamins A, D, E	Calcium, phosphorus
Fats and oils		Energy, vitamin D (fish oils)
Eggs	Calcium, phosphorus	Fat, avidin
Milk		Lactose
Cheese, cottage cheese	Calcium, phosphorus	
Liver	Calcium	Vitamin A
Vegetables	Calcium, phosphorus, protein, fat	
Cereals	Calcium, phosphorus	

[a] *Cooked and finely ground fish*

Maintenance

Nutritionally speaking, the stage of adult maintenance is considered to be the period of basal requirements. An adult animal is said to be **in maintenance** when it is not subjected to the additional physiological stresses of growth; pregnancy or lactation; regular work or high levels of activity; or extremes of environmental temperature. During this period, the diet must provide the correct amount, balance and availability of energy and nutrients required to maintain optimal health and activity and promote peak condition in the animal. Since animals eat to satisfy their requirement for energy, all essential nutrients must be present in the correct amounts relative to the energy content of the diet.

Dogs

Dogs are represented by a wide diversity of breeds of different body types, with adult bodyweights which range over 100-fold from 1 kg to 115 kg. Energy expenditure is directly related to the weight of actively metabolising tissue, so for animals with such widely differing body weights, energy requirements are more closely related to the animal's **metabolic bodyweight** than to bodyweight itself. For moderately active pet dogs, maintenance energy requirements may be calculated using the equation:

$$ME \text{ (kcal/day)} = 110 \text{ BW}^{0.75}$$

where BW is the dog's bodyweight in kilograms. For more active dogs, the allowance can be increased to $125\,W^{0.75}$. However, variations in body composition, shape and coat type are complicating factors in determining energy requirements, particularly for the larger breeds. For example, Newfoundlands tend to need less than the predicted amounts whereas Great Danes need more, despite these two breeds being of comparable bodyweight.

The amount of food needed to meet these requirements may then be calculated from a knowledge of the energy values of foods. Feeding recommendations are only ever given as guidelines and are subject to individual variability

between dogs and to differences in activity level and environmental conditions. If extra snacks, treats or table scraps are added to the diet, their energy content must be taken into account when calculating the daily food allowance. In addition, spaying may reduce the resting energy requirement of bitches by up to 10%. Regular weighing of the animal allows the owner to monitor the adequacy of the feeding regimen on a quantitative basis.

> Although the dog is a member of the order Carnivora, in a nutritional sense it is more accurately defined as omnivorous and, unlike the cat (see below), the dog is able to survive on a diet composed entirely of vegetable material, although a diet based on animal tissue is likely to be preferred.

Most adult dogs in maintenance are able to eat all they require in a single meal and it is perfectly acceptable to adopt a once-a-day feeding regimen. It is usually best to avoid late evening meals since dogs may need to excrete faeces or urine within a few hours of feeding and this can be inconvenient in the middle of the night. There is no disadvantage in feeding more frequently provided that the total daily intake is limited to the dog's daily needs, and feeding 2–3 times a day to coincide with family meals is a common practice. Whatever the frequency of feeding, a routine should be established and adhered to as far as possible (see Table 9.14).

Cats

Domestic cats show a relatively narrow range of adult bodyweights (from 2.5 to 6.5 kg) and their energy requirements may be calculated from a linear relationship. In normal circumstances, an adult cat requires 70–90 kcal/kg bodyweight per day, depending on its level of activity. However, large, overweight individuals and very inactive or caged cats (such as those in a hospital environment)

Table 9.14 Recommended nutrient requirements for the dog, according to physiological status

Status	Minimum ME density (kcal (kJ)/g)	Digestibility (%)	Protein (%ME)[a]	Fat (%ME)[a]	Fibre (%DM)[b]	Ca (mg/100 kcal (418kJ))	PO⁴ (mg/100 kcal (418kJ))	Na
Maintenance	3.5 (14.6)	>75	16–20	30–50	5	130–160	110–160	15
Growth Gestation Lactation	3.9 (16.3)	>80	22–28	30–50	5	280	200–250	23
Geriatric	3.75 (15.7)	>80	14–18	30–50	4	130–150	110–140	15
Stress: Environmental Psychological Physical	4.2 (17.6)	>82	20–25	30–50	4 max	150–250	130–230	23

[a] The proportion of metabolisable energy supplied by that nutrient
[b] g/100 g dry matter

have lower maintenance energy requirements and allowances should be based on 50–70 kcal/kg bodyweight per day.

Cats have the ability to regulate their energy intake from day to day and unless they are fed an exceptionally palatable diet or lead a particularly sedentary life, they will normally adjust the amount of food they eat to achieve the correct balance.

The cat exhibits a number of nutritional peculiarities which distinguish it from the dog and reflect its naturally predatory lifestyle. Several aspects of feline metabolism have evolved in adaptation to a strictly carnivorous diet which is typically high in protein and low in carbohydrate. In addition, the cat has a dietary requirement for a number of nutrients which are only found naturally in significant quantities in animal tissues.

Cats may be considered as **obligate carnivores**, since taurine, preformed vitamin A and arachidonic acid are only found in significant quantities in animal tissues. It is thus essential that the cat is supplied with at least some animal-derived materials in its diet. In view of these nutritional specialties, it should be noted that long-term feeding of dog foods to cats is unacceptable, since these diets may not meet the specific nutritional requirements of the cat.

When allowed continuous access to food, cats tend to adopt a pattern of small, frequent (usually 8–16) meals throughout the whole 24-hour period. However, cats readily adapt to different feeding schedules imposed by their owners and are commonly fed two meals per day. Nevertheless, if feeding time is restricted then sufficient food must be provided to satisfy their daily nutrient and energy requirements.

Special nutritional differences of the cat may be summarised as follows:
- A limited ability to regulate amino acid catabolism, resulting in a higher dietary requirement for protein than dogs and an inability to adapt to extremely low-protein diets (they also tend to find low-protein diets unpalatable).
- A high dietary requirement for taurine, partly because of an inability to conjugate bile acids with glycine instead of taurine and also because of a low rate of taurine synthesis *in vivo*.
- A particular sensitivity to arginine deficiency.
- A limited ability to synthesise niacin.
- An inability to convert β-carotene to retinol (vitamin A), resulting in a dietary requirement for preformed vitamin A.
- A limited ability to convert linoleic acid to arachidonic acid.
- A limited ability to metabolise carbohydrate, resulting in an intolerance of high-carbohydrate diets.

Environmental factors are known to affect the volume of food a particular animal will eat. Most cats do not relish cold food straight from the refrigerator and prefer to eat food that is close to their own body temperature and that of freshly killed prey. This response may reflect a behavioural strategy in the wild which ensures that only the freshest prey is eaten.

Cats do seek variety in their diet, as long as the new food is not *too* different from the familiar one, or the palatability too low. However, during times of stress, such as when hospitalised, a familiar diet is preferred. Repeated exposure to fresh supplies of a new food which is not initially acceptable to the cat may encourage the cat to overcome its reticence. Furthermore, cats can often detect and may reject diets that are deficient in certain nutrients, so it is important that any diet offered is nutritionally complete (see Table 9.15).

Status	Minimum ME density (kcal (kJ)/g)	Digestibility (%)	Protein (%ME)[a]	Fat (%ME)[a]	Fibre (%DM)[b]	Ca (mg/100 kcal (418kJ))	PO⁴	Mg	Na
Maintenance	3.7 (15.7)	>75	24–26	>25	5	130–200	120	80	15
Growth Gestation Lactation	3.9 (16.3)	>80	30–35	>40	5	160–250	120–200	150	30
Geriatric	3.75 (15.7)	>80	24–26	>34	5	130–150	120	80	15

Table 9.15 Recommended nutrient requirements for the cat, according to physiological status

[a] *The proportion of metabolisable energy supplied by that nutrient*
[b] *g/100 g dry matter*

Reproduction and lactation

The reproductive life stage is a nutritionally demanding time for the bitch or queen. During this period, her intake of energy and nutrients must be adequate not only to meet her own maintenance requirements but also to support normal growth and development of her offspring during pregnancy and, through milk production, during lactation. At peak lactation her energy and nutrient requirements may rise to up to three or four times the level required for maintenance. This may involve eating large volumes of food and, at times of high demand, achieving a sufficient intake can be a problem. This may be offset to some extent by feeding a diet which is:

- Concentrated with respect to energy and nutrient density.
- Palatable to encourage feeding.
- Highly digestible to reduce bulk.

The additional requirements imposed by pregnancy are relatively small and can usually be met by simply increasing the amount of the animal's normal food, provided that this is well balanced. In late pregnancy and particularly if the litter is large, the space occupied by the gravid uterus may be so great that the physical capacity for food intake is limited. In this case, feeding a concentrated diet can help to ensure an adequate intake and offering smaller, more frequent meals can also be beneficial. To meet the high demands of lactation a palatable, highly digestible, concentrated diet should be fed. Milk production is affected by protein quantity and quality in the diet and it is important that the extra food supplied is of good quality. It is not appropriate to simply increase the dietary energy content by adding fat or carbohydrate sources. Diets formulated for growth or specifically for gestation and lactation are suitable for feeding at this time.

During pregnancy and lactation, the content and balance of nutrients in the diet are critical and must be carefully regulated. Provided that a balanced diet is fed, the increased requirement for nutrients is met when food intake is increased to meet the energy needs of the bitch or queen. **Supplementation with vitamins or minerals is *not* required and could actually be harmful by causing an imbalance in the diet.**

Dogs

The average duration of pregnancy in the bitch is 63 days, but her energy requirements do not increase appreciably until the last third of gestation when most fetal weight gain occurs. It is important, therefore, to avoid overfeeding in early pregnancy, since this will lead to the deposition of unwanted fat and may predispose the bitch to problems at whelping. A gradual increase in food allowance over the second half of gestation is all that is required and a satisfactory regimen would be to increase the amount of food by 15% of the bitch's maintenance ration each week from the fifth week onwards. During the week before whelping the bitch should, therefore, be eating 60% more than when she was mated. Appetite may be reduced in the later stages of pregnancy, particularly with large litters, and it is sensible to divide the daily allowance into several small meals.

Lactation represents the most nutritionally demanding life stage for the bitch. During the first 4 weeks post whelping, she must eat enough to support both herself and her rapidly growing puppies which may double their weight within a matter of days. The extra energy and nutrients needed over and above her normal intake depends on the size and age of the litter but at peak lactation (3–4 weeks after whelping), she may need to eat anything up to four times her normal maintenance allowance. Failure of the diet to meet these demands means that the bitch will nurse her young at the expense of her own body reserves, with a resultant loss of weight and condition.

The food allowance should be increased steadily throughout the first 4 weeks of lactation (in accordance with the bitch's needs):
- A highly palatable, digestible and concentrated food should be offered in several small meals or *ad libitum*.
- Food should be made available throughout the night.
- An unlimited supply of drinking water should also be provided to cater for the large volumes involved in milk production.

Weaning of the litter should be accomplished gradually in order to prevent mastitis in the bitch and growth check in the puppies. Most puppies begin to take an interest in solid foods from about 3 to 4 weeks and once they are eating well, the bitch may be separated from the puppies for progressively longer periods to allow her milk supply to diminish. Weaning may be completed between 6 and 8 weeks of age and it may be advisable to cut the bitch's ration down to half her maintenance level immediately following total separation. Her food allowance may be gradually increased over a period of days and if she has lost condition during lactation, extra food may be introduced as soon as her milk supply has dried up.

If the litter is large and particularly if the bitch's milk supply seems inadequate, supplementary feeding of the puppies should be encouraged from about 3 weeks.

Eclampsia (post puerperal hypocalcaemia) is a condition which can affect lactating bitches, especially of small breeds, with larger litters. Lowered blood calcium concentrations lead to signs which range from restlessness and ataxia to muscle tremors and collapse with tetanic convulsions. **Treatment** involves the oral or intravenous administration of calcium, depending on the severity of signs, and puppies should be removed immediately from affected bitches and hand-reared.

Although some owners give calcium and vitamin D supplements to bitches in late pregnancy and lactation as an 'insurance policy', these do *not* prevent eclampsia and may, in fact, increase the risk of eclampsia or calcinosis in the bitch and produce developmental abnormalities in the puppies.

Cats

Gestation length for cats is similar to that of dogs and is in the region of 64 days. However, unlike dogs and most other mammals, pregnant queens start to eat more and gain weight within a week of conception. By the end of the third week of gestation, the pregnant queen will have gained almost 20% of the extra weight she will carry at term. Following parturition, only about 40% of this extra weight is lost (compared with almost 100% in the bitch) and the remaining 60% is lost during the course of lactation.

This unusual pattern of bodyweight gain in early pregnancy is thought to be due to the extra-uterine deposition of fat and protein reserves which may be mobilised in late pregnancy and lactation, when dietary intake of the queen may be insufficient to meet her greatly increased nutritional demands.

Throughout pregnancy, food intake of the queen rises continuously to fuel her extra weight gain and peaks at around 7–8 weeks of gestation. The food allowance may be gradually increased from 1 week of a successful mating and since cats rarely overeat, an *ad libitum* feeding regimen is perfectly acceptable. Voluntary intake may drop slightly just before and immediately after parturition, after which food consumption rises progressively to meet the increased demands of lactation. As with the bitch, energy requirements of the lactating queen vary with litter size and age and at peak lactation may be anything up to four times her maintenance level. Again, a highly palatable, digestible and concentrated diet should be fed as frequent small meals and *ad libitum* feeding is preferred to allow the queen to successfully control her energy intake. Food should be available throughout the night and an unlimited supply of fresh drinking water must be accessible at all times.

It is normal for the queen to lose weight during lactation as her body reserves are used up, but she should achieve her premating weight by the time the kittens are weaned at 6–8 weeks. Although kittens begin to take solid food from about 3–4 weeks of age and demand less of the queen, her energy requirements remain elevated to allow for restoration of her depleted body reserves. After weaning, the additional food allowance can be gradually cut back until the queen is eating her normal amount or adjusted to compensate for any observed weight loss or gain.

Growth

In relation to bodyweight, growing animals require a much higher plane of nutrition than their adult counterparts. For young animals, the diet must not only supply all the nutrients required for maintenance but also those required to fuel rapid growth and development and to support their active lifestyle. In particular, they have higher demands for energy, protein (which must be digestible and have an amino acid profile appropriate for growth), vitamin E and certain bone-forming minerals, such as calcium and phosphorus. Both the *amount* and *balance* of nutrients provided are critical for the growing puppy or kitten and dietary errors at this stage can have damaging effects, particularly on skeletal development, which may be long-lasting and potentially irreversible.

To meet these high demands, young animals must eat large amounts of food relative to their size, but their physical capacity to do so is limited by their small stomach volume. The daily food allowance should therefore be divided into several small meals to compensate for this and the diet itself should meet certain criteria. A suitable diet for growth is formulated to ensure an adequate intake of energy and nutrients in a relatively small volume of food.

Diets for growth should be:
- Concentrated.
- Nutritionally balanced.
- Highly palatable.
- Highly digestible.

For the first few weeks of life, all the nutritional needs of the puppy or kitten are met by their mother's milk and no supplementary feeding is necessary, unless the milk supply is inadequate. As their interest in solid food gradually increases, finely chopped soft foods or dry kibble moistened with milk or gravy may be provided in shallow bowls. The food may be the same as that offered to the mother or may be one designed specifically for growth.

> Contrary to popular belief, milk is not essential in the diet of weaned puppies or kittens.

After weaning, their ability to digest lactose becomes progressively less efficient and feeding large quantities of milk can result in diarrhoea. Nevertheless, milk remains a useful source of nutrients for individuals that can tolerate it, if fed in restricted amounts.

Puppies

Most owners are aware that correct nutrition is fundamental to achieving normal growth and development in the growing dog, but there is a common tendency to overfeed (to produce rapid growth rates) or to oversupplement the diet (to prevent classic deficiency syndromes). Excessive energy intake, however, is likely to cause obesity in the small breeds and rapid growth rates in the large and giant breeds, which may be detrimental to the animal. The aim should be to allow the puppy to grow sufficiently quickly to enable it to fulfil its genetic potential while the bones are still capable of growth. A more rapid increase in bodyweight can place undue stresses on the juvenile skeleton, particularly in the fast-growing large and giant breeds, and may predispose to a variety of disorders which are characterised by abnormalities of bone growth and development. Examples of these include **osteochondrosis syndrome**, **hip dysplasia**, **wobbler syndrome** and **enostosis (panosteitis)**. In some cases, excessive dietary calcium intake may also play a major contributory role. It is therefore unwise to overfeed growing dogs in an attempt to obtain the maximum possible rate of growth and a more advantageous approach is to moderately restrict their intake and allow them to take slightly longer to reach their adult weight (Fig. 9.3).

Oversupplementation with fat-soluble vitamins A and D may also result in skeletal and other abnormalities and care should always be exercised with supplements such as cod liver oil, which is a rich source of both these vitamins. A properly balanced diet which is formulated for growth does not need any form of supplementation and careless use of additives can result in serious dietary imbalances with deleterious consequences. This is true even of the large breeds, since their extra needs are catered for by their increased food intake to meet their energy requirements.

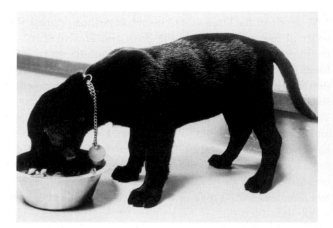

Fig. 9.3 Young animals should be fed diets specifically designed for their growing needs.

All puppies grow very rapidly in the early stages and by 5–6 months of age, most breeds will have reached about half their adult weight. However, because of the wide variation in adult bodyweight, different breeds continue to mature at different relative rates and in general, the larger breeds take longer to mature than the smaller breeds. Small and toy breeds may reach their adult weight at 6–9 months of age. Larger breeds will still be growing at this age and take longer to mature. Labrador Retriever or Newfoundland puppies, for example, may not reach their adult weight until 16 months or 2 years, respectively.

At weaning (between 6 and 8 weeks of age), the puppy's energy requirements are about double those of an adult of the same breed, per unit of bodyweight. As the puppy grows, this requirement declines progressively, and by the time it has reached 40% of its mature weight, the energy requirement is only 1.6 times that for adult maintenance. At 80% of its mature weight, the puppy needs only 1.2 times as much energy as an adult per unit of bodyweight.

> High levels of high-quality protein are also required for growth. Although it is often thought that large amounts of additional protein in the puppy diet will aid the development of good condition and muscle, this is not the case. Instead, protein eaten in excess of requirements is metabolised to produce energy or stored as fat.

Most puppies can be weaned onto a varied diet or a single, complete food between 6 and 8 weeks of age. At this stage, it is better to feed them four small meals a day than to allow continuous access to food. Commercial diets designed specifically for growth are ideal and it is recommended that a growth formulation is fed until the puppy attains at least 75% of its adult weight. Although such diets require no further supplementation, some owners may like to offer alternative foods from time to time. Meat, offal, cheese, eggs and bread are often fed to dogs, but only a few different food sources should be introduced gradually at any one time, to allow the digestive system to adapt. Nevertheless, if alternative foods are to form the major part of a home-prepared diet, food composition tables should be consulted and careful supplementation with vitamins and minerals will almost certainly be required.

Puppies should have their food allowance divided into four or five meals a day until about 10 weeks of age and then three meals a day until they have reached approximately 50% of their expected adult bodyweight. At this stage (5–6 months), the frequency of feeding can be reduced to twice daily. As the puppy approaches its adult weight, the daily food allowance can be gradually incorporated into a single meal, as in the adult. *Ad libitum* feeding is not recommended for growing dogs, since they tend to overeat and this can lead to obesity or skeletal developmental abnormalities. As a guide, feeding at a level of 85% of *ad libitum* feeding has been shown to result in optimal growth and body composition in dogs. Precise recommendations on the amounts to feed are difficult to give because of huge variations in individual requirements and in the caloric densities of the foods themselves. It is important, therefore, that the health and condition of growing dogs is regularly assessed 'by hand and eye' to monitor their progress and allow any necessary dietary adjustments to be made.

Kittens

Kittens weigh between 85 g and 120 g at birth and may gain up to 100 g per week in the early stages of growth so that at weaning, they should weigh between 600 g and 1000 g. Males grow at a faster rate than females and by 6 weeks of age they are already significantly heavier. At 1 year, male cats can be up to 45% heavier than females from the same litter.

At weaning, the energy requirements of kittens per unit of bodyweight are between three and four times that of an adult and reach a peak at about 10 weeks of age. Unlike puppies, kittens do not tend to overeat and are not prone to the same problems of obesity and skeletal developmental abnormalities as growing dogs. It is usual, therefore, to allow kittens unrestricted access to food during the rapid growth phase although multiple small feeds throughout the day (at least four or five per day at weaning) may also be offered. Moist food which is left uneaten should be discarded at least twice daily.

Concentrated diets designed for kitten growth are ideal at this stage to ensure an optimal intake of energy, protein, taurine and calcium, in particular. Growing kittens tend to have acidic urine due to the liberation of hydrogen ions during bone growth and it is important that urine-acidifying diets designed for the management of struvite-associated lower urinary tract diseases are avoided in young cats (up to a year of age).

Although male kittens take slightly longer to mature than females, most kittens will have attained 75% of their ultimate adult bodyweight by 6 months of age. Further weight

gains after this are attributable to developmental changes rather than skeletal growth and at this stage, the growth diet may be changed to an adult formulation. If desired, the frequency of feeding may be reduced to twice daily, but many people continue to offer multiple feeds throughout the day, even to adult cats. This pattern of feeding fits in well with the cat's natural preference to snack feed during both day and night rather than eat a small number of large meals. Total food intakes continue to rise between 6 and 12 months to coincide with continued slow growth, but tend to stabilise at an adult level towards the end of the first year.

Feeding orphaned puppies and kittens

Hand-rearing of puppies and kittens may be necessary if the mother has an inadequate supply of milk, if she is sick or if the litter is orphaned. The ideal alternative is to cross-foster the young on to a lactating bitch or queen whose young are old enough to be weaned, but this is not always a practical option. Motherless puppies and kittens have vital requirements in two main areas, that is, provision of a suitable environment and nutrition.

Care of orphaned puppies and kittens may be summarised as follows:
- Ideally, the environment should be controlled by an incubator. Alternatively, a heating pad with adequate insulation of the pen can be used.
- After they have been fed, the mother would normally provoke reflex defecation and urination in the puppies and kittens by licking the anogenital area. This action can be stimulated by applying a piece of damp cotton wool at the anogenital area or simply by running a dampened forefinger along the abdominal wall.
- Between 16–21 days, puppies and kittens no longer require stimulation to urinate and defecate and from 28 days, when they completely control their body temperature, they begin to explore their surroundings and become more independent.

The food supplied must be a concentrated source of nutrients based on the composition of normal bitch or queen's milk. Table 9.16 shows the average composition of milk from bitches, cows, goats and queens. It is clear that cow's and goat's milks are inadequate as a substitute for rearing puppies and kittens since the protein and fat levels are too low. Calcium levels are also considerably lower than that of bitch's milk. Many commercially available milk substitutes are now available for dogs and cats. They are usually based on cow's milk which has been modified to resemble bitch or queen's milk more closely. They can be administered by means of a small syringe or a puppy or kitten feeding bottle.

	% Nutrient as fed (g/100 kcal (418 kJ)) (ME)				
Nutrient	**Bitch's milk**	**Cow's milk**	**Queen's milk**	**Goat's milk**	**Evaporated milk + water**[a]
Water	77 (0)	88 (0)	81.5 (0)	87 (0)	80 (0)
Protein	8.2 (6.6)	3.2 (5.4)	7.4 (8.4)	3.5 (5.5)	5.3 (5.5)
Fat	9.8 (7.8)	3.7 (6.3)	5.2 (5.9)	4.2 (6.6)	6.1 (6.3)
Lactose	3.6 (2.9)	4.6 (7.8)	5.0 (5.7)	4.5 (7)	7.6 (7.8)
Calcium	0.28 (0.22)	0.12 (0.2)	0.035 (0.04)	0.13 (0.2)	0.19 (0.2)
Phosphorus	0.22 (0.18)	0.1 (0.17)	0.07 (0.08)	0.11 (0.17)	0.15 (0.16)
ME					
kcal/100 g[b]	125	59	88	64	97
kJ/100 g[b]	522	246	360	267	406

Table 9.16 Nutrient content of milk from different sources

[a] 3 parts whole evaporated milk diluted with 1 part water
[b] ME content as-fed was estimated using nutrient energy densities of 3.5 kcal (14.6 kJ)/g for protein and lactose, and 8.5 kcal (35.6 kJ)/g for fat

Dried milk feeds should be reconstituted daily and fed warm (38°C). Food must be given slowly and must not be forced into the animal. Frequent, small feeds (at least four) should be offered throughout the day. When feeding from a miniature bottle, the hole in the teat may need to be enlarged so that the flow is improved and the puppy or kitten does not suck in air. When they begin to explore their surroundings (at 3–4 weeks), a high-quality puppy or kitten food can be introduced. This can be mixed with a milk substitute to begin with and then offered separately.

Senior animals

As a general guideline, dogs and cats may be considered to be geriatric once they have reached the final third of their anticipated lifespan. The aim of feeding elderly but otherwise healthy animals is to slow or prevent the progression of metabolic changes associated with ageing and thus to increase longevity and preserve the quality of life. Old age is often, however, accompanied by clinical disease for which dietary management may constitute an important component of therapy. Chronic renal failure is a particular problem of middle-aged and old cats, whereas old dogs tend to be more susceptible to heart disease. There is a tendency towards obesity in older animals, especially dogs, and oral hygiene measures have particular significance in old age. Free access to a clean supply of water is essential to prevent dehydration.

Dogs

Most senior dogs have a maintenance energy requirement which is approximately 20% less than that of a younger adult of equivalent bodyweight. This decline in energy requirement appears to be linked to both a reduction in physical activity and a decrease in basal metabolic rate which is largely driven by changes in body composition (reduction in lean body tissue and concomitant increase in fat mass). To reduce the risk of obesity, therefore, older dogs should be fed to a lower energy requirement than younger dogs without restricting the intake of other essential nutrients. This means that reducing the amount of food offered is not an advisable way to achieve weight loss; reducing total energy intake is the safest practice. The majority of dogs maintain digestive efficiency as they age, making the determination of energy provision to senior dogs relatively straightforward to calculate. Nevertheless, it is probable that some individuals might exhibit a reduction in apparent digestibility of nutrients and/or have a reduced appetite and may be underweight if intake does not meet their energy requirements.

High levels of dietary protein may increase the renal workload when kidney function may already be impaired to some extent. Conversely, very low protein diets may be associated with a risk of protein malnutrition and tend to be unpalatable. Historically there has been a belief that reducing protein intake in older animals will relieve 'stress' on their renal function and may help to prevent or slow progression of renal disease. More recent data has shown, however, that this theory cannot be substantiated. Indeed, there is no scientific evidence to support restricting dietary protein in healthy, clinically normal dogs (and cats) as they age.

In general, healthy older dogs should have diets based on their individual needs which will be related to bodyweight, condition and physical activity. Early clinical and biochemical signs of chronic renal failure would support the introduction of a diet with a low phosphorus and moderately reduced protein content.

Protein sources for older dogs should be highly digestible and of high biological value.

Although restriction of dietary sodium or phosphorus may be indicated in old dogs with cardiac or renal diseases, respectively, there is no evidence that healthy individuals have altered requirements for these or other minerals. Similarly, vitamin requirements of healthy senior dogs are not thought to differ markedly from those of younger adults.

Cats

In contrast to dogs (and humans), the energy requirements of cats do not change with increasing age. Evidence suggests that there is no apparent change in body composition (lean:fat ratios) with advancing age. This is supported by the fact that obesity is not considered a significant problem in old cats and there is a greater tendency for geriatric cats to be underweight. The maintained lean:fat ratio probably reflects constant activity levels throughout life and suggests that basal metabolic rate probably does not decrease as cats age. Cats show a significant decline in digestive function with age, resulting in a significant decrease in the digestibilities of protein, fat and, hence, energy. Most healthy cats are able to compensate for this effect by increasing their food intake to maintain bodyweight but in some cases, provision of a more energy-dense food may be appropriate. In contrast to dogs, calorie provision to senior cats should not be reduced.

In view of the high protein requirements of the cat and reduced digestive efficiency in old age, restriction of dietary protein is not recommended in healthy individuals because of the associated risk of protein malnutrition. Again, highly digestible protein sources of high biological value should be employed for all healthy, clinically normal older cats. However, moderate restriction of dietary protein to alleviate clinical signs of uraemia may be implemented, together with dietary phosphorus restriction, in cats with evidence of chronic renal failure.

Careful monitoring of food intake is important in the senior cat and may help to identify conditions associated with altered food intake. For example, hyperthyroidism is characterised by weight loss despite an increased appetite, and prolonged inappetence may predispose an obese cat to hepatic lipidosis.

Table 9.17 summarises the age-related changes in dogs and cats and their effect on nutritional status.

Working dogs

Working dogs perform at a wide range of activity levels and in a variety of environmental conditions, from acting as guide dogs for the blind to pulling sledges in polar regions. The diet and feeding regimen employed in each case varies widely according to the role the dog is asked to perform and its individual work and training schedule. Any increase in physical activity requires extra energy to sustain the increase in muscular work but a further allowance must be made for

Table 9.17 Ageing changes in dogs and cats and their effect on nutritional status

Ageing change	Effect on nutritional status
Metabolism	
Reduced sensitivity to thirst	Dehydration
Reduced thermoregulation	Increased energy expenditure with extremes of heat
Reduced immunological competence	Increased susceptibility to infection
Decreased activity and metabolic rate (possibly due to decreased thyroid function)	Decreased energy needs predisposes towards obesity
Increased body fat	Predisposes towards obesity
Special senses	
Decreased olfaction	Reduced food intake which may
Decreased ability to taste	lead to a loss of weight and
Decreased visual acuity	condition
Oral cavity	
Dental calculus	
Periodontal disease	Reduced food intake which may
Loss of teeth	lead to a loss of weight and
Decreased saliva production	condition
Gingival hyperplasia	
Urinary system	
Decreased renal function	
Decreased renal blood flow	Decreased protein requirement
Decreased glomerular filtration rate	
Skeletal system	
Osteoarthritis	Decreased mobility reduces energy requirements
Reduced muscle mass	Decreased protein reserves
Cardiovascular system	
Congestive cardiac failure	Decreased salt intake

the element of stress that is associated with strenuous activity. Both physiological and psychological stresses further increase the demand for energy and certain nutrients in hard-working dogs.

The main fuels for muscular exercise in the working dog are fats and carbohydrates. Sprinting dogs, such as the racing greyhound, require short, but very intense bursts of energy. In these circumstances, the muscle fibres contract very rapidly and rely mainly on readily available glucose as an energy source. Muscle glycogen stores supply approximately 70–80% of the energy required for this type of exercise with fats providing the rest. For these working dogs, a diet which provides a relatively large quantity of carbohydrate may be appropriate, since this helps to maximise muscle glycogen reserves. Useful sources of carbohydrate include corn, oat flakes, rice and potatoes.

However, high-carbohydrate diets are not suitable for most other working dogs and may actually reduce performance. They may exacerbate the accumulation of lactic acid in muscles during prolonged exercise, leading to muscle damage and exhaustion. For working dogs which are active for long periods (endurance performers), energy for sustained muscle activity is produced through aerobic fatty acid oxidation with fat providing 70–90% of the energy and carbohydrates providing the rest. Dogs which perform this type of work may benefit from training on a high-fat diet. This also applies to dogs which operate in a hostile environment (such as sledge dogs or avalanche rescue dogs) where extra energy is required to maintain body temperature as well as for increased muscular activity. For most other working dogs, the optimal dietary fat:carbohydrate ratio falls somewhere between these two extremes.

The protein requirements of hard-working dogs may be slightly increased over maintenance levels, but there is no evidence to suggest that a high-protein diet will promote superior muscle development. Exercise stress may increase the demand for specific amino acids and has been associated with anaemia, so a good-quality protein source is essential for dogs in work. Suitable protein sources include meats, fishmeal, powdered whole egg and casein.

Little is known about the requirements of hard-working dogs for vitamins and minerals, but there may be a higher requirement for iron because of its involvement in haemoglobin production and oxygen transport. Similarly, vitamin E and selenium requirements may be increased, since they act as antioxidants and protect cell membranes, including red blood cells, from damage. If the diet is nutritionally balanced, however, these increased demands will be met when the dog consumes more to satisfy its energy requirements.

The amount of extra energy required by working dogs depends on environmental conditions, the amount of exercise and the nature of the work. A dog which travels long distances in the course of its work may need as much as two to three times the normal adult maintenance ration. Despite this, food intake may be reduced in some dogs due to fatigue and to offset this, the diet should be concentrated, palatable and highly digestible. This type of diet is also lower in bulk, which is a significant advantage to the working dog. As well as being an ideal energy source for most working dogs, fat is an excellent means of increasing the energy density of the diet and both fat and protein may be used to enhance palatability.

Where the type of work performed is not overly strenuous, the additional needs may be met by simply feeding more of the dog's nutritionally balanced maintenance diet. At higher levels of performance, a more concentrated source of energy and nutrients is recommended and complete diets formulated for active dogs are ideal. Alternatively, supplementary foods, such as fish or meat, may be added to the maintenance ration, but this strategy will require suitable vitamin and mineral supplementation. On rest or training days, the dietary requirements will differ and the amounts fed must be adjusted accordingly. A smaller allowance of the same meal is most appropriate.

Working dogs should receive only a small concentrated meal before working as a full stomach limits performance and increases the risk of bloat. If the working period is prolonged, a further small meal may be given during the rest period. The main meal should provide two-thirds of the daily ration and should be reserved until after work. A rest period of about an hour should be allowed before feeding if the work is strenuous. To prevent dehydration, working dogs should be given free access to water.

Clinical nutrition

Nutritional factors may affect the health of any animal in a number of ways. The provision of a nutritionally adequate diet is clearly important in the prevention of disease associated with deficiencies of imbalances of specific nutrients. Nutritional diseases are now rare in companion animals, thanks to the widespread feeding of nutritionally balanced commercial diets, but problems do occasionally arise:

- Where the animal's intake is reduced.
- When the diet is poorly formulated or stored.
- When an otherwise balanced diet is carelessly oversupplemented.
- Where the animal is unable to digest, absorb or utilise the nutrient as a result of disease or genetic factors.

Nutritional support at times of stress, disease or injury is a second area in which nutrition may impact on disease. Failure to consider this aspect of disease management may have a detrimental effect on the animal's recovery. Finally, dietary modification may form an integral part of the management of a variety of clinical conditions.

Nutritional support

The nutritional requirements of the stressed or traumatised patient differ markedly from those of the healthy animal and, coupled with this, there is often a reduced desire or physical ability to eat. Failure to address these altered needs can result in malnutrition of the critical care patient and will have an adverse effect on the animal's recovery.

Conversely, the therapeutic benefits of appropriate nutritional support for these animals may include:

- Increased survival rates.
- Improved tolerance to invasive procedures.
- Shorter hospitalisation periods.
- Decreased risk of infection.
- Earlier return to mobility.
- More rapid wound healing.

Altered nutritional needs of the stressed patient

In the healthy animal, short-term fasting results in a series of adaptive mechanisms which are designed to maintain blood glucose concentrations, preserve lean body tissue and promote survival. Because there is little or no intake of food, the body mobilises its own tissue reserves to provide essential nutrients and lowers its metabolic rate to reduce energy expenditure.

Most cells adapt to using fatty acids, instead of glucose, as an energy source, and within a few days, fat becomes the major source of fuel in the fasting animal. However, the cells of some tissues, such as the brain, kidney and red blood cells, still require a constant supply of glucose for energy. To meet this demand, tissue proteins are broken down to provide amino acids which can then be converted to glucose. In starvation, therefore, fat reserves are used to supply energy but even in the healthy animal, there is inevitably some loss of tissue protein. When feeding is resumed, amino acid mobilisation decreases and metabolism returns to normal within 24 hours.

In conditions of stress or trauma, however, these adaptive mechanisms to food deprivation are overridden. An initial 'ebb' or 'shock' phase lasts for a few hours up to 2 days, during which intravascular fluids are redistributed (**hypovolaemia**) to maintain tissue perfusion. Treatment during this phase is aimed at life-saving procedures. Metabolism *may* be lowered (**hypometabolism**) during this phase.

This phase is quickly followed by a 'flow' period of accelerated metabolism which is designed to support the healing of wounds and resistance to infection. This stage can last from days to several weeks, depending on the severity of the injury. During this period of **hypermetabolism**, energy requirements increase in accordance with the severity of the injury and are particularly high in cases of head trauma (because the brain has a particularly high energy requirement), septicaemia, extensive burns or following radical surgery. Even healthy animals undergoing minor elective surgery may experience a transient increase in energy requirements of up to 10% above normal.

In stressed animals, glycogen reserves are rapidly depleted and fat becomes the major and preferred energy source. In addition, healing tissues and some tumours require glucose as an energy source and the breakdown of tissue proteins increases markedly in order to maintain blood glucose levels to meet this demand. Nevertheless, high levels of dietary carbohydrate are contraindicated in hypermetabolic patients, since they commonly exhibit a peripheral insulin resistance and are unable to utilise glucose efficiently. An excessive intake of carbohydrate during this period can result in respiratory acidosis and other complications. Unlike the healthy animal, these metabolic changes are not immediately reversed when feeding is resumed.

Protein-energy malnutrition

The cumulative drain on tissues may continue for weeks and, if not corrected, can result in protein-energy malnutrition. During this time, nutritional support becomes a crucial part of the treatment. **Protein-energy malnutrition (PEM)** can have a number of adverse effects which, in combination, can delay recovery and increase the patient's susceptibility to infection and shock. The most obvious effects of protein-energy malnutrition are muscle wasting and weakness, but

other side-effects include reduced immune function, increased risk of infection and delayed wound healing. Impaired digestive function exacerbates the problem. In extreme cases, death can occur due to sepsis and failure of the heart, lungs and other organs.

Patient assessment

Some form of nutritional support is required for any animal that is unable or unwilling to eat voluntarily, but a thorough veterinary examination is necessary to assess the individual requirements of the patient and the most appropriate method of administering support.

Specific nutritional support is indicated if:
- Oral intake is reduced for 3–5 days or if it is anticipated to be interrupted for this length of time as a result of surgical or other in-hospital procedures.
- There is an acute weight loss of >5–10% of bodyweight (excluding fluid losses).
- Actual weight is 15% or more below ideal bodyweight.
- Body condition, as scored on a scale of 1 (cachectic) to 5 (obese), is below the optimal score of 3.
- Physical changes are accompanied by hypoalbuminaemia.
- Recent trauma, surgery or sepsis is accompanied by anorexia.

Patients who have recently undergone major surgery or trauma, especially when this is associated with head injuries, blood loss, sepsis, severe burns or open wounds, are prime candidates for nutritional support. Another group of patients are those which are physically unable to eat (with jaw fractures, for example) and those with chronic wasting diseases, such as cancer.

Once an initial assessment has been made, the degree and duration of nutritional support can be estimated and a nutritional plan formulated on an individual basis for each patient. For surgical patients, preoperative assessment is particularly important so that invasive tube placement can be performed at the time of the initial surgery (see Table 9.18).

Techniques for nutritional support

Nutritional support for small animals may be provided by either the enteral or the parenteral route. Total parenteral nutrition is the provision of nutrients by the intravenous route, but this technique is expensive with inherent technical

Table 9.18 Practices that may adversely affect the nutritional status of sick animals
Failure to record daily weight
Failure to observe, measure and record the amount of food consumed
Delay of nutritional support until the patient is in an irreversible state of depletion
Withholding food for diagnosis procedures
Failure to recognise and treat increased nutritional needs brought about by injury or illness
Failure to appreciate the role of nutrition in the prevention of and recovery from infection: unwarranted reliance on drugs
Prolonged administration of glucose and electrolyte solutions
Rotation of staff at frequent intervals and confusion of responsibility for patient care
Inadequate post-operative nutritional support
Limited availability of laboratory tests to assess nutritional status

problems and is usually reserved for a small number of patients with gastrointestinal failure.

Where there is a functional gastrointestinal tract, enteral nutrition is a more economical and physiologically sound option. Prolonged lack of enteral nutrition can result in intestinal mucosal atrophy, with an associated reduction in functional capacity and risk of intestinal bacterial translocation into the portal blood. A number of techniques are available for enteral feeding, the choice of which depends on various factors including type of injury, medical condition or surgical procedure, and should be based on individual patient assessment.

If voluntary intake is adequate, nutritional support may simply take the form of providing a more concentrated source of energy and nutrients. Other patients may be encouraged to feed by hand feeding, providing aromatic foods or heating the food offered to stimulate the appetite. Inappetent cats may respond to a pharmacological intervention such as intravenous administration of diazepam, or oral ciproheptadine but this method of appetite stimulation should not be continued for longer than 3 days and should be used with care as the diazepam has been associated with sporadic hepatotoxicity. It is important to check that adequate amounts are actually being consumed.

Where the patient's needs cannot be met through voluntary intake, some form of involuntary tube feeding must be considered. Force feeding by syringe, by daily orogastric intubation or by rolling the food into small balls and 'pilling' the animal are short-term options, but these methods can be stressful for the patient and may not satisfy the animal's nutritional needs.

Surgical placement of a **pharyngostomy tube** has been used successfully for feeding patients with prolonged anorexia and an inability to pick up or chew food. However, the popularity of this method of tube feeding has recently declined in favour of nasal feeding, oesophagostomy or gastrostomy tubes (see Chapters 22, Fluid Therapy and Shock, and 19, Surgical Nursing).

Naso-oesophageal or **nasogastric intubation** requires no sedation and is well tolerated by most cats and dogs. The tube may be left in place for several weeks, but since the tube size is limited, this method can only be used for feeding larger animals. It can, however, be used for long-term administration of fluids to any size of animal. Nasal feeding is recommended as an adjunct to voluntary feeding or where sedation or anaesthesia of the patient poses too great a risk for surgical placement of a gastrostomy tube (Fig. 9.4).

Gastrostomy tube feeding is indicated where long-term involuntary nutritional support is anticipated and the presence of pharyngeal or oesophageal lesions precludes the use of pharyngostomy tubes (Fig. 9.5). The use of gastrostomy tubes is increasing in small-animal medicine thanks to the development of a technique for percutaneous tube placement without the need for laparotomy. Percutaneous endoscopic gastrostomy (PEG) is a simple and well-tolerated procedure, but requires the use of a flexible endoscope. Alternatively, a large-bore Foley catheter can be placed into the stomach at laparotomy and secured to the abdominal musculature. Complications associated with this method include peritonitis and tube displacement or blockage. Gastrostomy tubes are of wide bore and so will accommodate most types of diet. The tube may be left in place for weeks to months, and tube feeding by this method can be continued by most owners at home.

Feeding directly into the small intestine by **enterostomy catheter** may be required when serious conditions of the upper gastrointestinal tract, such as pancreatitis or major gastric or small bowel surgery, are present. Animals fed in this way require liquid elemental diets that require little digestion and are readily absorbed from the jejunum and ileum. Parenteral nutrition would be an alternative if small-bowel function was not satisfactory.

Energy and nutrient requirements

Daily energy requirements of the hospitalised patient are based on basal energy requirements (BER) or cage-rest maintenance energy requirements (MER) multiplied by an

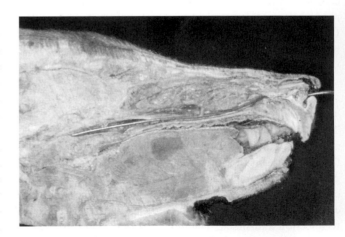

Fig. 9.4 Nasal feeding tube passing through the ventral meatus.

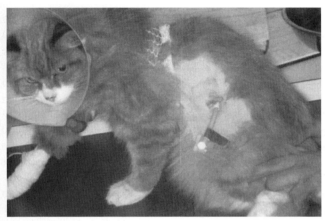

Fig. 9.5 Gastrostomy tube placed to provide nutrition to a cat with empyema.

arbitrary factor, the size of which varies according to the severity and nature of the illness (1.2 to 3 times). In some cases, energy requirements may be below normal because the animal is hypometabolic or because it is physically inactive as a result of the injury.

> Maintenance energy requirements (MER) are calculated using the formulas:
>
> MER (kcal/day) = 110 × BW$^{0.75}$ (kg) (dog)
>
> MER (kcal/day) = 70 × BW (kg) (cat)
>
> where BW is the animal's bodyweight.

The volume of food required is calculated by dividing the total daily energy requirement (kcal) by the energy density of the diet (kcal/ml) as recorded on the product label. The total volume required is divided into 4–6 feeds per day, depending on previous oral intake and individual animal tolerance. The normal stomach capacity is no more than 90 ml/kg in dogs and 50 ml/kg in cats. All dietary transitions should be made slowly and in the initial stages of nutritional support; the calculated amount of nutrients should be approached over a period of 48 hours to avoid vomiting, abdominal discomfort and diarrhoea. For animals that have been inappetent for prolonged periods, slow rates of administration (> 10 minutes) are recommended.

Weight and body condition score should be recorded on a daily basis to enable accurate calculation of the patient's energy requirements and to monitor its progress. Adjustments in food allowance can then be made on an individual basis according to observed changes in the animal's bodyweight, body condition and level of activity.

Stressed, hypermetabolic patients use fat, rather than carbohydrate as their main source of energy and most cells become progressively less able to use glucose efficiently. High levels of carbohydrate in the diet during this period can, in fact, give rise to serious metabolic disturbances which may lead to respiratory or cardiac failure. High-fat diets are therefore recommended and tend to be more pala-

table, digestible and calorie-dense, which are advantages for feeding potentially anorexic patients. Protein requirements of the stressed animal are higher than normal to maintain wound healing and immunity and to compensate for the higher rate of protein breakdown. However, some restriction of dietary protein may be indicated in certain specific conditions, such as chronic kidney or liver disease.

Supplementation of the diet with certain amino acids, including **glutamine** and **arginine**, may be beneficial in the nutritional management of **critical-care patients**. There may also be an increased requirement for water-soluble **B-complex vitamins**, and **zinc** may have an important role in wound healing. There is further evidence from the human field indicating that antioxidants may be beneficial in preventing the ongoing cellular damage which occurs following a trauma involving ischaemia, hypovolaemia and shock.

Suitable diets

In selecting a diet for enteral administration, it is important to consider the most appropriate dietary formulation, the caloric density of the diet and, where appropriate, the diameter of the feeding tube. Commercial liquid enteral diets or liquidised canned diets may be used for most purposes. Elemental diets containing amino acids or glucose may be useful if gastrointestinal function is compromised, or to supplement other diets.

Ideally, diets for the critical patient should be highly palatable, highly digestible and nutrient dense in order to ensure an adequate intake of nutrients in a reduced volume of food. Although healthy dogs (but not cats) can be maintained on a plant-based diet, such diets are unsuitable for the metabolically stressed animal and should be replaced by a meat-based diet for the duration of the dog's illness and convalescence. Following injury, the metabolism of the dog tends to revert to its more carnivorous origins and is more closely aligned with that of the cat. Thus, protein and fat utilisation is increased and carbohydrate is used with decreasing efficiency. In addition, plant-based diets are less digestible than meat-based diets and can cause digestive upsets in the stressed patient.

Complications of nutritional support

Following a period of food deprivation, all dietary transitions should be made slowly to avoid complications including the development of potentially serious metabolic derangements (Table 9.19). In the initial stages of refeeding, vomiting may occur due to gastrointestinal hypomotility and diarrhoea may result from reduced intestinal surface area, decreased enzyme activity. Normal digestive function is usually restored within a few days of appropriate enteral feeding.

Calorie intake has an important effect on convalescence. An insufficient intake can result in PEM, but overfeeding can be equally detrimental, particularly when the carbohy-

Table 9.19 Food reintroduction schedule for animals recovering from vomiting, diarrhoea or pancreatitis

Day	Percent of normal daily food quantity
1	33
2	66
3	100

Feed small, frequent meals (4–5 day) of a highly digestible, low fat (<15% DM; <30% ME), low fibre (<2% DDM 0.5 g/100 kcal (418 kJ) ME) diet

drate intake is excessive. In starved, hypometabolic patients, excessive carbohydrate can lead to insulin-induced transport of phosphorus and potassium into cells and subsequently, hypophosphataemia and hypokalaemia. The resultant respiratory and cardiovascular failure could prove fatal in some cases.

Other complications of nutritional support include mechanical problems or infections related to the feeding tube. Tube obstructions can be minimised by using liquid diets with fine-bore tubes, by sieving liquidised canned diets prior to administration via oesophagostomy or gastrostomy tubes, and by flushing with water after each feed. Occasionally, naso-oesophageal tubes may be regurgitated and pharyngostomy tubes can cause gagging, airway obstruction and related problems. Fewer complications are seen with oesophagostomy tubes.

Dietary sensitivity

The term **dietary sensitivity** describes any clinically abnormal response to a particular food item and may be further classified as either **food intolerance** or true **food allergy (hypersensitivity)**. True dietary hypersensitivity is an immune-mediated phenomenon whereas food intolerance denotes any other clinically abnormal response to a dietary component. Food intolerance can result from an impaired ability to digest the food (often because a specific enzyme is lacking) or from pharmacological, metabolic or toxic reactions. With the exception of certain specific conditions, the clinical signs associated with hypersensitivity reactions are often indistinguishable from those produced by food intolerance, and management protocols are identical for both.

In the dog and cat, dietary sensitivity usually manifests as skin or gastrointestinal disease, and a number of cases will present with signs involving both systems. Pruritus is the most frequently observed presenting sign, which is accompanied by a gradation of clinical signs associated with self-inflicted trauma. Dietary sensitivity has also been implicated in some cases of **otitis externa** in dogs and of **miliary dermatitis** and **eosinophilic plaque** in cats. Certain forms of food intolerance, notably **lactose intolerance** and **gluten-sensitive enteropathy of Irish setters**, usually manifest as diarrhoea. In addition, a number of chronic conditions of the gastrointestinal tract have been reported in which dietary hypersensitivity may play a role, including **inflammatory bowel disease** in cats and canine **idiopathic chronic colitis**.

Food sensitivity may be associated with any dietary ingredient, including additives (although extremely rare), but most reactions are caused by dietary proteins. In cats, reactions to cow's milk and beef account for more than half the reported cases, whereas reactions to cow's milk, beef and cereal (alone or in combination) are most commonly reported in dogs. The successful management of dietary sensitivity involves identification of the offending ingredient and its elimination from the diet. By examining the animal's detailed dietary history, it may be possible to identify foods which the animal has never eaten (or at least within the previous month) and these can be used to form the basis of an elimination diet which is 'hypoallergenic' for that individual. Such restricted diets should contain a minimum number of protein sources which, preferably are not commonly associated with sensitivity reactions. Elimination diets that have been used successfully in dogs and cats include chicken, lamb, rabbit, duck, venison and a variety of fish species which are typically fed with rice, tapioca or potatoes.

The elimination diet should be fed for a minimum of 3 weeks, although a trial period of up to 60 days may be necessary in some animals to achieve a complete remission of signs. Failure to respond within this time suggests that either dietary sensitivity is not involved, other factors may be contributing to the clinical disease or the animal is sensitive to the protein in the elimination diet.

> During the diagnostic period, there should be **no access to any other source of nutrients**, including treats, chews or nutritional supplements.

A small number of animals will react to commercially prepared elimination diets but not to home-prepared diets using the same ingredients and it may be preferable to use a home-prepared diet in the initial diagnostic stages.

If clinical improvement occurs, a diagnosis of dietary sensitivity may be confirmed by challenging with the original diet and demonstrating an exacerbation of clinical signs within 1–14 days. Reintroduction of the elimination diet should result in an improvement in signs and, at this stage, it may be possible to introduce a commercially prepared diet with the same ingredients. Individual protein sources can then be introduced at weekly intervals to identify specific dietary allergens that should be avoided. Once a diagnosis has been established, it is usually possible to manage cases of dietary sensitivity using commercial diets with selected protein sources of high digestibility. Alternatively, it may be possible to identify a range of standard products that the animal is able to tolerate.

Obesity management

Obesity is the most common form of malnutrition seen in companion animal practice, with an estimated incidence of

25–33% in dogs and 6–25% in cats. Although cats tend to be more efficient regulators of their energy intake, this ability may be overridden, and recent trends towards the free-choice feeding of palatable dry cat foods together with a more sedentary, indoor lifestyle may have increased the frequency with which feline obesity is observed in some parts of the world. Obesity may not only reduce the animal's enjoyment of life but a number of serious clinical problems have been linked to the condition.

Conditions associated with obesity:
- **Osteoarthritis**.
- Respiratory distress and reduced exercise tolerance.
- **Diabetes mellitus**.
- Circulatory problems.
- Lowered resistance to infections.
- Liver disease, including **idiopathic hepatic lipidosis** in cats.
- Dermatological problems which, in cats, may be linked to difficulties in self-grooming.
- Increased risk of **feline lower urinary tract disease**.
- Increased surgical and anaesthetic risk.

Obesity is a consequence of energy intake exceeding requirement at some stage in the animal's life. During this phase, excessive energy intake results in the deposition of fat in adipose tissue and is associated with an increase in fat-cell size (**hypertrophy**) in the adult, or fat cell numbers (**hyperplasia**) in the growing animal. Once fat-cell hyperplasia has occurred, the animal retains a lifelong predisposition for excessive weight gain and it is important that food intake of growing dogs, in particular, is controlled to avoid obesity in the adult. The initial dynamic phase of fat deposition is followed by a static phase in which the animal remains fat but its bodyweight is fairly stable. Appetite may be normal or even reduced and this apparent anomaly may be confusing for the owners.

An animal is considered obese if its bodyweight is 15% or more above the ideal. Breed standards may provide useful guidelines for determining the ideal weight of pure-bred dogs, but are of little value in crossbred dogs and cats. Practical assessment of the degree of obesity involves subjective evaluation of the animal's appearance and palpation of the subcutaneous fat deposits. In normal animals, the ribs should be palpable but covered with a moderately thin layer of fat and there should be a definite indentation, or waistline, behind the rib cage when viewed from above. Dogs also tend to accumulate fat around the tail head and obese cats may develop an 'apron' of fat in the groin. Accumulation of fat in the abdominal cavity must be differentiated from abdominal enlargement due to other causes, such as ascites, gas, pregnancy or abdominal organ enlargement.

Dietary therapy of obesity is aimed at moderate, controlled energy restriction. Rapid weight loss should not be attempted in obese cats, since this can lead to the development of **hepatic lipidosis,** which is potentially fatal. In general, it is recommended that an initial target weight is set which represents a 15% reduction in bodyweight. Further reductions can then be planned once this target weight has been reached. For dogs, this degree of weight loss can be achieved within 12 weeks by feeding 40–50% of the animal's energy requirement for maintenance at its target weight. In cats, a 15% reduction in weight can be safely achieved over 18 weeks by feeding 60% of the animal's target energy requirements.

Simply feeding less of the normal diet is not recommended, since prepared pet foods are balanced to a normal energy intake and by restricting energy intake, essential nutrients may also be restricted. This can produce deficiency states that may be dangerous or even lethal. In addition, this technique rarely forms part of a structured weight loss programme, and success rates tend to be low.

A more effective strategy is to **feed a prepared low-calorie diet which has been specifically formulated to achieve weight loss and ensures an adequate intake of essential nutrients**. This is particularly important when the diet is to be fed long-term. Dietary therapy should be combined with an increase in physical activity (where possible) and behavioural modifications which aim to produce lifelong habit changes and, therefore, permanent weight loss. A protocol for successful weight reduction in dogs and cats is provided in Table 9.20.

Gastrointestinal disease

Gastrointestinal disorders are common in dogs and cats. In most cases, dietary modification can form an important, sometimes essential, part of managing the condition. Although some acute gastrointestinal disorders can be life-threatening, most cases tend to be self-limiting and respond well to symptomatic treatment. The principle of 'bowel rest' in which food is withheld for 24–72 hours is commonly adopted while fluid and electrolyte status is maintained through the oral or parenteral administration of rehydration fluids. Subsequently, small amounts of a highly digestible, bland diet (such as boiled rice, fish or chicken) may be gradually reintroduced. In contrast, chronic conditions which persist for longer than 3–4 weeks are unlikely to resolve without first identifying a specific cause and implementing the appropriate therapy.

Oesophageal disease

Oesophageal lesions may necessitate feeding via gastrostomy tube to allow the oesophagus to heal, otherwise soft, moist or liquidised foods may be offered. Patients with megaoesophagus should be fed from an elevated position to allow food to enter the stomach with the help of

Table 9.20 Dietary management of obesity in dogs and cats

- Council the owner on the need to reduce the animal's body weight, stressing the medical implications of obesity
- Weigh the dog or cat and set a target weight. The planned reduction should represent no more than 15% of the animal's current weight
- Indicate to the owner how long it is likely to take to reach the target weight safely. The weight loss can usually be achieved in 10–15 weeks in dogs and 16–20 weeks in cats
- Calculate the amount to feed based on 40–50% (dogs) or 60% cats) of the maintenance energy requirements at target body weight
- Stress the concept of feeding the weight reduction diet to the exclusion of all other foods. The discipline and cooperation required of all who come into contact with the animal may be reinforced if they are encouraged to record the total daily food intake on a chart. It may be preferable to confine cats to the home to prevent supplementation from other sources
- Advise weighing the animal carefully on the same scales at the same time every week or fortnight and encourage the owner to record the weight on the chart supplied. Small and steady weight losses are more evident from the weight chart than from simple observation of the animal
- Careful monitoring of cats during weight reduction is recommended. Owners should be questioned to check that food intake matches expectations, and clinical examination should be performed at regular intervals. Periodic haematological and blood biochemical evaluation may also be appropriate
- If satisfactory weight loss is not occurring, then the daily food allowance may be reduced by 10%, whilst keeping a careful watch on the general health of the animal. If such a reduction is necessary, it should be maintained for the rest of the dieting period
- When a satisfactory weight loss has been achieved, the dog or cat should be changed to a normal high-quality diet. It is important to calculate and regularly reassess the daily amount of food required to maintain the target weight
- Follow up after 1 and 3 months, and then at six-monthly intervals
- At all times, give the owner adequate encouragement

gravity. Traditionally, slurries have been used but many cases are now thought to cope better when fed a more textured diet.

Gastric dilatation – volvulus

Although cereal-based dry foods have previously been linked to this condition in dogs, it is now thought that they may have been falsely incriminated. Gaseous distension of the stomach may result from swallowed air and may be associated with rapid food consumption and excitement or physical activity close to the time of feeding. General dietary recommendations are to feed small frequent meals of a highly digestible, meat-based diet which will encourage gastric emptying and reduce stomach distension. Dogs, particularly those at high risk, should not be fed or allowed to drink large volumes of water within 1 hour of exercise or excitement and should preferably be fed away from other dogs.

Chronic diarrhoea

Diarrhoea may be defined as an increase in frequency, volume or fluidity of faeces, but these characteristics should be considered in the context of the diet being fed. High-fibre diets, for example, will lead to a marked increase in faecal volume and frequency of defecation compared with 'normal' highly digestible foods. Diarrhoea may be classified as 'chronic' if it persists for longer than 3–4 weeks.

Large quantities of water are either consumed or secreted into the gastrointestinal tract every day and in normal circumstances, approximately 95% of this water is reabsorbed from the large intestine. A relatively small decrease in absorption (or increase in secretion) can readily result in increased faecal water content and diarrhoea.

Diarrhoea occurs as the result of one or more mechanisms:

- Interference with the digestion or absorption of nutrients. Nutrients retained within the intestinal lumen exert an osmotic effect leading to the retention of water and diarrhoea (osmotic diarrhoea). Osmotic diarrhoea is most commonly seen with nutritional overload, but it is also associated with any condition in which there is a deficiency of enzymes or enterocytes, including **exocrine pancreatic insufficiency (EPI)**, and **brush border enzyme** (such as lactase) **deficiency**.
- Increased secretion of fluid into the intestine by enterocytes (secretory diarrhoea), which may be stimulated by bacterial toxins and by the products of bacterial degradation of bile acids and dietary fat.
- Increased intestinal permeability due to mucosal damage, which can result from severe inflammation or as a consequence of other disease processes, e.g. cardiac disease, lymphatic obstruction. If the pore size is large, fluid and plasma proteins escape into the intestinal lumen, creating a protein-losing enteropathy and diarrhoea.
- Altered intestinal motility. Contrary to popular belief, most cases are due to a reduction in segmentation contractions rather than increased peristalsis, resulting in stagnation of intestinal contents, bacterial proliferation and degradation of nutrients. The increased faecal volume stimulates secondary peristaltic contractions which may give the impression of hypermotility.

Small-intestinal disease

Diarrhoea of small-intestinal origin tends to lead to an increase in faecal volume since this is the main site for digestion and absorption of nutrients and this, in turn, can lead to an increased frequency of defecation. Pale, fatty faeces (**steatorrhoea**) are seen when there is maldigestion or malabsorption of fat, as in EPI and some other small-intestinal disorders. Because nutrients are poorly absorbed into the body, weight loss is common, often despite a marked increase in appetite.

Diet plays an important role in the management of many small-intestinal diseases, generally in conjunction with appropriate pharmacological therapy. Although no single diet is appropriate for every condition, it is generally accepted that diets for the management of conditions involving the small intestine should be highly digestible, since many diseases are likely to interfere with digestive and absorptive function. In most circumstances, therefore, high-fibre diets are contraindicated for the management of small-intestinal disease.

Restriction of dietary fat is recommended in a range of small-intestinal diseases which disturb fat digestion or absorption, including **EPI, small-intestinal bacterial overgrowth (SIBO)** and **lymphangiectasia**. Pancreatic enzymes are reduced or absent with EPI, whereas SIBO adversely affects bile salts. In addition, bacterial metabolism of undigested fat may promote intestinal secretion and further aggravate the diarrhoea.

In some cases, medium-chain triglycerides (MCTs) may form a useful supplemental source of energy, since some MCTs can be absorbed intact from the gastrointestinal tract and can reach the circulation via portal rather than lymphatic channels.

- Restriction of dietary fat is less important in the cat than the dog and some diarrhoeic cats appear to fare better on moderate- to high-fat diets.
- Moderate to high quantities of good-quality protein are recommended for small-intestinal diseases, since protein malabsorption or protein-losing enteropathy may be a feature of some cases of chronic small-intestinal diarrhoea. Protein deficiency can further compromise a diseased intestinal tract.
- Protein is also important in relation to dietary sensitivity, since most 'allergens' are proteins. Gluten, a protein in wheat and other cereals such as barley (not maize), is responsible for a particular enteropathy of Irish setters in which poor weight gain or weight loss is usually accompanied by chronic diarrhoea. Where dietary sensitivity is the cause of diarrhoea, sources of dietary protein should be minimised to one or two ingredients, which are not normally associated with sensitivity reactions.
- Carbohydrate digestion and absorption can be impaired in all conditions that damage the lining of the small-intestinal wall. Nevertheless, starch presents a relatively low digestive challenge in comparison with fat and may be used to provide a greater contribution to the energy content of diets which are restricted in fat. Highly digestible sources of carbohydrate, such as rice, are recommended. Simple sugars such as lactose, which is found in milk, should be avoided because the enzymes required for their digestion may be lacking.
- Although dietary fibre is commonly used in the non-specific treatment of acute diarrhoeas, it is generally not suitable for use in chronic small-intestinal diseases. In the short term, fibre may improve faecal consistency, but in chronic cases it may interfere with digestion and absorption, thereby further compromising an impaired gastrointestinal tract. In particular, soluble fibre is contraindicated in EPI since this may interfere with pancreatic enzyme activity.

- Several small-intestinal diseases can result in deficiencies of water-soluble B-complex vitamins, especially cobalamin (vitamin B_{12}) and folate.

Large-intestinal disease

Animals with large-intestinal diarrhoea tend to show very frequent defecation and pass small quantities of faeces on each occasion. This may be associated with urgency, straining or pain on defecation. The presence of fresh blood and copious amounts of mucus are also characteristic of large-intestinal problems. Although weight loss is not usually a feature of large-intestinal disease, it can occur as a secondary problem if appetite is depressed over a long period of time.

- Dietary fibre may be beneficial in the management of some large-intestinal diarrhoeas. Bacterial fermentation of fibres within the large intestine yield short-chain fatty acids, which are important for maintaining the health of cells of the large-intestinal wall and promote acidification of the contents of the colon. The effects of non-fermentable fibre are primarily related to an increase in faecal bulk. This may help to exercise the smooth muscle of the colon and improve contractility and, in addition, may bind faecal water to produce more formed stools.
- Diets containing a mixture of both permeable and non-permeable fibres can, therefore, be valuable as non-specific therapy in a number of large-intestinal diseases, including certain infections and 'irritable bowel syndrome', which may be associated with stress.
- Since many cases of colitis and inflammatory bowel disease in dogs and cats are thought to have an immune component, single protein source 'hypoallergenic diets' may be of benefit in their management, at least in the initial stages of therapy.

Constipation

Constipation may be defined as an inability to pass, or difficulty in passing (**tenesmus**), faeces. Retained faeces in the rectum and colon become progressively harder as water is reabsorbed and the faecal mass becomes increasingly impacted. High-fibre diets are of benefit in the prevention, but not the treatment, of constipation. Insoluble fibre increases faecal bulk which is thought to increase colonic motility by stretching colonic muscles, resulting in more forceful, albeit less frequent, contractions. Soluble fibres may add further to faecal bulk, through their ability to retain water in the intestinal lumen. Fibres combining soluble and insoluble properties may be optimal for the prevention of constipation.

Pancreatic disease

Exocrine pancreatic insufficiency

Exocrine pancreatic secretions are reduced or absent in patients with **exocrine pancreatic insufficiency (EPI)** resulting in an inability to adequately digest fat and, to a lesser extent, protein and carbohydrate in the diet. Because there is poor digestion and malabsorption of nutrients, especially fat, weight loss is common despite a marked increase in appetite and affected animals produce large volumes of pale, fatty faeces (**steatorrhoea**).

Although enzyme replacement therapy improves digestibility in patients with EPI, their requirements for energy and nutrients are still higher than in the normal animal. Low-fat diets of high digestibility help to reduce the digestive challenge within the gastrointestinal tract and may reduce the daily requirement for enzyme replacer. High-fibre (particularly soluble fibre) diets are to be avoided, since they interfere with pancreatic enzyme activity. Requirements for cobalamin (vitamin B_{12}) are often raised with EPI, and those for zinc and copper may also be marginally increased. Cobalamin deficiency may also occur with EPI but can be corrected by parenteral supplementation.

Pancreatitis

The initial therapy of acute pancreatitis is aimed at preventing the secretion of proteolytic enzymes from the exocrine pancreas, which promote further tissue damage within the organ. This involves a strict policy of nil by mouth (food and water) for 2–5 days with the parenteral administration of fluid and electrolytes. If vomiting does not occur for 48 hours, oral electrolyte drinks may be given for 1–2 days before the gradual reintroduction of solid food.

High-carbohydrate foods (such as rice, pasta or potatoes), which have the least stimulating effect on pancreatic secretions, may be offered initially in several small feeds per day. If this is tolerated, a highly digestible, low-fat diet may be offered, in which the protein content is moderately reduced and of high biological value. This type of diet is useful in the recovery period of acute pancreatitis and may also help prevent recurrent bouts of chronic pancreatitis.

Liver disease

Hepatobiliary disease can lead to derangements in both the metabolism and storage of proteins, fats, carbohydrates and certain micronutrients, as well as in the detoxification of potentially hazardous by-products. **Hepatic encephalopathy (HE)** can occur where there is either critical loss of functional hepatic tissue (60–70%) or **portosystemic shunting**. In HE, a number of neurotoxic substances (mainly ammonia) may enter the peripheral and cerebral circulation, giving rise to a complex of neurological signs. These toxins are derived mainly from the alimentary tract, being synthesised by gastrointestinal flora or consumed in the diet, but ammonia is also produced as a by-product of protein catabolism and when amino acids are converted to glucose and energy via gluconeogenesis.

Nevertheless, the liver has a large functional reserve and a phenomenal capacity for regeneration following insult. Nutritional support during the period of hepatocellular repair can help to delay or prevent irreversible progression of the disease. For dogs, this can be achieved by modification of the diet in the following ways:

- Adequate energy provision, using non-protein sources. This limits ammonia production by avoiding the use of amino acids to provide energy and by preventing muscle wastage.
- Moderate restriction of dietary protein to help limit the amount of ammonia generated both in the intestines and from the use of amino acids for gluconeogenesis. However, dietary protein intake must be carefully balanced to meet the individual animal's needs, since an inadequate intake will promote the breakdown of structural proteins.
- High-quality proteins are recommended since they tend to be highly digestible and are likely to meet the animal's needs with minimal production of ammonia.
- Careful use of fat as an energy source, which increases the energy density of the diet and improves palatability. Both these effects are beneficial in the management of dogs with liver disease, since inappetence is a common problem. However, moderate fat restriction is indicated in dogs with an impaired ability to digest fat due to a lack of bile.
- Provision of complex carbohydrates, such as starch and fibre, in the diet to improve glucose utilisation by slowing down the delivery of glucose from the gut to the liver.
- Inclusion of dietary fibre, which may assist in the elimination of ammonia and other toxins in the faeces, inhibits ammonia production by bacteria in the colon and prevents constipation, which is also important in the management of HE.
- Supplementation with water-soluble vitamins (B-complex) to compensate for impaired synthesis and increased losses of these nutrients. Supplementation with vitamin E may be beneficial in limiting ongoing liver disease.
- Supplementation with zinc, which is involved in the detoxification of ammonia, can help to improve nervous signs associated with HE. Zinc reduces fibrosis and, by reducing the availability of copper, provides protection against liver injury associated with copper accumulation in the liver. This is particularly beneficial in patients with copper storage liver disease.
- Restriction of dietary copper intake.
- Moderate restriction of sodium intake, especially where liver disease is associated with hypoalbuminaemia or portal hypertension, since an excessive intake can precipitate or exacerbate ascites.

Diets for cats with liver disease must meet the normally high feline requirements for protein and essential amino acids. Protein-restricted diets are not recommended unless the disease is accompanied by HE, although this is rare in cats. The protein content of these diets should be of high biological value and ensure an adequate intake of arginine, taurine and carnitine. Diets formulated for the management of feline chronic renal failure may be appropriate in this minority of cases.

Most cats with liver disease, particularly those with **hepatic lipidosis**, may have increased protein requirements and the requirements for B-complex vitamins and fat-soluble vitamins K and E may be similarly raised. High-fat diets may be detrimental in feline hepatic lipidosis and in cats with other forms of hepatic disease. Highly digestible diets with a relatively high protein content, moderately reduced fat content and enhanced levels of zinc and vitamins B, K and E are likely to be of benefit in most cats with hepatic disease. For cats with hepatic lipidosis, enteral tube feeding will almost certainly be required.

Diabetes mellitus

Animals with **diabetes mellitus** have impaired production or release of insulin which may be combined with a tissue insensitivity to insulin (insulin resistance). This results in an imbalance in the metabolism of carbohydrate, fat and protein and is characterised by hyperglycaemia and an inability to regulate blood sugar levels. Successful long-term management of diabetes mellitus involves a combination of appropriate insulin replacement therapy and a suitable dietary regimen. The aim is to provide a consistent supply of nutrients to match the activity of exogenous insulin and thereby achieve relatively stable blood glucose levels. Consistency in the feeding regimen is essential and involves the standardisation of the quantity of food given, the dietary content (energy density and dietary constituents) and the timing of meals. The exercise routine, which may alter the animal's energy requirements, should also be carefully regulated. A schedule should be established that is compatible with the normal household routine.

Feeding a patient with diabetes mellitus should incorporate:

- Timing of feeding should be arranged such that maximal absorption and metabolism of nutrients coincides with maximal activity of administered insulin and may vary with the type of insulin preparation used. Insulins with an intermediate duration of action (such as lente or isophane preparations in dogs and lente or protamine zinc preparations in cats) are commonly used as single or, where insulin metabolism is faster, as twice daily injections.
- Increasing the number of meals daily reduces the degree of post-prandial hyperglycaemia and improves glycaemic control, provided that the meals are fed whilst the injected insulin is still active. In most cases, however, the daily food allowance may be divided into two meals. When insulin is injected once daily, one meal

may be fed at the time of injection with the second meal given 6–8 hours later. When insulin is given twice daily, meals should either be given at injection times (2 meals/day) or additionally at times of peak insulin activity (3–4 meals/day).

For *canine* diabetics, modification of the diet can help to improve glycaemic control and may reduce the requirement for replacement insulin therapy:

- Simple sugars, such as glucose, sucrose and lactose, are to be avoided (other than in the emergency treatment of hypoglycaemia resulting from insulin overdosage) since they are rapidly absorbed and promote wide fluctuations in blood sugar levels.
- Complex carbohydrates such as starch, however, are digested relatively slowly and result in a more gradual release of glucose into the circulation over a period of hours.
- Dietary fibre further slows down the rate of digestion within the gut, lumen therefore slows the rate of post-prandial nutrient uptake. When combined with the slow digestion of starch, this effect helps to reduce post-prandial glycaemic peaks which facilitates the control of blood glucose levels.
- High-fat diets should be avoided since diabetics tend to develop hyperlipidaemia and other lipid-related complications.

> The benefits of high-fibre, high-starch diets have not been clearly demonstrated in diabetic *cats*, which are poorly adapted to high-carbohydrate diets. Current recommendations are to feed diabetic cats a 'normal' feline diet, although semimoist foods, which are high in sample sugars, are contraindicated. As with dogs, meal times and the amount and type of diet must be standardised as far as possible.

If the diabetic animal is also obese, which can exacerbate diabetes, weight reduction measures should be incorporated into the diabetic regimen. Dietary therapy for other coexisting disease, such as chronic renal failure, hepatic disease, congestive heart failure or chronic gastrointestinal disease, may take priority over diets designed for improving glycaemic control, but again, consistency in the feeding regimen is the rule.

Chronic renal failure

Chronic renal failure (CRF) is a relatively common syndrome in older dogs and cats and represents the end stage of a number of renal diseases. It is a progressive condition in which existing renal damage is irreversible, but dietary measures can improve the clinical signs of uraemia associated with CRF and may help to slow progression of the condition. Clinical signs of CRF are not apparent until at least 65–75% of renal tissue is destroyed.

Since many of the clinical signs related to CRF are associated with the accumulation of toxic protein catabolites and failure to excrete phosphorus, the emphasis in dietary therapy is on modification of the phosphorus and protein contents of the diet. However, other dietary components to be considered include calcium, sodium, potassium and water-soluble vitamins, together with the dietary energy content and fat. Maintenance of normal hydration is also important, through the provision of unlimited access to drinking water or via fluid replacement in cases of persistent vomiting.

- Dietary **phosphorus restriction** is an important part of management of CRF which should be initiated early in the course of the disease. This helps to limit renal mineralisation and secondary hyperparathyroidism. In cats, feeding a diet low in phosphorus and protein content has been shown to double their lifespan as compared to cats with CRF fed normal diets. In dogs, this type of diet has been shown to slow progression of renal damage.
- **Restriction of dietary protein** is of clinical benefit in uraemic patients, since this minimises the accumulation of nitrogenous waste associated with protein breakdown; helps to limit the intake of dietary phosphorus; and reduces the protein-related solute load on the failing kidneys, thereby lessening the severity of polydipsia/polyuria. Nevertheless, excessive protein restriction is to be avoided, since this can result in protein malnutrition in both dogs and cats. The protein in diets for patients with CRF should be of high biological value.
- For dogs with CRF, a staged approach to management is recommended and early cases may benefit from phosphorus restriction whilst maintaining a 'normal' protein intake. More advanced cases which are showing clinical signs of uraemia should be fed diets which are restricted in both phosphorus and protein. Where possible, the degree of protein restriction should be individualised according to the dog's clinical and biochemical status.
- The potential risks of dietary protein reduction are greater in the cat than in the dog. It is currently recommended that well-hydrated cats with azotaemia (increased concentrations of urea, creatinine or other non-protein nitrogenous compounds in blood) and hyperphosphataemia (or hypoparathyroidism) should be fed diets which are restricted in phosphorus and moderately restricted in protein.
- Feeding an **energy-dense** diet, in which the energy content is derived from non-protein sources, avoids tissue catabolism and helps to reduce nitrogenous waste production. Appetite is often poor in affected animals, so the energy density of the diet should be high to enable the animal to obtain its nutritional requirements from a relatively small volume of food. Fat is particularly useful in this respect, since it increases energy density and aids **palatability** of the diet. For this reason, canned diets designed to support dogs and cats with CRF tend to be high in fat.

- Many cats with CRF are hypokalaemic and require some degree of dietary **potassium** supplementation. However, some cats (often those most severely affected) are hyperkalaemic, so serum potassium levels should be closely monitored in cats with CRF.
- Serum **calcium** levels may be low, normal or high in patients with CRF. Calcium supplementation may be required in hypocalcaemic individuals.
- **Sodium** balance may be disrupted in advanced CRF and systemic hypertension can occur in both dogs and cats. It is currently recommended that dietary sodium levels are either normal or moderately restricted, since excessive sodium restriction may also be detrimental.
- Requirements for **water soluble (B-complex) vitamins** may be increased in dogs and cats with CRF because of reduced intake (inappetence), increased urinary losses in polyuric cases and higher demands during the recuperative processes.

Urolithiasis

Urolithiasis is the disease which results from the formation of calculi (uroliths) within the urinary tract. Crystals form in urine when the concentrations of its constituents exceed a critical level of supersaturation. Dietary factors can profoundly influence urolith formation because dietary ingredients and feeding patterns influence the pH, volume and solute concentration of the urine.

Urolithiasis is an important cause of **feline lower urinary tract diseases (FLUTD)**, particularly in obstructed cases. Traditionally, struvite urolithiasis has been of greatest importance but although the incidence has declined in recent years, calcium oxalate urolithiasis is now seen with increasing frequency. Uroliths which are commonly found in dogs include struvite, calcium oxalate, cystine and ammonium urate. Mixed calculi may also occur in some cases. Various types of urolith may be found in both cats and dogs. In both species magnesium ammonium phosphate (struvite) and calcium oxalate form most frequently.

Struvite

Factors which decrease the risk of struvite (magnesium ammonium phosphate) crystal formation in urine include:
- Acidification of the urine (to between pH 6.0 and 6.5 in cats and between pH 5.5 and 6.0 in dogs).
- Increased urine volume to dilute solute concentrations and increase the frequency of urination.
- Moderate restriction of dietary magnesium and phosphorus.

Diets which achieve these goals may be used to dissolve struvite uroliths *in situ* or to prevent recurrence of the condition. Initial relief of obstructed cases may require surgical intervention.

Commercial diets are available which have been designed to achieve urinary undersaturation with struvite, although urinary acidifiers may be added to an animal's normal diet to achieve the appropriate effect. Diets of high moisture content and high digestibility are preferred, but water may also be added to dry foods if necessary. Moderate supplementation with sodium chloride (salt) may stimulate thirst and promote increased water turnover. Acidified diets are not appropriate for feeding to young animals or to pregnant or lactating females. Furthermore, levels of taurine and potassium should be enhanced when acidified diets are fed to cats.

The main difference between canine and feline struvite urolithiasis is that in dogs, struvite uroliths are usually associated with urinary tract infection, whereas most feline struvite uroliths are sterile. Urease-producing bacteria such as staphylococci and *Proteus* spp. create an increasingly alkaline environment and conditions which are ideal for the formation of struvite and, occasionally, other types of urolith. Where infection is present, prolonged antibiotic therapy is essential in addition to dietary and other measures. Dietary protein restriction may also be beneficial in these cases, since this reduces the available substrate in urine for urease-producing bacteria.

Calcium oxalate

It is not possible to dissolve calcium oxalate uroliths *in situ* by dietary or any other means, and surgery is currently the only method of removing them in dogs and cats. Nevertheless, dietary manipulation can help to prevent recurrence of the condition. The goal is to reduce urinary saturation with calcium oxalate. Diets designed for the management of calcium oxalate urolithiasis should promote increased urine volume, preferably through the addition of water to the food. Although restriction of dietary calcium and oxalate may be beneficial, restriction of only one of these components may increase intestinal absorption of the other. Although increased magnesium intake is sometimes recommended in the prevention of calcium oxalate urolithiasis, care should be taken to ensure that this does not predispose the animal to struvite urolith formation.

Cystine

Cystine urolithiasis occurs in dogs with an inherited defect in cystine metabolism, resulting in impaired reabsorption of the amino acid from the proximal tubule of the kidney and, hence, cystinuria. This leads to cystine urolith formation since cystine is relatively insoluble, particularly in acidic urine. Dissolution and prevention of recurrence of cystine uroliths can be achieved through:

- Increasing water intake to increase urine volume.
- Reduction of dietary protein to reduce cystine excretion.
- Alkalinisation of urine (with bicarbonate or citrate) to increase cystine solubility.
- Administration of compounds such as D-penicillamine or 2-mercaptopropionylglycine (2-MPG), which convert cystine to a more soluble compound.

Ammonium urate

Urate uroliths occur mostly in Dalmatians and in patients with portosystemic shunts, when hepatic conversion of uric acid (a product of purine metabolism) to allantoin is impaired. Allantoin is highly soluble but increased urinary excretion of uric acid may predispose the dog to urolith formation.

Surgical relief of obstruction may be required in some cases. In others, dissolution and prevention of recurrence of urate uroliths may be achieved by:

- Restriction of dietary protein to limit purine intake.
- Supplementation with potassium citrate to promote neutral or slightly alkaline urine.
- Increased water intake.
- Administration of allopurinol which inhibits uric acid production.

Idiopathic cystitis in cats

For a significant proportion of cats with non-obstructive lower urinary tract disease, a specific cause cannot be identified for this clinical sign and the condition is classified as 'idiopathic'. Although clinical signs resolve spontaneously within 5–7 days, many cases recur after a variable period. Studies have shown that the rate of recurrence can be reduced by feeding a canned diet formulated for the production of acidic urine, although the equivalent dry formulation has no impact on the biological behaviour of the disease.

Skin disease

Deficiencies of essential fatty acids, protein, zinc, vitamins A, E and certain B-complex vitamins may give rise to skin disease. In addition, supplementation with supraphysiological doses of certain nutrients, including vitamins A and essential fatty acids, have been used in the treatment of specific skin conditions where no apparent dietary deficiency exists. Essential fatty acids, particularly those of the omega-3 series found in marine fish oils, are currently thought to be of greatest value in the management of pruritic skin diseases associated with hypersensitivity reactions. A third area in which diet is related to skin disease is that of dietary sensitivity which, in dogs and cats, is commonly manifest as a pruritic skin disorder.

Cardiac disease

Congestive heart failure

Congestive heart failure is associated with retention of sodium and water. Restriction of dietary sodium is a useful dietary strategy which helps to decrease fluid retention. Renal function is often compromised in cardiac failure and so the transition to a low sodium diet should take place gradually (over at least 5 days) to allow the kidneys to adapt.

Weight loss is common in cardiac patients (**cardiac cachexia**) as a consequence of a number of factors. Patients are often anorectic and malabsorption may occur as a result of reduced intestinal perfusion. Furthermore, energy requirements may be increased which can accelerate the wasting process. It is essential to ensure an adequate energy intake and if voluntary intake is reduced, some form of nutritional support is necessary. Fat may improve palatability and increase the energy density of the diet, but high-fat diets may not be appropriate in all cases. Some cardiac patients may be obese and for these, controlled weight reduction can help to improve clinical status.

Some degree of renal and hepatic dysfunction is often associated with congestive heart failure. Diets in which the protein content is moderately restricted and of high biological value should be introduced for these patients, but in other patients with protein energy malnutrition an increase in protein intake may be necessary.

Diuretic agents can have a marked effect on nutritional requirements, particularly for sodium and potassium, and may increase urinary losses of water-soluble vitamins (B-complex). Long-term use of frusemide or thiazide diuretics may cause potassium depletion and may also promote urinary magnesium loss. Conversely, spironolactone tends to conserve potassium but sodium excretion is enhanced and in this case, low-sodium diets should be avoided. Low-salt diets should also be used with care when vasodilators such as captopril and enalapril are administered, since these drugs are also associated with sodium loss and potassium retention.

Dilated cardiomyopathy

Low myocardial concentrations of **carnitine** have been associated with **dilated cardiomyopathy** in some dogs, notably Boxers, and dietary supplementation with L-carnitine (not D-carnitine or a mixture of D- and L-carnitine) is recommended as an adjunct to conventional medical therapy. In cats, many cases of dilated cardiomyopathy have been linked to **taurine** deficiency and plasma taurine status should be determined in all cases, prior to supplementation. Where appropriate, the deficient diet should be replaced with a feline diet of adequate taurine content and additional taurine supplementation should be provided as necessary, usually for a period of 12–16 weeks.

Nutrition of small and exotic pets

Small mammals

Basic energy and macronutrient requirements for rabbits and rodents are given in Tables 9.21 and 9.22.

Rabbits

Rabbits are herbivores with a high dietary requirement for fibre. Most domestic rabbits are fed balanced commercial pelleted foods or coarse mixes which may be supplemented with hay (as bedding) and small quantities of a variety of green vegetables, carrots and fresh salad crops. Supervised browsing on grass and other plants may also be encouraged but grass cuttings should not be fed.

Rabbits have an unusual metabolism of calcium which necessitates careful regulation of the dietary calcium content. Excessive dietary calcium can give rise to urolithiasis, whereas dietary deficiency (often exacerbated by a vitamin D deficiency) is a common cause of osteodystrophy with associated skeletal and tooth defects. Problems can arise in some rabbits fed 'rabbit mixes' because rabbits are selective feeders and may reject the pellets and whole grain in the ration. Most vitamin and mineral supplements are incorporated in the pelleted portion of the diet and rejection of these can produce a diet which is seriously deficient in calcium, vitamin D and other nutrients. Owners should encourage the rabbit to eat all ingredients in the ration by offering smaller quantities and refilling the pot only when all food has been consumed.

Rabbits tend to adjust their food intake according to their energy requirements and the energy content of the diet, but adults are likely to eat approximately 30–60 g of dry food/kg BW per day. Free access to clean water in bowls or sus-

Table 9.21 Basic energy requirements for rabbits and rodents (ME (kcal/day) = 110–440 $W^{0.75}$)					
	Rabbits	**Guinea pigs**	**Hamsters**	**Gerbils**	**Rats and mice**
Body weight (W)	0.5–7.0 kg	0.75–1.0 kg	85–140 g	50–60 g	20–800 g
Maintenance	110.00	110.00	110.00	110.00	110.00
Growth	190–210	145.00	145.00	145.00	145.00
Gestation	135–200	145.00	145.00	145.00	145.00
Lactation	300.00	165.00	310.00	440.00	440.00

Table 9.22 Basic macronutrient requirements for rabbits and rodents (after Tobin, 1996)					
	Rabbits	**Guinea pigs**	**Hamsters**	**Gerbils**	**Rats and mice**
ME (kcal/g)	2–2.4	1.7–2.9	2.5–3.9	2.5–3.7	2.2–3
Protein (%)	12–18	18–20	18–22	17–18	13–20
Fat (%)	2–4	2–4	4–5	10–12	1–5
Fibre (%)	10–16	7–11	4–8	4.00	4.00

pended bottles should be provided and adults may drink 5–10 ml/100 g BW per day.

Guinea pigs

Guinea pigs are herbivorous animals and, like humans and other primates, require a dietary source of vitamin C. A deficiency can result in clinical signs of scurvy within 2 weeks of feeding a deficient diet. The main types of feed are pelleted foods or coarse mixes, but these should be formulated specifically for guinea pigs. Rabbit feeds are unsuitable since they are lower in protein and are not supplemented with vitamin C, and some products contain coccidiostats which can cause liver or kidney damage in guinea pigs. Some pelleted feeds for guinea pigs contain vitamin C at levels which only just meet the minimum requirements and prolonged storage (over 3 months) can deplete vitamin C levels in the food. Supplementary vitamin C may be administered in the drinking water (1 g/litre) or fresh fruit or leafy vegetables, which contain high levels of the vitamin, may be added to the diet. Any dietary changes should take place gradually to avoid gastrointestinal upset.

Relatively high levels of fibre are required and a shortage can cause caecal impaction and fur chewing which may result in the formation of hairballs. An adequate supply of good quality hay can usually prevent these conditions. Guinea pigs should be provided with a diet that requires gnawing to promote balanced wear of the teeth. Malocclusion can prevent feeding, drinking and swallowing of saliva (**slobbers**) and can prove fatal within 6 days of signs occurring.

Guinea pigs may eat 5–8 g/100 g BW per day. Food may be provided in open bowls on the cage floor, but may become contaminated with excreta. Average daily water intake is 10 ml/100 g BW but this may increase if no succulent foods are fed and free access to water should be provided. Open water bowls may be contaminated and so inverted water bottles with a small sipper tube are often suspended from the side of the cage slightly above floor level. Fresh water should be provided daily and the water bottle cleaned.

Rats and mice

Rats and mice are omnivorous and will eat almost anything. Their nutritional requirements are well documented and commercial pelleted foods or coarse mixes are widely available. The basic ration may be supplemented with small quantities of a variety of foods including biscuit, apple, tomatoes and chocolate (as a treat) and offering these may encourage handling by the owner. Most rats and mice will adjust their energy intake to match their requirements but overfeeding of highly palatable foods can lead to obesity. As a guide, adult rats require 10–20 g/day of dry food, whereas adult mice require 5–10 g/day.

Free access to water should be available from small bowls or suspended water bottles. Adult rats may drink 25–45 ml/day and adult mice may drink 5–7 ml/day.

Hamsters

Hamsters are omnivorous and although specific diets are available, most good-quality rat or mice diets will meet the requirements of the hamster. Commercial pelleted diets or coarse mixes can be supplemented with treat foods such as washed vegetables, seeds, fruits, crackers and small amounts of cheese or cooked meat. Diets rich in simple sugars (glucose, lactose, sucrose, fructose) are best avoided and hamsters fare better when the carbohydrate source is starch. **Malocclusion** and overgrowth of teeth can be prevented by providing hard foods that require gnawing, such as dog biscuits or whole cereal seeds, such as maize.

Most adults will eat 5–15 g of pelleted feed and drink 15–20 ml of water per day, although free access to water should be offered. Food and water should be provided in heavy dishes that are not easily overturned or contaminated or alternatively, hoppers may be used. Stale food should be removed from the cage to prevent hoarding by the hamster.

Gerbils

Gerbils are herbivorous or **granivorous** and their natural diet is based on grains and seeds, supplemented with fresh vegetables and roots when these are available. Commercial pelleted foods or seed and grain diets are available for gerbils, although adult gerbils can be fed good-quality rat or mice diets. Some mixes may contain large amounts of sunflower seeds which are very palatable to gerbils but have a high fat and low calcium content. Gerbils may therefore selectively eat sunflower seeds at the expense of other dietary ingredients but an excessive intake can result in obesity and calcium deficiency with associated skeletal problems. The diet should be supplemented with chopped green vegetables, roots and fruit and if pelleted food is given, an appropriate seed mix should also be provided. Average food consumption in the adult is 10–15 g daily. Like other rodents, gerbils need some hard foods or pieces of wood in their environment to gnaw and so prevent problems with tooth malocclusion.

Gerbils conserve water efficiently through their ability to concentrate their urine. Most of their water requirement is met from succulent foods and from metabolism of the diet. Nevertheless, free access to clean water should always be provided. Food dishes should be ceramic, since plastic dishes may be eaten. Water containers with drinking tubes are best placed outside the cage and should be checked regularly to ensure that they are working.

Chinchillas

In the wild, chinchillas eat a wide range of vegetables, but their diet is composed mainly of grasses and seeds. Commercial diets are available but good-quality rabbit or guinea pig diets are also suitable. Good-quality hay should be available *ad libitum* and the diet may be supplemented with small quantities of dried fruit, nuts, carrot, washed green vegetables and fresh grass. However, supplements should be provided in moderation to prevent obesity, bloat, diarrhoea or other gastrointestinal upsets. Some hard foods or objects should be available to gnaw and prevent teeth malocclusion problems.

Adults may eat approximately 20 g/day. Free access to water should be provided from hanging water bottles although it may be advisable to offer an additional water dish until the animal is used to drinking from a bottle.

Ferrets

Ferrets are essentially carnivores with high protein and fat requirements. High-fibre diets should be avoided. Pelleted diets for ferrets are commercially available, otherwise high-quality tinned or dry cat foods may be fed. Dog foods are not appropriate for long-term feeding. Whole carcasses (mice, rabbits, day-old chicks) or chicken heads may occasionally be offered to provide variety or to supplement the diet. Many ferrets will eat other foods and small quantities of raw carrot or apple, cooked meat, dried fruit and raw liver can be offered.

Food intake in adults may be 20–40 g per day and working ferrets are commonly fed twice daily. Food preferences are established early in life and some individuals may resent dietary change. Water intake is approximately 75–100 ml per day.

Reptiles

Chelonians

Land tortoises are herbivores or omnivores, whereas terrapins are mainly carnivores and scavengers. Feeding errors in captive chelonians are a common cause of shell defects and hypovitaminosis A so vitamin/mineral supplementation is usually required. Newly hatched tortoises start to feed properly once the yolk sac has been absorbed and may be offered a variety of finely chopped fruits, vegetables, cold hard-boiled eggs, sprats, day-old chicks and other sources of animal protein. This should be supplemented with vitamins and minerals and meals should be offered twice daily. Juvenile and adult tortoises may be fed the same range of foods but they do not need to be chopped up and they can be housed outdoors in summer, with access to grass and other plants. Food intake is reduced or will stop for up to several weeks prior to hibernation, which occurs when ambient temperature and daylight hours begin to decrease. Although most water requirements are met from their food, tortoises should be provided with regular access to water.

Young terrapins feed in water and their diet includes small insects, small crustaceans and amphibian eggs and larvae. Adult terrapins eat amphibians and fish in the wild so in captivity, whole fish or chopped portions of whole fish should be fed to prevent nutritional imbalance. Herring, sprat, whitebait, sardines, minnows, sand eels, tadpoles or froglets, fresh prawns, shrimps and snails are all suitable foods. It is also possible to feed tinned cat or dog foods, hard boiled eggs, cheese, earthworms or fresh liver or kidney rubbed in a vitamin/mineral supplement occasionally. However, feeding should take place in a separate container from the normal living quarters and the amount of food offered at any one time should not exceed that which can be eaten within 20 minutes.

Snakes

Snakes are carnivorous and in captivity will eat rabbits, rats, mice, gerbils, chicks, earthworms, fish, amphibians, lizards or even other snakes. The whole carcass is fed, to provide a balanced diet. For humane reasons and to prevent injury to the snake, food is generally offered as dead prey, which may be freshly killed or thawed from frozen. Certain types of fish, including whitebait, has high thiaminase activity and prolonged feeding without thiamine supplementation can result in thiamine deficiency. Water requirements of snakes are low but water should always be provided.

The quantity of food and frequency of feeding depends on the bodyweight and surface area of the prey. For example, small garter snakes may require feeding on a daily basis, whereas a large python feeding on antelope may only need to feed twice a year. As a guideline, adult snakes should be fed as often as is required to maintain normal bodyweight. Snakes may not eat for long periods of time and although this is normal at certain times of the year or before a slough, this can result in **inanition**. Regular weighing is advisable and excessive weight loss may indicate that nutritional support is required. Fluids and easily assimilated foods can be administered by stomach tube.

Lizards

The range of lizards kept in captivity are insectivores, carnivores, herbivores, fruigivores and omnivores and consequently, eat a wide variety of foods. Some species may change their feeding requirements as they mature. Insectivores (geckos, chameleons, skinks, anoles, lacertids) feed mainly on mealworms, silk moth larvae, crickets, locust, wingless fruit flies. However, these insects are relatively deficient in calcium and the insects themselves must be fed an appropriate nutritional supplement to ensure an adequate intake of supplement in the lizard. Common iguana are usually fed vegetables, fruit, chicken, pink mice or dog food. Monitors and tegus eat raw eggs, meat, dog food or rodents such as pink mice, mice or rats. Biotin deficiency can occur due to the avidin content of raw eggs. Vitamin and mineral supplementation is usually required in diets for captive lizards. All lizards should have access to fresh water. Some, such as chameleons, will only drink from water droplets on plants and it is important to mist the tank several times a day. Most lizards should be regularly sprayed with water to prevent skin problems associated with low humidity.

Amphibians

Amphibian species include the frogs, toads, salamanders and newts. Most adults are terrestrial but return to the water to breed and the larval stages are aquatic. Adult amphibians are carnivorous and since feeding is initiated by the movement of prey, live prey is usually required. However, some species may adapt to feeding on dead prey, meat, tinned dog food or even commercial pelleted diets. Raw meat must be supplemented with calcium (10 mg/g of meat). Captive amphibians should be fed twice weekly.

Adult frogs and toads feed on insects such as fruit flies, crickets and mealworms, and large toads will also eat mice. Aquatic species may eat fish and prepared fish diets. Salamanders eat earthworms, slugs, insects and prepared fish diets. Larval stages are herbivorous and feed on algae initially, or food sprinkled on the water. As they mature, aquatic prey (small crustaceans) and then larger insects or animals are eaten.

Ornamental fish

One of the difficulties in feeding ornamental fish is that, with a few exceptions such as the goldfish, they are rarely kept in a single species environment. Anatomical differences and variations in feeding strategies complicate the formulation of a single diet which will meet all the requirements of a mixed community, which may include representatives of herbivorous, omnivorous and carnivorous fish species (see Table 9.23).

An adequate delivery of nutrients is essential for the optimum health of the fish, but in a closed aquatic environment, overfeeding and poor diet formulation can have a detrimental effect on conditions in the aquarium. Waste, in the form of uneaten food, undigested food and the excreted metabolic breakdown products of protein, will directly pollute the living environment and can pose a serious threat to the health of aquarium fish. To minimise the risk of pollution-induced stress, the diet must be palatable, easily digested, nutritionally balanced and of high biological value. A number of commercial diets are available for ornamental fish. Nutritionally complete diets are marketed as pellets, flakes and granules and other, complementary, foods include certain pond foods and frozen insect larvae, bloodworms and cockles.

Incomplete foods should be fed with care and although they are useful 'treats' for aquarium fish, an excessive intake may result in dietary imbalance. Live aquatic food, such as *Daphnia* or *Tubifex* spp., is sometimes offered but may represent a disease risk and prefrozen packs are considered safer. Fish kept in an established pond may feed on the pond's natural flora and fauna, so complete diets are seldom required. Species which are kept in relatively bare display ponds, such as koi carp, will require a complete diet.

Of the complete diets available, flake formats offer versatility in that they can be floated on the water for surface

Table 9.23 Maintenance feeding requirement of five popular species of ornamental fish (after Pannevis and Earle, 1994)

Fish species	Fish size (g/fish)	Maintenance feeding requirement (% BW food/day)	Maintenance feeding requirement (mg food/(fish. day))
Goldfish	3.60	0.40	14.40
	4.80	0.20	11.50
	8.10	0.30	25.80
	11.70	0.20	18.30
Neon tetras	0.18	1.90	3.80
Leopard danio	0.31	≤ 2.4	≤ 7.2
Kribensis	1.10	≤ 1.0	≤ 10.2
Moonlight gourami	1.90	≤ 1.5	≤ 28.5

feeders or submerged to sink slowly for middle and bottom feeders. Since the flakes are easily broken up into smaller pieces, they provide an excellent single food for a range of species and sizes of fish. Granules offer lower leaching of nutrients because their surface area to volume ratio is larger, and different granule sizes and densities may be used to target different groups of fish in the aquarium.

As a general guideline, fish kept in a community tank should be fed to satiation two or three times per day. This allows close inspection of both the fish and tank on a regular basis. Feeding to satiation involves the continuous addition of small amounts of food to the aquarium until the fish stop feeding eagerly and normally is achieved in a few minutes or less, depending on the tank size and stocking density.

It should be emphasised that pollution from nitrogenous waste is a considerable threat to the health of fish held in a closed water volume. Correct diet formulation and feeding regimen can improve protein utilisation and help to minimise pollution, but water quality should be maintained through regular water changes or, in the larger aquaria, through the use of filter systems which must be properly maintained.

Cage birds

Passerine bird species, such as the canary and zebra finch, eat a wide variety of insects, fruit and small seeds to obtain a balanced diet in the wild. Captive birds should be fed a mixture of seeds and fruit which mimic the bird's natural feeding ecology. Similarly, *psittacine* birds, such as parrots, budgerigars, cockatoos, cockatiels, macaws and parakeets, seek out a natural diet containing a wide range of insects, fruit and seeds, but in captivity they are commonly fed only seed mixes which are composed predominantly of sunflower seeds that are high in fat but low in calcium and vitamin A. This type of diet may predispose the bird to obesity or nutritional disorders and the problem is compounded in some individuals that become addicted to sunflower seeds.

Commercial diets formulated to meet the needs of different types of bird are preferred to home-formulated diets. All-seed diets are unlikely to be nutritionally complete for birds and careful vitamin/mineral supplementation will be required. Although commercial, balanced diets need no supplementation, supplementary foods such as green vegetables (lettuce, chickweed, parsley, watercress), sprouted seeds, root vegetables, fruit (apples, plums, oranges, grapes, tomatoes) may be offered to provide variety and, in home-prepared diets, nutritional balance. These foods may be mixed with cooked egg, chicken, cheese or milk. Millet sprays are often fed to adult budgerigars, but if soaked in hot water and left for 24 hours, they can also provide a useful toy and food for young budgerigars and canaries.

Small birds have high metabolic rates and energy requirements, so it is important that a continuous supply of food is available. Empty husks should be blown from the top of the food on a frequent basis to avoid mistakes in judging how much the bird has actually eaten. Food may be provided in seed hoppers but young birds may be fed from the floor of the cage until they are familiar with alternative feeding systems. Fresh water or milk and water (for breeding and moulting birds) should be available at all times.

Two types of mineral grit, insoluble and soluble, are frequently offered to companion birds as a dietary supplement. Insoluble grit, such as quartz or other forms of silica, remains in the gizzard where it may assist in the mechanical digestion of food and, thus, improve digestibility of the diet. Soluble grit, such as oyster shell or cuttlefish, is usually completely digested by birds and provides a valuable supplementary source of minerals including calcium and phosphorus. However, oversupplementation with insoluble grit is potentially hazardous and may lead to gizzard impaction and eventual death. Canaries do not appear to need insoluble grit in their diet but a source of soluble grit is essential.

KEY POINTS

- Proper nutrition is essential for the maintenance of optimum health, well-being and activity in all living creatures.
- Each species has its own specific nutrient requirements.
- Some life stages require special dietary consideration. These include growth, gestation and lactation and old age.
- Water can be considered a nutrient, as the body cannot survive without it. All species should have continuous access to fresh, clean water.
- For dogs and cats, a balanced diet is best achieved by feeding a complete food that has been formulated specifically for the species, at a given life stage. No extra supplements are advisable. Home-prepared diets should not be advised.
- Particular care should be taken over the nutrition of exotic species, providing a wide range of food items and vitamin/mineral supplements as necessary.
- All animals should be fed to maintain optimum bodyweight – the ribs should be palpable.
- Many medical conditions will respond to modification of some aspect of the diet and nutritional support is particularly important at times of illness or other forms of stress.
- Many nutrients are now known to provide health benefits above and beyond simple nutrition, and are known as functional ingredients. An example is vitamin C, which has nutritional properties but is also an antioxidant.

Further reading

Agar, S. (2001) *Small Animal Nutrition*, Butterworth-Heinemann, Oxford.

Beynon, P. H. and Cooper, J. E. (1991) *Manual of Exotic Pets*, British Small Animal Veterinary Association, Gloucester.

Burger, I. (1993) *The Waltham Book of Companion Animal Nutrition*, Pergamon Press, Oxford.

Hand, M. S., Thatcher, C. D., Remillard, R. L. and Roudebush, P. (2000) *Small Animal Clinical Nutrition*, 4th edn, Mark Morris Institute, Kansas.

Harper, E. J. and Skinner, N. D. (1998) Clinical nutrition of small psittacines and passerines, *Seminars in Avian and Exotic Pet Medicine*, vol. 7, no. 3, pp. 116–127.

Kelly, N. and Wills, J. (1996) *Manual of Companion Animal Nutrition and Feeding*, British Small Animal Veterinary Association, Gloucester.

Markwell, P. J. (1994) *Applied Clinical Nutrition of the Dog and Cat*, Waltham Centre for Pet Nutrition, Melton Mowbray.

Pannevis, M. C. and Earle, K. E. (1994) Maintenance energy requirements of five popular species of ornamental fish. *Journal of Nutrition*, vol. 124, pp. S2616–2618.

Thorne, C. (1992) *The Waltham Book of Dog and Cat Behaviour*, Pergamon Press, Oxford.

Tobin, G. (1996) Small pets – food types, nutrient requirements and nutritional disorders. In Kelly, N. and Wills, J. (eds), *Manual of Companion Animal Nutrition and Feeding*, pp. 208–225, British Small Animal Veterinary Association, Gloucester.

Wills, J. (1996) Basic principles of nutrition and feeding. In Kelly, N. and Wills, J. (eds), *Manual of Companion Animal Nutrition and Feeding*, pp. 20–21, British Small Animal Veterinary Association, Gloucester.

Wills, J. and Simpson, K. W. (eds) (1994) *The Waltham Book of Clinical Nutrition of the Dog and Cat*, Pergamon Press, Oxford.

10

Genetics and animal breeding

S. E. Long and *L. Daniels*

Learning objectives

After studying this chapter, students should be able to:

- Define the terms autosome, sex chromosome, gene, gene locus, allele, dominance and recessive, epistasis, homozygous and heterozygous.
- Describe the structure of DNA.
- Explain X inactivation.
- Describe mitotic and meiotic cell division.
- List the differences between mitotic and meiotic cell division.

Genetics is the science of inheritance, i.e. the study of how characteristics are passed on from parents to offspring. These characteristics may be the colour of the eyes, type of fur or the type of enzyme that is produced by a cell.

Genetic information is located on the **chromosomes** in the cell nucleus. Chromosomes are usually considered in pairs because one of each pair is inherited from each parent. A chromosome pair is alike and therefore said to be homologous.

- Two of the chromosomes are called the sex chromosomes and are designated X and Y.
- The female has two X chromosomes (XX), and the male has one X and one Y chromosome (XY).
- The other chromosomes are called the **autosomes**.

> *SUPPORTING DATA*
> Each species has a characteristic number of chromosomes. For example, the number of chromosomes in the cat = 38 (Fig. 10.1), dog = 78, horse = 64. If you were to weigh all the chromosomes in a cell from each of the species you would find that the weight was more or less the same. They all have roughly the same amount of genetic material, but it is cut into a different number of pieces.

The chromosomes are composed of chromatin fibres, which are long molecules of **deoxyribonucleic acid** (DNA) and associated protein. DNA has a unique structure. It consists of two strands, joined together rather like a ladder. The 'steps' of the ladder are formed by two bases, either adenine (A) and thymine (T) or guanine (G) and cytosine (C). A

> *SUPPORTING DATA*
> **DNA** If, on one side of the ladder there is a sequence of, for example AGTAACGGC, then on the other side of the ladder the sequence must be TCATTGCCG. The structure of the base pairs is such that they cause the sides of the ladder to twist, forming a double spiral, or double helix. The DNA molecule is then very tightly folded and coiled to form the chromatin fibres of the chromosome.

always links with T, and G always links with C. Thus the steps of the ladder are a sequence of base pairs and it is this sequence which forms the genes.

Genes

Genes are particular sequences of base pairs along the chain structure of DNA and it is the genes that code for the characteristic of the cell and hence the individual. Each gene is located at a particular position on the chromosome. This is called the gene locus.

The genes that are located on the sex chromosomes are said to be **sex-linked** genes. There are many more genes on the X chromosome than the Y chromosome so that sex-linked genes are more likely to be on the X than the Y.

Genes that can only be expressed in one sex are said to be **sex-limited** genes. Some genes or gene combinations are not compatible with life and are said to be **lethal factors**. If an individual receives such a gene or genes, that individual dies.

> *SUPPORTING DATA*
> - **Sex linkage**: the orange coat colour gene in the cat, or the gene for haemophilia A in the dog are examples of **sex-linked** genes on the X chromosomes.
> - **Sex limited**: the genes associated with milk quality are **sex-limited** genes because, although they are carried by males and females they can only be expressed in the female.
> - **Lethal genes**: the *Manx* gene for taillessness is dominant and in the homozygous state, is lethal and the embryo dies *in utero*

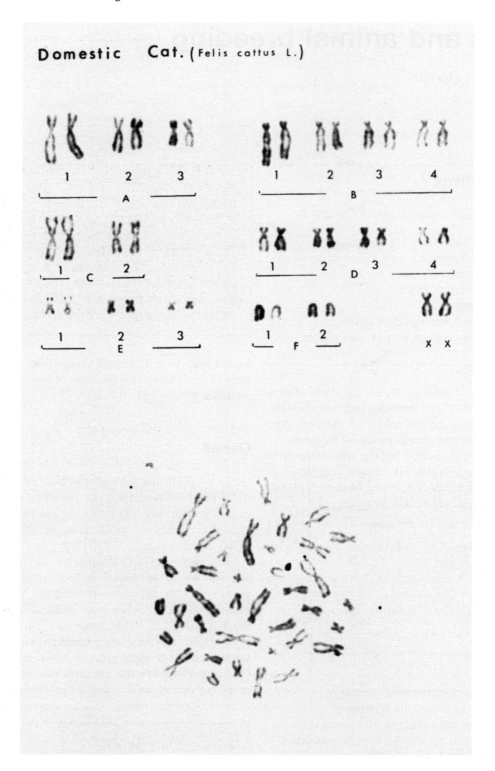

Fig. 10.1 Normal chromosome complement of a female cat. (*Top*: karyotype; *bottom*: spread.)

Sex chromosomes and X inactivation

The X chromosome is often one of the largest chromosomes and carries a number of genes that are important in the day-to-day metabolism of the cell. Since females have two X chromosomes and males have one X chromosome (and one Y chromosome) it follows that females must receive twice the number of those genes that are carried on the X compared to males. In order to compensate for this, only one of the X chromosomes in each cell of a female is activated. The other X chromosome becomes highly contracted and most of the genes are inactivated and non-functional. In some cells this contracted X chromosome is visible in the nucleus as a small dot and is known as the Barr body (after the person who first described it) or the sex chromatin. The Y chromosome is usually quite small and carries the genes that code for maleness. Very few other genes are carried on the Y chromosome.

If the chromosome is damaged at the site where the gene is located and there is misrepair, i.e. the sequence of base pairs is not the same as it was before, then one of two things may happen:

(1) The sequence is so different that the code no longer exists and so the gene is destroyed.
(2) The sequence allows coding for the characteristic but in a slightly different way, i.e. there is a gene mutation.

Alleles

Alleles are just slightly different versions of the same gene. They arise because of small mutations in genes which make their coded message slightly different from each other. There can be any number of mutations, and therefore alleles, but an individual can only have a maximum of two different alleles in a cell. This is because alleles have the same locus and there are only two loci in a cell for a gene, one on each homologous pair of chromosomes.

> The gene locus is the gene 'address' on the chromosome. Each gene has a different address and cannot 'live' at another address on the chromosome (which can be thought of as a block of flats with a series of different addresses). Since chromosomes come in homologous pairs there will be two 'blocks of flats' with the same addresses in each. Alleles are members of the same family which live at the same address, but only one allele can be 'at home' at the same time. Thus, even although there may be many members of the family (i.e. a whole series of alleles) only two alleles can be in the cell at the same time, one on each homologous chromosome at the appropriate locus.

Dominant and recessive genes

If there are two different alleles in a cell, it might be expected that both alleles would be expressed. In fact this does happen in many circumstances and the genes are said to be codominant (e.g. the genes coding for blood groups).

However, some alleles are only expressed if there are two copies of the same allele in the cell. These are said to be **recessive** genes. Genes that can be expressed when only one copy is present and which can suppress the other allele are said to be **dominant** genes.

The different actions of genes are symbolised by a capital letter for a dominant gene and a small letter for a recessive

gene. For example, the gene for black coat colour in the Labrador is dominant to the gene that codes for brown. If an animal has two copies of the same allele it is said to be **homozygous** for that allele. If an animal has two different alleles then it is said to be **heterozygous**.

> *GENE NOMENCLATURE*
> If black is dominant to brown, then the black gene is designated B and the brown gene is designated b. A black Labrador can have either BB or Bb genes because B will suppress the expression of the b gene. However, brown (i.e. chocolate) Labradors must be bb because brown is recessive and can only be expressed if two copies of the allele are present.
> • **Phenotype**: external appearance of the animal.
> • **Genotype**: genetic make up of the animal.

Epistasis

Some genes can suppress the expression of other genes that are not their alleles, i.e. they suppress the effect of genes on a different locus (e.g. the albino gene blocks the expression of all the coat-colour genes). These genes are said to show epistasis.

Cell cycle

When a cell is carrying out its normal functions, it is said to be in interphase or G1 (G stands for 'gap'). If it wants to replicate itself it has to first synthesise new genetic material and this is called the synthesis (or S) stage. This is followed by a resting stage, called G2 and then there is separation of the new genetic material into the two new cells. This is the nuclear division or M phase. The two new cells can then get on with their jobs so they are again said to be in interphase. There is thus a cell cycle (Fig. 10.2.)

Cell replication

Mitosis

When a cell replicates, it is important that the genetic material replicates exactly, otherwise new cells would not be exactly the same as the originals. Many cells are continually replicating (e.g. cells from the lining of the intestine) and it is important that the new cells can carry on the job of the old.

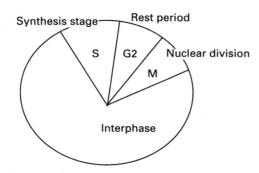

Fig. 10.2 The cell cycle.

The actual separation of the genetic material to the new cells is a dynamic process but for the purposes of description it has been divided into four stages:

- Prophase.
- Metaphase.
- Anaphase.
- Telophase.

Meiosis

A different type of cell division is necessary for those cells that are going to develop into gametes (ova and sperm). This is called meiotic division, and its stages are similar to those of mitotic division. However, it is a longer and more complicated process because the chromosomes have to be separated into different gametes in such a way that the total number is reduced by half and yet there is still one copy of each pair of alleles that was present in the parent cell. In this way, when the two gametes fuse at fertilisation to form a zygote, the new individual has the correct number of chromosomes and the right combination of genes in order that each cell can do its job. Thus, each individual receives half its chromosomes (and hence half the genes) from one parent and half from the other.

During the stages of meiotic division, new DNA is synthesised in the S phase of the cell cycle, as with mitosis, and the new chromosomes are held together at the centromeres. However, the prophase in meiosis is much longer than in mitosis.

DIFFERENCES BETWEEN MITOSIS AND MEIOSIS
- In meiotic prophase the homologous chromosomes lie side by side, whilst in mitosis they do not.
- In meiotic metaphase I the homologous chromosomes line up on the metaphase plate side by side, whilst in mitosis they line up one below the other.
- In mitosis the nuclear membrane reforms at telophase, but in meiosis this does not happen at telophase I.

Identification of animals carrying a recessive gene

Animals homozygous for a particular gene will always breed true when bred together, but heterozygous animals will sometimes produce offspring which are homozygous for the recessive gene. Usually (but not always), the recessive gene is unwanted, so that breeders would like to be able to identify those animals that are heterozygous carriers of a recessive gene and avoid breeding from them. Identification of the recessive carrier can be done by test mating to either a homozygous recessive animal or to a known heterozygous recessive carrier.

CROSSING TO A HOMOZYGOUS RECESSIVE ANIMAL

If you have a black Labrador and you want to know whether its genotype is BB or Bb then you can cross it with a chocolate (bb) Labrador.
- If the black Labrador is BB then all the offspring will be black, although their genotype will be Bb.
- If the black Labrador is Bb, it will still produce black puppies, but it is also able to produce chocolate (bb) puppies.

How this arises is demonstrated below.

Checkerboard for determining the genotype of offspring:
Bb (father) × bb (mother)

Sperm of father: Eggs of mother:	B	b	
b	Bb	bb	
b	Bb	bb	Offspring

It can be calculated mathematically that if a dog with a dominant phenotype produces seven phenotypically dominant puppies when mated to a homozygous recessive dog, then you can be 99% sure that its genotype is homozygous dominant. The more phenotypically dominant puppies that are produced the more sure you can be that the genotype is homozygous dominant. Of course, if only one recessive puppy is produced, irrespective of the number of dominant puppies, then you know the phenotypically dominant dog must be a carrier of the recessive gene. You do not have to mate your dog to the same homozygous recessive dog to get the offspring; it is the number of offspring that is important.

Crossing to a known heterozygous animal

If there are no homozygous recessive animals available it is possible to carry out the test mating with a known carrier of the recessive gene.

There are exceptions to this law due to **linkage**. Genes separate independently because of the processes during meiosis, in particular because of the phenomenon of crossing over. This causes genes on the same chromosome to be separated. However, the closer on the chromosome that two genes lie, the less likely it is that the crossing over will separate them. Therefore, genes lying close to each other on a chromosome are said to be linked, and if an animal inherits one of the linked genes it is very likely that it will inherit the other gene. This is an advantage if both genes are desirable but a big disadvantage if a breeder is trying to retain one gene and eradicate the other.

> ### CROSSING TO A KNOWN HETEROZYGOUS ANIMAL
>
> If a black Labrador has previously produced a chocolate offspring, then that black Labrador *must* be Bb, i.e. a known heterozygote. We can mate our unknown black Labrador with this known heterozygote. If our unknown black Labrador is really Bb then the checkerboard will be:
>
> | Sperm of father: | B | b |
> | --- | --- | --- |
> | Eggs of mother: | | |
> | B | BB | Bb |
> | b | Bb | bb |
>
> i.e. a chocolate Labrador (bb) *could* be produced.

This time, 16 phenotypically dominant (BB black) puppies would have to be produced before you could be 99% sure that the animal was homozygous dominant. Again, these puppies do not have to be produced from a single mating and the birth of only one recessive puppy will prove the dog to have been a carrier of the recessive gene.

Both these matings, i.e. to a homozygous recessive animal or a known heterozygous animal are called the **backcross to the recessive**. The animals that are mated are the parent generation and the offspring are the **filial** generation or F1 generation. If the offspring were to be mated they would produce the F2 generation and so on.

Multifactorial inheritance and the influence of environment

Some characteristics are governed by single genes but many others are controlled by the combination of a number of genes. Such characteristics are said to be **polygenic.** Variation in the genes controlling these polygenic traits will cause a variation in the characteristic.

Furthermore, the degree to which these genes can be expressed may be influenced by the environment. In other words the final production of a characteristic is **multifactorial** (i.e. having many causes). For example, the size of a dog will depend upon its genes but also on the amount of food that is available. There is great scope for variation, but such characteristics are difficult to control by selective breeding because of the number of different factors that are involved.

Inheritance of more than one pair of genes

Animals obviously have a large number of genes, but each is inherited without being influenced by the presence of other genes. This is Mendel's second law.

> Mendel (1822–1884) was an Austrian monk and a biologist. He did not know anything about chromosomes or the mechanism of cell division but he knew that the process was orderly and organised such that one could predict the outcome of different matings.
> - **Mendel's first law**: alleles separate to different gametes. This describes the outcome of meiosis.
> - **Mendel's second law states**: each pair of alleles separated independently of every other pair of alleles.

Breeding strategies

When breeders wish to ensure that animals breed true they try to make them homozygous for the genes governing the desirable characteristics.

- **Inbreeding** is the breeding of two individuals more closely related than the population as a whole. Related individuals are more likely to have the same alleles and so more likely to produce offspring which will be homozygous for the genes. The more closely they are related the more likely it is that they will have the same alleles. Therefore, the closer the inbreeding, the more likely is it that the offspring will be homozygous. Inbreeding is a very good way of 'fixing' a characteristic (i.e. creating homozygosity), but inbreeding will fix the 'bad' alleles as well as the good. This is why inbreeding is generally regarded as dangerous.
- **Line breeding** is a form of inbreeding which involves mating within a certain family or line and aims to maintain a relationship with a particular popular ancestor (e.g. show champion). In general, although the animals that are

mated are related, they are not so closely related as, for example, father and daughter or brother and sister. They are more likely to be grandparents and grandchildren or cousins. In this way it is hoped that the 'bad' alleles will be different in the two animals to be mated and so not be homozygous in the offspring.

- **Outcrossing** (or outbreeding) is the mating of two individuals less closely related than the population as a whole. This will mask the effects of recessive genes that are considered to be 'bad'. The rationale behind this is that such individuals are unlikely to have the same bad alleles and so the offspring will be heterozygous. This results in hybrid vigour or heterosis, which is when the offspring of an outcross seem to be 'bigger and better' than their parents. Unfortunately, such individuals will not breed true because they are heterozygous and not homozygous for their alleles.

Parentage analysis

When a dog breeder requires an analysis to prove the parentage of a puppy this may require several blood samples being submitted to the laboratory, e.g. the puppy, the two parents and even the grandparents in some situations. Cat parentage can also be determined by similar analysis.

PARENTAGE ANALYSIS

When looking at a number of different loci, e.g. those governing red cell surface antigens, the combination of different loci creates a unique picture of an individual. The combination of the alleles is inherited from the parents and so can be used for parentage analysis.

Modern techniques of parentage analysis now look at the sequences of base pairs in the DNA molecule itself. (This is a little like constructing a bar code similar to that on goods in the supermarket!) Patterns of sequences found in the DNA of the offspring must also occur in one or both of the parents. If enough sequences are examined, no two individuals will have exactly the same pattern (or bar code) and so a genetic 'fingerprint' can be made.

Breed variation

Selection for various different characteristics has resulted in a number of different breeds. This has been more extensive with dogs than with cats. Dogs can be divided into seven breed groups recognised by the English Kennel Club. The Governing Council of the Cat Fancy (GCCF) recognise and classify pedigree cats.

Deformities and malformations

Any deviation from the normal anatomy is described as a malformation or deformity. These can arise during foetal development or be acquired during life.

Congenital abnormalities

The term simply means that it was present at birth. Congenital abnormalities may or may not be genetic in origin.

The term **phenocopy** is one used to describe an abnormality that looks like a genetic defect but which has been caused by an environmental effect, such as nutrition or drug administration. This can make it extremely difficult to determine whether an abnormality is really genetic in origin.

Inherited defects are caused by the genes acquired from the parents or acquired due to mutations during gametogenesis. There are many genetic abnormalities and some are described in the books listed under Further reading.

Abnormalities caused by single gene defects for which there are tests available to identify heterozygous carrier animals:

- CLAD – Irish Setters, Irish Red and White Setters.
- Congenital stationary night blindness in Briards.
- Copper toxicosis in Bedlington Terriers.
- Fucosidosis in English Springer Spaniels.
- PRA in Irish Setters.
- Pyruvate kinase deficiency in West Highland White Terriers.
- Haemophilia.

Genetic abnormalities for which there are eradication schemes:

- Numerous eye defects.
- Hip dysplasia.
- Elbow dysplasia.

KEY POINTS
- Understanding of basic genetic principles will help the veterinary nurse in the administration of control schemes for the eradication of genetic abnormalities in animals.
- The genetic material is genes on the chromosomes within the cell nucleus.
- Slight variations of each gene are called alleles for that gene. There can be any number of different alleles of a gene but an individual animal can only possess a maximum of two alleles. Alleles interact either in a dominant or recessive manner, or they may be co-dominant.
- Genetically determined characteristics, and abnormalities, can be governed by single genes, a combination of a number of genes or by the interaction of genes and the environment.

Further reading

Animal Health Trust web-site: http://www.aht.org.uk

Nicholas, F. W. (1987) *Veterinary Genetics*, Clarendon, Oxford.

Robinson, R. (1990) *Genetics for Dog Breeders*, 2nd edn, Pergamon, Oxford.

Vella, C. et al (1999) *Robinson's Genetics for Cat Breeders and Veterinarians*, 4th edn, Butterworth–Heinemann, Oxford.

11

Exotic pets and wildlife

J. E. Cooper, C. J. Dutton and *J. Belle*

Learning objectives

After studying this chapter, students should be able to:

- Appreciate the wide range of less familiar animals that may be presented for veterinary attention.
- Understand the important biological differences between mammals, birds and reptiles and how these influence their care.
- Be able to advise on the choice of an exotic pet.
- Be aware in theory of methods of housing, handling, sexing and identification of different species, including fish and invertebrates.
- Realise the different approaches needed to anaesthetise and perform surgery on the diverse species that are being presented at practices.
- Be familiar with the available literature and relevant sources of information.

'Exotics', sometimes called the 'other' pets, are an important feature of veterinary practice in Britain and many other parts of the world. The definition of 'exotics' is imprecise. Strictly the term means 'foreign, bizarre' but in practice an exotic includes any small pet that is not a dog or a cat and encompasses wild animals brought in as casualties. They present an exciting challenge to the veterinary nurse, who is often the first and most immediate point of contact for the client.

Anatomy and physiology

Many exotic pets are **vertebrates** and share various anatomical and physiological similarities. **Invertebrates**, such as insects and spiders, are substantially different. The main groups of exotic pets and their features are given in Table 11.1.

Mammals and birds are **endothermic**, or 'warm-blooded'. An endothermic animal is able to maintain its own body temperature above that of its surroundings, within certain limits, using internal (physiological) control mechanisms. Thus a rabbit's body temperature is likely to be 39.5°C in both summer and winter.

Reptiles, amphibians and invertebrates are **ectothermic**, or 'cold-blooded'. With very few exceptions they are unable to control their body temperature by intrinsic (internal) means and so it will fluctuate depending upon the ambient temperature. However, an ectothermic animal uses external or behavioural means (e.g. basking, burrowing) to control its body temperature.

Mammals

The mammals that are most commonly kept as pets are set out in Table 11.2. which shows that they fall into three different groups (Orders): the Rodentia, the Lagomorpha and the Carnivora. Most of them can be considered domesticated species and many that have become popular as pets were first used as laboratory animals. Rabbits are now the third most commonly kept mammal in the UK and have attracted increasing interest from veterinary surgeons and veterinary nurses. Rabbits present many health and welfare challenges and it is often the nurse who is consulted over such matters. Other species are sometimes encountered in veterinary practice, such as the diminutive Roborovski's hamster or the large Shaw's jird, but knowledge of their close relatives means that they can be treated as if they were hamsters or gerbils although they are possibly a little less amenable to handling.

Although small mammals share many anatomical features, there are some differences that are relevant to the biological and veterinary care of these species (Tables 11.3 and 11.4). The veterinary nurse should take every opportunity to become familiar with the normal features, in order to be able to detect ill-health or abnormalities more easily.

Having once studied the anatomy and physiology of the dog and cat in detail (see Chapter 2, Anatomy and Physiology), veterinary nurses should be able to note the external features of the herbivorous and omnivorous small mammals (i.e. excluding the carnivorous ferret) where they differ:

- Both the herbivorous and the omnivorous small mammals have chisel-shaped incisors for gnawing; they also have flat tables of cheek teeth for grinding coarse vegetable matter. The rodents have one pair of incisors in both upper and lower jaws. Rabbits have one pair in the lower jaw but two in the upper (one large and a smaller pair directly behind them). All the teeth of rabbits and herbivorous rodents are what is known as **open-rooted**: they grow continually throughout life.
- The joint surfaces of the temporomandibular joint are flat compared with those of the dog and cat, allowing both

Table 11.1 Main groups of exotic pets and their features

Group	Features	Examples
Vertebrates		
Mammals (Mammalia)	Internal skeleton Endothermic ('warm blooded') Skin bears hairs Lungs Produce live young Feed young on milk Internal fertilisation	Rat (*Rattus norvegicus*) Mouse (*Mus musculus*) Guinea pig (*Cavia porcellus*) Chinchilla (*Chinchilla laniger*) Syrian hamster (*Mesocricetus auratus*) Mongolian gerbil (*Meriones unguiculatus*) Ferret (*Mustela putorius furo*) Rabbit (*Oryctolagus cuniculus*) Sugar gliders (*Petaurus breviceps*)
Birds (Aves)	Internal skeleton Endothermic Wings Skin bears feathers Scales on legs Lungs Eggs with hard shell Internal fertilisation	Budgerigar (*Melopsittacus undulatus*) African grey parrot (*Psittacus erithacus*) Amazon parrot (*Amazona* spp.) Canary (*Serinus canaria*) Cockatiel (*Nymphicus hollandicus*) Fowl (chicken) (*Gallus domesticus*) Pigeon (*Columba livia*)
Reptiles (Reptilia)	Internal skeleton Ectothermic ('cold-blooded') Dry skin with scales Lungs Oviparous (eggs with hard or soft shells) or ovo-viviparous (live-bearing) Internal fertilisation	Common iguana (*Iguana iguana*) Mediterranean tortoise (*Testudo* spp.) Box tortoise (*Terrapene* spp.) Garter snake (*Thamnophis* spp.) Corn snake (*Elaphe guttata*) Leopard gecko (*Eublepharis macularius*)
Amphibians (Amphibia)	Internal skeleton Ectothermic Moist skin with mucous and sometimes poison glands Oviparous, occasionally ovo-viviparous Lungs in adult, gills in larva (tadpole) Larval form External fertilisation	Common toad (*Bufo bufo*) Marine toad (*Bufo marinus*) European tree frog (*Hyla arborea*) Edible frog (*Rana esculenta*) Great-crested newt (*Triturus cristatus*) European salamander (*Salamandra salamandra*) Axolotl (*Ambystoma mexicanum*)
Fish (Pisces)	Internal skeleton Ectothermic Moist skin with scales Gills Oviparous (eggs without shells) or ovo-viviparous (live-bearing) Sometimes larval form Usually external fertilisation	Goldfish (*Carassius auratus*) Koi carp (*Cyprinius carpio*) Guppy (*Lebistes reticulatus*) Angel fish (*Pterophyllum scalare*) Platies (*Xiphophorus* spp.) Siamese fighting fish (*Betta splendens*) Discus (*Symphysodon discus*) Oscar (*Astronotus ocellatus*) Seahorse (*Hippocampus* spp.)
Invertebrates		
Arthropods (Arthropoda)	External skeleton (cuticle) Paired jointed limbs Segmented Open vascular system Oviparous or viviparous	Indian stick insect (*Carausius morosus*) Red-kneed tarantula (*Euthalus smithii*) Tree bird spiders (*Avicularia* spp.) Tree crabs (*Coenobita* spp.) Emperor scorpion (*Pandinus imperator*)
Molluscs (Mollusca)	Shell but no cuticle Ventral muscular foot Unsegmented Open vascular system Oviparous or viviparous	African land snail (*Achatina* spp.) Garden snail (*Helix aspersa*)

sideways and backwards-and-forwards movement of the lower jaw. Lower in the gastrointestinal tract they have a relatively large **caecum**, where bacteria break down the cellulose of plant cell walls to allow the animal to make use of this plant material as food.

- The rabbit and all the small rodents practise **caecotrophy**, which is the eating of faeces. The rabbit passes two different types of faeces: the dry pellets that we consider 'normal', and, at night, **caecal** pellets, which are dark in colour and covered with mucus so that they tend to stick

Table 11.2 Small mammal species commonly kept as pets

Order	Sub-order	Family	Species	English name
Rodentia[a]	Myomorpha	Muridae	*Rattus norvegicus*	Fancy rat
			Mus musculus	Mouse
		Cricetidae	*Meriones unguiculatus*	Mongolian gerbil
			Mesocricetus auratus	Syrian hamster
			Phodopus sungorus	Russian hamster[b]
			Cricetulus griseus	Chinese hamster[b]
	Hystricomorpha	Caviidae	*Cavia porcellus*	Guinea pig
		Chinchillidae	*Chinchilla laniger*	Chinchilla
	Sciuromorpha	Sciuridae	*Tamias sibiricus*	Siberian chipmunk
Lagomorpha		Leporidae	*Oryctolagus cuniculus*	Rabbit
Carnivora		Mustelidae	*Mustela putorius furo*	Ferret
Marsupialla		Petauridae	*Petaurus breviceps*	Sugar glider

[a] *Note the division of the family 'Rodentia', the rodents. The 'mouse-like' rodents are further divided into the rats and mice, and the gerbils and hamsters. All these small rodents are omnivorous. The Sciuromorpha or squirrels, like rodents that are also omnivores, and the Siberian chipmunk has a lifestyle very like that of the squirrels of Europe and North America. Hystricomorpha are the third group of rodents: they are herbivores and come from South America*
[b] *The Russian and Chinese are the dwarf hamsters. Unlike the Syrian hamsters they are social animals, living in family groups in the wild*

together and emerge in a mass. These caecal pellets are eaten directly from the anus and complete a second passage of the gut so that all possible nutrients are extracted from the food.

- The hamsters have cheek pouches, used for carrying food back to the nest when on extensive foraging expeditions. The chinchillas and the small pet rodents tend to hold their food in their front paws while feeding. They are able to do this as they can supinate their front paws – rotating the radius to twist the carpus and manus, as can cats (but not dogs).

There are also certain features to note regarding skin and glands:

- Rabbits have no footpads: their feet are covered with hair.
- Female rabbits have a **dewlap** (a large fold of skin under the chin) from which they pluck fur to line the nest.
- Gerbils have a large skin gland on the mid-ventral abdomen, which in old age may become hypertrophied.
- Syrian hamsters have glandular areas on their flanks, where the skin is darkly pigmented. Older hamsters often lose their hair in these areas.

Table 11.3 Anatomical differences in small mammals

	Mouse	Rat	Syrian hamster	Gerbil	Guinea pig	Rabbit	Ferret
Teeth	Well-developed incisors for gnawing (one upper pair, rodents; two upper pairs – one small, rabbit)						Well-developed canines for tearing
Dental formula	1003 / 1003	1003 / 1003	1003 / 1003	1003 / 1003	1013 / 1013	1033 / 1023	3131 / 3132
Ears	Hairless	Hairless	Sparse hair	Hairy	Sparse except tip	Hairy	Hairy
Cheek pouches	Absent	Absent	Present	Absent	Absent	Absent	Absent
Stomach	Simple, two distinct regions	Simple, two distinct regions	Simple, two compartments	Simple, two distinct regions	Simple	Simple	Simple
Intestine	Long	Long	Long	Long	Long	Long	Short
Gall bladder	Present	Absent	Present	Present	Present	Present	Present
Appendix	Small	Small	Small	Small	Large	Very large	No caecum or appendix
Mammary glands	No teats in male	No teats in male	No teats in male	No teats in male	Teats in male	Teats in male	Teats in male
Testes	Retractable	Retractable	Retractable	Retractable	Retractable	Retractable	Not retractable
Scent glands	None	None	On flanks	Ventral midline	Perineal	Perineal	Anal sacs
Tail	No hair, scales	No hair, scales	Hair	Hair	No tail	Hair	Hair

Table 11.4 General biology of small animals

	Average life expectancy	Maturity	Oestrus	Gestation period	Size of litter	Age at weaning	Adult weight (g)	Temperature (°C)
Rabbit	M 8 years+ F 6 years	3 months+	Induced ovulation Oestrus Jan–Oct/Nov	28–32 days	2–7	6 weeks	varies	38.5
Guinea pig	4–7 years	M 8–10 weeks F 4–5 weeks	15–16 day cycle	60–72 days (average 65)	2–6	3–3.5 weeks	750–1000	38–39
Rat	3 years	6 weeks+	Every 4–5 days	20–22 days	6–12	21 days+	400–800	38
Mouse	1–2.5 years	3–4 weeks	Every 4–5 days	19–21 days	5–1	18 days+	20–40	37.5
Gerbil	1.5–2.5 years	10–12 weeks	Every 4–6 days	24–26 days	3–6	21–28 days	70–130 (M > F)	38
Syrian hamster	1.5–2 years	6–10 weeks	Every 4 days	15–18 days	3–7	21–28 days	85–150	37–38
Russian hamster	1.5–2 years	6–10 weeks	Every 4 days	19–20 days	3–5	21–28 days		
Chinese hamster	1.5–2 years	6–10 weeks	Every 4 days	20–22 days	3–5	21–28 days		
Chinchilla	10 years (up to 15)	8 months	Seasonally polyoestrous Cycle 30–35 days Nov–May	111 days	2 or 3 (1–4)	6–8 weeks	M 400 F 500	38–39
Chipmunk	M 3 years F 5 years	1 year	Seasonally polyoestrous Cycle 14 days Mar–Sep 2 litters/year	28–32 days	2–6	6–7 weeks	80–130	38 (NB: hibernation)
Ferret	5–7 years	6–9 months	Induced ovulation Oestrus Feb/Mar–Sep	42 days	2–6 (up to 10)	8 weeks	500–2000	38.8

- Guinea pigs have a greasy glandular area just above the tail, which is quite normal and should not be considered pathological.
- Chinchilla fur is very dense. These animals were originally imported to be bred for their pelts (skins). The coat over the body has no guard hairs and there may be up to 70 fine downy hairs per skin follicle. The tail does have a covering of guard hairs and there are fewer downy hairs in this region.

Sexing small mammals

This is more difficult in some species than in others. In all female rodents, the genital and urinary orifices are separate so that there are three orifices (from the most dorsal: anal, genital and urinary); in the male there are only two. However, the genital orifice is not patent much of the time and is often only to be seen as a patch or strip of naked skin. It becomes patent when the animal is in season and prior to parturition. In any female rodent, the separate orifices make it easy to distinguish whether a discharge or bleeding is urinary or vaginal in origin.

Rabbits, and most rodents, have large, open inguinal rings which allow the testes to be retracted into the abdomen. In all the small pet mammals except the Russian hamster, the descended testes are obvious in the mature male. Otherwise the sexes can be distinguished by the presence of the vaginal membrane in the female and the greater anogenital distance in the male.

- **Rabbits** are not difficult to sex once the testes have descended, as they lie in scrotal sacs on either side of the penis, which is easily protruded in the adult rabbit, slightly less easily in the young. The vulva of the female is a slit, pointed at the front, whereas the prepuce is more circular.
- **Guinea pigs** are easy to sex from birth: the penis can be protruded with gentle pressure around the relevant orifice or can be felt through the skin.
- **Chinchillas** can be difficult to sex unless one is aware that there is a significant urethral prominence in the female, which may be mistaken for a penis. The ano-genital distance is greater in the male and the female has a vaginal membrane.
- In the **ferret**, the opening of the prepuce is on the belly, near the umbilicus. The testes are only within the scrotum during the breeding season. The penis contains the os penis (a bone) that can be easily palpated.

Birds

Birds may be kept either as pets (often individually, or in pairs, in cages indoors) or for breeding or exhibition. Larger species and most wild birds are bred in aviaries but the smaller domesticated species, such as budgerigars and canaries, are usually bred in custom-built bird-rooms.

Domesticated species are those that have been bred in captivity for long enough for significant genetic changes to be established – such as the development of different breeds (in domestic fowl and canaries) or different colour mutations (in the budgerigar and the peach-faced lovebird).

There are 28 different orders of birds but most of those presented for veterinary attention are likely to fall into one of the following:

- Order Psittaciformes – budgerigar, parrots, etc.
- Order Passeriformes – perching birds, including canary, finches.
- Order Falconiformes – diurnal (not nocturnal) birds of prey such as hawks, falcons.
- Order Strigiformes – owls.
- Order Galliformes – domestic fowl, pheasants, quail.
- Order Anseriformes – ducks, geese and swans.

Table 11.5 describes some of the birds commonly kept in aviculture and also some of the different groups of non-domesticated species. Table 11.6 shows the significance of some of the anatomical features of various species.

Although the anatomy of birds follows the basic vertebrate pattern, it also shows a number of important differences from mammals, including adaptations for flight – especially by keeping weight to a minimum.

Skeleton and muscles

- The bones have thin cortices and some of them (pneumatised) contain an air sac as an extension of the respiratory system.
- Throughout the skeleton the number of joints (Fig. 11.1) is reduced to facilitate flying. The fusion of many of the vertebrae reduces mobility in the trunk region but a long, very flexible neck allows the bird to reach most parts of its body with its beak.
- An enlarged sternum (keel bone) allows the attachment of very bulky flight muscles, which in some species may comprise up to one-quarter of the bodyweight of the bird.
- The pelvis is modified to allow the passage of a large egg. This is achieved by having an open pubis rather than a symphysis.
- The weight of the skull is reduced by cavities in certain bones, reduction of the maxillary region and there being no teeth.
- In many species the tongue is rigid, containing a lingual bone, whereas in many parrots the tongue is thick, fleshy and very mobile and is used to manipulate food.
- There is a **quadrate bone** lying between the maxilla and each dentary, producing two joints between upper and lower jaw. This allows a variable amount of backwards-and-forwards movement in some species (it is particularly well developed in the parrots). There is also a joint between the upper part of the beak and the rest of the skull – the **craniofacial hinge** – and again the amount of movement varies from species to species.

Table 11.5 Bird species commonly kept		
Name	**Origin**	**Description**
Domestic species		
Budgerigar (*Melopsittacus undulatus*)	Australia	Many colour varieties. 'Show' budgies are much larger than the wild type
Canary (*Serinus canaria*)	Canary Islands	Many different breeds, some judged on colour, some on colour and 'type' and some on their song
Cockatiels (*Nymphicus hollandicus*)	Australia	Many colour varieties
Peach-faced lovebirds (*Agapornis roseicollis*)	Africa	In the wild a green bird with a pink/orange face and blue rump. Now in many colour varieties. An aggressive species
Zebra finches (*Poephila guttata*)	Australia	A prolific breeder, now in many colour mutations
Bengali finch (*Lonchura domestica*)	East Asia	A finch kept in its own right or as a foster parent for species unwilling to care for eggs or young in captivity

Other species that may now be considered to be domesticated are the Indian ringneck parakeet and the Australian Gouldian Finch, both of which are produced in many colour mutations

Different groups of non-domesticated species commonly kept in aviculture	
Foreign finches	Usually Australian, African or East Asian species
Softbills	Such as Pekin robins, mynah birds, various starlings and thrushes
British birds	It is permitted to keep certain species of British birds in captivity, but they must not be taken from the wild without a licence, and any young that are to be sold or exhibited must have been aviary-bred and close-ringed (ABCR) during the first few days of life
Grass parakeets	Small Australian parakeets related to the budgerigar. Examples are the elegant, the splendid, and Bourke's grass parakeet
Parrots	Many species kept by enthusiasts and others by commercial breeders to supply the demand for English bred, hand-reared (EBHR) parrots as pets
Waterfowl and pheasants	Many species are endangered or threatened in the wild and are kept successfully by aviculturists. Birds that are to be kept 'free range' must not be allowed to escape into the wild and so may need to be pinioned or contained in some way

- The number of digits in the forelimb (wing) is reduced to two: digit III, and a much reduced digit I which forms the **alula** (bastard wing) that carries a few feathers which are important for control at take-off and landing. In some adult and many embryonic birds there may be a claw on the alula.

Feathers

The plumage, composed of keratin, provides lightweight but strong feathers which help to insulate the bird. The feathers are divided into several groups:

- **Flight feathers** of the wings and tail are long and rigid.
- **Contour feathers** are those that make up the outer layer of feathers over most of the body. They are shorter and more flexible than the flight feathers.

- **Down feathers** and **filoplumes** lie beneath the contour feathers and provide a layer of insulation. (Birds carry very little subcutaneous fat compared with mammals.)

All feathers have the same basic structure. In the majority of birds all the feathers are shed each year during the moulting season, which in most species occurs in late summer, at the end of the breeding season. The developing feather is covered by a keratin sheath; while it is growing, a blood vessel runs up the shaft (the feather is described by aviculturists as being 'in pin', by falconers as 'in the blood'), so that damage to a feather at this stage will result in haemorrhage.

Birds keep their feathers in good order by preening. Most birds use oil from the **preen gland** on the top of the tail to waterproof them, although not all birds have a preen gland. Some birds (notably the cockatoos and cockatiel) produce a fine dust from their feathers which helps to keep the plumage in good order. Most birds in the wild bathe regularly and will do so in captivity as well, especially if encouraged.

Table 11.6 Significance of anatomical features in birds

Feature	Significance
Beak – variation in shape and size	Related to feeding habits, e.g. parrots open fruit and nuts, canaries and finches peck at seeds, raptors tear meat. Many psittacine birds also use beak for climbing
Legs and feet – variation in appearance	Related to habits and habitat, e.g. parrots climb (two toes pointing forwards, two backwards), canaries and finches perch (three toes forwards, one backwards), raptors grasp prey with talons, ducks swim with webbed feet
Wings – variation in shape and size	Related to flying, e.g. falcons have long pointed wings for hunting prey from a height, hawks have short rounded wings for quick dash through undergrowth. Some birds, e.g. penguin, ostrich, do not fly
Plumage – variation in colour and structures (e.g. crests)	Related to behaviour, e.g. recognition of own species or a mate, threat or warning to predators. Some species show sexual dimorphism, i.e. plumage differs between male and female

It is important for all birds, but particularly for falconry birds and racing pigeons, to protect the feathers and to minimise damage to the plumage when a bird is hospitalised.

Captive birds, and in particular waterfowl, may be prevented from flying by being 'pinioned'. This technique involves amputation of the terminal phalanx of one wing, causing the bird to lose balance when it attempts to fly. Non-veterinarians may pinion their birds at 2–3 days of age, but veterinarians must pinion older birds.

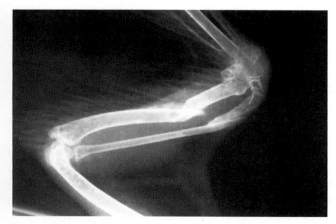

Fig. 11.1 Fractured radius and ulna in a Meller's duck (*Anas melleri*). (Good radiography facilitates diagnosis and treatment of skeletal problems in birds. Note that young growing feathers are visible on this radiograph – their vascular sheath is radiopaque.)

The gastrointestinal tract

The gastrointestinal tract in birds follows the basic vertebrate pattern of foregut, midgut and hindgut but with certain modifications (Fig. 11.2):

- There are no teeth. Some birds hold food with their feet and tear it with their beaks; others swallow food whole. In most species there is a diverticulum of the oesophagus in the ventral neck – the **crop**. This is used as a storage organ. In pigeons and parrots it produces a secretion known as **crop milk** that is used to nourish the young in the nest. There is no crop in the owls or in many diving birds.
- The stomach in most species is divided into a **proventriculus,** which is the glandular stomach, and the **ventriculus** or **gizzard**, which is a thick-walled chamber where food can be ground up and which may contain grit. There is no gizzard in birds that have a predominantly fluid diet, such as the nectar-eating (nectivorous) sunbirds and hummingbirds, and carnivorous birds, such as the birds of prey, tend to have a very thin-walled structure.
- The small intestine is short but otherwise unremarkable.
- The large intestine may or may not sport two large **caeca** (sing. caecum) from the junction between large and small intestines. This is the site for bacterial digestion in herbivorous and omnivorous species. Caeca are reduced or absent in carnivorous and nectivorous species.
- The digestive, urinary and genital tracts all open to the outside through one orifice, the **cloaca** or **vent**.

The respiratory system

The respiratory system of the bird is very different from that of the mammal and these differences have implications for anaesthesia in birds.

- The bird has no diaphragm. The main muscles of respiration are abdominal, which should never be restricted during restraint of the animal.
- The lungs are small compared with those of the mammal, and they are non-distensible. They lie close to the dorsal body wall in the cranial part of the body cavity.
- The air is drawn into and expelled from the body by the expansion and contraction of thin-walled air sacs, which are lined with serous membrane and extend throughout the body, even into some of the bones (pneumatisation).
- Air circulates through the lungs continuously, during both inspiration and expiration. This means that changes in depth of anaesthesia are likely to take place much more rapidly in birds than in mammals of comparable size.

Reptiles and amphibians

Table 11.7 shows some of the species most commonly seen in veterinary practice. Reptiles and amphibians are

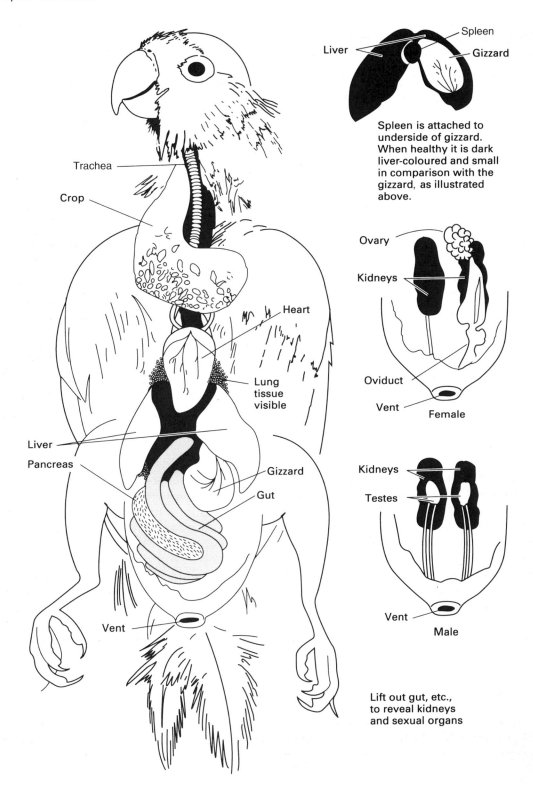

Fig. 11.2 Internal organs of a parrot.

ectothermic animals: although unable to control body temperature intrinsically, they can do so very effectively by behavioural means. For example, a lizard basks in the sun in order to raise its body temperature but it hides under a log or seeks the shade in order to lower its body temperature.

Ectothermic animals have their own **preferred body temperature** (PBT), which is the temperature range at which they can move about and feed and at which their digestive

enzymes, etc. are best able to act. Some species are tolerant of wide ranges of temperature; others come from very stable environments in the wild, where there is very little temperature variation. Examples of PBT for different reptiles are given in Table 11.8.

Some reptiles **hibernate** in cold weather. This is a complex physiological process and should not be confused with torpor induced by a sudden temperature drop. Other species

Table 11.7 Reptiles and amphibians kept as pets

	Type	Species	
Class Reptilia	Order Chelonia (tortoises, terrapins and turtles)	*Testudo hermanni*	Hermann's tortoise
		Testudo graeca	Spur-thighed tortoise
		Terrapene spp.	American box tortoise/'turtle'
		Pseudemys scripta elegans	Red-eared terrapin
	Order Squamata (snakes and lizards)	*Natrix natrix*	Grass snake
		Thamnophis spp.	Garter snake
		Elaphe guttata	Corn snake
		Elaphe obsoleta	Black rat snake
		Lampropecis spp.	King snake
		Python sebae	African rock python
		P. regius	Royal python
		P. molurus	Indian python
		P. reticulatus	Reticulated python
		Lacerta vivipara	Common lizard
		Anguis fragilis	Slow-worm
		Iguana iguana	Common or green iguana
Class Amphibia	Order Anura (frogs and toads)	*Bufo bufo*	Common toad
		Bufo marinus	Marine toad
		Xenopus spp.	Clawed toad
		Rana esculenta	Edible frog
		Rana pipiens	Leopard frog
		Hyla arborea	European tree frog
	Order Urodela (newts and salamanders)	*Triturus cristatus*	Great-crested newt
		Salamandra salamandra	European salamander
		Ambystoma mexicanum	Axolotl

aestivate, i.e. they become lethargic and they sleep because the temperature is too high and/or environmental conditions are too dry.

All reptiles have a dry skin, impervious to water and usually covered with scales. All of them shed (slough) their skins as they grow. Some, such as the tortoises, shed it in small parts; others, such as the snakes and some lizards, shed their skins at one time, often in one piece.

Some lizards can shed their tails (**autotomy**) if they are handled incorrectly, e.g. if the tail is grasped. This is a defence mechanism when it occurs in the wild: a predator's attention may be attracted to the discarded tail, allowing the lizard itself to escape unscathed. A new tail will grow but it is a poor cartilaginous replica of the original.

Although the basic anatomy of reptiles is similar to that of other vertebrates, the following special points should be noted:

- **Tortoises** and other chelonians have a modified skeleton: a bony 'box' composed of an upper part (**carapace**) and lower part (**plastron**), fused at the sides. The box consists of a modified vertebral column, ribs and sternum.
- Snakes and certain snake-like lizards have modifications related to their elongated shape: they have no limbs, or

Table 11.8 Preferred body temperatures of some reptile species (adapted from Cooper and Jackson, 1981)

Species	Activity range (°C)	PBT (°C)
Box turtle (*Terrapene ornata*)	22–35	27
Greek tortoise (*Testudo graeca*)	15–30	24
Green anole (*Anolis carolinonsis*)	30–36	34
Green (common) iguana (*Iguana iguana*)	26–42	33
Flap-necked chameleon (*Chamaeleo dilepis*)	21–36	31
Slow-worm (*Anguis fragilis*)	14–29	22
Boa constrictor (*Constrictor constrictor*)	26–37	32
Garter snake (*Thamnophis sirtalis*)	20–35	29

only vestigial limbs, and they have elongated lungs (only one functional in snakes), liver and intestine.

Reproduction

Reptiles produce eggs and they are either oviparous or ovo-viviparous:

- **Oviparous** reptiles lay their eggs within a calcareous shell (some are almost as rigid as a bird's egg but others are little more than a parchment-like membrane).
- **Ovo-viviparous** reptiles retain their eggs within the body of the female until the young are fully developed and capable of independent life.

This retention of the egg until hatching is not the same as true **viviparity**, because the developing reptile embryo is nourished only by the yolk of the egg, rather than by the mother via a placenta as is the case with viviparous mammals.

The young reptiles, whether hatched or born, emerge as small replicas of the adult and are immediately capable of feeding themselves.

Amphibians

Amphibians are often grouped and discussed with reptiles but they show many differences. In particular their skin is generally thin, mucous and permeable. Many amphibians can respire through their skin as well as using lungs (adults) or gills (larvae). The larvae metamorphose into adults.

Fish

There are three main groups of fish: the primitive Placoderms, the huge group of Osteichthyes (bony fish) and the Chondrichthyes (cartilaginous fish). Those of most relevance to veterinary practice are the bony fish (e.g. goldfish). Cartilaginous fish, such as sharks, are sometimes kept in captivity.

The type and temperature of water in which fish live are very relevant to their physiology and health, and Table 11.9 gives some examples.

Table 11.9 Water temperatures for fish

Type	Cold (up to 21°C)	Warm (21–29°C)
Freshwater	Goldfish	Guppy
Saltwater	Herring	Seahorse

Management and nutrition

Veterinary nurses are often asked for advice on the management of exotic pets, including suitable housing, feeding and general husbandry, and perhaps breeding. They are also asked which pets might be suitable in various circumstances. It is therefore important to have a good background knowledge on all aspects of pet care, as well as knowing how to handle the animals when they are brought into the practice and how to look after those that become hospitalised.

Choosing a pet

The choice of pet depends upon many factors and Table 11.10 suggests the main questions that should be asked of a potential owner who is considering an exotic as a pet. Clients may want pets for various purposes and these requirements have to be taken into consideration when making a choice. In all cases the animal must be easily handled and managed, relatively robust and unlikely to transmit disease. Examples of specific circumstances are given in Table 11.11.

Mammals

The housing, nutrition, general management and breeding of rodents, rabbits and ferrets are summarised in Table 11.12, and the species are looked at in more detail below.

Table 11.10 Advising on choice of pet: questions to ask

Question	Explanation
Are financial considerations important?	Some species are expensive to keep
What facilities do you have?	Avoid large pets such as rabbits and parrots if the owner has no garden or lives in a flat
How much spare time do you have?	Some pets, such as parrots, need considerable attention if they are not to become bored. Others, such as fish and invertebrates, need relatively little attention
What are your domestic arrangements?	Some pets are unsuitable for young children or elderly persons. Some animals are active at night, others by day
Are there any significant human health consequences?	People who are sensitive to fur or feathers should be wary of mammals and birds. Immunosuppressed persons should only have contact with pets of known health status
What other animals do you keep?	Some species may be incompatible or difficult to keep together, e.g. small birds and cats. Commensal bacterial and other organisms of some species may cause clinical disease in others

<table>
<tr><td colspan="2">Table 11.11 Advising on choice of pet: considerations</td></tr>
<tr><td>Requirement</td><td>Considerations</td></tr>
<tr><td>A pet for children</td><td>Diurnal</td></tr>
<tr><td>A pet (companion) for elderly people</td><td>Easy to feed
Food readily obtained and affordable
Temperature needs compatible with those of owner(s)</td></tr>
<tr><td>A family pet</td><td>No risk to babies
Compatible with family's lifestyle</td></tr>
<tr><td>For educational studies in the classroom</td><td>Weekend and holiday care need consideration
Heating may be switched off
Food supply must be reliable
Continuity in terms of care</td></tr>
<tr><td>Pets for educational talks and visits</td><td>Portability
Resilient to repeated handling
No special legal requirements</td></tr>
</table>

There is also useful information on cages for small mammals in the *How to Choose …* leaflets produced by the Universities Federation for Animal Welfare (UFAW), copies of which can be given to clients – preferably before they acquire a new pet. Much useful information on the management of small mammals has resulted from their use in laboratories, and contacts with these establishments, especially animal technicians who look after the animals, can prove beneficial.

Rabbits and guinea pigs

The domesticated rabbit is of European origin, whereas the guinea pig comes from South America. In addition to being popular pets, both species are used in research and as a source of food – in the case of the guinea pig, primarily in poorer parts of South America and Africa.

Husbandry and housing Rabbits and guinea pigs are usually kept out-of-doors, although many people now also keep them entirely as indoor pets ('house' rabbits). The standard housing for the rabbit or guinea pig is a hutch, with a covered sleeping area and a wire-fronted 'living' area. Owners should be encouraged to view a grassy outdoor run as essential for these species, or to allow regular 'free-ranging' in the garden.

Rabbits are hardy in the Northern European climate and suffer only if they are unable to keep dry, or from excessively high temperatures. With an underground burrow in the wild, they are always able to escape from the rain and from the heat of the summer sun.

Guinea pigs also dislike very hot weather and may suffer if they cannot stay dry.

Rabbits and guinea pigs may (but by no means must) be taken indoors during the winter, but care should be taken that the winter accommodation is well ventilated and not overheated, as poor ventilation and overheating may predispose to respiratory disease, particularly in rabbits.

Both species are social, living in colonies in the wild. Rabbits and guinea pigs can be kept together, although in some cases problems are encountered such as rabbits mounting cavies, or the cavies chewing the rabbit's fur. Owners should be encouraged to keep rabbits together, and to keep guinea pigs together, but with certain precautions:

- Two male rabbits will fight.
- Two female rabbits may live in harmony, or one may start to exert dominance over the other when she comes into season and starts to defend the 'nest burrow' as her own.

<table>
<tr><td colspan="5">Table 11.12 Small mammal husbandry: a summary</td></tr>
<tr><td></td><td>Rabbits and guinea pigs</td><td>Rats and mice</td><td>Gerbils and hamsters</td><td>Ferrets</td></tr>
<tr><td>Housing</td><td>Hutches or floor pens or outside runs</td><td>Cages or mouse/rat houses with opportunity to climb</td><td>Cages with deep bedding for tunnelling</td><td>As rabbit and guinea pig</td></tr>
<tr><td>Bedding[a]</td><td>Newspaper plus sawdust or woodchips and hay/straw</td><td>Sawdust, shavings, woodchips, well-shredded paper</td><td>As rats and mice</td><td>As rabbit and guinea pig</td></tr>
<tr><td>Diet</td><td colspan="3">Pelleted diets are available for all species but are best supplemented with:
vegetables, fruit, seeds
Some rodents will eat and apparently benefit from live invertebrates
Rabbits and guinea pigs need hay</td><td>Meat and eggs</td></tr>
<tr><td>Special care</td><td colspan="4">All species should be kept dry in a draught-free environment
A warm area is needed if rabbits, guinea pigs or ferrets are kept out of doors
Hygiene is important: cages should be cleaned thoroughly at least once a week</td></tr>
<tr><td>Vaccines, medicines[b]</td><td>Myxomatosis and VHD vaccine may be advisable for rabbits</td><td>—</td><td>—</td><td>Distemper vaccine may be advisable</td></tr>
</table>

[a] *Avoid synthetic fibres which can wrap around limbs or cause impaction of stomach*
[b] *Avoid unnecessary use of antimicrobial agents in all species but especially rabbits and rodents*

- A male and a female rabbit will live together, and either (or preferably both) can be neutered to prevent unwanted offspring. Rabbits in the wild will form pair bonds and so obviously this is the best and most natural arrangement for them in captivity.
- A group of female guinea pigs will live together without fighting.
- Male guinea pigs will live together without fighting if there are no females within sight, sound or smell.

Feeding   As rabbits and guinea pigs are grazing animals, the most important part of their diet is good-quality **roughage** – either hay or grazing. In the absence of sufficient roughage, both species (but particularly the guinea pig) may chew the fur of companions to make up the deficiency.

In the same way that puppies, kittens or breeding or working dogs are fed differently compared with a sedentary pet, so too a young or breeding rabbit or guinea pig requires a different diet from that of a sedentary adult animal. The amount of **protein** in the diet is as important for a young rabbit or guinea pig as it is for a young dog. The pellets used by rabbit breeders usually contain approximately 18% protein; commercial rabbit and guinea pig mixes vary in protein between 12.5% and 16.5%, and the higher level should be regarded as optimum for young and breeding rabbits.

Free access to good-quality grazing can make up a shortfall in the quality of the dry feed. Remember that during the winter the food value, particularly the **vitamin** content in greens that have been standing without growing for months, is quite low.

Guinea pigs have a specific requirement for dietary **vitamin** C: animals on free range, especially during the spring, summer and autumn, usually find enough vitamin C in the growing grass but otherwise the diet should be supplemented at a rate of 50 mg per guinea pig per day (more for pregnant and lactating animals). Some guinea pig mixes now contain this vitamin but otherwise it can be given in water, although this poses two possible problems:

- If given in a water bottle, it should be in one with a stainless-steel spout, as the soft metal of many drinking bottles will inactivate vitamin C.
- If given in a drinking bowl, vitamin C can be inactivated by organic matter – and guinea pigs are known to deposit their faeces in the bowls.

Some rabbit pellets and mixes contain **coccidiostats** and these should *not* be fed to guinea pigs due to the risks of toxicity. Coccidiosis is not a major problem in guinea pigs (though it can occur) and coccidiostats tend to reduce the efficiency of the gut, and cause poor growth in young animals.

Handling rabbits   Rabbits can be picked up by the scruff and supported under the rump. If they are then tucked under the arm, so that the eyes are covered, they can be carried safely using only one arm and (usually) without any struggling.

Handling guinea pigs   Guinea pigs can be picked up with a hand around the shoulders. They should also be supported under the rump, especially if large or pregnant animals.

Breeding rabbits   Rabbits are seasonally polyoestrous and are induced ovulators. They are mated by taking the female (doe) to the male (buck). She is then removed after mating, which takes place almost immediately. Pregnancy diagnosis by abdominal palpation can be performed at about 14 days. The gestation period is 28–32 days; the larger breeds take longer and have larger litters.

The doe spends very little time with her young, leaving them covered up in the nest and returning only once or twice every 24 hours to feed them. Owners may become anxious at the doe's apparent lack of interest in her litter and have to be reassured that this is normal. In the wild, the young are in danger every time the doe goes to them, possibly showing predators the way to the nest.

Young rabbits may be weaned from 6 weeks of age, preferably by removing the doe. The litter should then be kept together in familiar surroundings for a further week before they are sold.

Breeding guinea pigs   Guinea pigs have a long gestation period (63 days or more) and give birth to precocious young. Guinea pigs should be bred for the first time before they are a year old, as the large size of the young means that the pubic symphysis must open to allow them to be born. If the sow is too old before her first litter, the symphysis may not open and a caesarean section may be required. The opening of the symphysis, detectable by palpation, indicates that she is likely to give birth within a couple of days.

The age of puberty in the female guinea pig is only 4–5 weeks. The male should be removed in good time so that young females in the litter are not already pregnant by the time they are weaned.

Chinchillas

Husbandry and housing   Chinchillas are native to the Andes mountains but there are very few left in the wild. They were first imported for their skins but are now mainly bred as pets. The wild chinchilla is grey but many other colours have been developed by selective breeding.

Chinchillas are social animals and so are best kept in pairs. Ideally the pairs should be established while the animals are young. Females are more aggressive than males: if adults are to be introduced to one another, they should be kept in adjoining cages for a while and then the female should be introduced into the male's cage.

Although chinchillas can be recommended as pets for older children, they are nocturnal, and are very agile and active after dark. It is better not to house them in bedrooms where people are trying to sleep. They are normally kept indoors and so do not suffer extremes of cold, but with their very dense coats they are susceptible to overheating.

They are usually kept in all-wire cages, which should be as large as possible to allow plenty of exercise, and should include ledges and branches to climb on and chew and a nest-box for sleeping. They are very destructive animals and so all the food and water containers should be of earthenware or metal.

They keep their fur in order by dust-bathing. A shallow, non-chewable pan of commercial 'chinchilla dust/sand' should be put into the cage each day but should not be left there permanently as the animals tend to use it as a litter tray once they have dust-bathed.

Feeding A commercial chinchilla pellet contains about 18% protein. The animals must also be given good-quality hay; treats such as apple and carrot are acceptable. Too much of any high-fat foods such as peanuts or sunflower seeds may dull the coat and, if given to excess, may lead to fatty changes in the liver.

Handling Chinchillas should be picked up gently around the shoulders, if necessary using the base of the tail as further support. Breeders who exhibit their animals do not appreciate greasy hands spoiling the fur and a pair of light cotton gloves, a scarf or a towel can be used when handling such animals.

Breeding The breeding season in Northern Europe is from November to May. The gestation period is 111–114 days, and up to three precocious young are born. Owners sometimes ask whether to remove the male or to leave him in with the female and the litter. In most cases the male is very caring and protective but may tread on the young accidentally as he runs around the cage, particularly if no nest-box is provided.

Chipmunks

Husbandry and housing The Siberian chipmunk has become popular as a pet in recent years. Because they can become very stressed in the presence of electrical equipment such as televisions, videos and computers, these animals should be kept out-of-doors. They will live outside happily all the year round, as long as they have weather-proof nest-boxes and their enclosure is shaded to protect them from very hot weather. They do not hibernate for long periods but will sleep for short periods during very cold weather, becoming active again on warmer days.

They are usually kept in aviary-like accommodation, built with security in mind and always with a safety door. A weatherproof nest-box stuffed with hay should be provided for each adult, as they prefer not to share sleeping-quarters. They can be kept as a pair or, if the enclosure is large enough, as a group, although there may be aggression between males or between females, particularly during the breeding season. They usually have two litters a year, in about April and again in August. The young leave the nest-box at about 6 weeks of age but should be left with the parents for at least another 2 weeks.

Feeding Chipmunks are omnivorous and should be fed a diet that contains meat protein, fresh fruit and vegetables and a seed-and-nut mix. The animal protein can be provided by a complete cat food; the seed-and-nut mix can be a combination of birdseed with a commercial small rodent-mix.

Handling Unless they have been hand-reared, chipmunks are not easy to restrain and are best captured using a light net or trapped inside a nest-box and moved with the nest-box. If hospitalisation becomes necessary it should be for the minimum time possible; the veterinary surgery is likely to be a very stressful environment for them.

Small mammals (rats, mice, gerbils and hamsters)

The veterinary nurse is sometimes asked for advice about choosing small mammal pets for children and the following facts are worth bearing in mind:

- Hamsters are nocturnal; gerbils are diurnal; rats and mice are active at any time.
- All small mammals need to be handled regularly to keep them tame.
- Gerbils, when alarmed, leap in the air – and out of the owner's hands.
- Hamsters and gerbils are easily injured by falling.
- Rats and mice are climbers; they cling on to clothing, etc., and are less likely to injure themselves if they fall.
- Rats are probably the quickest learning of the small-mammal pets. They are more likely to form attachments to their owners. Fancy rats, handled regularly from weaning, are very unlikely to bite.

Husbandry and housing Syrian hamsters are solitary by nature. Dwarf hamsters will usually live in a pair if put together when young but it is unwise to attempt to introduce two adults to each other. Gerbils are social animals and live in extended family groups – do not attempt to introduce a non-family gerbil to a group, but make up pairs at weaning. Rats and mice are loosely social and very tolerant: two or more female rats or mice will live satisfactorily together; males will tend to fight but sometimes two or more males will live together if there are no females within sight, sound or smell.

Feeding All these small mammals are omnivores, thriving on a diet containing a proportion of animal-based protein. In the wild, hamsters and gerbils in particular will catch and eat invertebrates, while wild rats and mice will also eat carrion. A comparison of the nutritional content of most commercial 'hamster mixes' with that of a commercial laboratory animal pellet shows how poor the diet is on which these pets live. The diet, and thus their general health, can be improved by giving a daily helping of table scraps plus small pieces of fruit and vegetable.

Handling Tame hamsters and gerbils can be scooped up into two cupped hands, but be sure to support a gerbil so that it cannot leap away. Gerbils should never be picked up by the tail, as the skin may peel off.

In the case of aggressive small mammals, some authorities recommend scruffing (and this is standard in many laboratories). However, this can be distressing for the watching owner and is not easy to accomplish without being bitten. It may also be injurious for the Syrian hamster, with its protuberant eyes (the problems are similar when handling a Pekingese dog). It is best to pick up potentially aggressive small mammals with the aid of a small net or a towel: they can then be manipulated within the towel to expose the part required for examination or injection. In some cases, light (isoflurane) anaesthesia is helpful.

Mice may be picked up around the shoulders, or by the base of the tail, and then placed on a surface such as a rough towel. Pet fancy rats accustomed to being handled may also be picked up round the shoulders (Fig. 11.3a); a more anxious handler can put the thumb under the animal's lower jaw to hold the mouth gently closed. Awkward animals are best handled using a towel, after initially taking hold of the base of the tail. Rats may be scruffed to restrain them for injections but being rolled up in a light towel (Fig. 11.3b) is less stressful for an animal that is accustomed to only gentle handling at home.

Breeding Most small mammals can be induced to breed all the year round but in practice they tend to stop breeding during periods of decreasing day length, from late summer to the turn of the year. They all have a post-partum oestrus, which means that if male and female are kept together or have brief contact after parturition they will probably mate.

The solitary Syrian hamster female will usually be aggressive towards a male except when she is in oestrus, which occurs every 4 days. When ready to mate she exhibits lordosis (ventral curvature of the lower spine), as do most of the small mammals.

The young of most small mammals commonly kept as pets are born naked and blind. Many books, and folklore in general, claim that the young should not be handled for, say, a week after birth because it would induce the mother to eat her young. In practice this depends on such things as the tameness of the mother and her confidence in her usual handler. Many breeders handle young from birth.

Pet owners should be reminded that the mother will require several times as much food as usual while raising a litter, particularly a large litter. The usual diet can be supplemented with dry complete cat or dog food and baby-weaning foods.

Weaning should not be carried out too early. The young will start to eat solid food some time before they are ready to be weaned. To avoid stress at weaning, the female should be removed and the litter left together in the familiar environment for a few days before being sold or rehoused. In this way they lose their mother, siblings and familiar environment in easy stages rather than all at once.

Ferrets

Housing For at least 2000 years ferrets have been kept in Europe for hunting. Working ferrets are often kept in hutches or in a 'ferret court' which may be an outdoor enclosure with a shelter, or in an indoor area in a shed or barn where a number of ferrets live together.

Pet ferrets may live indoors (the standard in the US where hunting with ferrets is banned by law) or in a hutch outside. It is important to remember that ferrets are highly active carnivores and supreme escapologists, with an intelligence comparable to that of a cat. All pet ferrets should have

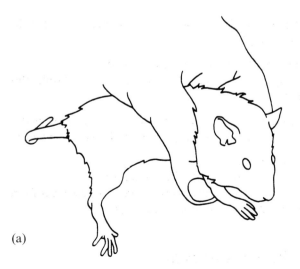
(a)

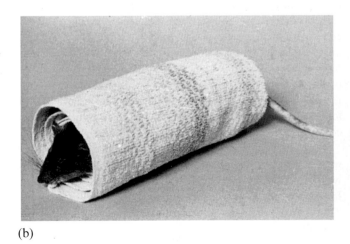
(b)

Fig. 11.3 Handling a pet rat. (a) Holding by grasping the shoulders. (b) Wrapped in a towel while recovering from anaesthesia (in this case, the towel is important in post-anaesthetic nursing care as small animals can quickly become hypothermic, but towel-wrapping is also useful as a restraint for an active rat).

regular exercise (mental as well as physical) in a stimulating environment and they have a great capacity for 'play'. Although solitary in the wild, they enjoy company and two or more will usually live together, though two males are likely to fight.

Feeding Working ferrets are often fed on their prey. The ferret's nutritional requirements are similar to those of cats but tinned cat foods tend to produce foul-smelling faeces (complete cat foods make them more acceptable). All ferrets, working or not, enjoy whole carcasses occasionally, such as those that are sold frozen for feeding to snakes and birds of prey. On no account should ferrets be restricted to the traditional diet of bread and milk, but milk alone will often be useful to tempt a sick or anorectic ferret to feed.

Handling Ferrets can be picked up around the shoulders, with a thumb placed under the lower jaw if there is any suspicion that the animal might attempt to bite (Fig. 11.4). Biting is more often through surprise than aggression, and it should also be remembered that ferrets have very poor eyesight but are highly efficient predators: a tentative finger is assumed to be edible prey. If a ferret does bite, its jaws tend to 'lock' and it can be difficult to remove though there are one or two tricks (including simply letting the animal find its feet if it is dangling in mid-air or immersing the ferret in water).

Breeding The breeding season for ferrets lasts from spring to autumn in Northern Europe. The testes of the male (hob) are withdrawn into the abdomen during winter and descend into the scrotum at the onset of the breeding season. When the female (jill) comes into season her vulva swells. She is an induced ovulator and is seasonally poly-oestrous (like the cat; see Chapter 18); if she is not mated she can remain in season until the autumn, which can be dangerous for her and can produce a potentially fatal anaemia. Unless jills are required for breeding, spaying is recommended. Some ferret keepers who want to postpone

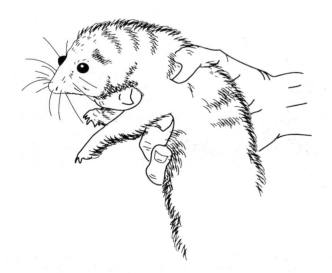

Fig. 11.4 Holding a tame ferret.

breeding in a young jill will 'mate' her with a vasectomised hob to take her out of season and into a pseudopregnancy.

Birds

An understanding of the biology and natural history of birds is important if one is to deal adequately with them in captivity and to provide them with optimum conditions when they are unwell. Some key points for hospitalised birds are as follows.

Birds are easily stressed, especially by close proximity of people, by loud noises and by violent movements:

- Reduce close contact by keeping birds some distance from people and other animals. An elevated position for the cage is ideal: most birds like to be in a high commanding position with a good view of their environment. Observe the bird from a distance before approaching it.
- Further reduce the stress of proximity by covering part of the cage or providing vegetation behind which the bird can hide.
- Reduce light intensity if a bird is frightened but remember that most birds must be able to see in order to feed.
- Avoid excess noises, including rattling of keys, banging of doors, barking of dogs. Discourage unnecessary visitors.

Birds must feed regularly, especially if they are small species with a high metabolic rate:

- Encourage feeding by providing the company of other birds or by offering moving or colourful food items such as mealworms, egg or berries (depending upon species).
- Acceptability may be enhanced if seeds are soaked before being offered, or if novelties are provided, e.g. a teasel head containing seeds.
- Food and water containers must be the correct shape; for instance, a heron needs a deep water container, not a shallow bowl.

Encourage normal behaviour to promote recovery from illness. For example:

- Social species will benefit from company.
- Preening behaviour may be stimulated if the bird's plumage is sprayed.

High standards of hospitalisation facilities promote better care of avian patients. Examples of good features include:

- Elevated cages.
- Dimmer switches to alter light intensity.
- A door that opens inwards (to discourage escapees from coming out) but that also closes naturally.

Choosing birds as pets

A veterinary nurse who is asked to give advice to novice bird-keepers should encourage them in the right direction (for the sake of the birds) with the following suggestions:

- Gain experience by keeping domesticated rather than wild species in the first instance.
- Those who would like a pet parrot but have never kept birds before: start with, perhaps, a pair of hand-reared cockatiels before attempting to keep the larger, non-domesticated species.
- Those who are determined to acquire large parrots as pets: spend a little more and acquire a British-bred, hand-reared parrot rather than an imported, wild-caught bird. Bear in mind that each species of large parrot has different inherent characteristics – in exactly the same way that different breeds of dog have different characteristics.
- Consult library books on the subject and talk to experienced bird-keepers before deciding to acquire a bird.
- Remember that a parrot might live for 40 or 50 years, or more.
- The young British-bred parrot that is sold just after weaning is a particularly demanding pet; it requires as much of its owner's time as would a new puppy.
- Most birds, and particularly the parrot species, are social and do much better when they have the company of their own species as well as that of humans. In the absence of contact with their own species, extensive human company is vital.

Cages and aviaries

Accommodation for pet birds can be divided into cages and the larger aviaries. In addition some tame birds may be allowed the freedom of the house, a practice that appeals to many people but the bird may damage furniture or other objects and can expose itself to hazards such as electric wires, ovens, poisonous chemicals and even lead pecked from leaded-light windows or old paint.

Cages   The two main groups of cage are the all-wire type or the box cage (with wire at the front but solid sides, roof and back wall). Their features are described in Table 11.13.

All-wire cages are acceptable for tame birds but they should always be placed at the side of the room or in a corner, reasonably high up, to give the bird a sense of security. Box cages are more suitable for wild and more nervous species, which feel less stressed when they cannot be viewed from all sides.

In the UK, any cage used for a captive bird (except poultry) should by law be large enough for the bird to stretch both wings fully in all directions. There is an exemption for birds that are being transported (e.g. to the surgery) or are under treatment by a veterinary surgeon but this does not necessarily apply to any bird in a veterinary practice or under the care of a non-veterinarian.

Cages for pet birds should be as large as possible, allowing room for parrots to climb and for canaries or finches to have a short flight between perches. Most commercial cages are fitted with ridged, plastic perches, which should be

Table 11.13 Cage design: box cages and all-wire cages	
Box	**Wire**
Open on only one side (front)	Open on all sides, unless covered
Often made of wood, not easily disinfected, subject to chewing	Easily disinfected, not likely to be chewed
Bird usually less easily frightened as it feels secure	Bird easily frightened unless one or more sides are covered
If illumination poor, inner recesses of cage may be too dark for feeding and other normal behaviour	Illumination good: facilitates clinical observation and encourages normal behaviour
Not liable to draughts but ventilation often poor	Liable to draughts but ventilation good

replaced by natural perching in several different diameters for the sake of the bird's feet. Fruit trees (unsprayed) and willows are reliable sources of non-poisonous wood but the branches should be scrubbed to remove any wild-bird droppings before they are placed in the cage.

Food and water receptacles should be placed where the bird can reach them easily (bearing in mind whether the bird normally feeds on or off the ground) but cannot defecate into them. Most parrots, whether large or small, appreciate 'toys' in the form of things to investigate, chew and destroy, but there should not be so many toys that there is no room for movement.

Hygiene is most important. Food and water containers should be cleaned daily. Cages should be emptied and thoroughly cleaned at least once a week.

Aviaries   Many people choose to keep birds in aviaries. They may have only one aviary as an ornament in the garden; or they may have a number and be keen aviculturists who try to breed birds in captivity. Most serious aviculturists are well aware of how to build and maintain an aviary but the amateur wishing to have one in the garden may ask for advice at the veterinary practice.

There are two components to an aviary:

- The mesh flight area – open to the air, wind, rain, snow and sun.
- The sheltered area – enclosed (other than an entrance), windproof, warmer, probably with windows to allow some sun to enter.

Each design should suit the intended occupants but the main points to be considered are as follows:

- Is planning permission necessary? In any case, as a courtesy, inform neighbours and do not keep noisy species if the neighbours are close or the garden is small.
- Avoid overhanging trees and strong winds.
- Try to position the aviary away from the road where disturbance and theft may prove a problem. Bird theft

is big business: keep only low-value species or invest in proper security.

- The smallest viable aviary size is about 1.8 m × 0.9 m but at this size it will be very difficult to keep clean. All aviaries should be protected against rats and mice by having deep foundations or a solid concrete base and also suitable wire around the room to exclude the rodents (e.g. 1 cm × 1 cm weld mesh).
- A frost-free shelter should be provided for all but the hardiest species. The shelter should have heat and light for any species likely to suffer during the winter without them.
- Roofing over the flight area will reduce the possibility of disease spreading from wild birds.
- Human entrance to the aviary is likely to be through a door. This should always open inwards (to discourage birds from flying out) and it is wise to have a double-door safety porch to minimise escape. At no time should both doors be open simultaneously.
- Seek advice from experienced bird-keepers about stocking densities and compatible species. Usually, only one pair of parrots can be kept in each aviary.
- Large parrot species may require heavy gauge wire to keep them contained (up to 12–14 g).

Disease control can be a problem in aviaries, especially if they cannot be fully cleaned because of the presence of soil, plants, etc. The following routines are important:

- Remove as much faeces, uneaten food, old feathers, soiled leaves and other debris as possible, preferably once a week.
- Ensure that the aviary is well watered and receives ample sunshine.
- At least twice a year turn over or replace soil and have faeces of birds checked for endoparasites.
- Ensure that aviary birds are kept under careful observation and can easily be caught or isolated if they appear to be unwell.

Handling birds

> All birds, except nocturnal species such as owls, are more easily caught and handled in the dark or in subdued light, which calms them.

Before removing a bird from a cage, always check that no doors or windows are open and no fans are in operation. Always transport birds in a secure box or basket, even over very short distances.

Small cage birds should be caught within their cage with as little chasing about as possible. Quietly remove toys and perches first.

Large birds, and those inclined to bite, can be caught using a towel or gloves (Fig. 11.5) – a towel is often prefer-

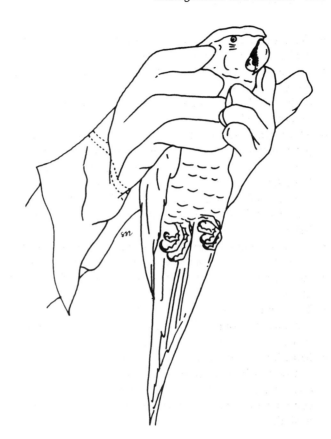

Fig. 11.5 Removing a parrot from its cage, using gloves.

able as it gives better control and does not restrict the handler's fingers once the bird has been caught. The large parrots should be grasped gently at the base of the skull with one hand, the other being used to support body and legs. A bird that clings to the bars of the cage with beak or feet should be detached gently by an assistant, not just pulled away. Pecking can be discouraged by putting an elastic band over the beak (but remember to remove it!) or by covering the bird's head with a light cloth bag.

Whatever the species, the aim when handling a bird should be to restrain its wings so that it can neither fly nor flap. Small birds can be held in one hand, with fingers around the neck, while larger birds are best grasped round the body (Figs 11.6 and 11.7).

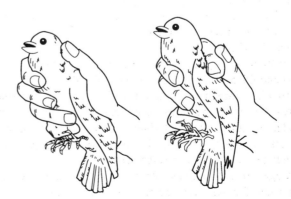

Fig. 11.6 Holding a small bird. Great care must be taken with these delicate animals, and no pressure should be placed on the abdomen.

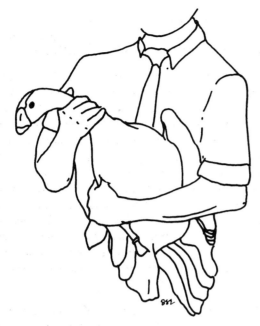

Fig. 11.7 Restraining a large bird: its neck is supported and it is unable to flap its wings.

Most pets are tame. This must be distinguished from **imprinting**, whereby a bird that has been hand-reared becomes imprinted upon humans rather than birds of its own species. Such individuals usually make affectionate and trusting pets but may react adversely to other birds and can develop other behavioural problems.

Feeding

The nutrition of birds is an important subject. Many non-specific diseases are due to or are exacerbated by nutritional deficiencies. Birds may be predominantly vegetarian, predominantly carnivorous or omnivorous (taking a mixture of foods). In practical terms several feeding groups of birds are recognised (Table 11.14).

In the wild, most birds have seasonal changes in their diet. Typical garden 'seed-eaters' often become almost entirely insectivorous during spring and summer and might enjoy a late summer/autumn glut of fruit before the leaner days of winter. Throughout the world, most birds time their breeding season to coincide with peak food availability to rear their young, be it the onset of warmer weather or the rainy season.

For captive birds, food should be fresh and of good quality and should be replaced regularly. Small birds (e.g. canaries) require ad lib feeding; they may eat 25% or more of their bodyweight per day. Large birds (e.g. owls) may need feeding only once a day and eat only 7–10% of bodyweight.

All captive birds should have a constant supply of clean drinking-water, though some species (e.g. raptors) will only drink infrequently or during certain periods such as egg-laying.

Seed-eaters (hardbills) Dry seeds are a convenient way to supply a very basic diet but there are very few birds that eat only dry seeds in the wild. No bird should be fed on dry seeds alone. However, birds that have been fed on one diet for a long time may be very reluctant to change, so that patience and determination are required to effect this. As with all animals, diet changes should be introduced gradually.

The veterinary nurse should be aware of the different seed mixes that are available for cage birds and should be able to distinguish between mixes for budgerigars, canaries, parakeets and finches, and be able to identify the seeds in them. The different types of seed have different food values, so that birds fed on one mix may be deficient in different nutrients from those fed on another mix.

Basic seed diets for small cage birds may be supplemented with:

- **Soft foods** – egg-based food that can be fed all the year round but particularly during the breeding season or moult or during convalescence.
- **Tonic mixes** – seed mixes giving a greater variety and more fat-rich seeds (useful during the winter when the need is for energy to keep warm, but feeding an excess of fat-rich seeds can lead to problems).
- **Greenstuff** – chemical-free weeds and vegetables from the garden increase the level of fat-soluble vitamins in the diet (always deficient in a seed-only diet).
- **Fruit**.
- **Vitamin/mineral supplements** – if the adequacy of the diet is in doubt.
- **Grit, cuttlefish bone and iodine blocks** – the last of these is essential for budgerigars that are not given iodine-supplemented seed.

Softbills The softbills are birds that feed naturally on 'soft' foods such as insects and fruit, in contrast to the hardbills that have beaks adapted to feeding on grain,

---

Table 11.14 Features of birds affecting feeding preferences

Group	Predominant food	Characteristic features	Examples
Hardbills	Seed	Strong broad beaks	Finches
Softbills	Fruit and/or insects	Pointed beaks	Thrushes, whydahs
Birds of prey	Dead animals (meat)	Hooked beaks	Falcons, hawks, owls
Nectar-feeding	Nectar, sometimes fruit	Long thin beaks and/or specialised tongues	Sunbirds, hummingbirds, lories, lorikeets

seeds and nuts. Softbills commonly kept as pets include the greater hill mynah and the Pekin robin as well as various indigenous aviary species. They are fed on proprietary softbill foods supplemented with fruit, vegetables, cheese, meat, insects, etc., according to the natural diet of the species in the wild. Those who care for wild-bird casualties sometimes breed suitable insects (such as grasshoppers and maggots) to provide a ready supply of fresh food for softbills.

Parrots and parakeets   Different parrot species are adapted to diverse habitats in the wild and so have disparate dietary preferences. None of them eats exclusively dry seeds. Some are nectar feeders (lories and lorikeets) and in captivity they are fed on a variety of commercial and home-made nectar substitutes with the addition of fruit. Most of the large parrots are omnivorous in the wild, eating a mixture of fruit, vegetables and seeds, plus insects and carrion to provide extra protein. A good diet for captive large parrots may include a good-quality parrot mix – but only up to about 20% of the total bulk of the diet. The rest will be made up of fruit, all sorts of vegetables and perhaps meat, dairy produce (yoghurt, fromage frais, cheese), brown bread, etc. Any bird that is not eating a very mixed diet will need a vitamin/mineral supplement.

Some pet parrots are encouraged to consume whatever the rest of the household is eating and, depending on that household's dietary habits, this can result in a well-nourished parrot. Parrots can be resistant to dietary change but are often willing to try foods if they see someone else enjoying them – either another parrot or the owner.

The birds tend to be wasteful feeders, taking one or two bites from a piece of fruit and then discarding the rest. This is sometimes interpreted by the owner as a dislike of a certain food. To minimise waste, it may be best to cut the food into small pieces before offering it.

Raptors

The diurnal (falconiform) birds of prey and owls are often brought into veterinary practices, perhaps as wild casualties or as birds belonging to falconers (kept either for hunting or for breeding). Falconry has become increasingly popular and while many people take a great deal of trouble to gain knowledge before acquiring a bird, others do not. Those who do show an interest should be encouraged by the veterinary nurse to go on a reputable falconry course and to join a falconry association before acquiring their own birds.

Raptors brought into the practice have special requirements that concern legislation as well as general handling and husbandry.

Legal position   In the UK, the Wildlife and Countryside Act 1981 makes it an offence to have in captivity certain falconiform birds of prey unless the bird has been ringed and registered. There is **an exemption for up to 6 weeks** for birds that are under the care of a veterinary sur-

geon, as long as proper records are kept. The current regulations should be checked with the Department for Environment, Food and Rural Affairs (DEFRA).

Handling raptors   The general rules of handling are as for other birds but owls are usually quieter in bright light rather than darkness. Gloves will protect the handler; alternatively, the bird can be wrapped in a towel. Falconers' birds are often relatively easy to handle, especially if they wear a hood; advantage can also be taken of their jesses and leash, which can be held or pulled tight.

Falconry birds that come to the surgery on the falconer's fist can be restrained for examination by being 'cast' – catching them by both hands around the body from behind, holding the wings against the body. The bird can then be laid on its sternum, preferably on a towel. The bird's head should be covered if it is not already hooded, so that it becomes quieter and more amenable.

Feeding raptors   The majority of birds of prey are wholly carnivorous but the preferred diet depends upon the species. Live food is not needed in captivity and may present legal and ethical problems. Most species will take butcher's meat, dead mice, or dead day-old chicks (hatchery waste) or quail. A regular supply of bone is important as a mineral source, especially for young birds. Feathers, fur and roughage will be regularly regurgitated as a pellet.

Water must be provided but is rarely taken, as the birds obtain moisture from their diet.

Reptiles and amphibians

Housing

Reptiles and amphibians vary greatly in their requirements but the main features of a captive environment are common to all and involve the following considerations:

- Ample **space** for normal behaviour including moving, climbing, swimming as appropriate.
- A **type** of environment matching that of the animal in the wild, e.g. damp areas for toads, pieces of bark (or artificial material) under which lizards can hide. Provision of choices.
- A **temperature gradient** (warmer at one end) so that the animal can select the temperature it favours. The heating element should be attached to a thermostat and monitored with a thermometer (ideally a maximum/minimum thermometer). The vivarium should be maintained at the inhabitant's preferred body temperature.
- Although some snakes can cope with poorer **lighting** conditions, lizards and land Chelonia require good lighting for activity and foraging. Various fluorescent tubes are made specifically for vivaria and will provide a good daylight spectrum, including some ultraviolet light.
- **Humidity** is important. Powerful heaters tend to dry the atmosphere. Regular water-spraying from a plant mister will maintain a reasonable degree of humidity and this

should be done regularly, even for desert species and of course very often for rainforest species.

- **Drinking-water** must be provided, though some species (e.g. chameleons) will drink only drops from moist foliage.
- **Ventilation** is important for maintaining health in the vivarium. If it is poor, it can be improved by introducing an airline powered by a small aquarium pump to encourage the circulation of fresh air, but this should be placed with care so that it does not cause draughts.

Vivaria may be glass aquarium tanks or they may be custom-built, often made from chipboard covered with melamine, the corners sealed with an aquarium sealant. Glass tanks are much harder to maintain at a reasonable temperature and are more difficult to service because the only access is from the top.

The furnishings of a vivarium will vary. Some herpetologists favour a clinically hygienic environment for snakes, with paper on the floor, a hide-box and a climbing branch for arboreal species. Others prefer a more natural design. Common substrates include bark chippings, peat, aquarium gravel and sand; the last of these tends to be used only for desert species of lizard but not for snakes as it can cause scale abrasions. Arboreal species should be given branches for climbing; burrowing species need sufficient depth of substrate for hiding. All species should have hiding areas or hide-boxes.

Hygiene is essential. Faeces should be removed as soon as possible, along with soiled areas of substrate. This is not easy in the 'natural' type of vivarium and tends to be done infrequently. Hypochlorite is a suitable disinfectant for the stripped-down vivarium, which must then be thoroughly rinsed and dried before being refurnished and its inhabitants returned.

Nutrition

Reptiles range from total herbivores (eating only plants) through omnivores (taking a mixture of plants and animals) to total carnivores (eating only animals). Some general guidelines are given in Tables 11.15 and 11.16.

Rodent-eating snakes
These include corn snakes, rat snakes and all the commonly kept pythons and boas. They should be fed on whole dead rodents – it is inadvisable in the UK to feed live vertebrate prey as it may make one liable to be prosecuted under the Protection of Animals Act 1911 (1912 Scotland). As a general rule, feed as much food as the snake will consume and then do not feed again until that meal has been digested and faeces passed. Captive-bred snakes are accustomed to feeding on dead prey; wild-caught snakes are sometimes more difficult to feed.

Fish-eating and invertebrate-eating snakes
These include garter snakes which can be fed on earthworms, small mice and pieces of fish. Frozen fish such as

---

Table 11.15 Feeding reptiles

Order	
Order Crocodilia	Crocodiles, alligators and caimans: predominantly carnivorous
Order Chelonia	Land tortoises: predominantly herbivorous but a number of species (e.g. box turtles) take food of animal origin Freshwater terrapins: predominantly carnivorous Marine turtles: predominantly carnivorous
Order Squamata	Snakes: predominantly carnivorous Lizards: predominantly carnivorous but a few species (e.g. iguanas) take food of plant origin

---

whitebait should be heat-treated in water at 80°C for 10 minutes in order to destroy thiaminase.

Insectivorous lizards
These can be fed on commercially produced insects such as crickets and locusts. It is important to dust the insects with a vitamin/mineral supplement first and to feed the correct size of insect for the animal. Lizards fed an unsupplemented diet tend to develop vitamin A deficiency and osteodystrophy caused by the poor Ca:P ratio in insects. Many insectivorous lizards in the wild also consume pollen, nectar and some fruit. Sweet, fruit substitutes should be offered from time to time.

Large omnivorous lizards
Lizards such as green iguanas are mainly insectivorous when young, becoming omnivorous as they grow. Their diet should contain a good amount of animal protein, as well as a good mixture of fruit and vegetables, and should be supplemented with calcium and vitamin D_3.

Basic husbandry

Mediterranean tortoises
Of the two common Mediterranean species, Hermann's tortoise (*Testudo hermanni*) has a horny spur on the end of its tail whereas the spur-thighed or Greek tortoise (*T. graeca*) has a short spur on the caudal aspect of each thigh.

Mediterranean tortoises can spend most of the spring and summer outside, with a shelter to sleep in at night. Indoor heated accommodation should be available for days when it

---

Table 11.16 Examples of reptile diets

Species	Staple diet
Greek (spur-thighed) tortoise (*Testudo graeca*)	Vegetable material
Garter snake (*Thamnophis* spp.)	Fish, amphibians, earthworms

is too cold for the tortoises to be active and feeding out of doors. Some people use greenhouses (heated or unheated) for this purpose.

Tortoises are herbivorous and the best diet for them is what they can find free-ranging over a large garden. If confined to a small pen, more food will have to be provided. Those that are kept over a period on one patch of ground may have high levels of roundworm infestation and need regular worming.

Male Mediterranean tortoises are most persistent in their pursuit of females. Courtship consists of butting the shell of the female and biting at her legs. A great deal of damage can be done to both animals if the female cannot escape from the male. It is best to keep males and females separate except when mating is required.

Mediterranean tortoises hibernate during the winter (and only those clearly unfit to do so should be kept awake). They should not be offered food for 3–4 weeks prior to hibernation, so that the intestines are empty before the animal becomes torpid. It is very difficult to keep a tortoise awake once day length starts to decrease; to keep it awake and feeding it is necessary to maintain artificial heat and also an artificial day length of 12 hours, with 'daylight' quality lighting.

Hibernation should be in a frost-proof and rodent-proof environment with good ventilation. The choice of insulation (e.g. hay, leafmould or shredded paper) does not matter as long as the tortoise is well protected. A healthy tortoise can lose up to 1% of its body weight per month in hibernation and anxious owners are known to weigh their pets regularly throughout the winter to monitor health. A sudden drop in weight indicates that something may be amiss and the tortoise should be awoken.

Young tortoises   Since import controls were applied, the average age of pet tortoises in the UK has been increasing steadily but many people now successfully produce hatchling tortoises. However, these enchanting little animals are very difficult to rear. They should be treated as adults as far as possible, i.e. they should graze outside and have access to sunlight, preferably in a cold-frame without its top to provide a draughtproof grazing area. On cold days they can be kept indoors in a vivarium. They should never be overfed: in the wild they would be active for much of the day in search of food, but in captivity they are inevitably less active and need less food to maintain optimum growth rate. Overfeeding and lack of supplementation of the diet lead to gross shell deformities in young tortoises that have grown much too fast.

Young tortoises would hibernate in the wild and should be allowed to do so in captivity.

Box 'turtles'   In the past the majority of land tortoises kept in the UK and other European countries were of the Mediterranean species. Large numbers were imported, often under unhygienic and inhumane conditions, and the mortality rate was very high.

Tighter controls on the capture and sale of Mediterranean tortoises has led to other species being imported and finding their way into homes and collections. These include the hinge-backed tortoises, *Kinixys* spp., and leopard tortoise (*Geochelone pardalis*) from Africa and the box 'turtles', *Terrapene* spp., from North America. The veterinary nurse should be familiar with the needs of box turtles (or tortoises), of which there are several species and subspecies, some of the latter being difficult to differentiate. It should be noted that their requirements in captivity are very different from those of the Mediterranean tortoises.

There are two main groups of these American tortoises. The Eastern usually has a uniformly dull brown plastron, sometimes smudged with darker brown; the Western has an intricate pattern of dark brown and yellow stripes on the plastron. The Eastern Box comes from the south-eastern states such as Florida and is adapted to a warm climate with a high relative humidity; the Western comes from the more arid states of New Mexico and Arizona and so prefers a drier climate.

In general, box tortoises should be kept all the year round in an indoor vivarium, in a warm environment and moist atmosphere but with good ventilation so that it never becomes stuffy. Species and subspecies vary in their temperature requirements and it is best to provide a temperature gradient of 20–30°C. During the summer, when the temperature is over 21°C, they enjoy being out of doors in a planted enclosure where they have access to water and shade – they do not fare well if left in the full sun.

The box tortoises are more closely related to freshwater terrapins than to true land tortoises. Most of them are omnivores, although youngsters may be largely carnivorous and some subspecies prefer insects. Many captive box tortoises are not given an adequate diet. Only one-third of the diet should consist of plant material, and of that 75% should be vegetable and 25% fruit. The remaining two-thirds of the diet should be of animal material, and examples of good sources of animal protein include crickets, grasshoppers, slugs, caterpillars, mealworms and sardines. Invertebrate food should be dusted with a calcium supplement to minimise the risk of metabolic bone disease. Small amounts of dog or cat food can be given but large quantities may cause nutritional disorders as they are not formulated for these species.

Most (but not all) box tortoises hibernate in the winter, though some can be kept awake in a warm cage with ample lighting. Only healthy box tortoises should be allowed to hibernate. The optimum conditions for hibernation are a temperature of 7–17°C, a draught-free and rodent-proof box and at least 40 cm depth of bedding – dry leaves, good-quality hay or shredded paper.

Health care of box tortoises is important and follows the general guidelines for captive chelonians. However, these animals can prove difficult to examine if they withdraw their head and all four limbs and close the shell.

Terrapins   The terrapin most commonly seen in captivity in the UK is the red-eared terrapin of North America. Hatchlings are sold at 3–5 cm long. The adult male is approximately 17–18 cm long and the female can grow to 28–30 cm.

Young terrapins require a vivarium with heated water and a basking area, with a basking spotlight, to help them dry out and to shed their scutes as they grow. They can be fed on a mixture of trout pellets, complete cat food, meat and fish. The latter should be supplemented with vitamins and minerals before feeding, and frozen fish such as whitebait should be heat-treated (as described for garter snakes). To minimise fouling of the water, it is best not to feed terrapins in their tank but in a separate container.

Large terrapins do well in an outdoor pond during the summer but it should be enclosed so that they cannot escape.

Mature males can be very aggressive and will attack other males (and sometimes females) if they are kept together in a small tank where the subordinate animal cannot escape.

Snakes

Snakes   The detailed requirements of snakes in captivity depend on the species. The North American group includes the corn snakes, rat snakes, garter snakes and king snakes.

Corn snakes and rat snakes are generally easy to maintain in captivity and easy to handle (particularly the corn snake). Captive-bred young of these rodent-eaters are commonly available and there are several colour mutations of the corn snake.

Garter snakes are relatively small and are good first snakes for well-informed children. In the wild they live in woodland and by watercourses, eating fish and dead invertebrates.

King snakes are more aggressive and they are reptile-eaters in the wild: they should be kept singly in the vivarium. Captive-bred individuals should have been brought up to eat dead mice but the feeding of wild-caught snakes can be a problem.

Royal (or ball) pythons are the smallest of the larger snakes commonly available and can be very reluctant to feed in captivity if caught in the wild. Veterinary practices often see long-term anorexics and these require lengthy treatment to rehydrate and then force-feed – some never feed voluntarily in captivity.

Indian (Burmese) pythons grow up to 4 m or more; they are strong snakes and, though some remain easy to handle, others can be belligerent. Many of them become too much of a handful for their owners, who offer them to zoos that may be already overstocked. Yet they continue to be bred regularly in captivity and hatchlings are commonly available.

Boa constrictors do not grow as large as Indian pythons: they have a slimmer build but they still tend to grow too large to be accommodated by the average household. They reproduce well in captivity and a snake that has been handled well when young usually remains amenable as it grows.

Reticulated pythons grow as large and as strong as Indian pythons, and are generally more aggressive.

Small lizards   Most lizards are territorial. There should be only one male of any species in a small vivarium, together with perhaps two or three females. The spe-

cies generally recommended as a beginner's lizard is the leopard gecko, a nocturnal lizard that has been bred in captivity for many generations and is relatively easy to handle.

Large lizards   The large lizard most commonly kept is the green iguana, often imported as young animals at 30–45 cm long. Many purchasers fail to appreciate that the males can grow up to 150 cm and that the species requires extensive heated accommodation: they are very demanding in time, space and money. In captivity they rarely reach their full potential size and often suffer from fibrous osteodystrophy (metabolic bone disease) due to an inadequate or poorly balanced diet.

Handling

Snakes   It is assumed that the snakes brought to a veterinary practice are not venomous. Venomous snakes are kept by some herpetologists, but in the UK many are covered by the strict regulations of the Dangerous Wild Animals Act.

All snakes are susceptible to bruising: they should be handled carefully and never held more tightly than necessary. Those that are normally quiet and easy to handle will become upset in a new and possibly threatening environment or as a result of maltreatment during clinical examination, injection or blood-testing.

Small snakes, unless they threaten and strike at the handler, should be lifted gently by a hand under their broadest part and then supported as they coil around the arm (Fig. 11.8). Aggressive small snakes can be caught with the aid of a towel or gloves and gently restrained behind the head.

To examine the head and mouth, the snake is supported just behind its head and then its mouth opened (if required) by gently inserting a flat instrument in the labial notch at the front of the mouth. Wooden lolly-sticks and pen-tops have been found useful for this task; there are doubtless many other possibilities.

Large snakes should be handled with care and never draped around the neck. Two or three competent people

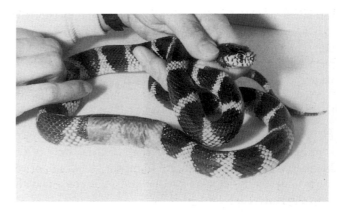

Fig. 11.8 Holding a king snake. This one has an adhesive dressing on a skin lesion, which needs careful nursing to avoid secondary infections.

should be present to help with really large snakes. Those known to be aggressive should be sedated before handling.

Lizards   Small lizards should be picked up round the pectoral girdle. Very small and delicate lizards can be trapped against the side of the vivarium with a soft cloth. Never catch a lizard by its tail: the shedding of the tail (autotomy) is a defence mechanism in many species (but not all).

Iguanas should be handled with care: they can inflict damage with their teeth, their short claws (particularly on the hindlimbs) and their long, lashing tails. It is best to use a towel or gloves, unless they can be grasped briskly in two hands with one hand round the shoulders and one holding the thighs along the side of the tail.

Fish

The health and welfare of fish depend very much upon the quality of the water in which they live. Important features of water quality are:

*   Temperature (less oxygen is present at higher temperatures).
*   pH (6–8 is the usual range for freshwater species).
*   Hardness/salinity (hard water is usually preferable).
*   Metallic salts in solution.
*   Ammonia and nitrate levels (deaths may occur if high – testing kits are available).
*   Bacteria levels.
*   Some species are very specific in their requirements.
*   Experienced aquarists can advise on these points.

Aquaria

Aquaria are usually made entirely of glass but tanks with frames are still in use. Setting up an aquarium needs planning and patience, and the following points are important:

*   Choose a site away from direct sunlight.
*   Ensure that the aquarium is properly supported – a tank full of water is heavy. Use pieces of polystyrene under all-glass tanks to minimise uneven pressures.
*   Install gravel on floor. It must be several centimetres deep if there is under-gravel filtration.
*   Add rocks and ornamental structures as necessary. Clean them first.
*   Add plants, ensuring that they come from a reputable dealer. Soak in 2 p.p.m. potassium permanganate for 48 hours before transfer.
*   Let the aquarium settle for 2 weeks before stocking with fish. Some people then add 'cheap fish' to test the water before introducing other species.
*   Tropical species need heating, either of the tank or of the whole room.

Feeding and maintenance

Proprietary food should be the staple diet, supplemented with live food if necessary, but the latter can introduce disease. Various supplements are available and can be useful. Never overfeed: assess how much is being eaten and give slightly less than this, provided once or twice daily.

Maintenance includes:

*   Regular observation of the fish and their environment.
*   Weekly cleaning (removal) of gross dirt from the bottom of the aquarium plus 10–15% of the water. Dechlorinate tap water before it is added.
*   Installing mechanical, biological or chemical filters for large tanks and the more sensitive species.
*   Taking prompt action if fish appear unwell or die or if the water changes in appearance.
*   Quarantining all incoming fish for at least 2 weeks.

Invertebrates

Invertebrates are increasingly being kept in captivity (Fig. 11.9). Their management differs according to their species, origin, age and other factors, and some examples are given in Table 11.17.

Wildlife

Space does not permit detailed discussion of the care of wildlife. Nevertheless, some basic information is important. Members of the public have traditionally brought wild mammals and birds that are in need of attention to veterinary practices and in recent years there has been an increased interest in work with such casualties. Wildlife organisations, including bat, badger, fox and hedgehog conservation groups, understandably expect an in-depth knowledge and commitment from practising veterinarians.

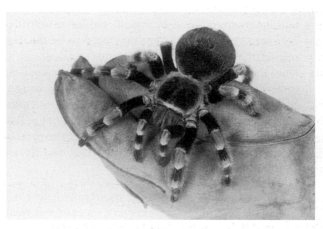

Fig. 11.9 A red-kneed tarantula on the hand. Gloves are not usually necessary but will reduce the risk of irritation from the spider's hairs (setae).

Table 11.17 Management and feeding of invertebrates		
Species	**Management**	**Main food**
Indian stick insect	Well-ventilated containers Temperate	Privet leaves
Giant millipedes	Containers with ample substrate Tropical	Dead leaves, fruit, vegetables, waste organic material
Giant snails	As above Tropical High humidity	Fruit, vegetables Calcium source
Red-kneed 'tarantula' spider	Spacious container with some substrate Tropical High humidity	Insects, other invertebrates

Specialist rehabilitation centres (some run privately, some by organisations such as the RSPCA) are also well established. An ability to deal with wildlife is, therefore, a useful skill for the veterinary nurse to acquire.

Wild animals are likely to fall into one or more categories:

- Those that have an infectious or parasitic disease (e.g. tuberculosis, tick infestation).
- Those that have an injury (e.g. a broken wing).
- Those that have been poisoned, intentionally or accidentally.
- Those that have been electrocuted or burnt, e.g. on power-lines or following a fire.
- Those that are oiled or have other chemical damage (see Chapter 4, p. 133).
- Those that are, or appear to be, orphaned.
- Those that have been displaced for some reason, e.g. birds that fly off-course on migration.

There are several questions that should be asked when dealing with a wildlife casualty:

(1) When and where was it found?
(2) What species is it? Some wild animals, particularly certain birds, are covered by special legislation (birds of prey in particular) and steps may need to be taken to register them or to keep appropriate records.
(3) Does the practice have the necessary facilities and staff to deal with the animal? Some species, such as badgers and herons, require a great deal of personal attention whereas others can be tended with a minimum of specialised accommodation or equipment. If the practice cannot cope, is there a wildlife centre that may be better able to assist?

From the outset it is necessary to ascertain whether it is in the animal's best interests to embark on care and treatment – and this can be a hard decision. Many factors have to be taken into consideration, of which the most important are:

- Is the animal so unwell or badly injured that it is unlikely to survive and is probably in severe pain?
- Even if the animal is likely to survive, will it be possible to return it to the wild when recovered? (With all wildlife casualties this must be the aim and is often a legal requirement.)
- If it cannot be rehabilitated in the wild, can it properly be retained in captivity? Will it have a reasonable quality of life?

Although the treatment of wildlife is challenging and stimulating, this must not be allowed to obscure the fact that the kindest approach to some casualties is euthanasia. Heroic surgery, expensive drug therapy and dedicated nursing have their place and will yield successful results in a proportion of cases but others, for a variety of reasons, fail to respond and are probably best humanely killed. Euthanasia is an option at each stage, as indicated in Fig. 11.10.

Assuming that the decision is made to attempt to keep the casualty, the following points are important:

- Keep proper records – species, date of arrival, diagnosis, treatment, outcome.
- Carry out all handling, examination and treatment with care – wild animals are easily stressed.
- Remember that nursing plays a very important part in the care of wild animals. Warmth, fluids and feeding, coupled with attention to wounds and discharges, will often go a long way towards keeping the patient alive and facilitating recovery.
- Getting the animal to eat voluntarily can prove difficult and needs a great deal of patience. Force-feeding may be necessary at first.
- Rehabilitation and release can prove time-consuming, difficult and sometimes impossible. Help can be obtained from people who specialise in wildlife care, e.g. those who run the reputable rehabilitation centres.

The British Wildlife Rehabilitation Council (BWRC) publishes a Code of Practice and can give advice.

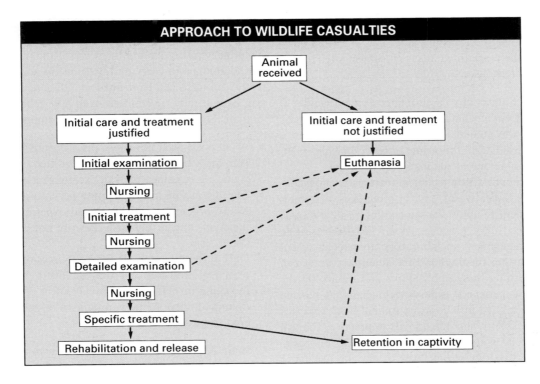

Fig. 11.10 Considerations in dealing with wildlife casualties.

Pain assessment and welfare considerations

An important part of the veterinary nurse's responsibility is to promote the welfare of the animal and to minimise pain and distress. It is best to assume that all animals are capable of feeling pain (the majority, including invertebrates, are certainly capable of *responding* to it) and to give them the benefit of the nurse's skill in practice.

It is helpful to consider this aspect of welfare under three headings: pain, discomfort and distress.

- **Pain** is a physical phenomenon, with which all humans are familiar. One assumes that exotic (and native wild) species can also experience pain of different degree (mild, moderate, substantial) and of different duration (acute or chronic).
- **Discomfort** is also a physical phenomenon but is milder than pain and may only be an inconvenience or irritation to the animal, e.g. a piece of bandage that has become loose and makes it difficult for the animal to walk or to lie down comfortably.
- **Distress** is a psychological phenomenon and may be associated with pain or discomfort, or can be entirely distinct. It occurs, for example, when a mother is separated from her young, or a social animal is kept alone. These and other 'stressors' can cause 'stress' in the animal. The terminology is important.

There are many ways in which the nurse can contribute to the relief of pain, discomfort and distress in exotic species. For example:

- Ensure that the animal receives the best possible care in terms of good feeding, handling and general management.
- Provide an environment that is appropriate to both the species and the particular individual.

    - Animals that like to burrow (such as gerbils) or to hide in a damp place (such as toads) should be permitted to do so.
    - Social species should not be kept alone.
    - Species that fight or strongly challenge one another should not be kept together in close confinement.

- Attend promptly to wounds, infections and other problems. Such attention must include supportive care (e.g. cleaning of ocular discharges, and handfeeding) as well as specific therapy.
- Make appropriate changes to management, e.g. use rubber mats to reduce pain and to minimise further damage to a rabbit with 'sore hocks' or a guinea pig with pododermatitis.
- Administer analgesics to prevent or minimise pain. These can include specific agents (e.g. buprenorphine) or general anaesthetics that have an analgesic effect (e.g. nitrous oxide).
- Administer other chemotherapeutic agents that, while not themselves analgesic, reduce the risk of further pain or distress (e.g. tranquillisers to prevent an animal from damaging itself in its cage).
- The question of euthanasia must never be overlooked. As with other species, the exotic or wild animal that is in substantial pain which is likely to persist may need to be killed on humanitarian grounds.

The veterinary nurse is likely to ask: 'But how do I know when an unfamiliar species is in pain?' This is a valid question, to which there are three answers: subjectivity, clinical indications and responses.

- **Subjectivity**. Subjectivity is probably a good guide. If under similar circumstances a human would be in pain, assume that the animal is also. Thus, if *any* species is anorexic and lethargic following surgery, consider post-operative pain as one of the likely causes.
- **Clinical indications**. Certain clinical features are now considered to be indicative of pain in laboratory mammals and it is prudent to apply the same criteria to these same species in veterinary practice. Much has been written about pain assessment in laboratory animals in recent years (see Further reading) and the veterinary nurse can gain from reading these publications and discussing the matter with experienced animal technicians. A scoring system is often used in laboratory animal work and this can be applicable to small mammals in practice. Clinical features can be common to all species (e.g. anorexia, dehydration, lethargy, weight loss) or may be specific to the type of animal (e.g. failure of rats to groom or a tendency for rabbits to press their heads against the wall of the cage). An observant veterinary nurse will quickly develop the ability to recognise signs that indicate pain, discomfort and distress.
- **Responses**. If in doubt, give the animal appropriate treatment (e.g. an analgesic) and see if there is a response. A ferret, for example, that looks dejected and is reluctant to move or feed following surgery on a broken leg may behave very differently after a subcutaneous injection of buprenorphine or flunixin.

Common problems and diseases

Diseases of exotic species can be infectious or non-infectious. Often there is an overlap and many apparently infectious diseases (e.g. respiratory conditions of rabbits, foot infections of birds) are due to, or precipitated by, poor management or inadequate diet. When taking a history, or discussing a problem with an owner, the veterinary nurse should obtain as much information as possible about the housing, feeding and general management of the patient. Ideally, the client's premises should be visited but in a busy practice this is not always practicable. Owners should therefore be encouraged to produce the animal in its own (uncleaned) cage together with samples of uneaten food. It can prove helpful if they also bring a photograph or drawing of the animal at home, in its own environment.

Common problems and diseases for different groups of exotic pets are summarised in Tables 11.18–11.20. Much useful information on the diseases of small mammals can also be obtained by reference to the literature on laboratory animals (see Further reading).

Zoonoses

Veterinary nurses should be aware of the potential of some exotic animals to carry and/or transmit zoonoses (Chapter 17). A zoonosis can be defined as a disease or infection that can be naturally transmitted from a vertebrate animal to a human. Each part of this definition is important:

- A zoonosis need not cause disease in its host: the organism may be present and transmitted without clinical signs, e.g. a guinea pig can excrete *Salmonella*.
- The disease or infection must be naturally transmitted. Many organisms can be spread experimentally, e.g. by injection, but in that case they are not considered to be zoonoses.
- Only vertebrate animals can be sources of a zoonosis. An organism transmitted from an invertebrate, such as a mosquito or tick, with no involvement of another animal (mammal, bird, reptile, amphibian or fish) is not considered to be zoonotic.

Some zoonotic diseases are common to a wide range of species: bacteria of the genus *Salmonella*, for example, can be acquired from animals ranging from ferrets to frogs. Others are more specific: for example, the virus of lymphocytic choriomeningitis (LCM) is only likely to be contracted from rodents. Animals with zoonotic infections need not show clinical signs of disease, since they may either be incubating the disease or carrying the organisms asymptomatically, and therefore the veterinary nurse's approach to zoonoses must be based upon other factors:

- **Awareness** that such infections exist and that apparently healthy animals may transmit them.
- **Reducing unnecessary exposure** to animals that may be a source of zoonoses. This may involve not handling an animal unnecessarily; or ensuring that, when it is handled, it is unlikely to bite or scratch or to contaminate wounds. Monkeys and other primates are a particularly potent source of zoonotic organisms.
- **Practising good hygiene** so that infections are less likely to spread. Hand-washing, protective clothing and other standard safeguards are usually adequate.
- **Taking prophylactic action** where this is available. For example, all veterinary nurses should be immunised against tetanus and those who come into contact with zoo animals, or captive primates should consider rabies and hepatitis vaccinations.

Common problems in pet mammals
Rabbits

- Overgrown claws.
- Malocclusion of front and cheek teeth – the teeth are not properly worn down, resulting in spikes and grossly over-long teeth that may require clipping or filing.

Table 11.18 Some diseases of small mammals

Species	Condition	Clinical signs	Treatment	Comments
All small mammals	Skin wounds and abscesses	Skin abrasions and lesions	Clean with appropriate disinfectant or cleansing agent. Suture where appropriate. Irrigate abscesses	Wounds may indicate fighting or other management problems. Rabbit abscesses may need to be excised *in toto*.
	Traumatic injuries	Incoordination, collapse, hyperpnoea, etc.	Warmth, fluids orally and/or by injection. Hand-feeding and nursing	Some species, e.g. hamsters, are prone to fall off surfaces. Damage may also be caused by poor handling (especially by children), cats, etc.
	Fractures	Locomotor disturbances, swelling, pain, etc.	Euthanasia may be necessary. Limb fractures can be fixed (externally or internally) but in small rodents often heal spontaneously. Nursing	Vertebral injuries are common in rabbits
	Dental problems	Excessive salivation ('slobbers'), dysphagia	Attention to overgrown teeth. Removal of plaque, attention to inflamed gingivae. Radiography to assess any bone involvement	Overgrowth of incisors and cheek teeth (malocclusions) is common in rodents and lagomorphs and may be associated with genetic factors, soft food, lack of wear, etc. Dental abscesses and periodontal disease are prevalent in ferrets
	Ectoparasites (flea, mite, tick or louse infestation)	Vary from inapparent infection to marked pruritus and skin lesions	Appropriate parasiticidal treatment of skin (and, in case of fleas, environment)	Skin lesions may also be due to environmental factors, nutritional deficiencies, or behavioural traits (barbering)
	Endoparasites (nematode, cestode, trematode, or protozoan infestation)	Vary from inapparent infection to diarrhoea. Rectal prolapse may be indicative of infestation with the pinworm *Syphacia*	Anthelmintic or antiprotozoal treatment. Various agents can be used orally including mebendazole (10 mg/kg), praziquantel (5–10 mg/kg) and for protozoa, sulphonamides or dimetridazole (1 mg/ml water)	Diagnosis of endoparasites will depend upon careful examination of faeces or (*post-mortem*) body tissues
	Respiratory disease	May range from mild respiratory signs, e.g. nasal discharge in rabbits, sneezing in rats, chattering in mice, to dyspnoea. Headtilt, due to labryinthitis, may be seen	Antimicrobial agents may be tried. Isolation of affected animals and attention to management (temperature and ventilation) are important	Difficult, if not impossible, to eliminate from a group or colony of rodents. Many different microorganisms may be involved but the primary pathogen in rodents is usually a virus or *Mycoplasma*. Secondary bacterial infection is common and may respond to chemotherapy

Table 11.18 (Continued)

Species	Condition	Clinical signs	Treatment	Comments
	Diarrhoea, enteritis (various types)	Loose faeces, fluid loss, electrolyte imbalance, etc.	Specific therapy plus fluids where appropriate	Many different causes, ranging from changes in diet to bacterial, viral and parasitic infections. Specific therapy will depend on cause, and laboratory investigation of faeces may be necessary. It is wise to check for *Salmonella*
Mouse, rat, guinea pig and rabbit	Ringworm	Hair loss, occasionally erythema and pruritus	Oral griseofulvin (25 mg/kg) for 4–5 weeks	Differential diagnosis in the rabbit includes plucking of hair for nest-building
Mouse and rat	Mammary tumours	Swollen, usually hard, mammary glands	Surgical removal	Often malignant, especially in rats. May be confused with mastitis.
	'Ringtail'	Raised corrugated (usually hyperkeratinised) lesions on tail	Raise relative humidity Lesions, which become infected can be treated topically	'Ringtail' and certain other non-specific skin lesions are associated with a low relative humidity (< 40%)
Mouse, rat, golden hamster, jird and guinea pig (occasionally rabbit)	Tyzzer's disease (*Bacillus piliformis* infection)	Diarrhoea, loss of condition, death	Rarely successful. Tetracyclines may be tried. Improve management	Stressors may be responsible for onset of disease
Golden hamster	Impacted cheek pouch	Swollen side(s) to face	Remove impaction manually or by irrigation with saline	Often caused by artificial foods, e.g. sweets, pellets
	'Wet tail' (proliferative ileitis)	Diarrhoea and perianal excoriation, especially in newly weaned animals	Rarely successful. Fluids by mouth or injection. Oral neomycin, kaolin preparations, etc. Nursing	Cause uncertain, possibly a form of colibacillosis. Often precipitated by stressors, e.g. change of diet or overcrowding. A similar condition may be seen in jirds but is probably not identical
Jird	'Fits' (epileptiform seizures)	Convulsions, lasting for 10–90 s	None necessary. Animal should be returned to cage and not disturbed	Cause and significance are uncertain. Often precipitated by stressors, e.g. handling
	Sebaceous gland disorders	Swollen gland on ventral surface of abdomen	If inflamed and/or infected use topical antimicrobial agent and/or corticosteroid. If neoplastic – surgical removal	
Guinea pig	Alopecia	Hair loss, usually without pruritus	Change of environment. Improved diet (including addition of vitamin C and hay)	Cause often uncertain. Common in female animals during pregnancy
	Scurvy (vitamin C deficiency)	Lethargy, swollen joints, weight loss, death. Often predisposes to infectious or parasitic disease	Vitamin C orally (50–100 mg/day per animal)	May occur even if diet contains vitamin C since deterioration of the latter can be rapid, especially at high temperatures
	Pregnancy toxaemia	Depression and anorexia during last 1–2 weeks of pregnancy or immediately after parturition	Corticosteroids by injection. Dextrose by mouth or injection. Avoidance of stress	Probably associated with heavy and long pregnancy, and obesity. Often only diagnosed post mortem

Table 11.18 (Continued)

Species	Condition	Clinical signs	Treatment	Comments
Guinea pig and rabbit	Pseudotuberculosis (*Yersinia* infection)	Diarrhoea, weight loss, enlarged mesenteric lymph nodes, death	Rarely practicable or wise. Culling and disinfection are preferable	Infection may be introduced by other animals (including wild birds and rodents) or contaminated greenfood
Rabbit	Ear canker (*Psoroptes cuniculi* infestation)	Inflammation of external ear canal: pruritus and self-inflicted damage	Soften exudate with liquid paraffin prior to cleaning and application of ear drops, for 5 days	Regular inspection of rabbit's ears will enable early infestation to be detected. In severe cases light anaesthesia will facilitate cleaning
	Sore hocks	Hair loss, swelling, ulceration and/or infection of hock(s)	Treat wounds. Provide soft bedding	Often follows trauma or prolonged periods on hard floor
	Hairball (gastric)	Anorexia, dehydration, sometimes diarrhoea. Hairball may be palpable	Liquid paraffin by mouth coupled with manual massage to break up hairball. Surgery may be necessary	Usually follows self-grooming and this may be due to boredom. Particularly prevalent in long-haired breeds, e.g. Angora
	Hepatic coccidiosis (*Eimeria stiedae* infestation)	Weight loss, anorexia, occasionally diarrhoea. Liver may be enlarged	Oral sulphonamides (e.g. 0.2% sulphadimidine or 0.3% sulphaquinoxaline) in water for 5 days	May be present in subclinical form – oocysts detectable in faeces. In severe clinical cases chronic hepatic damage may persist after treatment
	Enteritis complex	Depression, diarrhoea, fluid intestinal contents, dehydration, mainly in recently weaned animals (5–10 weeks old)	Food with high fibre content, e.g. hay. Nursing and supportive care. Antimicrobial agents may be helpful	Cause uncertain – probably multifactorial and associated with bacteria and change of diet. Differential diagnoses include coccidiosis and diarrhoea following a change in diet
	Myxomatosis	Conjunctivitis, blepharitis, subcutaneous swellings. Anorexia, depression, death	None specific. Nursing and supportive care, including hand-feeding	Vaccination can be used prophylactically. Control of the vector – the rabbit flea (*Spilopsyllus cuniculi*) – is also important
	Viral haemorrhagic disease	Lethargy, anorexia, haemorrhage, sudden death	None specific. Nursing and supportive care, including hand-feeding	Vaccination can be used prophylactically. Hygiene and isolation of affected cases
Ferret	Persistent oestrus	Swollen, sometimes abraded, vulva. May be severe – depression, anorexia, pale mucous membranes, death	Termination of oestrus by stimulation of vagina, mating (entire or vasectomised male) or hormonal therapy, e.g. proligestrone 0.5 ml SC Ovariohysterectomy and/or blood transfusions in severe cases	The mild syndrome is common but the more severe condition (oestrus-associated bone marrow depression) has only once been reported in Britain
	Canine distemper	Respiratory signs, conjunctivitis, diarrhoea, neurological signs, death	None specific. Nursing and symptomatic treatment	Vaccination can be used prophylactically

Table 11.19 Some diseases seen in birds

Condition	Clinical signs	Diagnosis	Treatment	Comment
Skin wounds	Skin abrasions and lesions, bleeding	Observation and examination	Clean with appropriate disinfectant. Control haemorrhage. Suture where appropriate	Wounds may indicate poor cage design, pecking by other birds, or predation (e.g. by cats). *See also* Abscesses
Traumatic injuries	Incoordination, collapse, hyperpnoea, etc.	Examination	Warmth. Fluids. Hand-feeding and nursing. Attention to wounds	As above
Fractures	Lameness, drooping wing, swelling, pain, etc.	Examination	External (splints, taping, plaster) or internal (pinning, wiring, plating) fixation. Nursing	Callus formation is rapid in small birds and fixation may not be necessary after 14–21 days
Feather conditions (various)	Feather loss or damage. Irregular or abnormal moult	Observation, examination of feathers	Depends on cause. If parasites present, parasiticidal treatment. If no parasites detected, improve diet, change environment, provide company and/or a mate. Some cases are due to hormonal imbalance and may respond to thyroxine or testosterone	A complex and often frustrating group of diseases
'Scaly leg' and 'scaly face' (*Knemidocoptes* infestation)	Raised keratinous lesions on feet and/or cere	Observation. Examination of crusts for parasites	Painting with liquid paraffin to soften scabs, followed (if necessary) by weekly painting of affected areas with 10% benzyl benzoate or 5% piperonyl butoxide	Deformity of the beak may be a sequel to 'scaly face'. Ivermectin may be effective against the mites
'Bumblefoot' (usually *Staphylococcus aureus* infection of foot)	Swollen, painful foot or digit	Observation. Examination. Aspiration of pus and bacteriology	Lancing, removal of pus and irrigation. Dressing of foot. Improved hygiene of perches	Differential diagnosis can include visceral gout (*see below*) and traumatic injuries
Articular gout	Swollen, painful joint(s)	Observation. Aspiration of urates	None, other than removal of urate deposits. Improve renal function by ensuring adequate water intake	Aetiology uncertain. May be associated with renal damage. Urates are deposited in joints and, in some cases (visceral gout) on the serosae of internal organs
Skin tumours	External swellings	Examination. Aspiration for cytology or biopsy for histopathology	Surgical removal	May be lipomas, fibromas, adenomas, or malignant equivalents. Differential diagnosis includes haematomas, feather cysts (*see below*) and abscesses (*see below*)
Abscesses	External swellings	Examination. Aspiration for bacteriology and cytology	Surgical removal or lancing and irrigation	Pus is usually caseous. Differential diagnosis includes haematomas, neoplasia (*see above*) and feather cysts (*see below*)

Table 11.19 (Continued)

Condition	Clinical signs	Diagnosis	Treatment	Comment
'Feather cysts' (*hyppteronosis cystica*)	External swellings, especially on wings	Incision or excision to demonstrate whorls of keratin	Surgical removal	Particularly prevalent in certain strains of canary. May be a genetic predisposition
Regurgitation	Food is regurgitated. In crop necrosis bird is unwell with fluid around beak and, sometimes diarrhoea	Eliminate 'normal' regurgitation (*see Comment*). Swab and smears of crop for bacteriology and mycology (*Candida*) and for direct examination for (e.g.) megabacteria	Nursing. Fluids. Clavulanate potentiated amoxycillin 12.5 mg/kg orally and/or nystatin orally. Vitamin B supplementation	Male budgerigars regurgitate food as part of courtship and may do this in captivity, even when kept alone. Crop necrosis is an infectious condition, possibly secondary to a nutritional deficiency or overuse of antibiotics. Megabacteriosis is increasingly being diagnosed in such cases.
Sinusitis	Swollen periorbital region	Observation and examination. Swabs for bacteriology	Parenteral antibiotics. Change of environment. In severe or intractable cases surgical drainage and irrigation of sinuses	Probably part of an upper respiratory disease syndrome, possibly precipitated or exacerbated by adverse temperature/relative humidity or prolonged exposure to smoke
Ectoparasites	May be none. Feather loss or damage, pruritus, anaemia	Observation. Examination of birds and cage/aviary for evidence of parasites	Pyrethrum-based powders or sprays. Dichlorvos strip in birdroom	In cases of mite infestation treat environment as well as bird. *See also* 'Scaly leg' and 'Scaly face' and feather conditions
Endoparasites	May be none. Loss of weight or condition, lethargy, anorexia, diarrhoea	Examination of bird and laboratory investigation of faeces and/or buccal/crop smears	Depends on parasite. Nematodes treated with levamisole 10 mg/kg orally or fenbendazole 100 mg/kg orally. Do not use latter in pigeons	Some parasites e.g. *Eucolous* may infest upper alimentary tract. Large numbers of ascarids can block intestine
Enteritis	Diarrhoea, loss of weight and condition	Observation and examination. Investigation of faeces may or may not prove helpful. Green staining often assists	Depends upon cause. Change of diet and/or oral antibiotics or sulphonamides (coupled with fluids and nursing) may be beneficial	'Enteritis' is a general term and probably refers to many conditions. Normal droppings consist of two portions – white urates and brown/black/dark green faeces. Very green faeces are usually indicative of reduced food intake and excess bile production
Respiratory disease	Noisy, difficult or exaggerated breathing. 'Clicking' or other sounds. Nasal or ocular discharge. Swollen sinuses	Observation and examination. Laboratory investigation	Depends upon cause. Antibiotics or sulphonamides – preferably by injection. Supportive care	There is a whole range of respiratory diseases. Many are due to or associated with bacteria but fungi and mites may also be involved. Chlamydiosis (chlamydophilosis) must always be considered: laboratory investigations (blood and faeces) will confirm. *See also* Sinusitis

Table 11.20 (Continued)

Species	Condition	Clinical signs	Treatment	Comment
	Dysecdysis	Difficulty in sloughing or abnormal in frequency	Attention to environment. Soaking of reptiles will facilitate sloughing	Underlying hormonal disturbances may also be involved
Amphibians and fish	'Fungus' (*Saprolegnia* infection)	Distinct fungal growth (like cotton wool) on body surface	Treat underlying factors. Topical therapy with povidone–iodine or malachite green	Usually secondary to other factors – e.g. skin lesions, poor water quality
	Leech infestation	Leeches visible. Anaemia. Secondary infection	Sodium chloride baths	Often introduced with live food or vegetation
	'White spot' (*Ichthyophthirius*) infection	Pinhead-size white foci on skin	Proprietary treatment – usually malachite green	Parasites can complete lifecycles rapidly in warm water. Often fatal if untreated
Fish	'Fin rot'	Damage and necrotic fins and tail	Depends on cause but attention to water quality essential. Antibiotics. Parasiticides	Environmental factors often responsible. *Saprolegnia* may supervene (*see* 'Fungus' *above*)
	External parasites: Protozoa, Monogenea, Crustacea	Various. Parasites may be visible on skin or gills. Hyperaemia and/or ulceration may occur	Depends on cause. Large parasites (e.g. *Argulus*) may be removed manually. Others may require parasitic baths	Detection of gill parasites may prove difficult in live fish. Skin parasites can lead to ulceration and bacterial septicaemia (*see earlier*)
	Tuberculosis	Various. Weight loss, skin lesions, ascites	Best to isolate/cull affected fish but treatment can be attempted. Hygiene	Common causes are *Mycobacterium marinum* and *M. fortuitum*. Zoonotic. Often only confirmed after death, but skin (and other) biopsies may permit ante mortem diagnosis

- External parasites – *Psoroptes cuniculi*, the rabbit ear mite, and *Cheyletiella parasitivorax*, the fur mite.
- Internal parasites – including roundworms (*Passalurus ambiguus*).
- Coccidiosis – most commonly seen in litters reared in unhygienic conditions. Signs are diarrhoea, poor growth, weight loss. Hepatic coccidiosis may be seen in adults.
- Abscesses – usually round the head, sometimes associated with tooth-root infection.
- Gastrointestinal problems – anorexia; diarrhoea; faeces matted around the anus (possibly if rabbit fails to eat its 'night faeces' because it is too obese to reach its anus); furballs; gastric dilatation (an emergency). Rabbits that have been anorectic and had gastrointestinal upset can often be tempted to feed with fresh, coarse greenstuff such as long grass, raspberry or dandelion leaves.
- 'Snuffles' – purulent nasal discharge or pneumonia. Most pet rabbits develop some lung damage during their lives. The incidence of respiratory disease increases in poorly ventilated or too warm an environment.
- Myxomatosis – a viral disease still widespread in the wild population, carried by the rabbit flea, which can reach the pet rabbits via a cat or dog passing through the garden. Vaccination is recommended for all pet rabbits.
- Viral haemorrhagic disease (VHD), first reported in China in 1984, has spread rapidly and reached the UK in 1992. It is highly infectious and can be spread from rabbit to rabbit or mechanically. An inactivated vaccine is available and rabbits should be immunised regularly.
- Fly-strike, or myiasis, is a common problem of rabbits kept in poor sanitary conditions. Literally the fly larvae will eat away at the flesh of the living animal. Larvae should be removed, wounds thoroughly cleaned, antibiotics and pain control commenced, and cases carefully assessed with respect to the extent of the injuries. Anaesthesia may be necessary for treatment and the animal may need to be euthanased on humane grounds.
- Traumatic injuries – falls, attacks by dogs/cats. Rabbits have very powerful hindlegs and a sudden leap in fear can result in spinal injury.

Many rabbits bought as pets for young children end up unhandled and largely ignored because of the development of behavioural problems, usually related to the onset of sexual maturity. Males often become aggressive and may bite or urine spray; females will bite and stamp in defence of their 'nest-burrow'. Neutering of both sexes is recommended: it will avoid these problems and will also reduce the incidence of uterine adenocarcinoma, a major cause of death in female rabbits.

Guinea pigs

- In the case of any sick guinea pig, ascertain the likely vitamin C status – low dietary values are likely to hamper recovery from skin and other diseases.
- Malocclusion – occurs but probably less commonly than in rabbits. Salivation may be a sign – commonly called 'slobbers'.
- Skin disease – may be caused by sarcoptic mange mite (*Trixacarus caviae*) and less frequently by ringworm. Lice are also sometimes seen. Poor hutch hygiene may lead to pododermatitis (sore feet). Hair loss may be due to 'barbering' by other guinea pigs.
- Nutritional disease – guinea pigs may 'barber' (chew) each other's hair if there is insufficient roughage in the diet. Vitamin C deficiency shows in young animals as poor growth, reluctance to move, swollen joints; skin wounds take a long time to heal.
- Diarrhoea – a number of causes.
- Impaction of the anus – quite common, particularly in males. Faeces may be normal or softer than usual and accumulate just inside the anus.
- Cystic and urethral calculi – not uncommon in guinea pigs.
- Respiratory disease – common in guinea pigs.
- Pregnancy toxaemia – quite common in the last 2 weeks of pregnancy; more likely in obese or stressed animals. The disease tends to have a rapid course. Sometimes the animal is found dead by the owner.

Chinchilla

Common problems include malocclusion ('slobbers'), abdominal pain (often gastric dilatation), fur-chewing (where not enough hay is supplied) and, less commonly, ringworm.

Rats, mice, gerbils and hamsters

- Malocclusion may occur in all the small pet mammals.
- Respiratory disease – all are susceptible and they may contract some infections from owners with sore throats and colds.
- Parasitic diseases – including various mange mites (*Demodex* species in hamsters, commonly *Notoedres* in mice and rats).
- Nutritional disease – more likely to be subclinical than an obvious nutrient deficiency, but a great many clinical problems in small-mammal pets can be helped by improving the diet. Animals allowed unlimited amounts of sunflower seeds may develop osteodystrophy.
- Impacted pouches – all species of hamster may suffer; the pouches may become impacted with either food or unsuitable bedding material (such as cotton wool).
- Traumatic injuries – not uncommon in the small pets (they may be dropped accidentally). The protruding eyes of Syrian hamsters are sometimes damaged and may require enucleation.
- 'Wet tail' disease in hamsters – seen in young, recently weaned animals which develop diarrhoea and quickly become dehydrated; often fatal. If the hamster was

recently acquired, owners should not purchase a replacement from the same source.

Many small-mammal pets develop behavioural problems, especially as a result of living in an inadequate unstimulating environment – often both too small and inadequately furnished. Gerbils without much to dig in will scrabble obsessively at one corner of the cage. Some will eat too much or drink too much or gnaw at the bars if there is nothing better to chew. Others exhibit stereotypical behaviour, performing a series of actions over and over again. Chipmunks kept in small cages indoors often repeatedly somersault in one corner of the cage.

Ferrets

The most common problems in ferrets are fleas, abscesses (which require veterinary attention) and endoparasites. They can also contract distemper (vaccination may be recommended if the disease is locally prevalent) and can catch colds or influenza from humans. Owners might also require advice about oestrus control, spaying, vasectomy and castration. Working ferrets, kept for hunting, tend to be susceptible to different diseases – many of them related to an outdoor life – from those kept as pets. American publications refer only to the latter.

Common problems in birds

Nutrition and environment

General poor health in birds is often associated with suboptimal accommodation and poor nutrition. Only with experience can the distinction be made between a really healthy, fit and active bird with glossy plumage and one that is surviving but in suboptimal health. However, there are certain specific deficiencies:

- Iodine deficiency – common in budgerigars, often presents as respiratory distress caused by pressure of the enlarged thyroid gland on the trachea.
- Vitamin A deficiency – very common in all cage birds, particularly those that have very little fruit or vegetable in their diet. Clinical signs may be those of mild to moderate upper respiratory disease, with swellings around the eyes, nasal discharge and blocked nostrils. More severe cases have small abscesses on the palate.
- Calcium deficiency – may occur in any species but is a particular problem in African grey parrots. Initially inactivity, drooping wings and general discomfort, progressing in severe cases to fits. Also seen in birds that have been laying constantly over a period.
- 'Stuck in the moult' – a state of constant moulting. Birds normally moult in response to decreasing day length at one end of the summer but some birds kept indoors moult constantly under the influence of artificial lighting. There may be a nutritional factor as well; increasing the protein content of the diet has helped in some cases.

Infectious and parasitic disease

- Roundworm infestation – common in aviary birds, particularly ground-feeding grass parakeets. Birds should be dewormed twice a year, before the breeding season starts in spring and after the moult in the autumn.
- Trichomoniasis – commonly transmitted to aviary birds (usually budgerigars) via the faeces of wild birds, especially pigeons. It is caused by a protozon that infects the upper part of the digestive tract, particularly the oesophagus and crop, resulting in inappetence and regurgitation.
- Salmonellosis – not uncommonly diagnosed in birds showing gastrointestinal signs. The serotypes isolated may or may not be those that commonly cause disease in humans. May be spread to aviaries by wild birds.

The two major infectious diseases in birds are (chlamydiosis now called chlamydophilosis) and PBFD (see below) is caused by a *chlamydophila* and may produce either respiratory or gastrointestinal signs. Suspect birds should be isolated. There is a danger to human health: the disease is spread in dry faeces. Nurses caring for such birds should wear gloves and masks, and should dampen the paper at the bottom of the bird's cage before moving it (to minimise the spread of the spores). The disease can be treated but pet birds that are confirmed carriers are sometimes euthanased because of the danger to human health. A health and safety risk assessment is essential when dealing with possible cases (COSHH).

Psittacine beak and feather disease (dystrophy) (PBFD), a viral disease affecting the integument, is seen in many different species but most commonly in cockatoos. Birds often present as 'feather pluckers': in severe cases the birds have very few feathers and those that remain are broken and greasy-looking, while the horn of the beak is soft and crumbly. Affected birds eventually die of the effects of secondary bacterial and fungal infection of the damaged skin and feathers. This is a very infectious disease and could pose a serious threat in a breeding colony of rare or valuable parrots. Rapid diagnosis is advisable.

Reproductive disorders

Persistent egg-laying may occur in any species but is particularly common in cockatiels. In the wild, birds continue to lay eggs until they have a full clutch. If an owner removes unfertilised eggs from a captive bird, it will lay more and may suffer severe depletion of stored calcium and protein. If a bird is 'broody' (wishing to lay eggs and then sit on them), it is far better that the owner should give her a nest-tray or box and allow her to sit, not removing the eggs (or putting in dummy eggs) until she has finished with them after a couple of weeks of fruitless incubation.

Egg-binding may occur with a first egg, or after a period of egg-laying. The bird may collapse and become anorectic: it will need supportive therapy as well as specific treatment to remove the egg.

Tumours and 'lumps'

Tumours are common in pet budgerigars. Lipomas occur over the breast in obese pet birds and tumours may also affect internal organs, particularly the gonads. This can result in pressure on the sciatic nerve, causing difficulty in perching. Feather lumps, or feather cysts, are particularly common in canaries. They are caused by deformities of a feather follicle, which eventually forms a large mass.

Behavioural problems

Behavioural problems are common in the larger pet birds. They include:

- Feather plucking.
- Nail chewing.
- Self-mutilation.
- Excessive screaming.

Stress-inducing factors that may contribute to such problems include:

- Poor diet.
- Boredom.
- Lack of companionship (bird or human).
- Lack of privacy.
- Sexual frustration (or wishing to breed).
- Lack of sleep (parrots need 8–10 hours of undisturbed sleep to remain healthy).
- Hot, dry atmosphere (often made worse by cigarette smoke or fumes). Rainforest species in particular prefer a high relative humidity.

Common problems in reptiles and amphibians

Failure to feed (in an otherwise healthy animal) may be because of an inadequate environment (temperature too low, poor lighting) or unsuitable food (a wild-caught snake may not recognise a dead white mouse as food).

Failure to slough (shed the skin) may occur in any reptile but is most important in snakes. When a snake is ready to shed, the skin becomes dull, the eyes appear milky and the animal will not feed. Sometimes the failure to shed is total but more often parts of the shed remain on the snake, including the eyelids or the tip of the tail. It is important that these are removed, and with great care, particularly the 'spectacles' over the eyes by gently wiping with a moistened cotton-bud. Increasing the humidity or allowing the snake to bathe will often help.

Other problems include:

- Stomatitis ('mouth rot') – infection within the mouth. This is common in snakes and also in debilitated tortoises (particularly after hibernation).
- Necrotic dermatitis ('scale rot') – common in snakes. Predisposing factors may be too low a temperature, or

too moist a vivarium so that the snake cannot dry out after being in water.

- Regurgitation of food – occurs for a number of reasons: the temperature in the vivarium may be too low for digestion; the snake may be suffering from endoparasites or a gastric infection; and some snakes will regurgitate if they are handled too soon after feeding.
- Hypovitaminosis A – not uncommon in lizards and Chelonia. The signs include swelling of the eyes, epiphora and unwillingness to feed. Hypervitaminosis A can also occur, usually as a result of over-supplementation, and causes skin lesions (usually a moist dermatitis).

Land tortoises may develop **post-hibernation anorexia (PHA)**, a blanket term to cover all those that do not start eating within a week or so of emerging from hibernation. They may have stomatitis, liver failure or kidney failure; or they may simply have exhausted their vitamin reserves or be dehydrated. The kidneys barely function during hibernation, so that waste products build up in the circulation and blood tests may reveal a very high blood uric acid. Some tortoises with PHA respond well to basic fluid therapy and vitamin supplementation.

Other land tortoise problems include:

- Roundworms – particularly where a number of tortoises are kept, or where they have been on the same piece of ground for a number of years.
- Infectious rhinitis – a very infectious and debilitating viral disease affecting the spur-thighed tortoise and certain other species; it may take a year or more to clear and carriers may remain.
- Osteodystrophy (MBD) in young animals fed a diet low in calcium or with a poor calcium/phosphorus ratio.

Nursing and anaesthesia

Animals that are sick and debilitated may need to be hospitalised and nursed within the surgery. Sometimes there is merit in housing the patient in its own cage; at other times special accommodation may need to be constructed. The practice should ensure that it is always prepared for emergencies involving exotic pets by having one or more of each of the following:

- 'Hospital cages' – designed for birds but equally useful for small mammals and sometimes reptiles and amphibians.
- Glass or plastic aquaria – primarily used for fish but easily modified to accommodate other species.
- Other suitable containers, e.g. bird cages (preferably with solid sides), buckets.

Important aspects of nursing exotics include:

- Provision of warmth/maintenance of the patient at its preferred body temperature or within its preferred optimal temperature zone (POTZ).
- Maintenance of fluid balance.

- Ensuring adequate nutrient intake.
- Minimising stress.
- Relief/control of pain.

Nursing of exotics and wildlife can, as with other species, be broadly divided into (a) medical nursing, and (b) surgical nursing. The former includes assisted/oral therapy (different species need different sizes of tube and qualities of food and fluids) and the calculation of drug doses based on the patient's metabolism. Surgical nursing relates to both major and minor procedures that may be carried out on animals. Wound management is a particularly important part of the nurse's responsibility.

The nurse may also be consulted on such issues as the choice of a pet (see earlier) and legal or ethical considerations relating to the tending of sick and injured wildlife. Some knowledge of the law – and where correct information can be found – is increasingly important. The nurse should also be aware of Codes of Practice – for example, that produced by the British Wildlife Rehabilitation Centre (BWRC) – for casualty animals.

Veterinary nurses may also be asked to collect samples from their exotic patients, to monitor the health of an individual or help in the diagnosis of disease. Faeces may be collected off a clean surface for gross and microscopic examination or for bacterial culture. Bacteriology swabs may also be taken directly from the rectum or cloaca, or sometimes (particularly in snakes with infrequent defecation) a cloacal wash of sterile saline may be used. Likewise, stomach or crop washes may be useful. Urine can be collected for analysis or urates examined for changes in colour or consistency. Snake skins can be examined for the presence of mites, and feathers collected to look for ectoparasites or to test for specific infectious diseases. The taking of blood samples and often their examination is increasingly the responsibility of the veterinary nurse, and it is important that the nurse knows the commonly used sites, and the appropriate techniques for its preservation and storage. There are a number of good texts (Mader, Fudge, etc., see Further reading) that provide this information in depth.

Anaesthesia of mammals, birds and reptiles

Diagnostic or surgical interventions often require manipulation or restraint. Simple, non-invasive procedures, such as radiography or ultrasonography, may sometimes be possible using physical methods alone, provided humane considerations are met. Examples of such methods are described in Table 11.21 and Fig. 11.11.

More invasive procedures (in terms of duration, levels of pain, etc.) will generally require chemical restraint. Variation in biology, including anatomy, physiology or behaviour, makes anaesthesia of exotic species a particularly interesting and challenging task. Fundamentals, however, remain the same as for domestic species, and it is important to emphasise that the needs and well-being of an animal during the pre- and post-operative periods are an integral part of the anaesthetist's responsibilities. Thought must be given to a reduction in pain, distress and mortality rate,

Table 11.21 Physical methods of restraint

Tools	General	Mammals	Birds	Reptiles
Diminish sense perception	Light if nocturnal Dark if diurnal Reduced physical contact Reduced noise	Cloth bag over head of (for example) a roe deer	Hooding a bird of prey/ ostrich	Lower temperature[a] Hooding
Allow safe confinement and examination	Bag Towel Net	Crush cage Anaesthetic induction chamber	Guillotine restraint device Specially designed harnesses, e.g. Velcro swanwrap	Snake tube Sandbag
Lend added strength or extend the arms	Net	Rope Snare	—	Snake hook or grab[b]
Subdue the animal	Physical restraint (with or without gloves)[c]	—	Towel wrap	Lower temperature[a]
Special techniques	Several methods are available[c]	Hypnosis of rabbits	Tonic immobility (galliforms)	Tonic immobility (dorsal recumbency) in lizards or crocodilians Vaso-vagal response in lizards[d]

[a] *No analgesia*
[b] *Care must be taken not to cause injury (do not handle sloughing reptiles)*
[c] *The greatest protection of all is a detailed knowledge of the biology and behaviour of the species*
[d] *Pressure on the eyes causes hypotension and bradycardia – recovery is spontaneous or follows a tactile or sonic stimulus (Malley, 1997)*

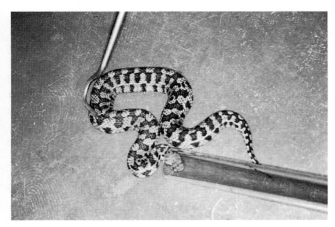

Fig. 11.11 Aggressive or venomous snakes (such as this Milos viper, *Macrovipera schweizeri*) can be safely restrained and examined using a Perspex snake tube.

as well as to improvements in the speed and quality of recovery.

Pre-operative preparations

Pre-operative assessment is important. The species *must* be identified. It should then be maintained at its preferred body temperature (PBT). This is particularly vital in reptiles due to their ectothermic nature. The PBT of an individual reptile can be taken to be its body core temperature (usually measured as the cloacal temperature) at which its heart rate is as close as possible to that calculated by the following allometric formula (Malley, 1997):

$$\text{heart rate (pulse)} = 34 \text{ (bodyweight [kg])} - 0.25$$

Temperatures for common species are suggested in a number of texts (e.g. Jackson and Cooper, 1981; McKeown, 1986) and examples are given in Table 11.8. In practice, given a choice, reptiles will select their own PBT and so it is generally simpler and safer to offer a thermal gradient (Davies, 1981), for example, by use of a heat-lamp or heat-pad at one end of the vivarium.

Patients should be allowed to acclimatise to their environment. During this period, food and water intake, bodyweight, urine and faecal loss, and other biological parameters, can be measured. For the more sensitive patient or where facilities for hospitalisation are inadequate, resulting in increased stress or risk of cross-infection, time away from the normal home environment should be minimised. These biological data may instead be provided by the owner.

Body condition must be assessed. Weight-to-length ratios (e.g. weight to cube of carapace length in chelonians; weight to ulnar ('carpal') length in birds) are useful indicators, as is the simple evaluation of pectoralis musculature in birds. Blood samples may be taken for routine biochemistry and haematology. It is important to note that reptiles are very susceptible to bacterial infections introduced through the skin and so the site of any injection must first be thoroughly scrubbed with povidone–iodine solution. Hydration status should be assessed and corrected, if necessary (see Chapter 22, Fluid Therapy and Shock). Methods of fluid replacement are described in Table 11.22. All fluids should be given at the PBT.

Ideally, animals should be free from clinical disease. Subclinical disorders, such as chronic respiratory diseases, are also important because they may cause respiratory depression, leading to anaesthetic complications. Normal liver and kidney function is essential for many anaesthetic agents and should be assessed or such agents avoided.

The duration of pre-anaesthetic fasting (withdrawal of food) depends on the species and is summarised in Table 11.23. Fasting is necessary in some species, e.g. chelonians, to avoid compression of the lungs, and in many other species, particularly some mammals and all snakes, to prevent vomiting (with its associated risks of an aspiration pneumonia). It is also important for some diagnostic procedures. Fasting in small mammals and birds, which have a high metabolic rate, can result in hypoglycaemia and is contraindicated.

Pre-anaesthetic handling and medication

Experienced animal handling is vital. Great care must be taken to minimise stress to the patient at all times, particularly during anaesthetic induction. Lighting and noise levels should be reduced, mobile phones and pagers switched off. It is often beneficial to minimise physical contact. This may be achieved by use of an anaesthetic induction chamber or by using fast methods of induction. Animals may also be habituated beforehand to the various anaesthetic techniques, e.g. trained to tolerate a facemask.

Pre-anaesthetic medication is often useful. It may allow a reduction in fear or apprehension leading to stress-free induction, a reduction in the dosage of anaesthetic agents, a reduction in salivation or reflex bradycardia, a smoother

Table 11.22 Methods of fluid replacement	

Species	Method
Mammals	Oral administration of proprietary rehydration fluids Parenteral administration – saline or Hartmann's solution. Given subcutaneously, intraperitoneally, intraosseously or intravenously
Birds	Oral administration of proprietary rehydration fluids Parenteral administration – saline, dextrose saline, or Hartmann's solution. Given subcutaneously, intramuscularly, intraosseously or intravenously
Reptiles	Immersion in potable water at preferred body temperature Oral administration of proprietary rehydration fluids – prepared as for mammals then diluted a further 10% with potable water Parenteral administration – a mixture of one part each of non-lactated dextrose saline. Ringer's solution, and water for injection. Given epicoelomically, intracoelomically, intraosseously or intravenously

Table 11.23 Duration of pre-anaesthetic fasting

Species	Time
Mammals (Flecknell, 1997)	Small primates or ferrets – 12–16 hours Small rodents or rabbits – unnecessary
Birds (Forbes, 1998)	< 200 g – rarely required (never more than 3 hours), crop should be empty Granivorous birds – rarely required Waterfowl and carnivores – 4–10 hours
Reptiles (Malley, 1997)	Chelonians or lizards – 18 hours Snakes – 72–96 hours

recovery, and a reduction in pre- and post-operative pain. A variety of agents is used, which include anticholinergics (e.g. atropine and glycopyrronium), phenothiazines, butyrophenones and benzodiazepines.

It is important that all anaesthetic and surgical equipment is prepared and checked prior to the start of any procedure.

General anaesthesia

Methods of induction depend on the species of animal, its size and ability to be physically restrained, its demeanour, for example, whether it is alert and aggressive or sedated and sleepy, the anaesthetic requirements, i.e. whether or not a surgical plane of anaesthesia is required, the presence of any concurrent diseases, the anaesthetic equipment available and the drugs available. Details are given in Table 11.24.

Topical anaesthetic agents (local analgesics) may sometimes be used and can reduce general anaesthetic requirements. Particular care is required in birds, in view of their susceptibility to the toxic effects of these agents.

Once the animal has been anaesthetised, it is important to position it correctly. In general, it is best to avoid dorsal recumbency in birds and reptiles; the weight of viscera on the lungs can reduce the tidal volume and accentuate respiratory embarrassment.

Maintenance of anaesthesia may be achieved by the use of inhalation agents, continuous intravenous infusion or

Table 11.24 Common methods and drugs of induction

Species	Oral	Inhalation	Injection Intramuscular	Injection Intravenous
Mammals	Generally unpredictable. Ketamine has been used in primates	Anaesthetic induction chamber or face mask Isoflurane (Isoflo; Schering-Plough) or Sevoflurane (Abbott)[a] are agents of choice	Fentanyl/fluanisone (Hypnorm; Janssen) and midazolam, both given intraperitoneally in small mammals, intramuscularly in large mammals; reversed with butorphanol Ketamine and medetomidine (Domitor; Pfizer), both given intramuscularly or intravenously; reversed with atipamezole (Antisedan; Pfizer)	
Birds	Rarely used Tiletamine 5% and zolazepam 5% (Zoletil; Virbac) in birds of prey	Anaesthetic induction chamber or face mask Isoflurane (Isoflo; Schering-Plough) or Sevoflurane (Abbot)[a] are agents of choice	Ketamine and medetomidine (Domitor; Pfizer); reversed with atipamezole (Antisedan; Pfizer) Alphaxalone and alphadolone (Saffan; Schering–Plough) Ketamine with diazepam or xylazine or midazolam. Avoid xylazine in pigeons	Ketamine and medetomidine (Domitor; Pfizer); reversed with atipamezole (Antisedan; Pfizer) Alphaxalone and alphadolone (Saffan; Schering–Plough) Ketamine with diazepam or xylazine or midazolam
Reptiles	Not used	Facemask, isoflurane (Isoflo; Schering–Plough) in lizards only Tracheal intubation in conscious patient, isoflurane (Isoflo; Schering–Plough) in chelonians, snakes and lizards	Alphaxalone andalphadolone (Saffan; Schering–Plough) Metomidate in snakes (also intracoelomically) NB: no analgesic properties Ketamine and medetomidine (Domitor; Pfizer) in Chelonia	Propofol (Rapinovet; Schering–Plough) commonly used (also intraosseously in Chelonia and squamates) Alphaxalone and alphadolone (Saffan; Schering–Plough)

[a] *No product licence in the UK*

repeated intramuscular injections – the last method being the most variable and unreliable.

Inhalation agents may be administered via a close-fitting facemask, particularly in small mammals and birds.

High gas flow rates (3–4 times the respiratory minute volume) are usually required. Once induction has been achieved, it is preferable to intubate the animal with an endotracheal tube and to use an appropriate anaesthetic circuit. Intubation is particularly important for operations on the head and mouth, or for situations where respiratory monitoring or mechanical ventilation may be required (especially in reptiles). Intubation may be complicated in some species, e.g. it is important not to bypass the lung of small snakes, leading to intubation of the non-absorptive air sac, or not to bypass the carina of chelonians, resulting in insufflation of only one lung. It may also be impossible to intubate very small animals without a significant risk of saliva obstructing the air flow. An Ayre's T-piece is probably the most useful anaesthetic circuit, since most patients will be less than 10 kg in weight. This circuit is best modified with the addition of an open-ended bag to the reservoir tube (Jackson–Rees modified T-piece), thus allowing assisted ventilation. The reservoir volume should be equal to approximately one-third of the animal's tidal volume and the fresh gas flow rate should be about 2–3 times its respiratory minute volume. The use of intermittent positive-pressure ventilation (IPPV) throughout anaesthesia may be necessary in reptiles, especially when premedicants are used. In birds, on occasions where access to the trachea is required, an air sac breathing tube may be inserted through the abdominal wall and used for the maintenance of anaesthesia. In mammals, birds and reptiles, isoflurane (Isoflo; Schering–Plough) or sevoflurane (Abbott) (no product licence) is the inhalation anaesthetic agent of choice.

Total intravenous anaesthesia is possible, e.g. using alphaxalone and alphadolone (Saffan; Schering–Plough) or propofol (Rapinovet; Schering–Plough), but often an additional opioid may be required for its analgesic properties. An infusion pump should be used.

Anaesthetic management

Methods of assessing the depth of anaesthesia are listed in Table 11.25. In addition to the reflexes, it is important to monitor respiration and the cardiovascular system. The depth, rate and pattern of respiration should be recorded. Methods include simple observation of the reservoir bag, use of an oesophageal stethoscope, or use of an electronic apnoea alarm. Cardiovascular parameters, such as the heart rate, rhythm, quality of pulse or tissue perfusion are also important. Techniques include observation of a carotid pulse, estimation of the capillary refill time, use of an oesophageal stethoscope, use of an electrocardiogram or use of a Doppler probe to monitor peripheral perfusion. Pulse oximetry is also used to monitor anaesthesia, the lingual clip being applied to the tongue or mucous membranes, or across a toe, footpad or tail, or a small rectal probe being

Table 11.25 Methods of assessing the depth of anaesthesia

Species	Method
Mammals	Heart rate
	Respiratory rate
	Righting reflex
	Response to painful stimuli:
	Toe or tail pinch
	Ear pinch
	Palpebral reflex (some species)
	Eyeball position
	Pupillary dilatation
	Nystagmus
Birds	Heart rate
	Respiratory rate
	Pedal reflex
	Corneal reflex
	Cloacal reflex
Reptile	Heart rate
	Respiratory rate
	Movement (A)
	Serpentine (slithering) movement (S)
	Muscle relaxation (A)
	Righting reflex (A)
	Tongue withdrawal reflex (S)
	Head-raising reflex (S)
	Response to painful stimuli:
	Skin prick (A)
	Tail pinch (S)
	Pedal (L)
	S-form (strike) posture (S)
	Jaw tone (Ch)
	Bauchstreich reflex (S)
	Laryngeal reflexes in alligators

S = snakes, L = lizards, Ch = chelonians, A = all species

inserted into the rectum, cloaca or oesophagus, as appropriate (Fig. 11.12). Despite such techniques, a good observer (such as a veterinary nurse) is *the* most important form of monitoring.

Body temperature should be monitored, preferably via an oesophageal or rectal electronic thermometer (contraindicated if using radiosurgery), and kept within the preferred range.

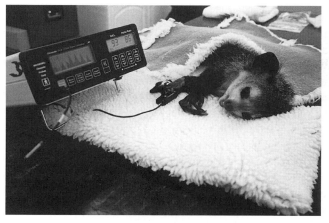

Fig. 11.12 Monitoring anaesthesia is important: use of a pulse oximeter on an anaesthetised patient.

Fluid balance should be maintained. As a routine, fluid should be replaced at a rate of 10–15 ml/kg of bodyweight/hour of general anaesthesia, administered parenterally. Details are given in Table 11.22.

If vomiting or regurgitation occurs, the animal must be placed in a head-down position, and the vomit aspirated from the mouth and the pharynx.

Reversal of anaesthesia

As soon as the procedure is complete, recovery from anaesthesia can begin. In many cases, this simply involves turning off the supply of isoflurane (Isoflo; Schering–Plough), while maintaining oxygen flow. With some of the injectable anaesthetic agents, such as the alpha-2-agonists (e.g. medetomidine) or the opioids, an antagonist may be used. Rapid recovery is advantageous, especially in patients with high metabolic rates; however, analgesia must be administered where relevant.

Post-operative care

The demarcation between intra- and post-operative care is often not clear, and many of the monitoring procedures and routine therapeutic regimes should be continued until the animal has recovered. In reptiles, this may not be considered to be the case until the righting reflex has fully returned, with normal locomotion.

Warmth and comfort must be provided. The patient should be kept at its preferred body temperature. If possible, an animal incubator should be used. Respiratory depression must be prevented. Cardiorespiratory stimulants, such as doxapram hydrochloride (Dopram-V; Fort Dodge), may be routinely used, particularly in reptiles. Intermittent positive pressure ventilation (with 10% carbon dioxide and 90% oxygen, or with air) can be necessary (and in reptiles, essential) right up until the removal of the endotracheal tube. In mammals, tube removal should occur when the swallowing and cough reflexes return, whereas in reptiles, it may not be appropriate until the animal is fully recovered. Maintained intubation also reduces the risks of an aspiration pneumonia and, in reptiles, where the glottis is normally closed in the relaxed state, intubation can prevent suffocation. Once again, dehydration status should be assessed and corrected, with anticipation of a period of reduced voluntary fluid uptake following anaesthesia. Consideration of analgesia is also important, particularly if agents such as propofol (Rapinovet; Schering–Plough) and isoflurane (Isoflo; Schering–Plough) have been used, with their minimal post-recovery analgesic properties.

The recovery environment is critical. The veterinary nurse must consider potential stressors to the patient and try to eliminate them accordingly. Simple improvements in the surroundings might include: reduced noise and light levels; reduction of draughts; positioning away from busy entrances and passageways; positioning at a suitable height (birds feel more secure in a high position); positioning away from other animals, e.g. barking dogs, birds should not be placed near cats or other predatory birds; provision of a nest box; provision of a suitable substrate; avoidance of unnecessary obstacles and perching before the animal is fully recovered. With careful planning, a number of injuries will undoubtedly be avoided.

Following anaesthesia, food and fluid intake, faecal and urine production, and the animal's demeanour should be monitored. Small patients, with a high metabolic rate, must eat soon after recovery. The total period of starvation should not exceed 3 hours. Low light levels may subdue, but may also prevent feeding. If the patient does not eat voluntarily, gavage feeding should be used. Should *any* problems occur, then assistance from a veterinary surgeon must be quickly sought.

Anaesthesia of amphibians and fish

Common anaesthetic agents of amphibians and fish include dilute solutions of tricaine methane sulphonate (MS222; Sandoz) or benzocaine (Scott, 1991).

For induction, fish are immersed and amphibians submerged up to their nostrils in one of these solutions, preferably within an induction tank (Fig. 11.13). The rate of induction is very variable, and the patient must be carefully monitored. The aim is to reach a stage of minimal activity, essentially sedation, rather than anaesthesia. Once this stage is reached, then the patient is removed from the induction tank and placed on a damp cool towel. Head and tail are covered. Depth of anaesthesia can be varied by syringing either oxygenated water or anaesthetic solution onto the animal and, in particular, its gills, if present. Gills should be kept wet. For recovery, fish are immersed and amphibians submerged up to their nostrils in clean oxygenated water and, in species with gills, encouraged to move with their mouth open, so that water flows over the gills.

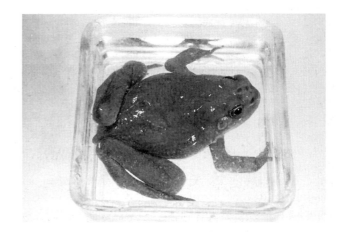

Fig. 11.13 Non-domesticated species may need special equipment or techniques for anaesthesia: this frog is being anaesthetised in water in a glass dish, using a water-soluble agent (benzocaine).

Acknowledgements

The authors would very much like to thank Paul Flecknell MRCVS, Neil Forbes FRCVS, Dermod Malley FRCVS and Martin Lawton FRCVS for their constructive criticism of, and specialist input into, this chapter.

Further reading

Barnett, J. (1998) Treatment of sick and injured marine mammals. *In Practice*, vol. 20, no. 4, pp. 200–211.

Beynon, P. H., Forbes, N. A. and Harcourt-Brown, N. H. (eds) (1996) *Manual of Raptors, Pigeons and Waterfowl*, BSAVA, Cheltenham.

Beynon, P. H., Forbes, N. A. and Lawton, M. P. C. (eds) (1996) *Manual of Psittacines*, BSAVA, Cheltenham.

Coles, B. H. (1997) *Avian Medicine and Surgery*, 2nd edn, Blackwell, Oxford.

Cooper, J. E. (1986) Animals in schools. *Journal of Small Animal Practice*, vol. 27, pp. 839–850.

Cooper, J. E. (1990) Feeding exotic and pocket pets. *Journal of Small Animal Practice*, vol. 31, pp. 482–488.

Cooper, J. E. (2002) *Birds of Prey: Health and disease* Blackwell, Oxford.

Davies, P. M. C. (1981) Anatomy and physiology. In Cooper, J. E. and Jackson, O. F. (eds), *Diseases of the Reptilia*, vol. 1, pp. 9–73, Academic Press, London.

Flecknell, P. A. (1997) *Laboratory Animal Anaesthesia*, 2nd edn, Academic Press, New York.

Flecknell, P. A. (1998) Developments in the veterinary care of rabbits and rodents. *In Practice*, vol. 20, no. 6, pp. 286–295.

Forbes, N. A. (1998) Avian anaesthesia. In Seymour, C. and Gleed, R. (eds), *Manual of Anaesthesia*, 4th edn, BSAVA, Cheltenham.

Frye, F. L. (1992) *Captive Invertebrates: A Guide to Their Biology and Husbandry*, Krieger Publishing, Melbourne, FL.

Fudge, A. M. (ed.) (2000) *Laboratory Medicine, Avian and Exotic Pets*, W. B. Saunders Company, Philadelphia.

Hillyer, E. V. and Quesensbury, K. E. (eds) (1997) *Ferrets, Rabbits and Rodents, Clinical Medicine and Surgery*, W. B. Saunders Company, Philadelphia.

IATA (Annual) *IATA Live Animal Regulations*, 20th edn, International Air Transport Association, Montreal, Canada.

Jackson, O. F. and Cooper, J. E. (1981) Nutritional diseases. In Cooper, J. E. and Jackson, O. F. (eds), *Diseases of the Reptilia*, vol. 2, pp. 409–428, Academic Press, London.

Lewington, J. (2000) *Ferret Husbandry, Medicine and Surgery*, Butterworth–Heinemann, Oxford.

Mader, D. R. (ed.) (1996) *Reptile Medicine and Surgery*, W. B. Saunders, Philadelphia.

Malley, D. (1997) Reptile anaesthesia and the practising veterinarian. *In Practice*, vol. 19, no. 7, pp. 351–368.

Mattison, C. (1987) *The Care of Reptiles and Amphibians in Captivity*, 2nd edn, Blandford Press, Poole.

McKay, J. (1989) *The Ferret and Ferreting Handbook*, Rowood Press, Avon.

McKeown, S. (1986) General husbandry and management. In Mader, D. R. (ed.), *Reptile Medicine and Surgery*, pp. 9–19, W. B. Saunders, Philadelphia.

Meredith, A. and Redrobe, S. (2002) *BSAVA Manual of Exotic Pets*, BSAVA.

Scott, P. W. (1991) Ornamental fish. In Beynon, P. H. and Cooper, J. E. (eds), *Manual of Exotic Pets*, pp. 272–285, BSAVA, Cheltenham.

Williams, D. L. (1991) Amphibians. In Beynon, P. H. and Cooper, J. E. (eds), *Manual of Exotic Pets*, pp. 261–271, BSAVA, Cheltenham.

Journals and magazines

Animal Welfare
Aquarist (The)
Journal of Herpetology
Cage Aviary Birds
Exotic DVM
Fur and Feather
Journal of Association of Avian Veterinarians
Journal of Herpetological Medicine and Surgery
Racing Pigeon Pictorial
Symposia of the British Wildlife Rehabilitation Council
Tropical Fish Hobbyist

Societies

Bat Conservation Trust
British Chelonia Group
British Falconers' Club
British Herpetological Society
British House Rabbit Association
British Rabbit Council
British Veterinary Zoological Society
British Waterfowl Association
British Wildlife Rehabilitation Council
Commercial Rabbit Association
Federation of British Aquarists' Society
Hawk and Owl Trust (The)
National Cavy Club
National Council for Aviculture
National Fancy Rat Council
National Ferret School (The)
National Hamster Council
National Mouse Club
Royal Pigeon Racing Association
World Pheasant Association

Addresses and details of these can be obtained from websites or through the authors.

12

Medicines: pharmacology, therapeutics and dispensing

J. Elliott and *E. Reubens*

Learning objectives

After studying this chapter, students should be able to:

- Categorise drugs used in routine veterinary practice into their therapeutic groups.
- List the routes by which drugs can be administered and explain the effect that drug formulation and route of administration has on the rate of absorption of a drug into the body.
- Calculate drug dosages accurately, regardless of the units of drug concentration used in describing a particular formulation.
- List the legislation that governs the storage, handling, use and supply of medicines used in veterinary practice.
- Discuss the implications that the legislation has for the working of a veterinary practice.

Pharmacology, the science of drugs, can be divided into two parts. First, it is concerned with the study of the way in which the functions of the living body are affected by drugs (**pharmacodynamics**) and, secondly, with the absorption, metabolism and excretion of drugs by the body (**pharmacokinetics**). Much of our understanding of the pharmacology of drugs is derived from studies in normal healthy animals; the study of **clinical pharmacology** attempts to transpose this information to the diseased clinical patient.

Therapeutics can be defined as the rational and optimal use of drugs in the management of disease states or in the manipulation of physiological functions. In order to use drugs in a 'rational' and 'optimal' way, an understanding of the nature of the disease process and of the pharmacology of the drugs to be used is required. Without such an understanding, the clinical use of drugs is 'empirical'.

The subject of **pharmacy** can be defined as the **preparation** of drugs and their formulation into medicines followed by their **dispensing** (giving out) to the owner of a sick animal. Nowadays, most medicines are formulated by the pharmaceutical companies ready for dispensing. In many veterinary practices, medicines are dispensed to owners of sick animals from the practice premises. They can also be dispensed by pharmacists when presented by the owner of the animal with a written instruction (**prescription**) from the veterinary surgeon who is responsible for the care of the animal in question.

Drug classification

Definitions

Drugs are often classified according to:

(1) The way in which they bring about their effect on the body.
(2) Which body system (or infective agent) they affect.

This is the most useful form of classification for the practice pharmacy as, in many instances, it determines what the drugs are used for in clinical cases (i.e. their **major desired effect** on the body). In addition, a knowledge of the mode of action of drugs may enable the prediction of **side-effects** (effects which occur in addition to the desired therapeutic effect). However, it is important to recognise the side-effects of drugs cannot always be predicted from the way in which they cause their desired effect. When the side-effects of a particular drug compromise the health of an animal they are termed **undesirable** or **adverse drug** reactions. Any suspected adverse drug reactions encountered in veterinary practice should be reported to the Veterinary Medicines Directorate on special (yellow) reporting forms. Any drug which is administered at dosages above those recommended for therapeutic use (accidentally or deliberately) may cause **toxic effects** in the animal. The **therapeutic index** of a drug is the ratio between the dose which causes toxic effects and the dose required to produce the desired therapeutic effect. The lower this ratio the more dangerous a particular drug may be to use and the smaller the margin of error allowed when determining the dose for a particular animal.

Most drugs produce their desired effects by interacting with a defined target in the body or in the infective organism. This target may be a receptor for a naturally occurring hormone or neurotransmitter, which the drug may **mimic** by stimulating the receptor (receptor agonist) or **block** by occupying the receptor without stimulating it (receptor **antagonist**). Other targets for drugs include enzymes which serve physiological functions in the body or the infective organisms and which may be inhibited by drugs.

The categorisation of drugs set out in the rest of this section is used by both veterinary and medical formularies and would be a logical way of organising a practice pharmacy into groups of drugs. In each case, examples of drugs used in small animal practice are given. The name used is always the **generic** (approved or official) name rather than a **proprietary** (brand or trade) name. Where possible, examples will be given where a product exists which has been approved (**authorised**) for use in small animals.

Drugs used in the treatment of infections caused by micro-organisms

The micro-organisms include bacteria, fungi, viruses and protozoa. Drugs used to treat infections caused by these organisms can be termed **antimicrobial agents**. If the drug is a natural product of another micro-organism (as many are) then it is called an **antibiotic**. These drugs show the property of **selective toxicity**, targeting and damaging processes which are essential to the micro-organism but which do not take place in animal cells.

Antibacterial drugs

These are some of the most commonly used drugs in small animal practice. If they are capable of killing bacteria they are described as **bactericidal**; whereas if they just prevent division of bacteria they are called **bacteriostatic**. An antibacterial drug is described as **narrow spectrum** if it is active against a narrow range of bacteria (usually either Gram-positive or Gram-negative organisms) and **broad spectrum** if it is active against a wide variety of bacteria (or other micro-organisms such as protozoa). Some antibacterial drugs when used in combination produce more than the additive effects of the two drugs when used alone. In these cases, the drugs are said to **potentiate** each other (e.g. *potentiated sulphonamides are a combination of a sulphonamide plus trimethoprim or baquiloprim*). Antibacterial drugs are classified into families of drugs which are chemically related. The family of *penicillins*, for example, have the same mode of action and so are all bactericidal and share common side-effects (all can induce allergic reactions in sensitive animals

or people) for the animal being treated. Small changes in structure, however, may change their spectrum of activity. Table 12.1 summarises the main families of antibacterial drugs used in small animal practice, giving examples of each. Selection of appropriate antibacterial drug therapy depends on a number of factors (e.g. the bacterium involved, the site of infection and the immunocompetence of the patient). Good prescribing practice would be to have first-line antibacterial drugs for certain routine uses (e.g. prophylactic use in orthopaedic surgery) and to reserve some drug groups (e.g. the fluoroquinolones) for treatment of difficult life-threatening bacterial infections.

Antifungal drugs

These will kill or stop the growth of fungi (and could be described as **fungicidal** or **fungistatic**). *Griseofulvin* is used to treat dermatophytosis ('ringworm') in the dog and cat and *nystatin* is contained in some topical ear preparations to treat yeast infections. Recent evidence suggests that the flea product *lufenuron* also has good efficacy against feline dermatophytosis.

Antiviral drugs

These are infrequently used in veterinary medicine. *Aciclovir* is used topically in the eye to treat feline herpes virus infection.

Antiprotozoal drugs

These are used to treat infections caused by protozoal organisms such as *Toxoplasma gondii*. Example: *pyrimethamine*.

Table 12.1 Antibacterial drug families

Family	Example	Spectrum of activity	Bactericidal or bacteriostatic
Penicillins[a]	Benzyl penicillin	Narrow (Gram-positive)	Bactericidal
	Amoxycillin	Broad	Bactericidal
Tetracyclines	Oxytetracycline	Broad	Bacteriostatic
Aminoglycosides	Neomycin	Narrow (Gram-negative)	Bactericidal
Lincosamides	Clindamycin	Narrow (Gram-positives and anaerobes)	Bacteriostatic
Sulphonamides	Sulphadiazine	Broad	Bacteriostatic
Potentiated sulphonamides	Sulphadiazine plus trimethoprim	Broad	Bactericidal
Nitroimidazoles	Metronidazole	Narrow (anaerobes)	Bactericidal
Chloramphenicol	Chloramphenicol	Broad	Bacteriostatic
Fluoroquinolones	Enrofloxacin	Broad	Bactericidal

[a] *Penicillins and cephalosporins (e.g. cephalexin) are related chemically and collectively called β-lactams*

Drugs used in the treatment of parasitic infections

Endoparasiticides

These are used to treat infections of internal parasites. The majority of such infections in veterinary medicine are caused by helminths (nematodes, cestodes and trematodes) and so the drugs are termed **anthelmintics**. The internal parasites of the dog and cat are **nematodes** (round worms) and **cestodes** (tape worms). As with antibacterial drugs, anthelmintics can be broad or narrow spectrum. Table 12.2 gives examples of commonly used drugs and their spectrum of activity.

Ectoparasiticides

Ectoparasiticides are used to treat infestations of fleas, lice, ticks and mites, and are often administered topically in the form of sprays, baths, dusting powders or impregnated collars. The organophosphate compounds (e.g. *dichlorvos*), synthetic pyrethroids (e.g. *permethrin*), *fipronil, imidacloprid* and *selamectin* are commonly used in small-animal medicine. Other ectoparasiticides are given orally to dogs and cats and rely on the parasites ingesting the drug with a blood meal (e.g. *Lufenuron*). *Lufenuron* has a unique action, inhibiting chitin development and so preventing adult fleas producing viable eggs and larvae and so contributes to environmental control of fleas within a household. An understanding of the life cycle of the parasite involved is important for the successful treatment of parasitic infestations (see Chapter 15). Treatment of the environment may be appropriate to try to prevent re-infestation as the eggs and larvae develop within the house. Some forms of synthetic pyrethroids are formulated for application to carpets and furnishings to provide persistence of the drug in the environment and are not for application to the animal. These can be co-formulated with the insect growth regulator, *methoprene*, which inhibits the development of eggs and larvae into adult fleas.

Drugs acting on the gastrointestinal system

These are shown in Table 12.3.

Drugs used in the treatment of disorders of the cardiovascular system

These work primarily on the heart, the blood vessels, the blood coagulation system or the kidney.

Drugs acting on the heart

The heart can be stimulated to beat more strongly by drugs which are called **myocardial stimulants** (or positive inotropes) – examples include *digoxin* and *pimobendan*. Other drugs also increase the rate at which the heart beats and may be used in an emergency to treat complete heart block. The **sympathomimetic** *isoprenaline* (mimics the action of the sympathetic nervous system on the heart) is an example of such a drug. When the heart beats very fast with an abnormal rhythm it is said to be *arrhythmic*. Cardiac arrhythmias can be suppressed by **antidysrhythmic drugs** such as *lignocaine* (for ventricular arrhythmias) and *diltiazem* (for atrial arrhythmias). (NB: The preparation of lignocaine used to treat ventricular arrhythmias must **not** contain epinephrine/adrenaline.)

Finally, in some forms of heart disease, the heart muscle fails to relax properly to allow adequate filling during diastole. In this circumstance (e.g. hypertrophic cardiomyopathy in cats), drugs which reduce the force of contraction and/or slow the heart rate to improve diastolic filling are used (e.g. *diltiazem* and the beta-blocker *atenolol*).

Drugs acting on the blood vessels

Vasodilators relax the smooth muscle of blood vessels and lower resistance to blood flow, so reducing the work the heart has to do. Some act primarily on arterial smooth muscle (**arterial dilators**; *hydralazine*), some act primarily

Table 12.2 Examples of anthelmintics

	Tape worms			Round worms		
Drug	*Echinococcus*	*Taenia*	*Dipylidium*	*Toxocara/ Toxascaris*	Whip worms (*Trichuris*)	Hookworms (*Uncinaria*)
Fenbendazole	0	2	0	2	2	2
Mebendazole	1	2	0	2	2	2
Nitroscanate	1	2	2	2	2	0
Piperazine	0	0	0	1	1[a]	0
Praziquantel	2	2	2	0	0	0
Selamectin	0	0	0	2	2	2

[a] *Effective at 1.5 times the normal dose*
2, excellent activity; 1, very good activity; 0, poor or ineffective

Table 12.3 Drugs acting on the gastrointestinal system

Main drug class	Class	Mode of action	Examples
Antidiarrhoeal agents		*Suppress diarrhoea non-specifically*[a]	
	Adsorbents	Coat the gut wall, adsorb toxins	Charcoal, kaolin, bismuth
	Modulators of intestinal motility	Reduce gastrointestinal motility	Loperamide, diphenoxylate
	Chronic antidiarrhoeals	Anti-inflammatory agents	Sulphasalazine, prednisolone
Anti-emetic drugs		Prevent or suppress vomiting (emesis)	Metoclopramide (vomiting due to gastritis) Acepromazine (motion sickness)
Emetic drugs		Stimulate vomiting	Washing soda (orally) Xylazine (by injection)
Laxatives		*Increase defecation*	
	Lubricant laxatives	Lubricate faecal mass	Liquid paraffin
	Bulk-forming laxatives	Increase volume of faeces	Isphagula husk
	Osmotic laxatives	Hypertonic solutions, poorly absorbed	Phosphate (enemas)
	Stimulant laxatives	Stimulate local reflex gut motility	Danthron
Antacids		Neutralise acid secreted in stomach	Aluminium hydroxide
Ulcer-healing drugs		Inhibit acid secretion in the stomach and allow ulcers to heal	Cimetidine
Pancreatin supplements		Contain protease, lipase and amylase activity to aid digestion in EPI[b]	

[a] Specific treatment relies on identifying the underlying cause. In some cases, for example, antibacterial drugs or anthelmintics may be indicated.
[b] Exocrine pancreatic insufficiency

on venous smooth muscle (**venodilators**; *glyceryl trinitrate*) and others act on both sides of the circulation (**mixed dilators**; *enalapril*). A potential side-effect of these drugs is excessive lowering of arterial blood pressure (*hypotension*). Indeed, some are used in man to treat hypertension and are called **antihypertensive** drugs. Recently, hypertension has been recognised as occurring in cats, often secondary to diseases such as chronic renal failure. The vasodilator drug, *amlodipine*, which is a calcium channel blocker with selectivity for vascular smooth muscle, has proved an effective antihypertensive agent in cats.

Drugs acting on the kidney

Diuretics increase the volume of urine produced by an animal and the amount of salt excreted. Many are used in the treatment of congestive heart failure because in this condition the kidney tends to retain salt and water which contributes to the problem. The loop diuretics (e.g. *furosemide*) and the thiazide diuretics (e.g. *hydrochlorothiazide*) are most commonly used. Both give rise to excess potassium loss. Use of potassium-sparing diuretics (e.g. *spironolactone*) with these drugs will counteract this effect. Angiotensin-converting enzyme (ACE) inhibitors, which block the formation of angiotensin II and, thus, the secretion of aldosterone, can be regarded as potassium-sparing diuretics, but also have balanced vasodilator activity as mentioned above (e.g. *benazepril* and *enalapril*).

An ACE inhibitor has also recently been approved for use in cats with chronic renal failure (CRF). The ability of ACE

inhibitors to lower glomerular capillary pressure is thought to be one way in which they may slow the progression of CRF.

Drugs acting on the blood-clotting system

Anticoagulants prevent blood clotting (*heparin, warfarin*) whereas **fibrinolytic agents** break down clots once they have formed (e.g. *streptokinase*). **Haemostatics** arrest haemorrhage and are usually applied topically to local bleeding areas (e.g. *calcium alginate*).

Drugs used in the treatment of disorders of the respiratory system

Inhalation of infective agents or allergens (e.g. pollen) stimulate inflammation and tissue damage leading to reflex stimulation of coughing and bronchoconstriction. The sites at which drugs may counteract some of these disease processes are shown in Fig. 12.1. Examples of the drugs acting at these sites are given in Table 12.4.

Drugs acting on the nervous system
Sedatives

Sedatives produce calmness, drowsiness and indifference of the animal to its surroundings, and are often used as **pre-**

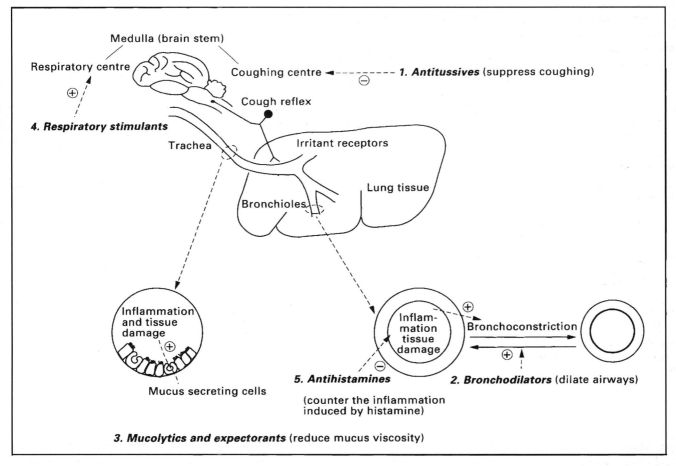

Fig. 12.1 A schematic representation of the respiratory system showing the sites at which drugs act in the treatment of respiratory disorders (⊕ = stimulation, ⊖ = inhibition of the processes indicated). Inhalation of allergens or infective agents initiate inflammation, bronchoconstriction, increased mucus secretion and coughing (via the cough reflex which stimulates the coughing centre in the medulla).

medicants for animals which are to be anaesthetised. Examples include *acepromazine* and *medetomidine*. The action of medetomidine can be reversed by the **sedative antagonist** *atipamezole*. The degree of drowsiness produced depends on the particular agent or agents used, the dose and the route of administration. A mild sedative is sometimes referred to as a **tranquilliser**, whereas drugs used to produce deep sedation (*narcosis*) can be called **narcotics**. See also Chapter 23, p. 649.

Opioid analgesics

These relieve pain by acting on opioid receptor sites in the brain and spinal cord. Examples are *morphine* and *buprenorphine*.

Combinations of sedatives and opioid analgesics can be used to produce deeper and more reliable sedation than sedatives alone. Such combinations are termed **neuroleptanalgesics**, an example being *fentanyl* and *fluansinone*. Sedation can then be reversed using an **opioid antagonist** such as *naloxone*.

General anaesthetics

These produce unconsciousness so that surgical or other procedures can be carried out painlessly. Pre-anaesthetic medication with sedatives and analgesics will allow a reduction in the dose of general anaesthetic required and produce a smoother induction and recovery from anaesthesia. **Injectable general anaesthetics** may be used for induction of anaesthesia (e.g. *thiopentone*) and maintenance of anaesthesia is often achieved by the use of **inhalational** (or **gaseous**) general anaesthetics (e.g. *halothane*).

Table 12.4 Drugs used in the treatment of disorders of the respiratory system	
Drug class	**Example**
Antitussive	Butorphanol
Antihistamine	Diphenhydramine
Bronchodilator	Theophylline, terbutaline
Mucolytic/expectorant	Bromhexine/ipecacuanha
Respiratory stimulant	Doxapram

Antimuscarinic drugs may be given before anaesthesia to counteract the salivation and increased bronchial secretions which, in small dogs and cats, may obstruct the airway. In addition, some surgical procedures may increase vagal nerve stimulation of the heart, reducing heart rate (causing bradycardia). Antimuscarinic drugs will prevent bradycardia. Examples: *atropine, hyoscine*.

Muscle relaxants

These prevent the message from the nerve reaching the skeletal muscle and so paralyse the muscle. *Pancuronium* is an example of such a drug which is used with general anaesthesia for intrathoracic surgery. Its effects can be reversed by the **muscle relaxant antagonist** *neostigmine*.

Local anaesthetics

These temporarily prevent conduction of an impulse along a nerve fibre. Tissues are infiltrated with drug around sensory nerve fibres to produce analgesia of an area. Motor nerve fibres can also be affected if the injection is made around them. Vasoconstrictors are often included in such preparations to reduce blood flow to the area and so prevent the local anaesthetic being removed from its local site of action. Example: *lignocaine* with *epinephrine* (*adrenaline*).

Anti-epileptics

These drugs are used to treat epilepsy, a condition of the central nervous system characterised by the spontaneous occurrence of convulsions or seizures. Examples: *phenobarbitone, diazepam*.

Drugs used in the treatment of disorders of the endocrine system

Disorders of the endocrine system result either from lack of production or overproduction of a hormone. Drugs are used either to replace the natural hormone or to prevent overproduction of the hormone in question (Table 12.5). Anterior pituitary hormones (or their analogues) are used in diagnostic tests for endocrine diseases. For example *tetracosactrin* (an adrenocorticotrophin analogue) is used in the ACTH stimulation test which is performed in the diagnosis of both Cushing's disease and Addison's disease.

Steroid hormones share a common chemical structure and are produced by the adrenal cortex (**adrenal cortiscosteroids**) or by the ovary and testes (**sex steroids** – see below). **Anabolic steroids** are derivatives of the male sex hormone, testosterone, and are used to increase muscle mass and to promote tissue repair in convalescing animals. Example: *nandrolone*.

Drugs acting on the reproductive and urinary tract

Table 12.6 describes sex hormones (sex steroids), luteolytic agents (prostaglandins), myometrial stimulants (ecbolics) and drugs used to treat urinary tract disorders. Drugs used in the management of disorders of urination are presented in Fig. 12.2.

Table 12.5 Drugs used in the treatment of endocrine disorders

Gland	Disease state	Drug class	Example
Adrenal gland	*Deficiency:* Hypoadrenocorticism	Adrenal corticosteroids Mineralocorticoids (sodium conserving) Glucocorticoids	Fludrocortisone Prednisolone, dexamethasone
	Excess: Hyperadrenocorticism (Cushing's disease)	Adrenolytic agent Glucocorticoid synthesis inhibitor	Mitotane ketaconazole
Thyroid gland	*Deficiency:* Hypothyroidism	Thyroid hormone replacement	Levothyroxine
	Excess: Hyperthyroidism	Antithyroid agent	Carbimazole
Endocrine pancreas	*Deficiency:* Diabetes mellitus (hyperglycaemia)	Insulin Oral hypoglycaemic agent	Protamine zinc insulin Glipizide
	Excess: Hypoglycaemia (low blood glucose)	Glucose (intravenous) Anti-insulin agents	Dextrose solution Dexamethasone (glucocorticoids)
Posterior pituitary gland	Diabetes insipidus (deficiency of ADH)	Posterior pituitary hormone (ADH analogue)	Desmopressin

Table 12.6 Drugs used in the treatment of reproductive and urinary tracts		
	Example	**Uses**
Sex hormones (sex steroids)		
Oestrogens	Diethylstilboestrol Oestradiol benzoate	Prevent implantation following accidental mating (misalliance) Treat urinary incontinence* Reduce the size of an enlarged prostate gland and anal adenomas
Progestogens Steroids which mimic the actions of progesterone	Megestrol acetate Delmadinone Proligestone	Postpone or suppress oestrus in the bitch and queen Management of some behavioural problems (aggression in male dogs)
Androgens Esters or analogues of the male sex hormone, testosterone	Methyltestosterone	Hormone alopecia in dogs and cats Deficient libido in males
Luteolytic agents (prostaglandins)	Dinoprost	(unlicensed use) Synchronisation of oestrus in cattle and sheep Induction of parturition in pigs
Myometrial stimulants (ecbolics) Stimulate the uterus to contract	Oxytocin (extract of posterior pituitary gland)	Dystocia due to weakness of the uterine muscle (uterine inertia)
Drugs used to treat urinary tract disorders		
Urinary acidifers Lower the pH of the urine	Ethylenediamine	In the management of urolithiasis (struvite calculi) Cystitis (aid action of antibacterials and urinary antiseptics)
Urinary alkalinisers Raise the pH of the urine	Sodium bicarbonate	In the management of urate uroliths
Urinary antiseptics Hydrolyse in acidic urine to release formaldehyde	Hexamine	Prophylaxis and long-term treatment of recurrent urinary tract infection

* *First line drug for the medical management of urinary incontinence secondary to urethral sphincter mechanism incompetence would be phenylpropanolamin (see Fig 2.2).*

Drugs used to treat malignant disease

Cytotoxic drugs kill actively dividing cells and are used in the **chemotherapy** of some forms of cancer which cannot be removed surgically (e.g. malignant lymphoma). As normal cells in the body are actively dividing, these drugs have a low therapeutic index and need to be used with great care. **They are also a hazard to people handling them** (as are some other drugs already discussed). Examples: *cyclophosphamide, vincristine*.

Drugs used to treat disorders of the musculoskeletal system and joints

Anti-inflammatory drugs

Anti-inflammatory drugs are considered here, although they can be used to reduce or suppress inflammation wherever it occurs in the body. The value of such drugs is to relieve the pain, swelling and fever caused by acute inflammation.

Corticosteroids of the glucocorticoid group will suppress inflammation and, at high doses, can produce **immunosuppression** which is required in the treatment of immune-mediated diseases which sometimes cause polyarthritis in the dog.

Non-steroidal anti-inflammatory drugs (NSAIDs) mostly inhibit the formation of prostaglandins and related compounds, which are important mediators of acute inflammation. These drugs will reduce pain and swelling following surgery or in a number of acquired inflammatory conditions such as osteoarthritis. Examples: *phenylbutazone, flunixin meglumine, aspirin*. Currently there is much interest in producing NSAIDs that are selective for enzymes that produce prostaglandins in the inflamed tissue but not those that produce protective prostaglandins in the stomach and kidney. Two drugs used in veterinary practice with a degree of selectivity for the enzymes found in inflamed tissues are *carprofen* and *meloxicam*. Currently, these are the only NSAIDs approved for pre-operative administration as part of a pre-emptive analgesic protocol.

Chondroprotective agents

These prevent further breakdown of cartilage and stimulate the synthesis of new articular cartilage. Example: *pentosan polysulphate sodium*.

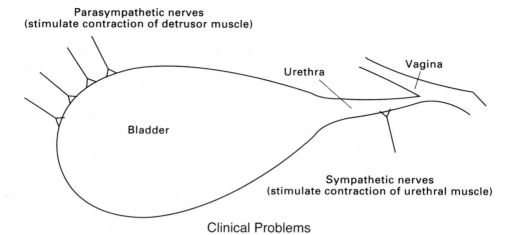

Clinical Problems

Clinical problem	Signs	Drug class and action	Example
Atonic bladder	Bladder overfills and may leak (overflow incontinence)	Parasympathomimetic (stimulates detrusor muscle to contract)	Bethanechol
Weak bladder neck (intra-pelvic bladder)	Dribbles urine particularly at rest	Sympathomimetic (increases urethral tone)	Phenylpropanolamine
Urethral spasm	Unable to pass stream of urine	Sympathetic antagonist (lowers urethral tone)	Phenoxybenzamine (α-adrenoceptor antagonist)

Fig. 12.2 The bladder and drugs which affect urination. The process of urination is brought about by parasympathetic stimulation of the detrusor muscle and inhibition of sympathetic tone to the urethral smooth muscle, allowing the bladder to contract and empty through the relaxed urethra. When the bladder fills, the sympathetic nervous system is active, maintaining continence by closing the urethra; the parasympathetic system is inactive, allowing the detrusor muscle to relax and the bladder to fill.

Drugs acting on the eye

Antimicrobial and anti-inflammatory agents can be applied topically to the eye in the form of drops or ointments. Local anaesthetics can also be formulated for topical application to the eye. Other drugs with actions on the eye include the following:

Mydriatics and cycloplegics

These dilate the pupil (mydriasis) and reduce spasm in the ciliary muscle. Examples: **antimuscarinic agents**, *atropine, homatropine.*

Drugs used in the treatment of glaucoma (raised intraocular pressure)

Miotics constrict the pupil and thus open the drainage angle for ocular fluid. Drugs which mimic stimulation of the parasympathetic nerve supply to the eye (**parasympathomimetics**) have this effect. Example: *pilocarpine.*

Carbonic anhydrase inhibitors will reduce the formation of aqueous humour. Examples: *dorzolamide* (given topically), *acetazolamide* (given orally).

Drugs used in keratoconjunctivitis sicca (dry eye)

These replace the tear film, which is deficient in this condition. *Hypromellose* drops are the most commonly used artificial tears. A **mucolytic**, *acetylcysteine*, may be beneficial when the tears are particularly mucoid and viscous. **Parasympathomimetics** (*pilocarpine*) administered by mouth may stimulate lacrimal secretion in some cases.

Drugs acting on the ear

Topical preparations containing antimicrobial, ecto-parasiticide and anti-inflammatory agents are all available. **Sebolytics** dissolve wax and cleanse the ear canal. Many different preparations are available using solvents such as *squalene* or *propylene glycol* and incorporating *benzoic acid* and *salicylic acid.*

Drugs acting on the skin

The skin can be treated with drugs given orally or parenterally, which reach the skin via its blood supply, or by topical application of preparations of drugs directly to the affected area. Topical drugs are usually formulated as creams, ointments, lotions, powders, shampoos or sprays. The vehicle or base of these may be selected to suit the type of lesion and location being treated, as described later. The active drugs contained in such preparations may be antibacterials, ectoparasiticides or anti-inflammatory agents. Drugs which have not been mentioned elsewhere which are used for disorders of the skin include the following:

- **Keratolytics** which loosen the horny layer of the epidermis causing it to separate away from the deeper epidermis. Examples: *benzoyl peroxide, salicylic acid.*
- **Astringents** precipitate protein on the surface of the skin to produce a protective coating. Examples: *zinc oxide, calamine.*
- **Disinfectants** in the correct concentration can be used topically to cleanse the skin and chemically destroy surface bacteria. Example: *chlorhexidine gluconate.*
- **Essential fatty acids** are given orally to animals and have potential *anti-inflammatory* properties with some evidence of beneficial effects in inflammatory skin conditions. Examples: *gamolenic acid* (GLA), *eicosapentanoic acid* (EPA). There are many proprietary preparations available containing these essential fatty acids, some of which also contain vitamins and minerals.

Drugs affecting nutrition and body fluids

Electrolyte and water replacement solutions (crystalloid fluids)

These are used to treat animals suffering from dehydration. **Oral rehydration solutions** consist of mixtures of sodium, potassium, chloride ions and an anion which is metabolised by the liver to form bicarbonate (e.g. citrate). In addition, glucose and amino acids such as glycine are included, not for nutritional purposes, but because they help the transport of sodium and water across the gut wall and into the bloodstream. **Parenteral solutions** are used to replace fluid losses in cases where the oral route is unsuitable and a parenteral route (usually intravenous route) is chosen. The composition of the fluid used depends on the type of losses sustained. For example, *replacement* of extracellular fluid volume requires a fluid with plasma concentration of sodium (about 140 mmol/l). When parenteral fluids are given to *maintain* hydration in an animal that is unable to drink, fluids which are much lower in sodium are more appropriate. Isotonicity of such fluids is maintained by the addition of glucose (e.g. 4% glucose and 0.18% sodium chloride). **Concentrated additives** such as potassium chloride, glucose (dextrose monohydrate) and sodium bicarbonate are available for addition to commercially available fluids so that the composition of the fluid can be adjusted to suit the requirements of the animal being treated. Nutrient solutions are available to provide nutrition by the intravenous route (parenteral nutrition). They consist of concentrated solutions of glucose or emulsions of lipid to provide calories and amino acids. They should only be administered through the jugular vein as the risk of phlebitis and infection when given through a small peripheral vein is high.

Hypertonic saline (e.g. 7.0% sodium chloride) is a special type of crystalloid fluid used in the treatment of hypovolaemic and endotoxaemic shock. Small volumes are given for the pharmacological effect this has on cardiac output and arterial blood pressure. Volume replacement with conventional isotonic crystalloid fluids or colloids (see below) should still form part of the treatment of such patients.

Plasma substitutes

Plasma substitutes are large-molecular-weight **colloids** in solution which are retained in the circulation rather than leaving capillaries and distributing into the whole extracellular fluid volume (as is the case with crystalloid fluids). Thus, a smaller volume of such colloid preparations will restore the circulating fluid volume in an animal suffering from haemorrhagic shock when compared with the volume of replacement crystalloid solutions required. Example: *gelatin.*

Blood substitutes

A recent addition to the parenteral fluids available for use in veterinary practice is a product that is both a colloid and has oxygen carrying capacity. It is a cross-linked bovine haemoglobin solution called *Oxyglobin* (Biopure Corp.) which can be used for animals requiring oxygen-carrying capacity. Indications for its use include acute blood loss or haemolytic crises where a source of cross-matched blood is not available.

Vitamins and minerals

These can be used as supplements for sick and debilitated animals, and, as such, would be regarded as medicines. Nutritional deficiencies may occur but are uncommon in the dog and cat nowadays with the use of commercial pet foods. Specific indications for a mineral would be eclampsia in the bitch where *calcium gluconate* would be given intravenously. *Phytomenadione* (vitamin K_1) is the specific antidote to warfarin poisoning.

Vaccines and immunological preparations

Vaccines are given to animals to stimulate immunity against an infectious disease (e.g. canine distemper). The body responds to antigens in the vaccine and the immunity produced is termed **active immunity.** **Live vaccines** consist of living organisms of a slightly different strain from that which causes the natural disease making them non-pathogenic (no signs of disease result) but still able to stimulate a protective immune response. The organisms in live vaccines multiply inside the host after administration and stimulate a long-lasting immune response. **Inactivate vaccines** contain sufficient antigen to stimulate an immune response and no multiplication of the organism in question is possible following administration of an inactivated vaccine. **Toxoids** (e.g. *Tetanus toxoid*) are forms of inactivated vaccines where toxins produced by organisms have been extracted and heat-treated to render them harmless. Inactivated vaccines usually contain adjuvants such as aluminium hydroxide or mineral oil which help to enhance the immune response to the antigens in the vaccine which is generally not as long-lasting as that obtained with live vaccines. An **autogenous vaccine** is prepared from material collected from an individual animal for administration to the same animal.

Immunoglobulins (antibodies, antisera) can be administered to animals to confer **passive immunity**. Example: *tetanus antitoxin*. These consist of serum containing antibodies raised in another animal (usually of the same species). They can have a neutralising effect on the organism or toxin in question and therefore give some immediate protection in the face of infection. Passive immunity only persists for about 3 weeks.

A polyvalent immunoglobulin raised against the Gram-negative outer cell membrane (lipopolysaccharide) is authorised for use in dogs. This form of passive immunity can be useful in protecting animals at risk of developing septic shock (e.g. puppies with parvovirus or bitches with pyometra).

Formulation and administration of drugs

Systemically administered drugs

If a drug cannot be applied locally (topically) to the site at which its action is desired, it must first be administered in such a way that it is **absorbed** into the blood circulation (systemically) from which it **distributes** to the place in the body where it acts. The rate and extent of absorption of the drug from its site of administration will depend upon its route of administration and the physical and chemical form in which it is administered (see below). The body gets rid of (**eliminates**) the drug by converting it into a different chemical compound by a process of metabolism followed by excretion of the drug from the body. The liver is the major organ where drug **metabolism** occurs and excretion of the drug itself or of its metabolites is into the bile or urine. Some volatile agents are excreted from the body via the respiratory tract.

Oral preparations

Administration of medicines is covered in Chapter 3, Observation and Care of the Patient.

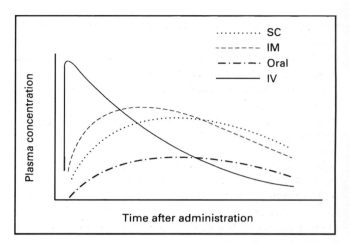

Fig. 12.3 Plasma concentration versus time curve for a 'typical' drug following its administration by: intramuscular injection (IM), intravenous injection (IV), subcutaneous injection (SC) and oral administration.

The oral route is the most convenient route for many drugs used in small animal veterinary practice as owners can dose their own pets at home. There are a number of problems with oral dosing, however, which are listed below:

- The absorption of the drug from the gut into the blood stream is often slower and less complete than when drugs are injected (given by a parenteral route, Fig. 12.3). It may take time for a tablet to dissolve and release its contents: some drugs are absorbed primarily in the small intestine rather than the stomach and so their absorption only occurs once the stomach empties.
- If the animal is vomiting, the oral route is not reliable. Some drugs are unstable in gastric acid or are destroyed by the enzymes of the gut, so the oral route cannot be used (e.g. penicillin G, insulin).
- Some drugs are broken down very rapidly and efficiently in the liver after absorption from the gut and so do not reach the general circulation (e.g. lignocaine, glyceryl trinitrate) or a higher dose is required when the drug is given orally (e.g. propranolol).
- Food in the gastrointestinal tract may affect the absorption of the drug by delaying its entry into the blood stream (e.g. digoxin) or reducing the amount of the drug absorbed (e.g. ampicillin). In other cases, fatty food helps the absorption of some drugs across the gut wall (e.g. griseofulvin, lufenuron or mitotane).
- Some drugs are not absorbed when given orally and remain in the gastrointestinal tract. They can be used as a form of local therapy but will not have systemic effects (e.g. neomycin can be used orally to treat enteric infections but not urinary tract infections).

Tablets   Many oral medications are in the form of **tablets** containing the active drug and some inert ingredients (binder and excipients) which bind the compressed mass together. Tablets may be coated for a number of reasons:

- To protect the tablet from the atmosphere, particularly moisture.
- To delay disintegration of the tablet and so protect the active drug from the acidic environment of the stomach or to protect the stomach from irritant effects of the drug (e.g. aspirin).
- To hide the bitter taste of the drug and so facilitate dosing (e.g. erythromycin).

Grinding up tablets will destroy the properties which the outer layers of the tablet provide. Before this measure is recommended or undertaken it is important to check with the manufacturer that such action can be taken without altering the properties of the medication. Some tablets are scored to facilitate breaking them in half for dosing.

Capsules Other oral medications are formulated as **capsules** which contain either powder or granules. The outer case of the capsule is made of hard gelatin and comes in two halves which slot together. The outer case prevents the drug, which may have a bitter taste, contacting the oral mucosa. Some capsule formulations of drugs contain granules of differing sizes and composition which will dissolve at different rates and so provide a sustained release of drug from the gastrointestinal tract (e.g. slow-release formulations of *theophylline* or *diltiazem*). This reduces the frequency of dosing required. The rate of release of an active drug from these formulations will vary between species depending on the conditions within the gastrointestinal tract and its rate of transit through the tract. Empirical use of slow-release formulations manufactured for human use in dogs and cats could lead to problems of poor absorption (and therefore lack of effect) or too rapid absorption (and therefore toxicity).

Mixtures Liquid medication (or **mixtures**) can be given by mouth and may contain the drug completely in solution if it is freely soluble or in suspension if it is insoluble (e.g. *kaolin* in water). Suspensions require thorough mixing before dosing and should always be labelled with the instruction: 'Shake well before use'.

- **Syrup/linctus** – drugs contained in a concentrated sugar solution.
- **Emulsion** – a mixture of two immiscible liquids.

Parenteral preparations

Strictly speaking, a parenteral route of administration means any route other than the oral route. It is generally taken to mean routes by which drugs are injected into the body of an animal. All preparations for parenteral use must, therefore, be sterile and pyrogen free. The most common routes of injection of drugs in small animal practice are:

- Intravenous – directly into venous blood.
- Intramuscular – into muscular tissue, usually of the leg or back.
- Subcutaneous – into the tissue beneath the skin.

Occasionally the intraperitoneal route of injection is used, particularly in small rodents. The peritoneal membrane provides a large surface area for drug absorption.

Intravenous route The **intravenous route** will provide the fastest distribution of the drug to its site of action that is possible since the drug is placed directly into the bloodstream. The peak plasma concentration of the drug achieved is higher than can be achieved by any other route but the drug concentration often decreases rapidly (depending on the rate at which the body metabolises and excretes the drug) as absorption of the drug from the site of administration is instantaneous and does not continue over a period of time as is the case for the oral route and other parenteral routes (Fig. 12.3).

Preparations for intravenous use must be true solutions where the drug to be administered is dissolved in sterile water (aqueous solution) or another type of solvent. It is important to make any intravenous injections slowly as a rapid (bolus) injection can result in a very high concentration of the drug (or solvent) reaching the heart or brain and causing detrimental effects. Suspensions of drugs cannot be administered intravenously as the particles in a suspension may block capillaries in the lungs causing death.

Drugs which may be irritant to the tissues should preferably be administered by the intravenous route as the drug is rapidly removed and diluted in the circulating blood (if the injection is made slowly). If irritant drugs are given (e.g. sodium thiopentone, vincristine) it is important to ensure that the injection is indeed made into the vein. Accidental injection into the tissues around the vein (perivascular injection) may cause severe damage.

Intramuscular route **Intramuscular injection** of drugs may be more convenient for less cooperative patients and drugs in suspension can be given by this route. After inserting the needle into a muscle to make the injection, it is important to draw back on the syringe to ensure that the tip of the needle is not in a blood vessel within the muscle.

Intramuscular injections may be painful; the severity of the pain depends on the volume of the injection, the viscosity of the material being injected and the chemical nature of the compound (how irritant it is to the tissue). The drug diffuses from the injection site by dissolving in the tissue fluid surrounding the muscle cells and is then absorbed into the blood capillaries and lymphatics supplying the muscle.

Subcutaneous route **Subcutaneous injections** can be made into any area of the body where there is loose skin – usually over the neck or back. Formulations of drugs for subcutaneous injection should be approximately of blood pH and blood fluid tonicity, and should not be irritant or cause vasoconstriction as this will impede the absorption of the drug into the bloodstream. Larger volumes can be administered by the subcutaneous route rather than by the intramuscular route.

Absorption rates In general, the rate of absorption of drugs given by the intramuscular route is faster than those given by the subcutaneous route since muscle receives a larger blood supply than subcutaneous tissue (Fig. 12.3). However, the physical and chemical properties of the drug formulation affect the rate of absorption from both of these sites. Formulations of drugs can be produced which contain a combination of different salts of the same drug, one of which is highly soluble (e.g. sodium salt of penicillin G) and so rapidly absorbed from the intramuscular injection site, another which is more slowly absorbed (e.g. procaine salt of penicillin G) and a third which is absorbed very slowly indeed because of its extremely low solubility (e.g. benzathine salt of penicillin G). This principle is used to produce long-acting injections of drugs which are sometimes called *depot preparations*. Insulin is also prepared in different physical forms which give different time to onset of action and duration of effect based on the speed of absorption of insulin from the injection site. Some formulations of insulin (protamine zinc insulin or insulin zinc suspension) may have a duration of action which make them suitable for once daily administration whereas other formulations (isophane insulin) have a shorter duration of action such that two injections per day may be necessary. *Implants* are an extreme example of a depot preparation where a small disc or cylinder of relatively insoluble drug (often a hormone) is inserted beneath the skin in a sterile manner using a special injection device. The drug can then be released over an extended period of time preventing the need for repeated administration.

Other injection sites Other sites of injection of drugs include

- *Intradermal* – into the dermis (allergy testing in dogs).
- *Intra-articular* – into a joint cavity.
- *Intrathecal* – into the cerebrospinal fluid (contrast media for myelography; therapeutic agents are not given by this route in veterinary medicine).
- *Epidural* – into the vertebral canal outside the dural matter (used to produce spinal analgesia when local anaesthetics are injected).
- *Intraperitoneal* – into the abdominal cavity.
- *Subconjunctival* – under the conjunctival membrane of the eye.

These are all forms of local therapy as the injection site is the site at which the drug is desired to produce its effect.

Other ways of administering drugs to produce systemic effects

Inhalation of drugs into the respiratory tract is a means of supplying drugs to this site of the body and for drugs to be absorbed into the bloodstream (e.g. gaseous anaesthetics). Formulation of drugs for inhalation is more difficult for administration to domestic animals than to man, where inhalation is a common way of administering drugs such as bronchodilators. In some university hospitals, drugs in solution can be produced in a very fine mist of liquid droplets which are inhaled by the animal. This process is called *nebulisation* and has obvious safety implications for the operators (see below).

Drugs can be absorbed across other mucous membranes of the body and produce systemic effects. For example, desmopressin is supplied in the form of drops, which in man are instilled into the nose. In the dog, it is more convenient to place these drops into the conjunctival sac. Absorption of the drug from this site into the bloodstream occurs and the systemic effects (antidiuretic action) become evident. As this drug is a peptide (small protein), its absorption following oral administration is reduced by enzymic breakdown of the drug within the gastrointestinal tract.

Some drugs are able to penetrate the skin and so be absorbed from the surface of the skin and have systemic effects. An example used in small-animal medicine is the nitrovasodilator, glyceryl trinitrate. This drug cannot be given by the oral route as it is removed so effectively by the liver. The organophosphate insecticide, fenthion, is another example of a drug which, when applied to a discrete area of skin, is absorbed into the bloodstream and distributed systemically.

Topically administered drugs

Topical preparations are applied directly to the site at which the drug is required. The most common sites to be treated topically in small-animal medicine are the skin, eyes and ears. Enemas could be considered a form of topical therapy where fluids are infused into the rectum to soften the faecal mass. In large-animal practice, topical applications of drugs are to the mammary gland (*intramammary preparations*), the vagina and uterus (*vaginal suppositories* or *pessaries*). It is important to remember that drugs can be absorbed across mucous membranes and even intact skin – particularly drugs that are lipid soluble (such as corticosteroids) – and so these drugs should not be assumed to be without systemic effects.

Examples of formulations of topical preparations include:

- *Creams* – semi-solid emulsions of oil or fat, and water (which usually contains the drug). They spread easily without friction and penetrate the outer layers of the skin, particularly if the fat used is lanolin. Water-soluble drugs are more active in creams than in ointments.
- *Ointments* – semi-solid greasy, insoluble in water and the drugs are present in a base of wax or fat (usually petroleum jelly). They are non-penetrating and more occlusive than creams and are most suitable for dry chronic lesions.
- *Dusting powders* – finely divided powders for application to the skin containing usually ectoparasiticides or antibacterials.

- *Wettable powders* – applied to the skin as a suspension after mixing with a large quantity of water. The animal is then dried by warmth leaving the powder in the coat (i.e. it is not rinsed off).
- *Lotions* – liquid preparations which consist of solutions of the drugs in water (e.g. calamine lotion).
- *Medicated shampoos* – aqueous solutions or suspensions of drugs which have a detergent base which gives good penetration of the coat. Shampoos are left in contact with the skin for the recommended period of time and then rinsed off thoroughly.
- *Aerosol sprays* – a way of applying liquid solutions or suspensions of drugs in fine droplet form. The liquid is packaged in a metal container under pressure and pressing the nozzle of the container causes the liquid to be expelled.
- *Eye medications* can be in the form of ointments or drops. Ophthalmic ointments tend to be more liquid (than the ointments described above), having a soft paraffin base, and when applied to the surface of the cornea they melt to form a thin film which covers the whole surface of the eye. Eye drops are aqueous solutions of drugs for instillation to the eye. In general, drops tend to be shorter acting than ointments and require more frequent application. Both forms of medication should be sterile and, once opened, should be stored only for the length of time recommended by the manufacturers.

Calculations of drug dosages

The responsibility for ensuring that the correct dosage of drug is administered to an animal under their care lies with the veterinary surgeon in charge of the case. However, veterinary nurses should understand how to calculate dosages of drugs.

Weights, volumes and concentration

The active ingredients in the preparation of a drug is expressed in terms of its weight. The standard units for weight are kilograms (kg), grams (g), milligrams (mg) and micrograms (no abbreviation used). These weights are related as follows:

1 kilogram (kg) = 1000 grams

1 gram (g) = 1000 milligrams

1 milligram (mg) = 1000 micrograms

If the weight relates to a tablet or capsule, then each tablet or capsule contains the stated weight of active drug. When considering liquid formulations of drugs (solutions or suspensions), the weight of active drug is related to a unit of volume of the suspension or solution. Standard units of volume include litres (l) and millilitres (ml) where

1 l = 1000 ml. Some drugs are relatively unstable in solution and so are supplied as a solid in a vial and the solvent (often water for injection) supplied separately. The drug is reconstituted by adding the solvent to the vial. Unless all the drug is used immediately, it is important to write on the vial the concentration of the solution of the drug you have just made (usually in terms of milligrams of drug per millilitre of solution) and the date on which it was reconstituted. The reconstituted drug may be stable if kept in the refrigerator for several days, so it is important to know the concentration of the solution which has been made.

Percentage solutions

Another way of expressing the concentration of a drug in solution is as a percentage of weight (*w*) of the drug per volume of solution (*w/v*). If 1 g of the active drug is dissolved into a total volume of 100 ml this produces a **1% solution**. If this fundamental fact is remembered, **percentage solutions can be readily converted into concentrations in terms of milligrams per millilitre**, which is usually a more convenient form when it comes to calculating dosages.

Exceptions to standard weights and volumes

Some drugs, such as insulin, oxytocin and heparin, are extracted from animal tissues and are not produced in a completely pure form. The concentration of the drug in the product is determined by its effect in a laboratory test system (bioassay) against an international standard. In most cases, the concentration of such preparations is given in terms of international units (i.u.) or simply units per standard volume (usually per millilitre). So, for example, all formulations of insulin for human use are produced at a concentration of 100 units/ml. There is now an insulin preparation licensed for veterinary use in this country which contains insulin at a concentration of 40 i.u./ml. Insulin is administered using special syringes which are graduated in units rather than in millilitres. It is important to use a 40 unit syringe for insulin of concentration 40 units/ml and a 100 unit syringe for insulin preparations of 100 units/ml.

Dosages

Drug dosage rates are usually expressed in terms of weight of drug per weight of the animal to be dosed (most often in milligrams of drug per kg bodyweight of the animal). Some drugs (particularly those used for cancer chemotherapy) are dosed on a weight of drug per body surface area (milligram per square metre body surface area). Conversion charts are available which give body surface area from the animal's weight in kilograms. The worked examples will illustrate some of the principles in calculation of dosages.

EXAMPLE 1

You are asked to dispense enrofloxacin tablets for a dog weighing 20 kg at a dose rate of 2.5 mg/kg twice daily for 7 days. The drug comes in tablet sizes of 15, 50 and 150 mg. Which tablet sizes would be most appropriate, how many tablets would you dispense and what instructions for dosing would you give to the owner?

Amount of drug required (mg)

$$= \text{dose (mg/kg)} \times \text{bodyweight in kg}$$
$$= 2.5 \text{ (mg/kg)} \times 20 \text{ (kg)}$$
$$= 50 \text{ mg}$$

Thus, the most appropriate tablet size to use would be 50 mg and the owners should be instructed to give one tablet twice a day for 7 days. The number of tablets required will be 14.

TIPS FOR CALCULATIONS

(a) Please note that it is important to be sure of the position of the decimal point in all drug calculations, so always write 0.01 rather than simply .01.

(b) In addition, the dose required in Example 2 is slightly lower than the convenient tablet size. Digoxin is a drug with a lower therapeutic index and care should be taken not to overdose an animal. In this case, the inaccuracy was deemed so small as to be of no consequence but judgement should always be made by the veterinary surgeon in charge of the case.

(c) In dosing with digoxin, food can interfere with the rate of absorption of digoxin from the gut, so an instruction to give the medication before meals is important.

(d) In Example 2 the total daily dose rate was given and had to be divided into two equal doses. An alternative way of expressing this would be to say the dose required is 0.005 mg/kg to be given twice daily, which was the way the dose rate in Example 1 was expressed.

EXAMPLE 2

A 6 kg miniature poodle requires digoxin for treatment of congestive heart failure. The dose rate **required** is 0.01 mg/kg each day which should be divided into two equal doses (0.01 mg/kg divided twice daily). The tablet sizes available are 62.5, 125 and 250 micrograms. What tablet size would you use, what would your dosing instructions to the owners be and how many tablets would you dispense for a 30-day course?

Daily dose required (mg)

$$= \text{dose (mg/kg)} \times \text{bodyweight in kg}$$
$$= 0.01 \text{ (mg/kg)} \times 6 \text{ (kg)} = 0.06 \text{ mg}$$

To convert milligrams to micrograms multiply by 1000:

Thus 0.06 mg = 0.06 × 1000 micrograms

$$= 60 \text{ micrograms}$$

This dose should be divided into two equal daily doses, so each dose should contain:

60/2 micrograms = 30 micrograms

Thus, the most appropriate tablet size to use would be the 62.5 microgram tablets, and the owners should be instructed to give half a tablet every 12 hours before food. For a course of 30 days the owners would require 30 tablets.

EXAMPLE 3

For injection, you are given a drug in solution which is 7.5% w/v. The dose required for the dog you are treating is 10 mg/kg and the dog weighs 18 kg. What volume of the drug should be given to this dog by injection?

Concentration of drug in solution

$$= 7.5 \text{ g in 100 ml (7.5\% w/v)}$$
$$= (7.5/100) \text{ g in 1 ml}$$
$$= 0.075 \text{ g in 1 ml}$$
$$= (0.075 \times 1000) \text{ mg in 1 ml}$$
$$= 75 \text{ mg/ml}$$

Amount of drug required

$$= \text{dose (mg/kg)} \times \text{bodyweight in kg}$$
$$= 10 \text{ (mg/kg)} \times 18 \text{ (kg)} = 180 \text{ mg}$$

Volume of drug required (ml)

$$= \text{Amount of drug (mg)/concentration (mg/ml)}$$
$$= 180 \text{ (mg)/75 (mg/ml)}$$
$$= 2.4 \text{ ml}$$

TIP

To convert the concentration of a solution expressed in percentages into mg/ml, multiply the percentage figure by 10.

Legal aspects of medicines and prescribing

The legislation which governs the storage, handling, use and supply of medicines in veterinary practice includes:

- The Medicines Act 1968.
- The Medicines (restrictions on the administration of veterinary medicinal products) Regulations 1994.
- The Retailer's Records for Veterinary Medicinal Products Regulations 2000.
- The Misuse of Drugs Act 1971.
- The Misuse of Drugs Regulations 1985.
- The Health and Safety at Work Act 1974.
- The Control of Substances Hazardous to Health Regulations 1998.

They have also been considered in Chapters 5 (Occupational Hazards) and 8 (The Law and Ethics of Veterinary Nursing).

The Medicines Act 1968

The Government ensures the quality, safety and efficacy of medicines for human and animal use by a system of licences approved by the Department of Health and the Department for the Environment, Food and Rural Affairs (DEFRA), respectively. Before a product can be manufactured, imported and distributed widely, the company or person who devises it has to gain a marketing authorisation by showing that the drug is safe, efficacious (produces the effects which the data sheet claims) and that the manufacturing process ensures a consistent quality of the product. Manufacturers and wholesale dealers of medicinal products require *manufacturer's* and *wholesale dealer's marketing authority*, respectively. As part of the licensing procedure, the company may need to perform a clinical trial of the drug in question and for this purpose they apply for an *animal test certificate*. An exemption to this law is that veterinary surgeons do not require a product licence to prepare a medicinal product themselves (or to request another veterinary surgeon to prepare such a product for them) for a particular animal or herd under their care. The veterinary surgeon is only allowed to stock a very limited supply of a medicine prepared in this way (2.5 kg of solid and 5 l of liquid). It is not permissible for vaccines (other than autogenous vaccines) to be prepared in this way.

Use of unlicensed products in veterinary medicine

The Medicines (restrictions on the administration of veterinary medicinal products) Regulations became law in December 1994. In non-food-producing animals, the regulations state that a product, which has a veterinary marketing authorisation for the species and the condition to be treated, or is authorised for another condition or another veterinary species should, if possible, be chosen before a product which is only authorised for human use. Products authorised only for human use may be used if no veterinary licensed alternative exists. Special products made by the veterinary surgeon or by a pharmacist for the veterinary surgeon, which have no marketing authorisation at all, should be used only if a veterinary or human authorised product does not already exist. These regulations (commonly referred to as the '*Medicines cascade*') have been produced to protect the consumer of animal products from drug residues. Their application to small animal veterinary practice has been clarified by guidance notes issued by the Veterinary Medicines Directorate (AMELIA 8).

Legal categories of medicines

When granting a marketing authorisation for a drug the licensing body places the medicine into one of three main categories. In order of decreasing strictness of controls over their supply to the public, these are:

- Prescription-only medicines (POMs) including Controlled Drugs (CD).
- Pharmacy-only medicines (P) including Merchant's List and Saddler's List medicines (PML).
- General sales medicines (GSL).

More detailed information of these categories and their subdivisions is given in Table 12.7. In summary, the only category of medicine which can be sold direct to the public by a veterinary practice without the owner having consulted with a veterinary surgeon are GSL products. For all other categories of drugs, the animals for which they are intended should be *under the care of a veterinary surgeon in* the practice and his or her authority should be sought before these drugs can be supplied by a qualified veterinary nurse.

Storage of medicines

The manufacturer's recommendations should be carefully followed for each medicine in terms of storage temperature and the sensitivity of the compound to light and humidity. The part of the building in which the medicines are stored should not be accessible to the general public. Well-designed shelves are essential to allow easy access to the drugs required and to reduce the possibility of breakage, spillage or misplacement of stock. There should be a work surface, which should be easy to clean, and adequate refrigeration space.

It is convenient to store the medicines on the shelves in their classification groups. Products in large containers should be stocked near ground level for safety. Effective stock control will save time and money, ensuring that old stock is used before new so that medicines in stock do not exceed their expiry date and that the pharmacy does not run out of a particular medication. In conclusion, a clean and tidy pharmacy makes for efficient and safe dispensing of medications.

Table 12.7 Legal categories of medicines			
Legal categories	**Subcategory**	**Definition**	**Examples**
Prescription-only medicines (POM)	Controlled drugs General POM drugs	A subcategory of POM where the regulations for supply and storage are even more stringent than general POM medicines (see text) Can only be described and dispensed by a veterinary surgeon or dispensed by a pharmacist against a prescription written and signed by a veterinary surgeon	Morphine (S2) Phenobarbitone (S3) Many veterinary medicines such as Antibacterial drugs Vaccines Any drug intended for parental administration
Pharmacy-only medicines (P)	General P medicines	Any drug in this category may be sold over the counter by a registered pharmacist to the general public. A veterinary surgeon may supply drugs in this category for the treatment of animals under his/her care	Most P medicines are human products Veterinary examples: Dermisol (Pfizer Ltd)
	Pharmacy Merchants List (PML)	Drugs in this subcategory, in addition to the general regulations described for P medicines, may also be sold by agricultural merchants registered with the Royal Pharmaceutical Society to persons whose business involves animals (e.g. farmers)	Large animal anthelmintics Ectoparasiticides
	Saddler's List (PML)	Saddlers who are registered with the Royal Pharmaceutical Society may sell certain anthelmintics to horse owners	Anthelmintics for horses
General sales list (GSL)	—	Medicinal products where the hazard to health or the need to take special precautions is sufficiently small that they can be sold without a prescription by pet shops or merchants who are not subject to special regulations. A number of veterinary products are GSL only when produced for external use or, when formulated for oral administration, a maximum strength which may be sold is stipulated	Piperazine citrate Permethrin flea spray Piperonyl/butoxide

Dispensing and labelling of medicines

The containers listed in Table 12.8 are recommended by the Council of the Royal Pharmaceutical Society for the dispensing of medicines from bulk packs. Note that paper envelopes and plastic bags are unacceptable forms of container.

The Medicines Act and the Medicine Labelling Regulations state the legal requirements for labelling of dispensed medicines. These regulations apply whether the medicines are dispensed in the manufacturer's original container or dispensed from bulk into smaller packages. Labels should be legible and indelible (written in biro or felt pen, not a washable ink or pencil). Printed labels can be generated by computers used in modern practices. The specimen label shown in Table 12.9 indicates essential information which has to be provided by law and also optional (but desirable) information.

If the medication is for external use the words 'For external use only' should appear on the label. In addition, any safety precautions the owners should take when handling the drugs should be added. When the drug is to be used in food-producing animals, the label must also include the withdrawal period (the time between the last dose of the drug and the use of meat, milk or eggs from the animal for human consumption).

The Misuse of Drugs Act 1971 and The Misuse of Drugs Regulations 1985

This legislation controls the production, supply, possession, storage and dispensing of drugs where the potential exists for abuse by humans. These are the controlled drugs (CD), a special category of POM products, and there are five schedules:

Table 12.8 Recommended containers for different medicines

Container	Medicine
Coloured flute bottles	Medicines for external application Examples: shampoos, soaps, lotions Enemas and eye and ear medications should be similarly dispensed if not already packaged in a suitable plastic container
Plain glass bottles	Oral liquid medicines
Wide-mouthed jars	Creams, dusting powders, granules
Paper board cartons/wallets	Sachets, manufacturer's strip or blister-packed medicines
Airtight glass, plastic or metal containers (preferably childproof)[a]	All solid oral medicines (tablets and capsules)

[a] *Discretion can be exercised with childproof containers. Some aged and infirm clients may request screwtop containers*

- **Schedule 1 (S1)** – addictive drugs such as *cannabis* and hallucinogens *mescaline* and *LSD*.
- **Schedule 2 (S2)** – the opiate analgesics *morphine, etorphine, fentanyl* and *pethidine* plus *cocaine* and *amphetamine*.
- **Schedule 3 (S3)** – the barbiturates *pentobarbitone* and *phenobarbitone* plus the opiate analgesics, *buprenorphine* and *pentazocine*.
- **Schedule 4 (S4)** – benzodiazepines such as *diazepam* and *chlordiazepoxide*.
- **Schedule 5 (S5)** – certain preparations of cocaine, codeine and morphine that contain less than a specified amount of the drug. (Examples: *codeine cough linctus, kaolin* and *morphine antidiarrhoeal suspension*.)

A veterinary surgeon does not have any general authority to possess or supply drugs from Schedule 1. Some of the other controlled drugs are subject to more stringent regulations than general POM medications, as detailed below:

Purchase Purchase of S2 requires a handwritten (in indelible ink) requisition from the veterinary surgeon to a wholesaler, manufacturer or pharmacist which includes the veterinary surgeon's signature, their name and address and profession, the purpose for which the drug is required and the total quantity of the drug required. If a messenger is sent to collect the drug, written authority has to be given by the veterinary surgeon for the messenger to receive the drug on their behalf. S3 drugs also require a written requisition for their purchase. This does not have to be handwritten but must be signed by the veterinary surgeon making the request. (See below for further information on prescriptions written for S2 and S3 drugs.)

Storage S2 drugs and buprenorphine and temazepam (from S3) must be kept in a locked cupboard which is attached to a wall. The veterinary surgeon is responsible for the key to such a cupboard which should only be opened with his or her authority.

Records A bound register of all transactions involving S2 drugs must be kept. Details of incomings (purchases) of S2 drugs and their outgoings (drugs given to animals on the practice premises or dispensed to an owner to give to their animal) should be recorded in separate parts of the register, with a section for each individual drug in both parts of the register (i.e. the records for pethidine should be separated from those for morphine). Record books should be retained for 2 years from the last entry. Such registers for controlled drugs are available commercially. In addition, any S2 drug which is no longer required by the veterinary practice can only be disposed of in the presence of a Home Office Inspector. A record has to be made in the register which the Inspector is required to sign.

There is no legal requirement for veterinary practices to retain records of other drugs they dispense which do not fall into the Controlled Drug category but it would be considered to be good prescribing practice. However, the Retailers' Records for Veterinary Medicinal Products Regulations 2000 requires veterinarians dealing with food-producing animals to keep records of all PML, P and POM products received from wholesalers and of each outgoing transaction involving the sale of these products to clients. The manufacturer's batch number of the product dispensed is one of the items that has to be recorded. These practices are expected to be able to conduct an audit each year so that incoming and outgoing products can be reconciled with those held in stock within the practice. Whilst these regulations do not apply to

---

Table 12.9 Label details, including information required by law and additional desirable details

Essential	Owner's name Owner's address Veterinary practice name Veterinary practice address For Animal Treatment Only Date Keep Out of Reach of Children
Optional	Quantity and strength of drug Instructions for dosing Total quantity of drug dispensed Initials of person dispensing

small-animal practice, most of the information required for outgoing transactions will form part of the clinical recording system for most practices. Recording of batch numbers, is, however, problematic, yet if a manufacturer has to recall a batch of product for any reason, practices should be able to identify to whom they have dispensed a particular batch of a given product. It should be possible to devise systems within a practice pharmacy whereby a record is kept of the start and end of use of batches of given products.

Special prescription requirements for controlled drugs

These apply to those drugs in S2 and S3. An example of a prescription is shown in Table 12.10. The format is the same for any drug which the veterinary surgeon would like a pharmacist to dispense to one of his/her clients. In the case of S2 and S3 drugs, the name and address of the client, the date and the quantity (in numbers and words) and strength of the preparation should be written in the veterinary surgeon's own handwriting. The prescription must not be dispensed later than 13 weeks from the date of issue (whereas prescription for general POM drugs can be dispensed for up to 6 months from the date of issue) and no repeat prescriptions are permitted (whereas for general POM drugs one can stipulate the number of times the prescription can be repeated).

The practice of issuing repeat prescriptions is one that should be done at the discretion of the veterinary surgeon in charge of the case, taking note of the stability of the animal's condition and the need for re-examination of the animal. Each practice should decide on its own policy for animals on long-term chronic medication so that nurses can inform clients of this policy.

Table 12.10 Example of prescription form for a controlled drug

Mr J. Fishwick, MA, VetMB MRCVS
50 High Street, Comberton, Cambridge CB4 1RL
Tel: 01223 849623

25th September 2002
Mr J. R. Fox's dog 'Smarty'
23 The Green,
Barton, Cambridge

Rx
Tablets Pethidine 50 mg
Send 10 (ten)

Label: Given half a tablet twice a day for 5 days

For Animal Treatment Only

This animal is under my care

No repeats

The Health and Safety at Work Act 1974 and The Control of Substances Hazardous to Health (COSHH) Regulations 1998

When common sense is used and a few general ground rules followed, the medicines used in most veterinary practices present a relatively small hazard to the health of employees. All data sheets of licensed medicines will discuss any hazards the medicine might pose to the operator (the person dispensing and administering the drug). The practice you work for should also have produced a COSHH Assessment for the substances (including drugs) which you come into contact with during the working day (see Chapter 5, Occupational Hazards). It is important that these documents are read and the safety measures followed to contain any risk to the absolute minimum.

Drugs can get into the body by accident and have systemic effects in the operator in a number of ways.

Absorption across the skin

This can occur with certain drugs such as prostaglandins (luteolytic agents), insecticides, nitrovasodilators and compounds containing the solvent DMSO (dimethyl sulphoxide) which aids penetration of substances which are dissolved in it across the skin. When handling such substances or when handling any substances when you have cuts or abrasions on your hands, gloves should be worn to prevent absorption across the skin. As a general principle, hands should be washed after handling any veterinary medicine and splashes or spills of medicines should be washed from the skin immediately.

Absorption across mucous membranes

The membranes of the eye (conjunctiva), nose and oral cavities are sites where drugs may reach if aerosols from liquid formulations or dust from powders containing the drug are formed. An aerosol is formed by very fine droplets of liquid which can be accidentally sprayed into the eyes or mouth. They are formed most often when reconstituting (dissolving) drugs for injection in the diluent supplied and when expelling air bubbles from a syringe. Care should be taken not to pressurise the contents of vials when reconstituting drugs. In addition, if the needle cover is kept on the needle when expelling air bubbles from the syringe, potentially dangerous aerosols will be avoided. Cytotoxic drugs should only be reconstituted by trained personnel and this should be carried out in designated areas. Should accidental contamination of the eyes, nose or mouth occur, washing or flushing with copious amounts of water should be the initial first aid measure and further medical help should be sought depending on the drug involved.

Accidental ingestion of drugs

This can occur through aerosols or dust, as described above, or through eating contaminated food. Food and drink must not be consumed or stored in areas where drugs are being handling, including areas where topical sprays (e.g. flea sprays) are applied to animals. Smoking should also be prohibited from these areas.

Inhalation

Inhalation of volatile substances such as gaseous anaesthetics (e.g. halothane), dust from powders and droplets from aerosols may cause irritation of the respiratory tract or the drugs can be absorbed and cause systemic effects. Hazards from inhalational anaesthetics can be minimised by the use of an adequate scavenging circuit attached to the anaesthetic circuit and by providing good ventilation of the operating room. Dust masks and eye protection should be worn when dispensing powders from bulk packs where a large amount of dust is inevitable, and insecticidal sprays should only be used in well-ventilated areas.

Accidental injection

This is the final way in which drugs may get into the body. This risk may be minimised by keeping all needles covered until the injection is made and disposing of the used needle in a safe way immediately after use. The quantity of drug which enters the body following penetration of the skin with a needle is very small. Oil-based vaccines can, however, produce very severe reactions. Some drugs, such as etorphine, are extremely toxic to man such that even these minute quantities are hazardous.

Hazardous drugs used in veterinary practice

The groups of drugs mentioned below carry special risks and so are worthy of note. It is important to realise that whilst some drugs may produce acute effects on the operator which are obvious shortly after exposure, other drugs can have cumulative effects, when exposure to small quantities occurs over a long period of time, which can be just as detrimental. For this reason it is good practice to keep your exposure to all drugs you handle to an absolute minimum by following the ground rules mentioned above.

- **Etorphine** – highly toxic following accidental injection or exposure of skin or mucous membranes to the drug.
- **Halothane** – repeated inhalation may damage the liver and has been incriminated in increasing the risk of miscarriages.
- **Cytotoxic drugs** – many are mutagenic (damage genetic material), carcinogenic (cause cancer) and teratogenic (damage the unborn foetus).

- **Prostaglandins** – may cause asthma attacks, have serious effects on the cardiovascular system and cause uterine contraction. Should not be handled by asthmatics or women of child-bearing age. The British Veterinary Association has drawn up a code of practice for using prostaglandins in cattle and pigs.
- **Antimicrobial agents:**
  - *Griseofulvin*, the antifungal drug, is teratogenic and should not be handled by women of child-bearing age. Protective clothing, impervious gloves and a dust mask should be worn when handling the powdered form and adding this to feed.
  - *Penicillins and cephalosporins* may cause hypersensitivity on exposure in operators who are allergic to these drugs. The reaction can range from mild skin rash to swelling of the eyes, lips and face with difficulty breathing, symptoms which would require immediate medical attention. You should not handle drugs in these two families if you have a history of allergy to them.
  - *Chloramphenicol* can cause a fatal aplastic anaemia in man, a reaction which is not related to the dose received and occurs in a very small number of people exposed to the drug when prescribed for them by doctors. Nevertheless, it is wise to avoid unnecessary exposure to this drug by taking the precautions mentioned above, including avoiding direct contact of the drug with the skin.

It can be seen from the above discussion that hazards are greatest from drugs which are formulated in a liquid or powder form where aerosols, accidental injection or dust can lead to significant exposure of the operator. Many capsules and tablets can be safely handled with minimal or no contact with the drug, provided they are not broken or ground up to release the contents in a powdered form. For all tablets it is good practice to wear gloves when handling them (e.g. cyclophosphamide, mitotane and griseofulvin). The use of a triangular metal or plastic tablet counter facilitates the counting of tablets and reduces any contact between the operator and the tablets to a minimum.

PRACTICAL TIPS WHEN DISPENSING DRUGS TO OWNERS
- Make sure the owner is aware of any special storage conditions that apply to the drug product (store in the fridge or out of direct sunlight). Label the product accordingly.
- If dispensing a suspension, make sure the owner is aware that the product should be shaken well before use – label accordingly.
- Go through the dosing instructions with the owner and make sure they understand them.
- If dispensing products containing penicillins (any members of the penicillin family), ask if the owner

has a penicillin allergy and alert the veterinary surgeon to this fact.
- If dispensing products which are potentially harmful to owners (cytotoxic drugs, mitotane, griseofulvin, chloramphenicol ointments for example) make sure the veterinary surgeon has discussed the safe handling of these products with the owner and ask if protective gloves are to be given out with the drug products.
- Encourage the owner to administer the full course of medication prescribed, make sure they are aware of when the animal needs to be seen again.
- If dispensing tablets, ask the owner how they will give the tablets.
- If they propose to give them with food, check with the veterinary surgeon that this will be acceptable.
- If they propose to crush the tablets, check whether this will be acceptable; drugs with film coatings or capsules, generally should not be crushed.
- When using childproof bottles, check that the owner is able to open these containers.
- Always advise owners to bring back the containers (with any unused drugs) to their next consultation.
- Do not re-use empty containers that clients have returned unless you are sure these have **not** been washed out. Residual moisture will damage most products.

DISPENSING AND PRESCRIPTION WRITING ABBREVIATIONS

ad. lib.	Without restraint
amp.	Ampule
aq.	Water
b.i.d.	Twice daily
cc.	Cubic centimetre
cap.	Capsule
disp.	Dispense
et	And
g or gm	Gram
h	Hour
IM	Intramuscular
IP	Intraperitoneal
IV	Intravenous
mg	Milligram
ml	Millilitre
o.m.	Every morning
o.n.	Every night
p.c.	After meals
PO or per os	By mouth
p.r.n.	As required
q4h	Every 4 hours
qd	Once daily
q.i.d.	Four times a day
q.s.	A sufficient quantity
rep.	Repeat
s.i.d.	Once a day (not universally accepted)
tab	Tablet
tbs	Tablespoon
tsp	Teaspoon
t.i.d.	Three times daily
u.i.d.	Once a day (not universally accepted)

Recognition of significant adverse drug reactions

Nurses are often consulted by owners for advice about adverse drug effects and, if in doubt, should consult the veterinary surgeon about specific cases. Examples of significant potential adverse drug effects where immediate veterinary attention should be sought are given below. This list is by no means exhaustive.

- Vomiting, anorexia and lethargy with non-steroidal anti-inflammatory drugs and with digoxin.
- Skin lesions, lameness and lethargy with potentiated sulphonamide preparations.
- Mucoid ocular discharge in dogs taking sulphonamide-containing preparations.
- Weakness and incoordination in animals taking vasodilator and other cardiac medications.
- Lethargy, anorexia and depression in cats taking antithyroid drugs (e.g. carbimazole griseofulvin or diazepam).
- Any vague signs of illness in animals taking cancer chemotherapy agents should be taken seriously.
- Haematuria in dogs taking cyclophosphamide.
- Loss of balance, nystagmus and circling in animals prescribed ear medications.

Further reading

AMELIA 8 (1995) *The Medicines (restrictions on the administration of veterinary medicinal products) Regulations 1994. Guidance to the Veterinary Profession*, The Veterinary Medicines Directorate.

Animal Medicines: A Users Guide (1995) Published by the National Office of Animal Health (ISBN 09526638 2 1).

Bishop, Y. (2000) *BVA Code of Practice on Medicines*, BVA Publications, London.

Bishop, Y. (ed.) (2001) *The Veterinary Formulary*, 5th edn, The Pharmaceutical Press, London.

Brander, G. C., Pugh, D. M., Bywater, R. J. and Jenkins, W. L. (1991) *Veterinary Applied Pharmacology and Therapeutics*, 5th edn, Baillière Tindall, London.

Wilkins, S. (1991) Hazards of handling veterinary medicines: Part 1. *Veterinary Nursing Journal*, vol. 6, pp. 15–17.

Wilkins, S. (1991) Hazards of handling veterinary medicines: Part 2. *Veterinary Nursing Journal*, vol. 6, pp. 53–55.

13

Laboratory diagnostic aids

P. A. Bloxham updated by Joy Venturi Rose

Learning objectives

After studying this chapter, students should be able to:

- Describe the management requirements for a veterinary practice laboratory.
- Explain the use and maintenance of laboratory equipment.
- Describe how samples are collected.
- Explain how samples are processed and examined.

Introduction

Veterinary nurses are able to provide the practice with the technical skill and ability to operate a small in-house laboratory. They need to understand the equipment currently available and know how to use it to produce good-quality, reliable results. They must perform basic diagnostic tests safely.

The RCVS's Guide to Professional Conduct, relating to Practice Standards, advises that veterinary practices must:

Either provide laboratory facilities; or have access to one or more other laboratories which are adequately equipped to perform routine clinical pathology rapidly and accurately.

If the practice provides laboratory facilities it must ensure that:

- Laboratory procedures are performed in a room or a designated area used specifically for that purpose.
- Laboratory procedures are undertaken only by designated person or persons under their supervision.
- Persons designated to undertake laboratory procedures are adequately trained for the tasks performed by them.
- Local rules are drawn up to cover cleanliness, tidiness, disinfection, first aid boxes, outbreaks of fire, the safe handling of equipment and clothing, the dispatch of specimens by post, the disposal of laboratory waste, and that the rules are displayed on a notice board in the laboratory.

This chapter is divided into two parts. The first section ('Running a Small-Animal Practice Laboratory') considers the management of a practice laboratory, understanding, use and maintenance of its equipment. The second section ('Diagnostic Tests') explains how to collect and examine specimens, or how to prepare them for submission to a pathology laboratory for professional examination.

Running a small-animal practice laboratory

Laboratory apparatus

Cleaning and disposal

Chemically clean glassware is essential, and although more glass is being replaced by disposable plastic, it is important to know how to clean and dry glassware. The use of commercial laboratory detergents is advisable and instructions should be followed carefully.

As a matter of routine, put all reusable glassware into disinfectant containers as soon as it has been used.

The cleaning procedure is as follows:

- Soak any dirty glassware in suitable disinfectants.
- Using disposable gloves, remove any surface material with the aid of test-tube brushes or other soft bristle brushes so as not to scratch the glass.
- Transfer to fresh solution of detergent and leave to soak, or use an ultrasonic bath.
- Once the glassware is physically clean, rinse it thoroughly in distilled/deionised water, with two or three changes of fresh water, to ensure complete removal of any residue detergents.
- Allow to drain.
- Then dry in a drying oven or in air, ensuring that the atmosphere is free from dust and chemicals.

CHECKLIST
- Soak in disinfectant.
- Remove debris.
- Soak in detergent.
- Rinse 2–3 times in distilled/deionised water.
- Drain and dry.

It should be routine practice to clean all equipment and work-surfaces daily following use. Equipment should be wiped down with suitable disposable cloths impregnated with disinfectant. Any tubes, curettes and pipes should be flushed through with disinfectant solutions. Some manufacturers recommend and supply special cleaning and flushing solutions for their machines and they should be used as appropriate.

Put disposable 'sharps' into sharps bins and all other disposable waste into yellow bin bags as soon as they have been used. They should then be disposed of as clinical waste.

Pipettes

Graduated pipettes have a series of lines or marks engraved on the side to indicate the volume of their contents. A 10 ml pipette of this type is graduated in 1 ml divisions; each 1 ml is subdivided into ten 0.1 ml units. The meniscus of the fluid in the pipette should be at the level of the line required.

One-mark volumetric pipettes have only a single mark on them, indicating the level for a specific volume.

For safety reasons it is preferable to attach a large-volume rubber bulb and apply gentle suction to fill rather than attaching rubber tube only and mouth sucking. Care is needed not to draw up the fluid beyond the mark. Cotton plugs may be inserted into the top of the pipettes to restrict fluid into the tube.

Micropipettes come in various styles, with single or adjustable volumes and disposable pipette tips. For some (particularly the very small volume types), positive displacement is achieved using a probe which comes into contact with the fluid; other micropipettes operate on the principle of air displacement. The disposable tips are usually colour coded for the various volumes. Accurate and reproducible pipetting requires care and practice. Tips should be discarded into sharps bins and most pipettes have an ejection system so that the tips do not need to be handled.

Automatic pipettes are two of basic types:

- **Single-shot reservoir** – dial the volume required and fill the reservoir; an electronic button then dispenses the required volume, one shot at a time.
- **Multihead pipettes** – often used for ELISA (enzyme-linked immunosorbent assay) plate work and normally have eight tips so that eight wells can be filled at the same time (electronically) with the same amount of fluid from a single reservoir.

Pasteur pipettes are now mostly made of moulded flexible plastic with integral bulbs, although they were originally made from soda glass and used by attaching a rubber bulb. The bulb is pressed and then the pipette tip immersed in the selected liquid; as the bulb is released, fluid passes up the capillary section of the pipette into the lumen of the tube. The fluid in the tube can then be released into a separate container by squeezing the bulb again. This system is commonly used for the manual removal or separation of serum or plasma from a blood sample.

Bottles

Chemicals and reagents are often supplied in plastic containers or in glass bottles. The original amber glass Winchester, a tall bottle, has been replaced by a more dumpy, wider-based bottle with a lower centre of gravity, which is less likely to be knocked over. Many acids are supplied in this type of bottle and should be kept in a metal safety cupboard with lockable doors and at floor level. Never put bottles of concentrated acid on high shelves.

Common reagent bottles for use in the laboratory have either a screw top or a glass stopper and are made from clear glass, clear or opaque plastic, or amber glass. If making up reagents it is important to label the bottles clearly (using a waterproof marker) showing details of contents and date made, together with any storage details. Any hazardous substances should be clearly identified with the correct symbols and stored in accordance with the Control of Substances Hazardous to Health (COSHH) regulations. Various adjustable volume dispenser systems are available to aid in the transfer of fluid from the bottles.

Smaller reagent bottles with integral pipettes in the lid are used for dispensing reagents and stains. Some dropping bottles have grooved glass stoppers so that drops can be dispensed. Many modern versions of the dropping bottle are of polythene, with an elongated, tapering nozzle that may be cut at the tip to allow a single drop at a time or, if cut lower down at a wider diameter, to dispense a stream.

Universal bottles are small, wide-mouthed, screw-top plastic or glass 30 ml bottles, often used for urine or faeces samples. They are usually supplied as sterile containers.

Microscopes

A good **compound light microscope** (Fig. 13.1) is an essential piece of equipment for every veterinary practice. By definition it consists of two separate lens systems: the ocular and the objective system. It is advisable to use a **binocular microscope** with an integral light source (usually a 6 volt halogen filament bulb). A **transformer** controlled by a **rheostat** modifies the intensity of the light source. The light passes through a **lens** and **field diaphragm** to a **mirror** that directs the light up from the foot to the **substage condenser**. The condenser consists of two lenses that focus the light source on the object being viewed: the condenser is moved up or down by turning the **condenser control knob.** Before the light reaches the condenser it passes through the **iris diaphragm**, which is a lever-controlled aperture that modifies the amount of light passing through the condenser. Below the iris there are often glass filters, e.g. a blue daylight filter to reduce the amount of red or yellow components of the light spectrum.

Above the substage condenser is the **stage**, which holds the slide being examined. It is mounted on a mechanical assembly referred to as the **mechanical stage**. This enables the slide holder to be moved left or right, up or down.

Above the stage is the **nosepiece**, with a **rotating turret** holding normally three or four **objective lenses**, each with a different magnification. The most common objective lenses are: ×4 (scanning), ×10 (low power), ×40 (high dry) and ×100 (oil immersion). The stage is racked up and down by means of an outer **coarse focus** and an inner **fine focus** knob on the **limb** of the microscope.

As light passes through the selected objective lens it travels up the **optical tube** mounted in the **body** of the microscope to a series of **prisms** in the **binocular head (body)** which deflect the light path through the **ocular lenses** mounted in

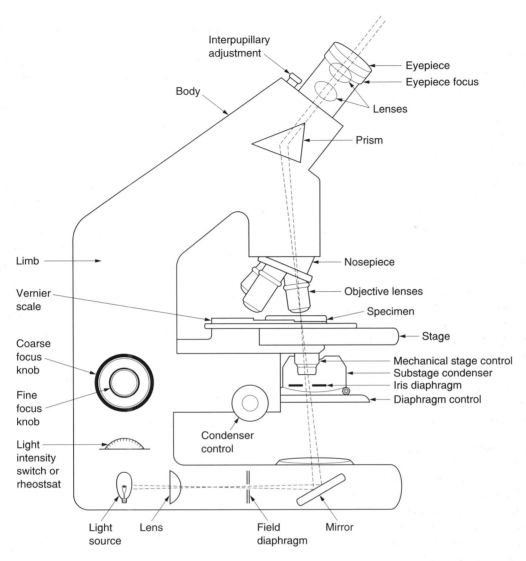

Fig. 13.1 Parts of and light paths through a compound light microscope.

the **eyepieces.** The eyepieces may be adjusted to the interpupillary distance of the person using the microscope and one of the ocular tubes in the eyepieces is adjustable to correct for individual differences between the two eyes. The **inclined binocular head** may increase the actual magnification 1.5 times, and the factor is engraved on the head. The lenses in the eyepieces are usually low powered with a magnification of 4 or 6, while 8 is the maximum for practical use.

Some binocular microscopes have interchangeable bodies so that a monocular photographic tube can be attached. Others have a permanent photographic tube as well as the binocular head. Specially designed teaching heads have two binocular sets.

The purpose of a microscope is to magnify and the size of the object can be measured if a measuring scale is put into one of the eyepieces. The amount of magnification is calculated by multiplication of the magnification of the eyepiece, magnification of the binocular head (if known) and the objective magnification.

Care, cleaning and maintenance of the microscope

- Locate in a convenient position and do not move unnecessarily.
- Carry using both hands, one under the base or foot and the other holding the limb.
- Do not place near centrifuges or other sources of vibration.
- Keep away from water and direct sunlight.
- Keep covered when not in use.
- To maximise the life of the bulb, turn the rheostat down before switching it off or if the light is left on for any period when not in use.
- Keep extra light-bulbs in stock but do not handle the actual bulb when replacing it.
- Only lens paper should be used to clean the lenses and eyepieces to avoid scratching the lenses.
- Remove oil from the oil-immersion objective after use and ensure that solvents do not remain in contact with the objective as they may loosen the cement holding the lens in place.

- When finished with the microscope, turn off the light (after turning down the rheostat), then lower the stage and turn the lowest power objective into position. Clean the oil-immersion lens and cover the microscope.
- If dirt appears in the field of study it is likely to be on the eyepiece. Rotate it: if the dirt also rotates, clean the eyepiece with a lens paper.

Using the microscope

(1) Check that the lowest power objective is clicked into position over the stage and that all lenses and eyepieces are clean.
(2) Check that the rheostat is down low and switch on then increase rheostat to medium setting.
(3) Ensure substage condenser is fully raised and iris diaphragm is fully open.
(4) Rack the stage down using the coarse focus knob and place the slide or counting number chamber firmly into the mechanical stage and centralise below the object lens.
(5) Adjust the distance between the two eyepieces so that each field appears identical and that both fields are viewed as one.
(6) Using the coarse focus, and before looking down eyepieces, rack the stage up until it is 2 mm away from the slide. This is to avoid inadvertently racking up too far and smashing the slide, particularly if the microscope's stop does not work correctly.
(7) Look down eyepieces and coarse focus (lowering the stage) steadily, immediately the object comes into view fine focus as required to bring it into clear view.
(8) Adjust the position of the condenser and iris diaphragm for optimal illumination, if required, according to manufacturer's instructions.
(9) Using the mechanical stage control knobs, examine the field on the slide under low power.
(10) If a specific area under view requires higher magnification, rotate the objective nose turret until the ×40 high dry objective lens clicks into place (most correctly adjusted microscopes do not require you to lower the stage to do this) and then adjust using the fine focus to obtain a clear image. The diaphragm and condenser may require readjustment as more light may be needed at the higher magnification.

To view an object under oil immersion:

(1) First view the field under low power, then swivel the objective half-way between the oil of the immersion high-power lens.
(2) Then place a drop of immersion oil on the slice over the field and rotate the oil immersion objective into position.
(3) If the field does not come into view, stop looking down the eyepieces and look directly at the position of the oil-immersion lens in relation to the surface of the slide and the oil. The lens of the objective should be in the oil but not touching the slide; return to the

eyepieces and slowly adjust the fine focus to bring into view.
(4) Adjust the iris diaphragm and condenser to ensure adequate illumination.

Never allow the high dry or other non-oil immersion lenses to come into contact with the oil. When finished with the oil-immersion viewing, lower the stage, rotate the lenses so that the lowest power is in position, turn the light down and then off, clean the oil-immersion lens and remove the slide from the stage.

TIP
When viewed through a compound microscope an object appears to be upside down and reversed. Movement of the mechanical stage is also reversed, so that as the stage is moved to the left the image moves to the right. Some microscopes enable the eyepieces to be swivelled to "correct" this.

Recording specimen positions   Each **axis** (there are two of them) has a **vernier scale** on it so that the position of any particular item on the object slide may be recorded. The main scale has a series of lines at intervals of 1 mm with numbers for identification. The vernier is a short scale with ten lines and figures. In use, the reading is the zero point of the vernier. If for example, the zero line lies between 14 and 15 on the main scale it means the reading is more than 14 but less than 15 to record. The first part of the recording will therefore be 14. The vernier is then examined and it will now be found that just one of the vernier lines will coincide more or less exactly with one of the lines of the main scale (all other lines being slightly separate from a main scale line). If the line in closest alignment is 7 then the reading will be **14.7**. The procedure is carried out for both the north and south axis of the verniers to finish up with two numbers with decimals. Record this on a label on a known side of the slide. To find the same field of view on a subsequent occasion, we select the same objective, place the slide on the stage with the label to the left or right as recorded and then preset both scales and verniers to the recorded figures in order to locate the specimen.

Colorimeter

Colorimetry is the measurement of light **absorbed** or **transmitted** by a substance. A colorimeter is the apparatus or analyser which measures the light absorbed (inverse or visual colorimetry) or transmitted (direct or potometric colorimetry) by a solution at a wavelength. The selection of a wavelength in a colorimeter is achieved by use of filters; however, most modern analysers are in fact spectrophotometers, which use prisms or monochromatic gratings to separate the light path into a single wavelength. This is then passed through the solution (normally held in a cuvette) and the emergent light is then detected and converted into electrical energy and displayed by means of an analogue meter or, more commonly, by means of digital readout.

Colorimeters and spectrophotometers are 'wet' chemistry systems that require the use of various liquid reagents which are commercially available in kit form. Detailed methodology for use of the kit in conjunction with a particular analyser is provided by the manufacturer or supplier. Systems may be manual or semi-automated, enabling one test to be performed on one sample at a time or larger automated ones allowing a variable number of tests to be performed on batches of samples.

Many practices however, use 'dry' chemistry systems which have less user variability. Several tests can usually be performed on the sample which is placed on to prepared slides or reagent strips using an integral automated pipette. The analyser determines the **reflective light** (usually as the reaction occurs) and displays the results. Whichever system is used, it is important to follow the manufacturer's operating rules fully and to ensure that the machine is kept clean, serviced and quality checked regularly. Often biochemistry analysers can include endocrine readers and can also be linked by a computer system to automated haematology and electrolyte analysers to enable a global print-out for each animal.

Temperature control Enzymes are totally dependent on temperature. The recommended temperature for performing determination of enzyme activity is 30°C; however, almost all laboratories have moved to the temperature of 37°C, as most chemical reagent systems are optimised at this temperature. It is essential that the temperature is controlled. Machines should not be placed in positions with direct exposure to sunlight and the ambient operating temperature must be maintained constantly.

Quality control Storage of kits, reagents and samples must be carefully monitored and regular use of internal quality control samples and external quality assessment samples as advised by the manufacturer is essential if accurate and reliable results are to be obtained. Operators should be adequately trained by the supplier and if necessary receive further professional training in order to become and remain competent.

Centrifuges

These machines spin at high speed to produce a large gravitational force referred to as the **relative centrifugal force (RCF)**, which is measured in *g* **forces**. Acceleration due to **gravity** (*g*) is 981 cm/second/second.

The objectives are:

• To separate the cells from fluid.

• To partition different density (size and mass) of material.
• To concentrate the material.

The deposit is termed the **sediment**; the fluid is the **supernatant**.

Standard centrifuges are of two types according to the style of **rotor head**: a **swing-out** and an **angle-head** (Table 13.1). A swing-out head consists of a rotor with specimen buckets suspended vertically from the arms of the rotor. As the rotor turns, the buckets swing out into a horizontal position. When the rotor slows down and stops, they fall back into a vertical position. An angle-head rotor has a series of holes drilled around the rotor at a fixed angle (normally 52° from the perpendicular). Samples are placed in these holes.

The inner bowl of the centrifuge is a solid piece of metal designed as a guard to retain the rotor buckets and samples should they become detached, or if metal fatigue leads to fracture of the rotor. It is good laboratory practice to wipe out, clean and disinfect the entire bowl as a matter of routine.

Modern centrifuges have a number of inbuilt safety devices, including an integral lid-lock that prevents opening of the centrifuge while the rotor is still spinning; nor can the rotor begin to operate until the lid is securely closed. A safety plate is present on many machines either as a separate screw-on lid behind the main lid or as an integral part of the main lid; like the guard bowl, it prevents penetration from inside in case of accidents.

Samples, usually in plastic or glass tubes, are put into buckets or carrier tubes which usually have rubber cushions at the bottom to prevent the bases of the sample tubes from damage or breakage. Ideally, for safety, the buckets should be removable for washing (and if necessary autoclaving) in case of breakage or spillage. To prevent aerosol dissemination, especially from potentially pathogenic samples, always use bucket guards or lids (these are autoclavable). It is important to ensure that buckets are balanced and so tubes of equal volume and weight should be placed opposite each other. Water-filled tubes may be used to balance the buckets if necessary.

Centrifuges can have variable speed control and a gauge to show the speed, a timer to dial up the required period of

Table 13.1 Performance comparison of the two types of centrifuge	
Swing-out	Generates air friction and heats up at speed
	Restricts speed of operation
	Samples can be remixed slightly at end of centrifugation
Angle-head	Can operate at higher speeds without heat build-up
	Deposit laid down at fixed angle of head may be disturbed as the centrifuge tubes are removed and stood upright in test tube racks

centrifugation and a brake to slow down the rotor once the timer switches off. To increase the gravitational force, the rotor's turning speed is controlled and so is the duration. If the radius of the centrifuge from the centre of the shaft to the tip of the bucket is R (cm) and the number of revolutions of the rotor per minute (r.p.m.) is N, then relative centrifugal force (RCF) in g forces is calculated using the following equation:

$$RCF \text{ (in } g) = 1.118 \times 10^{-5} R N^2$$

CENTRIFUGE CARE, HEALTH AND SAFETY, CLEANING AND MAINTENANCE
- Always follow the manufacturer's instructions.
- Keep a log of centrifuge usage and relate this to regular servicing and lubrication.
- Use on a firm dry surface away from water and preferably on a rubber mat to prevent excessive vibration.
- Check electricity cable and plug for cracks, looseness or damage.
- Always use the correct type of plug fuse.
- In the case of excessive vibration turn off immediately.
- Keep removable parts and inner surfaces clean and disinfected as necessary.

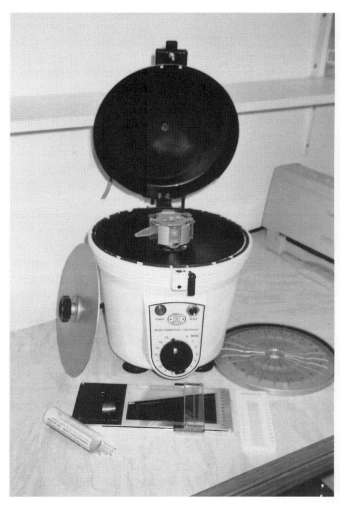

Fig. 13.2. Centrifuge with removable angle head, and to the right an adapter for microhaematocrit use which screws in, replacing the angle head. Also, from left to right: safety lid for use with microhaematocrit adapter, capillary tubes, microhaematocrit reader, plastic sealant for the capillary tubes.

Microhaematocrit This is a special type of centrifuge (see Fig. 13.2) for separating whole blood in capillary tubes to enable assessment of **packed cell volume (PCV)**. It has a special type of rotor consisting of an almost flat, horizontal surface with slots for capillary tubes. There is a rubber cushion on the outside of the lip of the rotor. A safety plate is screwed down on top of the rotor to hold the tubes in place and then the lid is closed to operate. Sometimes capillary tubes do not seal properly or may break. The rubber cushion may be covered with blood or be damaged by fragments of capillary glass. It should be wiped clean after use and the rubber replaced regularly. The entire head, rubber cushion and the safety plate should be disinfected as a matter of routine.

Incubator

Electric incubators are used to culture bacteria. These enclosed units of various sizes have removable shelves and impervious smooth surfaces of metal or plastic. They are well insulated with a gasket-sealed door so that the air inside is maintained at a set temperature ($37°C$ is the optimal temperature for almost all pathogenic bacteria). It is important to check the wiring and thermo-

stat and to maintain a daily record of the temperature to ensure consistent operation. Potentially dangerous bacteria may be grown, therefore it is essential to have a set procedure for cleaning and disinfecting or perhaps fumigating the incubator.

General safety in the laboratory

The laboratory can be a dangerous place. Training and complete understanding of the Health and Safety at Work Act 1974 as it relates to laboratories is essential, as is knowledge of the Control of Substances Hazardous to Health (COSHH) regulations (discussed in Chapters 5 and 8). Attendance at a specialist Laboratory Health and Safety training course is ideal as well as competence in simple first aid procedures. See Chapter 5, p. 143. Always refer to a more experienced person or authority if in any doubt about laboratory practices or procedures.

SAFETY IN THE LABORATORY
- Ensure adequate laboratory training and access only to authorised people.
- Smoking, eating or drinking must be prohibited.
- Protective laboratory coats should be donned on entry and removed on departure from the laboratory area.
- Disposable gloves should be worn and goggles as necessary.
- Keep the laboratory and all work surfaces clean, neat and tidy.
- Clean up and disinfect working surfaces immediately after use.
- Provide suitable labelled containers of disinfectant solution for immediate soaking of contaminated equipment, e.g. glassware.
- Books and papers should be kept away from the working bench area and separate from any samples or reagents being handled.
- Follow the local Health and Safety rules.
- Bunsen burners must not be left with a blue flame in between stages of use and should be turned off immediately they are not needed.
- Dispose correctly of clinical waste, used reagents and old equipment.
- Act immediately to control spillage.
- Record any accident (see 'Accident Book').

Dealing with spillages and disposal of clinical waste

It is possible that significant pathogens may be isolated in the practice laboratory. Attention to Health and Safety codes is important at all times, particularly when working with bacterial samples. Attention to the control and disposal of clinical waste is very important and current legislation places the responsibility for it on the person who generates the waste (see also p. 143).

The laboratory has a responsibility to ensure all material is made as safe as possible and that clinical waste is collected regularly and transported by licensed clinical waste carriers to approved incineration facilities and disposed of correctly under the legislation. Record-keeping and adherence to the regulations are important.

NB: Clinical waste disposal containers and bags are normally coloured yellow but in certain parts of the country other colours are used.

All the preceding aspects are very important. Quality results depend on good working practices; safety and care in the laboratory also depend on adherence to standard operating procedures.

SPILLAGES AND DISPOSAL PROCEDURES (TABLE 13.2)
- Restrict volumes handled to avoid large spills.
- Report to a senior person if in doubt.
- Wear protective clothing including face and eye protection if necessary.
- Record all incidents.

Accidents

All but the most minor laboratory accidents should be immediately referred to a trained first aider or the emergency medical service. See Table 13.3 for some first aid procedures.

All accidents should be reported to a responsible person and entered into an accident book in a standard format. See also Chapter 5, 'Occupational Hazards'.

ACCIDENT BOOK
The minimum information to be recorded in relation to accidents at work, in order to satisfy the regulations in the Management of Health and Safety at Work Regulation (amended 1999), cover emergencies and Reporting of Injuries, Diseases and Dangerous Occurrences Regulations 1995 (RIDDOR).
(1) Give full name, home address and occupation of the person who had the accident.
(2) The person filling in the book must sign and date it. If they did not have the accident then they must also give their name, home address and occupation.
(3) Record time and date of accident and where it happened.
(4) State how the accident happened. Give the cause if you can. If any personal injury, state what it is.
(5) If the accident is reportable under RIDDOR then employer must initial and report.
(6) Accident books must be retained for 3 years after the date of the last entry.

Diagnostic tests

Collection of specimens

Good-quality samples are essential for good-quality laboratory results. Collection methods and containers used all contribute to this.

Table 13.2 Spillage safety

Spillage or disposal problem	Action
Corrosives and liquid chemicals	Mixed with a commercially produced chemical binder spills powder, collect into plastic bucket, label and arrange for special disposal
Flammable liquids	Absorb into sand, transfer to buckets, remove to safe open area to evaporate, wash area thoroughly with water and detergent
Biological fluids/substances	Disinfect and wipe down with paper towels or for larger spills use a commercial lab spills powder Dispose of as clinical waste Disinfect area
Cultures and contaminated equipment, e.g. culture plates, used samples	Autoclave in sealed autoclave bags and then treat as clinical waste

Table 13.3 First aid procedures

First aid situation	Emergency action
Contamination by biological agents:	
Skin	Wash thoroughly with soap and water Do not scrub skin. Use antiseptic wipes
Mouth	Rinse out thoroughly with water
Wounds from sharp injuries	Irrigate wound immediately with running water and wash with soap/antiseptic and water. Dress wound
Eye splashes	Wash out immediately with sterile in-date eye wash solution for at least 10 minutes (failing this running tap water or deionised water). Do not rub eye
Contamination by chemicals:	
Skin	Flood area with copious amounts of water for at least 10 minutes
Eye	Flood eye as above, ensure affected eye is downwards so substance not washed to other eye
Inhalation	Remove to fresh air if possible and refer to hospital immediately
Ingestion	Medical attention ASAP. Do not induce vomiting

Blood

Venipuncture is normally by syringe and needle but a vacutainer kit can also be used. The needle size should be the largest practical for the animal to avoid clotting inside the needle or the necessity to suck hard and collapse the vein around it, potentially damaging blood cells. Length needs to penetrate comfortably into the vein lumen. The syringe size will be sufficient to correctly fill the selected collecting con-

tainer. The vein of choice is the **jugular** where possible but the **cephalic** vein is also commonly used.

The animal is safely and securely restrained (see Chapter 1) and the handler normally raises the vein. Clip the hair and clean and swab with a topical alcohol wipe.

Collection from the **jugular** can be with the animal sitting and head twisted up and to one side or with a cat on its side or back and the head extended. The vein is raised by pressure below the point of venipuncture. Penetrate the lumen and up the inside of the vein. Slowly pull back on the syringe and let the blood flow into it without applying undue pressure. When sufficient blood has been collected release pressure on the vein, then remove the needle gently. Quickly apply direct light pressure to the venipuncture site using a sterile swab of cotton wool. Immediately remove the needle from the syringe (to avoid clotting or blood cell damage) and smoothly fill the collecting pot. Avoid forced expulsion of blood which may damage the blood cells.

> **TIP**
> When collecting from the **cephalic vein** slight flexion and extension of the carpal joint can assist blood flow. After collection, tape over the animal's swab to prevent further bleeding. If working alone with an anaesthetised or calm animal raise the vein with the left hand under the leg and the thumb on top, or apply a quick-release tourniquet, and approach the vein from the side.

Vacutainer systems   A 'vacutainer' is an evacuated tube (i.e. with a vacuum) as part of a complete system incorporating a double-ended needle screwed into a holder. The small vacutainers have a 3 ml volume but only a 2 ml draw, in order to minimise the amount of pressure put on the red cells. It is important to collect blood with the complete vacutainer system. Never inject blood from a syringe into a vacutainer.

It is sometimes possible to insert a needle into the vein and collect the blood directly into a container drop by drop. However, clotting is more likely to occur. The animal should ideally be standing and the collection tube is held beneath the shank of the needle.

Type and condition of blood   When blood clots and clot retraction takes place, the fluid is referred to as **serum**. **Plasma** is that fluid separated from non-clotted blood. To prevent clotting **anticoagulants** are used, the most common being heparin, ethylene diamine tetra-acetic acid (**EDTA**), oxalate fluoride and sodium citrate.

If the red cells become broken or lysed they release their contents into serum or plasma. This is referred to as **haemolysis**. If serum or plasma is reddish in colour after separation, then haemolysis has occurred. This might result from:

- Excess pressure when pulling back the syringe plunger.
- Too vigorous mixing of samples.

- Osmotic pressure because the skin or the needle/syringe has water on or in it.
- The use of too fine a needle, damaging red cells.
- Failing to separate the plasma for transit.

Lipaemia is the presence of lipids/fats in the blood. This is often a physiological condition which occurs after feeding (especially ingestion of fatty foods) and so it is advisable to sample fasted animals, not ones just fed. Lipaemia may also be a pathological condition associated with metabolic conditions.

Icteric samples are those with significant amounts of bilirubin in the blood. The level of 'normal range' bilirubin varies between species: equine serum, for example, will always appear more icteric than feline because of the much higher level of bilirubin in the horse due to the lack of a gall bladder.

Chromatins are colour agents and they may interfere with colorimetric or spectrometric biochemical determinations by influencing the colour of serum and plasma. They include the carotene intake in the diet: the serum and plasma colour of grazing animals ingesting high carotene levels, such as dairy cattle, is more yellow than in other species.

Coagulants and colour codes   Table 13.4 shows the colour codes and the appropriate anticoagulants for specific tests. The general principle is that **EDTA** whole blood is used for haematology. **Oxalates** are usually used as either sodium, potassium, ammonium or lithium salts, but currently the only useful routine salt is the potassium oxalate salt with sodium fluoride (**OXF**) which is used for glucose determination. **Heparin whole blood** is used for lead determination, while **sodium citrate** is used for clotting times and special coagulation studies. **Clotted blood with serum taken off** is used for most routine biochemistry or serology but **heparin plasma** may be used in many (but not all) cases, as an alternative to serum.

Storage of serum and plasma   If serum or plasma is to be stored rather than immediately tested or posted to a laboratory, label the sample clearly with indelible marker and then store at $-20°C$ in a suitable deep-freeze. Do not keep at room temperature for any length of time, but samples can often be retained in a reasonably stable state for a few hours at $+4°C$ in a refrigerator.

Serum and plasma should never be exposed to extremes of heat. If frozen, samples that have been thawed should not be frozen again: they should only be frozen and thawed once.

Urine

Collection methods will depend upon the reason for the sample and the type of animal to be sampled. In general, sufficient urine of a representative sample (e.g. not the first few drops, which may contain mucoid material from other parts of the urinogenital tract), free of contaminants, is required. However, samples fulfilling all these criteria are usually those that are more invasive to the animal and may sometimes require sedation or even anaesthetic. Often, as a quick and convenient way of obtaining some initial diagnostic information easier methods but ones which are more likely to produce contaminated samples are used. Urine should be collected into a sterile universal container.

The preferred methods for bacterial examination are:

- **Cystocentesis** – can be performed in dogs and cats. A sterile 1- to $1\frac{1}{2}$-inch needle is inserted into the bladder through the surgically prepared abdominal wall. The bladder should be full to avoid damage to other internal organs. As much urine as possible is removed to prevent leakage of urine through the needle hole created by the procedure. The sample obtained is free of external contamination.
- **Catheterisation** – sterile gloves and catheter are used and the external genitalia are cleaned. Maintain sterility by feeding the **urethral catheter** gradually out of its protective pack whilst being fed into the urethra where it should pass easily. Performed easily in male dogs and in male cats. Sedation may be required. A **Jackson's cat catheter** can be used for cats and a **Foley catheter** is required for bitches. Female cats are rarely catheterised.

Other samples can be collected by **manual expression of the bladder,** with the animal standing or in lateral recumbency. The external genitalia should be cleaned and hair dampened back out of the way. Gentle pressure on the

Table 13.4 Vacutainer and universal tube colour codes, their anticoagulants and applications

Vacutainers	Collecting pots	Anticoagulant	Type of sample	Application
Red	White	None	Clotted blood/serum	Biochemistry, serology
Green or green and orange	Orange	Heparin	Whole blood and plasma	Biochemistry, lead, electrolytes
Lavender	Pink	EDTA	Whole blood	Haematology
Grey	Yellow	Oxalate Fluoride	Whole blood	Glucose
Light blue		Sodium citrate	Whole blood and plasma	Coagulation tests
Dark blue		None	Clotted blood/serum	Trace elements
	Brown	(Serum gel)	Serum	Serology

Always check colours as manufacturers may change them. Vacutainers are not advisable in some smaller animals as the vacuum can collapse the vein

bladder is carried out. The initial urine is allowed to pass out (and with it any surface bacteria) and a midstream sample is collected. This is most easily performed with smaller animals but contraindicated in any with possible urinary tract obstruction.

Metabolic cages for urine collection are sometimes available, as is special non-absorbent cat litter or resorting to collecting a mid-stream sample as it is voided by the animal.

Table 13.5 lists the preservatives used in urine and details the reasons for using them. However, in a practice laboratory it is better to test a urine sample immediately rather than use any preservative. Urine should not be stored frozen but kept at refrigerator temperature, unless some specific analytical requirement calls for freezing.

Spun-down (centrifuged) sediment should be examined as soon as possible, but formalin may be used to preserve the material.

Faeces

Use a wide-mouthed universal container or faeces pot, which must be sterile, and bear the following points in mind:

- It is preferable to collect fresh faeces per rectum with a gloved finger or hand rather than use a stale defecated sample picked up from the ground or litter tray.
- Ensure that the animal is securely restrained so that it is unable to bite, scratch or wriggle while the procedure is carried out.
- It is best to collect urine before collecting faeces, as collection per rectum may cause voiding of urine.
- Long fingernails may damage the mucosa.
- Do not use force to collect faeces from the rectum. It is important that the area around the anus is cleaned and lubricated to prevent skin flora being introduced into the faeces sample, and to prevent damage to the anal/rectal mucosa.

Table 13.5 Urine preservatives and their applications

Hydrochloric acid (HCl)	Biochemical analysis of urea, ammonia, calcium, total nitrogens and uric acid (mix well before testing, as deposits form)
Thymol crystal	Biochemical analysis
Acetic acid	For ascorbic acid determination
Boric acid	Similar to HCl plus microbiological examination
Chloroform	Cannot use for glucose, is a COSHH risk
Toluene	Is a COSHH risk
Formalin 40%	One drop as above but not glucose
Sodium bicarbonate	For porphyrins
Refrigeration (up to 6 hours)	Most satisfactory method

All urine preservatives are used to prevent bacterial action, chemical decomposition, or to stabilise constituents

- The faeces should fill the pot, to prevent too much air getting into the sample (which may kill off any anaerobic bacteria or lead to desiccation of the faeces and any parasites present).

Faeces should be kept at room temperature for only a short period before being examined, and should be kept out of sunlight. If examination of the faeces has to be delayed for a few hours, take a transport swab of the sample for bacteriology and place the labelled pot, with its lid screwed on securely, in the refrigerator. Do not freeze it. Be aware that stored faeces may ferment in the pots: lids may blow off if not secured.

To summarise:

- Collect fresh rectal samples.
- Fill sterile screw-top universal containers.
- Examine immediately.

Skin

Collection of **plucked hairs** for examination for ringworm infection should be made at the active edge of the lesions. Pluck individual hairs, including the root. If not examined immediately, place in a paper envelope for examination later.

A **tape technique** may be used to examine an area of skin for surface mites, melassezia and bacteria:

(1) Take a section of clear adhesive tape.
(2) With the sticky face down, press the tape against the hair and skin.
(3) Pull off and repeat over the area to be investigated.
(4) Place the tape on to a microscope slide for examination.

To obtain samples of **coat brushing** for mite examination, use a toothbrush or similar bristle brush (this method is unlikely to identify ringworm, which affects the root shaft):

(1) Work a small area at a time in the one direction, brushing the coat.
(2) Tap the brush into a Petri dish or on to a glass slide.
(3) Use forceps or tweezers to pick out the hairs.
(4) Do not put hair samples into plastic bags, as static electricity builds up and the samples are then very difficult to handle and examine.

For **skin scrapes**, use a scalpel blade to remove the surface layer of skin. It is important to go sufficiently deep to achieve **petechial** blood oozing (pinpoint clusters of surface capillary bleeding) (see Chapter 15):

(1) Place a drop of paraffin oil on the clipped skin area to be examined.
(2) Gently squeeze the skin into a fold to bring any bacteria or parasites nearer to the surface.
(3) Scrape with the scalpel blade.

(4) Carefully scrape the scalpel on to a microscope slide for examination.

If the sample is to be submitted to a laboratory, put a clear warning that a scalpel blade is included (especially if it is unprotected).

To prevent desiccation (i.e. when a sample is to be looked at later):

(1) Place some filter or blotting paper in the lid of a Petri dish and wet it with sterile water.
(2) Place two stick applicators or matchsticks on top.
(3) Suspend the slide on the sticks.
(4) Put the base on as a lid, seal with tape and label the dish.
(5) Place in a cool, dark place.

Some refrigerators may be suitable for storage but be warned that some of them extract moisture as they cool and therefore the period of storage should not be too long (as the seal on the dish is not totally airtight).

For longer storage, use airtight jars with a moist bed – but all must be prepared aseptically. For material under a cover slip on a slide, the area may be protected from desiccation by sealing the edges with nail varnish or epoxy resin.

Pustules may be sampled with a sterile needle on a small 1 or 2 ml syringe:

(1) Suck the contents of the pustule into the needle.
(2) Express on to a glass slide.
(3) Make either a **squash preparation** (by placing a second slide on top at right angles to the first and squashing) or a **smear** (by use of a spreader).
(4) Samples may then be examined fresh under low power or stained and examined under high power.

Cerebrospinal fluid (CSF)

The examination of CSF may be very useful in diagnosing some neurological conditions. The animal must be anaesthetised before the fluid is collected. The area of the spine that is tapped is normally either the atlanto-occipital or the lumbosacral space.

- Prepare the selected area by shaving and full sterile/aseptic precautions, as for any surgical procedure.
- Insert a suitable spinal tap needle into the subarachnoid space of the spinal column, taking care not to advance the needle too far (which could damage the spinal cord).
- Normally the animal is placed in lateral recumbency and the fluid is collected into an EDTA tube for cytology, by means of free flow.
- Do not aspirate the fluid.

It is possible to collect a second, plain tube sample (with no anticoagulant added) for biochemical tests after the sample has been centrifuged to spin down any cellular material.

Synovial fluid

Synovial fluid is collected by means of **arthrocentesis** from the joint in order to investigate a particular joint problem such as arthritis or in some cases of shifting lameness. Collection may be made on a conscious animal or following anaesthesia, depending on the animal and the joint. Arthrocentesis is made aseptically with a syringe and needle after the site has been prepared surgically.

Thoracic fluid

The pleural cavity contains only enough fluid for adequate lubrication of the intrathoracic organs and the cavity lining. The main reason for collection and examination of thoracic fluid (by means of **thoracocentesis**) is to find the cause of an increase in fluid volume. Collection is performed aseptically into EDTA tubes and plain tubes.

Abdominal fluid

The amount of peritoneal fluid in the abdominal cavity is only sufficient to provide lubrication of the abdominal organs and peritoneum. Any increase in volume may be investigated by means of **abdominocentesis**. Aseptic collection is usually performed via the most dependent part of the ventral midline in the standing animal following normal skin surgical preparation. Some of the fluid sample is transferred into EDTA for cytology, while the rest should be transferred into plain tubes or sterile containers for biochemistry and perhaps bacteriology.

Tissue samples, tumours and abdominal organ biopsy

Biopsy techniques relate to the sampling of a section of tissue, tumour or organ for cytological or histopathological examination.

FORMALIN

Formalin is a strong antiseptic and disinfectant that has the ability to preserve tissue samples by '**fixing**' or hardening them. It is commercially prepared from a pungent gas, formaldehyde, as a solution of 40% strength in water, i.e. a **40% formaldehyde** solution. Formalin is a hazardous substance (it gives off a gas that irritates eyes and nose) and it is important that local COSHH and Health and Safety rules are understood and adhered to.

Containers or pots for formalin-fixed tissues should be wide-mouthed and screw-topped to aid removal as the fixing process hardens the tissue.

For routine cases, tissues for histopathology are fixed in **10% formal saline**, which is made by diluting formalin in a buffered saline solution so that it contains 10% formalin (Table 13.6). This buffered solution is preferred but it is possible to use normal saline (sodium chloride in sterile distilled water), though the specimen is likely to be affected by cellular and histochemical changes because, with the lack of a buffer, there is no control of pH.

Fresh tissues need to be transferred immediately into the fixative, as the process of **necrosis** (cell death and lysis) can occur very rapidly. The container should allow a minimum of 10 parts fluid to one part tissue, by volume, which will ensure sufficient formalin penetration into the tissue for rapid fixation.

When submitting tissue to a laboratory, ensure that the container is labelled and securely sealed, and that there is an indication of the original location of the tissue.

Toxicology specimens

- All specimens should be collected free from any extraneous contamination. They should not be washed.
- Each sample must be collected and submitted in separate leakproof, airtight, sterile and chemically clean plastic or glass containers.
- Each container must be labelled with the owner's name, animal identification, type of sample, date of collection and the name and address of the practice.
- All samples must then be placed together in one large container.
- Unless tissues are to be examined histologically, samples are best collected fresh and then frozen. They should then be dispatched to the toxicology laboratory on ice.
- Consult the laboratory prior to packing and submitting as they may have special requirements.
- In cases of poisoning, it is essential that accurate records are kept at all stages, as evidence may be needed for possible litigation.

Submission of pathological samples to laboratories

In order to maximise the potential for diagnostic information, the intention is that material should arrive at the laboratory in a condition as similar as possible to that when it was actually collected. Correct preservation, properly completed paperwork, clear labelling and good packaging are all essential.

Preservation for transit

Tissue, once it has been removed from an animal, immediately starts to die. Cell membranes break down, leading to destruction or lysis of cells, and this process of **autolysis** is hastened by increased temperatures and humidity. 'Fixing' and freezing are methods of preventing or reducing autolysis. Tissues for standard histological examination should *not* be frozen.

Haemolysis is a form of cell degeneration in blood cells. Red blood cells are likely to be damaged if exposed to heat, cold or violent shaking. If possible, separate serum from the clot by centrifugation before dispatch. Whole-blood samples should be gently but adequately mixed with the correct amount of anticoagulant to avoid clotting (which would make them unsuitable for examination). Pack whole-blood samples and serum in a way that minimises temperature variation and physical damage in transit.

Labelling and paperwork

If samples are being sent away, the name of the veterinary surgeon and the practice's name and address should be recorded. All request forms should also contain:

- Name of owner.
- Name of animal (or some reference number relating to that animal).
- Animal's species, breed, age, sex, and whether intact or neutered.
- Date of sampling and time of collection.
- List of samples collected, including type of anti-coagulants used (if applicable).
- Clinical history, including any specific presenting signs and any current treatment.
- Details of site or sites (if swabs, skin scrapings or biopsy material are submitted) with a schematic diagram to show the position.
- Indication of tests or examinations required.

Submit the completed forms in plastic envelopes to protect them from possible contamination. Each sample relating to the case should be individually and clearly labelled with the name of the owner and the animal, and should be in agreement with details on the submission form.

Packaging

Most commercial laboratories supply special postal packs for submitted samples. All samples must be packed in compliance with postal regulations (Table 13.7).

Always assume that if something can be broken in transit, it will be. Packing should be such that:

Table 13.6 Buffered 10% formal saline: to make 1 litre	
Formalin (40% formaldehyde solution)	100 ml
$NaH_2PO_42H_2O$	4.5 g
Na_2HPO_4	6.5 g
Distilled water	900 ml

Table 13.7 Postal regulations and packaging requirements for pathological specimens

Packaging requirements for pathological samples (from January 1999):
Any diagnostic specimen sent through the Royal Mail has to be packaged in containers conforming to United Nations Regulation 602. The main points concerning the packaging are as follows.

(1) Water-tight primary container(s) such as a glass tube. This has to be surrounded by sufficient absorbent material and placed inside a secondary container. The secondary container and absorbent material must be capable of containing all the contents of the primary container(s)
(2) An itemised list of contents, and details of the sender, must be attached to the secondary container.
(3) The secondary container must be placed inside a UN-approved outer container – usually cardboard. This must be labelled with an appropriate hazard designation.
(4) The packaging has to meet UN requirements with regard to pressure and impact. Because of this it is likely to be more expensive than current packaging used to send diagnostic material through the post.

In addition, the following postal regulations should be adhered to:

(1) Use First Class or Datapost. DO NOT USE PARCEL POST.
(2) Label the outside with the words:
    PATHOLOGICAL SPECIMEN – FRAGILE. WITH CARE.
    As well as the laboratory address it must show the name, address and telephone number of the sender who will be contacted in case of leakage or damage.
(3) Every specimen must be in a primary container which is securely sealed. Maximum of 50 ml volume unless Post Office-approved multi-specimen packs.
(4) Primary container must be wrapped in sufficient absorbent material to absorb all of the sample if leakage or breakage occurs.
(5) The container and absorbent material must be sealed in a leakproof plastic bag.
(6) The plastic bag must then be placed in one of the following:
    (a) Plastic clip-down container.
    (b) Cylindrical lightweight metal container.
    (c) Strong cardboard box with full depth lid.
    (d) Two-piece polystyrene box with special grooved join.
(7) It is recommended that this complete package is placed in a padded (Jiffy) bag.
(8) Other packaging systems must be Post Office approved.

- Sample material is not damaged.
- Containers do not break or leak.
- Samples do not contaminate each other or the accompanying paperwork, or anybody who handles the package in transit or on receipt.

Containers should be secure, leakproof and protected from breaking but not so bound up in cling-film, cotton wool, bubblepack and sticky tape that the laboratory staff are unable to open them on receipt.

Transport swabs should be used with the correct media in them to prevent desiccation of microbial material. Fixed tissue should be in secure formal saline containers.

(2) Place a spreader slide just in front of the drop of blood and angle the slide at about 25–45° with the surface of the first slide.
(3) Draw the spreader slide back into the drop of blood, causing the blood to run along the interface between the two slides but not right to the edges.
(4) Push the spreader slide steadily with an even, rapid motion towards the far end of the other slide. This will draw the blood along behind the spreader slide and make a thin, even blood film.
(5) Allow to air dry.
(6) Clean the edge of the spreader slide.

Haematology

Blood smears

Clean, washed, oil-free glass microscope slides are required for the preparation of blood smears (Fig. 13.3). The most useful slides have a frosted area at one end on which sample identification can be recorded. For a spreader slide, select a slide with a smooth edge and chip off the corner.

(1) Place a drop (10 microlitres) of well-mixed EDTA whole blood at one end.

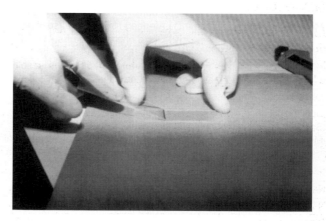

Fig. 13.3 Making a blood smear.

(7) Once the film is air-dried, it may be stained to examine cell morphology using **Romanowsky stains** (various alkaline methylene blue stains combined with eosin) such as Leishman's stain, or Wright's (or a modified Wright's/Giemsa to include some haemoparasites). **Supravital stains** such as brilliant cresyl blue or new methylene blue can be used for **reticulocyte** counts also to detect inclusions and other cellular material such as blood parasites, including *Haemobartonella* spp. and *Babesia* spp.

Instructions for staining techniques can vary between different texts as clarity of results will influence decisions on, for example, the time a stain is left on the slide. Individual operators develop their own preferences. Table 13.8 shows some methods.

Examination of blood films

The blood film is used to perform a **differential white blood cell count (WBC Diff.)**. The aim of this important procedure is to estimate the relevant proportions (as percentages) of the different types of white cells in a sample.

(1) The film should be scanned under low power to note the quality of the film and stain and the cell numbers.
(2) Then scan the feather end of the film for platelet clumps and large abnormal cells.

(3) Finally, under low power, select an area of the film at least one-third from the end of the film at the side edge which is to be examined under high-power oil immersion for cell counting.
(4) Swing out the low-power objective, place a drop of oil on the area and then swing in the oil-immersion lens; focus and count using the battlement technique.

Battlement technique   Rather than count each cell of each type (though the greater the number counted, the greater the accuracy), technicians often use the battlement technique (Fig. 13.4) to cover a reasonable area of the sample and to counteract distribution bias:

(1) Move two fields along the edge of the field, two fields up, two fields along and two fields down.
(2) Continue the sequence until 100 cells have been counted.
(3) Record the numbers of each type of cell.
(4) Express these as percentages of the total WBC count or in absolute numbers.

Poor-quality films   These can result from a number of problems:

- Too thick, therefore impossible to identify the cells due to poor separation. Correct by using smaller drop of blood.
- Too thin with insufficient cells found. A larger drop of blood required.
- Uneven thickness caused by jerky or hesitant spreading technique.

Table 13.8 Common blood smear staining methods		
Giemsa staining method		
Solution 1 (Analar)	Methyl alcohol, absolute	
Solution 2	Giemsa stain consisting of:	
	Azure 11-eosin	3 g
	Azure 11	0.8 g
	Glycerol	200 ml
	Solution 1	300 ml
Solution 3	Buffer solution (pH 7.0) consisting of:	
	Disodium hydrogen orthophosphate	9.47 g
	Potassium dihydrogen orthophosphate	9.08 g
	Distilled water	1 litre
	(can obtain as buffer tablets to dissolve in the distilled water)	
Method	(1) Air-dried films fixed in solution 1 for 3 minutes	
	(2) Dilute one volume of solution 2 with nine volumes of solution 3. Flood slide and stain for 15 minutes	
	(3) Wash and differentiate with solution 3, until cells are identifiable microscopically	
	(4) Drain and air dry	
Leishman's staining method		
Solution 1	Leishman's stain	
Solution 2	Buffered distilled water	(pH 6.8)
Method	(1) Cover smear with Leishman's stain and fix for 2 minutes	
	(2) Add to the slide twice the volume of solution. Allow to mix but avoid spillage	
	(3) Allow to stand for approximately 15 minutes when a metallic scum will be visible on the surface of the solution	
	(4) Wash gently with buffered with solution 2 and allow to dry.	

Note: There are also available commercially produced quick stain kits which are simple to use but may not give as clear cellular definition as Leishman's stain

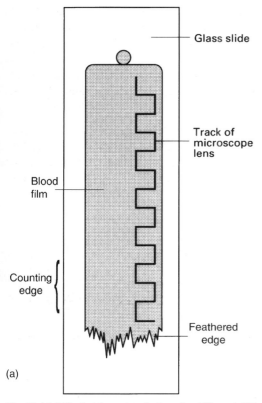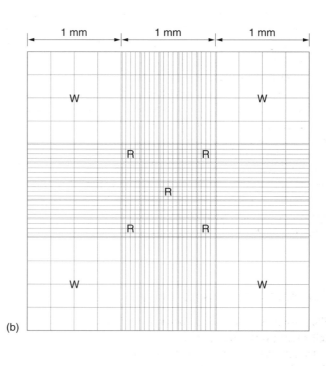

Fig. 13.4 (a) The battlement technique for differential blood counts. A good blood smear will be thumb shaped and about half the length of the slide without touching the sides. (b) Haemocytometer slide counting area as seen under the microscope. Total white blood cells are counted in the areas marked W and total red blood cells are counted in the areas marked R.

- Holes caused by greasy slide.
- Streaks caused by dirty or jagged spreader slide.

Stains should be filtered, as often debris and deposits prevent adequate staining and cellular differentiation.

Production of good-quality smears requires practice. Uniform staining may best be achieved by use of autostaining machines.

When examining the WBCs seen in a blood film, it is important to remember that red cells are also present and that they too should be looked at and commented upon. Figure 13.5 shows the various aspects of red cell development and morphology.

The total WBC count   The most common, of various methods, are either by automated haemotology analyser (preferred) or manually by using a Unopet haemocytometer kit which contains diluting reservoirs and capillary pipettes for making a 1:100 dilution of blood in ammonium oxalate or acetic acid, both of which lyse erythrocytes. Cells are counted using a haemacytometer and cover glass (Fig. 13.4b).

Table 13.9 shows the normal reference haematology data for a number of species.

Red cells: morphology and terminology

Erythrocytes (red blood cells, RBCs) are non-nucleated biconcave discs that are pale greenish-yellow when unstained. They take up eosin when stained by Romanowsky stains, and become pinkish.

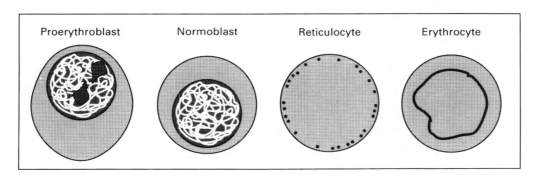

Fig 13.5 Erythrocyte development and morphology.

Table 13.9 Haematology reference ranges for domesticated animals

Parameter	Units	Canine	Feline	Equine	Thoroughbred	Bovine	Ovine
RBCs	10^{12}/l	5.0–8.5	5.5–10.0	5.5–9.5	7.0–13	4.5–9.0	5.0–10.0
Haemoglobin	g% (100 ml)	12–18	9.0–17	8.0–14	10–18	9.5–14.5	8.0–14
PCV	% (1/1)	37–57	27–50	24–44	32–55	30–40	22–38
MCV	fl	60–77	40–55	39–52	37–50	40–60	23–48
MCH	pg	19–23	13–17	15.2–18.6	13.3–18	14.4–18.6	9–13
MCHC	g% (100 ml)	31–34	31–34	30–35	31–38	26–34	29–35
WBCs	10^9/l	6–15	4–15	6–12	7–14	3.5–10	4–10
Lymphocytes	10^9/l	1–4.8	1.5–6.5	1–6	1.7–9.8	1–4.6	2.6–7.2
	%	12–30	25–33	15–50	25–70	40–60	65–72
Mature neutrophils	10^9/l	3.6–10.5	2.5–12.5	2.1–9	2.1–9.1	0.7–4.9	0.7–3.2
	%	60–70	45–75	35–75	30–65	21–49	18–32
Band neutrophils	10^9/l	0–0.3	0–0.45	0–0.24	0–0.28	0–0.2	0–0.1
	%	0–2	0–3	0–2	0–2	0–2	0–1
Eosinophils	10^9/l	0.1–1.5	0.1–1.8	0.1–1.4	0–1.5	0–1.6	0–1.0
	%	2–10	4–12	2–12	1–11	0–16	0–10
Monocytes	10^9/l	0.18–1.5	0–0.6	0.12–1.2	0–1	0–1	0–1
	%	3–10	0–4	2–10	0.5–7.0	2–10	0–10
Basophils	10^9/l	0	0	0–0.3	0–0.4	0	0–0.2
	%	rare	rare	0–3	0–3	rare	0–2
Platelets	10^9/l	200–500	200–600	90–500	100–300	200–300	200–700

Source: Bloxham Laboratories Ltd, Teignmouth, Devon

Proerythroblasts are the first stem cells of **erythropoiesis** or red cell production. They have a large nucleus with nucleoli and a rim of blue-stained cytoplasm. Haemoglobin synthesis commences on cell division within the cytoplasm and the cells become smaller. These are referred to as **nucleated RBCs (NRBCs)**. NRBC cytoplasm changes from purple to greyish pink as the cells get smaller through stages of cell division (**normoblasts**). When the cell is completely haemoglobinised, the small dense nucleus is extruded leaving a greyish-blue or polychromatic cell with a reticular structure which stains blue with supravital stains such as brilliant cresyl blue or new methylene blue. These cells have no nucleus and are referred to as **reticulocytes**. Within normally 12 days in the peripheral blood stream, these lose their polychromasia and are adult red cells. **Crenation** is a term applied to cells showing irregular margins and prickly points due to shrinkage. It is usually found in association with too slow air-drying of blood films.

Howell–Jolly bodies are basophilic nuclear remnants seen as the NRBCs change to young erythrocytes. They are found in response to anaemia and splenic disorders or after splenectomy.

Target cells are RBCs with a central rounded area of haemoglobin surrounded by a clear zone, with a dense ring of haemoglobin around the perimeter of the cell due to increased membranes or decreased volume. They are often found in non-regenerative anaemia.

Rouleaux is a type of red cell arrangement used to describe grouping of RBCs in stacks. This is common in healthy horses but is otherwise associated with increased fibrinogen or globulin concentration in the blood.

White blood cells (leucocytes)

WBCs are nucleated cells consisting of various types (Fig. 13.6) which may be classified into three morphological forms: **polymorphonuclear (PMNL) granulocytes**, **lymphocytes** and **monocytes** (both agranulocytes).

PMNL granulocytes have a single nucleus consisting of a number of lobes. They have granular cytoplasm and can be differentiated by the staining reaction of these granules into **neutrophils**, **eosinophils** and **basophils**.

The nucleus of a **neutrophil** will stain purple-violet. The immature or juvenile cell is shaped first like a kidney-bean and then like a horseshoe, at which stage it is often termed a **metamyelocyte** or later 'banded'. As the cell matures it forms lobes, the number of which increases with increasing maturity. The cytoplasm stains a light pink; the granules are violet although often under the microscope appears clear. A rise in immature neutrophils is termed '**shift to the left**'.

Neutrophilia is an increase in neutrophils and is found in infectious inflammatory conditions and under 'stress' or conditions induced by steroids.

Eosinophils are similar to neutrophils but they do not usually become as multilobular and their cytoplasmic granules will stain orange-red or pink. In each species of animal, the shape and colour of stained eosinic granules are slightly different: some are small and oval, others are larger (such as in the horse), while cats tend to have large rod-shaped granules.

Eosinophilia is an increase in the number of these cells and is often found in association with allergy and parasitism. **Eosinopenia** is a lack of these cells and is often found in the dog in association with steroid usage and Cushing's disease (hyperadrenocorticism).

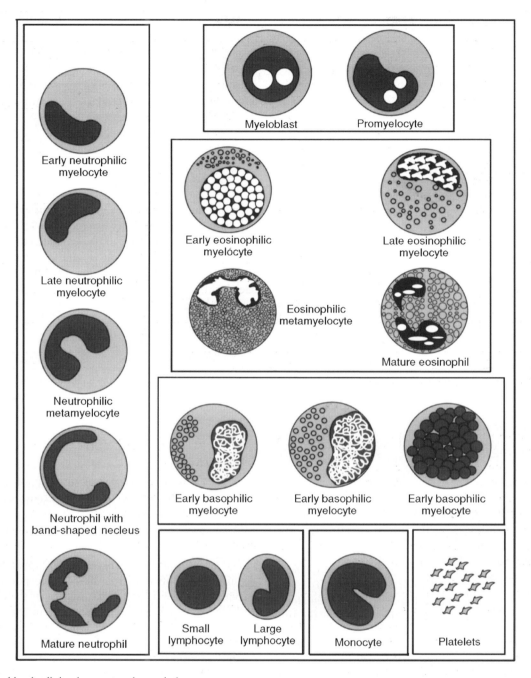

Fig. 13.6 White blood cell development and morphology.

Basophils are often slightly smaller than neutrophils (8–10 micrometres in diameter). The nucleus is usually shaped like a kidney-bean and the cytoplasm contains a mass of large granules that stain deep purple and may obscure the nucleus. They contain histamine and heparin, which are released at the site of inflammation. They are rarely found in normal films for most animal species but may be present in conditions of chronic tissue damage and myeloid leukaemias.

Lymphocytes are of two types. The nucleus of the smaller (7–10 micrometres in diameter) is round and will stain deep purple; it occupies most of the cell so that the cytoplasm, which stains a pale blue, is seen only as a rim around the nucleus, often only to one side. This is the most common form. The nucleus of the larger type (12–20

micrometres in diameter) stains slightly lighter and has more light blue cytoplasm, which may contain a few reddish granules.

Lymphocytes play an important protective role and are associated with the production of antibodies and recognition of 'foreign' substances such as bacteria and viruses, or the body itself in autoimmune conditions. **Lymphocytosis** is found in some viral conditions and leukaemias. **Lymphopenia** is a decrease in lymphocyte cells that is found in some viral conditions, after steroid use and in some chemotherapy patients. It is important to note that many lymphomas and other neoplastic conditions do not produce a lymphocytosis and may in fact show up as a lymphopenia.

Monocytes are large cells (16–20 micrometers in diameter) with a variably shaped nuclei often elongated and lobulated, occasionally kidney bean shaped. The cytoplasm is blue-grey containing vacuoles and sometimes pink granules. They are macrophages (carry out phagocytosis).

Thrombocytes (platelets) very small cells which stain blue/pink. Involved in the repair of damage to blood vessels: they adhere to the damage and to each other to plug the 'leak' and are then involved in the clotting process (coagulation) to produce fibrin. **Thrombocytopeenia**, a reduction in the number of platelets, may result in internal or external haemorrhage, while an increase (**thrombocytosis**) may follow haemorrhage or surgery and can occur in some cancerous conditions.

Packed cell volume (PCV)

The PCV, also referred to as the **haematocrit**, is that percentage of whole blood composed of red blood cells. For whole blood collected in EDTA vacutainers:

(1) Mix adequately by hand or on a roller mixer.
(2) Fill a plain capillary microhaematocrit tube to about three-quarters full by capillary action.
(3) With a finger on the top, seal or plug the bottom end with a clay or plastic material.
(4) Place in a microhaematocrit centrifuge with the plugged end facing out and resting on the rubber rim cushion. Give 5 minutes' centrifugation. (Fresh blood samples, collected directly from the patient by means of a lancet-type puncture or from a drop of blood at the time of venipuncture, contain no anticoagulant and it is necessary to use a **heparinised microhaematocrit capillary tube**. These tubes are internally coated with heparin: as the blood flows up the tube, the anticoagulant mixes with the blood to prevent clotting.)
(5) After centrifugation, place the tubes in a **haematocrit reader**. This has a linear scale: the bottom of the tube contents is at zero and the top of the plasma meniscus is at 100. From the scale, read off the level of the top of the RBCs (the **red supernatant layer**). This percentage is the **PCV**.
(6) A white-to-grey layer sitting on top of the red cells and below the plasma is referred to as the **buffy coat** and consists of white blood cells and platelets.
(7) The clear-to-yellow layer at the top is the **plasma**.

Normal PCV ranges for various species are shown in Table 13.9. A decrease in PCV is often found in anaemia, haemorrhage, etc., while increases may be found in cases of dehydration.

Total red cell counts

These are commonly carried out by machine and are an essential part of the haematological examination. Manual red cell counting is still required for avian and reptile bloods because their nucleated red cells are not differentiated readily by automated machine counting systems. A Unopette system is available using Isotonic saline 0.85% to dilute the blood. There are also other methods that use either phosphate buffered saline, Hayems solution or Dacies formal citrate. Refer to standard haematological texts for details of these procedures.

Haemoglobin and calculated RBC parameters

Haemoglobin estimation is a routine part of any haematology examination, generally by colorimetric or spectrophotometric chemical reactions and calculated either manually or by an automated haematology analyser. Calculated values include mean corpuscular volume (MCV), mean corpuscular haemoglobin (MCH) and mean corpuscular haemoglobin concentration (MCHC).

Biochemistry

This section covers the main biochemical tests involved commonly in practice laboratory investigations using simple wet or dry chemistry systems.

Urea and BUN

Urea is a nitrogenous waste product that is formed in the liver from two molecules of ammonia as the end product of amino acid utilisation. It is then transported in the plasma fraction of the blood to the kidneys, where it is excreted in the urine.

The term **blood urea nitrogen (BUN)** expresses the amount of nitrogen atoms in the blood incorporated to urea. Laboratory analysis and measurement of the concentration of BUN and of urea have been used in the evaluation of renal function but are not the same. There is a difference of 2.144 times in magnitude between the weight (in mg/100 ml plasma or serum) of urea and that of BUN.

In the international system (SI) of units, these substances are expressed in terms of **molecular** or **molar** concentration, a **mole** (mol) being the unit of amount of the substance. The multiplication factors to convert the old units, expressed in mg/100 ml, to the SI units of millimoles per litre (mmol/l) are 0.17 for urea and 0.36 for BUN.

Increased urea may be associated with several conditions:

- High levels of urea in serum or plasma are usually assumed to be due to renal failure but there are other considerations.
- Chronic heart failure combined with poor renal perfusion will reduce the amount of urea taken to the kidney in the circulation and hence lead to an increase of the amount in the blood. Obviously if severe renal hypoxia occurs due to the poor circulation, renal failure will ensue and urea levels will rise even more.

- High-protein diets may increase the level of urea.
- Low-carbohydrate diets may lead to breakdown of body proteins or catabolism and then increase in urea.
- Dehydration may cause an apparent increase in urea.
- Urethral obstruction and ruptured bladder both may lead to increased urea concentrations.
- Other systemic and metabolic conditions may also increase urea.

Table 13.10 shows the normal reference values for urea and a number of other biochemical parameters.

Blood glucose

Many laboratories continue to refer to 'blood glucose' but the correct term is now 'plasma glucose'. Modern glucose methods are performed on plasma, whereas in the past whole-blood samples were used. As the level of glucose in RBCs is low, blood glucose values quoted in older texts may be lower than those found by current methods.

The level of glucose in the blood is an indication of carbohydrate metabolism and a measure of the pancreatic endocrine function, as it is controlled by insulin and glucagon:

- **Insulin** increases the cellular utilisation of glucose from blood.
- **Glucagon** production causes an increased production and release of glucose from tissue to the bloodstream.

Table 13.11 shows some of the conditions that cause increase or decrease in plasma glucose.

In the practice, it is possible to determine glucose by means of reagent strips or dip-stick methods. Newer reagent strips use whole blood: glucose levels can then be reliably measured by means of a small reflectance meter or by comparing the colour change on the pad with reference colours that indicate the relevant concentration. A number of systems are available and the manufacturer's methodology supplied with the system should be followed.

Other biochemical estimations

Determination of total serum protein, albumin, globulin, creatinine, cholesterol, bilirubin and various enzymes assists in the diagnosis of several common conditions (Table 13.12). Various 'dry' or 'wet' chemistry systems are available and a **refractometer** (see Fig. 13.7) might be used to determine total serum protein as well as urine specific gravity.

In determining enzymes, controlled temperature conditions are important: in animal biochemistry a temperature of 30°C is recommended. However, it should be noted that some laboratories and some texts quote enzyme activity at either 25 or 37°C. In the last few years most laboratories have now moved to the use of 37°C, as the commercial reagents have become optimised for this temperature.

Examination of the skin

Examination of samples for external parasites such as insects (fleas and lice) and arachnids (ticks and mites) depends on collection of suitable samples by means of skin scraping, pustular collection, ear wax collection or hair brushing. The samples are mounted on slides and examined under the microscope.

Parasites might be detected in the sample by the presence of eggs, larvae, nymphs, adults, or just faeces. Therefore understanding of their life cycles to recognise the various stages of development is necessary. These are described in Chapter 15. Table 13.13 gives some of the features to look for in identifying evidence of lice, fleas, Dipteran maggots and mites.

Ringworm

Ultraviolet light from a Wood's lamp may be used to examine hair samples from animals possibly infected by dermatophyte fungi such as *Microsporum* spp. (see Chapter 15). Affected material may fluoresce a bright yellow-green.

Table 13.10 Biochemical reference ranges for domesticated animals

Parameter	Units	Canine	Feline	Equine	Thoroughbred	Bovine	Ovine
Albumin	g/l	25–37	21–39	23–38	21–34	27–37	24–32
T. protein	g/l	54–77	54–78	57–84	43–67	70–88	65–78
T. globulin	g/l	23–52	15–57	16–50	22–50	32–56	27–50
Urea	mmol/l	1.7–7.4	6–10	2.5–8.3	2.8–6.1	2–6.6	3–8
Creatinine	μmol/l	0–106	80–180	60–147	106–168	44–165	44–150
T. bilirubin	μmol/l	< 16	< 10	10–40	10–40	< 9	< 8
Glucose	mmol/l	2–2.5	4.3–6.6	2.8–5.5	3.4–5.9	2–3	2–3
Cholesterol	mmol/l	3.8–7	1.9–3.9	2.3–3.6	2.3–3.6	1–3	1–2.6
ALT	U/l@30°C	< 25	< 20	< 25	< 25	< 40	< 50
SAP	U/l@30°C	< 80	< 60	40–120	40–160	< 80	< 40
γGT	U/l@30°C	< 20	< 20	< 25	< 40	< 15	< 20
CK	U/l@30°C	< 100	< 80	< 150	< 150	< 50	< 50
AST	U/l@30°C	< 25	< 35	< 130	< 212	< 100	< 50

Source: Bloxham Laboratories Ltd, Teignmouth, Devon

Table 13.11 Conditions associated with increased and decreased blood glucose

Increased glucose:
Post-feeding sample
Increased glucocorticoids (stress, Cushing's)
Administration of corticosteroids
Diabetes mellitus
Pancreatitis
Glucose treatment
Use of morphine

Decreased glucose:
Hepatic disorders
Insulin treatment or
Insulinoma
Starvation/malabsorption
Hypothyroid/hypoadrenal
Severe renal glucosuria
Idiopathic in some toy breeds
Artefact in old sample

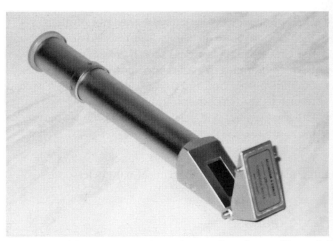

Fig. 13.7 A Refractometer can be used to test for urine specific gravity and serum protein.

However, only about 60% of cases of *M. canis* show this fluorescence and its lack does not rule out ringworm infection. Fluorescing hairs should be plucked out and examined under the microscope. Non-specific bluish-white fluorescence is not due to ringworm but is commonly found due to scales of flaky skin, mud, dirt, nail surfaces and any petroleum-based materials, including many detergents and paraffin oil.

WARNING
Ultraviolet light is potentially dangerous and can damage the conjunctiva of the eye. Long exposure burns the skin, rather like sunburn (which of course is due to UV rays). Both the operator and the animal must be protected by careful use of the Wood's lamp.

If there is no relevant fluorescence:

(1) Pluck hairs from the edge of any lesion and together with a skin scraping, place on a microscope slide with a few drops of 10% potassium hydroxide (KOH) (20% KOH digest is sometimes used but often damages the hairs too much). Put on cover slip.

(2) Heat the slide over a Bunsen flame, for a few seconds only, to assist in clearing the hairs so that details of the hair shaft may be seen with the microscope under high dry.

In cases of ringworm, the fungal spores or arthrospores will appear as small, spherical, refractile bodies occurring in chains or as a complete sheath around the hair shaft and totally invading the keratinous epithelium. **Hyphae** may be seen as filaments infecting the hair from which the arthrospores are produced.

The standard medium for ringworm culture is Sabouraud's dextrose agar, which is incubated at 25°C for up to 2 weeks. Plucked hairs or skin scrapings are pushed

Table 13.12		
Parameter	**Increased values**	**Decreased values**
T. protein	Dehydration, lactation, infection and neoplasm	Liver disease, renal disease, malabsorption, immunodeficiency
Cholesterol	Hypothyroidism, Cushing's, post-feeding, diabetes mellitus, pancreatitis, nephrotic syndrome	Liver disease, lipoprotein deficiency
Bilirubin	Intra- and extra-hepatic icterus, pre-hepatic icterus or haemolysis	Of no diagnostic significance
ALT	Hepatic anoxia, metabolic disorders, hepatoxins, hepatitis	Of no diagnostic significance
SAP	Liver and bile duct damage, bone growth in young, steroids (in dogs)	EDTA sample, haemolysis
GT	Cholestasis and cirrhosis	No diagnostic significance
CK	Myositosis, muscular trauma, myopathy, haemolysis, myocardial infarct	No diagnostic significance
AST	Myopathies, hepatic damage and haemolysis	No diagnostic significance

Table 13.13 Identification of ectoparasites*		Eggs	Nymphs	Larvae
Lice Sucking	⎧ ⎨ Dorsoventrally flattened, ⎩ wingless Grey to red No eyes Membranous abdomen with hair on segments	Biting lice Yellower	(Nits): Oval white, plug/ operculum at one end	Similar to adults but smaller and no reproductive organs
Biting	⎧ Pincer claws ⎪ Elongated head ⎨ Piercing mouthparts ⎪ Clasping or running legs ⎩ Rounded head Mandibular mouthparts			
Fleas	Small wingless (4–5 mm long) Laterally compressed body Large hindlegs Adults have piercing/sucking mouthparts	(Cat flea): Oval, white, glistening, 0.5 mm long		White to brown (creamy yellow on hatchings); small, maggot-like; very active, light-shy; 2–5 mm long; sparse hairs Pupae: very sticky
Flies (Diptera)	Large adults with wings	Small (1 mm long), elongated, creamy white		House fly maggots can grow up to 12 mm long in less than 1 week
Mites	Almost circular body or cigar shaped Four pairs short legs, perhaps with suckers (only front two pairs project beyond body) Adult female 400–600 × 300– 400 μm *Cheyletiella* larger, less rounded; legs longer with combs; horn-like hooks either side of head	Oval	Four pairs of legs	 Three pairs of legs; 'orange-tawny'

* See Chapter 15, p. 375

into shallow cuts made in the agar. Dermatophyte identification is based on colony morphology and pigmentation together with microscopic examination of the macroconidia or macroaleuriospores (Table 13.14).

There is also a modified commercial Sabouraud's agar with added pH indicator (phenol red): the pathogenic fungi usually grow faster than saprophytes and they produce alkaline metabolites, so that the indicator in the agar turns from yellow to red. Cultures should be examined at 7, 10 and 14 days if an indicator is used.

Faecal examination

Visual examination

- Consistency (hard, soft, fluid).
- Colour (yellow; brown; green; red, due to blood; or black, due to digested blood).
- Whether fatty or mucoid.
- Presence of worms (round or tape), bones, hair, fur or some other foreign bodies.

Table 13.14 Morphological identification of dermatophytes		
Dermatophyte	**Colony identification**	**Microscopic identification**
Microsporum canis	Flat, white and silky centre. Bright yellow edge. Reverse of culture yellow	Eight- to fifteen-celled macroconidia or macroaleuriospores, knobby end. Thick walled
Microsporum gypseum	Flat powdery irregular fringe. Brown colour with reverse yellow/brown	Symmetrical thin-walled three- to eight-celled macroconidia. Pointed ends. Boat-shaped
Trichophyton mentagrophytes	Flat, granular, tan coloured or heaped white colony. Reverse yellow-red/brown	Cigar-shaped, two- to six-celled. Heaped colonies may have no macroconidia
Trichophyton verrucosum	Small velvet white	Macroconidia seldom seen

Microscopic examination

Direct faecal smear for initial assessment of parasite burden looking for worm eggs and protozoan oocytes (Fig. 13.8a).

Direct wet preparation for initial assessment of partially or undigested material:

(1) Place a drop of saline on to a microscope slide.
(2) Add an equal amount of faeces.
(3) To assist in contrast, various stains can be used to indicate signs of possible pancreatic deficiency (see Table 13.15).
(4) Mix thoroughly, make a thin smear and place a cover slip on top.

Table 13.15 Stains used to indicate possible pancreatic deficiency	
Stain	**Use**
Lugol's iodine or iodine	Starch granules appear blue black
New methylene blue	Undigested muscle fibres–nuclei and striations visible
Eosin	Undigested muscle fibres
Sudan III or IV	Undigested muscle fibres Fat globules stained orange or red

Stains for faecal smears. Use one drop of selected stain per slide

(5) Use low power to examine the field for the presence of worm eggs.
(6) Use medium power to look for protozoa.

Alternatively, instead of putting on a cover slip, allow the slide to dry; then flame-fix and stain for more detailed high-power or perhaps oil-immersion examination.

Faecal flotation

Faecal flotation is based on differences in specific gravity. Water has a specific gravity of 1.000; parasitic eggs are heavier at 1.100–1.200; and many solutions of salts or sugar have a higher specific gravity of 1.200–1.250. Faeces placed in such solutions will partition: heavy debris will sink but the lighter eggs will rise to the surface. The most common solutions used for this procedure are sugar solution, zinc sulphate, saturated sodium chloride or sodium nitrate.

Standard flotation method:

(1) Mix faeces and the solution to break them up.
(2) Push the mixture through a fine sieve or muslin cloth or gauze.
(3) Transfer to a test tube so that the solution fills the tube completely, forming a meniscus at the top.
(4) Place a cover slip on and leave to stand upright, undisturbed for 10–20 minutes.
(5) Carefully lift the cover slip off vertically and place it on to a microscope slide, ensuring that the fluid is trapped between the slide and the coverslip.
(6) Examine the slide under a low-power microscope objective.

Centrifugal flotation is normally performed rather than standard flotation. The tubes are spun at low speed (1000–1500 r.p.m.) in a centrifuge for 3–5 minutes, then the top fluid meniscus is removed and examined.

Commercial kits are based on the standard flotation technique but they consist of a plastic vial containing a filter, so that the sample does not need to be filtered or sieved in advance.

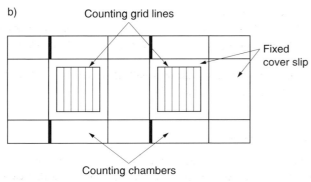

Fig. 13.8 (a) Worm eggs and oocysts: (1) *Trichuris* spp., (2) *Toxascaris* spp., (3) *Toxocara* spp., (4) *Uncinaria* spp., (5) *Taenia* spp. and (6) *Isospora* spp. (b) McMaster's counting slide for worm ova.

Faecal sedimentation

Faecal sedimentation concentrates eggs by centrifugation in water but microscopic detection is difficult because of the presence of faecal debris.

(1) Mix about 2 g of faeces with tap water and then strain.
(2) Half-fill a centrifuge tube with the strained fluid.
(3) Spin for about 5 minutes at 1500 r.p.m.
(4) Pour off the supernatant.
(5) With a Pasteur pipette, transfer some of the sediment on to a microscope slide and put on a cover slip.
(6) Lugol's iodine may be mixed with the sediment prior to examination under low power.

McMaster technique

The standard quantitative technique used to determine the number of eggs per gram of faeces is the McMaster technique, which requires a special counting chamber (Fig. 13.8b). Table 13.16 describes one of several modified methods based on this technique (see Chapter 15, for various parasite ova found in dog and cat faeces).

Occult blood

Occult ('hidden') blood is evidence of insidious chronic bleeding from ulcers, neoplastic lesions or parasitism in the digestive tract. Dramatic bleeding is usually obvious: faeces are either black (melaena), containing partially digested blood, or they show frank blood (haematochezia). Confirmation of the presence of occult blood requires biochemical detection. The reagents orthotoluidine or benzidine react with haemoglobin peroxidase in faeces with occult blood to yield a colour change which is detected visually. However, both reagents are so sensitive that they will react with any dietary haemoglobin or myoglobin; hence the animal must be placed on a totally meat-free diet for 3 days before its faeces are collected for occult blood testing. Commercial test kits are available.

Table 13.16 Modified McMaster's protocol

(1) Weigh 3 g faeces. Put into 120 ml wide-mouthed glass-stoppered bottle with glass beads. Add 42 ml tap water and shake well
(2) Pour faeces suspension through wire mesh screen, collecting filtrate in clean bowl
(3) Mix and transfer to 10 ml centrifuge tube. Fill to within 10 mm of top
(4) Centrifuge for 2 minutes at 1000 r.p.m. (800 g)
(5) Discard supernatant and emulsify packed sediment
(6) Fill to within 10 mm of top with saturated NaCl
(7) Invert tube several times until even suspension
(8) Fill both McMaster counting chambers
(9) Count oocysts and worm eggs under 10× objective and 10× eye piece
(10) Count/gram of faeces = total number from both chambers × 50

Other procedures that may also be carried out as part of a faecal examination include faecal trypsin (protease) tests to determine presence or absence of pancreatic trypsin faecal activity, although these have been largely superseded by serological tests (see Chapter 17, pp. 427).

Urine examination

Gross examination should start with the amount produced. The normal dog will produce 25–60 ml/kg bodyweight while a cat normally voids 10–20 ml/kg bodyweight every 24 hours. **Polyuria** is production of excess urine; **oliguria** is a reduction in the amount voided. Colour, turbidity, odour and specific gravity should also be checked.

Colour

Normally yellow, the intensity of the colour may give some indication as to the specific gravity or concentration of the urine: the darker it is, the more concentrated.

- If the urine is browny-yellow and on shaking a slight greenish foam appears on the surface, then bile pigments are likely to be present.
- Red or red-brown coloration is likely to indicate the presence of red blood cells, haemoglobin or myoglobin. Drugs may alter the colour of the urine and so will some foods, such as beetroot.

Turbidity

Normal urine should be clear. If it is cloudy (turbid), sediment is likely to be present and this should be harvested by centrifugation for microscopic examination.

Red and white blood cells, crystals, epithelial cells, casts, bacteria, yeasts and fungi may cause increased turbidity of urine and can be identified microscopically.

Odours

Ammonia is produced in stale urine, due to bacterial activity, and an odour is given off.

- This same odour in freshly voided urine may be due to urease-producing bacteria involved in cystitis.
- Male cats and the males of many other species tend to produce strong urine odours in order to mark their territory.
- The typical sweet acetone smell of peardrops is found in urine from ketotic animals.

Specific gravity

Specific gravity is the density or weight of a known volume of a fluid compared with an equal amount of distilled water. Distilled water has a specific gravity of 1.000. Factors affecting the specific gravity of urine are shown in Table 13.17.

Table 13.17 Factors affecting the specific gravity of urine

Factors increasing specific gravity:
Dehydration
Fluid loss
Reduced water intake
Acute renal failure
Shock

Factors decreasing specific gravity:
Excess water intake (polydipsia)
Diabetes insipidus
Pyometra

Refractometer   The specific gravity of urine may be determined by using a refractometer (see Fig. 13.7) to assess the fluid's refractive index: the higher the concentration, the higher the refractive index. Density is also influenced by temperature and the determination should be made at a constant temperature, or the refractometer should be corrected to compensate for the operating temperature.

Only a few drops of urine are required for determination using a refractometer. They are placed on the glass of the chamber and the lid is closed. The refractometer is held up to the light and the specific gravity is read from the scale. If the reading goes off the top end of the scale, the urine is very concentrated: dilute it with an equal volume of distilled water and measure again. In this case multiply the actual scale reading after the decimal point by 2 to give the correct final specific gravity of the urine.

Hydrometer   Specific gravity may also be determined by using a hydrometer, which floats in water. The bottom of the meniscus reads zero on the scale of the stalk. The urine volume required may be 10–15 ml and the accuracy is not as good as that of the refractometer. Temperature is much more critical using a hydrometer.

Chemical determination   Commercial reagent urine dip-stick methods are useful for an initial indication but chemical constituents in all types of dog and cat urine may produce inconsistencies, so a follow-up test using either of the methods above is recommended.

Other tests using chemical determination

Commercial reagent test strips are plastic mounted with a variable number of test reagent pads. For example, a 10-determination urine stick can be used for determination of pH, specific gravity, blood, protein, glucose, bilirubin, ketones (acetoacetic acid), urobilinogen, nitrate and leucocytes. They are best used with fresh urine and should never be used on preserved samples. Stale samples are likely to have bacteria growth from the environment or skin or faecal contamination which may affect glucose pH and blood determination. The older the sample, the more the ketones,

bilirubin or urobilinogen present will decrease in the urine. Some strip systems enable a reflectometer determination of the end result rather than relying on visual determination. Table 13.18 gives reference values for pH and specific gravity in the urine of domestic animals.

Determination of pH   The pH of a solution is the expression of its hydrogen ion concentration. A pH above 7.0 is alkaline, while below 7.0 is acidic. Stored samples tend to become more acid as CO_2 is lost to the air and false results may occur if the samples are not kept cool and covered.

- Urine pH is affected by diet: vegetarian diets produce more alkaline urine, while carnivorous animals have acid urines.
- Acidic urines (decrease in pH) may be due to pyrexia (fever), starvation, acidosis, high protein diets, muscle catabolism or some drugs.
- Alkaline urines (increase in pH) may be due to high vegetational content of the diet, urinary retention, urinary tract infections, alkalosis or certain drugs.

The pH may be determined simply by means of pH papers or with multi-reagent dip-sticks/strips. It is important to realise that the colour of urine may itself colour the detection strip and cause an artefact in the visual determination. Electrode pH meters are available as small stick-type instruments with digital readout: they are inexpensive and should be considered as a more reliable method.

Blood in urine   This is detected by means of a similar principle to the detection of occult blood in faeces. Red blood cells, haemoglobin and myoglobin cause oxidation of the reagents, turning them from yellow-orange to green and then to dark blue as the amount of haemoglobin or myoglobin increases. Spots of green are likely to indicate whole RBCs, while solid colour suggests the presence of haemolysed blood. Ascorbic acid may inhibit the detection, giving false negatives, and high specific gravity and high protein levels in the urine may reduce the reactivity. Oxidising agents such as hypochlorites and bacterially produced peroxidases may give false positives. Myoglobin from muscle breakdown will also yield a positive reaction. Any positives found on dip-sticks should be examined microscopically to confirm the presence of blood.

Haematuria is the presence of whole blood in the urine. The presence of lysed blood is referred to as **haemoglobinuria;** and **myoglobinuria** indicates the presence of myoglobin in the urine.

Table 13.18 Reference ranges for urine pH and specific gravity		
Species	**pH**	**Specific gravity**
Canine	5.2–6.8	1.018–1.045
Feline	6–7	1.020–1.040
Equine	7–8.5	1.020–1.050
Bovine	7–8.5	1.005–1.040
Ovine	7–8.5	1.020–1.040

- The most common causes of haematuria are cystitis and associated infection or inflammation of the urinary tract, urolithiasis, acute nephritis, thrombocytopenia and various coagulopathies which cause bleeding.
- Haemoglobinuria is associated with haemolysis of blood in the blood stream or haemoglobinaemia. Conditions such as autoimmune haemolytic anaemia (AIHA), systemic lupus erythematosus (SLE), *Leptospira haemorrhagica* infection, babesiosis and poisoning should be considered as causes.
- Myoglobinuria occurs due to muscle breakdown in cases such as azoturia (rhabdomyolysis) in horses.
- If no haemoglobinaemia is detected in blood but the urine is red-brown and the dip-stick indicates the presence of blood in the urine, then it is more likely to indicate myoglobinuria than haemoglobinuria. Haemoglobin precipitates in ammonium sulphate while myoglobin does not and so confirmatory testing is possible.

Protein in urine

This is normally present in only very small amounts, but collection methods associated with free collection or expressing of the bladder are likely to contain more due to production of secretions from the urinogenital tract. The main cause of increased proteins, however, is associated with decreased reabsorption of proteins by the tubules and leakage from the glomerular part of the kidney. The dip-stick protein reagent primarily detects albumin, not total proteins, and is less sensitive to globulins, mucoproteins and monoclonal proteins. Alkaline urines, and those contaminated with some antiseptic or detergents, may show up as false positive for protein.

True **proteinuria** is found in acute and chronic nephritis, congestive heart failure, other causes of renal damage or nephrosis, cystitis, urethral inflammation, vaginitis and other conditions of the genital tract and traumatic catheterisation. Following parturition or during oestrus the level of protein may rise and be detected, but normally any protein detected by the dip-stick is suggestive of **urogenital damage**.

Glucose in urine

This is referred to as **glucosuria** and the amount present depends on the amount in the blood and the ability of renal filtration and reabsorption. The so-called **renal threshold** is the blood level of glucose above which the normal kidney cannot filter or reabsorb (see Chapter 17).

- Strip-test reagents use a double enzyme reaction system to detect glucose and the test is very specific.
- Tablet reagent systems use a copper reduction method, which is less specific and detects any sugars.

The normal minimum detection level is around 5.0 mmol/l. Ascorbic acid may give false negative results and the presence of ketonuria may reduce the detectable level of glucose in such urine. Stale or bacterially contaminated urine may also have false negative glucose due to the presence of glucose-using organisms.

Glucosuria may occur in diabetes mellitus and occasionally in cases of adrenal hyperplasia (Cushing's disease), hyperthyroidism, chronic liver damage, stress, general anaesthesia and in specific renal conditions in which the tubules are unable to resorb glucose.

Ketones in urine (ketonuria)

Ketones are detected by means of dip-stick or reagent tablets, but these primarily detect one ketone body – that of acetoacetic acid – and are less sensitive to acetone, while they do not detect beta-hydroxybutyric acid (BHB).

Ketonuria may indicate liver damage, diabetes mellitus or ruminant ketosis.

Bile pigments

Bilirubinuria is the presence of bile pigments (urobilinogen and conjugated bilirubin) in the urine. It is found in a number of conditions including obstruction of bile flow into the intestine, bowel changes, cholangitis, bile duct obstruction, liver damage due to release of conjugated bilirubin from hepatocytes and in cases of haemolytic anaemia. Bilirubin may be detected by the multistrip dip-stick but this is not as sensitive as reagent tablets which incorporate a diazo reagent:

(1) Urine is placed on a supplied pad.
(2) A tablet is placed on the pad.
(3) Two drops of water are placed on top of the tablet so that they run down on to the pad.
(4) If the area of the mat around the tablet turns blue, bilirubin is present in the urine.

Urobilinogen is an intestinal bacterial breakdown product of bilirubin. Some of it is absorbed from the intestine into the blood stream and then small amounts are excreted from the kidney into the urine. It is therefore normal to find some urobilinogen in the urine (urobilinogenuria) and a lack of it may indicate bile duct obstruction. However, oxidation occurs rapidly and the oxidised form is not detected. It is essential to test fresh samples of urine. Increased amounts occur in haemolysis and some cases of hepatocyte damage.

Microscopic examination of urine

Normal urine does not contain much sediment, but a few epithelium cells, some mucus and blood cells may be found. Bacteria may be present due to contamination at the time of collection or during subsequent storage. Reagent sticks provide some information, but examination of spun-down sediment in urine is a very useful diagnostic aid.

(1) Place 5 ml of fresh mixed urine into a conical centrifuge tube and spin at 1500 r.p.m. (around 100 *g*) for 5 minutes.
(2) Pour off the supernatant, leaving the sediment with a little urine in the bottom of the tube.
(3) Flick the base of the tube to resuspend the sediment and withdraw some by Pasteur pipette.
(4) Make an unstained wet preparation by placing a drop on a slide and placing a cover slip on top.

(5) Examine by microscope with the condenser down and the iris diaphragm partially closed so that only a little light passes through.

It is possible to add a stain such as 0.5% new methylene blue to aid examination prior to putting on the cover slip. If high-power oil-immersion examination is required, make a smear similar to a blood film; air-dry and then stain by Gram stain for bacterial examination, or by Giemsa or modified Wright's stain for cellular study.

Commercial urine microscopic analysis chambers similar to McMaster worm-egg slides and manual blood cell counting chambers are available and these may be used instead of the standard microscope slide and cover slip method.

- **Pyuria** is the presence of large numbers of WBCs (usually neutrophils) in urine and suggests inflammation in the urinogenital tract.
- **Haematuria** is the presence of large numbers of RBCs in urine and indicates bleeding into the urinogenital tract. In concentrated urine the cells shrivel up and are crenated. In dilute urine they swell and lyse, leading to haemoglobinuria – the empty cells are referred to as ghosts and must be distinguished from yeasts, fat globules or crystals.
- **Epithelial cells** are flat, irregular squamous cells with a small nucleus. They are shed from the surface of the urethra, vagina or vulva in naturally voided urine.
- **Transitional cells** are rounder and smaller; they come from further up the tract and in voided urine they indicate cystitis or pyelonephritis. Catheterised samples are likely to have higher numbers than voided urine.
- **Tubular epithelial cells** are the same size as WBCs and are easily confused with them. They tend to be round with a large nucleus and their presence is suggestive of tubular damage.
- **Casts** are formed in the tubules and consist of precipitated proteins due to the acidic condition of the lower (distal) collecting tubules of the kidney. They are classified into various types depending on the other material incorporated with the protein. They dissolve in alkaline urine and should be looked for in fresh urine. High-speed centrifugation may break them up and so it is important to prepare the sediment carefully.
- **Hyaline casts** are clear, cylindrical, colourless and refractile and they rapidly dissolve in alkaline urine. An increased number is found with mild tubular inflammation, pyrexia and poor circulation.
- **Cellular casts** may contain RBCs, WBCs, epithelial cell, or a mixture of cell types.
- **Granular casts** are hyaline casts with granules in them. These granules are remnants of epithelial cells and WBCs. They are associated with significant inflammatory change.
- **Waxy casts** are more opaque than hyaline casts and usually wider with square rather than round ends. They are often found in more chronic degenerative renal tubular changes.

- **Mucus threads** are thinner, without definite walls, and are usually twisted strands or ribbons. They are not casts and are normal products of the lower urinogenital tract.
- **Spermatozoa** may be found in entire male urine and are of no diagnostic significance.
- **Bacteria, fungi** and **yeasts** may be found as contaminants of urine but their presence is only likely to be significant if accompanied by large numbers of leucocytes and if the sample was collected aseptically by catheterisation or midstream void and examined fresh. Yeasts in particular are likely to be urine contaminants from the external genitalia.

Crystals

Crystals in urine may be associated with clinical conditions such as cystitis, urolithiasis and haematuria, but may also be found in apparently normal animals.

Alkaline urines tend to contain phosphates and calcium carbonates, which dissolve in acid urine. Acid urine may contain urates, oxalates, cystine, leucine and tyrosine crystals.

Crystals are more likely to be found if freshly collected urine is allowed to stand and cool. Figure 13.9 shows the typical morphological pattern of some common crystals seen microscopically in urines.

Uroliths are calculi composed of crystals in the urine and they may cause blockage or damage to the urinary tract. The condition is referred to as **urolithiasis** and chemical analysis of the 'stones' may be performed to identify the materials involved and to assist in the treatment and control of them.

Bacteriological examination

Bacteria may be examined by means of microscopic study using stains. They may be grown on culture media plates (usually a mixture of nutrients and blood in agar): their colony growth may assist in identification and their particular fermentation ability may be used alone or in conjunction with serological tests to confirm their identity.

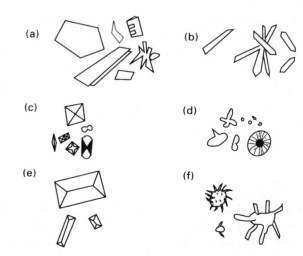

Fig. 13.9 Urine crystals: (a) urates, (b) hippuric acid, (c) calcium oxalate, (d) calcium carbonate, (e) struvite and (f) ammonium urate.

Sampling

The first stage in any bacterial examination is to obtain suitable samples. Swabs from open wounds, pus or orifices such as the buccal cavity, vagina and ears may be obtained using commercial sterile cotton-tipped swabs.

- If posted to a laboratory, it is essential that they are placed into **transport media**. Most commercial laboratories supply the transport media and swabs for postal submission.
- For use in the practice, dry swabs may be perfectly acceptable, especially in the preparation of smears.

The collection of body fluids has been described earlier in this chapter. **Vesicles** and **abscesses** are best sampled by means of a needle and syringe. Sampling of **post-mortem organs** is best achieved by heat-searing the surface with a spatula that has been flamed over a Bunsen and placed on the surface to sterilise it. The surface is then cut with a sterile scalpel and a swab of the cut internal surface is taken.

In all cases, it is important to ensure aseptic collection of microbiological samples.

Smears

The making of bacterial smears requires only a thin application of material on to a slide.

- For **direct smears from swabs**, lightly roll the end on to the middle of a clean microscope slide.
- For **fluid samples**, a drop of the fluid is transferred aseptically with a Pasteur pipette or by means of a flamed and cooled bacterial wire loop.
- **Colonies from agar plates** may be picked off individually by a wire loop and mixed with a drop of sterile saline on the slide.

It is also possible to smear directly from tissue or pus.

Heat-fixing

When the sample has air-dried, the smear is passed through a Bunsen flame 2–3 times with the sample side up. This achieves heat-fixing and prevents the sample from being washed off, provided that the smear is not too thick. It kills the bacteria but preserves the cell morphology for staining. It is important not to overheat: the back of the slide should feel warm but should not burn the back of the hand. When the slide has cooled it is ready for staining.

Staining

Methylene blue
A simple stain which shows up the presence and morphology (shape) of bacteria. A specific aged and oxidised version referred to as polychromatic methylene blue is used for staining anthrax bacilli in blood smears and for demonstrating McFadyean's reaction.

Freshly made or **new methylene blue** should never be used when polychromatic methylene blue is required.

Shape

Round bacteria are **cocci**; they may be single or in pairs (**diplococci**), clusters or bunches (such as staphylococci) or chains (streptococci). Rod-shaped bacteria are termed **bacilli**; some are rods with enlarged round ends (**coccobacilli**) and others may be spiral in shape (**spirochaetes**). Bacteria that have variable shapes are referred to as **pleomorphic**

Gram stain
The standard staining method that separates bacteria into two types: Gram-positive and Gram-negative organisms, based on the structure of the cell wall. It consists of a **primary stain** of crystal violet which is treated with a **mordant** iodine (1.0 g iodine crystals, 2.0 g potassium iodide and 200 ml of distilled water). The next stage is to **decolourise** with alcohol and then **counterstain** with carbol fuchsin.

- **Gram-positive** bacteria resist decolourisation and remain blue-violet in colour.
- **Gram-negative** bacteria are decolourised; they take up the counterstain and become red in colour.

A procedure for performing a Gram stain is illustrated in Table 13.19.

Table 13.19 Gram-stain protocol

Solutions
Crystal Violet
Gram's Iodine or Lugol's Iodine
Methanol or Acetone
Dilute Carbol Fuchsin (ZN carbol fuchsin diluted 1/10 with distilled water) or Safranin 0.5% in distilled water

Procedure
1. Prepare a thin smear
2. Allow to dry naturally and then fix over a flame
3. Flood the slide with Crystal Violet solution. Leave for 30–60 seconds (time not critical)
4. Gently rinse with water and drain
5. Immediately flood with Gram's Iodine or Lugol's Iodine (**the mordant**) and leave for 60 seconds
6. Gently rinse with water and drain
7. Flood side with **Decolouriser**. Methanol for Gram's Iodine – decolourise until the colour ceases to come out of the smear normally about 30 seconds. OR Acetone for Lugol's Iodine – immediately wash with water. This is an important step as acetone is a harsh decolouriser and although it produces better contrast than other decolourisers it may be too severe for some bacteria such as bacillus and clostridia
8. **Counterstain** with dilute Carbol Fuchsin or Safranin for 30–60 seconds. Prolonged staining with dilute carbol fuchsin may cause Gram+ve organisms to be mistakenly considered as Gram+ve
9. Rinse and shake off excess water and air dry
10. Examine under oil immersion

Lugol's iodine   Lugol's iodine is more concentrated than Gram's iodine: the same amount of stain is combined with only 100 ml of distilled water. Lugol's is used rather than Gram's for a darker colour, giving less chance of excessive decolourisation.

Ziehl–Neelsen stain   This is another commonly used stain, which detects acid-fast bacteria such as **mycobacteria** (tuberculosis and Johne's disease). They are stained with carbol fuchsin and heated; they are then resistant to decolourisation with acid alcohol and so retain the red colour when counterstained with methylene blue.

Culture media

Culture media for routine bacteriology are available from various commercial suppliers, as either prepoured plates, dry powder or dehydrated media. Some of the most commonly used media – blood agar, MacConkey's, selenite broth and Sabouraud's agar – are described in Chapter 14 along with simple (basal) and enriched media, and biochemical media.

Inoculation of agar plates to cultivate potentially pathogenic bacteria

Whatever the origin of the sample, once it has been aseptically collected it is spread along one edge of the agar plate (the inoculation well) and must then be spread on the plate and diluted so that individual colonies can be grown. The most common procedure is by **streaking.** One method is shown in (Fig. 13.10).

(1) Take a platinum bacterial loop; flame it until it is red-hot and then allow it to cool. Touch it on to the agar to ensure that it has cooled.
(2) From the point of application A of the sample on the plate (inoculation well), streak in a zigzag over part B of the plate.
(3) Remove the loop and flame it again, using a hooded bunsen to prevent dissemination of bacteria.
(4) Cool, and then place the loop on agar.
(5) Streak through part C of the plate, picking up the edges of part B.
(6) Flame again, and repeat the process at point D.
(7) The loop should then be flamed and put away. Place the Petri dish lid on top of the inoculated agar dish.

Incubation of cultures

Culture plates should be placed upside down in an incubator to prevent moisture accumulating on the bacteria and agar surface. Most common pathogenic bacteria can be grown aerobically at 37°C. The incubator temperature must be constant and the correct temperature must be maintained at all times.

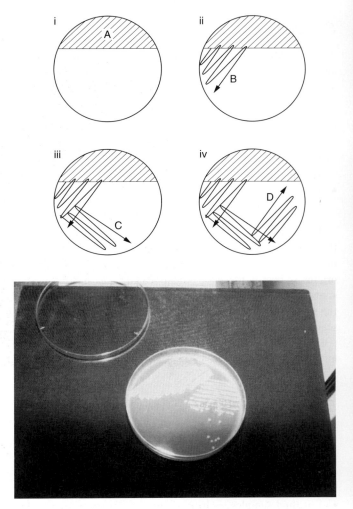

Fig. 13.10 A method for plating out bacterial samples onto an agar plate.

Following incubation (usually for 18–24 hours) the growing bacteria should be seen as separate colonies at the end of the streak (Fig. 13.11). Any growth that is not associated with the streak lines is likely to be due to contamination of the media, either when being poured or while inoculation was taking place. There may be many airborne yeasts and fungi in the environment and these can become contaminants of the culture plates if sufficient care is not taken.

Identification of bacterial growth on blood agar starts with recording the colony characteristics, such as:

• Any zone of haemolysis in the blood agar around the colony (haemolytic or non-haemolytic).
• The size of the colony – pinpoint, medium, large – and the measurement in millimetres (mm).
• The colour of the colony (grey, cream, yellow, white, etc.).
• If opaque, translucent or transparent. The shape and consistency (either irregular or circular, raised, flat, convex, mucoid, flaky, sticky, hard and crusty).
• The odour (sweet, musty, pungent, etc.).

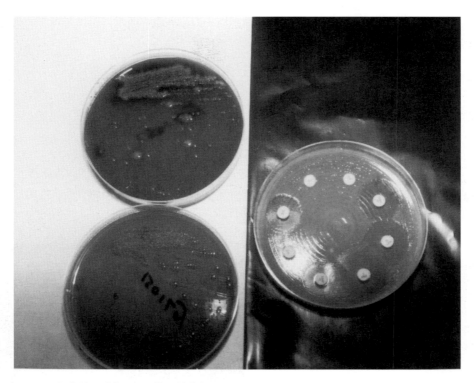

Fig 13.11 Culture plate growth (left) and Sentest plate (right).

Antibiotic sensitivity testing

After a bacterium has been cultivated and identified as a potential pathogen involved in a disease process, antimicrobial treatment of the animal is ideally based upon *in vitro* sensitivity of the bacterium, so that the most relevant antimicrobial agents can be selected. A specific medium is preferred for performing sensitivity testing and is usually an agar-based medium such as Mueller–Hinton or Sentest agar.

(1) The specific bacterial colony is selected and transferred with the flamed loop to another agar plate. Using a small amount of sterile water it is plated out (streaked evenly) to cover the whole of the agar.
(2) Antimicrobial discs containing various antimicrobial agents are placed on the surface of the agar. The discs may be placed individually by means of sterile tweezers or loaded into commercial cartridge disc dispensers that can dispense up to eight different antimicrobial discs at a time on to the inoculated plate.
(3) Following incubation, zones of inhibition around some discs indicate that the antimicrobial substance has prevented the growth of the bacterium and the isolate is therefore sensitive to that drug.
(4) If the bacteria grow to the edge of the disc, they are resistant to the particular agent on that disc.

Disposal

The important subject of disposal of clinical waste, including culture plates, is discussed earlier (p. 335).

Further reading

Baker, F. J. and Silverton, R. E. (1998) *Introduction to Medical Laboratory Technology*, 7th edn, Butterworth-Heinemann, Oxford.

Cowell, R. L. and Tyler, R. D. (1989) *Diagnostic Cytology of the Dog and Cat*, American Veterinary Publications, Santa Barbara.

Doxey, D. L. and Nathan, M. B. F. (1989) *Manual of Laboratory Techniques*, BSAVA Publications.

Hawkey, C. M. and Dennett, T. B. (1989) *A Colour Atlas of Comparative Veterinary Haematology*, Wolfe Medical Publications, London.

Jain, N. C. (1993) *Essentials of Veterinary Hematology*, Lea & Febiger, Philadelphia.

Kaneko, J. J. (1989) *Clinical Biochemistry of Domesticated Animals*, 4th edn, Academic Press, London.

Knottenbelt, C. M. and Busby, W. (1999) Laboratory tests. In Moore, M. and Simpson, G. (eds) *Manual of Veterinary Nursing*, BSAVA Publications.

Pratt, P. W. (1992) *Laboratory Procedures for Veterinary Technicians*, 2nd edn, American Veterinary Publications, Santa Barbara.

Simpson, G. (1994) *Practical Veterinary Nursing*, 3rd edn, BSAVA Publications.

Soulsby, E. J. L. (1982) *Helminths, Arthropods and Protozoa of Domesticated Animals*, 7th edn, Baillière Tindall, London.

Willard, M. D., Tvedten, H. and Turnwald, G. H. (1989) *Small Animal Clinical Diagnosis by Laboratory Methods*, W. B. Saunders, Philadelphia.

14

Elementary microbiology and immunology

M. Fisher and *H. Moreton*

Learning objectives

After studying this chapter, students should be able to:

- Discuss the concept of disease, and the inter-relationship between micro-organisms and animals.
- Discuss the morphology of the important groups of micro-organisms causing disease in mammals, with particular reference to companion animals.
- Describe the theoretical and practical skills necessary to identify microbial infection in animals.
- Explain how the interaction between infectious agent and animal determine the outcome of exposure to disease.
- Describe the measures used to control and treat infectious diseases.

Introduction to disease-causing organisms

- **Health** – a state of physical and psychological well-being and productivity.

- **Disease** – an abnormality of structure or function that impairs performance and has a recognisable syndrome of clinical signs.

The group of living things known as micro-organisms or **microbes** includes the bacteria, viruses, fungi, algae and protozoa. Microbiology is the study of microscopic organisms, too small to be seen by the naked eye, deriving its name from the Greek words: *mikros* (small), *bios* (life) and *logos* (science). Most micro-organisms are **unicellular** (i.e. they consist of only one cell which carries out all the functions necessary for life but a few, e.g. some fungi, are **multicellular**). Viruses differ from other micro-organisms in that they have no cellular structure. Micro-organisms vary in size from the relatively large protozoa to viruses that can only be seen with an electron microscope (Fig. 14.1).

The most common concept that people have of micro-organisms is of those that cause disease, which are called **pathogens**. With few exceptions, pathogens are parasites, living on or in the host and interfering in some way with the host's metabolism, to cause clinical signs of disease. The parasite may feed on the host's tissues or body fluids or it may use the host's own food supply.

Parasites can be divided into three main categories: pathogenic, commensal and mutualistic. The term **symbiosis**,

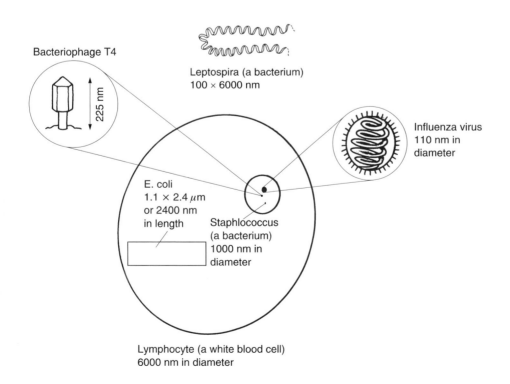

Fig. 14.1 Relative sizes of various micro-organisms, plus a white blood cell for comparison.

meaning 'living together', is sometimes used to describe any close, permanent association between different organisms, both beneficial and harmful. Therefore, commensalism, mutualism and parasitism are all examples of symbiotic relationships, as shown by Fig. 14.3. The macro-organisms affecting cats and dogs that are commonly referred to as parasites are covered in Chapter 15.

Pathogens harm the host, causing disease, but parasitism is not always harmful. In fact, the more successful parasites cause little or no damage to the host because if they are to survive then the host must survive too. Even within a species of bacterium some strains may be much more pathogenic and/or virulent than others, as recent food-poisoning outbreaks involving *Escherichia coli* O157 have illustrated.

When a micro-organism invades a host and starts to multiply, it establishes an infection. If the host is susceptible to the infection then disease results.

In order to cause infectious disease, a pathogen must:

- Gain entry into the host.
- Establish itself and multiply in the host tissue.
- Overcome the normal host body defences for a time.
- Damage the host in some way.

Some micro-organisms cause disease by secreting or releasing poisonous substances called **toxins** which disrupt specific physiological processes in the host. Others invade tissue cells and damage or destroy them. Viruses, for example, cause cell damage because they interfere with the normal cell metabolism and many leave the host cell by rupture of the cell membrane. Once they have entered the tissues of the host, some micro-organisms are localised and remain at the site of entry. For example, *Staphylococcus intermedius*, which causes skin disease, generally attacks in this way. Others spread through the body (systemic spread), usually via the lymphatic system and blood circulation. Once they have invaded the host, some micro-organisms can grow and multiply in any tissues of the body but many are more selective and localise in a particular tissue or organ. If these more demanding organisms do not reach the particular cells in which they can live, they will not produce disease. Viruses in particular often have an affinity for a specific tissue or organ.

TERMS USED TO DENOTE THE PRESENCE OF INFECTION-RELATED MATERIAL IN THE SYSTEMIC CIRCULATION
Bacteraemia: the presence of bacteria in the blood.
Viraemia: viruses in the blood.
Toxaemia: the presence of toxins in the bloodstream.
Septicaemia is used when bacteria are actively multiplying in the blood.
Pyaemia describes the presence of pus in the blood.

In some diseases, symptoms occur because of an over-reaction of the host's own defence mechanisms. This can lead to cell damage or an allergic reaction.

Parasites vary greatly in their ability to cause disease, or their pathogenicity. Some will almost always cause serious disease, while others are less pathogenic and cause milder illnesses. Whether disease develops or not depends on various factors such as the ability of the host to resist infection and the virulence of the pathogen, i.e. the degree of pathogenicity.

Many produce toxic enzymes to assist in the process of invasion and tissue destruction. For example, the enzyme hyaluronidase helps the pathogen to penetrate the tissues of the host by breaking down the 'tissue cement' which holds the cells together. Another enzyme, lecithinase, lyses or disintegrates tissue cells, especially red blood cells. Virulence is determined by factors such as:

- The ability of the parasite to invade particular cells and tissues and cause damage (its **invasiveness**).
- Its ability to secrete toxins which disrupt physiological processes in the body (its **toxigenicity**).

Toxins

Toxins are poisonous substances that have a damaging effect on the cells of the host. The effects of the toxin are not only felt in the affected cells and tissues but elsewhere in the body as the toxin is transported through the tissues.

Two types of toxin are recognised:

- **Exotoxins** which are manufactured by living micro-organisms and released into the surrounding medium.
- **Endotoxins** which are part of the micro-organism and only liberated when it dies.

Exotoxins

Exotoxins are proteins produced mainly by Gram-positive bacteria during their metabolism. They are released into the surrounding environment as they are produced. This can be into the circulatory system and tissues of the host or, as in food poisoning, into food that is then ingested. Microbial toxins include many of the most potent poisons known to man and may prove lethal even in small quantities. The body responds to the presence of exotoxins by producing antibodies called **antitoxins** that neutralise the toxins, rendering them harmless. Exotoxins, as they are proteins, are destroyed by heat and some chemicals. Chemicals such as formaldehyde are used to treat toxins so that they lose their toxicity but not their ability to elicit an immune response. These treated toxins are called **toxoids** and if injected into the body will stimulate the production of antitoxins. For example, tetanus toxoid is used to provide immunity to tetanus.

Infoldings of the cell membrane, known as **mesosomes**, give the membrane a larger surface area which is and controls the passage of substances into and important since mesosomes are thought to be the site of cell respiration. Mesosomes may also be involved in cell division by serving as the site of attachment for the bacterial chromosome.

Cell membrane (plasma membrane) lies just inside the cell wall. It is selectively permeable and controls the passage of substances into and out of the cell. In many bacteria, folds of the cell membrane called mesosomes project into the cytoplasm.

Inside the cell membrane is the **cytoplasm**, a thick fluid containing dissolved substances such as nutrients, waste products, and enzymes. Within the cytoplasm are numerous small rounded bodies called ribosomes. It also contains various inclusion granules, some of which function as food reserves.

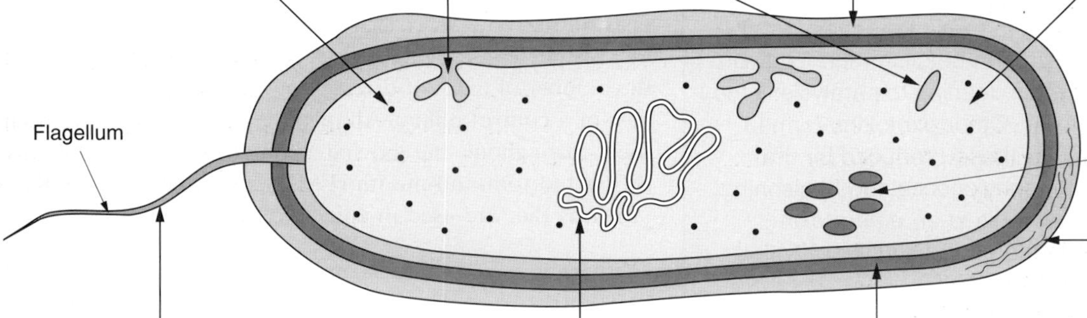

Many bacteria also contain one or more **plasmids**. A plasmid is a small, 'extra' piece of DNA which can replicate independently from the chromosome.

Ribosomes contain ribonucleic acid (RNA) and are the site of protein synthesis.

Flagellum

Storage granules.

Many species of bacteria move by means of one or more thread-like structures called **flagella** (singular: flagellum). Flagella are long, hollow tubes of a contractile protein which extend from the plasma membrane and through the cell wall. They function by rotating in a corkscrew fashion, moving the bacterium through liquid sometimes as fast as 10 μm per second or about 3000 body lengths per minute.

Most bacteria have a **cell wall**: this is a rigid structure made mainly of a substance called peptidoglycan (sometimes called murein). It maintains cell shape and prevents the cell from bursting. Cell walls vary in thickness and in composition and it is these differences that determine how the bacteria appears following staining with the Gram stain.

The **bacterial chromosome** is suspended within the cytoplasm of the generic material of the bacterium. A bacterial cell, unlike the cells of other organisms, lacks a distinct membrane-bound nucleus. Instead, the nuclear material or nucleoid consists of a single chromosome. The chromosome is a circular, extensively folded molecule of deoxyribonucleic acid (DNA) and contains the hereditary information of the cell.

Capsules and slime layers
Some bacteria secrete a gelatinous capsule outside the cell wall. These capsules can vary considerably in thickness. Other species produce a more fluid secretion called a slime layer which adheres less firmly to the cell. Capsules and slime layers can serve a number of functions. They act as a barrier between the bacterium and its environment, protecting the cell from hazards such as drying out and chemicals. The presence of a capsule may protect pathogenic bacteria from being engulfed by the host's phagocytic white blood cells because the phagocyte is prevented from forming close enough contact with the bacterium to engulf it. The chances of infection are therefore increased. Capsules assist the adherence of bacteria to surfaces and may also serve as a food reserve.

Many bacteria, particularly those that are Gram-negative, have numerous straight hair-like appendages called **pili** (singular: pilus) or fimbriae (singular: fimbria) which have nothing to do with movement. Different types of pili have different functions. Some play an important part in enabling bacteria to stick to host cells. For example, in infection, pili help pathogenic bacteria to attach to the cells lining the respiratory, intestinal or urinary tracts, thus preventing them from being washed away by bodily fluids. Other pili, sometimes called sex pili, are involved in the transfer of genetic material from one bacterial cell to another during bacterial conjugation. Some microbiologists now use the term fimbriae to refer to the appendages involved in attachment and restrict the term pili to those involved in the transfer of DNA during conjugation.

Fig. 14.2 Components of a generalised bacterial cell and their functions.

> **EFFECTS OF TOXINS**
> The effects of toxins are usually very specific. For example, when spores of the anaerobic tetanus bacilli, *Clostridium tetani*, get into a wound which provides favourable conditions, they may germinate and grow in the tissues. The bacteria do not spread through the tissues but secrete an exotoxin which travels along peripheral nerves to the central nervous system where it interferes with the regulation of neurotransmitters that control the relaxation of muscle. This leads to uncontrollable muscle spasms and paralysis. Tetanus toxin is called a **neurotoxin** because of its activity in the nervous system. Unlike tetanus, which is caused by exotoxins produced while the organism is growing within the host, botulism, caused by the saprophytic bacteria, *Clostridium botulinum*, is the result of ingestion of food containing the toxins. In botulism, the exotoxin affects the nervous system leading to paralysis; it too is therefore a neurotoxin. Other exotoxins formed outside the body include those produced by the bacteria which cause staphylococcal food poisoning, *Staphylococcus aureus*. This is an enterotoxin because it functions in the gastrointestinal tract causing vomiting and diarrhoea.

Endotoxins

Endotoxins are part of the cell wall of certain Gram-negative bacteria and are released only when the cells die and disintegrate. Compared with exotoxins, they are less toxic, cannot be used to form toxoids and are able to withstand heat. Blood-borne endotoxins are responsible for a range of non-specific reactions in the body such as fever. They also make the walls of blood capillaries more permeable, causing blood to leak into the intercellular spaces, sometimes resulting in a serious drop in blood pressure, a condition commonly called **endotoxic shock**. They are also responsible for the change in capillary blood flow in equine hooves that leads to laminitis.

Aflatoxin

Toxins are not made exclusively by bacteria. The saprophytic fungus, *Aspergillus flavus*, produces a toxin called aflatoxin. The fungus grows in warm, humid conditions and contaminates a variety of agricultural products such as peanuts, cereals, rice and beans. Aflatoxin has been implicated in the deaths of many farm animals that have been fed on mouldy hay, corn or on peanut meal.

Transmission

In addition to infecting an individual host, in order to be successful, an agent must in some way infect other suscep-

tible individuals. Spread may occur directly, from dam to offspring, for example, or indirectly via contact with contaminated bedding, grooming equipment or even on the air. In some diseases 'carriers' are important. These are animals that have previously been infected and still carry infection but do not show clinical signs. These animals can then provide a source of infection for other susceptible animals. Disinfection and other biosecurity measures are aimed at preventing transmission. More details on transmission can be found in Chapter 17.

Epidemiology

Epidemiology is the study of the occurrence, spread and distribution of a disease. It can be used, for example, to identify the cause or the source of an infection, to monitor the number of cases of disease and to monitor the effectiveness of a control policy. All of these applications have been used throughout the bovine spongiform encephalopathy (BSE) and foot-and-mouth (FMD) epizootics in the UK.

Terms that are used in epidemiology include:

- **Endemic** – a disease is present at a normal level in a country or area, e.g. myxomatosis is endemic in wild rabbits in the UK, as is cat flu in the cat population.
- **Epidemic** – a pronounced increase in the level of infection. Recent examples of epidemics include parvovirus infection in dogs after its first appearance, BSE in the UK and AIDS infection of humans worldwide.
- **Epizootic** – more specifically, an animal disease 'epidemic'.

(Thrusfield, 1997)

Bacteria

Size and shape

Bacteria (singular: bacterium) are single-celled organisms (Fig. 14.2) and most range in size from $0.5\,\mu$m (micrometre or micron; 1000th of a millimetre; 10^{-6} m) to $5\,\mu$m in length, though there are some exceptions. Three basic shapes are generally recognised, and these are sometimes used as a means of classification and naming of bacteria (Fig. 14.4):

- Cylindrical or rod-shaped cells called **bacilli** (singular: bacillus). Some bacilli are curved and these are known a **vibrios**.
- Spherical cells called **cocci** (singular: coccus). Some cocci exist singly while others remain together in pairs after cell division and are called **diplococci**. Those that remain attached to form chains are called **streptococci** and if they divide randomly and form irregular grape-like clusters they are called **staphylococci**.

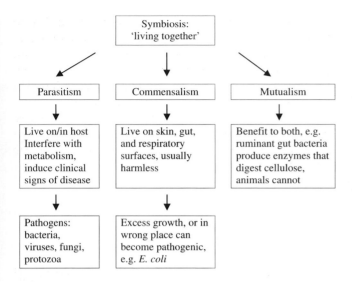

Fig. 14.3 Relationship between micro-organisms and animal hosts.

are only present in certain species or under certain environmental conditions. Table 14.1 shows the shapes and some characteristics of some bacteria that cause disease in dogs.

> **NAMING BACTERIA**
> All bacteria, in common with plants and animals, are named according to the binomial system; the first word, the generic name, starts with a capital letter and indicates the genus to which they belong, such as *Escherichia*, followed by a species name, that is specific, such as *coli*. Thus *Escherichia coli* is one of the species of the genus *Escherichia*, *Homo sapiens* (modern man/woman) is one of the species of the genus *Homo*. The generic name is frequently shortened, e.g. (*Escherichia*) *E. coli* and (*Staphylococcus*) *Staph. aureus*.

- Spiral or helical cells called spirilla (singular: spirillum) if they have a rigid cell wall or spirochaetes if the cell wall is flexible.

Structure

As already mentioned, the morphology of bacteria can affect their physiology and pathogenicity. The shape and physiology of bacteria present in infections are used to identify their species and thus assess prognosis and suitable treatments. Figure 14.2 shows the structure of a generalised bacterial cell. Some of the structures are common to all cells; others

Endospores

Some species of bacteria produce dormant forms called **endospores** (or simply spores), that can survive unfavourable conditions. They are formed when the vegetative (growing) cells are deprived of some factor, e.g. when the supply of nutrients is inadequate. It is important to note that endospore formation (or sporulation) is not a method of reproduction; one vegetative cell produces a single spore which, after germination, is again just one vegetative cell. Spore formation is most common in the genera *Bacillus* and *Clostridium*. These genera contain the causative agents of tetanus, anthrax and botulism. These diseases are zoonoses, commonly affecting domestic and farm animals. Species susceptibility to each varies, e.g. dogs only infrequently suffer from tetanus, whilst horses are very susceptible and require routine vaccination, as do humans.

Many endospore-forming bacteria are inhabitants of the soil but spores can exist almost everywhere, including in dust. They are extremely resistant structures that can remain viable for many years. They can survive extremes of heat, pH, desiccation, ultraviolet radiation and exposure to toxic chemicals such as some disinfectants. The reason why endospores are so resistant is not completely understood but heat resistance is thought to be due to the fact that a dehydration process occurs during spore formation which expels most of the water from the spore. The spore develops within the bacterial cell and under the microscope appears as a bright, round or oval structure.

The fact that spores are so hard to destroy is the principal reason for the various sterilisation procedures which are carried out in veterinary practice. Common techniques employed to kill spores include **autoclaving**: moist heat 121°C under pressure 6.9 kPa for more than 15 minutes; **Tyndallisation**: repeated steaming; **dry heat**: 160°C for at least 2 hours.

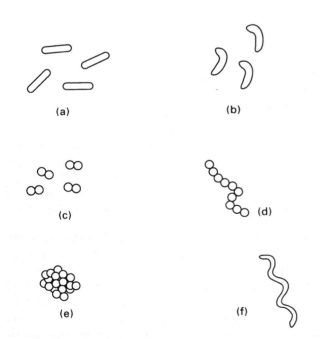

Fig. 14.4 Classification of bacteria by shape. (a) Bacilli. (b) Vibrios (curved bacilli). (c) Diplococci. (d) Streptococci. (e) Staphylococci. (f) Spirochaete.

Table 14.1 Bacterial diseases of dogs				
Name of bacteria	Disease caused	Gram stain	Shape	Aerobic?
Salmonella spp.	Diarrhoea, etc.	−ve	Rod/bacillus	Yes
Campylobacter spp.	Diarrhoea, etc.	−ve	Curved rods	Yes (but prefer less oxygen than in air)
Bordetella bronchiseptica	Kennel cough	−ve	Short rods/bacilli	Yes
Leptospira spp.	Leptospirosis	−ve	Helically coiled (spirochaete)	Yes
Staphylococcus spp.	Pyoderma	+ve	Cocci	Yes
Clostridium tetani*	Tetanus	+ve	Long rods (bacilli)	No

*Rarely a cause of disease in dogs, much more common in horses

Conditions necessary for bacterial growth

Bacteria can grow and reproduce only when environmental conditions are suitable. The essential requirements for growth include:

- A supply of suitable nutrients.
- The correct temperature. The temperature at which a species of bacteria grows most rapidly is the optimum growth temperature. Most mammalian pathogens grow best at normal body temperature.
- The correct pH. The majority of mammalian pathogens grow best at pH 7–7.4.
- Water.
- The correct gaseous environment. Many species of bacteria can grow only when oxygen is present. Bacteria which must have oxygen for growth are called strict or obligate aerobes. Some, the **obligate anaerobes**, can only grow in the absence of oxygen, while others, the **facultative anaerobes** grow aerobically when oxygen is present but can also function in the absence of oxygen. A few species, the **microaerophiles**, grow best when the concentration of oxygen is lower than in atmospheric air.

Reproduction of bacteria

If their environment is suitable, bacteria can grow and reproduce rapidly. The time interval between successive divisions is called **the generation time**. In some bacteria the generation time is very short; for others it is quite long, e.g. under optimum conditions the generation time of *E. coli* is 20 minutes, whereas for the tuberculosis bacterium, *Mycobacterium tuberculosis*, it is approximately 18 hours. Given appropriate conditions, growth is exponential, i.e. one bacterium produces 2, then two produce 4 and so on.

Bacteria reproduce asexually by simply dividing into two identical daughter cells, a process called **binary fission**. Prior to cell division, the cell grows; once it has reached a certain size, the circular chromosome or nucleoid replicates to form two identical chromosomes. As the parent cell enlarges, the chromosomes are separated and the cell membrane grows inwards at the centre of the cell. At the same time, new cell

wall material grows inwards to form the septum and this divides the cell into two daughter cells (Fig. 14.5). These may separate completely, but in some species, e.g. streptococci and staphylococci, they remain attached to form the characteristic chains or clusters. Replication of pathogenic bacteria usually takes place outside the host's cells, unlike pathogenic viruses where reproduction is intracellular.

Conjugation

The process of conjugation involves the passage of DNA from one bacterial cell, the donor, to another, the recipient, while the two cells are in physical contact. The cells are pulled together by an appendage called the sex pilus which is formed by the donor cell. Once contact has been made, the pilus retracts so that the surfaces of the donor and reci-

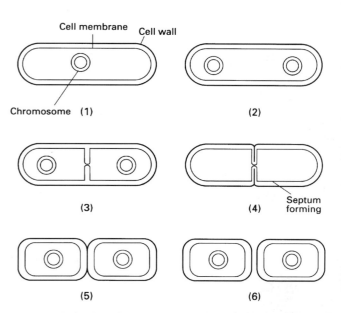

Fig. 14.5 Replication of bacteria by binary fission. (1 and 2) The cell grows and the chromosome replicates to form two identical chromosomes. (3) As the cell enlarges, the chromosomes are separated and the cell membrane grows inwards at the centre of the cell. (4) At the same time, new cell wall material grows inwards to form the septum. (5 and 6) The cell divides into two daughter cells.

pient are very close to each other. The cell membranes fuse forming a channel between the two cells and DNA then passes from the donor to the recipient (Fig. 14.6).

Frequently, a plasmid is transferred from the donor to the recipient but sometimes part of the donor cell chromosome, or even the whole chromosome, is transferred. Conjugation is important because the recipient acquires new characteristics. For example, one plasmid, the R plasmid, carries genes for resistance to antibiotics.

Conjugation is rare among Gram-positive bacteria but common among those that are Gram-negative. It is sometimes regarded as a primitive type of sexual reproduction but this is misleading because unlike sexual reproduction in other organisms, it does not involve the fusion of two gametes to form a single cell.

Bacterial cultivation in the laboratory

The cultivation of bacteria in the laboratory requires an appropriate nutrient material or culture medium. This term is used to describe any solid or liquid on or within which bacteria can be grown. A culture medium must contain a balanced mixture of the essential growth requirements, namely carbon, nitrogen and water. Culture media can also be used as a method of bacterial identification as many bacteria have specific individual requirements for optimal growth. Table 14.2 summarises the uses of common media, and their role in diagnosis is described in Chapter 13.

Media are of two basic types:

- Liquid media or **broths** in which all the required nutrients are included in a fluid.

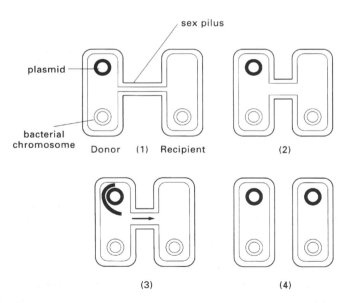

Fig. 14.6 Sequence of events in conjugation. (1) Donor and recipient cells are pulled together by the sex pilus, which is formed by the donor cell. (2) The pilus retracts, bringing the two cells very close to each other, and the cell membranes fuse to form a channel between the two cells. (3) The plasmid replicates and one strand passes through the channel to the recipient. (4) The two cells separate. The recipient becomes a donor because it now has the plasmid.

- Solid media consist of a nutrient solution hardened to a jelly-like consistency by the addition of a substance called agar (this is used as bacteria cannot utilise it as a food source), a substance which is derived from seaweed.
- **Solid** media are usually used in flat dishes with lids called Petri dishes; a Petri dish containing the solid medium is called a plate. Solid media have the advantage that differences in size, shape and colour of bacterial colonies (i.e. a visible growth of bacteria) can be used for identification and individual colonies can be separated.

All these media can be bought ready prepared as broths or on Petri dishes, or can be bought dried for reconstitution in a practice laboratory.

Respiratory requirements

The different respiratory requirements of bacteria can be used to help identify bacterial pathogens, as can their detailed biochemical pathways used to provide energy. A lot of bacteria will grow in the amount of oxygen in the air, so may be cultured in an incubator; others will not grow in oxygen (anaerobes). Petri dishes containing appropriate culture media can be placed in an **anaerobic jar** to minimise atmospheric oxygen and encourage the growth of anaerobes. Respiratory mechanisms of any particular bacteria can be identified in a similar way to that mentioned for sugar fermentation (Table 14.2), by testing for the presence of **enzymes** involved in oxidative processes, such as the enzymes **catalase** and **cytochrome oxidase**.

The smaller organisms

Infections can be caused by a number of organisms that are a little or a lot smaller than most bacteria. In order of decreasing size these are:

- Rickettsias, mycoplasmas and chlamydias.
- Viruses.
- Prions.

The first three organisms, rickettsias, mycoplasmas and chlamydias, are classified as bacteria and are considered first. The subsequent sections will examine viruses and prions, and the diseases that they cause.

Both rickettsia and chlamydia possess a cell wall like other Gram-negative bacteria but both of these organisms need to live inside other cells, that is they are obligate intracellular organisms. These bacteria are responsible for a number of diseases in animals including:

- Chlamydia: Various strains of *Chlamydia psittaci*, the cause of psittacosis in psittacene birds (parrots, parakeets) and mammals. Psittacosis is a zoonotic infection which humans can acquire by inhaling chlamydia in the airborne dust or cage contents of infected birds. Feline pneumonitis is caused by *Chlamydia psittaci* and the

Table 14.2 Summary of the uses of common bacterial media

Medium		Type	Use	Examples
Plates	Nutrient agar	Simple	Growth of nutritionally undemanding species, e.g.	*E. coli*
	Blood (add 5–10% blood)	Enriched	supports the growth of most pathogens and used to detect haemolysis	Most mammalian pathogens
	Chocolate agar (heat blood agar to 80°C, so cells release haemoglobin)	Enriched	suitable for certain more fastidious pathogens	*Neisseria* species
	Deoxycholate-citrate	Selective	Inhibits growth of certain bacteria but not others	For growing *Salmonella*.
	MacConkey's	Selective and differential	To distinguish those enteric species which ferment lactose from enteric species on same plate which do not	*E. coli* is acid producing, so colonies are red, but most strains of *Salmonella* show colourless colonies
	Sabouraud's	Selective	For growing fungi	Dermatophytes
	Peptone water/ nutrient broth or solid medium + biochemical + indicator	Biochemical	Some species in genera can ferment different sugars To detect pathogens that produce urease	Different species of *Salmonella* Increase in pH from breakdown of urea to ammonia turns indicator red
Broths	Nutrient broth	Standard	For growth of bacteria in fluid	
	Peptone water	Simple	Provides basic growth requirements	
	MacConkey's	Selective	Contains bile salts to isolate enteric from nonenteric bacteria	
	Selenite broth	Enrichment	Favours and encourages growth of small numbers of wanted species in mixed sample	For growing *Salmonella*
Transport		Simple	Do not support growth, but ensure survival of organisms	Swabs sent for lab analysis

organism may be the cause of conjunctivitis in the cat. They are transmitted by inhalation of infectious dust and droplets and by ingestion. There is also evidence to suggest that vector-borne infection may occur.

- Rickettsias: They are transmitted by vectors such as the tick, louse, flea and mite from an infected individual. For example *Haemobartonella felis*: infectious feline anaemia. Another rickettsial infection is caused by *Ehrlichia* spp. A particularly pathogenic species is *Ehrlichia canis*, endemic in much of France and the Mediterranean basin (Trees and Shaw, 1999).

Generally, the identification of rickettsia and chlamydia is more difficult and thus more specialised than that of most bacteria. Diagnosis of infection may be based on demonstration of the organisms themselves or on the demonstration of increased titres in paired serum samples (see later section on Immunity). The rickettsiae are smaller than most bacteria and are barely visible under the ordinary light microscope. They can only be cultivated in tissue culture or in the yolk sac of embryonated eggs. Typically, they are rod shaped, about $0.8–2.0\,\mu$m long.

Mycoplasma are tiny bacteria-like organisms but unlike other bacteria do not possess a cell wall. They include:

- *Mycoplasma felis* – a cause of chronic conjunctivitis in cats.
- *Mycoplasma* species have been implicated in complicating respiratory tract infections in a number of species, notably calves.

Mycoplasma will grow on agar-based media but, as they are so fragile, isolation and identification are specialised skills.

More information about the diseases caused by these small bacteria may be found in Chapter 17.

Viruses

Structure and naming

Viruses are extremely small and are sometimes not classified as living organisms as they are incapable of reproduction without a host cell. A virus particle or virion is little more than a package containing instructions for the recreation of further virus particles. Each virus particle is composed of two parts:

- **Nucleic acid**: RNA or DNA (never both) forming a central core.
- **A protein coat**: the capsid (Fig. 14.7).

Together, these two parts form the nucleocapsid. For some viruses, this is all that an individual virus particle will consist of. Various shapes of virus nucleocapsid have been identified:

- Helical (Fig. 14.8a and b).
- Icosahedral (Fig. 14.8c and d).
- Complex (poxvirus).
- Composite – some bacteriophages (Fig. 14.1).

Some viruses have an additional envelope around the outside, often formed of the host cell membrane (Fig. 14.7c). Each of the helical or icosahedral shapes of the nucleocapsid could be enveloped or non-enveloped (Fig. 14.8), giving four possible basic shapes for viruses. In fact, there are no animal viruses (only plant viruses) that are helical and non-enveloped, so cat or dog viruses can be grouped by and large into the other three types. Viruses have been classified together on the basis of structural similarities so, for example, the group of viruses causing true flu are the influenza viruses (unlike equine and human flu, the disease that we call cat flu is caused by two viruses, neither of which is influenza virus), and horse flu is caused by equine influenza virus.

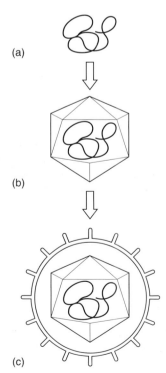

(a)

(b)

(c)

Fig. 14.7 General virus components: (a) central core of nucleic acid; (b) capsid surrounding the nucleic acid to form the nucleocapsid with icosahedral symmetry; (c) in addition, some viruses possess an outer envelope.

Viral replication

A virus is only able to attach to cells that carry a compatible receptor. So, for example, influenza viruses can only attach to ciliated epithelial cells in the respiratory tract. This specificity of viruses for specific tissues is known as tissue trophism. Viruses normally have only one or two host species that they are able to infect. So, parvovirus in dogs does not infect cats and measles virus will only infect humans and apes. Once attached, virus particles are taken into the host cell [Fig. 14.9(2)] by fusing the virus envelope with the host cell membrane or, in the case of non-enveloped viruses, by causing the host cell to engulf the virus particle into the cell. Once inside the cell, the virus is able to switch the cell's normal metabolism to obey the instructions of the virus. The virus may cause this to happen immediately, so the cell begins to produce the constituents of new virus particles within hours of infection [Fig. 14.9(4)]. Alternatively, as in the case of AIDS, the virus may join with the host cell's own nucleic acid for an extended period before making any changes to cell metabolism (more details of retrovirus replication may be found in Chapter 17). New virus particles are then assembled and released from the cell [Fig. 14.9(6)]. Depending on the virus, this may leave the host cell intact or may cause its rupture and destruction.

Transmission

Viruses are transmitted from host to host either directly (e.g. by a cat licking feline calicivirus in nasal secretions off the face of another cat) or indirectly (e.g. a dog licks the floor of a kennel that had been occupied by a dog with parvovirus infection and that had not been adequately cleaned). Different viruses have adapted their means of transmission according to their structure (which affects their ability to survive in the environment) and their location in the host. So, for example, a respiratory tract virus is often transmitted by sneezing virus particles from one host into the air breathed in by another host. This is ideal for influenza virus as these enveloped viruses are not very robust so do not survive for extended periods in the environment. An ability to survive in the environment for longer periods is beneficial for canine parvovirus. The virus must be licked up and ingested by another dog for infection of the gastrointestinal tract to occur.

Think about the viral diseases that you know that infect dogs, cats and other species, and work out how they are likely to be transmitted. Transmission of disease is discussed in more detail in Chapter 17.

Incubation

Once a host animal has been infected with a small number of virus particles, there is a time lag before the symptoms that are associated with the infection are seen; this is the incubation period. During this time, the virus reaches the cells that it can invade and initially infects a small number of cells in

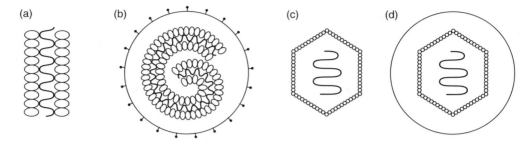

Fig. 14.8 Four types of viral structure: (a) helical naked; (b) helical enveloped; (c) icosahedral naked; (d) icosahedral and enveloped.

order to increase the number of virus particles. Symptoms (or signs) are seen once large numbers of virus particles infect a large number of cells.

Viral diseases

Some infections in dogs and cats that are caused by viruses are shown in Tables 14.3 and 14.4. More details of viral diseases may be found in Chapter 17.

Diagnosis of viral infections

Viral infections may be diagnosed on the basis of their symptoms and the animal's history. Often, however, there are several infections that may cause similar signs and it may be important to be able to confirm the particular virus present. This may be carried out in a number of ways, e.g.:

- Virus particles are too small to be seen with the light microscope but they may be seen with an electron microscope.
- Large numbers of virus particles may clump together in cells; the clump may then be seen with the light microscope. Large groups of rabies virus are seen in cells of animals infected with rabies; these are known as Negri bodies. An animal can only be examined for these and a number of other virus-related changes at post mortem.
- Serology may be carried out to detect virus antigen or the antibody produced by the host in response to infection.

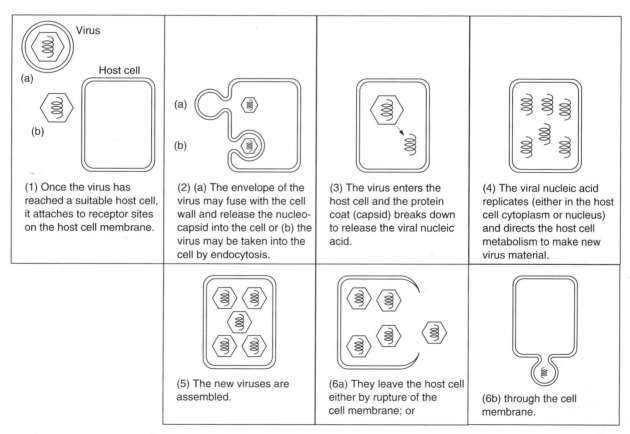

Fig. 14.9 Replication of animal viruses.

Table 14.3 Some viral diseases of dogs

Name of virus	Disease caused	Nucleic acid type	Shape of nucleocapsid	Enveloped
Parvovirus	Parvovirus	DNA	Icosahedral	No
Canine adenovirus 1 (CAV-1)	Infectious canine hepatitis	DNA	Icosahedral	No
Canine adenovirus 2 (CAV-2)	Infectious canine tracheo-bronchitis	DNA	Icosahedral	No
Canine distemper virus	Distemper	RNA	Helical	Yes
Canine parainfluenza virus	Part of kennel cough syndrome	RNA	Helical	Yes
Rabies virus	Rabies	RNA	Helical	Yes

Treatment of viral infection

Viral infections can be combatted in a number of ways:

- Treatment of animal virus infections normally involves supportive nursing, for example:

    - Fluids to prevent dehydration in the case of canine parvovirus infection.
    - Tempting foods for cats with cat flu.
    - Antibacterials to limit secondary infection.

- Animals may be vaccinated in order to stimulate an immune response.
- There are now some specialised treatments for a few viral infections in humans, such as AIDS, the shingles form of chickenpox and herpes simplex (the cause of cold sores). Some antiviral treatments are also used in companion animals, though this is mainly confined to ophthalmic treatment, e.g. trifluridine for the treatment of feline herpes virus conjunctivitis.

Prevention of viral infection

As virus infections are difficult to treat once the animal is infected, control has been aimed at preventing infection, particularly of severe virus diseases. This can be done at a number of levels:

- A country can have a border policy to prevent entry of diseases that are not present in a country, e.g. countries seek to prevent entry of rabies by quarantine or vaccine policies.
- Catteries may be designed so that airborne viruses are not readily transmitted from cat to cat.
- Suitable disinfectants can be used to kill viruses that may be present in animal cages between occupants.
- Individual animals may be protected by vaccination, e.g. **canine distemper** and **parvovirus, feline leukaemia**, etc. More details about vaccination may be found in Tables 17.3 and 17.5 and in the section on Immunity.

Table 14.5 shows the major similarities and differences between the different types of micro-organism.

Prions

These are very small protein infectious particles that cause infections within the central nervous system that lead, eventually, to the death of the affected animal. The incubation period is usually long – taking from 2 months to 20 years before signs of disease become apparent. Until relatively few years ago, the study of prion diseases was extremely specialised work carried out by a few people. Researchers had investigated scrapie, a prion infection of sheep that has

Table 14.4 Some viral diseases of cats

Name of virus	Disease caused	Nucleic acid type	Shape of nucleocapsid	Enveloped
Feline parvovirus (panleucopenia)	Feline infectious enteritis	DNA	Icosahedral	No
Feline herpesvirus	Feline rhinotracheitis cat flu	DNA	Icosahedral	Yes
Feline calicivirus		RNA	Icosahedral	No
Feline coronavirus	Feline infectious peritonitis (FIP)	RNA	Helical	Yes
Feline leukaemia virus	Retrovirus causing feline leukaemia	RNA	Icosahedral	Yes
Feline immunodeficiency virus	Retrovirus	RNA	Icosahedral	Yes
Rabies virus	Rabies	RNA	Helical	Yes

Table 14.5 Major similarities and differences between different types of micro-organism					
Characteristic	**Bacteria**	**Viruses**	**Fungi**	**Protozoa**	**Algae**
Size	0.5–5 µm	20–300 nm	3.8 µm (yeasts)	10–200 µm	0.5–20 µm
Cell arrangement	Unicellular	Non-cellular	Unicellular or multicellular	Unicellular	Unicellular or multicellular
Cell wall	Present; mainly peptidoglycan	Absent	Present; mainly chitin	Absent	Present; mainly cellulose
Nucleus	No true membrane-bound nucleus	Absent	Membrane-bound nucleus	Membrane-bound nucleus	Membrane-bound nucleus
Nuclei acids Reproduction	DNA and RNA Asexual by binary	DNA or RNA Replicate only within another living cell	DNA and RNA Asexual and sexual by spores, budding in yeast	DNA and RNA Asexual and sexual	DNA and RNA Asexual and sexual
Nutrition	Mainly heterotrophic – can be saprophytic or parasitic; a few are autotrophic	Obligate parasites	Heterotrophic – can be saprophytic or parasitic	Heterotrophic – can be saprophytic or parasitic	Autotrophic
Motility	Some are motile	Non-motile	Non-motile except for certain spore forms	Motile	Some are motile
Toxin production	Some form toxins	None	Some form toxins	Some form toxins	Some form toxins

been recorded in Europe for the last 200 years. Interest and research in prion infections increased greatly following the outbreak of BSE (bovine spongiform encephalopathy), which was first identified in the UK in 1985. It appears that BSE may be transmissible to humans as a result of eating infected beef. There have been over 100 deaths attributed to a new variant (vCJD) of a human encephalopathy, CJD. Around 20 cases of a similar disease in cats (FSE, feline spongiform encephalopathy) have been recorded in the UK since 1990. Affected cats exhibit incoordination. It is thought that these SEs may originally have derived from scrapie. A lot of research effort is aimed at being able to confirm disease in the live animal. At present, diagnosis is based on the appearance of brain tissue at post mortem examination, although several potential tests on live animals are being evaluated.

Immunity

Animals survive injury and potential infection due to the effectiveness of their defence systems against pathogens, foreign or 'non-self' invasion. This capacity to distinguish foreign material from self, and to neutralise, eliminate or metabolise it is termed **immunity**. Throughout early gestation, the foetus learns to recognise what constitutes itself so that later in life it can identify foreign material, in order to eliminate it. There are several lines of defence, the first innate (natural) defences include:

- Barriers such as skin, hair, tears, saliva.
- Lysozyme in saliva and tears – kills Gram-positive bacteria.

The second lines of defence include the non-specific immune responses such as inflammation, phagocytosis, pyrogen and interferon. Phagocytic cells that are specialised at identifying and removing foreign material, e.g. neutrophils and macrophages. Details of the structure of different WBCs are given in Chapter 13.

The most specific mechanisms that each animal has are termed **acquired immunity**. Acquired immunity, as its name suggests, is not present at birth but is acquired through life. The process begins with the presentation of foreign material or **antigen** to lymphocytes in lymph nodes (Fig. 14.10a). There are two main types of lymphocyte, **B** maturing mainly in the bone marrow, and **T**, maturing in the thymus gland. Some lymphocytes will recognise the material and will respond in a number of ways. B lymphocytes react by producing specific **antibodies (immunoglobulins, Ig)** (Fig. 14.10b) that bind tightly to antigens in the foreign material (Fig. 14.10c). This is termed humoral immunity, and the antibody is specific to each individual antigen. Once covered with antibody, the rest of the immune system can readily remove the foreign material (Fig. 14.10e).

T lymphocytes produce a number of substances known as cytokines or lymphokines, which are cell messengers. Lymphokines, unlike antibody, do not bind specifically with antigen, but direct cell functions and responses. There are four main types of T cells, one type of which, the T helper cell, is attacked by the retroviruses that cause AIDS-like diseases such as feline immunodeficiency virus. Another type, **cytotoxic**, acts as a killer cell, eliminating body cells infected by intracellular pathogens such as viruses.

The process of recognition and antibody production is a process that goes on continuously, so that an animal acquires, through exposure to infections, a repertoire of antibodies to protect it from the range of infections in its

ANTIGEN

An antigen is a foreign material that the immune system can recognise. Not everything that is foreign to the animal will be recognised as foreign, e.g. a metal implant such as a pin or plate will be accepted. Biochemical markers, such as proteins, are the usual indicators of 'foreignness'.

environment – this is termed **natural immunity**. The process takes a little time to become fully effective against any particular infection. During this time lag, some very pathogenic (an organism that is capable of causing severe disease) organisms may have already caused irreversible damage to

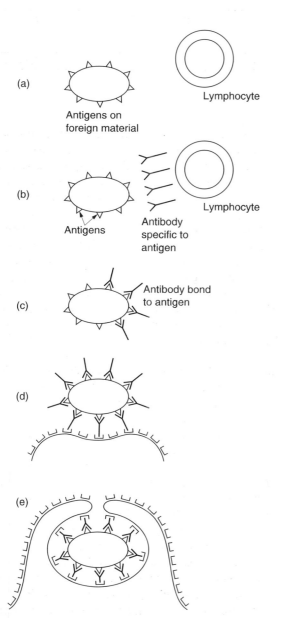

Fig. 14.10 (a) Antibody production following recognition of antigen by B lymphocyte. (b) The lymphocyte produces specific antibody. (c) Antibody binds to antigen. (d) Antibody facilitates adherence to phagocytic cell. (e) Foreign material engulfed by phagocytic cell.

the animal (e.g. rabbit myxomatosis or distemper in a dog) or even caused its death (e.g. parvovirus infection in a puppy). There are several ways in which the animal may be assisted to acquire an immune response to infection:

- The animal's mother can pass antibodies to its offspring. This protects the very young animal during the period immediately after birth and prevents it from succumbing to infection. In most domesticated mammals these antibodies are passed in the first milk or colostrum and there is a limited period after birth when the newborn animal's intestine allows the antibodies to pass into the bloodstream. In humans, the structure of the placenta allows transfer of antibodies to occur before birth, thus colostrum is not so important for human babies. This type of transfer of immunity is known as **passive immunisation** as the recipient is not producing its own antibodies. In order to maximise the antibody levels in maternally derived immunity, the dam can be vaccinated just before pregnancy or perhaps even during pregnancy, depending on the recommendations of an individual vaccine.

- Another type of passive immunisation is carried out to protect an animal temporarily from an infection or toxin. Here, **antisera** or **antitoxins** to the specific infection or toxin are administered. The antibodies within the preparation bind to the infectious agent or toxin in the animal and stop its damaging effects. Examples of the use of antitoxins include administration of tetanus antitoxin to a horse that is suspected of having tetanus or to a horse that is not protected from tetanus and that had been cut. Antiserum may be administered to a dog that has been bitten by an adder to prevent the venom exerting its adverse effects on the dog.

- **Active immunisation** is carried out more commonly. Here, the animal is presented with a specific antigen in a safe form – this may be in the form of a killed virus, a modified or attenuated virus or bacteria, heat-treated toxin (toxoid), just the part of a virus that is recognised by the immune system without the pathogenic part or a bacterial strain that is without virulence. The antigen (or vaccine) is administered when the animal is healthy so that its lymphocytes can respond to the antigen by producing antibody. Importantly, in addition to producing antibody, some **memory B lymphocytes** are stored so that the next time the animal meets the same antigen it can respond rapidly and effectively.

- A vaccination schedule for a young pup or kitten usually starts when the pup or kitten is about 8–10 weeks of age. Before this the presence of colostrally derived immunity may prevent the animal from producing its own antibodies.

- A vaccination schedule often consists of two initial priming doses (in pups and kittens spaced 2–3 weeks apart, and in horses 4–6 weeks apart), then regular boosters to keep reminding the memory cells of the antigen. Some antigens, thus vaccines, are very effective at producing a long-term memory (such as distemper vaccine or tetanus); the memory of others fades more quickly (particularly influenza vaccine in horses) so may need boosting more frequently.

- Because vaccines may contain viruses or bacteria and because it is imperative that the animal is presented with undamaged antigen, it is important that vaccines are stored as directed on the data sheet and that they are not used past their expiry date. It is also important that they are administered as directed and not mixed with unrelated products, e.g. other vaccines or antibacterials, as these may adversely affect the integrity of the vaccine.
- Vaccination **certificates** are used to demonstrate that an animal has received appropriate vaccine. It may be used locally to demonstrate that a pet is vaccinated before entry into kennels or may be used to verify that an animal has been appropriately protected prior to export. Certification of rabies vaccination is an integral part of the Pet Travel Scheme, whereby pets can travel back from the European mainland to the UK without the need for quarantine. More information about the requirements for the scheme can be found at www.defra.gov.uk.

Allergy

Allergy or hypersensitivity occurs when the immune system reacts in an inappropriate way following exposure to an antigen. Allergic reactions occur after one or more exposures to an allergen. There are four main types of allergic reaction: of these immediate (Type 1) and cell-mediated (Type 4) are readily identified in veterinary practice. Type 1 hypersensitivity occurs when the immunoglobulin IgE is produced, this results in the release of histamine from mast cells. Clinical signs include hay fever, wheals following flea bites and anaphylactic reactions. Delayed or cell mediated hypersensitivity, involving T cells, occurs as a late reaction in flea-bite hypersensitive dogs, for example. More examples can be found in Chapter 17.

Immune-related disease

The immune system is highly effective when it functions well but in some circumstances, as in hypersensitivity, the immune system reaction can be inappropriate. Examples include glomerulonephritis caused by the deposition of immune complexes in the kidney glomeruli, and the skin lesions in canine leishmaniasis caused by cell-mediated immune reponses.

Autoimmunity

Autoimmunity can be one of the most destructive of these inappropriate immune responses. This occurs when the immune system, for some reason, turns on 'self' tissue and begins to destroy it, such as occurs in haemolytic anaemia and pemphigus.

Transplants

Transplanting tissues or organs from one human to another is commonly carried out. However, without careful tissue matching and the use of immunosuppressive treatment, the transplant would fail as the body's immune system attacked the transplanted material having recognised it as 'foreign'.

Diagnostic use of antibodies

Antibody–antigen binding is recognised to be highly specific; it has therefore been utilised in a number of diagnostic tests, to detect, for example:

- The presence or absence of an antibody.
- The level of an antibody.
- The presence of an antigen (Fig. 14.11).

Pregnancy diagnosis kits often also utilise this technology.

> **KEYPOINTS**
> - Bacteria and viruses are important causes of disease in companion animals.
> - Understanding the transmission of bacteria and viruses is essential in order to prevent spread of disease from animal to animal.
> - Bacteria and viruses can be identified by a variety of laboratory tests.
> - Understanding the disease-causing agent and the way that it causes illness allows the development of rational treatment and control regimens.
> - The immune system has a protective role in animals. Protection against specific infections can be provided by vaccination.

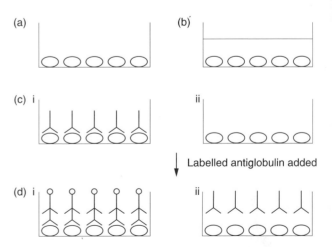

Fig. 14.11 Diagrammatic representation of ELISA. (a) Antigen in base of well; (b) test serum added; (c) (i) test serum contains specific antibody which binds to antigen, (ii) does not contain antibody, therefore no binding; (d) labelled antiglobulin added, (i) binds to antibody and produces colour change, (ii) no binding, thus no colour change.

In veterinary practice, enzyme-linked immunosorbent assays (ELISAs) are used to assess the success of transfer of passive immunity in neonates such as calves or foals. Test kits may also be purchased for diagnosis of other infections such as feline leukaemia.

Further reading

Epidemiology

Thrusfield, M. (1997). *Veterinary Epidemiology*, 2nd edn, Blackwell Science.

Microbiology

Gillespie, S. and Bamford, K. (2000). *Medical Microbiology and Infection at a Glance*, Blackwell Science.

Heritage, J., Evans, E. G. V. and Killington, R. A. (1996). *Introductory Microbiology*, Cambridge Univ. Press.

Quinn, P. J. et al. (1994). *Clinical Veterinary Microbiology*, Wolfe Publishing.

Trees, S. and Shaw, S. (1999). Imported diseases in small animals. In *Practice*, vol. 21, pp. 482–491.

Immunology

Day, M. J. (1999). *Clinical Immunology of the Dog and Cat*, Manson Publishing.

Playfair, J. H. L. and Chain, B. M. (2001). *Immunology at a Glance*, 7th edn, Blackwell Science.

15

Elementary mycology and parasitology

M. Fisher and *V. Walsh*

Learning objectives

After studying this chapter, students should be able to:

- Describe the ecto- and endoparasites that affect dogs and cats.
- Describe the geographic distribution and zoonotic potential of parasites.
- Discuss how the lifecycle of a parasite determines the possible routes of infection.
- Identify parasites on the basis of their location on or in the host and their morphology.
- Discuss treatment options for parasite control.
- Describe options for prophylaxis to prevent parasite infection.

DEFINITIONS
- **Parasite**: one eukaryotic organism living off another (the **host**) to the advantage of the parasite.
- **Ectoparasites** live on the outside of the host.
- **Endoparasites** live inside the host.
- **Eukaryote**: organism in which the chromosomes are enclosed in a nucleus (e.g. animals, plants, fungi).

Fungi

There are many different fungi – as one can see by looking at a mouldy slice of bread. Only a few specific fungi, however, are able to infect animals. Fungi can be divided into unicellular yeasts and multicellular moulds, and the fungal pathogens seen in small animal veterinary practice include both categories:

- **Moulds** (Fig. 15.1a): the 'ringworm' dermatophytes ('skineaters').
- **Yeasts** (Fig. 15.1b): *Candida albicans*, the 'thrush' yeast, is often present in the intestinal tract of animals without causing disease but it can become pathogenic in certain circumstances.

Fungi grow aerobically and gain their energy from the organic substances on which they grow.

Dermatophytes

Fungal infections of **keratin** (the horny tissue that forms nail, hair and skin) can affect cats, dogs, rabbits and guinea pigs. The condition broadly known as **ringworm** is caused by dermatophytes, such as the species *Trichophyton mentagrophytes* (dog, cat, rabbit and guinea pig) and *Microsporum canis* (dog and cat), amongst others.

In its most obvious form, ringworm appears as circular areas of hair loss with active fungal infection around the edge of the lesion. The lesions may be small and discrete or large and coalescing, with an irregular outline. Some infections are not very inflamed and cause little irritation, whilst others may cause severe inflammation. A more marked reaction is common in dogs.

Transmission may be directly from affected animal to animal, or to humans (many dermatophytes are zoonotic). Long-haired cats, in particular, may appear normal but may be carriers of infection. There may also be indirect transmission via bedding, cages, etc. Ringworm spores can remain viable in the environment for prolonged periods (see Chapter 13, p. 329).

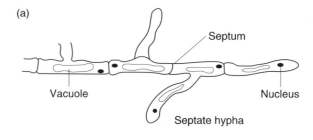
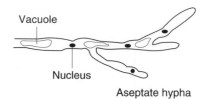
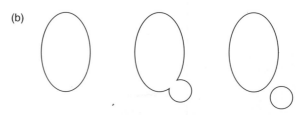

Fig. 15.1 Different forms of fungi; (a) moulds; (b) yeast, e.g. *Candida albicans*, showing budding.

Diagnosis

Place hair pluck or skin scrape on a slide and stain, for example, with lactophenol cotton blue. Affected material, including hair shafts, will stain blue (Fig. 15.2).

Using a Wood's lamp in a darkened room, examine the animal's hair. Once the lamp has warmed up sufficiently, it produces ultraviolet light and some 60% of *Microsporum canis* isolates will usually fluoresce and appear apple-green in colour. (Other things, e.g. surface scale, may fluoresce but it will not be apple-green.)

Culture a sample of the suspect hair and/or scale on specialist medium, e.g. Sabouraud's or dermatophyte test medium (DTM). The latter contains a colour indicator that turns from yellow to red in the presence of dermatophytes. The culture should be incubated at room temperature and any dermatophytes should grow within 2 weeks.

Treatment
Topical

- Fungicidal wash such as enilconazole.
- Paint the affected area with povidone–iodine.

Topical treatment is usually repeated after an interval to effect a full cure. It may be possible to treat the area of a discrete lesion only or it may be necessary to wash the whole animal. In severe or non-responsive cases, e.g. some long-haired cats, it will be necessary to clip the affected part or even the entire animal to facilitate treatment.

Systemic
Itraconazole or ketoconazole can be administered orally for the treatment of dermatophytes in dogs and cats. Griseofulvin is administered in tablet form and has to be given for a prolonged period as the levels build up gradually in the skin. Care, including the wearing of gloves, should be taken when handling griseofulvin as it is **teratogenic** (i.e. it can cause malformation of a fetus).

Candida albicans

Candida infections are usually opportunistic, that is they take advantage of a young, debilitated or immunocompromised animal and cause infection. Infection may also be seen after prolonged antibacterial treatment. The infection is known as 'thrush' and is commonly seen on mucous membranes, e.g. in the mouths of puppies or kittens.

Identification is by means of the appearance of a white growth on the affected area. Infection of the mouth in a puppy or kitten may be associated with unwillingness to suck. Very rarely it may infect the skin, though *Candida* is not usually included in the dermatophytes. Treatments for candidiasis include amphotericin and flucytosine.

Malassezia pachydermatitis

Malassezia pachydermatitis (Fig.15.3) is a yeast that may be found on normal skin. In some situations, particularly seborrhoeic conditions, overgrowth may cause pruritic dermatitis or otitis in dogs. Infection can be treated with a shampoo containing chlorhexidine and miconazole.

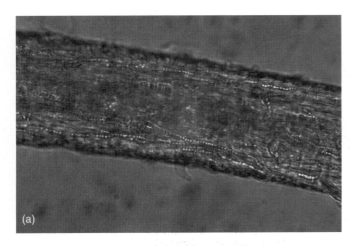

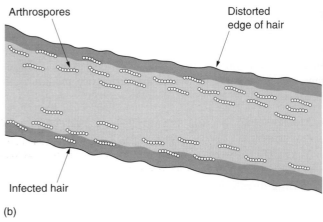

Fig. 15.2 (a) Dernatophyte infected hair. (Photograph courtesy of Mark Craig.) (b) Diagram of Dernatophyte infected hair.

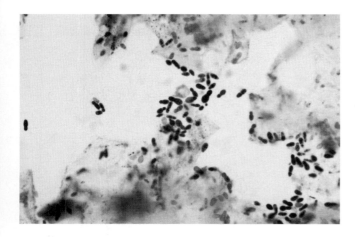

Fig. 15.3 Bottle-shaped yeast, *Malassezia pachydermatitis*. (Photo courtesy of Mark Craig)

Other fungal infections

Occasionally dogs or cats develop internal fungal infections. A number of different fungi can be responsible, for example *Aspergillus fumigatus* can infect the nasal passages of the dog.

Ectoparasites

Except for certain important fungi mentioned previously, most ectoparasites belong to the animal kingdom and have a hard chitinous outer shell or exoskeleton. They include:

- **Insects**, where the adult has three pairs of legs and the body is divided into head, thorax and abdomen (e.g. lice, fleas).
- **Arachnids**, where the adult has four pairs of legs and the body is divided into two parts only: cephalothorax and abdomen (e.g. mites, ticks).

Usually it is the adult stage, often together with the immature stages, that is parasitic. There are two cases where it is only an immature form that is parasitic: the first is a mite, *Trombicula autumnalis*, and the other is the larva of the blowfly (see Chapter 17, p. 427).

Insects

The diagnosis and control of insect ectoparasites are given in Table 15.1.

Table 15.1 Diagnosis and control of insect ectoparasites

	Diagnosis	Control
Lice	Demonstration of the eggs attached to hairs. Visualisation of the adult louse. The adult lice may be seen with the naked eye on close examination of an animal's haircoat or may be seen in a skin scrape/brush	Thorough cleaning Topical surface treatment with an insecticidal wash spray or spot-on.
Fleas	Demonstration of an adult flea or their faeces in the coat of a dog or cat by combing the coat thoroughly, preferably with a very fine toothcomb (ideally a human louse comb). The animal may be brushed over a sheet of damp white paper. Flea faeces will be seen on the paper as small black dots. Since they contain a large amount of undigested blood, a ring of red is seen around the black spot when moistened. There is also a skin test for allergy to fleas	Control of the environment at stages: – Hoovering, particularly around where the pet sleeps – Applying an environmental insecticide and/or an insect growth regulator such as methoprene or pyriproxyfen, for example, to kill the immature stages. Depending on the formulation these products may be applied to the animal or directly to the environment. The chitin synthesis inhibitor (lufeneuron) is given orally to the dog or cat or by injection to the cat. It prevents eggs hatching and/or larval development Control of adult fleas on the animal: – Thorough grooming, e.g. using a human louse comb – Applying an insecticide in the form of, for example, a spray, impregnated collar, powder, shampoo or spot-on. The active ingredient in insecticides is now less often an organophosphate or a carbamate as these have been replaced by synthetic pyrethroids, phenylpyrazole (fipronil), chloronicotinyl nitroguanidine (imidacloprid) or avermectin (selamectin)
Dipteran fly larvae	An affected animal will often stop eating and appear restless and later depressed. The animal should be thoroughly examined to find the larvae and thus diagnose the problem	In order to treat the infestation, the first step is to remove the larvae: – Wash the affected area with a mild antiseptic solution, ensuring that the larvae are removed in the process – Lightly towel-dry the area. Apply antiseptic ointment Any underlying problem (e.g. diarrhoea) that may have predisposed the animal to becoming 'fly blown' should be investigated and treated

Lice

Infection with lice is also known as pediculosis. Lice are subdivided into biting lice (Figs 15.4 and 15.5) and sucking lice (Fig. 15.6), reflecting their manner of feeding.

Infection is transmitted by close contact as the louse spends its entire life cycle on the host. Alternatively, infection may be transferred by eggs collected onto grooming equipment. However, lice are highly **host specific** and will not survive if transferred to another host. (Other parasites, such as the cat flea, are more ubiquitous and will be found on a number of different hosts.)

Cats, dogs, rabbits, rodents and birds may be affected with lice. Often young or debilitated animals are the worst affected. Large numbers of lice cause intense irritation and concomitant self-inflicted injury. In addition, the sucking lice may cause anaemia if they are present in large enough numbers.

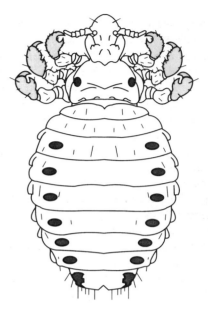

Fig. 15.6 Dorsal view of the sucking louse (approximately 2 mm long). *Linognathus setosus* is the sucking louse of the dog. Sucking lice tend to have elongated, narrow heads.

Life cycle

Adult female lice lay their eggs individually and cement them to hairs. The eggs ('nits') are just visible to the naked eye (Fig. 15.7). When these hatch, immature lice that are identical to the adult emerge and, after several moults, become adults. The whole life cycle takes about 2–3 weeks.

Fleas

Adult fleas bite the host in order to take a blood meal. The area that has been bitten shows something of an

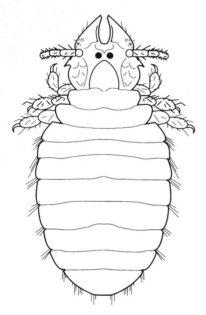

Fig. 15.4 Dorsal view of the biting louse (2 mm long, light to dark brown in colour). If viewed from the side, the louse would appear dorsoventrally flattened. This is the cat louse, *Felicola subrostratus*.

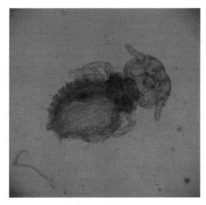

Fig. 15.5 The species of biting louse found in dogs is *Trichodectes canis*. Biting lice tend to have shorter, broader heads than sucking lice.

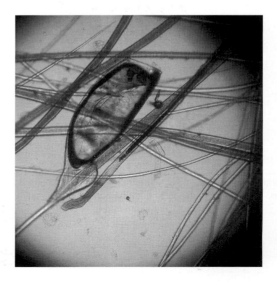

Fig. 15.7 Louse egg ('nit') attached with 'cement' to the shaft of hair.

inflammatory reaction and causes some irritation. A heavy flea infestation may cause anaemia. Fleas can transmit disease as they feed and fleas appear important in the spread from cat to cat of *Bartonella henselae*, the agent responsible for cat scratch disease in humans. It is believed that a cat's claws may be coated in the bacteria, probably derived from the cat grooming infected flea faeces out of its coat.

Some animals become sensitised to **allergens** (particles that an individual may become sensitised to on repeat exposure) in flea saliva and develop severe lesions after just a few bites. This is known as **miliary dermatitis** in the cat and **flea allergic dermatitis** in the dog.

The species of flea may be identified by the appearance of the head (Fig. 15.8). Most fleas on cats and dogs are the 'cat flea' *Ctenocephalides felis felis* (often abbreviated to *C. felis*) but dogs in a dog-only situation (e.g. greyhound kennels) may be infected with the dog flea *Ctenocephalides canis*. Infrequently other fleas, e.g. hedgehog fleas, are found on cats or dogs.

Birds have their own species of flea, the immature stages of which live in the bird's nest.

Life cycle of the cat flea

The life cycle of the cat flea is shown in Fig. 15.9. The adult is laterally compressed, which allows the flea to move readily between the host's hairs. The female flea feeds, then mates on the host and then lays eggs. These are smooth and fall off into the environment, particularly around where the animal

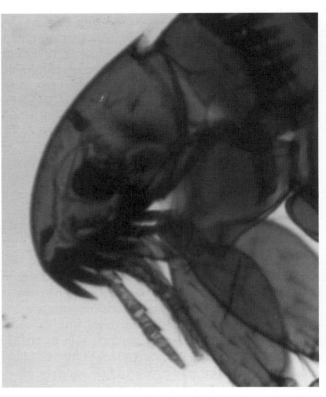

Fig. 15.8 Lateral view of the head of a cat flea, showing combs whose absence or presence and appearance are used in species identification.

usually lies. After 2–14 days these hatch out into larvae that look like small maggots. These feed on skin debris, the faeces of adult fleas and other organic matter in the environment. After about a week, each matured larva spins a cocoon

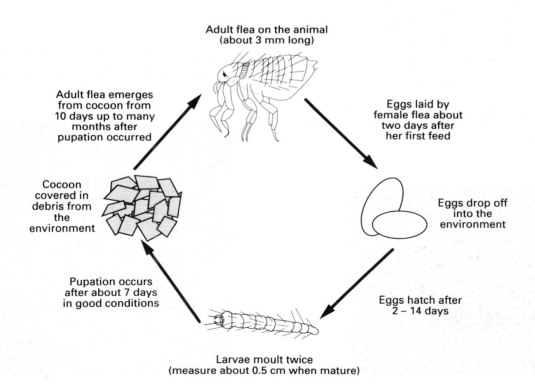

Adult flea on the animal
(about 3 mm long)

Adult flea emerges
from cocoon from
10 days up to many
months after
pupation occurred

Eggs laid by
female flea about
two days after
her first feed

Cocoon
covered in
debris from
the
environment

Eggs drop off
into the
environment

Pupation occurs
after about 7 days
in good conditions

Eggs hatch after
2 – 14 days

Larvae moult twice
(measure about 0.5 cm when mature)

Fig. 15.9 Life cycle of the cat flea.

and pupates. The outside of the cocoon is sticky and so bits of debris from the environment stick to it. After a further 10 days (though this can be considerably longer in cold or dry conditions) the adult flea is fully developed inside the pupa. Before it emerges, it waits for signs of a host being available, e.g. pressure. (This is one explanation for the stories that occur of occupants going into an empty house and being bitten by fleas within hours.) Once emerged from the pupal case the flea will locate a host and jump onto it.

Dipteran flies

Myiasis is defined as parasitism by larvae of the dipteran flies (green-, blue- and black-bottles).

The life cycle is shown in Fig. 15.10. The flies lay their eggs on a suitable site, which might be, though is not necessarily, on an animal, e.g. in the fleece of a sheep or around the anus of a rabbit. Flies are particularly attracted to a smelly animal, such as one that is soiled with diarrhoea. Attraction can be minimised by ensuring animals are kept clean. The larvae (maggots) hatch after as little as 12 hours and begin to traumatise the skin surface and feed off the damaged tissue. Laval development can be prevented by treating the animal with a laval growth inhibitor such as cyromazine. After several moults the larvae drop to the ground. Here they may overwinter as larvae before pupating or they may pupate immediately. Eventually the adult fly emerges from the pupal case.

Arachnids

The arachnids of veterinary importance are the ticks and the mites. The immature larvae that emerge from the eggs appear like a smaller version of the adult, except that they have only three pairs of legs, whereas the nymph and adult stages each have four pairs of legs.

Mites

The mites are all **permanent ectoparasites** (they spend their entire life cycle on the host), except for *Trombicula autumnalis,* where it is only the larva that is sometimes parasitic. Mites may be subdivided into the burrowing and the surface mites. Both types of mite cause dermatitis, which may or may not be itchy, depending on the type of mite present. Diagnosis is usually by inspection of coat brushings, skin scrapes or hair plucks; specific guidance on diagnosis and treatment of each mite is given in Table 15.2.

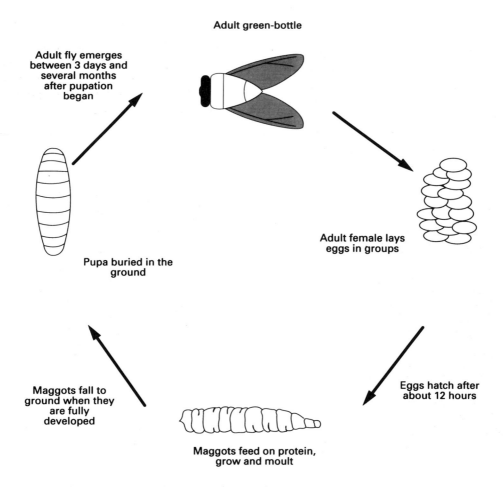

Adult green-bottle

Adult fly emerges between 3 days and several months after pupation began

Pupa buried in the ground

Adult female lays eggs in groups

Maggots fall to ground when they are fully developed

Eggs hatch after about 12 hours

Maggots feed on protein, grow and moult

Fig. 15.10 Life cycle of the blow fly.

Table 15.2 Diagnosis and treatment of mites		
Diagnosis	**Presence of mite in:**	**Treatment**
Sarcoptes scabiei *Notoedres* *Cnemidocoptes* *Demodex* *Cheyletiella*	Skin scrapes or blood test Skin scrapes Skin scrapes Skin scrapes or hair plucks Coat brushings or sellotape strips (adult mite and/or eggs)	Mite infections may be treated with a suitable acaricide such as amitraz or selamectin. Where no licensed product is available, treat with, e.g., fipronil. Where no prolonged activity, repeat treatments after 10–14 days to ensure all immature stages killed. Also treat the environment in *Cheyletiella* infection.
Otodectes cynotis	Ear wax	Clean the ear canal; instil ointment containing suitable acaricide, often in combination with antibiotic. Also treat in-contact animals to clear reservoir of infection. Alternatively, in cats, selamectin spot-on may be used

Burrowing mites

Burrowing mites live in small tunnels within the surface layers of the skin. They lay their eggs within small nests within these tunnels. There are three genera of burrowing mites typically seen in domestic pets:

- *Sarcoptes scabiei* var. *canis*.
- *Notoedres* sp.
- *Cnemidocoptes* spp.

Sarcoptes scabiei var. *canis* (Fig. 15.11) This

mite affects dogs and, very rarely, cats. (*Sarcoptes* species may also cause mange in rodents.) Often the tips of the ears, elbows and then the face are the first areas affected but large areas of the body may be infected in severe cases. Affected areas become hairless, thickened and inflamed. This is partly due to the effect of the mites themselves and partly due to the trauma that the animal causes by rubbing and scratching the affected area – the condition is very itchy. *Sarcoptes* infection in dogs will infect humans but normally the lesions are small and self-limiting. A separate type of *Sarcoptes* is responsible for causing scabies in humans, and another species may cause mange in rodents.

Notoedres   This, the burrowing mite of the cat (Fig. 15.12), is seen very rarely in the UK but it causes similar signs to *Sarcoptes* in the dog. *Notoedres* species infection also occurs in rats.

> **PRACTICAL TIP**
> Look at the antiparasitic treatments in your practice and your local pet shop and familiarise yourself with the trade names containing the active ingredients mentioned in the text.

> **EXAMINATION OF COAT BRUSHINGS**
> Surface brushings are most readily examined in a Petri dish under a low-power dissecting microscope. A portion of the sample may also be prepared and examined as for skin scrapes.

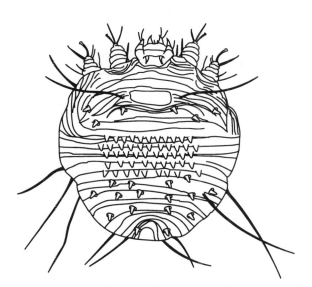

Fig. 15.11 Dorsal view of an adult *Sarcoptes* mite (0.4 mm long). Note the short, stubby legs that barely project beyond the body, spines and pegs, terminal anus, and pedicles at end of legs with suckers on ends.

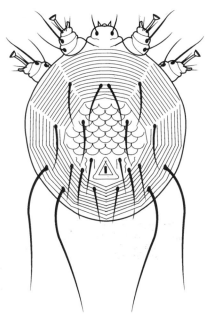

Fig. 15.12 Dorsal view of adult female *Notoedres* mite (0.36 mm) long showing concentric circles on body; dorsal anus.

Cnemidocoptes spp. These mites (Fig. 15.13) are the cause of 'scaly leg' and 'scaly face' in birds, particularly budgerigars.

Demodex This small, cigar-shaped mite (see Fig. 15.14) may be found in normal hair follicles without necessarily causing any problem. In some individuals, particularly young dogs belonging to short-haired breeds, the number of *Demodex* increases dramatically and causes a dermatitis that is characteristically an area of non-itchy alopecia. Often the area around the eyes is first affected. It can be trickier to find than the other burrowing mites as it is smaller and dwells deep within the hair follicle. Hair plucks are often useful to find this mite.

Demodex may also cause mange in hamsters and gerbils. The burrowing mite found in the guinea pig is *Trixacarus caviae*.

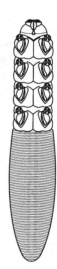

Fig. 15.14 Ventral view of *Demodex* mite showing cigar-shaped body (0.2 mm long).

Surface mites

Otodectes cynotis These are the small ear mites in dogs and cats (Figs 15.15, 15.16). They live within the ear canal, often stimulating a dark brown waxy discharge. Mites may be seen on the surface as small white moving dots. Secondary bacterial infection may result in a pus-like discharge.

Many cats are infected, often without showing clinical signs. Some cats and most dogs show clinical signs of head shaking and ear rubbing when infection is present. This may result in trauma to the ears and haematoma formation in the ear flap.

Ear 'canker' in rabbits is caused by *Psoroptes cuniculi*.

Cheyletiella Animals affected with this fur mite are often said to be affected with 'walking dandruff', since infection often leads to the production of excess scale and since the mites are just visible with the naked eye (they are almost 0.5 mm long; Figs 15.17 and 15.18). Infection does not usually cause any marked loss of hair. Often the mites will move onto humans handling the animals and, though they will not survive for long periods, they will often bite. Small raised red spots appear in the affected areas of the human body.

Trombicula autumnalis This mite (also known as *Neotrombicula autumnalis*) normally becomes a problem in late summer and autumn, particularly in chalky areas of southern England. The larval mites (Fig. 15.19) attach themselves to the legs of passing animals, including dogs or cats, and feed, causing intense irritation to the host.

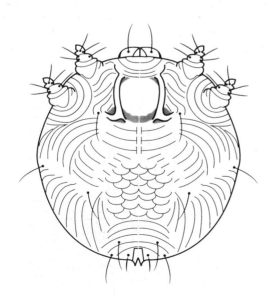

Fig. 15.13 Dorsal view of a *Cnemidocoptes* mite (0.2 mm long).

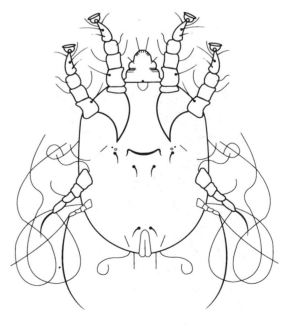

Fig. 15.15 Dorsal view of *Otodectes* mite (0.4 mm long). Note the longer legs protruding from the body and unjoined pedicles (stalks) with suckers on the ends.

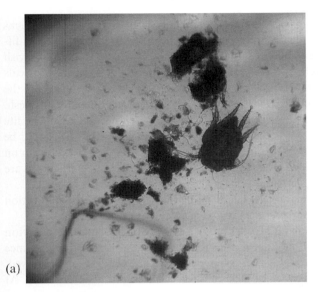

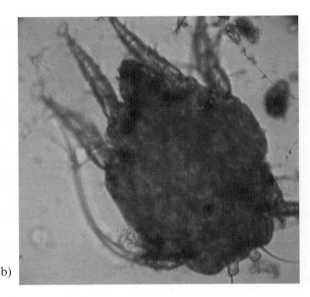

Fig. 15.16 (a) Debris from ear canal. (b) Increasing magnification of a single mite (0.4 mm long).

Dermanyssus This is the 'red mite' that sucks blood of chickens and occasionally other animals. All stages live off the host, e.g. in the eaves of poultry houses. The mites visit chickens to feed, particularly at night. Infection causes irritation and debility, with anaemia in heavy infections. Control is by cleaning the hen-house and treatment with an acaricide.

Ticks

Ticks on livestock are important in many parts of the world as carriers or vectors of disease. (A **vector** is a carrier of disease where development of disease may or may not

occur in the carrier – it may simply transfer the infection from one host to the next or a developmental stage may occur in the tick.) A heavy tick burden may cause anaemia. In small animal practice it is more usual to encounter just one or two ticks on a cat or dog, with an owner who is concerned about how to get rid of them. However, even in these low numbers, ticks can transmit infections such as the Lyme disease agent, *Borrelia burgdorferi*, to dogs. Since the advent of the Pet Travel Scheme, there is an increased opportunity for some of the tick-transmitted diseases present in mainland Europe to be introduced into the UK. In order to prevent infected ticks entering the UK it is mandatory for dogs or cats to be treated with an approved acaricide before their return to the UK. Details of the latest requirements may be found on the DEFRA website at www.defra.gov.uk.

Several species of ticks may affect dogs in the UK and one of these (*Ixodes canisuga*) is host specific to the dog. However, by far the most common ticks seen on small animals are the sheep tick (*Ixodes ricinus*) (Fig. 15.21), particularly in country dwellers, and the hedgehog tick (*Ixodes*

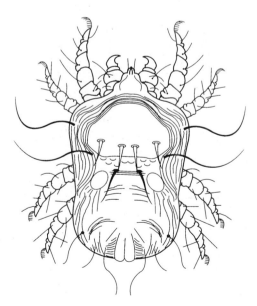

Fig. 15.17 Dorsal view of *Cheyletiella* mite (0.4 mm). Note the 'comb' on the end of each leg and the large palps on either side of the head, each with a large claw.

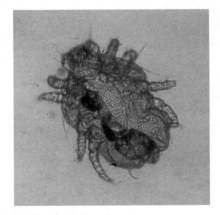

Fig. 15.18 Cheyletiella mite (0.4 mm).

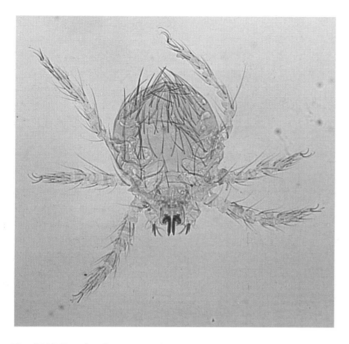

Fig. 15.19 *Trombicula autumunalis* (Harvest mite) larva (1 mm long, orange-brown in colour). Note that there are only three pairs of legs.

hexagonus), common especially in urban areas. These ticks are remarkably cosmopolitan and will attach to many different hosts. Initially all that is visible is a small greyish swelling, firmly attached to the animal. Inspection reveals pairs of legs close to the attachment with the host; the mouth parts (Fig. 15.22) are buried into the animal's flesh. Once the tick has fed fully it will drop off its host. The life cycle of the sheep tick is shown in Fig. 15.20. It should be noted that some other ticks, such as the dog tick, remain on the host from larva to adult and only drop off once they are fully fed adults.

Diagnosis is based on finding the ticks. The identification of the species of tick is a specialised skill.

Individual ticks may be removed by dabbing a cotton wool bud that has been treated with an acaricide (substance that is toxic to ticks). Once dead they can be gently removed. A number of tick removal devices are also available. At times of tick challenge it may be worthwhile carrying out prophylactic treatment to ensure any ticks are repelled from the dog or cat and/or that any that do attach are killed soon afterwards. There are a number of products available to achieve this, some of which will protect against flea infestation at the same time.

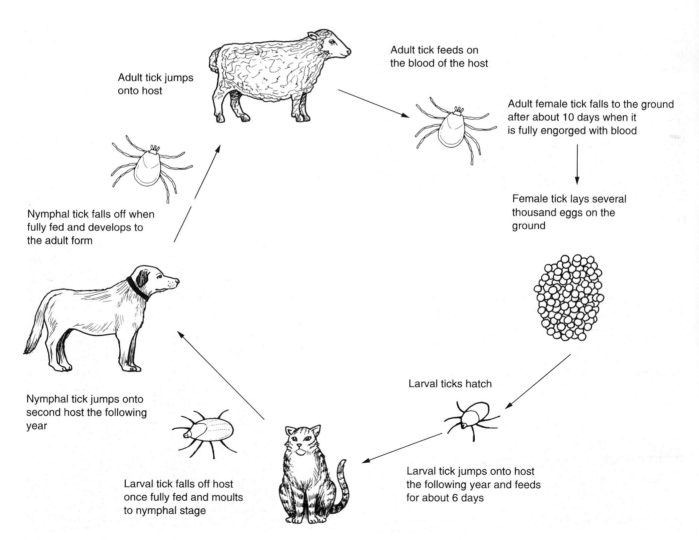

Fig. 15.20 Life cycle of the sheep tick.

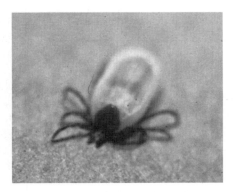

Fig. 15.21 Engorged adult female sheep tick *Ixodes ricinus*, measuring approximately 7 mm. Note the small dark brown scutum or plate near to the head.

> *PRACTICAL TIP*
> Never try to pull off a live tick unless using an effective 'tick remover', as its mouthparts may be left embedded in the animal and may become a focus for infection.

Endoparasites

Endoparasites may be further subdivided into helminths and protozoa. The **helminths** are the worms and are further subdivided into three types: the **flukes** (which are found in the liver of sheep and cattle but do not normally affect dogs or cats in the UK), the tapeworms or **cestodes**, and the round worms or **nematodes**. The **protozoal parasites** are small unicellular organisms. Table 15.3 lists the species in each category seen in small animal veterinary practice.

Helminths

Cestodes (tapeworms)

A cestode is tape-like and has no alimentary tract. It is composed of three parts: the head or scolex, an area behind this where segments or proglottids form and finally the maturing segments (Fig. 15.25).

Each tapeworm has an immature stage that develops in a separate or intermediate host; the exact structure varies according to the species of tapeworm.

The tapeworms in cats and dogs are *Echinococcus granulosus* (dogs), *Dipylidium caninum* (dogs and cats) and the *Taenia* species (one species in cats and several species in dogs). Their presence is not normally any problem to the final host, though the sight of tapeworm segments is repugnant to owners. There is more often a problem with infec-

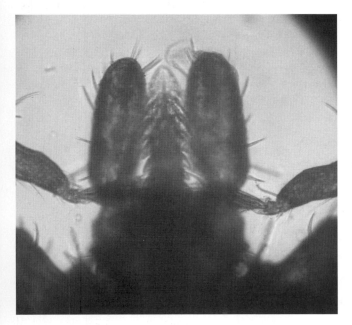

Fig. 15.22 Mouth parts of tick.

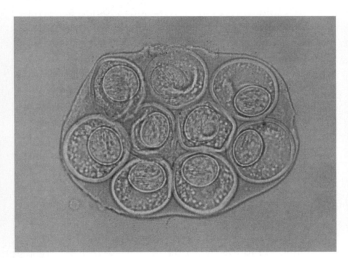

Fig. 15.23 A *Dipylidium caninum* 'egg packet'.

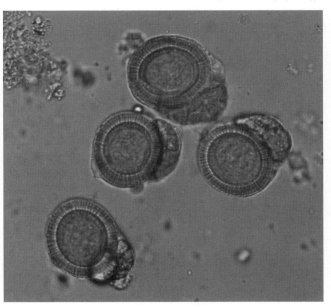

Fig. 15.24 *Taenia* spp. eggs, each approximately 40 μm in diameter.

Table 15.3 Species of endoparasite

	Species	Affects
Helminths		
Flukes		
Cestodes	*Echinococcus granulosus granulosus*	Dogs
(tapeworms)	*Echinococcus granulosus equinus*	Dogs
	Echinococcus multilocularis	Dogs and cats[a]
	Dipylidium caninum	Dogs/cats
	Taenia spp.	Cats/dogs
Nematodes		
(roundworms)		
Ascarids	*Toxocara canis*	Dogs
	Toxascaris leonina	Cats/dogs
	Toxocara cati	Cats
Hookworms	*Uncinaria stenocephala*	Dogs
	Ancylostoma tubaeforme	Cats[b]
	Ancylostoma caninum	Dogs
Whipworm	*Trichuris vulpis*	Dogs
Heart worm	*Dirofilaria immitis*[c]	Dogs
Capillaria	*C. plica*	Dogs
	C. hepatica	
Lungworms	*Aelurostrongylus abstrusus*	Cats
	Angiostrongylus vasorum	Dogs
	Oslerus osleri	Dogs
Protozoa		
Coccidia	*Eimeria intestinalis*	Rabbits
	E. flavescens	Rabbits
	E. stiedae	Rabbits
Isospora		Dogs/cats
Cryptosporidium parvum		Dogs/cats
Sarcocystis spp.		Dogs/cats
Toxoplasma gondii		Cats
Neospora caninum		Dogs
Hammondia		Cats
Giardia		Dogs
Babesia		Dogs[d]

[a] *Mainland Europe only*

[b] *Hookworm infection occurs rarely in cats in the UK*

[c] *Not UK – endemic in the Mediterranean area*

[d] *Not in the UK, though infected dogs may be imported from the southern part of mainland Europe*

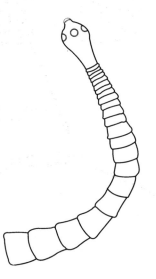

Fig. 15.25 Typical adult cestode.

TAPEWORM DEFINITIONS

Adult tapeworm:

- **Scolex**: head of a tapeworm – used for attachment to the host's intestine using suckers and the rostellum (where present) for attachment.
- **Strobila**: the chain of individual segments.
- **Rostellum**: the anterior part of the scolex, present in most tapeworms. It is a protrusible cone and is armed with hooks in some species.
- **Proglottid**: name for each individual segment that makes up the strobilia.

Immature tapeworms (**metacestodes**)

- **Cysticercus**: fluid-filled cyst containing a single invaginated scolex attached to the cyst wall.
- **Cysticeroid**: single evaginated scolex (this is the form found in invertebrate intermediate hosts).
- **Hydatid cyst**: large cyst containing many scolices, some loose in the fluid inside and some contained within 'brood capsules'.
- **Coenurus**: a cyst with many invaginated scolices attached to the cyst wall.

tion of the intermediate host, either because the presence of the tapeworm cysts causes disease or because affected meat is condemned as unfit for human consumption.

Dipylidium caninum

This is probably the most common tapeworm of cats and dogs in the UK. The intermediate host is the flea, and the biting louse in the case of the dog. It is normally diagnosed by the presence of motile segments (shaped like rice grains) around the anus or in the faeces of a cat or dog (see Fig. 15.23). The life cycle is shown in Fig. 15.26.

> **PRACTICAL TIP**
> Control depends on treating the existing infection then eliminating any flea or louse problem to break the transmission cycle. *D. caninum* occasionally infects man.

Taenia spp.

Dogs and cats are affected with the taeniid tapeworms when they eat raw meat, either in the form of uncooked meat or offal or through catching and eating prey containing the intermediate stages. The life cycle of *Taenia hydatigena* is shown in Fig. 15.27, and the names of the specific tapeworms with their final and intermediate hosts are shown in Table 15.4.

Diagnosis is based on seeing segments passed by the animal. More rarely eggs, liberated from the segments, are seen during microscopic examination of a faecal sample. These are smaller than *Toxocara* eggs (see Fig. 15.24), measuring about 40 μm in diameter.

Control is based on treating the current infection, then preventing the animal having access to uncooked flesh, which is something that is easy to do where the animal is fed by the owner but more difficult if the infection is derived from wild prey.

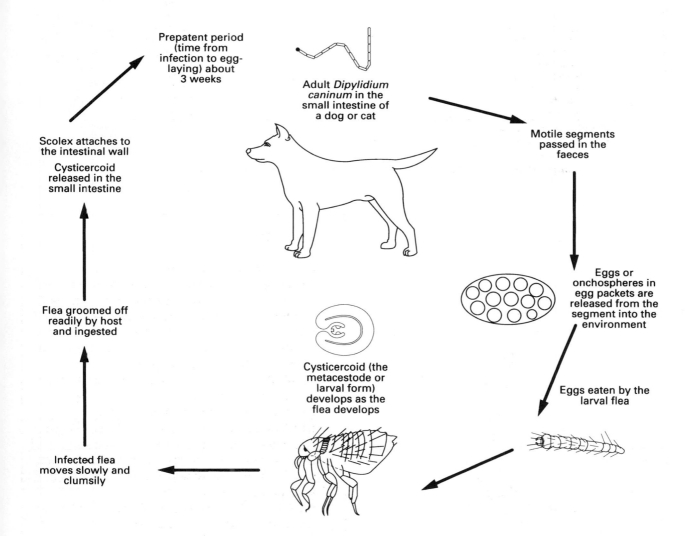

Fig. 15.26 Life cycle of *Dipylidium caninum*.

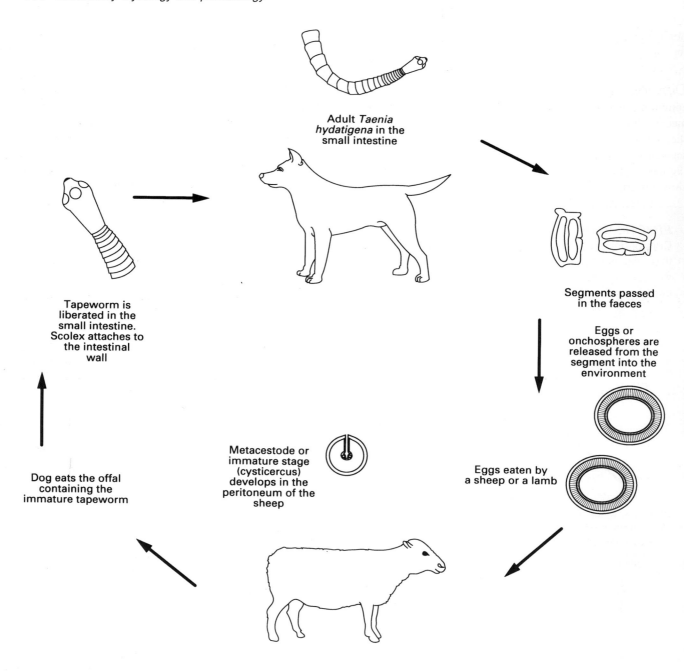

Fig. 15.27 Life cycle of *Taenia hydatigena*.

Table 15.4 Hosts of *Taenia* tapeworms		
Name of *Taenia* species	**Final host**	**Intermediate host**
T. taeniaeformis	Cat	Rat or mouse (*Cysticercus fasciolaris* in the liver)
T. serialis	Dog	Rabbit (*Coenurus serialis* in connective tissue)
T. pisiformis	Dog	Rabbit (*Cysticercus pisiformis* in the peritoneum)
T. ovis	Dog	Sheep (*Cysticercus ovis* in muscle)
T. hydatigena	Dog	Sheep/cattle/pig (*Cysticercus tenuicollis* in the peritoneum)
T. multiceps	Dog	Sheep/cattle (*Coenurus cerebralis* in the central nervous system)

Echinococcus granulosus granulosus. This organism has a dog-to-sheep life cycle (Fig. 15.28). It is an important zoonosis that occurs in the UK but is fortunately fairly rare – it is most common in rural areas, such as parts of Wales, where dogs have the opportunity to feed on sheep carcasses on the hills. Following accidental ingestion of eggs, hydatid cysts can develop in man, particularly in the liver or lungs.

The adult parasite is very small, only about 6 mm long, and several thousand may be present in the intestine of a single dog. Dogs in affected areas should be regularly treated with an effective anthelmintic and denied access to sheep carcasses.

If a human ingests a proglottid or individual eggs, then a hydatid cyst may develop in the liver or lungs in the same way as it will develop in the sheep. This forms a space-occupying lesion that may grow to some considerable size. Treatment of affected people is based on anthelmintic treatment followed by draining the cyst then surgically removing the wall of the cyst. This is quite a hazardous procedure for the patient.

Echinococcus granulosus equinus is a separate tapeworm that has a dog-to-horse life cycle. It occurs particularly where hounds are fed on horse offal. It is not believed to pose a zoonotic risk.

Echinococcus multilocularis is a related tapeworm found in continental Europe, where it is particularly recognised in Switzerland. The intermediate stage, a multilocular invasive cyst, is normally found in rodents but man can be infected. Dogs, foxes and cats can act as final hosts, though cats are considered to be a poorer host. This parasite is the reason for the necessity to treat animals returning to the UK with praziquantel. Up-to-date information about this and other requirements of the pet travel scheme may be found at www.defra.gov.uk/animalh/quarantine/index.htm.

Cestode infections in other animals

Birds and other animals such as rabbits, mice, rats and hamsters may all be infected with adult tapeworms specific to the host species. In most cases infection has no effect on the host.

Occasionally a heavy tapeworm burden in hamsters may be associated with weight loss and perhaps intestinal blockage. In each case the intermediate host is an invertebrate such as a beetle or mite.

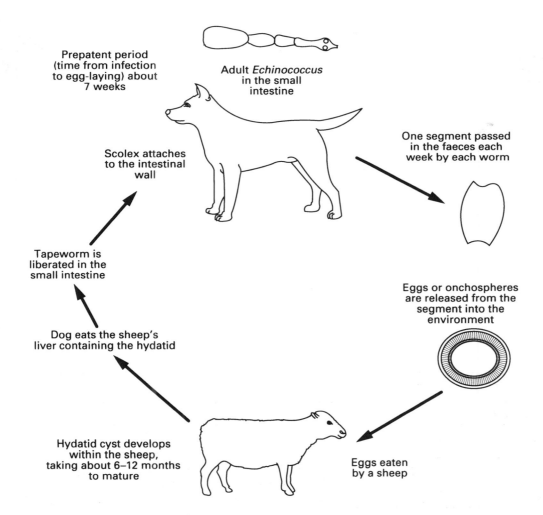

Fig. 15.28 Life cycle of *Echinococcus granulosus granulosus.*

Treatment of cestode infections

The adult tapeworm can be killed with a number of anthelmintics; these may be products that only have activity against tapeworms, in which case they are known as cestocides. Alternatively, the preparation may have activity against other helminths, particularly nematodes, as well as tapeworms; these are known as broad-spectrum anthelmintics. The active ingredients that have cestocidal activity are shown in Table 15.5.

It is much more difficult to kill the immature tapeworm infections in the intermediate hosts and this is not usually carried out.

Nematodes

Nematodes are round worms with a proper digestive tract. Most have a direct life cycle, though some (e.g. the lungworms) have a slug or snail intermediate host. Others may be carried by a **paratenic host** (one that acts as carrier only – no development of the parasite occurs in this host).

Major groups of nematodes

Important nematode groups seen in small animal veterinary practice include:

- Ascarids (especially *Toxocara canis, Toxascaris leonina* and *Toxocara cati* in dogs and cats). Large, fleshy worms (Fig. 15.29), most numerous and frequent in young animals. Ascarids occur commonly in other animals including reptiles (e.g. tortoises) and birds (especially parakeets); in each case the ascarid species is host specific. Heavy burdens may be associated with poor growth or intestinal impactions.
- Hookworms (*Uncinaria stenocephala* and *Ancylostoma caninum*).
- Whipworm (*Trichuris vulpis*).
- Heart worm (*Dirofilaria immitis*) (not in UK).

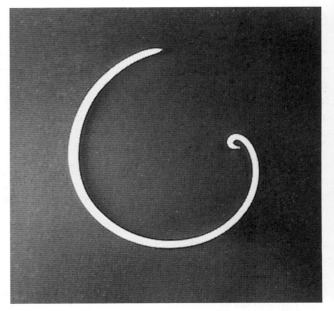

Fig. 15.29 Typical appearance of adult ascarid (approximately 6 cm long).

- Bladder and liver worms (*Capillaria* spp.).
- Lungworms (*Aelurostrongylus abstrusus, Angiostrongylus vasorum, Crenosoma vulpis* and *Oslerus osleri* – formerly known as *Filaroides osleri*).

Toxocara canis This is a very important worm, since it is a zoonosis and can also cause disease in young pups. Its life cycle is shown in Fig. 15.30.

Pups are first infected before birth by **larvae** that pass from the bitch's muscles to her uterus after about the 42nd day of pregnancy. These larvae migrate through the liver and lungs of the young pups and are then coughed up and swallowed. They remain in the small intestine where they develop to **adult worms** by the time that the pups are 3 weeks of age. The pups can also receive further infection from infective eggs in the environment and by infective larvae that pass in the mother's milk. Usually the majority of

Table 15.5 Anthelmintics

Name of active ingredient	Trade name	Animal	Activity
Dichlorophen	Numerous	Dog, cat	C
Praziquantel	Droncit	Dog, cat	C
Fenbendazole	Panacur/Zerofen	Dog, cat	NC
Mebendazole	Telmin KH	Dog	NC
Nitroscanate	Lopatol/Troscan	Dog	NC
Piperazine	Numerous	Dog, cat	N
Pyrantel	Strongid	Dog	N
Pyrantel/febantel	Drontal	Puppy dog	N
Pyrantel/praziquantel/febantel	Drontal plus	Dog	NC
Pyrantel/praziquantel	Drontal Cat	Cat	NC
Selamectin	Stronghold	Dog, cat	N
Lufeneuron/milbemycin oxime	Program Plus	Dog	N

N, nematodes; C, cestodes. This indicates that those preparations have activity against some, though not necessarily all, nematodes or cestodes. The reader is directed to the NOAH Compendium for further details on individual products

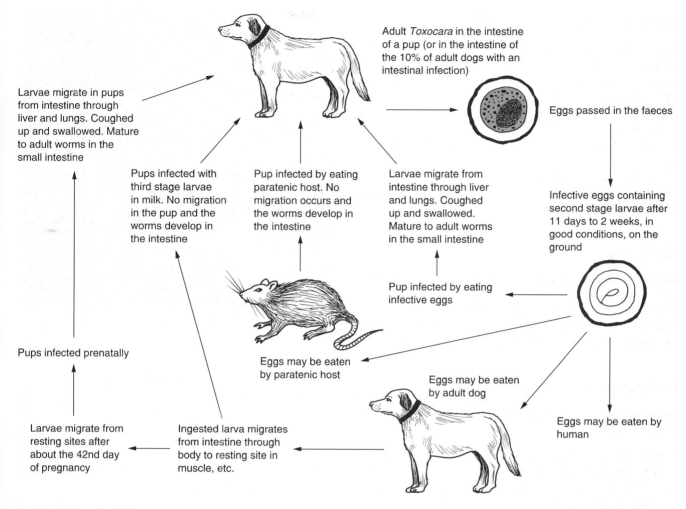

Fig. 15.30 Life cycle of *Toxocara canis*.

the infection will have occurred across the placenta. Pups that have a heavy *Toxocara* burden will typically be stunted with distended bellies; they may vomit and/or have diarrhoea, and severe infections may lead to a total blockage of the intestine.

As immunity develops following exposure, and possibly related to an increase in age, pups begin to expel their *Toxocara* infection spontaneously from about 7 weeks of age. Most have expelled all of their adult worms by 6–7 months of age. Normally further larvae that are ingested pass from the intestine to muscle where they enter a resting state.

Adult worms pass large numbers of **eggs** (as many as several thousand eggs per gram of faeces in a 3-week-old pup). Each egg is surrounded by a thick wall (Fig. 15.31) which is very resistant to either physical or chemical damage. The eggs are not immediately infective but require time for a larva to develop inside. In ideal conditions this will take about 14 days, but may take much longer in low temperatures. Since the larva remains in the shell until eaten by an animal, the eggs may remain infective in the environment for at least 2 years.

Larvae that are accidentally eaten by **other animals** (including humans), migrate from the intestine and enter a resting state in other tissues. If a **human** ingests a large number of infective eggs and these all migrate together through the body, a condition known as 'visceral larval migrans' may develop, associated with signs of damage to the organs through which the larvae are migrating. If only a few larvae are ingested, they will usually migrate through the human

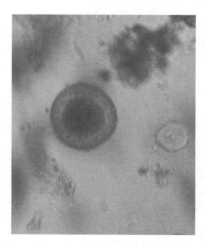

Fig. 15.31 *Toxocara canis* egg (approximately 80 µm diameter). Note the dark contents and dark shell with pitted edge.

body without any signs of illness, except in the rare case where they come to rest in the eye, when sight disfunction or even blindness may result. Infection is usually seen in children, as they are the most likely to have unhygienic habits. If the animal that ingests the eggs happens to be a *bitch*, the larvae remain in this resting state until she becomes pregnant; some of the larvae will migrate to infect her pups; and others will remain to infect her subsequent litters.

To perpetuate their life cycle, dormant larvae in the tissues of birds or animals other than dogs depend upon their paratenic host being eaten by a dog.

In about 10% of **adult dogs**, for one reason or another, including a low level of challenge, adult worms will develop in the small intestine. Lactating bitches are particularly likely to have a patent infection, probably due to the change in their hormonal status. Their infection may come from a number of sources including young worms passed by the pups that the bitch ingests as she cleans up around the nest. Usually the bitch expels her remaining infection shortly after the pups are weaned.

CONTROL OF TOXOCARA CANIS
The aims are:
- Control of infection in the dog to prevent disease in pups, and eggs put into the environment.
- Prevention of infection in children.

Control in dogs is based on:
- Prenatal infection in the pups may be controlled by treating the bitch, prior to whelping, with a product that will kill the migrating larvae, e.g. fenbendazole from the 42nd day of pregnancy to 2 days post-whelping.
- Alternatively, the pups may be treated at regular intervals with a suitable anthelmintic, starting from 2 weeks of age; the bitch should be treated at the same time.
- Reducing the number of eggs in the environment is very difficult once the eggs are present. Scorching with a flame-thrower has been found to be the most effective method, but education of the dog-owning public is the best way to reduce egg output in the future.

The most important methods of preventing children from becoming infected are to ensure that:
- Dogs defecate in specified areas in parks.
- Children wash their hands before eating.
- Children are discouraged from handling young pups unless the animals have been thoroughly wormed.
- Use 'pooper scoopers' or other means of appropriate faeces disposal.

Toxascaris leonina   This ascarid will infect both cats and dogs. Its life cycle is shown in Fig. 15.32. It has rarely been implicated as a zoonosis.

There is no prenatal infection; therefore infection is usually first seen in adolescent animals. The worm is not normally associated with clinical signs, since large burdens are reasonably well tolerated.

The egg (Fig. 15.33) can be distinguished by the smooth outer wall to the shell.

Toxocara cati   This organism is responsible for ascarid infection in cats, particularly kittens. It is transmitted to kittens by their mothers' milk; infection also occurs through infective eggs in the environment and ingestion of paratenic hosts (Fig. 15.34). A heavy infection may cause stunting of kittens and a pot-bellied appearance.

The adult worm can be distinguished by the appearance of the alae or 'wings' either side of the head end (Fig. 15.35). The egg is grossly indistinguishable from that of *T. canis*.

Control is by regular treatment of kittens from about 3 weeks of age until they are several months of age (kittens are infected via the milk so will be 6 weeks old or more before the first infection becomes patent).

Hookworms   Hookworms are short, stout worms (Fig. 15.36) with hooked heads. *Uncinaria stenocephala* and *Ancylostoma caninum* occur in the small intestine of the dog. *U. stenocephala* is the more common of the two in the UK and is known as the northern hookworm; it is particularly seen in greyhounds or hunt kennels.

The two species may be distinguished by the appearance of the head: *A. caninum* has three pairs of large teeth. *A. braziliense* (Fig. 15.37) has two pairs of similar teeth, whilst *U. stenocephala* has plates in the mouth cavity. The life cycle is shown in Fig. 15.38.

The worms attach to the intestinal mucosa by their mouthparts. They use their teeth to damage the surface and then feed off the tissue fluids, particularly blood in the case of *A. caninum*. A heavy *Uncinaria* spp. burden may cause a dog to be thin and *Ancylostoma* spp. may cause anaemia. Eggs produced by the adult female worms are passed in the faeces.

The infective larvae of both worms may penetrate the skin. *Uncinaria* spp. larvae simply cause a dermatitis as the larvae are incapable of travelling further, whereas *Ancylostoma* spp. larvae may travel to the intestine and develop to adults. Bitches may infect their pups with *Ancylostoma* spp. larvae via their milk. Cats can be infected with hookworm but infection appears rare in the UK.

Whipworm   *Trichuris vulpis*, the whipworm of the dog, has a whiplike appearance (Fig. 15.39). The worms burrow into the mucosa of the large intestine, leaving the thicker caudal end in the intestinal lumen. A low burden is well tolerated but a heavy infection may be associated with a bloody, mucus-filled diarrhoea.

The eggs in which the larvae develop are characteristic (Fig. 15.40) and are covered in a thick shell which makes them resistant to damage in the environment. Eggs containing infective first stage larvae may survive for several years in the ground. *T. vulpis* therefore tends to cause problems when dogs have access to permanent grass runs but clinical signs are rarely seen in the UK.

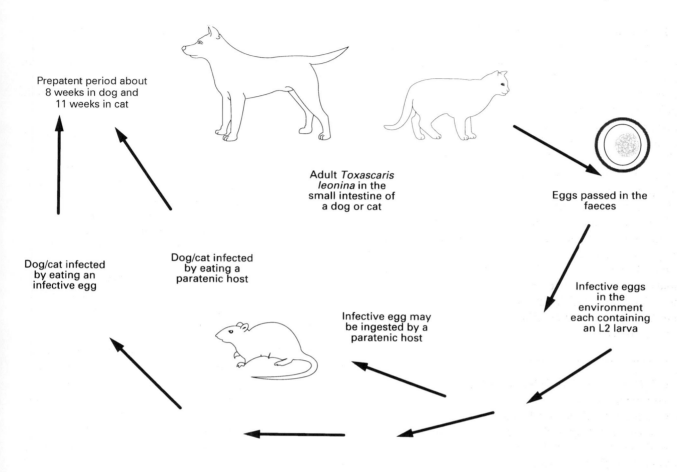

Prepatent period about
8 weeks in dog and
11 weeks in cat

Adult *Toxascaris
leonina* in the
small intestine of
a dog or cat

Eggs passed in the
faeces

Dog/cat infected
by eating an
infective egg

Dog/cat infected
by eating a
paratenic host

Infective eggs
in the
environment
each containing
an L2 larva

Infective egg may
be ingested by a
paratenic host

Fig. 15.32 Life cycle of *Toxascaris leonina*.

The heartworm

Dirofilaria immitis does not occur in the UK but may be seen in dogs that are imported from warmer countries. The adult worms live in the heart and the immature larvae are known as microfilariae. These are dispersed in the host's blood and transmission occurs when a mosquito transfers the microfilariae from one host to another. A light infection in a dog may be well tolerated but a larger burden can lead to right-sided heart failure. Infection in cats is somewhat less common but clinical effects of just a single worm can be severe in cats. This is another parasite to consider when owners are planning to take their pet to mainland Europe, as heartworm is endemic from the Mediterranean area of France southwards. Prophylactic treatment should be carried out by owners, using one of the treatments now licensed in the UK, following data sheet instructions.

Bladder and liver worms (*Capillaria* spp.)

Adult worms of *Capillaria plica* live in the bladder and so the eggs are passed in the urine of affected dogs. The eggs appear very like *Trichuris* eggs, but are smaller with less distinct plugs. Infection is rarely seen in the UK.

Capillaria hepatica is a parasite of rats, particularly wild rats. The adult worm lives in the liver of the host, where it lays its eggs. These are only released when the rat dies or is eaten by another animal. Cats, dogs and man may be infected, but this occurs very rarely.

Other *Capillaria* species specific to birds may cause diarrhoea in pigeons.

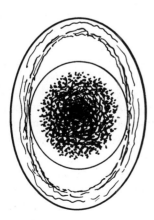

Fig. 15.33 *Toxascaris leonina* egg (approximately 85 μm long). Note the smooth outer wall. Contents are paler than those of *Toxocara* species.

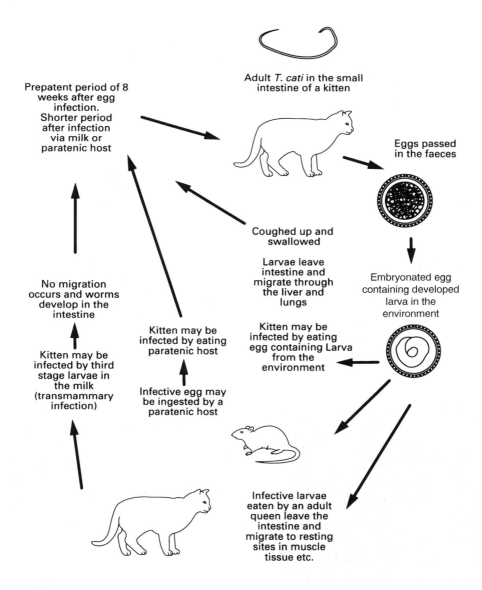

Fig. 15.34 Life cycle of *Toxocara cati*.

Lungworms   Cats become infected with *Aelurostrongylus abstrusus* (cat lungworm) by eating a slug or snail containing the infective larvae. The adult worm lives within the lung tissue of the cat. Infection with many worms may cause coughing, but a few worms often go unnoticed.

Adult females produce larvae (rather than eggs) that are coughed up and swallowed. Diagnosis is confirmed by finding larvae in the faeces using the Baermann technique.

Dogs acquire *Angiostrongylus vasorum* infection through eating a snail containing the infective larvae. Transmission of this infection in England was confined to Cornwall and South Wales, but it is now being seen in southern England as well.

The slender adult worms live in the pulmonary artery of the dog. The adult females produce eggs that travel to the alveoli, hatch and the larvae then penetrate through the alveolar walls. The larvae are then coughed up, swallowed and passed in the faeces. Clinical signs include coughing and dyspnoea.

Faeces may be examined for presence of the larvae using the Baermann technique.

Oslerus osleri (formerly Filaroides osleri)   The adult worms live in small nodules at the bifurcation of the trachea (in dogs, particularly greyhounds). The nodules can be seen on endoscopy and they may cause coughing in some dogs but others tolerate their presence without showing symptoms.

The adult female worms produce larvae that are coughed up and swallowed. The life cycle is direct (i.e. the parasite passes directly from one host to the next without having to infect an alternative or intermediate host) and the bitch may infect her pups as she grooms them.

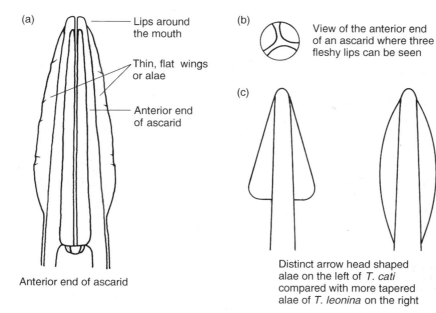

(a) Lips around the mouth

Thin, flat wings or alae

Anterior end of ascarid

Anterior end of ascarid

(b) View of the anterior end of an ascarid where three fleshy lips can be seen

(c) Distinct arrow head shaped alae on the left of *T. cati* compared with more tapered alae of *T. leonina* on the right

Fig. 15.35 Anterior end and alae of adult ascarid.

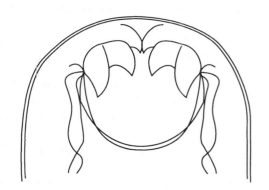

Fig. 15.36 Hook worm next to one pence piece.

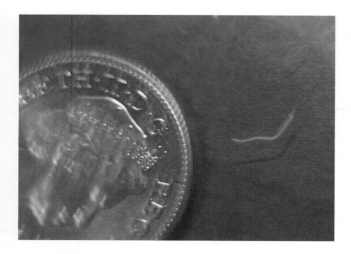

Fig. 15.37 Head of *Ancyclostoma braziliense*, showing two pairs of teeth at the entrance to the buccal capsule. *Uncinaria stenocephala* has a similar sized buccal capsule but with cutting plates instead of teeth. *A. caninum* has three pairs of teeth.

Diagnosis of nematode infections

It is important that faecal samples are fresh and are quickly picked up from the ground, otherwise the sample can become contaminated with free-living nematodes and their eggs from the environment. The main diagnostic methods are modified McMaster techniques to detect nematode eggs in faeces and the Baermann technique to detect larvae.

Treatment of nematode infections

Treatment of nematode infections is carried out in three main situations:

- Regular treatment to remove any infections that may have accumulated since the animal was last wormed. A broad-spectrum anthelmintic with additional cestocidal activity is often used. Adult dogs and cats will usually be treated at 3–6-month intervals. There is now an option to control nematodes and fleas at the same time using either selamectin (Stronghold) in cats and dogs or lufenuron and milbemycin (Program Plus) in dogs; both treatments are administered at monthly intervals. Control of tapeworms, where necessary, has to be carried out separately.
- Control of *Toxocara* infections in puppies and kittens. Since these infections occur in the vast majority of litters it is normal to treat all puppies and kittens regularly.
- Treatment of an animal where the presence of a nematode infection has been diagnosed as the cause of a clinical problem. Here the product with the best activity against that infection will usually be chosen.

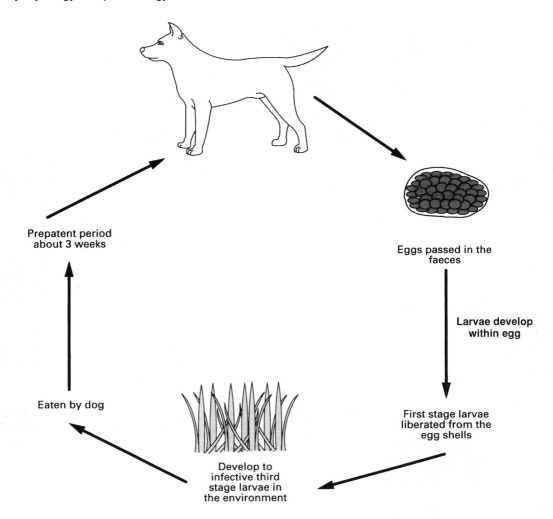

Fig. 15.38 Life cycle of *Uncinaria stenocephala*.

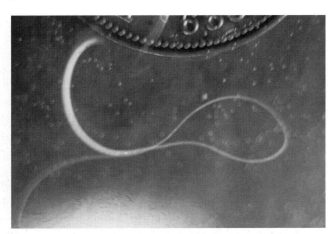

Fig. 15.39 Whipworm (*Trichuris vulpis*). Note the wide posterior end and the narrow anterior end normally buried in the mucosa of the largest intestine (1–3 cm).

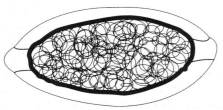

Fig. 15.40 *Trichuris vulpis* egg (approximately 70 μm long). Note plugs at both ends.

Protozoal parasites

Major protozoal parasites

Coccidia   Coccidia may cause marked diarrhoea in young animals, particularly lambs, birds and rabbits.

Rabbits may be infected with three *Eimeria* spp., all of which have the typical coccidian life cycle (Fig. 15.41).

- *Eimeria intestinalis* and *E. flavescens* infect the caecum, causing diarrhoea and emaciation.
- *E. stiedae* infects the bile ducts in the liver, causing wasting, diarrhoea and excess urine production.

Diagnosis is based on finding oocysts present in the faeces (Fig. 15.42). The small rod-like organisms found in the faeces of sick rabbits are not coccidia and are not believed to be significant.

Treatment such as sulphonamide may be given in the rabbits' drinking water, or to pet rabbits on an individual basis. Control is based on making sure that the rabbits have clean bedding and that droppings and/or diarrhoea are not allowed to build up in the feeding area.

Isospora   This protozoan is also known as *Levineia*. Two species infect cats and another two infect dogs.

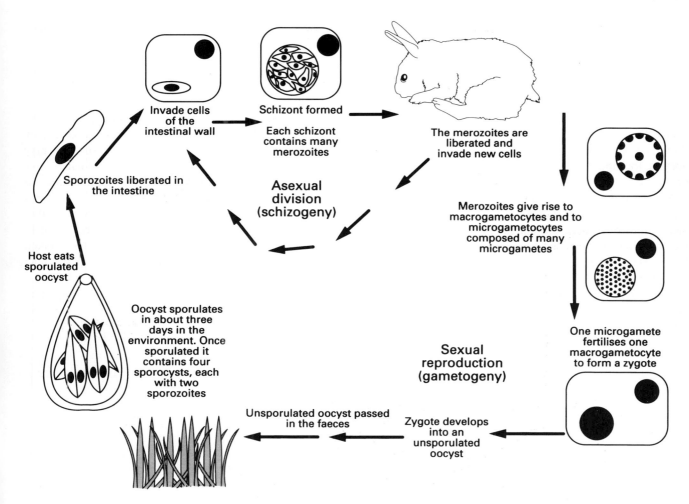

Fig. 15.41 Life cycle of *Eimeria* spp.

The animals are infected when they ingest either sporulated oocysts (oocysts are not sporulated until a few days after they were passed in the faeces) or infected intermediate hosts. Reproduction occurs in the cells lining the small intestine.

Infection is usually associated with few clinical signs – but there may be transient diarrhoea. Heavy infection may cause severe diarrhoea in puppies and kittens.

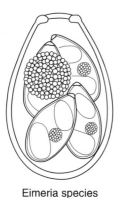

Eimeria species

Fig. 15.42 Sporulated oocyst of *Eimeria* spp.

Cryptosporidium parvum   This is a small protozoan that parasitises epithelial cells in the small intestine. Both asexual and sexual reproduction occurs in the intestine and small oocysts, the result of sexual reproduction, are passed in the faeces. Infection occurs by ingesting sporulated oocysts; this has been associated with diarrhoea in young puppies and kittens and the young of other domestic animals. Humans may be infected, usually only causing a transient diarrhoea, though severe diarrhoea may be associated with infection in immunocompromised individuals.

Diagnosis is based on finding the oocysts (4.5–5 μm diameter) in the faeces. Identification may be assisted by staining with Ziehl–Neelsen, as the oocysts are acid fast, or by immunofluorescence techniques. There is currently no licensed treatment for the infection in small animals.

Sarcocystis   This organism has a more complex life cycle than the coccidia and therefore is classified separately. The intermediate hosts are ruminants, pigs or horses. Large unsightly cysts are formed in muscle, so infected meat is condemned. In addition, infection may result in marked illness in the infected animal. The final host for each species is the dog or the cat. For example, *Barcocystis tenella* (also known as *Sarocystis ovicanis*) is a parasite of sheep and dogs.

Reproduction occurs in the small intestine without clinical signs. The oocysts, measuring approximately 10–15 μm, are already sporulated when passed.

Toxoplasma gondii

The final host for *T. gondii* is the cat (Fig. 15.43). Sexual reproduction occurs in the epithelial cells of the small intestine. Oocysts are produced that are passed in the faeces. The cat usually shows no sign of infection and normally, after excreting oocysts for about 10 days, becomes immune and stops production.

Asexual reproduction occurs in the extra-intestinal (outside the intestine) tissue of almost any animal. Following ingestion of oocysts or asexual stages the sporozoites leave the intestine and travel to tissue, particularly muscle or brain. Here they divide to form **tachyzoites**. Once an immune response is started by the host these undergo slower division; they are then known as **bradyzoites**. These remain in the tissue in the hope that they will one day be eaten by a cat.

These cysts in tissue are minute and cause little problem except in certain circumstances:

- An ewe is infected for the first time during pregnancy. Some cysts may occur in the placenta and may cause abortion.
- A woman is infected for the first time during pregnancy, e.g. by eating meat containing bradyzoites or accidentally swallowing sporulated oocysts. Infection of the fetus may result and, depending on the stage of preg-nancy, this may result in abortion, severe abnormalities or no clinical signs at all. Fortunately, infections during human pregnancy are not common. Further information and information leaflets can be obtained from Tommy's, The Baby Charity, who have taken over the work of the Toxoplasmosis Trust in the UK: www.tommys.org/website.
- Infection in humans may be associated with malaise and 'flu-like symptoms that vary in severity from individual to individual.

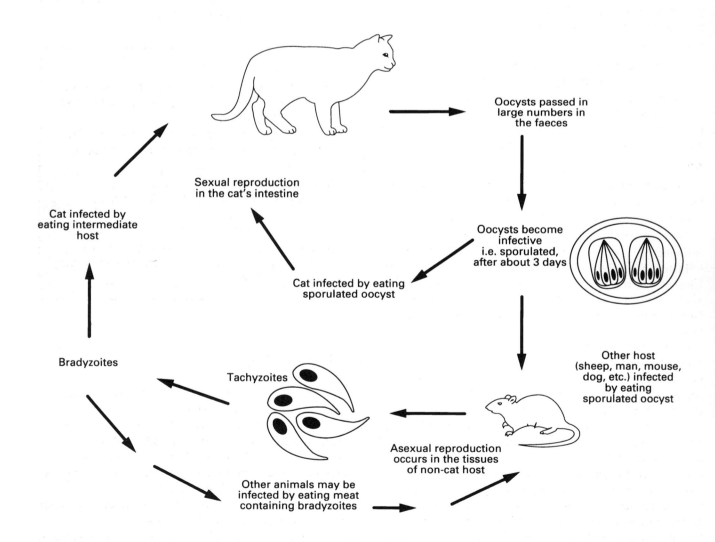

Fig. 15.43 Life cycle of *Toxoplasma gondii*.

• Cysts in immunosuppressed individuals may once again begin to undergo rapid division and cause severe tissue lesions.

In order to try and prevent these infections occurring:

• Farmers are advised to prevent cats, particularly young cats, from getting into food stores intended for sheep. There is now a vaccine against *Toxoplasma* for sheep.
• Pregnant women are advised to take precautionary measures. For example, they should not clean out cat litter trays, they should wear gloves when gardening and they should ensure that all meat is thoroughly cooked before eating it.

Neospora caninum There is no effective treatment to prevent oocyst shedding in the cat. Children that have been infected prenatally are treated with antiprotozoals to prevent any long-term effects.

This parasite causes incoordination in young dogs and abortion in cattle. In the past, infection was normally ascribed to *Toxoplasma gondii*. It is believed that the dog is the final host for this parasite. Treatment of affected puppies may be necessary. Breeding bitches can be screened serologically for signs of infection.

Hammondia This is another protozoan parasite where the cat is the final host. Infection is not normally associated with clinical signs. Sexual reproduction occurs in the intestine of the cat and oocysts are produced that appear similar to those of *Toxoplasma*. The intermediate hosts for *Hammondia* are rodents, so the presence of these oocysts does not provide a human health risk.

Giardia spp. This flagellate protozoan may parasitise the small intestine of man and domestic animals. It is still unknown how important *Giardia* infection in pet animals is as a source of human infection, but it may cause death in cage birds such as cockatiels and budgerigars.

Infection may be asymptomatic or may be associated with transient or chronic diarrhoea. Puppies are at greatest risk. Diagnosis is based on demonstration of the cysts (Fig. 15.44), which are small (approximately 10 μm) and may be passed intermittently in the faeces. Even when a sample is positive, cysts may be present in low numbers, so a sensitive detection technique is used, such as centrifugal flotation using saturated zinc sulphate solution. The cysts can then be stained with Lugol's iodine to increase visibility. It is suggested that collecting samples for 3 days and pooling the sample may help overcome intermittent excretion.

Some protozoal infections are not endemic in the UK, but clinical disease may be seen in animals that are imported from, for example, parts of Europe, where the disease is endemic. These include *Babesia*, a parasite that infects the red blood cells of dogs, thereby causing anaemia. This is a tick-transmitted infection endemic in southern Europe. Leishmaniasis is caused by a flagellate protozoan and is transmitted by sandflies. It occurs in many warmer parts of the world, including the Mediterranean area. Incubation can be particularly long and it is often extremely

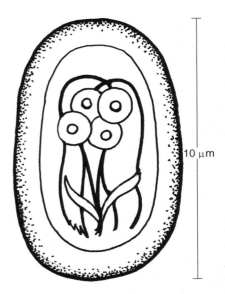

Fig. 15.44 Cyst of *Giardia* spp.

difficult to completely clear the infection with treatment. More information about these diseases may be found in the review by Trees and Shaw (1999).

KEY POINTS
• Parasites of dogs and cats are important causes of disease in these animals and many can infect man (i.e. they are zoonotic).
• Some ectoparasites (those on the skin) can be recognised grossly, others require microscopic examination.
• Most endoparasites can be identified by examining samples taken from the animal, particularly faeces.
• Protection against parasites may be carried out in a preventive manner or by treating when the infection causes clinical signs, depending on the parasite and the circumstances.

Further reading

Bishop, Y. (2001). *The Veterinary Formulary*, 5th edn, Pharmaceutical Press, London.

Bowman, D. D. (2000). *Georgi's Parasitology for Veterinarians*, 7th edn, W. B. Saunders, Philadelphia.

Overgaauw, P. A. M. (1997). Aspects of *Toxocara* epidemiology: toxocarosis in dogs and cats. *Critical Reviews in Microbiology*, vol. 23, pp. 233–251.

Trees, A. and Shaw, S. (1999). Imported diseases in small animals. *In Practice*, vol. 21, pp. 482–489.

Urquhart, G. M., Armour, J.A., Duncan, J.L. and Jennings, F. W. (1996). *Veterinary Parasitology*, 2nd edn, Blackwell Science, Oxford.

16

General nursing

S. Chandler

Learning objectives

After studying this chapter, students should be able to:

- State the methods of assisted feeding.
- Identify the complications associated with assisted feeding.
- Calculate the nutritional requirements for tube feeding.
- Describe the special nursing requirements for a range of patients including the vomiting, soiled and recumbent.
- Describe the special nursing considerations for the geriatric patient.
- Prepare the equipment for carrying out an enema.
- Describe the various forms of physical therapy.

Assisted feeding

The importance of maintaining nutrition during the recovery of patients from surgery or disease cannot be overemphasised. Convalescent periods can be radically reduced when adequate nutrition is provided. Feeding tubes are readily available and have become more frequently used when per os feeding is impossible or contraindicated. It is essential that the veterinary nurse becomes familiar with the management of these tubes.

Assisted feeding should only be instigated when all attempts to induce the animal to eat voluntarily have failed. Anorexic patients may be tempted to eat by:

- Improving palatability, i.e. warming, wetting.
- Hand-feeding.
- Offering odorous foods, e.g. pilchards.
- Offering favourite food (liaise with owners).
- Freshly cooked food.
- Smearing food on lips.
- Stroking/company.
- Privacy feeding.

Reasons for assisted feeding are:

- Failure to entice voluntary eating.
- Physical inability (e.g. fractured jaw).
- Following injury or surgery to oral cavity, or where feeding is contraindicated (e.g. oesophageal trauma).

Methods of assisted feeding

Methods include:

- Placing food on back of tongue and encouraging the animal to swallow (Fig. 16.1), as in per os administration of medicines.
- Syringe feeding of liquid food.
- Tube feeding.

Tube feeding

- Pharyngostomy tube – less popular now due to the high incidence of epiglottic entrapment and interference with the larynx or numerous nerves in this area.
- Naso-oesophageal tube (Fig. 16.2).
- Nasogastric tube – not recommended due to high incidence of gastric reflux and resultant osesophagitis and stricture formation.
- Oesophageal – not commonly used in the UK but reportedly has few side-effects than pharyngostomy tube.
- Gastrostomy tube, surgically placed in the stomach (Fig. 16.3).
- Enterostomy tube (either duodenostomy or jejunostomy tube).

(See also Chapter 9, p. 215).

> *WARNING*
> Aspiration pneumonia is a real risk with syringe feeding. Ensure that the patient's head is in a natural position – *not* raised – and that the animal swallows between the administration of each bolus. Give 0.5–5 ml at a time, depending on the size of the patient.

> *TUBE FEEDING – METHOD*
> - Start gradually – introduce food over 2–3 days.
> - For tubes placed surgically there are rarely complications feeding 6 hours following placement (although some texts advise no use for 24 hours).
> - Prepare the total amount of food to be fed at a single feed (day one will aim to supply one-third of the calculated kcals).
> - Ensure food is at room temperature or slightly higher (cold food may induce vomiting or rapid stomach emptying).

- Ensure appropriate connectors/syringes are available.
- With naso-oesophageal tubes: if there is any evidence of coughing/choking **stop**. Check tip of catheter is correctly beyond 7th rib in the oesophagus before continuing.
- Divide one-third of the calculated food requirement into 5–6 feeds, administer one of these portions, e.g. in a 30 kg Labrador this will be approximately 50 ml/feed on day one.
- Observe your patient's reaction; a strange sensation may be experienced as the stomach has had no preparation for the arrival of food. It is common for patients to lick their lips – this is not because they think it's tasty but because they feel nauseous!
- Give food **slowly**.
- Finally flush the tube with 5–30 ml of water in order to clear debris and maintain patency (depending on size of patient).
- Clean and redress area as required.

Considerations when tube feeding

- If no problems arise with initial feeds, volumes given can be increased to meet calorific (kcal) requirements.
- If prior to a feed, stomach contents are expelled from the tube. Do not feed as the stomach has not emptied sufficiently.
- If the patient begins to vomit, reduce the volumes of feed.
- The total calculated feed should be administered in at *least* four separate feeds. Avoid feeds during the night unless absolutely necessary – most patients don't eat continuously!

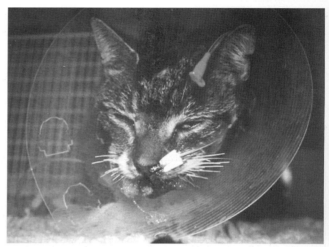

Fig. 16.2 A naso-oesophageal tube (placed under light sedation) in a cat with a fractured jaw.

- Some food can be administered through infusion pumps via giving sets; this may be preferable in smaller patients or those that continue to vomit with bolus feeds.
- Diets should be balanced so that they supply the correct amount of all nutrients (including water) and meet the patient's calorific requirement (see later).
- It is important to keep the tube free from blockage. In practice the complete milks cause the fewest problems, having the added advantage of less preparation time, less mess and higher digestibility.

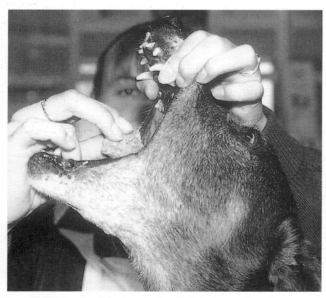

Fig. 16.1 Placing food, by hand, directly into the oral cavity may encourage animals to begin eating after a period of illness or major surgery.

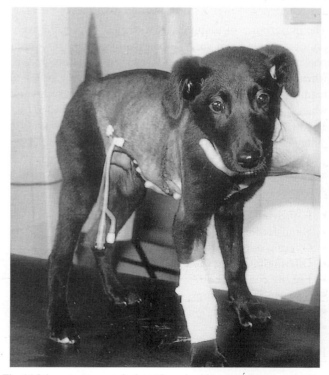

Fig. 16.3 A gastrostomy tube in a 12-week-old puppy after removal of an oesophageal foreign body. Partial thickness oesophageal damage necessitated tube placement. Tube feeding (including all water requirements) as maintained for 5 days. Antibiotics were also given by this route.

- Some veterinary authorities recommend carbonated drinks to flush tubes. The bubbles help to loosen any solid food particles that collect on the inside of the feeding tube. This method should be used cautiously as large amounts of fizzy fluid can make patients feel unwell and possibly induce vomiting. (It is not recommended by the author.)
- All liquidised foods should be the consistency of whole-fat milk to ensure easy passage down the tubes. Most tinned foods require a large amount of water added to them.

All the diets in Table 16.1 and Fig. 16.4 are concentrated and easily digested. This is important because normal dog and cat food when liquidised becomes bulk limiting, i.e. the amount of fluid food that needs to be fed to reach the patient's daily kilocalorie (kcal) requirement is enormous and cannot physically be administered over a 24-hour period without the risk of vomiting.

The enterostomy tubes are less frequently placed and due to their position (duodenum or jejunum) predigested and very simple nutritional units must be delivered (simple sugars, amino acid complexes and emulsified fats). If normal food is supplied severe digestive tract complications will arise.

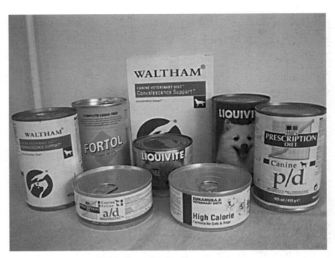

Fig. 16.4 Foods available for tube feeding.

Calculation of kilocalorie requirements

This should be carried out for all tube-fed patients. The basic energy requirement (BER) is measured in metabolisable kcal/day (see Chapter 9, Nutrition) and calculations depend on the patient's bodyweight (in kg):

- **Patients over 5 kg**: BER = 30 × bodyweight + 70.
- **Patients under 5 kg**: BER = 60 × bodyweight.

Taking disease factors into the calculation:

BER × disease factor = kcal requirement

The factors are

- Cage rest: 1.2.
- Surgery/trauma: 1.3.
- Multiple surgery: 1.5.
- Sepsis/cancer: 1.7.
- Burns: 2.0.

Geriatric nursing

Geriatric nursing involves nursing the ageing animal in both health and disease. Geriatric patients must be treated with extra care, for whatever reason they are admitted. They are less able to adapt to change and recover from medical or surgical interference more slowly (**for each 5 years of a pet's age, allow 24 hours longer to recover**).

The key to nursing the geriatric patient is good information (history, medication), the provision of security (own blanket, etc.), comfort (soft bedding), the correct type of food and an adequate source of water.

The changes of old age can be physical or mental (Table 16.2). Many of the mental alterations are related to physical change, e.g. disorientation is made worse when the patient is blind or deaf. Ageing changes and the accumulation of any injuries the patient may have sustained result in a loss of functional reserve, i.e. organs of the body become less

Table 16.1 Foods suitable for tube feeding

Food	Manufacturer
Concentrated liquidised tinned food	Various: Hills p/d Waltham Convalescent Support diet Eukanuba High Calorie diet Hills a/d Liquivite
Liquid complete foods Convalescent support	Waltham Fortal Arnolds

Table 16.2 Physical and mental changes in geriatric animals

Physical	Mental
Greying of muzzle, etc.	Lowered response to stimuli
Thickening of the skin	Less adaptable
Coarse coat	Fussy about food
Loss of musculature	More likely to develop food
Loss of stamina and strength	preferences
Weakening of bone	Less interested in activity
Lowered tolerance to change	Less obedient
Loss of sight	Disorientation
Loss of hearing	
Poor tolerance to lack of fluid intake	
Impaired temperature regulation	
Arthritis and joint stiffness	
Higher susceptibility to infection	

capable of dealing with extra demands placed on them for repair of tissue, assimilation of substances, etc.

Disease

Changes due to disease must be carefully distinguished from those of old age, although disease can become more obvious or affect a patient more rapidly when they become old. Very few sick, elderly patients suffer from a single disease. Many conditions are subtle and multiple. Commonly found disorders of geriatric animals include:

- Cancer.
- Chronic renal disease.
- Cardiac disease (cardiomyopathy).
- Osteoarthritis (degenerative joint disease – DJD).
- Cataracts.
- Dental disease.
- Constipation.
- Incontinence (see below).

Apparent **incontinence** is not always due to a total inability to control micturation but rather where patients lose bladder muscle/sphincter tone. This may result in 'leaking' of urine during sleep, relaxation or long periods of confinement. These patients cannot be left alone for long periods without the opportunity to urinate. They urinate in the house or while asleep and may appear incontinent to their owners.

Nursing considerations

Ensure that the patient's history is known. This includes any current treatment, the preferred food and conditions they suffer from. Remember that they may be suffering from diseases other than those for which they have been admitted. Specific conditions are dealt with in Chapter 17 (Medical Disorders and Their Nursing). The following points are general guidelines.

Drugs

All patients should be weighed, however, it is particularly important to weigh the geriatric patient so that accurate drug dose calculations can be made. Drug dosage is the veterinary surgeon's responsibility but anaesthetic drugs may well be prepared by nursing staff and accurate calculations are essential. Young patients may have the capacity to survive mild medication overdosage; **geriatrics may not**.

Feeding

Geriatric patients generally need fewer calories but simply feeding them less can result in a lowered intake of protein, vitamins and minerals.

Dietary considerations in the absence of any disease includes a highly digestible, well-balanced proprietary food. There are many available and some companies produce diets specifically formulated for the older dog. Cats tend to stay active for longer and special diets are less available. To avoid digestive upsets, any changes in diet should be introduced gradually. Lack of interest in food is rarely due to true anorexia in the previously appetant hospitalised geriatric patient. It is more likely that the patient is offered different food, finds the amount offered too great, has dental disease resulting in pain or has difficulty in standing when eating.

Obesity

This is common in the geriatric patient and management is achieved through client education. Emphasise to the owners that excess weight is potentially *dangerous* to their pet, extra strain being placed on the heart, kidneys, liver and musculoskeletal system in obese patients. This may help to persuade owners their pet would be happier and healthier if it lost weight. Give them target weights, being careful to check all diets with a veterinary surgeon thereby ensuring increased exercise (if possible) and diet changes are not contraindicated.

Fluid balance (water and urine)

> **WARNING**
> Do not restrict water intake in the geriatric patient unless they are vomiting.
> This is particularly important in relation to the withdrawal of fluids prior to surgery.

No patient should be deprived of water for more than an hour before induction of anaesthesia. Water does *not* need to be withdrawn the night before; this can be extremely dangerous. Younger patients will tolerate the insult, but geriatric patients can be pushed over the fine dividing line of renal compromise and may well suffer irreparable damage to renal function that will only be noticeable weeks later.

If the amount of water being consumed by a geriatric is in doubt, then measuring fluid intake may be necessary to ensure adequate quantities are being provided. Urine output will indicate adequate fluid provision and this too can be measured. Remember that many elderly patients will be suffering from various degrees of renal compromise and may drink and urinate in excess of normal calculated volumes (2 ml/kg/day urine, 40–60 ml/kg/day maintenance fluids). If vomiting is present, ensure that intravenous fluids are administered. Observe urine for normal colour and passage (i.e. no straining).

Exercise

Little and often is recommended. Elderly dogs enjoy 'pottering'. Even hospitalised dogs should be given time to wander, maybe in an outside run. Frequent walks will help to exercise stiff joints and ensure plenty of opportunities to urinate (which may save time on cleaning out kennels). Elderly cats often sleep for long periods of time. Encouraging them to move around can be beneficial to circulation and joint health. Take special care if the patient is blind or deaf. Many owners will not have previously experienced an elderly pet, so discuss considerations on discharge or at consultation.

Defecation

Constipation is more common in the elderly dog and cat. Observe defecation where possible to enable elimination of any suspected tenesmus or difficulty in evacuation of faeces. Faecal examination should be on a regular basis to detect any abnormalities.

Bedding and kennelling

Blankets and soft bedding should be provided, along with foam mattresses for those with osteoarthritis. Keep geriatrics out of draughts and if possible somewhere not too noisy. Encourage frequent light exercise to improve peripheral circulation and maintenance of peripheral temperature. External additional heat sources may be required. Core temperature should be monitored if there is any suspicion that the patient is cold.

Grooming

Groom elderly patients regularly, as they are less likely to keep themselves clean. It helps to give a feeling of well-being and provides an opportunity to check the coat and skin, and to clean discharges from eyes and nose. The human contact is also beneficial.

If the patient has lost its sight or hearing, move slowly and talk reassuringly at all times. This will help to prevent the bite of surprise that elderly dogs so often attempt when suddenly touched or frightened.

Vaccination

Geriatric animals are less responsive to vaccination – they probably have sufficient acquired immunity. However, annual boosters are still advisable.

Convalescence

This will take more time and effort than in younger patients. Have patience and allow a longer period for convalescence.

Maintenance of normal body temperature is especially important pre-, intra- and post-operatively. Thermoregulation in geriatrics is often compromised.

If patients are discharged before they have fully recovered, inform the owners that it will take some time for a pet to complete its recovery. Adequate water intake is very important; ensure that patients can reach water bowls and add water to food if necessary. Exercise should be gentle. Physiotherapy, especially massage, may be used to improve circulation to the extremities.

Care of the vomiting patient

Vomiting (**emesis**) is the forcible ejection of contents of the *stomach* through the mouth. It should not be confused with regurgitation, which is the return of undigested food from the *oesophagus* (see Chapter 17, p. 427, Medical Disorders and their Nursing).

Nursing of the vomiting patient can be very straightforward (e.g. in the case of scavenging) or much more complex (e.g. as a result of metabolic imbalances). Some of the common causes of vomiting are shown in Table 16.3.

Table 16.3 Causes of vomiting		
Mechanical/functional disorders	**Metabolic disorders**	**Miscellaneous**
Pyloric stenosis	Motion sickness	Kidney disease (nephritis)
Pyloric stricture	Scavenging	Liver disease
Gastric foreign bodies	Pain	Metabolic alkalosis
Other gastrointestinal foreign bodies	Drug reactions	Electrolyte imbalances, e.g.
Intussusception	Neurological disorders	hyponatraemia,
	Food allergies	hypokalaemia
	Distasteful smells	Diabetes mellitus
		Toxaemia
		Poisoning

Mechanical and functional disorders

Patients suffering from mechanical or functional disorders are usually admitted for surgical correction of the condition. Dietary management is usually simple.

Foreign bodies

Food is generally withheld until surgery has been carried out. If water induces vomiting, it too should be withheld but replaced by intravenous fluids. Most vomiting patients have some degree of dehydration and in these cases an intravenous drip is set up to provide fluid.

The reintroduction of food and water after surgery will vary in each individual case but the following are basic guidelines.

In some cases nothing will be allowed by mouth for 24–48 hours. Intravenous fluid therapy must continue to supply calculated daily requirements. Feeding during this time should not be neglected and hopefully some form of enteral feeding will be available, e.g. gastrostomy tube (Fig. 16.3), naso-oesophageal tube (Fig. 16.2) or jejunostomy tube (surgically placed into the small intestine).

Tube feeding allows the surgical site a chance to heal whilst still providing a route for nutrition, which is essential to rapid recovery.

If fluids by mouth are allowed, initially offer small amounts frequently (50–100 ml every hour). If these are not vomited, then the amounts can be increased over the next 8 hours. Intravenous fluids may be continued during this time as total fluid requirements will not be achieved initially.

Reintroduction of feed begins once fluids are retained, usually over 24–72 hours. Food offered will vary: usually it will be a bland diet of soft small chunks of moist food, offered little and often. Liquidised food may be specified in some cases, e.g. in the management of pyloric stenosis. Bland foods include chicken, fish or a commercially prepared diet.

Feeding of patients after intestinal surgery (enterectomy or enterotomy) should begin immediately after recovery from anaesthesia, this helps to prevent intestinal stasis.

Megaoesophagus

Patients with megaoesophagus regurgitate rather than vomit. Food becomes lodged in the oesophagus cranial to a stricture or narrowing, so that only a limited amount of food reaches the stomach.

Dietary management (even after surgery, if performed) will involve varying degrees of liquidised/semi-solid food fed from a height (Fig. 16.5). Feeding from a height helps to prevent regurgitation and the possible development of aspiration pneumonia – gravity helps the passage of food to the stomach. Passage of food can also be aided after feeding by gentle coupage whilst the patient is in an upright position (see p. 412).

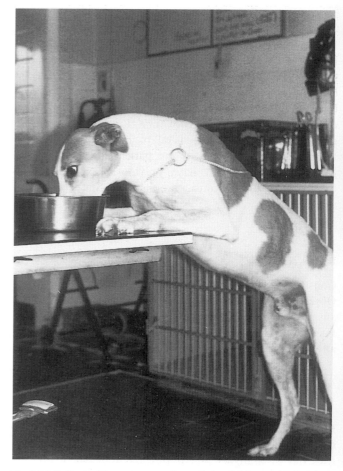

Fig. 16.5 Patient with a megaoesophagus being fed from table-height to aid passage of food to the stomach.

Metabolic disorders

Patients that vomit due to metabolic disorders are generally more challenging to the nurse. If vomiting has been prolonged, they will be dehydrated and require fluid therapy in combination with other treatment. The percentage of dehydration can be estimated clinically (Table 16.4).

It is pleasant for the patient to have moist cotton wool wiped around the mucous membranes of the mouth, especially if water has been withdrawn. This not only freshens the mouth but also removes excess saliva.

If water is not vomited, oral electrolyte fluids may be useful (Chapter 22 discusses fluid therapy).

Antiemetic drugs, such as metaclopramide, are frequently prescribed. They must be administered by intravenous administration as per os is usually contraindicated in these patients. For continuous effect, the veterinary surgeon may request drugs to be placed in the drip fluid.

When vomiting ceases, water and then food can be reintroduced.

Reintroduction of food

The following is a general guide for the reintroduction of food to a patient that has been vomiting. It assumes that

Table 16.4 Recognition of dehydration*

Grade	Per cent dehydration	Clinical signs
Slight	<5	Not detectable
Mild	5–6	Slight decrease in skin turgor
Mild	6–8	Delay in skin fold return Slight increase in capillary refill time (CRT) Dry mucous membranes Sunken eyes
Moderate	10–12	Tenting of the skin Sunken eyes Increased CRT Tachycardia Cold extremities Early signs of shock
Severe	12–15	Clinical signs of shock, i.e., tachycardia, weak pulse, pale mucous membranes and cold extremities These may lead to coma and death

water does not cause vomiting. **If at any stage vomiting reoccurs, return to the previous day's protocol**.

- **Day 1**: Offer small amounts of bland food 3–4 times daily. Total amount offered should equal one-quarter to one-half of normal daily kilocalorie requirement.
- **Day 2**: Offer small amounts of bland food frequently, to total one-half to three-quarters of daily requirement.
- **Days 3–6**: As for days 1 and 2 but total amount offered should be equal to normal requirement.
- **Days 7–14**: Reintroduce normal diet by mixing increasing amounts with the bland diet.

Patients that have had a single acute vomiting episode due to scavenging will need to be starved for 24–48 hours before the reintroduction of food. In these cases the above regime can be followed and can be given as advice to owners over the telephone. For any other reason it is only a guideline. Specific types of food may be required, longer periods of starvation necessary or placement of feeding tubes. A veterinary surgeon will give instructions on the course to be followed.

General points to remember

- Nausea is unpleasant. It can be identified in dogs and cats by:
    - Restlessness.
    - Salivation.
    - Repeated swallowing.
    - Retching.

Bring these signs to the attention of the veterinary surgeon.

- Clean away any excess vomitus and clean the mouth. If not contraindicated, offer small amounts of cool, fresh water (10–15 ml) to allow rinsing of the mouth.
- Handle gently. Lift only if absolutely necessary, ensuring that no pressure is placed on the patient's abdomen.
- Hand-feeding and encouragement may be required during the recovery period.
- **If syringe feeding of fluids is instituted at any time, remember the potential for the development of aspiration pneumonia. It is surprisingly easy to cause pneumonia, especially in smaller dogs and cats.**
- When patients are discharged, give the owners **written** instructions regarding the type of food, the amounts to be offered, its consistency and the method of feeding.

The soiled patient

Hospitalised patients may become soiled at some time during their stay. It is the nurse's responsibility to ensure that all soiling is cleaned efficiently, effectively and quickly.

Regular walking of in-patients may seem time consuming but it may conserve time spent in cleaning kennels and soiled patients. Cats must be supplied with litter trays; check with owners regarding types of litter used, as some cats are fussy.

Animals may become soiled by:

- Urine.
- Faeces.
- Blood.
- Vomit.
- Food.
- Other body fluids.

Reasons for soiling include:

- Confinement to a small area.
- Disturbed routine
- Medical or surgical condition.
- Untrained puppies.
- Recumbency.

Action when soiling occurs

(1) Clean as quickly as possible.
(2) Choose shampoos carefully. Take into consideration patient's coat length, reason for hospitalisation and area to be cleaned or bathed. Chlorhexidine gluconate or povidone–iodine are preferable if the patient has any surgical or open wounds. Dry dog shampoos are available, but they are inadequate if soiling has occurred.
(3) Once the area has been cleaned, dry it thoroughly. Most patients will tolerate a hair dryer after a towel rub down. All knots in the coat should be removed since they may harbour faeces. Conditioners will make the process much less tiresome for nursing staff and the patient, especially in long-haired breeds.

(4) Whilst grooming, check for any area of soreness, especially if the patient is recumbent. If necessary, clip hair away from these areas.

(5) It is best to clip heavily contaminated areas, especially if further contamination is expected (e.g. under drainage tubes). Ensure that client permission has been given. White petroleum jelly can be applied around these areas after clipping, preventing soreness and to make cleaning easier. There are also barrier film sprays (like a plastic skin), e.g. Cavilon (3M), that can be used to protect skin surfaces from urine and faecal scalding.

(6) Cats generally keep themselves very clean. If bathing is necessary, use mild shampoos and avoid products based on coal tar (phenol is poisonous to cats – see Chapter 3). Regular grooming of hospitalised long-haired cats is essential.

(7) Cats with oral lesions or fractured jaws are unable to clean themselves and regular cleaning of the lips, chin and paws will be required.

Enemata

An enema is a liquid substance placed into the rectum and colon of a patient. The enema is not intended to flush colonic contents but to distend the rectum and distal colon gently, initiating normal expulsive reflexes.

Reasons for performing an enema

Emptying the rectum

- To relieve constipation or impaction.
- As preparation for radiographic studies. The colon and rectum overlie abdominal structures and will obscure them if they are not emptied.
- As part of a radiographic contrast study.
- To enable the administration of drugs.
- In preparation for endoscopic examination.

As a diagnostic aid

Barium sulphate enemata can be given to outline the rectal and colonic walls. Remember, however, that the patient needs to evacuate the barium after radiography – a quick retreat to the outside is strongly advised!

Administering medication

The colon has a large capacity for absorption. For this reason it is a good route for the administration of soluble drugs although, it is rarely used in veterinary medicine due to lack of patient cooperation.

Solutions used for enema administration

The choice of solution depends on the purpose of the enema.

Water

Warm tap water is the preferred solution. It is readily available, non-toxic and non-irritant. In addition, any cleaning of the perianal area is reasonably straightforward.

Liquid paraffin

This is readily available and reasonably cheap. Cleaning the patient after the enema can be difficult, since liquid paraffin is oil-based and not water-soluble. The patient needs to be bathed with shampoo to remove this substance.

Mineral oil

This suffers the same disadvantages as liquid paraffin and is more expensive. However, oil-based substances are an advantage when treating a constipated patient. The oil helps to soften and lubricate the faecal masses and allows easier evacuation of the bowel.

Saline (phosphate enema)

This is usually available as manufactured sachets with phosphate included. They promote defecation by being osmotically active, promoting water retention in the colon. These enemata should be used with care in small (below 15 kg) and young patients because their excessive use can result in unwanted absorption of certain ions resulting in system toxicity.

Ready-to-use mini enemata

A proprietary brand of miniature enema is introduced into the rectum by an attached nozzle. It is extremely useful in cats, the procedure being no more stressful than using a rectal thermometer.

Gastrointestinal cleaning agents

One such agent is Klean Prep.

These are laxatives rather than enemata but can be used for bowel clearance for all the same indications. These agents are given per os and defecation occurs rapidly after administration. Stomach tubing may be required to administer the fluid as they are flavoured for the human market and dogs are usually unwilling to drink them.

Miscellaneous substances

- Glycerine and water.
- Olive oil and water.
- Obstetrical lubricant.
- Soft soap.

These variations are either more expensive, or largely outdated and have no advantages over solutions already mentioned. In addition, soap may cause mucosal irritation.

Equipment

The basic equipment includes enema solution, gloves, lubricant (e.g. K-Y jelly) and any of the following: can and tubing, Higginson syringe, prepared barium bag, syringe and catheter (Fig. 16.6).

> **ADMINISTRATION OF AN ENEMA**
>
> Table 16.5 gives guidance of the volumes of solution. The method for dogs, which requires two people, is as follows.
>
> (1) Prepare all equipment.
> (2) The assistant restrains the patient in a suitable area, preferably outside where cleaning will be easier.
> (3) Lubricate the end of the tube or nozzle.
> (4) Elevate the patient's tail and place the tube into the anus. Rotate gently until access to the rectum is achieved (this is easy in the dog but occasionally more difficult in the cat).
> (5) Advance the tube into the rectum.
> (6) Stand to the side of the patient and allow fluid to run into the rectum by gravity or gently pump in fluid.
> (7) Allow dogs free exercise to evacuate bowels and supply cats with litter trays and an adequately sized cage.

The recumbent patient

An animal that is lying down and unable to rise is described as recumbent. A large number of conditions might result in recumbency, the more common being:

- Fractures (e.g. pelvis, limbs).
- Spinal trauma (e.g. disc protrusion).
- Electrolyte imbalances, head injuries, shock.
- Weakness due to medical disease (e.g. Cushing's syndrome, cardiac disease).
- Neurological disease (e.g. coma).

Kennelling

Bedding

Bed the patient on thick, waterproof (PVC-covered) foam mattresses, with 'Vetbed' or similar on the top. If these are unavailable, use thick layers of newspaper with blankets on top. Beanbags, although very comfortable, become soiled very easily and are difficult to clean; they are normally impractical in the hospital situation.

Size

Previously active animals attempt to drag themselves around (especially fracture and spinal cases in which pain has been relieved). The kennel should be large enough for such a patient to lie in lateral recumbency comfortably, but not so big that it has room to cause damage to itself.

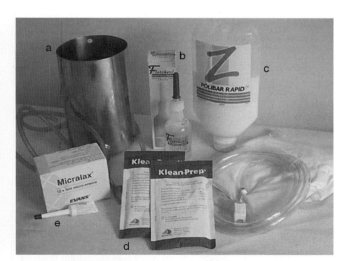

Fig. 16.6 Products/equipment for carrying out an enema. (a) Can and tubing. (b) Proprietary phosphate enema. (c) Prepared barium. (d) Klean Prep Sachets. (e) Micralax.

Table 16.5 Enema solutions and volumes

Solution	Volume used (ml/kg)	Frequency
Water	5–10	Every 20–30 minutes if necessary
Liquid paraffin	2–3	Every 1–2 hours
Saline solution	1–2	Do not repeat for 12 hours
Barium sulphate	5–10	Not necessary
Klean Prep	20	Should not be necessary
Laxative fluids		Not usually required

Position

Most recumbent patients benefit from being nursed in a kennel sited in an area of activity. This stimulates them and relieves boredom since nursing staff inevitably talk to them more frequently. Ensure kennels are not in direct sunlight, since these patients may be unable to move to a shady area.

Food and water

Ensure that both food and water are within easy reach. Patients who are recumbent due to a medical condition may be depressed and hand-feeding necessary.

Patients who fail to drink sufficiently can have water added to their food or be encouraged to drink by syringing water into the side of their mouths.

Most recumbent patients require a concentrated, highly digestible diet to meet the extra nutritional needs of stress due to kennelling or continuing tissue repair. Highly digestible diets have the added advantage of producing less faecal material. **The energy requirement supplied by carbohydrates is generally lower during recumbency and the amount of carbohydrates offered may need reducing. Sick animals may have an *increased* nutrient requirement, since these are necessary for tissue repair, i.e raised protein**.

If the recumbent patient fails to eat, seek advice from the owner regarding preferences and favourite foods.

Obesity may be an existing problem or weight may be gained during the period of recumbency due to less energy being used. It may be necessary to introduce reducing diets, but only in consultation with the veterinary surgeon.

Urination and defecation

If possible, recumbent patients should be taken outside. The change of environment and fresh air are beneficial to their mental attitude. In addition, natural urination and defecation are always preferable to catheterisation and enemata. Help patients to stand since many are unwilling to urinate lying down. Towel support is useful (Fig. 16.7); even tetra/quadraplegics can be managed in this way, using crossed towels to support the chest. When an animal is supported, apply gentle pressure to the bladder to encourage urination (Fig. 16.8).

WARNING
Placement of urinary catheters is invasive and should not be carried out casually. Antibiotic cover will be required and the potential for temporary bladder function problems after removal of indwelling catheters must be recognised. The raised possibility of urinary tract infections is also a major consideration.

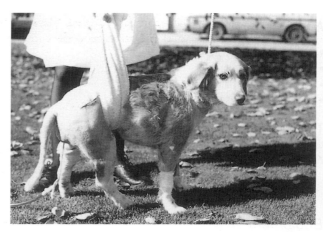

Fig. 16.7 Assisted walking for the recumbent patient supported by a towel. This method can be adapted using crossed towels over the chest when tetraplegia is present.

Indwelling Foley catheters can be used. They are beneficial in keeping the patient dry by preventing soiling from urine overflow 24 hours a day. Indwelling Foley catheters with a bag attached have the added advantage of enabling urine output to be easily measured.

In dogs, plastic dog catheters can be sutured to the prepuce or catheterisation can be carried out 2–3 times daily. There are also Foley catheters made from silicone that can be passed up the male urethra and remain in the bladder in exactly the same manner as the latex Foley (see p. 417). The silicone is so smooth that the catheter advances up the curved male urethra without the aid of a stylet, although wire-guide stylets are available and may make the procedure even easier.

Cats' bladders can generally be manually expressed, although catheterisation may also be performed.

Ensure a record of defecation is kept. It is easy for 3–5 days of non-production to go unnoticed. If the patient becomes constipated, a laxative may be required.

Any diarrhoea in the recumbent patient increases the risk of sores, infection in any wounds, fly-strike in the summer and discomfort to the patient. Inform the veterinary sur-

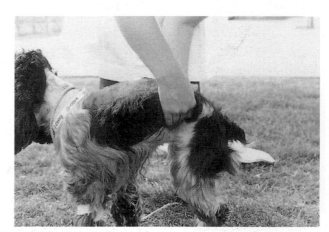

Fig. 16.8 Manual bladder expression whilst supporting a recumbent patient.

geon. Clip excess hair in the perianal/anal area. Cleaning as quickly as possible after contamination occurs is extremely important.

Decubitus ulcers and urine scalding

Prevention

It is better to prevent both decubitus ulcers (Fig. 16.9) and urine scalding, rather than treat them after they have occurred.

- The use of soft bedding with absorbable blankets (e.g. 'Vetbed'), together with regular turning of the patient (every 4 hours), will help to lessen the occurrence of sores.
- Bony prominences are most likely to suffer (e.g. elbows and ischial wings). These areas can be padded with foam rings from the top of tablet pots (Fig. 16.10) or the patient can be encouraged to lie laterally for *short* periods (a balance between lateral and sternal recumbency needs to be found – see 'Hypostatic Pneumonia').
- Massage is beneficial and can be performed while the patient is recumbent.
- Slings to raise patients for longer periods are used in the US and at larger veterinary establishments in the UK (Fig. 16.11).
- Catheterisation (indwelling or repeated) enables bladder drainage without soiling. Otherwise assisted walking is essential to provide opportunities for urination.
- Waterbeds may be useful but are rarely used in the UK.

Management

Any patients which are dirtied by urine should be checked for the presence of urine scalds. They begin as innocent-looking red patches and, if treated at this stage, are very easily managed. There is no excuse for them getting worse if nursing care is adequate.

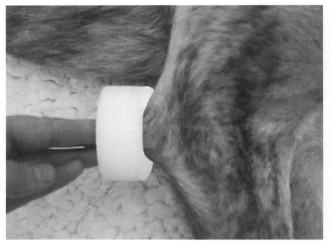

Fig. 16.10 Padding of bony prominences with foam can help to prevent occurrence of decubitus ulcers.

Urine scalding is relieved by:

- Regular washing with a mild antiseptic shampoo (e.g. dilute chlorhexidine gluconate or povidone–iodine). Both must be rinsed off thoroughly.
- Clipping off hair and the application of soothing healing or barrier creams.
- Catheterisation. This is no longer considered good practice by some clinicians. Simple urine management is sufficient, unless the patients condition expressly requires catheterisation. (See warning regarding complications of indwelling catheters.)

Decubitus ulcers are far more serious and can be extremely difficult to resolve.

Treatment:

(1) Clip the area around the sore.

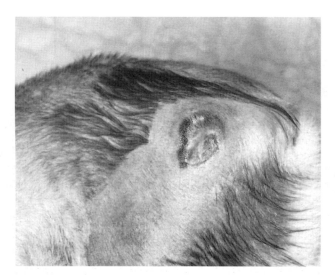

Fig. 16.9 Decubitus ulcer on the skin overlying the ilium.

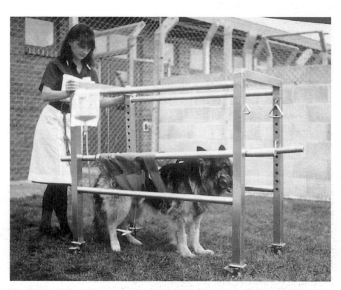

Fig. 16.11 Wheeled 'total support' walking frame systems assist mobility of heavier patients and enable effective physical therapy with the patient in a normal walking position. (The urinary catheter in this figure has been clamped during motion to prevent back-flow of urine whilst the collection bag is suspended above the bladder!)

(2) Clean with a mild antiseptic solution (e.g. dilute povidone–iodine or chlorhexidine gluconate).
(3) Dry thoroughly.
(4) Apply an appropriate cream or protective barrier film (e.g. Cavilon; 3M).
(5) If it is summer, and the position of the ulcer allows, cover with a dressing to prevent fly strike and contamination.
(6) If on lower limb consider bandage use.

WARNING
Hardening of areas prone to decubitus ulcers with spirit is *not* recommended.

Hypostatic pneumonia

Hypostatic pneumonia is caused by the pooling of blood and a consequent decrease in viability of the dependent lung. It is more likely to occur in an old, sick and debilitated animal that has been in lateral recumbency for a long period. Turning the patient at least every 4 hours – 24 hours a day – is essential nursing. Encourage sternal recumbency by using sandbags, water/sand-filled containers or X-ray cradles and remember to support the head.

Regular **coupage** (the external impact massage of the thorax with cupped hands) 4–5 times daily for 5 minutes will improve thoracic circulation; by promoting coughing it also aids removal of secretions that build up in the bronchial tree. **Check with a veterinary surgeon before using coupage** to ensure that there are no contraindications such as fractured ribs.

WARNING
It is important to realise that serious secondary chest infections may result if hypostatic pneumonia is allowed to develop. This alone can cause *death*.

If hypostatic pneumonia with a secondary infection is present, continue all the above guidelines for prevention. In addition, treatment (e.g. antibiotics) will probably be prescribed.

Signs of hypostatic pneumonia are:

- Fast/frequent shallow breathing.
- Increased respiratory effort.
- Moist noises when breathing, possibly even gurgling.
- Depressed attitude.

If you suspect hypostatic pneumonia, inform a veterinary surgeon immediately. Auscultation of the lung fields and radiography may be required to confirm the diagnosis.

Passive physiotherapy

Physiotherapy helps to maintain and improve peripheral circulation. It is of benefit to all recumbent patients, even if only for the extra human contact and attention.

Massage

This is particularly useful for the limbs. Massage from the toes towards the body to encourage venous return to the heart.

Supported exercise

Towel-walking is the most common (and cheapest) method. Make sure that adequate staff are available, as both the patient and the staff member can be injured if the patient is heavy.

Hydrotherapy

Swimming is very useful physiotherapy for dogs (cats generally do not appreciate it!). Small dogs can be swum in large sinks and baths in the hospital; larger patients need pools. Swimming enables patients to move their limbs freely without weight-bearing forces.

Check the temperature of the water before immersing the patient. *Constant* support and observation are essential to prevent panic and possible drowning.

Passive joint movement

Manually moving joints within their normal range helps to prevent stiffness and improves circulation.

Coupage

As previously described.

Body temperature

Recumbent patients expend very little energy; therefore heat production is lower than normal. Body temperature may fall to a subnormal level. Blankets to cover the patient may be sufficient. Other heating methods include:

- Veterinary duvet-type covers with reflective filling.
- Veterinary instant heat pads, which should be wrapped initially: when activated, they heat to 52°C.
- Hot-water bottles, which should be wrapped to prevent burning of the patient.
- Heated waterbeds – use only if the patient is very debilitated and will not bite or scratch. They are expensive pieces of equipment to replace if punctured.

- Bubble packaging – cheap and effective.
- Silver foil is good for extremities. Remove if patients become active, especially young ones (it is 'edible').
- Silver reflective survival blankets.
- Infrared lamps.
- Incubators.

> **WARNING**
> Electrically heated beds are *not* recommended unless the patient is under *constant supervision*. Some varieties have been implicated in causing serious burns when patients were placed directly on top of them. A blanket should always be between the heated pad and the patient.

Home nursing

Recumbent patients are generally managed in a hospital environment. Some will inevitably be recumbent for a longer period and may be nursed at home. Most owners are quite capable of learning how to nurse their own pet but remember that tasks which come automatically to a nurse need to be pointed out to an owner. It is helpful to write clear instructions which owners can refer to once they are home. Reassure owners that they can phone at any time if they are worried. Arrange weekly checks at the surgery to check for signs of decubitus ulcers, urine scalding or hypostatic pneumonia.

Comatosed patient

In this context, 'comatosed' is interpreted as a long-term coma rather than simple recovery from anaesthesia. This may occur in conditions such as tetanus, neurological disease or after major convulsions. In reality these patients are rarely nursed in general practice – they really need an intensive care unit and a large number of personnel.

The nursing of a comatosed patient is essentially similar to that for a recumbent one and all the nursing points made for the care of the recumbent patient can be implemented for the comatosed patient – with the exception of eating, drinking and exercise. Nutrition is best provided by either total parenteral nutrition (TPN) via a jugular catheter or by a jejunostomy tube, fluid intake being by intravenous fluids.

In addition, the following points should be considered when nursing the comatosed patient:

- Keep a patent airway – pull the tongue forward and consider endotracheal intubation.
- Clean any secretions from the oral cavity – use a sucker or swabs and lower the head to encourage drainage by gravity.
- Monitor at 15-minute intervals:

  - temperature, pulse and respiratory rate and rhythm;
  - mucous membrane colour;
  - capillary refill time;
  - urine output;
  - drip rates;
  - drug administration.

Constant 24-hour observation is essential for the comatosed patient.

Urinary catheterisation

A catheter is a tubular, usually flexible instrument passed through body channels for the withdrawal of fluids from (or the introduction of fluids into) a body cavity.

Reasons for urinary catheterisation

- To obtain a (sterile) urine sample when:

  - A patient will not urinate when required (this may be because the patient is only at the surgery for short periods, e.g. at consultation, or timed urine samples are required, e.g. water deprivation test).
  - Obtaining a midstream urine sample (MUS) is impossible because the amount produced during exercise is little (e.g. the male dog that squirts 2 ml at every tree). A culture and sensitivity examination is requested (it is essential that urine is collected in a sterile manner for this examination: MUS samples become contaminated at the prepuce and vulva and provide meaningless results).

- To empty the urinary bladder:

  - Before abdominal, vaginal and urethral surgery.
  - Before a pneumocystogram.
  - When there is a partial obstruction or inability to urinate but a catheter can be passed into the bladder (e.g. due to prostatic enlargement).

- To introduce contrast agents for radiographic procedures.
- To maintain constant, controlled bladder drainage (indwelling catheters):

  - In the recumbent or incontinent patient to prevent soiling.
  - After bladder surgery, to avoid overdistension of the bladder, thereby reducing tension on the suture line and helping to provide optimum healing conditions for the operative site.

- In **hydropropulsion** (the use of water pressure to dislodge particles causing an obstruction: a urinary catheter is placed caudal to the particle and water pressure is used to dislodge the calculi from the urethra back into the

bladder). Hydropropulsion can be used to relieve a partial blockage in an emergency situation. It is nearly
always followed by surgery (e.g. cystotomy or urethrostomy).

- To maintain a patent urethra:

  - In male cats suffering from feline lower urinary
    tract disease (FLUTD) – a catheter may be placed
    to maintain bladder drainage whilst treatment or
    dietary management is initiated; catheter place-
    ment also allows flushing of the bladder with solu-
    tions which may dissolve struvite crystals (e.g.
    Walpole's solution, although this is an older tech-
    nique which is now rarely used).
  - Where dysuria or anuria is present but surgery is
    delayed due to the patient being in a poor condi-
    tion for surgery (e.g. raised blood urea levels, elec-
    trolyte imbalance, etc.).

- To monitor urine output:

  - Where a patient with renal compromise is on large
    volumes of intravenous fluids.
  - If the patient is in intensive care.
  - After renal surgery to ensure adequate production
    of urine.
    **N.B. Minimum urine output = 1–2 ml/kg body-
    weight/hour**.

- Introduction of drugs.

Complications associated with catheterisation

Complications which might arise include infective cystitis,
reactive cystitis, urethral damage, failure to catheterise the
urethra, resistance by the patient, blockage of indwelling
catheters or removal of indwelling catheters by the patient.
Reasons for these complications are described below, and
Table 16.6 outlines methods of preventing them and the
action to be taken should they arise.

Infection

Urinary tract infection (UTI) can easily be caused by catheterisation if bacteria present in the urethra are pushed into
the bladder by the catheter. In most circumstances the bacteria are rapidly eliminated and cause no further concern.
The risk of infection is increased when:

- The bladder is traumatised.
- A preputial or vaginal discharge is present.
- Indwelling catheters are used or repeated catheterisation
  is carried out.
- The patient is immunosuppressed, i.e. its immune system
  is compromised in some way and the body's natural
  defences are not operating correctly.

Cystitis after catheterisation

This is associated with indwelling catheters. It is rarely seen
otherwise, unless repeated catheterisation has been carried
out.

Urethral damage

This is most likely to occur in the male dog, due to the
ischial curve of the urethra – some epithelial damage is
inevitable as the catheter is passed around the curve. (This
is why a small amount of blood may be present in the tip of
the catheter on removal from the urethra, be gentle!)

Urethral damage in the bitch is usually due to excess force
being used to advance the catheter into the bladder.

> The increase in resistance of organisms to antibiotic
> treatment is well documented. Therefore prophylactic
> antibiotic cover for catheterisation (especially where
> indwelling catheters are in place) is less acceptable
> than in the past. As a result many establishments
> support a reluctance to place indwelling catheters,
> preferring to use frequent visits outside or bladder
> expression.

Failure to catheterise the urethra

Failure to catheterise the urethra may occur in the bitch if
the urethral orifice is passed and the catheter cannot be
advanced because it meets the cervix. Catheterisation of
the cervix is a rare occurrence and is easily identified:

- By viewing the urethral orifice with a lighted speculum.
- Because no urine flows through the catheter – but note
  that catheters can be placed correctly and still not produce urine, due to either an empty bladder or an obstruction to urine flow (e.g. excessive lubricant blocking the
  drainage holes).

Patient resistance

This is common in bitches, queens and tomcats. Sedation or
general anaesthesia may be required.

Blockage of indwelling catheters

Urine will cease to flow from the catheter. Flushing of catheters at regular intervals (2–3 times per day) is advisable.

Table 16.6 Complications associated with catheterisation

	Prevention	Action
Infection	Use only new or re-sterilised catheters. Use sterile gloves to handle catheters or employ the 'no touch' technique described for dog catheterisation. Use sterile lubricants. Clean penis or vulva thoroughly before catheterisation; clip surrounding hair if necessary Catheterisation should be carried out in a clean environment, not in the patient's kennel. Ensure that systemic antibiotics are prescribed by the veterinary surgeon. A single (long-acting) dose may be sufficient after just one catheterisation of a healthy patient Patients with indwelling catheters should receive systemic antibiotics whilst catheterised and continue the course for 5–10 days after removal.	If infection becomes evident, treatment will consist of systemic antibiotics and, in some cases, soluble antibiotics flushed directly into the bladder
Cystitis after catheterisation	Gentle introduction of the catheter – no force should be necessary. Use of lubricants is beneficial – they help to limit the epithelial damage to the urethral mucosa, thereby reducing inflammation Trauma is less likely if an experienced person catheterises debilitated patients	With indwelling catheters there is inevitably some degree of cystitis after removal of the catheter. If it is significant: • Encourage the patient to increase its fluid intake, either as water or by adding water to the food. • Walk the patient frequently to allow urination; observe colour and amount of urine passed. If catheterisation of the cervix does occur, remove the catheter and begin with a new one.
Patient resistance		Sedate or, in extreme cases, anaesthetise the patient.
Blockage of indwelling catheters	General hygiene and cleaning Encourage increased water intake (this helps to maintain a continuous flow of urine through the catheter) If bags are attached, check regularly to ensure that urine is able to drain freely	Flush with sterile saline or water.
Urethral damage	Never use force. Use adequate lubrication. If an obstruction or difficulty occurs, stop and inform a senior member of staff.	If trauma caused by catheterisation is suspected, a veterinary surgeon will have to decide what further action is to be taken. Minor trauma will be treated with a course of antibiotics.
Failure to catheterise the urethra in the bitch	The only prevention is to gain experience in bitch catheterisation, which can only be achieved with practice. The easiest way for the student nurse to appreciate the position of the urethral orifice is the use of a lighted speculum to provide viewed introduction of the catheter.	

Removal of indwelling catheters by patients

Adequate suturing (tomcat, dog) and the application of Elizabethan collars should prevent catheter removal by the patient.

Types of urinary catheter

Most catheters (Table 16.7) manufactured for the veterinary market, are supplied individually, double wrapped, with an inner nylon and outer paper or plastic sleeve. The catheters are ready for use, having been sterilised by either ethylene oxide gas or gamma radiation. Silicone Foley catheters come non-sterile and require sterilisation by autoclave or ethylene oxide. Metal bitch catheters may be autoclaved although they are now rarely in use.

With the exception of silicone catheters (which may be re-sterilised in the autoclave), urinary catheters are designed for single use only. The cleaning and re-use of catheters (other than silicone varieties) is not recommended.

Dog catheters

Plastic dog catheters
These have a rounded tip behind which are two oval drainage holes (one at each side) (Fig. 16.12a). They are designed for single use in the male dog and can be used as indwelling catheters.

Type	Species	Sex	Material	Indwelling	Sizes (FG)	Length (cm)	Luer fitting
Dog catheter	Dog	Male and female	Flexible grade of nylon (polyamide)	No but can be adapted to be indwelling	6–10	50–60	Yes
Silicone Foley	Dog	Male and female	Flexible medical grade silicone	Yes	5–10	30 and 55	No
Tieman's	Dog	Female	PVC (polyvinyl chloride)	No	8–12	43	Yes
Foley	Dog	Female	Teflon-coated latex	Yes	8–16	30–40	No
Cat catheter	Cat	Male and female	Flexible grade of nylon	No	3 and 4	30.5	Yes
Jackson cat catheter	Cat	Male and female	Flexible grade of nylon	Yes	3 and 4	11	Yes
Silicone cat catheter	Cat	Male	Medical grade silicone	Yes	3.5	12	Yes
Slippery Sam catheter	Cat	Male	PTFE (Teflon)	Yes	3–3.5	14 and 11	Yes

Table 16.7 Types of urinary catheter

Choose the largest gauge appropriate for patient size. If too small a catheter is used, the tip of the catheter has a tendency to 'catch' in the urethral epithelium and bend. This may cause significant urethral trauma.

The only exception is where the urethra is narrowed due to a partial obstruction such as enlarged prostate, or a stricture. In these cases, there is no option other than to use a catheter that would otherwise be too small for the patient.

A second disadvantage of using small catheters in large patients is that the patient is stimulated to urinate when the catheter is introduced into the urethra, and urine will flow around the catheter as well as down the lumen.

Many people prefer to use dog catheters to catheterise bitches. They have no curved tip but are much firmer, providing more control for insertion into the urethral orifice, particularly when digital catheterisation is used. This extra rigidity far outweighs the advantage of the curved tip of the Tieman's catheter (Fig. 16.12b).

Foley silicone catheter   In design these catheters (Fig. 16.12d) are exactly the same as a standard latex bitch Foley. For dogs a longer length is obviously selected. The catheter is very flexible but despite this will advance up the curved male urethra into the bladder where the retaining balloon can be inflated, thus creating an indwelling male dog catheter. Wire-guide stylets are available that pass up the centre of the catheter, to assist in catheter introduction if required. Silicone catheters have the added advantage of being autoclavable and therefore can be re-used (this may make their relatively high cost more acceptable). It is the microscopic 'smoothness' of the medical grade silicone that enables these catheters to be passed up the male urethra. Silicone is inert and causes no mucosal irritation.

All lubricants are compatible with these catheters.

Bitch catheters

Tieman's catheter   Designed for catheterisation of the human male, these catheters (Fig. 16.12b) became popular for use in the bitch due to their curved tip. The moulded tip was found to be advantageous when placing it into the urethral orifice. However, the rest of the catheter is so soft and flexible that the amount of control over the tip is negligible. This makes placing the catheter into the urethral orifice a very difficult task. The excessive length of the catheter is a further disadvantage.

Latex Foley indwelling bitch catheter   Foley catheters (Fig. 16.12c) incorporate an inflatable balloon behind the drainage holes at the tip of the catheter. The balloon is inflated after placement of the catheter into the bladder, making it an indwelling catheter.

Foley catheters are produced for the human market, but suitable sizes are available for use in most bitches except very tiny puppies. They cannot be used in cats or the male dog (unless in conjunction with a urethrostomy). The balloon is inflated (usually with sterile water or saline) via a channel built into the wall of the catheter which ends in a side arm and a one-way valve. The catheter is removed by deflating the balloon through the same side arm. The latex catheters *must not be re-used*: the balloon is weakened after use and cannot be relied upon to function correctly if re-used.

Latex Foley catheters are very flexible – this provides maximum patient comfort but causes a problem when introducing them. Placement is achieved by the use of a rigid metal stylet or probe laid beside the catheter with the point secured in one of the drainage holes at the catheter's tip (Fig. 16.13). The stylet is removed once the balloon is inflated.

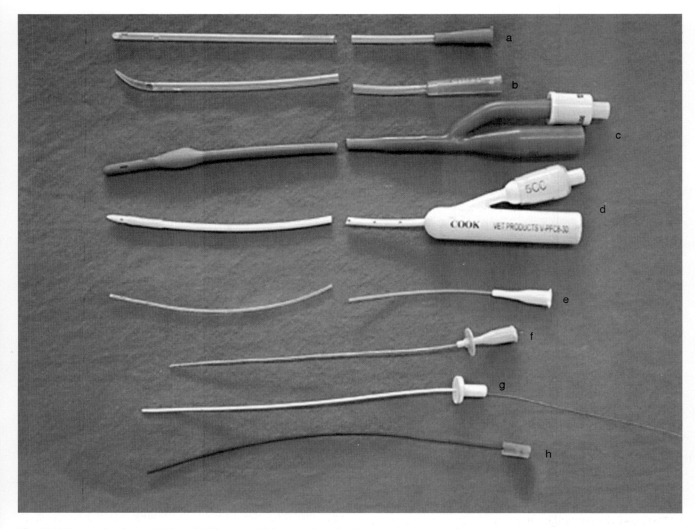

Fig. 16.12 Types of catheter: (a) dog; (b) Tieman's; (c) latex Foley; (d) silicone Foley; (e) cat; (f) Jackson cat; (g) silicone cat; (h) Teflon cat.

Latex Foley catheters must not be lubricated with petroleum-based ointments or lubricants, which will damage the latex rubber so that the balloon may burst on inflation.

The absence of a Luer mount in this catheter may cause problems for continuous collection of urine, but urine collection bags with appropriate connectors are available from medical suppliers. If these bags cannot be supplied, the catheter must have an adapter placed so that drip bags can be used for urine collection (Fig. 16.14a). Unless 3-litre drip bags are employed, frequent emptying will be required in most dogs. It would be unwise to leave a large dog with only a 1-litre collection bag attached overnight.

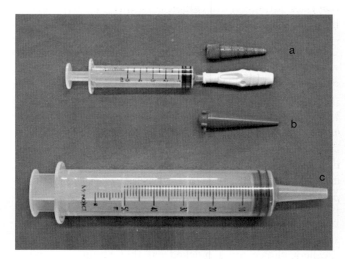

Fig. 16.14 (a) Spigot: metal or plastic, to provide a Luer connection for the Foley catheter enabling empty drip-bag attachment (to collect urine) or to allow bladder drainage with a Luer side attachment syringe.
(b) Bung: to prevent continuous drainage and therefore soiling of the patient, when a urine collection bag is not in use. (c) 50 ml catheter-tipped syringe.

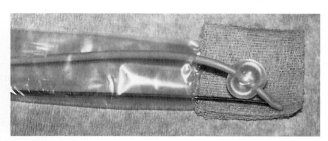

Fig. 16.13 Correct placement of the stylet in the tip of the Foley catheter. The balloon is inflating correctly and therefore the catheter is ready for use.

An alternative is to bung the catheter and drain the bladder at regular intervals with a spigot or a catheter tip 50 ml syringe (Fig. 16.14b). This method may be acceptable for a recumbent patient but not, for example, after bladder surgery.

Silicone indwelling Foley These can be used in the bitch (at shorter lengths) as for the male (Fig. 16.12d). They still require a stylet for correct placement in the bitch. Their use in bitches is still low due to their cost, the existing latex Foley being adequate in nearly all cases. The silicone Foley is inert, causing little mucosal irritation and may be preferable for use in patients with wounds near to the urethral opening.

Cat catheters

Conventional These straight catheters (Fig. 16.12e), with a Luer connection are compatible with all lubricants and are for single use. They are basically a small version of the dog catheter.

Jackson Jackson catheters (Fig. 16.12f) were designed primarily for use in male cats suffering from feline lower urinary tract disease. They can be used in any male or female cat.

A fine metal stylet, lying in the lumen of the catheter, gives extra rigidity and provides better control for insertion into the urinary bladder. It also helps to displace any loose obstruction (e.g. protein plugs or crystals in the urethra). A normal catheter would be too flexible to achieve this. The stylet is removed once the catheter is in place.

The Jackson is much shorter than the other cat catheters. This is to enable the entire length of the catheter to be placed in the patient, thereby allowing the flange to be sutured to the prepuce. The circular plastic flange is present just behind the Luer fitting of the catheter. In this way the catheter becomes indwelling.

Silicone tomcat catheters A silicone catheter with distal side holes (Fig. 16.12g), very similar in design to a standard Jackson cat catheter. A wire guide is supplied to assist introduction. The proximal fitting enables syringe attachment, and suture holes in the baseplate allow suturing to the prepuce.

Teflon tomcat catheters In appearance it is very similar to the conventional cat catheter (Fig. 16.12h). The very smooth catheter shaft material ensures ease of catheter placement. The material is also inert and causes no mucosal irritation. Suture holes in the silicone hub allows securing of the catheter to the prepuce. It is therefore an excellent choice for a blocked cat that requires a longer-term indwelling catheter. These catheters are designed for single use only.

All lubricants are compatible. Re-use is not recommended.

Equipment

Specula

A speculum is an instrument which assists cavities to be viewed. Specula assist catheterisation of bitches by holding back the vaginal tissue and allowing good visualisation of the urethral orifice. This is of great aid to the student nurse: digital catheterisation can be difficult without a visual knowledge of the urethral position.

It is preferable for all specula to be sterile and it is often cheaper in the long run to invest in a metal speculum that can be autoclaved, rather than using the home-made variety that needs gas sterilisation. If no specula are available, bitch catheterisation is still possible digitally.

There are several varieties of speculum, most of which are not specifically designed for catheterisation.

Nasal speculum There are many slight variations, the adult size being the most appropriate. All have two flat blades which separate when the handles are closed together (Fig. 16.15a). Some have a retaining device; others have to be held open. A light source may be attached to one of the blades to illuminate the vagina. If this is not available, a pen torch held by an assistant is an effective alternative.

Rectal speculum This is used rarely, mainly due to expense. Rectal specula (Fig. 16.15b) are conical in shape and, once in place, a section of the conical arm slides out to allow viewing of the urethral orifice. The main problem is to align the removable section with the urethral orifice – easy in theory, but difficult in practice.

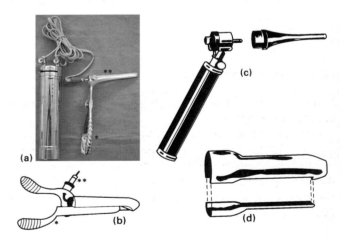

Fig. 16.15 (a) Nasal speculum, suitable for use as a bitch vaginal speculum. Pressing together the handles* causes the blades** to move apart and open the vestibule. (b) Rectal speculum, suitable for use as a bitch speculum. The lower sliding panel* is removed after insertion into the vestibule to expose the urethral opening. The lighting attachment**, which is connected to a battery, provides a self-contained light source. (c) Catheterisation speculum for attachment to an auriscope resembles an ear speculum except that a segment of its wall is absent. (d) A speculum made from the container of a Monojet disposable syringe by cutting away a segment of the plastic.

Auriscope This is a normal auriscope handle and light but the attachment used has a section removed from its wall (Fig. 16.15c).

Home-made speculum Monojet syringe packing cases are ideal rigid plastic specula and they are cheap. Simply remove one section of the cover, file the edges smooth and use an external light source (Fig. 16.15d).

Batteries and transformers

Ensure that these are electrically tested and working correctly. Spare batteries should always be in stock. Transformers are usually away from the vulva and do not require sterilisation.

Speculum bulbs

These are best stored separately as they break easily. They cannot be sterilised in the autoclave and therefore need gas or, more realistically, chemical sterilisation.

Stylets

Stylets can be made or bought. Ensure that they are long enough for easy use – they need to be at least two-thirds the length of the longest Foley catheter stocked.

Stylets can be packed and autoclaved or chemically sterilised.

Metal guide wires are supplied for use with silicone Foleys – these are placed up the centre of the catheters and therefore need to be longer than the length of the Foley. They can be autoclaved.

Urine collection bags

Manufactured varieties come prepacked and sterile; they are designed for single use.

Previously used drip-bags can be used with a giving set attached. Ensure that the end of the giving set is thoroughly cleaned and chemically sterilised before being attached to the urinary catheter. Attach a screw attachment bung to the end of the giving set during storage to keep it clean from dust and dirt.

Bungs and spigots

Plastic bungs are supplied in multipacks requiring sterilisation or individually packed sterile units. Chemical sterilisation is the only practical method for these bungs. Metal spigots can be autoclaved or placed in chemical sterilising solution until needed.

Three-way taps

These are invaluable when draining bladders via a catheter. They avoid leakages by controlling urine flow whilst syringes are emptied.

Catheter storage and checking

Catheters should be stored in a dry environment and laid flat without any pressure on top of them. Unless a suitably long drawer is available, urinary catheters are best left in their boxes and removed only when required.

All catheters have a shelf-life, after which sterility is no longer guaranteed by the manufacturer. Make regular checks, especially if the practice's use of catheters is infrequent.

Cleaning and sterilisation of catheters

Practice policy regarding re-use of catheters is rarely the nurse's decision; however, the process of cleaning and sterilisation is time-consuming and is *not* recommended for urinary catheters. Silicone catheters are the only variety marketed as autoclavable.

Cleaning

(1) Flush, with force, copious amounts of cold water through the catheter immediately after use. This is usually done with a syringe. Cold water prevents coagulation of any protein that may be present.
(2) Remove any blockage with a wire stylet and repeat step (1).
(3) Wash the exterior and interior of the catheter with a mild detergent. Rinse thoroughly, as in (1).
(4) Check catheter for kinks, holes, etc. If any damage is found the catheter *must* be discarded.
(5) Dry in a warm, dust-free atmosphere.

Sterilisation

Pack appropriately (autoclave bags or ethylene oxide). Autoclaving is the best method for nylon catheters. The COSHH Regulations have made the use of ethylene oxide in most practices difficult and expensive. There are no short cuts and therefore it is unlikely that any but the largest of veterinary establishments will continue to sterilise equipment by this method on their own premises.

Methods for urinary catheterisation

Actual procedures for urinary catheterisation of dogs, bitches (three methods), tomcats and queens are set out in Table 16.8. Several general points apply to all methods.

Table 16.8 Methods for urinary catheterisation

	Equipment	Method
Dog catheterisation	Catheter Lubricant Swabs for cleaning Syringe to assist urine drainage Three-way tap (if required) Sample pot Gloves Urine bag or a bung Kidney dish *If the catheter is to be made indwelling:* Suture material Zinc oxide tape For silicone male Foley catheters, water sufficient to fill balloon Guide wire Syringe	1. Wash hands and put on gloves 2. Clean prepuce 3. Extrude penis; if not experienced, get an assistant to do this two-handed (Fig. 16.17) 4. Clean prepuce 5. Remove catheter from the outer wrapping and cut a feeding sleeve from the inner sterile packaging (Fig. 16.18). This allows easy feeding of the catheter from the packaging into the urethra using a no touch technique For silicone male Foley catheter placement, feed guide wire up the center of the catheter 6. Lubricate the catheter and insert the tip into the urethra (Fig. 16.17) 7. Advance the catheter up the urethra. Resistance may be met at the os penis, where there is a light narrowing of the urethra, at the ischial arch and area of the prostate gland if enlarged Steady but gentle pressure should overcome this resistance. If the catheter cannot be passed, re-evaluate catheter size 8. Inflate balloon once tip of catheter is in bladder if silicone male Foley in use 9. Proceed according to reason for catheterisation (e.g. drain bladder, collect sample, hydropropulsion) To provide an indwelling dog catheter from a polyamide catheter (Fig. 16.19): 1. Place zinc tape around catheter near to prepuce 2. Stitch to prepuce; or 3. Stick to prepuce Neither of these options is ideal because dog catheters are not designed to be indwelling. Best to use silicone indwelling male Foley
Bitch catheterisation Method 1: Urethra viewed in dorsal recumbency	Speculum (with or without light source) Alternative light source if required Catheter Lubricant Swabs for cleaning Gloves *If a Foley catheter is being placed:* Stylet Sterile water/saline to inflate cuff Urine bag Syringe	1. Wash hands and put on gloves 2. Ensure the bitch is in a straight dorsal recumbent position with the hindlimbs flexed and drawn forward (Fig. 16.16). The tail needs to be under control too 3. Clean vulva 4. Remove catheter from outerwrapping and expose tip only from inner sleeve 5. If a Foley catheter is being used, insert the stylet 6. Place lubricated speculum blades between the vulval lips as caudally as possible to avoid the clitoral fossa (Fig. 16.20) 7. Insert *vertically* into the vestibule and turn handles cranially (Fig. 16.20) 8. Open the blades of the speculum. The urethral opening will be visible on the cranial side of the vertically oriented vestibule, approximately half way between the vulva and cervix (Fig. 16.21) 9. Insert the tip of the catheter into the urethral orifice (Fig. 16.21). **Draw the hindlimbs caudally**. This straightens the urethra, making it easier to push the catheter into the bladder 10. Proceed depending on reason for catheterisation. If a Foley catheter is being used, inflate balloon, withdraw stylet, attach bag and place Elizabethan collar (Fig. 16.22)
Bitch catheterisation Method 2: Urethra viewed standing	As in Method 1 Generally only one assistant is required	1. Wash hands and put on gloves 2. Ensure tail is well restrained 3. Clean vulva 4. Place speculum between vulval lips and advance at a slight angle towards the spine, then horizontally (Fig. 16.23) 5. Open blades and identify urethral orifice. This will be on the ventral floor of the vestibule 6. Insert catheter at a slightly ventral angle so as to follow the direction of the urethra into the bladder 7. Proceed as for Method 1

	Equipment	Method
Bitch catheterisation Method 3: Digital	Sterile gloves Catheter Lubricant Swabs for cleaning Collection pots *If a Foley is being placed*: additional equipment is as in Method 1	1. Restrain in preferred position, lateral or standing (standing is generally easier) 2. Scrub hands and put on sterile gloves in an aseptic manner 3. Ask an assistant to clean the vulva (gloved person having sterile hands) 4. Assistant removes outer wrapping from catheter and the inner package is removed by the scrubbed person 5. Holding the sterile part of the packaging, place stylet if necessary 6. Lubricate first finger of *non-writing* hand 7. Place finger into vestibule and feel along ventral surface for a raised pimple (Fig. 16.24) 8. Place finger just cranial to this raised area, which is the urethral orifice (Fig. 16.24) 9. Raising hand and finger dorsally, digitally guide catheter, tipped slightly ventrally (as in Method 2) into the urethral orifice The catheter will run past the fingertip if the orifice is missed 10. Proceed as for Method 1. The digital method may be difficult or even impossible in smaller breeds
Tomcat catheterisation	As for dog catheterisation	1. Wash hands and put on gloves 2. Restrain patient and have control of the tail 3. Pull patient's hindlimbs slightly cranially 4. Prepare feeding sleeve as for the dog catheter and lubricate tip 5. With one hand extrude penis by applying gentle pressure each side of the prepuce with two fingers (Fig. 16.25) 6. Introduce catheter into the urethra gently 7. Collect sample or drain bladder 8. If a Jackson catheter is being placed for continuous drainage, stitch flange to prepuce
Queen catheterisation This is rarely carried out but is quite straightforward if required (e.g. for contrast studies)	As for dog catheterisation	1. Restrain patient 2. Wash hands and put on gloves 3. Remove outer wrapping and cut a feeding sleeve 4. Lubricate tip of catheter 5. The catheter is placed between the vulval lips and 'blindly' introduced into the urethra. Angle the catheter ventrally, placing gentle pressure until the catheter slips into the urethra 6. The catheter is not designed to be indwelling

Check that (1) there are no splits, tears, holes, etc., in the packaging and no kinks are visible; (2) the balloon inflates before placement of a Foley catheter; (3) the stylet moves freely in the lumen before using a Jackson cat catheter

Physical restraint

Most patients will allow urinary catheterisation under gentle physical restraint without resistance. If necessary, use a muzzle on a dog. Ensure that the patient is at a comfortable working height.

Dogs and cats can be restrained in a standing position or in lateral recumbency.

Bitches can be restrained in dorsal recumbency (Fig. 16.16).

Chemical restraint

Sedation

- Dog: rarely required unless the patient is aggressive or very nervous.

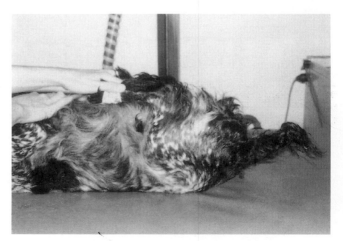

Fig. 16.16 Correct hindlimb position for the introduction of a Foley catheter with the patient in dorsal recumbency.

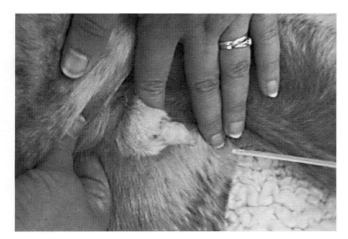

Fig. 16.17 Two-handed method for penis extrusion for introduction of a catheter into the urethra.

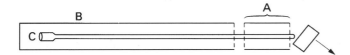

Fig. 16.18 Creating a feeding sleeve for easy introduction of urinary catheters. A: feeding sleeve; B: outer packaging; C: catheter.

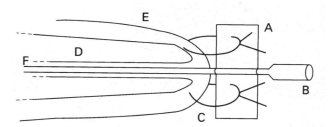

Fig. 16.19 Suturing of polypropylene catheter to prepuce, to create an indwelling male urinary catheter. A: zinc tape butterfly; B: Luer tip catheter; C: suture; D: penis; E: prepuce; F: catheter in urethra.

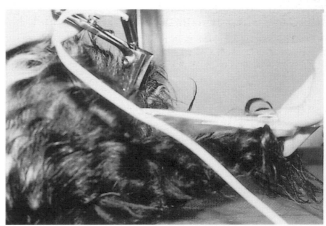

Fig. 16.20 Correct speculum angle in the vestibule and the horizontal position of the Foley catheter as it is advanced into the bladder.

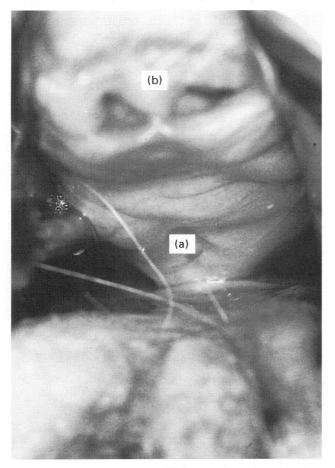

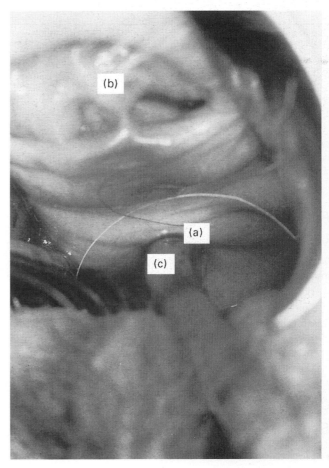

Fig. 16.21 Close-up view of the position of (a) the urethral orifice, (b) clitoral fossa and (c) catheter in position.

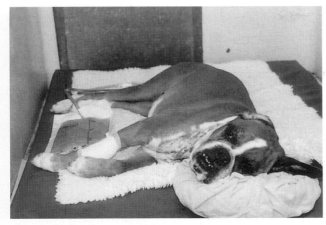

Fig. 16.22 Recumbent patient with Foley catheter in place and urine collection bag attached. (This patient was unable to raise her head; therefore no Elizabethan collar was necessary.)

- Bitch: most bitches will accept catheterisation more readily if lightly sedated, especially if dorsal recumbency is chosen. Standing catheterisation is best done without sedation, otherwise the patient tends to keep sitting down – which can be tiring for the assistant.

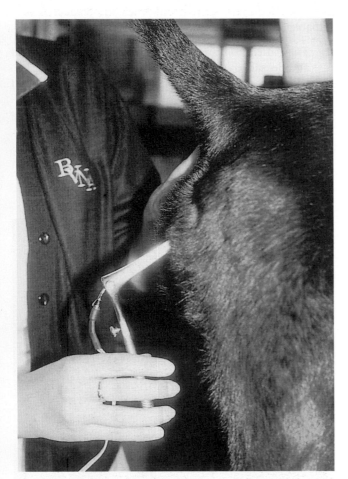

Fig. 16.23 Angle of speculum for introduction between lips of vulva in standing bitch. The speculum handle is then raised to insert the blades fully into the vestibule, avoiding painful interference with the clitoral fossa.

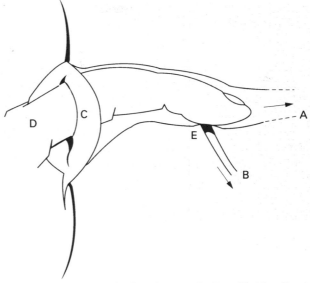

Fig. 16.24 Digital catheterisation: A: to cervix; B: to bladder; C: vulva; D: finger; E: raised area (urethral orifice).

- Cat: catheterisation of the cat is generally less stressful for all concerned if the cat is sedated.

General anaesthesia (GA) This is rarely indicated or necessary unless the patient has sustained other trauma which makes catheterisation under sedation humanely unacceptable (e.g. fractured pelvis, vaginal mass). It is sensible to catheterise during general anaesthesia if this is required for other treatment (e.g. catheterise a paraplegic patient whilst under GA for a myelogram).

Equipment preparation

Prepare all equipment *before* restraining the patient. Patient cooperation will be greater if prolonged restraint is avoided.

Lubricants

There is some debate over the necessity for the use of lubricants. Urinary catheterisation can be done without but

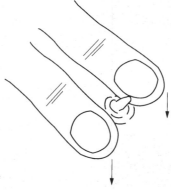

Fig. 16.25 Extrusion of tomcat penis.

lubricants aid passage of the catheter and help to avoid abrasive trauma.

- Check contents of lubricants before using them with Foley catheters; most are water-based and are compatible with commonly used catheters.
- Make sure that lubricants are sterile. Xylocaine gel (Astra) and K-Y jelly (Johnson and Johnson) are ideal choices. Xylocaine gel has the added advantage of desensitising the urethra, penis or vestibule.

Cleaning

- Clean the area with an antiseptic solution to remove any discharges and surface dirt.
- Clip around the area if necessary, especially in long-haired breeds. (Remember to check that permission for this has been obtained from the owner.)

Gloves

The use of gloves is recommended for health and safety of personnel. In general, multiple packs of non-sterile gloves are adequate because the catheter will be fed from its package using a 'no touch' technique. Gloves are therefore used to prevent contamination of staff with urine, rather than protection of the patient from infection.

Sterile gloves will be required when digital catheterisation is performed, as the catheter tip is inevitably touched by the finger.

Length of catheter

Measure a dog or cat catheter against the patient before unpacking the catheter. This measurement gives a rough estimate of the length of catheter to insert into the patient.

Stop inserting once urine flows. Overinsertion can result in the catheter bending and re-entering the urethra or, even worse, knotting in the bladder and requiring surgical removal.

Other methods of emptying the urinary bladder

Natural micturition

This is non-invasive and usually easy to achieve by nurse or owner. In most circumstances it is the preferred method for emptying the bladder but there are several disadvantages:

- The sample is always contaminated and therefore useless for culture and sensitivity evaluation.
- If the patient is unable to urinate normally, another method has to be employed.

- Patients often refuse to produce urine when convenient and required.

If not required for culture, then collection of samples from the environment may be acceptable in some cases, e.g. urine can be retrieved from litter trays that have been left empty or filled with non-porous beads (so-called 'washable' litter!).

Manual expression of the bladder

In cats this is probably the most common method. Dogs, especially recumbent ones, can also be encouraged to urinate in this way.

As long as the bladder is of a reasonable size, this task becomes easier with practice. Pressure should be applied steadily and slowly – do not use sudden pressure as this may cause trauma to the bladder. Generally very little pressure will initiate a free flow of urine. Excessive pressure should never be required as the bladder can become bruised or even ruptured.

Cystocentesis

This should only be carried out when the bladder is of a palpable size (Fig. 16.26). The method is as follows:

(1) The patient is restrained in a position between lateral and dorsal recumbency.
(2) Clip an area about 5 × 5 cm on the midline caudal abdomen.
(3) Prepare the skin aseptically, and manually immobilise the bladder, through the abdomen wall.
(4) Using a syringe (5–20 ml) with a needle attached (23 gauge ×1 inch), insert through the abdominal wall and into the bladder.

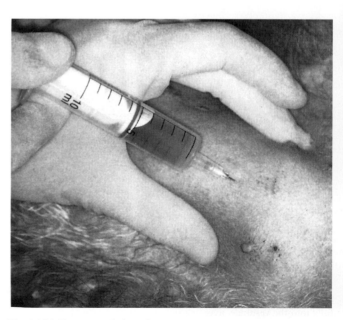

Fig. 16.26 Cystocentesis in a dog.

(5) Remove urine.

(6) Apply gentle pressure at the injection site as the needle is quickly removed. The use of larger gauge needles is to be discouraged because it increases the possibility of urine leakage from the bladder after needle removal.

This technique is fairly straightforward and generally without complications, as long as an aseptic technique is used. It may be the only method available for urine drainage in an obstructive emergency. As this procedure involves entering a body cavity it must only be carried out by a veterinary surgeon.

KEY POINTS

- Aspiration pneumonia is a real risk with syringe feeding.
- For 5 years of a pet's age, allow 24 hours longer to recover.
- Young patients may have the capacity to survive mild medication overdose, geriatrics may not.
- Do not restrict water intake in the geriatric patient unless they are vomiting.
- Minimum urine output should equal 2 ml/kg/day in the normal cat and dog.
- Feeding of patients after intestinal surgery should begin immediately after recovery from surgery, to prevent intestinal stasis.
- Sick recumbent animals may have increased nutrient requirement (protein rather than carbohydrate) for tissue repair.
- Placement of urinary catheters is invasive and should not be carried out lightly.
- Prophylactic antibiotic cover for indwelling urinary catheters is necessary, but with an increasing occurrence of antibiotic resistance, other methods of urine control need to be considered.
- Serious secondary chest infections may develop as a result of hypostatic pneumonia.
- Electrically heated beds are potentially dangerous, take care with their use in recumbent patients.
- Constant 24-hour observation is essential for the comatosed patient.

17

Medical disorders and their nursing

C. George and *L. A. Slater*

Learning objectives

After reading this chapter, students should be able to:

- Identify how micro-organisms can affect the animal and what the pathogenic effects are.
- Explain how infection can be transmitted and methods of control.
- Compare innate and acquired immune defences, indicating factors that may influence them.
- Describe the common complications and nursing requirements of medical disorders.
- Understand how to nurse and care for patients with medical disorders.

Infectious disease

Infectious diseases are caused by micro-organisms, commonly **bacteria**, **viruses**, **fungi** and **protozoa**.

A contagious disease is a disease that is capable of transmission by direct or indirect contact from one animal to another. This includes all those diseases listed below, together with internal and external parasitism.

A non-infectious disease is one that does not involve micro-organisms.

Infectious/contagious diseases found in the UK in the dog include the following:

- Distemper.
- Infectious canine hepatitis.
- Kennel cough complex.
- *Leptospira canicola* and *icterohaemorrhagiae*.
- Lyme disease.
- Parvovirus.
- Rabies.
- Salmonellosis.

Infectious/contagious diseases infecting cats in the UK include:

- Chlamydiosis.
- Feline leukaemia virus (FeLV).
- Feline infectious anaemia (FIA).
- Feline infectious peritonitis (FIP).
- Feline immunodeficiency virus (FIV).
- Feline upper respiratory tract disease (FURTD).
- Rabies.
- Salmonellosis.
- Toxoplasmosis.
- Feline panleucopaenia.

How contagious diseases are spread

To understand how these diseases cause such widespread problems it is important to understand the way the infective organism leaves the animal, how another comes into contact with it and then the route the organism takes to infect that new animal.

Exit routes for organisms

The key exit routes for infectious organisms are the body secretions and excretions:

- Oral, nasal and ocular discharges.
- Urine.
- Faeces.
- Vomitus.
- Blood.
- The skin.
- *In utero*, in milk.
- Venereal contact, semen and parturition.

Especially important are organism-laden saliva and droplets suspended in an aerosol.

Saliva is important with diseases such as rabies, infectious canine hepatitis, FeLV and FIV – bite wounds, as a result of animal-to-animal fighting, are the commonest method for saliva to gain access and cause infection. An important consideration for infectious disease control in this case would be reduction in conflict by neutering, as well as vaccination if available.

The spread of infection by droplets is a significant hazard, as it is exceptionally difficult to limit aerosol distribution. Droplets released can affect a significant area and large number of animals – especially when the population is housed close together, as seen in rescue and breeding environments and air exchange is poor. Droplets are an important factor in the spread of canine distemper, kennel cough complex and feline upper respiratory tract disease.

Ocular discharges may spread disease such as chlamydia, where cat-to-cat grooming can enhance disease spread.

Urine

Infected urine plays a significant role in the spread of disease such as leptospirosis and infectious canine hepatitis. In some diseases the organisms target specific organs and tissues, in others distribution is a little more haphazard and depends on the site of infection. However, where there is kidney involvement the urine may contain high concentrations of the organism.

Faeces and vomitus

If the organism infects the gastrointestinal tract the cells are often invaded and become damaged. With a GI tract that is unable to perform its normal tasks, diarrhoea and/or vomiting will occur and the organism is passed out, leading to an infected environment.

Diseases where this poses a threat of infection include canine parvovirus, bacterial enteritis and feline panleucopaenia.

Blood

This is important with the rickettsial parasite, *Haemobartonella felis*, the cause of feline infectious anaemia, and involves the infection of a vector – the flea. The flea picks up a meal of infected blood from the host cat, moving on to the next cat and so transmitting the disease.

Skin

Ectoparasites such as ringworm, lice, fleas and mites are spread this way, some by direct contact (lice), others by direct or indirect contact, such as fleas, mites and ticks, which can exist in the environment.

Fomites, such as grooming equipment and bedding may play a role, e.g. ringworm and fleas.

In utero *and via milk*

Many diseases are spread to potential offspring across the placenta or later to newborn puppies/kittens via the milk. These include feline leukaemia virus and *Toxocara* infections, feline panleucopaenia, feline infectious anaemia and feline immunodeficiency virus.

Venereal, semen and parturition

Infection may occur at mating or via the placenta and fetal fluid at birth. Feline panleucopaenia FIV are examples of this route.

Transmission routes between animals

Contagious diseases are transmitted either by direct or indirect contact.

- Direct contact requires immediate physical contact between the infected animal and another susceptible animal.

- Indirect contact involves spread of infection between hosts via the environment, objects (**fomes:** singular, **fomite**: plural) or by another animal (**vector**).

Environmental contamination may be the surrounding land and buildings, airborne contamination as a result of droplets suspended in an aerosol (e.g. after sneezing) or may be contamination of food and water.

Poor handling hygiene and cooking methods can result in *Salmonella* and *Campylobacter* infection, and water is an important dispersal agent for leptospirosis. *Toxoplasma gondii* is spread by eating infected meat – either mice/birds or uncooked 'bought' meat.

Routes of infection of a new host

Ingestion

This is one of the most common routes of access. This may occur through direct ingestion of the organism or through ingestion of a vector.

Sources of contamination include food, water, coprophagia and consuming fleas during grooming. Mutual grooming activity and licking others will also allow cross-contamination as it brings susceptible animals in contact with any body secretions. Vectors and fomites have a role.

Inhalation

This could be inhalation of contaminated fluid droplets, e.g. following sneezing/coughing or inhalation of infected particles of dust. The risk of infection through inhalation is reduced by providing adequate air exchange and avoidance of overcrowding. The greater the concentration of organism in the air space the greater the risk of infection and the risk of a more severe disease.

Through the skin

This protective layer is most commonly a route of access to infectious organisms when it is broken by biting or scratching, during fighting activity. Inoculation with the organism can also occur with insect (flea) bites, scratching and with the use of unsterile needles. All these are incidences where the healthy, intact skin has been damaged and infection is introduced.

A secondary bacterial infection can occur when the skin has been traumatised and the body's protective barrier is damaged, such as after a burn or self-inflicted injury, or at the site of a surgical or traumatic wound.

Ectoparasites such as lice, mites and fleas are transmitted across the skin surfaces following direct or indirect contact between hosts.

Some parasites penetrate the skin surface by active burrowing through intact, healthy skin – hookworm larvae and sarcoptic mites are examples.

Mucous membranes

Systemic infection frequently occurs across the gastrointestinal and respiratory membranes. Micro-organisms also cause infection by contaminating other membranes – the conjunctiva, associated with *Chlamydia psittaci*, vaginal mucous membranes in connection with bacterial and fungal infections and the prepuce/penis with balanitis and venereal diseases.

Congenital route

Micro-organisms already present in the bitch/queen, or infected during the course of the pregnancy can pass through to the fetus. This is an example of **vertical transmission** and is an important route, especially in the following infectious diseases:

- *Toxocara canis*.
- *Toxoplasma gondii*.
- FeLV.
- Feline panleucopaenia.

Depending on the organism and the severity of the disease its effect may be:

- Fetal death – resorption, mummification, abortion or stillbirth.
- Born infected and showing clinical signs of disease.
- Born without outward signs of disease but remains a carrier.
- Fading kitten syndrome.
- Sudden death.

In some diseases infection via the milk poses a serious threat. For example, newborn kittens should be removed and hand-reared at birth, in FIV infection, to minimise the infection across the milk and tested at a later stage to identify any presence of the virus.

Introduction to viral diseases

Viruses are named either by the type of disease they produce, e.g. feline **immunodeficiency** virus, or by their classification to other viruses, e.g. feline **calici** virus.

Viruses are grouped and classified according to similarities in their physical, biochemical and genetic properties. The broadest description groups viruses into two groups, the DNA virus and the RNA virus, depending on which type of nucleic acid is involved in the viral particle. Further classifications describe viruses as single stranded, double stranded, segmented or non-segmented and whether the virus is enveloped or 'naked'.

The **retrovirus** family, the *retroviridae,* is a large group of RNA viruses that share particular features of a physical, biochemical and genetic nature.

The retrovirus family is further divided into three sub-groupings – the *spumavirinae, oncornavirinae* and the *lentivirinae*. Examples include FIV (lentivirus) and FeLV (oncovirus).

The *coronaviridae* are a large family of RNA viruses. An example of a coronavirus is Feline infectious peritonitis.

Modes of transmission of viruses

Most viruses collect in the body secretions of the infected animal. The more concentrated the micro-organisms the more chance infection will be successful. Viruses that can establish an infection by ingestion or aerosol contact are usually more easily transmitted than those requiring inoculation.

Introduction to bacterial diseases

Bacteria are micro-organisms lacking in nuclear membrane and with a cell wall of unique composition. Most bacteria are unicellular. They are classified according to shape (see Chapter 13).

Method of transmission

Bacteria can cause primary disease but are most often associated with a secondary infection following the initial introduction of disease caused by viruses.

Some bacteria are **commensal** – that is, they exist within the host without causing clinical disease (but have the potential to do so). If conditions alter, perhaps the animal becomes stressed as a result of going into boarding kennels, or following corticosteroid injection, the bacteria becomes active and causes infection. Examples of this are *Pasteurella* spp. and *Pseudomonas*. Existing asymptomatically in most cats' mouths, *Pasteurella* causes cellulitis following innoculation of the micro-organism by cat bite wound.

Obligate pathogens are those that always cause clinical signs and ill-health. An example here would be *Clostridium tetani*, which always causes disease once contracted.

Terminology and definitions
Preventive medicine

Methods taken to attempt to reduce or control the spread of infection. These include:

- Pet owner education – vaccination, pet hygiene, e.g. faecal collection, worming and flea prophylaxis.
- Vaccination programmes – see Table 17.1.
- High levels of hygiene – food preparation, human personal hygiene, correct use of disinfectants.

Table 17.1 Vaccination programmes

Disease	Type of vaccine	Age at which vaccines may be used	Booster required
Canine distemper	Modified live	8–9 weeks 1st injection 2nd injection 3 weeks later*	Annually or as advised
Infectious canine hepatitis	Live CAV-2	As above	Annually
Kennel cough complex	Covers *Bordetella bronchiseptica*, CAV and CP1V	10–14 days prior to risk Given intra-nasally	4–6 monthly*
Leptospirosis	Killed virus	9 weeks 1st injection 2nd injection 3 weeks later	Annually
Canine parvovirus	Attenuated live	As above A dose at 6 weeks is indicated for puppies at high risk	Annually
Feline panleucopaenia	Killed or modified live	9 weeks 1st dose with 2nd due 3 weeks later	Annually
FURD	Modified live or dead	As above	Annually
Chlamydia	Attenuated live	As above	Annually
FeLV	Cultivated	As above	Annually

* *Depending on vaccine manufacturer*

- Use of isolation facilities – suspected cases or quarantine for animals of unknown status.
- Improving animal conditions – control of feral/stray population, neutering programmes, minimise stress, maintain general health and nutritional state.

Direct/Indirect contact

Where a disease requires **direct contact** between an infected animal and a susceptible animal to achieve infection. This may occur by:

- Multi-animal housing, repeated contact and especially mutual grooming behaviour.
- Free-roaming animals or animals in contact during exercise.
- Sexual contact.
- Biting, i.e. innoculation.

Diseases spread by **indirect contact** require an organism that can survive away from the host, as the animals do not come into physical contact at any time. The length of time an organism can survive in the environment varies from hours to years.

The infected animal contaminates the environment in some way, which the susceptible animal then comes into contact with. Environmental contamination is usually as a result of loss of a body secretion such as saliva, urine, faeces, etc.

Fomites are inanimate objects that are part of the overall environmental contamination and remain a site for contamination unless they are disinfected appropriately or until the organisms ability to exist in the environment has ceased. Many fomites can move, e.g. bedding, feeding bowls, thermometers, and so can easily disperse around the animal's

location acting as a reservoir of the organism and able to widely contaminate that area. Correct barrier nursing is essential to ensure those animals in a veterinary environment are adequately isolated from others (see Table 17.2), as even insignificant items can spread infection – personnel's shoes, pens used to record patient details, door handles, etc.

Vectors

Some organisms can survive between hosts by existing in a living, or **animate carrier**. These are known as **vectors** and include flies, ticks or mites.

- **Biological vectors** or **intermediate host.** The organism undergoes some development within the biological host but this is not the host that final development of the disease will occur in and it is not usually shed. The next animal to become infected with the organism ingests the vector to do so. The organism that causes Lyme disease, *Borrelia burgdorferi*, is carried by deer ticks, prior to infecting dogs.
- **Definitive host.** The susceptible animal of the species that the infection development is completed in, i.e. shed, such as *Toxoplasmosis gondii*.
- **Mechanical hosts.** These simply transmit the disease from the infected animal to the susceptible animal. These are described as **transport** or **paratenic** hosts:

  - **Transport hosts.** The transport host is not affected by the infectious agent. It can pass on the infection to susceptible animals at any time and does not have to be ingested to do so. An example might be the flea carrying feline panleucopaenia – the infection is passed on when the flea bites a susceptible animal.

Table 17.2 Methods of control of spread of infection	
Principles	**Practice**
Encourage good prevention methods	Client education of the need for vaccination of all dogs Run an efficient repeat vaccination scheme Ensure adequate ectoparasite and endoparasite treatment/prevention
Maintain strict import control to prevent/minimise introduction of disease to UK	Strict adherence to PETS scheme Maintain quarantine scheme for animals entering UK from other countries
Maintain very high levels of kennel/ward hygiene	Remove insect vector method of transmission by regular treatment of environment Perform sterilisation or disposal of potential fomite items Establish efficient air exchange system within environment Avoid overcrowding
Identification and treatment of infectious disease	Avoid contact (direct/indirect) between animal and possible infected animal Deliver early and effective treatment of infected animals Practice efficient barrier nursing
Essentials of barrier nursing	Remove infected/suspected infectious animal to isolation quarters Isolation unit to be a clearly definable area with independent air exchange, feeding facilities and wash/cleaning provisions. The unit should be kept adequately stocked at all times to avoid any possible breakdown in isolation techniques Introduction of adequate protective clothing for personnel, i.e. preferably waterproof overalls or arm length gloves, aprons with sleeves, leg covers and covers for shoes or dedicated foot wear. These should be removed and disposed of into clinical waste All pieces of equipment should be dedicated to the isolation unit Where possible all items that come into contact with the animal, e.g. bedding, equipment, etc. should be disposable and should be discarded into clinical waste. Where this is not possible, e.g. scissors, fluid pumps, etc., efforts should be made to seal these inside protective packaging prior to use or for them to be cleaned and then soaked in appropriate disinfectant following completion of nursing the case The animal should remain in the isolation unit until either: (a) it is categorically cleared of any infectious disease by blood analysis; (b) it is considered to no longer be contagious, as determined by appropriate analysis; (c) it is euthanased/dies

- **Paratenic hosts**. The organism lives within the tissues of this host and so it must be ingested for infection to occur. There is no development of the organism. An example of the **paratenic** host is *Toxoplasma gondii*; the cat must eat the infected mouse (or uncooked meat) to become infected.

Carriers

These are animals that have been infected with an organism but do not display the clinical disease – they are **asymptomatic.**

A **healthy carrier** is an animal that has been exposed to the organism but has never become ill or had symptoms of the infection. The animal's immune system will have fought off the infection but the animal carries the infection and sheds it into the environment. Examples of this are *Haemobartonella felis* and *Chlamydiosis*.

The **convalescent carrier** is an animal that has recovered from the clinical disease but continues to shed the infective agent into the environment for some time following recovery. The period of time shedding continues varies with each disease. Examples include *salmonellosis,* cat flu and infectious canine hepatitis.

Open carriers are those animals that continuously shed the organism into the environment. **Closed carriers** are infected animals that carry the infection but do not release

it into the environment. This may be permanent or shedding may be triggered by factors such as stress or corticosteroid treatment.

When an animal has an active viral infection with a presence in the blood circulation this is known as **viraemia.** It is once the virus is in the systemic circulation that widespread disease is possible throughout the body. The animal that carries this and is permanently shedding the virus is termed **persistently viraemic.**

When the organisms are bacteria, their presence in the blood circulation is termed **bacteraemia.**

Vertical and horizontal transmission

- **Vertical** – transmission of disease to the fetus via the placenta during pregnancy.
- **Horizontal** – transmission of disease by direct or indirect contact.

The incubation period

This is the term used to describe the time interval between the susceptible animal coming into contact with the micro-organism and the presence of clinical disease – the clinical signs. This is usually given as a range (of days usually) and varies with each disease.

Factors that affect the incubation period include:

- The dose of micro-organisms.
- The immune system status of the susceptible animal.
- The general health and nutritional status.
- Animal's age.
- Route of entry.

The severity of the infection will depend on the following:

- The dose of micro-organisms.
- The state of the animal's immune system.
- Vaccination history or degree of acquired immunity with presence of antibodies.
- Animal's stress levels.
- Concurrent disease.
- Administration of corticosteroids.
- Animal's general health and nutritional state.

The most frequent route of infection is across the mucous membrane of the respiratory and or digestive tract, following either inhalation and/or ingestion. Once there, the factors seen above will determine whether the animal becomes infected, either without ever showing clinical signs (carrier) or becoming ill with the disease, or if the organism will be eliminated without causing infection.

If infection occurs the micro-organism will invade the epithelial cells of the respiratory or intestinal tract and local lymph nodes, where it will replicate. Some organisms provoke an immune reaction at this stage, others do not see a response from the immune system until the organism is in the circulation and the animal is viraemic. If the animal becomes viraemic, other tissues and organs will become affected by the organism as it is distributed around the body. Most viruses will target the organs that are rapidly dividing; once these have been invaded, clinical signs will be observed associated with the damage inflicted.

Separation of the infected animal and disease control

Isolation is the physical removal of the animal suspected or proved to have a contagious, infectious disease, thus eliminating the opportunity for contact, direct or indirect, to be made with other susceptible animals or people if the disease is zoonotic. An isolation area should be established with self-sufficient amenities such as wash facilities, general stock, drugs and means of disposal of infected items. Personnel should be suitably attired to protect contamination of themselves (especially if the disease is zoonotic) and also of their clothing.

Routes of transmission should be considered and protocols established to avoid contact. Droplets in aerosols are particularly difficult to avoid, but shared air space should be minimised with a good rate of air exchange or flow.

Quarantine is the compulsory isolation, with associated strict protocols, of animals with notifiable diseases. In the case of small animals this is when an animal comes from a country out of the PETS travel scheme, and is a method of guarding against the introduction of rabies to the UK. Under these conditions the animals do not come into contact with any other animals for a 6-month period.

The subject of quarantine, kennel management and the PETS travel scheme is covered in more detail in Chapter 6.

Barrier nursing is the term used to describe the methods involved in nursing an isolated animal.

Zoonosis

A zoonosis is a disease that can be transferred from animals to humans, some with potentially fatal consequences (rabies).

Avoidance of cross-infection includes:

- Good, routine personal hygiene, washing hands after handling animals and before touching anything that will be brought up to be in contact with mouth, etc. for example, holding/chewing pens, smoking cigarettes, handling food, etc.
- Do not allow animals to lick humans, particularly on the face/mouth, especially children who will be more susceptible and have a lower personal hygiene awareness.
- Always keep separate utensils for animal food preparation and human use and use separate areas for their washing up, etc.
- Pregnant females should be extra vigilant about personal hygiene after contact with animals.
- Clear up faeces, vomit, etc. immediately after deposited.
- Wear protective clothing all the time and change once soiled.
- Seek medical advice if contamination is suspected.

Canine infectious diseases

The canine infectious diseases considered in this section are summarised in Table 17.3, and their clinical signs in Table 17.4.

Distemper (hard pad)

Canine distemper is an infectious viral disease of the dog. It has a high morbidity rate and a variable mortality rate depending on the body systems affected and immune system efficacy of the infected animal.

It is most frequently seen in young dogs between the ages of 3 and 9 months, when the maternal antibody levels fall and if acquired immunity cover is inadequate. Distemper is also seen in other animals that have insufficient protection, i.e. those not vaccinated. Other species such as fox, badger, mink and ferret are also susceptible to distemper infection.

As droplets in aerosols play a major role in infection distribution, most outbreaks occur where there is a high density of dogs, such as rescue centres, housing estates and cities generally, as opposed to rural locations, etc.

Table 17.3 Canine infectious diseases

Disease	Agent	Incubation period	Major organs affected	Main method of transmission	Zoonotic	Diagnostic methods	Major nursing needs	Control/ prevention
Distemper	Virus	7–21 days	Respiratory Gastrointestinal	Inhalation	No	History and clinical signs Blood analysis Post mortem	Rehydration Symptomatic	Vaccination Client education
Infectious canine hepatitis (ICH)	Virus	5–9 days	Lymphatic system Liver	Inhalation/ ingestion	No	History and clinical signs Blood analysis	Pain management Fluid therapy Symptomatic	Vaccination Client education
Kennel cough complex	Bacteria/virus mixed	5–7 days	Upper respiratory tract	Inhalation	No	History and clinical signs Pharyngeal swabs	Symptomatic Antibiotics	Vaccination
Leptospira canicola and *Ictero-haemorrhagia*	Bacteria	5–7 days	Kidneys Liver	Urine	Yes	History and clinical signs Blood analysis	Fluid therapy Antibiotics	Vaccination
Lyme disease	Bacteria	Variable: acute–extended	Commonly joints	Vector – deer tick	Yes	History – especially geographical	Antibiotics NSAID	Avoidance of risk environment
Parvovirus	Virus	3–5 days	Myocarditis Gastrointestinal system	Faeces	No	Clinical signs Vaccination history CITES test	I/V Fluids	Vaccination
Rabies	Virus	1 week–1+ year Normally 3–8 weeks	Nervous system	Saliva to skin wound	Yes – fatal	Clinical signs History Post-mortem examination	N/A	Vaccination
Salmonellosis	Bacteria	2–3 days following a stressful episode	Gastrointestinal system	Faeces	Yes	Sterile tissue or body fluid examination	I/V fluids +/– antibiotics	Hygiene Disinfection

Table 17.4 Major clinical signs of canine infectious disease

	Clinical signs particular to this disease (see text for details)
Distemper	Hyperkeratosis of nose leather and foot pad Permanent dentition damage Nervous signs
Infectious canine hepatitis	Abdominal pain Corneal oedema Jaundice
Kennel cough complex	Dry, non-productive cough Serous/mucopurulent nasal discharge
Leptospira	Kidney pain
Lyme disease	Episodic polyarthritis
Parvovirus	Foul smelling dark brown/red diarrhoea Sudden death in young puppies Young puppies in heart failure
Rabies	Behavioural changes Excessive salivation Stupor Ataxia/paralysis
Salmonellosis	Follows period of stress Abdominal pain

Table 17.5 Canine distemper virus – nervous signs

Site	Symptoms
Cranial nerve defects	Poor night vision Blindness
Cerebral	Ataxia Circling Pacing Seizures
Cerebellar	Ataxia Dysmetria Hypermetria Head tilt Nystagmus
Spinal	Weakness Paresis or occasional paralysis of the hindlimbs Faecal and/or urinary incontinence Chorea or twitching associated with any group of muscles, often those of the limbs or flanks

Clinical signs

Clinical signs of **acute** distemper infection include some or all of the following:

- Depressed mental state.
- Anorexia.
- Pyrexia.
- Tonsilitis.
- Pharyngitis with a dry cough.
- Conjunctivitis.
- Rhinitis – initially serous changing to mucopurulent due to a secondary bacterial infection.
- Vomiting, diarrhoea, dehydration, loss of body condition.
- Hyperkeratosis of nose and foot pads – this is where the colloquialism for distemper, **hard pad**, comes from. The foot pads become thickened, with deep fissures and eventually exfoliate.
- Exudative pneumonia associated with a secondary *Bordetella bronchiseptica* infection.
- Tachypnoea and dyspnoea.
- Skin rash progressing to pustules, especially on abdomen. Thought to be part of an immune mediated response as animals that develop rashes often recover.
- Nervous signs (see Table 17.5).
- In infected puppies less than 6 months of age damage to the permanent dentition (enamel and dentition exposure) is likely ('distemper rings').

The severity of symptoms experienced will depend on:

- The degree of protection provided by maternal antibodies, acquired protection or vaccination.
- The intensity of the viral challenge.
- The nutritional status of the dog.
- Concurrent infections including parasitism.

In approximately 50% of the animals that contract acute disease, presentation of **nervous signs** will occur. These vary in type and severity but all result in a grave prognosis (see Table 17.5). Canine distemper is considered the most common cause of convulsions in dogs less than six months of age.

Some animals only display nervous symptoms with all the other signs of distemper infection absent. Some animals do not even demonstrate the disease until some years after infection with the virus. Dogs that develop late onset neurological signs often show immunity to canine distemper virus. This may be due to the protective blood–brain barrier mechanism – sealing in the viral infection in the central nervous system when otherwise throughout the body the immune system has eliminated it.

Nervous signs present in two different forms:

- One is referred to as **multi-focal encephalitis**. Clinical signs include incoordination, weakness in hindlimbs (paresis), menace reflex defects, head tilts, nystagmus, facial paralysis and head tremors. Affected dogs remain mentally alert. It is a slow progressive disease, occurring in dogs 4–8 years, and possibly taking more than a year to reach maximum severity.
- The other form of chronic distemper encephalitis is referred to as **old dog encephalitis**. It is a rare, progressive disease found in dogs over 6 years of age. As the disease progresses symptoms develop from generalised visual impairment to mental depression, circling, head pressing and being unresponsive to normal stimuli.

Recovery from either form is unlikely and most animals suffering from these symptoms will eventually be euthanased.

Distemper infection is also experienced as a **mild or sub-acute** form. It frequently goes unnoticed by the owner and often undiagnosed as its presenting signs are vague and recovery is rapid. Symptoms experienced may include a transient period of depression and mild pyrexia of less than 40°C. Secondary bacterial infection is rare. Dental hypoplasia of enamel may be seen.

Aetiology and pathogenesis

Canine distemper virus (CDV) is caused by a morbillivirus, related to measles in humans and rinderpest virus in ruminants. The virus is labile off the host and is very susceptible to ultraviolet light, desiccation, heating and disinfection.

The virus is shed in urine, faeces, saliva, vomitus, nasal and ocular discharges.

Due to the gastric acid and bile salts destroying the virus, the gastrointestinal system is not an important transmission route. Inhalation is the most common route for transmission, as droplets in aerosol, spread between dogs in close contact or by direct contact between dogs.

Once the animal has been exposed, the virus initially replicates in macrophages and lymphocytes. If the body's immune system mounts a sufficiently vigorous response, as a result of maternal antibodies or acquired or vaccine protection, the infection will end there.

If the animal fails to raise sufficient immune system activity then the virus will move on to the epithelial cells of the gastrointestinal and/or respiratory systems.

Other sites for replication include the lymph nodes from where infected macrophages and lymphocytes enter the systemic circulation via the lymphatic vessels, going on to invade other lymphoid tissues and the bone marrow.

Other tissues now infected by the disease include the respiratory system, conjunctiva, gastrointestinal system, nose and pads of feet and the nervous system.

The virus may be found within the central nervous tissues within 10 days of exposure of the virus. It may remain there for long periods.

It is common for a secondary bacterial infection to occur with CDV as a result of immunosuppression – particularly *Streptococci* spp., *Staphylcocci* spp., *Mycoplasma* spp., and *Bordetella* spp. These result in a significant increase in the clinical signs.

Due to the high incidence of contact within the dog opulation to CDV it may appear as a concurrent infection with other diseases such as Infectious canine hepatitis, leptospirosis, parvovirus or toxoplasmosis.

Diagnosis

- History.
- Analysis.

  - Epithelial cells with eosinophilic bodies.
  - Antibody titre rising at least fourfold.
  - Immunofluorescence for virus in lymphoid tissue.

  - Detection of antibody in CSF.

- Post mortem.

Treatment

Treatment of the infected animal is purely symptomatic. This involves broad-spectrum antibiotics to counter the secondary bacterial infection and intravenous fluid therapy to rebalance water and electrolyte losses. Anti-convulsants for nervous signs along with antiemetics and antidiarrhoeal drugs are also part of the drug therapy protocol. Good standards of nursing care along with strict isolation techniques are vital. Even if all other dogs in the immediate environment are assumed to be protected due to a full vaccination history, isolation and barrier nursing is essential as no vaccination is 100% reliable.

Nursing care

The nursing requirements of the CDV-infected animal are centred on managing the symptoms.

- Managing the infectious patient – see barrier nursing (Table 17.2).
- General nursing of the symptoms suffered, removal of crusted ocular and nasal discharges, etc.
- Management of nutritional status.
- Disinfection of environment.
- Vaccination protocol for any other dogs in the infected dog's household.

Infectious canine hepatitis (ICH)

Infectious canine hepatitis (ICH) is an infectious viral disease of the dog. The mortality rate can be high when affecting unweaned puppies; however, this declines with the older dog as the severity of signs diminish with age. Foxes are also affected by ICH.

The virus targets three types of tissue:

- The liver.
- Lymphoid tissue.
- Vascular endothelium.

Recognised complications include:

- Nephritis.
- Corneal oedema or blue eye.

Clinical signs

ICH presents most commonly in its **acute form**. Signs include:

- Sudden onset depression of mental state.
- Anorexia.
- Pyrexia.

- Shock.
- Pale mucous membranes.
- Jaundice.
- Tonsilitis and generalised lymphadenopathy.
- Abdominal pain with praying position, with vocalisation just prior to death.
- Haemorrhagic diarrhoea.
- Hepatomegaly.

The disease may also present as **sudden death**, especially affecting neonatal puppies with most dying without any other signs. Others die following a brief period of anorexia, pyrexia and shock and occasionally haemorrhagic diarrhoea, abdominal pain and crying.

With **sub-acute** presentation of the disease symptoms include depression, anorexia and mild pyrexia. A temporary corneal oedema may also occur.

Aetiology and pathogenesis

Adenovirus 1 or CAV-1 is associated with ICH.

As adenoviruses are more resilient than the distemper virus, this poses a risk by environmental contamination as well as direct contact between dogs. The virus can remain viable off the host for up to 10 days – yet is still susceptible to destruction by heat, desiccation and disinfection.

The virus is excreted from the infected animal in the saliva, faeces and urine.

Another contamination risk is from the convalescent carrier – the animal that has recovered from the infection who continues to shed the virus for up to 6 months post infection, in their urine.

For CAV-1, ingestion is the main mode of transmission.

The virus replicates in local lymph nodes, possibly also intestinal Peyer's patches and mesenteric lymph nodes.

A viraemia follows within 5–9 days associated with infected lymphocytes. At this point, one of two effects will result:

- An immune response elicits release of antigen–antibody complexes into the circulation – these may then cause glomerular nephritis as they become deposited in the renal glomeruli. The virus will also attack the renal tubular cells, leading to an interstitial nephritis in about 70% of cases.
- Where the animal is unable to produce a sufficient immune response the virus targets the bone marrow, liver, other lymphoid tissue as well as vascular endothelium.

The mortality rate can be high, particularly in unweaned puppies. Here ICH often presents as sudden death, however infection in older animals results in less severe symptoms with sudden deaths rarely occurring in dogs older than 2 years of age.

Immunosuppression is less of a problem in this disease, compared to CDV and so a secondary bacterial infection is less of a complication.

Diagnosis

- History.
- Clinical signs.
- Blood analysis including:

  - Haematology (leucopaenia).
  - Biochemistry (elevated salt, bilirubin and blood urea).
  - Urine analysis (proteinuria).
  - Rising antibody titre.
  - Intranuclear inclusion bodies found within hepatocytes.
  - Virus isolation from major organ tissues such as liver and kidney.

- Post mortem.

Treatment

Care of the ICH patient is based on management and nursing care of the symptoms. This includes intravenous fluid therapy, including whole blood transfusion if bleeding has been severe. In addition antibiotic drug therapy is also indicated along with B-vitamins. Analgesics are indicated to control abdominal pain.

Approximately 20% of dogs develop uni- or bilateral corneal oedema (blue eye) post recovery. This is as a result of a localised immune reaction as the virus comes into contact with the corneal endothelium, leading to leakage of fluid into the aqueous humour. These corneal changes may remain as a complication leading to permanent visual impairment but in the majority of cases these are temporary.

Nursing care

- Managing the infectious patient – see barrier nursing (Table 17.2).
- General nursing of the symptoms suffered.
- Management of nutritional status.
- Vaccination protocol for any other dogs in the infected dog's household.
- Disinfection of the environment.
- Management of the potential convalescent carrier and the risk posed to others.

Kennel cough complex

Kennel cough (or virus-induced tracheobronchitis) is a highly infectious disease of the dog affecting any age group. It is caused by a mixture of virus, bacteria and mycoplasma and involves the lower respiratory tract with an incubation period of 5–7 days.

Whilst morbidity is high, the mortality rate is low, with most animals recovering from the complex within 3–7 days after the onset of clinical signs. The cough may persist for weeks or months if untreated.

It is a highly infectious disease affecting dogs, especially affecting high-density populations such as those found in boarding and breeding kennels and rescue centres.

Clinical signs

These include:

- The classic dry, non-productive cough. A hacking cough often with a retching sound, owners may report as if the animal has 'something stuck in its throat'. The cough can be reproduced by gentle, external pressure on the trachea (this is also possible into the recovery phase). The animal may be settled without symptoms until times of high excitement, exercise or environmental temperature change.
- Retching, sometimes leading to vomiting due to over-coughing.
- Animal remains otherwise bright and alert.

Aetiology and pathogenesis

Bordetella bronchiseptica is the most important cause of kennel cough but other viruses, bacteria and *Mycoplasma* are also involved, usually in conjunction with *Bordetella* spp.

Viruses associated with the complex include CDV, CAV-2 and canine parainfluenza virus (CPI). Others that have been linked to the condition but have been shown to have little real impact are CAV-1, canine herpesvirus and reovirus.

Most viruses cause a kennel cough infection with a very low mortality rate; however, a complicated CAV-2 infection can result in a fatal outcome, as secondary bacterial infections gain opportunities due to an inflammatory reaction.

Infection is achieved by direct dog-to-dog contact or by very effective aerosol transmission. Within 4 days of contact with the infectant material the animal will display full clinical signs as a result of the micro-organisms establishing colonies within the respiratory epithelium.

The canine parainfluenza virus is relatively labile, not surviving long off the host and is easily inactivated by chemical disinfectants. CAV-2 is moderately resistant and can survive for months in the environment. It is, however, sensitive to heat and humidity. Steam cleaning is an effective means of disinfecting the environment and potential fomites.

Quaternary ammonium disinfectants are effective against CAV-2 and CPI viruses.

Diagnosis

- Diagnosis and subsequent treatment are focused on history and clinical signs.
- Blood analysis is rarely performed as practical treatment remains symptomatic.

Treatment

Used to reduce the severity and duration of clinical signs treatment involves antibiotics to reduce the risk of secondary bacterial infections. **Antitussants** are also indicated to reduce the desire to cough – preparations including codeine and butorphanol.

Nursing care

- Managing the infectious patient – see barrier nursing (Table 17.2), in this case with particular regard to air exchange.
- General nursing of the symptoms suffered.
- Management of nutritional status.
- Vaccination protocol for any other dogs in the infected dog's household.
- Disinfection of the environment.
- Vaccination of other in contact dogs.

Leptospirosis

This is a zoonotic disease – ensure effective precautions are taken when nursing these cases.

Leptospirosis is an infectious disease caused by bacteria (Gram negative). The disease affects many animals – domestic and wild – of no particular age, with some animals acting as reservoirs for others, whilst not actually contracting full clinical signs themselves (for example rats and cats).

With an incubation period of 5–7 days, the disease is mainly spread by contact with infected animal's urine. Mortality rates can be high with sudden death or rapid deterioration rapidly resulting in death within a few hours is common.

There are two serotype leptospira responsible for the disease in dogs. These are:

- *Leptospira canicola*.
- *Leptospira icterohaemorrhagiae*.

Weil's disease in humans is caused by infection with the *Leptospira icterohaemorrhagiae*. This is sometimes referred to as 'the yellows' as it produces jaundice.

Clinical signs

In reality it is difficult to differentiate between the serotypes on presentation. Broadly speaking the two strains may display the signs described below.

Sub-acute leptospirosis is rarely diagnosed as it presents with vague symptoms including anorexia, lethargy and pyrexia.

L. icterohaemorrhagiae is especially associated with damage and inflammation of the liver. In young puppies with per-acute presentation, sudden death will occur without any obvious earlier signs of disease.

In the **acute** form the following may be seen:

- Sudden onset pyrexia.
- Anorexia.
- Severe depression.
- Jaundice.
- Vomiting.
- Polydipsia.
- Haemorrhagic diarrhoea.
- Petechial haemorrhages.
- Generalised bleeding possible, including epistaxis.

The condition may deteriorate within hours, even with rapid treatment, with rapid onset of dehydration, shock and collapse, often death.

L. canicola is associated with interstitial nephritis. In the **acute** form symptoms are:

- Sudden onset pyrexia.
- Depression.
- Pyrexia.
- Vomiting.
- Oliguria.
- Dehydration.
- Kidney pain and swelling.
- Halitosis and oral ulceration as a result of azotaemia.
- Jaundice may develop with liver involvement.

Routes of possible infection:

- Through the intact mucosal membranes of the gastrointestinal or respiratory tract. The dog's habit of licking urine is a major risk factor.
- Penetrating intact skin.
- Entrance through cuts and abrasions to skin.
- Transplacental and venereal transmission.

Aetiology and pathogenesis

Following contact and infection with the bacteria the animal will suffer a leptospiraemia of about 7 days duration.

It is mainly spread through direct contact between animals, via contaminated environment, especially through urine contaminated water. Where the urine acidity would damage the bacteria, the diluting effect of an environmental water source encourages their survival.

Once transmitted and within the systemic circulation the leptospiras rapidly multiply, damaging many organs as the disease progresses. The renal tubular epithelial cells are a particular focus as a site for colonisation and therefore the kidneys are a common site for damage to occur along with inflammation caused to the liver.

In particular, *L. canicola* targets the kidneys, damaging the proximal tubules, causing tubular cellular death and inciting a local inflammatory response, with inflammatory cellular invasion. This leads to marked kidney pain and swelling.

L. icterohaemorrhagiae focuses on the liver, resulting in hepatocellular damage and perivascular haemorrhage, further involving the lungs and gastrointestinal tract.

Blood coagulation may be affected with generalized bleeding.

Recovery is dependent on an increased specific antibody level in the blood circulation.

Dogs recovering from leptospiral infection continue to shed organisms in their urine for long periods into the convalescent phase.

Leptospiral organisms are readily destroyed by desiccation, disinfection and ultraviolet light.

Diagnosis

- History.
- Clinical signs.
- Serological detection of rising antibody titre.
- Urine or blood culture of bacteria.
- Biochemical blood analysis.

  - Elevated blood urea and creatinine.
  - Hyperphosphataemia.
  - Elevated salt, bile acids, bilirubin.

- Urine analysis.

  - Proteinuria.
  - Haematuria.
  - Granular casts.

- Leucocytosis.
- Post mortem.

Treatment

Intravenous fluids are provided to tackle dehydration and overcome shock. Whole blood transfusions may be indicated with *L. icterohaemorrhagia*, if perivascular damage is determined and anaemia is present.

Antibiotics immediately inhibit the multiplication of the organism and have a direct impact on the mortality of the animal, as damage to the liver and kidneys will be reduced. Important antibiotics are penicillin, streptomycin and tetracycline as they are effective and not contraindicated in conditions where renal damage is expected. Tetracyclines and aminoglycosides are used to prevent the disease being spread by the carrier state.

Nursing care

- **Zoonotic** disease.
- Managing the infectious patient – see barrier nursing (Table 17.2).
- General nursing of the symptoms suffered.
- Management of nutritional and fluid status.
- Vaccination protocol for any other dogs in the infected dog's household.
- Disinfection of the environment, with particular care taken with exposure to and disposal of infected urine.

Lyme disease

Lyme disease, or Lyme borreliosis, is a zoonotic bacterial infection, caused by the spirochaete *Borrelia burgdorferi*. It occurs worldwide and has been recognised for several decades.

The main vectors for this disease are deer, with dogs and humans becoming infected as a result of tick bites in a contaminated environment. It is not naturally occurring in cats.

The bacteria-carrying ticks have a long life cycle and the bacterial organism has the ability to survive long periods in body tissues so complete eradication can be very difficult.

Clinical signs

- Polyarthritis – episodic lameness or acute limb pain.
- Fever.
- Inappetence.
- Lethargy.
- Lymphadenopathy.

Aetiology and pathogenesis

The deer tick, *Ixodes damini*, is the main vector. This is a three-host tick with a life cycle of 2–3 years. Within its life cycle, larvae and nymphs feed primarily on rodents and small mammals (including dogs and cats) with adult ticks feeding on deer or larger mammals.

The clinical signs displayed are produced as a reaction to the organism generally but also its location and are usually associated with infection. Where the organism affects the kidneys, azotaemia may develop, with proteinuria, haematuria, pyuria and tubular casts.

If the organisms are located in a joint, then synovial fluid analysis will demonstrate a suppurative polyarthritis.

Diagnosis

- Geographical history – endemic habitat visitation.
- Clinical signs.
- Immunofluorescent assay and enzyme immunoassay analysis.
- Simultaneous IgG and IgM antibody titre measurement.

Treatment

Antibitoics are used to treat the bacterial infection – those used are tetracyclines, ampicillin or erythromycin.

Non-steroid anti-inflammatory drugs such as aspirin may be indicated for pain relief during periods where polyarthritis is a clinical sign.

Nursing care

- **Zoonotic** disease.
- Barrier nursing.
- General nursing and medication administration, including analgesia.
- Client education regarding avoidance of endemic areas or advice regarding tick repellents.

Parvovirus

Canine parvovirus (CPV) infection was first recognised in 1978 when it is thought to have developed as a mutation from the feline parvovirus associated with feline panleucopaenia. It is thought that a few years later, in 1981 a further mutation occurred, making the virus even more specific to dogs.

Parvovirus is one of the most resistant viruses, surviving off the host and in the environment for months or even years. Specific parvovirus disinfectant products have been produced since the disease's first appearance to enable environmental disinfection. Dogs are susceptible at any age – if they have insufficient or an absence of antibodies – either as a result of insufficient maternal antibodies or as a result of non-vaccination.

It is spread by direct or indirect contact with infected dogs or their faeces.

Severity of the disease depends on the age, immune/antibody status of the recipient animal, as well as its levels of stress and any other existing disease or concurrent infection with parasites. The virus targets replicating cells and, depending on those factors, either cardiac or gastroenteritis tissues will be affected.

Clinical signs

- Sudden death in young puppies.
- Young puppies in heart failure.
- Depression.
- Anorexia.
- Persistent vomiting – food in the early stages but then bile-stained or blood-stained fluid.
- Diarrhoea – liquid, red-brown in colour with a foul smell.
- Dehydration, shock, hypothermia, leading to death if untreated.

Aetiology and pathogenesis

Dogs become infected either by ingestion or inhalation of CPV. The virus is taken up by the lymphatic system – the tonsils, regional lymph nodes and gut associated lymphoid tissue – depending on its route of admission. It is here that primary replication occurs and within a 3–5 day period a viraemia is present.

The target for further replication now depends on the age of the dog – CPV targets rapidly dividing cells.

If the dog is 7 weeks of age or under the myocardial cells are rapidly developing and these are the focus for CPV, leading to myocardial infections in this age group.

Immunosuppression will also occur as the rapidly dividing cells of the bone marrow and lymphoid tissue are also invaded.

In dogs older than 7 weeks the myocardial development is complete and so the virus targets the continually dividing cells of the gastrointestinal tract. These animals will demonstrate the clinical signs associated with this organ along with immunosuppression associated with the lymphatic system invasion.

In 1978, when CPV 2 was first identified both myocardial and intestinal symptoms were seen, as no dog held any antibody protection against the new virus. Nowadays maternal antibody levels are good as breeding bitches are generally vaccinated and so the myocardial presentation is much less commonly observed.

Diagnosis

- History (general and vaccination) and clinical signs, especially presence of foul smelling haemorrhagic, fluid diarrhoea.
- Severe leukopaenia with white cell count less than 1.0×10^9/litre.
- CPV antigen capture CITE test.
- Histopathology of affected tissue.

Treatment

Myocardial CPV therapy is rarely successful and owners should be given a very guarded prognosis – symptomatic treatment includes cage rest, diuretics and nutritional support.

Treatment of CPV associated with the intestinal tract involves intensive intravenous fluid therapy. If vomiting is protracted and/or haemorrhagic diarrhoea is severe, the prognosis becomes more cautious.

Whole blood or plasma expanders may be indicated for animals in shock whilst crystalloids should be administered to balance electrolyte and fluid loss.

Antiemetics are important to reduce electrolyte and fluid losses as well as the debilitating effect of persistent vomiting.

If secondary infections are a concern then a broad spectrum antibiotic may be administered.

Once the dog has overcome the initial stage of the disease and can take small amounts of fluid orally, e.g. water or a rehydration fluid, the nutritional status of the dog can be assessed.

Many dogs recover with some degree of malabsorption so a low fat diet may be required into the convalescent period or permanently.

Nursing care

- Barrier nursing.
- Management of fluid status and nutritional requirement.

- General symptomatic nursing including management of vomiting.
- Administration of appropriate medication.
- Disinfection using preparations effective against parvovirus.
- Vaccination of other in-contact animals.

Diseases affecting both dogs and cats

Rabies

Rabies is a virally induced neurological disease. It has an exceptionally high fatality rate and is an important fatal, **zoonotic** disease.

The disease is widely spread around the world with a few island country exceptions and has existed for many, many years. Records as far back as the 20th century B.C. contain information on mad dogs biting people.

All warm-blooded animals are susceptible to infection with the rabies virus, although there are ranges of susceptibility. For example, birds are highly resistant to the disease, while dogs, cats, horses, sheep and humans are moderately resistant. Amongst the least resistant are bats and cattle.

Wild animals are considered the principal reservoir for the virus but domestic pets represent a direct threat for transmission as they are in contact with humans.

Although some infected dogs and humans have survived it is generally regarded as a fatal disease.

In countries where rabies is present, effective vaccination of domestic pets is directly linked to a fall in the number of humans infected with the virus.

The rabies virus is quite labile and does not exist in the environment. Sunlight, warm temperatures, desiccation, heat and disinfectants will all destroy it.

Clinical signs

There are three stages of rabies – prodromal, excitative and paralytic.

Prodromal This is essentially displayed as a change in the animal's characteristic behaviour. Wild animals become fearless of humans, moving around open territory during the day. Pets become hypersensitive to their surroundings, becoming fearful and apprehensive or alternatively overly affectionate. This period may last 1–3 days.

Excitative stage This is the stage that bites become a danger to people in contact with the animal. Animals that display hypersensitivity may bite out at anything including wood, metal and imaginary objects. This is the 'mad dog' stage of the disease. If the excitative signs are a prominent feature of the behaviour the animal is said to have 'furious' rabies. This may last 3–4 days.

Some animals, however, may not display the hypersensitive, excitative signs, or they may be of very short duration.

These animals will instead be oblivious to their surroundings and be mentally dull. This is known as 'dumb' rabies. The most obvious symptoms with these animals are the signs of paralysis and facial expression changes as the nerves are affected.

Paralytic Incoordination is one of the first signs of the paralytic stage of the disease. The virus damages motor neurons resulting in a hindlimb ataxia ascending to paralysis. Other nervous injuries include damage to the muscles of swallowing (**deglutition**) leading to drooling of saliva and an inability to swallow. Other nerves are also damaged by the virus, resulting in facial expression changes – drooping eyelids, sagging jaw and squinting eyes. Changes also occur to the respiratory nervous system, resulting in the animal's death by respiratory arrest. The animal may otherwise die as a result of a seizure, as the virus affects the brain. This stage may last 1–2 days.

From onset of clinical signs in pets, death usually occurs within 2–7 days.

Recovery rates following rabies infection are low. As the risk of further contamination poses serious risk to human life animals with signs of rabies are euthanased.

Humans infected with the virus display similar symptoms as described here, but with **hydrophobia** being a classic sign.

Aetiology and pathogenesis

The virus must come into contact with nerve endings for infection to occur. This usually comes about by injection of saliva as a bite but could also occur with infected saliva coming into contact with a fresh wound, conjunctiva or olfactory mucosa.

The location of the bite or contaminated wound has some bearing on the onset of clinical signs, as does the quantity of virus. As the virus migrates towards the central nervous system to reach full effect and clinical signs, the closer the contact to the CNS is, the quicker the onset of clinical signs. Ultimately affecting the CNS itself and neurons, signs are nervous in nature – abnormal behaviour and paralysis.

Diagnosis

Clinical signs and history will provide important information. The personnel involved in examining any animal suspected of the virus, or one which has come into contact with an infected animal, should take great care in the approach of such an animal, especially one that is reported to be exhibiting excitative signs (the use of 'noose poles' and 'syringe poles' is indicated where handling or injections are required). Transmission routes should be borne in mind and any abrasions, especially to the face or hands should be covered. Masks with visors should be worn to avoid infection via the mucous membranes.

As rabies cannot be confirmed by any reliable antemortem test, the diagnosis is based upon clinical signs and relevant history.

Post-mortem diagnosis is achieved through examination of portions of the brain and brain stem. This is performed by a DEFRA veterinary officer, within a recognised laboratory. The brain is examined for Negri bodies which represent accumulation of virus protein in the neurons.

Treatment

Treatment is not recommended for animals showing signs of rabies due to the risk to human life. Handling of any suspect cases should be avoided.

Dogs with clinical signs should be placed in strict isolation, pending further symptom identification and euthanasia.

Rabies vaccination for pets

Rabies is not present in the UK and so the only animals that will have been vaccinated against it are those entering the country from overseas where rabies is endemic or those returning to the United Kingdom under the Pets Passport Scheme (see Chapter 6).

Rabies vaccination for humans

Only those people deemed at risk are vaccinated, i.e. staff working in quarantine kennels or veterinary hospitals where animals mid-quarantine would be taken if they should become ill.

Salmonellosis

Salmonellae are commonly occurring bacteria, found in the intestinal tract of healthy mammals, birds, reptiles and insects. Under certain circumstances these can cause systemic disease.

This is a **zoonotic** disease and is spread principally by faecal contamination.

Clinical signs

These are variable and will be evident a few days after a stressful episode. Dependant upon:

- Quantity of bacteria.
- The immune status of the host.
- Concurrent disease.

The focus of the bacterial infection will also affect the presentation of the disease – whether this be gastroenteritis, bacteraemia/endotoxaemia, organ focus or associated with the symptomless carrier.

Signs progress as follows as the disease intensifies:

(1) Fever.
(2) 'Off colour'.

(3) Anorexia.
(4) Vomiting.
(5) Diarrhoea.
(6) Abdominal pain.
(7) Weight loss.
(8) Dehydration.

Where there is a severe bacteraemia or endotoxaemia the animal may show signs of shock or exhibit central nervous system signs. *In utero* infections may lead to abortions, still-births or the birth of weak puppies.

Aetiology and pathogenesis

The species that are of major significance in the dog and cat are *S. typhimurium* and *S. anatum*. These are not host specific.

The bacteria move on to create systemic signs when the infected animal is placed under stressful conditions such as hospitalisation or boarding/quarantine, especially if overcrowding is apparent. Anaesthesia, medical and surgical procedures or immunosuppressive treatments will also encourage the infective agent.

Faecal contamination is the most important method of contamination. The most frequent method of cross-contamination is via food, water or fomites. The bacteria can survive long periods off the host.

Following a successful recovery, 'shedding' becomes a concern. The salmonellae target the tips of the intestinal villi; it is here that they multiply. From this site, and local lymph nodes, they continue to infect the environment on an intermittent basis, lasting from 3 to 6 weeks each time.

With excessive production and intestinal colonisation, it is possible for an endotoxaemia or bacteraemia to develop.

Diagnosis

This is founded on clinical signs and historical evidence. Haematological and biochemical analysis are non-specific and faecal analysis will be equally unhelpful.

Specific culture and typing of salmonellae from faeces samples is the best available method of definitively reaching the diagnosis of salmonellae positive. Samples for culture, taken at the time of surgery or post mortem should include liver, spleen, intestinal tract and mesenteric lymph node. A sample of the lung tissue is also required, although usually this would only be carried out as part of a post mortem.

Treatment

Treatment of salmonellae is dependent on the severity of the symptoms. Intravenous fluid therapy is likely to be a requirement of all infected animals.

Antibiotic drugs such as chloramphenicol, erythromycin, ampicillin and enrofloxacin are useful, although drug resistance can be an issue. Antibiotics are normally only indicated where there are signs of systemic diseases as gastrointestinal salmonella is usually self-limiting.

Nursing care

- Barrier nursing – **zoonotic** disease.
- Management of fluid status and nutritional requirement.
- General symptomatic nursing including management of vomiting and diarrhoea.
- Administration of appropriate medication.
- Strict hygiene measures to be followed, especially with cooked/uncooked food/processed food preparation and faecal collection/disposal.
- Advise owners of appropriate hygiene measures, especially food handling and faecal disposal. Special care should be paid to households with small children and/or where puppies are present as there is an increased risk of faecal contact here.

Feline infectious diseases

The feline infectious diseases considered in this section are summarised in Table 17.6, and their clinical signs in Table 17.7.

Chlamydiosis

A world-wide recognised condition, *Chlamydia psittaci* is considered to be the cause of over 30% of conjunctivitis cases in the UK.

The bacterium targets the conjunctiva and affects all ages of cats with kittens being the most severely affected. It is a highly species-specific organism rarely if ever, affecting other animals.

It is thought it may also infect the reproductive tract of queens resulting in abortions and possibly a cause of infertility, however this remains to be proven clinically.

As the organism is very short lived off the host, transmission occurs via direct contact between animals.

Clinical signs

Early disease:

- Pyrexia initially with cat remaining bright.
- Chemosis or conjunctivitis with discharge, serous in nature initially.
- Rhinitis with discharge.
- Blepharospasm with hyperaemia.
- Sneezing.
- Occasionally a pneumonitis may develop.
- Discharges may become purulent.
- Newborn kittens may become infected before their eyes are open, resulting in ophthalmia neonatorum.

Table 17.6 Feline infectious diseases

Disease	Agent	Incubation period	Major organs affected	Main method of transmission	Zoonotic	Diagnostic methods	Major nursing needs	Control/prevention
Chlamydiosis	Bacteria	< 7 days	Upper respiratory tract	Direct contact	Very slight risk	Conjunctival scraping	General care	Vaccination Owner education
Feline leukaemia virus	Virus	Months/years	Immune system	Saliva	No	Blood analysis	General and symptomatic	Vaccination
Feline infectious anaemia	Bacterial parasite		Red blood cells	Unknown, but fighting and fleas implicated	No	Blood analysis – smear/stain	General	Flea control Cat fight control
Feline infectious peritonitis	Virus	Variable	Severe inflammation of body tissues	Unclear – probably inhalation/ingestion, linked to faeces	No	Tissue biopsy	General	Unknown
Feline immunodeficiency virus	Virus	Variable – may not show clinical signs for years	Immune system	Cat bites – saliva	No	Blood analysis	General	Unknown
Feline upper respiratory tract disease	Viruses – Feline calici virus Feline herpes virus	2–10 days	Upper respiratory tract	Saliva Ocular and nasal discharges	No	Clinical history Swab analysis	Antibiotics I/V fluids Nutritional support	Vaccination
Toxoplasmosis	Coccidian parasite	3–10 days	Intestinal tract Throughout body	Faeces	Yes	Tissue biopsy Serology	Antibiotics	Limit ingestion of wild animals
Feline panleucopaenia	Virus	2–7 days	Gastrointestinal tract Immune system	Body excretions	No	Vaccine history Blood analysis	I/V fluids Antibiotics	Vaccine

Table 17.7 Major clinical signs of feline infectious disease

	Clinical signs particular to this disease (see text for details)
Chlamydiosis	Conjunctivitis Rhinitis
Feline leukaemia virus	See main text
Feline infectious anaemia	Anaemia Tachypnoea Tachycardia
Feline infectious peritonitis	Severe tissue inflammation Peritoneal or thoracic cavities leading to fluid accumulation Major organs – signs depend on which organ is affected and therefore are very variable
FIV	Initial mild illness followed by apparent recovery After time a multitude of symptoms will develop
FURD	Nasal and ocular discharges Fits of sneezing Mouth ulceration Dyspnoea
Toxoplasmosis	Respiratory disease Ocular disease
Feline panleucopaenia	Sudden death Praying position Bowl hugging

Chronic disease:

- Thickened conjunctiva.
- Minimal exudates.

Aetiology and pathogenesis

The method of transmission is not known; however, direct contact between cats appears to be important – especially with ocular or nasal discharges.

Carriers of the disease remain an outlet for further infection as they continue to shed the organism without displaying signs clinically themselves. The organism may also be harboured in the gastrointestinal and genital tract.

The incubation period is 4–10 days following infection. The animal may suffer the symptoms for several months; however, improvement can normally be expected within 2–3 weeks.

Diagnosis

- Clinical signs and history.
- Examination of conjunctival swabs – culture.

Treatment

Treatment with topical or systemic antibiotics are indicated, doxycycline being the drug of choice. In cases of multi-cat households the whole cat population should be treated at the same time.

Treatment should continue for a further 2 weeks following absence of clinical signs.

Nursing care

- Maintain strict levels of hygiene to avoid cross-contamination to other animals.
- Administration of appropriate medication.
- Owner advice, especially regarding multi-cat households.
- Application of basic hygiene standards will prevent any slight possibility of cross-transmission to humans.

Feline leukaemia virus (FeLV)

FeLV is a species-specific retrovirus, affecting both domestic and wild cat populations and is widely distributed around the world.

It is a frequently occurring viral disease with estimates suggesting that as many as two-thirds of the cat population have been exposed to the virus within their lifetime. It is estimated that 1–2% of healthy cats are FeLV positive, in multi-cat households up to 30% may be FeLV positive. The occurrence is so high that FeLV should be high on the list of differentials of causative agents for any ill cat – it is estimated that 18% of all sick cats will be positive for the virus.

Whilst the morbidity of this disease may be high the mortality rate is quite low with many animals being asymptomatic for years or suffering the disease and recovering to good health.

Its main effect is upon the immune system, damaging or destroying the cells of the immune system, thereby diminishing the animal's ability to fend off other diseases and infections.

The FeLV virus is from the same viral family as feline immunodeficiency virus.

The virus is labile off host – infection is therefore achieved via prolonged and close contact between cats, saliva being the most concentrated source of the virus.

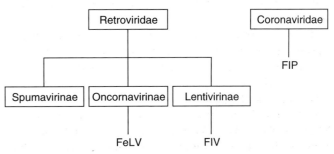

Fig. 17.1 Feline virus groups.

Clinical signs

Clinical presentation of FeLV falls into two groupings – neoplastic disease or non-neoplastic disease (degenerative). Non-neoplastic diseases are usually associated with immunosuppression. There is an overall deterioration in the cat's general health and body condition.

Neoplastic (15% of cases):

- Lymphosarcoma is the most common FeLV associated disease. It may be described as thymic, multicentric, alimentary or miscellaneous depending on its location.

Non-neoplastic – degenerative disease (85% of cases):

- Thrombocytopaenia.
- Immune-mediated haemolytic anaemia.
- Non-regenerative anaemia.
- Glomerulonephritis.
- Myeloproliferative disease.
- Immunosuppression:
  - FIP.
  - FIV.
  - Cat flu.
  - Feline enteritis.
  - Toxoplasmosis.
  - Oral infections.

- Immune system diseases:
  - Glomerular nephritis.
  - Polyarthritis.
  - Polyneuritis.

- Reproductive system disease:
  - Fetal resorption.
  - Abortion.
  - Stillbirths.
  - Thymic atrophy (fading kittens).

Aetiology and pathogenesis

The mortality rate is most severe with very young kittens. Young kittens infected *in vitro* suffer a persistent viraemia and die. Kittens 8 weeks of age and younger are 70–80% likely to become persistently viraemic while only 10% of adults becoming infected are likely to be persistently viraemic.

The virus can be transmitted along a number of routes. A queen can infect her kittens either by the *in vitro* route or across via her milk. Saliva is heavily laden with virus and so dense populations of cats, where direct contact with saliva is possible, either by grooming each other or via bite wounds, account for the increased morbidity rate with this group. Cats fed from the same food bowl can be infected. The virus is also present in mucus, urine and faeces, as well as milk.

There are five overlapping stages to the pathogenesis to this disease – clinically indistinct but important dividers regarding the immune responses seen.

(1) After oronasal exposure the virus replicates in the tonsils and pharyngeal lymph nodes, or if the virus has been inoculated via a bite, the virus will replicate at a regional lymph node.
(2) The virus then infects a small number of circulating lymphocytes and macrophages which move on to spread the virus around the body.
(3) The virus moves on to infect and further replicate in the spleen, gut-associated lymphoid tissues, lymph nodes, intestinal crypt epithelial cells and bone marrow precursor cells.
(4) FeLV-infected neutrophils and platelets from the bone marrow are then released into the circulatory system.
(5) FeLV infects epithelial and glandular tissues, including tissues of the salivary gland and bladder – which promotes the subsequent shedding of the virus in saliva and urine.

Invasion of the bone marrow leads to anaemia, leukaemia and immunosuppression. The invasion of the intestinal crypt epithelial cells – the Lieberkuhns – leads to enteritis. The virus is excreted following invasion of the salivary, lacrymal and pancreatic glands, and when the urogenital system is affected by the virus, abortions, stillbirths and infertility occur.

If infection with the virus elicits an adequate immune response (within the first 4–8 weeks following exposure) then the infection activity will be halted at stage 2 or 3. The virus is then eliminated or forced into a latent state. Approximately 40% of cats exposed to the virus will eliminate the virus and recover, approximately 30% will maintain a latent infection.

A latent infection may act as a reservoir for intermittent release and further infection with the virus. This may occur following periods of stress, during a concurrent infection or after the administration of a corticosteroid drug. It is also possible that the virus will be slowly eliminated without becoming actively shed.

Where the virus is not fended off, the FeLV infection will progress through all five stages with the cat becoming persistently or permanently viraemic and therefore infectious. This may occur as speedily as 4–6 weeks after infection.

Cats that do become persistently viraemic will usually die of an FeLV-related disease within 2–3 years of infection.

Diagnosis

- History and clinical presentation.
- Serum/white blood cell/bone marrow cells examination for viral protein.
- ELISA test.

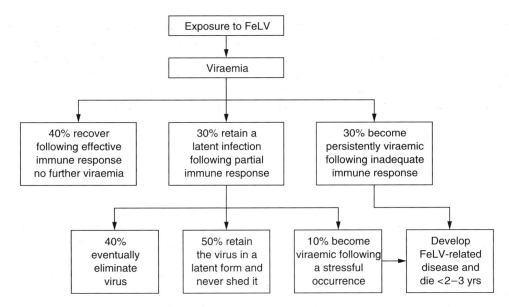

Fig. 17.2 FeLV exposure flow chart.

Treatment and nursing care

Where there is an active viraemia the prognosis remains very guarded and any treatment and nursing care is based on symptomatic management of signs and antibiotics to ward off any secondary bacterial infection.

If supportive therapies are to be successful, drugs such as corticosteroids, anabolic steroids and multivitamins will be required, along with prolonged courses of antibiotic drugs to manage/prevent secondary infections. Any response to the therapies described above will be much slower and less successful than may normally be experienced in other conditions.

When managing cats with the disease, care must be taken to avoid any incidences that may affect their immune status – e.g. by maintaining good anti-flea protocols – to reduce the possibility of contracting *Haemobartonella felis*. Regular worm treatments should be performed as well as routine vaccinations, especially against cat flu and infectious enteritis, and the avoidance of feeding raw meat due to the risk of *Toxoplasmosis gondii* infection.

Known FeLV positive cats should not be housed in multi-cat households, even if the other cats are vaccinated as no vaccine is guaranteed 100% effective. Infected cats should be kept indoors to prevent possible contact with other cats in the area.

Feline infectious anaemia

This disease is otherwise known as haemobartonellosis and is caused by the bacterial parasite *Haemobartonella felis*. Infection with the parasite may be achieved by cat bites, flea infestations, across the placenta or via the queen's milk.

H. felis is another disease which may develop when the host cat's immune system is affected by stress or concurrent illness. Those cats positive to FeLV or that are not vaccinated for the routine cat infectious diseases are at an increased risk of contracting the disease. Feline immunodeficiency virus (FIV) has also been associated with FIA; however, it is also seen in previously healthy cats.

Clinical signs

- Anaemia.
- Tiredness.
- Depression.
- Inappetence.
- Pale gums.
- Weight loss.
- Splenic enlargement.
- Enlarged lymph nodes.
- Pyrexia.
- Tachypnoea and tachycardia.

Aetiology and pathogenesis

The bacteria live on the surface of red blood cells. These organisms damage the structure of the red blood cells, leading to their destruction and their eventual death – thereby producing anaemia. This damage and destruction may be further exacerbated by the cat's immune system as it attempts to eradicate the parasite.

The method of transmission is unclear; however, cat bites seem to be a key route as young male cats engaged in regular fights are commonly infected. A heavy flea burden also appears to increase the incidence. Infection with the parasites is transmitted across the placenta and milk.

Cats that are FeLV positive, unvaccinated, outdoor roaming and/or frequently engaged in cat fights are all at greater risk of contracting the disease.

Once infected the animal will suffer cycles of parasitaemia – where complete absence of signs may occur in between bouts of profound anaemia. During the times of asymptomatic disease the animal remains infective.

The clinical signs displayed are seen as a result of the anaemia caused by the effects of the organism's activities. Some cats will not be anaemic because they are asymptomatic carriers, others because they are only mildly infected by the disease.

Once cats have been infected with FIA they will remain carriers for life.

Diagnosis

Blood analysis is performed as the main diagnostic tool, however the cyclic nature to the organism's presence in the blood circulation can lead to identification problems. Blood analysis is performed using Wright–Giemsa stained thin blood smears (see Chapter 13). The parasites should then be visible on the surface of the blood cells. Blood for examination should be collected at intervals over time to compensate for the fluctuating parasitaemia.

Routine haematology shows a high reticulocyte count indicating a regenerative anaemia. As the red blood cell destruction occurs as a result of the bacteria, the bone marrow is triggered to releasing more red blood cells – and as the destruction of the mature cells picks up the younger and less mature reticulocytes are released in an attempt to keep the circulating red blood cells at a suitable level.

Haemobartonella felis organisms may be seen in cats who are clinically well due to carrier states or infection with a mild strain of the bacterium.

Treatment

Antibiotics are indicated to manage the disease – doxycycline is the drug of choice, administered over a 2–3 week period.

In conjunction with the antibiotics, corticosteroids may be given to reduce the immune-system triggered destruction of the red blood cells.

Cats with severe anaemia may require whole blood transfusions.

Nursing care

- Intravenous fluid therapy where dehydration is presented.
- General nursing, including encouragement with feeding.
- Administration of drugs prescribed by veterinary surgeon.

Feline infectious peritonitis

Feline infectious peritonitis (FIP) is a severe disease of the cat, caused by a coronavirus. Although the incidence is low (1–5%) it is difficult to treat effectively and is usually fatal.

It occurs most commonly in multi-cat households and amongst pedigree cats, especially the Burmese, and is seen most frequently in young cats under 2 years of age, those with concurrent disease or stressed cats.

The virus is present in faeces and may be shed for extended periods by infected cats.

Clinical signs

Clincial signs are varied, dependent on the areas and organ(s) targeted by the coronavirus. In the early stages, signs will be vague and may include inappetence, intermittent pyrexia, and diarrhoea with weight loss. As the virus then targets particular sites, clinical signs then become more specific – relating to either 'wet' or 'effusive' FIP, or 'dry' or 'non-effusive' FIP.

- **Wet, effusive FIP.** Fluid accumulates in the thoracic or abdominal cavity – this is due to inflammation of the blood vessels lining the tissues of these body cavities. The clinical signs reflect the anatomy affected – abdominal swelling (ascites) and/or increased respiratory effort/dyspnoea.
- **Dry, non-effusive FIP.** The virus has targeted other areas and so there is little or no fluid accumulation in the thoracic or abdominal cavity but there will be severe inflammation at one or more other sites, e.g. internal organs such as the liver, kidneys, the eyes, the intestines or the brain. A persistent pyrexia is often seen.

Aetiology and pathogenesis

The mode of transmission is not fully understood and the incubation period appears very variable.

Cats are usually infected through inhaling or ingesting the virus – via direct contact or by indirect contact through an infected environment. Although the virus may last for some time in the environment it is fairly easily destroyed by routine disinfection and good standards of hygiene.

There are many different strains of the virus – most leading to mild signs only (90%), probably a short episode of diarrhoea, as the animal's immune status fights off the virus. In those animals where the immune response is poor the virus will progress towards full FIP infection (10%).

The virus replicates in macrophages. Infected macrophages then disperse around the body, via the circulation targeting the vascular beds of the peritoneum, pleura, eye, meninges or kidneys.

Antibodies to coronavirus result in the formation of perivascular antigen/antibody complexes, which then cause vasculitis. If the virus has targeted the peritoneal or pleural vessels, this leads to fluid leakage and accumulation within the cavity.

Diagnosis

- Blood sample analysis – examination of blood samples for the presence of antibodies will demonstrate an antibody response to coronavirus. Unfortunately it is not possible to differentiate between the different strains of coronavirus or between previous or current infection, so all these tests establish is that the cat has at some point, recently or in the past, been exposed to the virus.

    It is possible to also perform blood analysis to identify the virus but these are also unable to define which type of coronavirus.

    Routine haematology and biochemistry will show a number of disorders that can be associated with FIP and these will be additional indicators towards the disease.
- Exudate collection and analysis (if present).
- Tissue biopsy.
- Post-mortem examination.

The veterinary surgeon will often have to gather the collective evidence of clinical signs, routine blood analysis results, coronavirus serology and exudates analysis to reach a presumptive diagnosis of FIP.

Treatment

This is essentially **palliative** (i.e. gives temporary or partial relief) as the disease is invariably fatal. Antibiotics are helpful against secondary infections and corticosteroids may slow the deterioration of the cat's condition. Reducing the extent of abdominal distension by aspiration of the exudates may relieve the animal's discomfort for a short period, as will the respiratory effort be eased with thoracocentesis.

Nursing care

Supportive care includes administration of any drugs, general nursing care and encouraging good nutritional intake.

Owners should be advised about vaccination protocols if there are more cats in the household. The diagnosis of FIP should be confirmed by tissue biopsy, or by post-mortem examination, so that the risk to the other cats can be determined – although this is just an indicator as FIP is often not transmitted amongst groups of cats.

Following the discovery of FIP in the household the remaining cats should be vaccinated to maintain good health and enhance the immune system, undue stresses should be avoided (boarding, overcrowding or major changes to household/routine) and several months should elapse before any new cats are introduced to the group.

No vaccine specifically designed for FIP is currently available in the UK.

Feline immunodeficiency virus

FIV is an RNA retrovirus, affecting both domestic and wild cat populations worldwide. Known colloquially as **feline AIDS** it is found in around 7% of the UK population. It is a species-specific virus.

FIV is a fatal condition; however, just as in human HIV infection, carriers may be symptom free for years before succumbing to the virus. During the asymptomatic period there is a gradual decline in the animal's immunity as the virus infects, damages and ultimately destroys the animal's white blood cells. The animal will then show clinical signs of the virus and its effects as the immune system fails to fight off diseases and infections.

Clinical signs

There are generally four stages to FIV, similar to those seen in human HIV infection:

- First stage – acute infection. The animal may be 'under the weather' with a mild fever, loss of appetite, diarrhoea and lymphadenopathy. This stage may go unnoticed by the owner. This stage begins about 4 weeks after infection and could last for up to 4 months.
- Second stage – asymptomatic carrier. This may last several months or years, depending on the animal's immune status, stress levels and nutritional state.
- Third stage – persistent generalised lymphadenopathy. In humans these are the only signs of this stage; however, in cats, most will show other signs of general illness.
- Fourth stage – AIDS-related complex. These cats will suffer from chronic respiratory disorders, with gastrointestinal conditions and skin complaints, in addition to the persistent generalised adenopathy. There may be a fever, generalised lethargy and weight loss. Recurrent gingivitis, rhinitis and conjunctivitis are common. Anaemia, renal disease, uveitis and nervous system diseases will also be possible.
- Fifth stage – this is signalled by the occurrence of opportunistic infections, lymphoid depletion and severe emaciation leading to the animal's death. In cats there are no clear distinctions to be made between the final two stages of the disease.

Aetiology and pathogenesis

Infection is rare in cats less than 1 year old, increasing to a peak at 8 years of age. It is 30 times more commonly seen in outdoor cats and three times more likely to be a male cat that is infected. This indicates that fighting and the resultant cat bites are an important route of transmission. Saliva contains significant quantities of the virus. Other potential avenues for transmission include fomites (shared feeding bowls), mutual grooming activities and via the placenta in pregnant queens (the virus may also contaminate kittens via milk). Sexual transmission is not thought to be significant. It is possible that fleas could play a role, therefore an appropriate preventative protocol should be adopted.

The geographical areas of the UK where FIV is found in its highest numbers are Northern Ireland, Scotland, south and south-east England.

There are no vaccines for FIV and the virus cannot be eliminated by a normal immune response elicited by infection. The animal will produce antibodies but these are ineffective.

The virus is labile off the host and is susceptible to destruction in the environment by routine disinfection, heat and desiccation.

Diagnosis

- Clinical history of chronic or recurring infections with poor recovery record, seen in a cat that is lethargic, thin and in poor, general condition.
- Blood sample analysis – for detection of antibodies to viral protein.
- ELISA test or more sophisticated and more reliable tests such as polymerase chain reaction (PCR) or immunofluorescence Western blot test.

The ELISA-based tests provide a diagnosis but can be unreliable:

- Some FIV-positive cats produce different antibodies to those detected on the test, leading to a false negative result.
- It is possible for samples to be contaminated during processing.
- FIV antibodies are not produced in the first 8 weeks of the infection.
- Negative test results should be repeated after an 8–12 week interval.
- Mother cats transfer antibodies to their newborn kittens via milk. These FIV antibodies are then detected when the kittens are tested for FIV antibodies. FIV is usually only passed on to about one-third of the litter; however, all the kittens will have these maternally derived antibodies present at the time of sampling as they may remain in the kittens' immune system for up to 4 months. Kittens that have been infected with the virus do not usually produce their own antibodies to the virus for a further 2 months. Therefore, to avoid false positives, kittens born to FIV positive mothers should not be tested until they are at least 6 months of age.

Identification of the virus, isolated from the lymphocytes confirms the diagnosis.

Treatment

There is no specific treatment except for symptomatic care to promote the best health possible.

Managing the healthy FIV positive cat:

- Routine vaccination is recommended to shield the cat from immune system infection that may provoke the FIV virus to become active.
- A regular flea treatment protocol will minimise the risk of *Haemobartonella felis* infection and a regular worming routine should also promote overall good health.
- FIV positive cats should be prevented from eating raw meat due to the risk of *Toxoplasma gondii* infection.
- Virus-positive cats should be prevented from further transmitting the disease by physical restriction, such as enclosing the garden or building a pen. This also increases the protection afforded to the infected cat from infection of other diseases from other cats.
- The cat should also be neutered. In the male this is to reduce the likelihood of cat fights, and thus transmission through biting. In the female, neutering should be undertaken to prevent reproduction. Infected queens that do go on to produce a litter should have the kittens removed at birth and these should be hand-reared, to eliminate viral transmission across milk. These kittens should be tested at 6 months.
- As social contact is a low-risk method of transmission it is still possible for this cat to remain in its multi-cat household; however, it is wise to bear in mind the important role of saliva and so feeding bowls should be kept separate and mutual grooming should be discouraged. Litter trays and food bowls should be disinfected carefully after each use.
- Cats that are antagonistic to others should be separated to avoid conflicts leading to bite wounds.

Nursing care

Care of the cat ill with FIV is based on generalised symptomatic care:

- Attention to nutritional status.
- Administration of intravenous fluid therapy.
- General nursing care.

Feline upper respiratory tract disease

Feline upper respiratory tract disease (FURD), otherwise known as 'cat flu' is a highly contagious disease involving two viruses:

- Feline herpes virus 1 (FHV-1). May also be known as feline viral rhinotracheitis (FVR).
- Feline calici virus (FCV).

The symptoms of cat flu may be caused by infection with one or both of these.

It is commonly seen where there are large groups of cats; it is spread principally by inhalation of droplets held in aerosols. Other methods of transmission include direct contact with a cat displaying signs of flu, by indirect contact with fomites or the environment, or by contact with an asymptomatic carrier cat that is shedding the virus.

The virus is present in large amounts in saliva, tears and nasal discharges. Environmental contamination remains a threat for up to a week following the presence of an infected cat.

The cats most at risk are those that are not vaccinated or are immunosuppressed and kittens and elderly cats. Purebred cats, especially Siamese, are prone to a more severe infection.

The disease has a very high morbidity rate; however, its mortality rate is fairly low, although it can be fatal (as a result of secondary infections).

Clinical signs

Feline herpes virus causes the most severe form of the disease, potentially leading to a fatal outcome in some cases. The majority of cats do go on to make a full recovery, although this may take several weeks. Many will be left with residual, permanent effects of the damage caused by the virus, such as chronic rhinitis or ocular discharge.

Feline calici virus usually causes a less severe complaint with less dramatic nasal discharges. For this virus, oral ulceration is a key sign (and may be the only sign), found on the tongue, roof of the mouth or nose. Sometimes this virus may cause lameness or fever in young kittens.

- Paroxysmal sneezing.
- Serous nasal and ocular discharge.
- Anorexia.
- Depression.
- Pyrexia.
- Nasal and ocular ulceration.
- Hypersalivation.
- Loss of voice.
- Coughing.

Secondary infections begin to play a role in the downward spiral of the cat's health. The ocular and nasal discharges become mucopurulent, with an increased risk of keratitis and corneal ulceration as the eyelids often get stuck together. The nasal passages become blocked and the cat's sense of smell is diminished and then lost. Mouth breathing occurs.

Anorexia occurs, probably as a result of pyrexia, oral ulceration and loss of olfaction. Hypersalivation is probably as a result of mouth pain due to the oral ulceration.

Where the disease is not sufficiently severe to become fatal, the cat will show signs of recovery within 7–21 days, depending on the breed, age and degree of secondary infection.

Aetiology and pathogenesis

Feline herpes virus is a DNA virus that is fairly resistant, surviving in the environment for up to 8 days off the host.

Feline calici virus, a RNA virus, is more easily destroyed away from the host.

Following inhalation the viruses replicate in local lymph nodes before targeting the epithelial cells of the respiratory tract and conjunctiva.

Most cats that recover from FURD become carriers of the virus. In a carrier state each virus behaves differently.

FHV-1 can become latent, or dormant, with shedding only occurring at intervals associated with periods of stress, concurrent infection or following corticosteroid treatment. It is possible that mild clinical signs of the disease will also become evident. Cats carrying the FHV-1 virus remain carriers for life.

FCV carriers shed the virus continuously – some over a long period of time following clinical recovery, i.e. years, but many shed for just a short period and then viral shedding stops completely.

Diagnosis

- Clinical history and presentation.
- Oropharyngeal swabs examined for the presence of the viruses.

Treatment

Once again supportive, symptomatic treatment is indicated. This may include intravenous fluid therapy, antibiotics to control secondary infections and attention to the cat's nutritional state.

Nursing care

- Barrier nursing.
- General care, with particular attention to feeding and easing breathing difficulties.
- Administration of medication and fluid therapy.
- Owner guidance regarding carrier state.

Toxoplasmosis

Toxoplasmosis is caused by *Toxoplasma gondii*, a coccidian parasite affecting both domesticated and wild felines. It is widely spread around the world, with many species of vertebrates performing the role of the intermediate hosts, including fish, amphibians, reptiles and all warm-blooded animals, including man.

Cats are the only species in which the parasite can complete its life cycle (definitive host) and the only species that shed oocysts.

Transmission can occur by one of three potential methods:

(1) Carnivores most commonly become infected by ingestion of an infected intermediary host containing encysted bradyzoites.

(2) Herbivorous intermediary hosts are most frequently infected by ingestion of sporulated oocysts shed into the environment by infected cats.
(3) During pregnancy, via the trans-placental route. Tachyzoites actively multiply within the placenta and spread to the fetus.

Infection rates are dependent on the degree of infestation and subsequent ingestion of infected prey (intermediate hosts, such as rodents and birds) by cats. Therefore it is the stray and feral cat population who maintain the highest concentration of infection as they rely most heavily on this source of food. The prevalence (20–60%) increases with age as well as type population, although shedding of the organism into the environment is as low as 1%, due to the fact that infected cats do not re-shed oocysts in subsequent infections with *T. gondii*. Young cats (< 2 years of age) appear more susceptible to infection.

Clinical signs

Infection with *T. gondii* may be asymptomatic. Cats that are likely to become ill with the infection and exhibit signs are the very young, the old, immunosupressed and those with concurrent disease. The number of organisms ingested is a factor. Infection with this organism is common; however, it is rarely the cause of significant disease in any species.

When clinical signs are manifested, these will be associated with the organs affected by the organism and could be any of the following:

- Anorexia.
- Lethargy.
- Pyrexia.
- Weight loss.
- Diarrhoea.
- Vomiting.
- Icterus.
- Respiratory disease.
- Muscle hyperaesthesia.
- Lameness.
- Pancreatitis.
- Ascites.
- Stillborn kittens/fading kittens.
- Nervous system signs.
- Myocardial dysfunction.
- Sudden death.

The organs most commonly infected are the eyes and the lungs.

Clinical signs are normally seen soon after infection, as the tachyzoites are actively multiplying in host cells.

A dormant infection may be reactivated if the animal becomes ill with another disease, such as FIV, or following glucocorticoid administration or immunosuppressive drugs.

Aetiology and pathogenesis

Cats usually become infected by ingestion of an infected intermediate host. The encysted organism is held within the prey's tissues. Following ingestion, the cyst wall is digested by the cat and the infectious organisms are released into the cat's intestinal tract.

The parasite then moves through the intestinal wall and replicates throughout the body as rapidly dividing tachyzoites. This is known as the extra-intestinal cycle.

The organism is also invading the epithelial cells of the intestine – the entero-epithelial cycle, culminating in the formation of oocysts, which are passed out of the intestinal tract in the cat's faeces.

The cat ultimately develops an immune response preventing further shedding of oocysts. Tachyzoites production is halted with bradyzoites formed instead. These are the slowly replicating form and are retained within the tissue cysts. Tissue cysts are present throughout the body in multiple sites, each cyst containing large numbers of bradyzoites.

(See also Chapter 15.)

Nursing care

- **Zoonotic** disease.
- Appropriate care and use of disinfectants when handling faeces or cleaning litter trays.
- Administration of drugs.
- Advise clients regarding safe practice:

  - Prepare pets' food in a separate area, using separate utensils and feeding bowls.
  - Do not allow pets to lick bowls, utensils, or cooking items used by humans.
  - Empty cat litter trays daily and disinfect with boiling water and then disinfectant products. If a cat is excreting oocysts, by cleaning out the tray this regular sporulation will not have occurred and therefore will not be infectious.
  - Pregnant females should wear protective gloves (i.e. waterproof) when gardening; hands should be washed thoroughly prior to any contact with others, own face or items that come into contact with the mouth, e.g. drink cups or cigarettes.
  - Cook all meat thoroughly to at least 70°C.
  - Wash all vegetables thoroughly.
  - Cover children's play areas and sand pits to prevent them becoming cat litter trays.

Risk to humans

Toxoplasmosis is an important zoonotic disease principally because it can affect newborn babies – if a previously unaffected pregnant female acquires toxoplasmosis during her pregnancy. In this situation there is a 40% chance that the fetus will acquire the infection. In 10% of these cases severe neurological or ocular disease is present at birth.

Around 30% of the adult population in the UK have serological evidence of infection with *T. gondii*. The vast majority are either asymptomatic or have only mild clinical disease. Most surveys show that owning or coming into contact with pet cats does not constitute an increased risk of contracting the disease. It is stray and feral cats that hold the risk of infection.

In humans it appears the main risk of contracting the disease is to adolescents and adults and is linked to ingestion of infected meat, through poor meat hygiene and eating undercooked meat.

Feline panleucopaenia

Feline panleucopaenia is an acute and severe viral disease of domesticated and wild felids, affecting the animal systemically but especially the intestinal tract. It is caused by the feline parvovirus, which is related to canine parvovirus.

The disease has a high morbidity and high mortality rate. It is spread by direct contact or by indirect contact via an infected environment. The virus can last many months in the environment and is resistant to heating and routine disinfectant products. Parvocidal products are, however, effective in destroying the virus.

It is shed via all body secretions and excretions during the acute phase of infection.

The highest infection rates occur where heavy population of unvaccinated cats exist in close proximity – rescue centres and feral colonies. Young cats are more susceptible to infection with the virus.

Clinical signs

The type and extent of clinical disease vary, depending on the degree of virus transmitted and the extent of cytolysis as a result of the replication virus.

(1) **Per acute**: An acute, severe form of the disease.

- Severe depression.
- Sub-clinical temperature.
- Death within 24 hours.

(2) **Acute**: This is the most common presentation of the disease. There is a sudden onset of signs.

- Pyrexia.
- Anorexia.
- Depressed mental state.
- Vomiting.
- Severe and foul diarrhoea.
- Severe dehydration and electrolyte imbalance.
- Cats adopt 'praying' position.
- May remain close by their food and water bowls, with their heads hanging over the bowl, but will refuse to eat or drink.
- Hypothermia.
- Coma, death.

An affected cat that survives about 5 days of illness will often go on to recover as the immune system (kicks in) to quash the active infection.

(3) **Sub-acute or mild infection**:

- Mild depression.
- Mild fever.
- Mild enteritis.

The cat will be ill for about 2–3 days and will go on to make a rapid, uncomplicated recovery.

(4) **Sub-clinical infection**: Common in older cats, who go on to develop a lifelong immunity, following recovery.

- Lack of clinical signs.
- Mild leukopaenia.
- Mild fever.

(5) ***In utero* infection**:

- Fetal death.
- Fetal resorption.
- Fetal mummification.
- Stillbirth.
- Cerebellar hypoplasia.

Aetiology and pathogenesis

In susceptible cats, exposure to the virus results in replication of the virus locally, depending on the transmission route – in the oropharynx, tonsils, and/or within the Peyer's patches in the small intestine.

Viral replication only occurs in rapidly dividing cells. The viral growth results in rapid cytolysis, destroying the infected cell and releasing large quantities of the virus.

This results in a transient viraemia, leading to the infection of other mitotic target cells throughout the body, including the crypt cells of the jejunum and ileum and the lymphopoietic cells of the bone marrow, thymus and spleen. In neonatal kittens, this also includes the cells of the developing retina and cerebellum. The cat shows signs of severe gastroenteritis and immunosuppression. There are no cardiac signs with feline panleucopaenia, compared to the canine equivalent.

The virus is then released systemically once again, by these target cells, leading to a secondary viraemia, and accompanying pyrexia. This phase lasts around 7 days until the virus-neutralising antibodies appear in the blood. The virus is then neutralised and controlled and the animal makes a rapid recovery from the clinical signs.

Where pregnant females are infected rapid fetal death occurs.

Diagnosis

- Clinical history.
- Information of poor vaccination status.
- Routine haematology – marked leukopaenia.
- Detection of the virus in faeces.
- CITE test.

Treatment

Supportive and symptomatic treatment includes intravenous fluid therapy and broad-spectrum antibiotics to help the damaged immune system fend off secondary infection.

Nursing care

- Barrier nursing.
- Administration of fluids and medications, as prescribed.
- Owner advice regarding other cats within household.
- Nutritional support – may require long-term special diet to account for severe damage to the small intestine – a low fat, high-digestibility diet is recommended.

Respiratory tract diseases

The respiratory system comprises the nasal cavities, pharynx, larynx, trachea, bronchi, bronchioles and alveoli. Respiratory tract disease may involve any of these organs and can be classified as either upper (affecting the upper airway, i.e. nose, pharynx, larynx and trachea) or lower (affecting the lungs, i.e. bronchi, bronchioles and alveoli).

Acute respiratory failure

Respiratory failure occurs when the lungs are unable to function adequately, i.e. when they can no longer transfer oxygen to the circulation and eliminate carbon dioxide from the body. Clinical signs of acute respiratory failure include dyspnoea, cyanosis, open mouth breathing, orthopnoea, hypoxia, increased respiratory effort, collapse and tachycardia. Upper airway obstruction, lower airway disease and extra-pulmonary disorders such as diaphragmatic hernia, pneumothorax or pleural effusion may lead to respiratory failure.

Immediate nursing care

Dyspnoea is an emergency that requires immediate veterinary attention if the animal's life is to be saved. On presentation of a dyspnoeic patient, the veterinary nurse should administer oxygen by any means that the animal will tolerate. Table 17.8 shows the different methods of oxygen administration available. The patient should be placed in a stress-free environment and be continually observed. If the patient is to receive long-term oxygen therapy, the oxygen should be humidified to prevent drying of airways.

If the patient is collapsed it should be supported in sternal recumbency to allow inflation of both sides of the lungs. The airway must be kept clear of secretions, such as saliva or blood and the head should be positioned with the neck extended and the tongue pulled forward. If the patient is unconscious an endotracheal tube should be placed.

Resuscitation equipment should be prepared in case the animal deteriorates. Equipment required for endotracheal intubation includes an endotracheal tube, local anaesthetic spray (cats), laryngoscope, cuff inflator, bandage for securing the tube, circuit/ambu bag, and an oxygen supply. If respiratory arrest occurs, the patient should be intubated and intermittent positive pressure ventilation (IPPV) performed at 10–20 breaths per minute. Vital signs should be continually monitored.

Table 17.8 Methods of oxygen administration		
Method	**How to set up**	**Comment**
Mask	A close-fitting mask should be used to prevent rebreathing of carbon dioxide	Easy and quick to set up, but often poorly tolerated by dyspnoeic patients
Flow by	Involves placing an oxygen supply in front of the nose/mouth	Easy and quick to set up. Very useful in animals that will not tolerate other methods of oxygen supplementation
Nasal oxygen tube	Involves placing an infant feeding tube into the nose (see Table 17.9)	More difficult to set up than other methods. Good for long-term oxygen therapy
Buster collar/cling film	Involves placing a relatively large buster collar on the patient, covering the front with cling film (leaving a small gap at the top for carbon dioxide to escape) and piping oxygen in at the back	Easy to set up but should be used with care, as animals which pant excessively may become hyperthermic
Oxygen cage	An oxygen cage can be set up by covering the front of a kennel with cling film and piping oxygen into it. An incubator can also be used as an oxygen cage	A good way of administering oxygen without stressing the patient, but only suitable for cats and small dogs. Access to the patient should be minimal because each time the cage is entered all the oxygen escapes. Difficult to monitor patient because not easily accessible. Patient may overheat
Endotracheal tube	Intubation	Used in animals which are unconscious or that have respiratory arrested. Only method suitable for performing IPPV

Table 17.9 Placement of a nasal oxygen tube	
Equipment needed	Infant feeding tube Local anaesthetic drops Lubricating gel Suture material/superglue
Procedure	(1) Instil local anaesthetic drops into nostril (2) Allow 1–2 minutes for analgesia effect (3) Measure tube from nares to medial canthus and mark (4) Put lubricating gel on the tip of the tube (5) Gently push into nostril into a medioventral direction (6) Stop when the mark is reached (7) Secure in place with suture or glue

Extra-pulmonary causes of dyspnoea

Diaphragmatic hernia

Rupture of the diaphragm allows abdominal organs to pass into the thoracic cavity. The abdominal organs prevent lung expansion causing tachypnoea and dyspnoea. Usually caused by trauma (e.g. road traffic accident), but can be congenital. Surgery is required to repair the diaphragm. The patient may suddenly deteriorate on handling as more of the abdominal viscera enter the thorax.

Pneumothorax

A pneumothorax occurs when air accumulates in the thoracic cavity, outside the lungs. It can be classified as open or closed. An open pneumothorax occurs when the thoracic wall is penetrated, e.g. by a stake or stick. As the animal breathes, air is sucked through the hole into the thoracic cavity. A closed pneumothorax occurs when an airway is ruptured, allowing air to leak from the lungs into the thoracic cavity. A closed pneumothorax is common after trauma, such as a road traffic accident, but other causes include bullae, foreign bodies and neoplasia. If the leak is small it may seal itself, but larger leaks lead to a massive accumulation of air in the thoracic cavity, preventing lung expansion. This is known as a **tension pneumothorax**.

Pleural effusion

Accumulation of fluid in the thoracic cavity is known as a pleural effusion. Different diseases produce different types of fluid. The fluid can be classified into different categories, i.e. blood, chyle, transudate, modified transudate or exudate. A sample of fluid should be sent for cytology and culture to help determine the cause of the pleural effusion. If blood is suspected, a packed cell volume should be performed to distinguish it from other fluids. If the fluid is milky in appearance a triglyceride level will determine whether it is chyle. Table 17.10 shows how to distinguish between a transudate and an exudate; there is significant overlap between the categories and the classification also depends on the cell type present. Pure transudates are produced by hypoproteinaemia. Modified transudates may be caused by congestive heart failure, neoplasia or a long-standing pure transudate. Exudates are produced with feline infectious peritonitis, bacterial infection (pyothorax) or again, neoplasia.

Accumulation of air or fluid in the thoracic cavity reduces the space for lung inflation. The severity of clinical signs depends on the volume of air or fluid present and the degree of lung collapse.

In the early stages clinical signs include tachypnoea and shallow respirations. As the condition worsens, the animal will show signs of severe respiratory distress, such as dyspnoea, cyanosis and orthopnoea, and signs of shock, i.e. tachycardia, weak peripheral pulse, pale mucous membranes, collapse, decreased awareness and hypothermia.

Chest percussion will show increased resonance with a pneumothorax and decreased resonance in the ventral thorax with a pleural effusion. Heart sounds will be muffled if a pleural effusion is present.

Nursing care

- Monitor vital signs.
- Provide oxygen supplementation.
- Assist veterinary surgeon in performing thoracocentesis (see Table 17.11).
- Keep patient warm and quiet.
- Support in sternal recumbency.
- Provide intravenous access.
- Administer intravenous fluids.

Table 17.10 Comparison of transudates and exudate				
	Appearance of fluid	**Protein content (g/litre)**	**Nucleated cell count (1×10^9/litre)**	**Specific gravity**
Pure transudate	Colourless and clear or slightly opaque	<25	<1	<1.018
Modified transudate	Straw coloured or pink and slightly opaque	<35	<7	1.018 (approx.)
Exudate	Thick, coloured (yellow–brown) Often foul smelling	>30	<5–300	>1.018

Table 17.11 Thoracocentesis	
Equipment required	Clippers Cotton wool and skin disinfectants Local anaesthetic Sterile gloves For dogs: intravenous catheter, extension set, 3-way tap and 50 ml syringe (or larger) For cats: butterfly catheter, 3-way tap and 20 ml syringe Bowl Sample pots (plain and EDTA tubes)
Procedure	(1) Place patient in sternal recumbency (2) Clip lateral thorax over 7th/8th intercostal space (3) Inject local anaesthetic and wait for a couple of minutes (4) Prepare thoracocentesis site (5) Veterinary surgeon to put on sterile gloves (6) Hand VS thoracocentesis equipment in a sterile manner (7) VS to hand nurse syringe (8) VS to insert catheter into thoracic cavity (9) Nurse to gently withdraw plunger (10) Once the syringe is full, turn the 3-way tap off to the patient and empty the fluid into the bowl (11) Turn 3-way tap off towards the air and continue draining (12) Continue procedure until no more air or fluid is withdrawn (13) Repeat for the other side if necessary (14) Send fluid for analysis

Note: drainage of one side of the thorax is usually adequate, but occasionally both sides will need to be drained

Thoracocentesis should be sufficient to stabilise a patient and provides fluid samples for analysis. However, if the fluid or air rapidly accumulates again after thoracocentesis, an indwelling chest drain is indicated. Indwelling chest drains are indicated in most cases of pyothorax and chylothorax.

Laryngeal problems

Laryngeal problems include laryngitis and laryngeal paralysis. Owners often report a change in bark and animals with laryngeal paralysis may show signs of exercise intolerance or dyspnoea.

Nursing care

- Use a harness.
- Avoid stress and excitement.
- Place in a quiet environment.
- Monitor vital signs.
- Keep cool.

- Sedate if necessary.
- Administer oxygen if dyspnoeic.

In severe cases of laryngeal paralysis it may be necessary to anaesthetise and intubate the animal, so equipment should be set up ready.

Coughing

There are many causes of coughing in the dog and cat including: kennel cough, tracheal collapse, airway foreign bodies, pharyngitis, tracheitis, bronchitis, feline asthma, pneumonia, lung worm, pulmonary oedema (e.g. heart failure), neoplasia and pulmonary haemorrhage.

There are many diagnostic tests available:

- Blood tests for haematology and biochemistry.
- Faecal analysis for lung worm larvae.
- Thoracic radiographs.
- Bronchoscopy.
- Bronchoalveolar lavage (BAL) for cytology and culture (see Table 17.12). This is performed by passing a sterile tube (e.g. dog urinary catheter, infant feeding tube or special BAL tube) into a lung lobe. The tube may be directed into a particular lobe through a bronchoscope or passed blindly through the endotracheal tube. The latter technique is favoured in small patient or if a suitable endoscope is not available.

Antitussives are used to suppress coughing but should only be used when coughing is persistent and unproductive or when the animal's welfare is compromised, e.g. tracheal collapse. Other drugs used to treat respiratory disorders include anti-inflammatories to reduce inflammation, bronchodilators to treat airway-narrowing, expectorants to encourage removal of secretions, mucolytics to reduce mucous viscosity, antibiotics to treat specific bacterial infections and anthelmintics for lung worm infections.

Nursing care

- Monitor vital signs.
- Use a harness.
- Restrict exercise.
- Diet if obese.
- Avoid dry, dusty or smoky atmospheres.

Table 17.12 Bronchoalveolar lavage	
Equipment	Sterile tube Sterile saline Syringes Sample pots (EDTA and plain tubes)
Procedure	(1) pass the sterile tube into a lung lobe (2) inject the saline, then aspirate (3) send samples for cytology and culture

Note: Coupage can be performed during a bronchoalveolar lavage to aid sample collection

- Isolate and barrier nurse if an infectious disease is suspected.
- Administer medications as per the veterinary surgeon's instructions.
- Perform nebulisation.
- Perform coupage.

Nebulisation and coupage aid removal of secretions in patients with pneumonia and should be performed for 5–10 minutes, three to four times daily. Nebulisation forms tiny droplets of water, which are breathed in and moisten respiratory secretion, making them less viscous. Coupage is performed by percussing the chest wall with cupped hands; it helps loosen secretions and stimulates coughing.

Humidification is another technique that can be used to moisten secretions in the respiratory tract, making it easier for the animal to cough them up. It can be easily performed by the owner at home, by taking the pet into the bathroom with them two to three times daily.

Nasal discharge

Nasal discharge may be seen with upper respiratory tract diseases and may be serous, mucoid, mucopurulent or haemorrhagic (epistaxis). The discharge may be unilateral or bilateral. Other signs of nasal disease may include sneezing, facial swelling, dyspnoea, snorting, facial rubbing and anorexia.

Causes of nasal discharge include viral infections, e.g. canine distemper, feline upper respiratory disease; fungal infections, e.g. aspergillosis; secondary bacterial infections, allergies, tumours and foreign bodies, such as grass seeds. Animals with nasal foreign bodies are often distressed and will paw at their face or rub their nose on the ground. Epistaxis may be caused by trauma, hypertension, coagulopathies and neoplasia.

The following tests may be useful in investigating nasal disease:

- Blood tests including haematology, biochemistry, clotting profile and serology for aspergillus or viral antibody titres.
- Radiography of the nasal cavities and thorax.
- Rhinoscopy (anterior and retrograde examination).
- Nasal biopsy for histopathology.
- Nasal flush for cytology (see Table 17.13).
- Bacterial and fungal culture.

Treatment involves specific therapy dependent on the cause of the nasal discharge, e.g. removal of nasal foreign bodies, antibiotics to treat bacterial infection, topical antifungals to treat aspergillus and surgery or radiotherapy for neoplasia.

Nursing care

- Monitor vital signs.
- Bathe discharge from nose as necessary.

Table 17.13 Nasal flush	
Equipment required	Sterile saline Syringe (use 20 ml Luer tip for cats/small dogs and 50 ml catheter tip for large dogs) Laryngoscope Bandage to pack pharynx Bowl
Procedure	(1) General anaesthetic (2) Pack pharynx with bandage (3) Place patient with head hanging over the edge of the table (4) Hold bowl under mouth to catch the saline (5) Flush up both nostrils with saline (6) Remove bandage and examine for pieces of tissue/foreign bodies (7) Examine back of mouth for pieces of tissue/foreign bodies (8) Send off sample of flush for cytology

- Keep clean, bath and groom as necessary.
- Encourage animal to eat.
- Isolate and barrier nurse if an infectious disease is suspected.

Heart disease

Heart disease can be classified as congenital, i.e. present at birth, or acquired, where the disease develops over time. Heart disease leads to congestion and heart failure. Heart failure may be classified as acute (sudden onset) or chronic (develops over a long period of time).

Chronic heart failure

Heart failure can be described as left- or right-sided. Clinical signs depend on which part of the heart is affected. Heart disease can affect both sides of the heart, causing signs of left and right heart failure.

Left-sided heart failure causes pulmonary venous congestion and pulmonary oedema. Clinical signs include lethargy, exercise intolerance, coughing, tachypnoea, dyspnoea and orthopnoea. Syncope may occur with arrhythmias or hypotension.

Right-sided congestive heart failure causes systemic venous congestion. This leads to abdominal distension due to ascites and hepatomegaly, and dyspnoea due to pleural effusion. Exercise intolerance or syncope may occur due to poor cardiac output.

Treatment for chronic heart failure is aimed at alleviating clinical signs. Drugs used to treat cardiac failure include diuretics, vasodilators, antidysrhythmics and positive inotropes (see Chapter 12 for more information).

Nursing care

- Restrict exercise.
- Avoid stress.
- Monitor vital signs.
- Diet if obese.
- Feed a low-sodium diet (avoid salty treats).
- Administer drugs as per veterinary surgeon's instructions.

Congenital heart defects

Patent ductus arteriosus

In the fetus, the ductus arteriosus connects the pulmonary artery to the aorta, allowing blood to bypass the lungs. The ductus arteriosus should close soon after birth, but sometimes it remains patent, allowing shunting of blood from the aorta into the pulmonary artery. This leads to left-sided heart failure.

Patent ductus arteriosus is the most common congenital heart defect in dogs. A machinery-type murmur is heard on auscultation of the heart and is usually detected by the veterinary surgeon at the time of the first vaccination. Treatment involves surgery to ligate the ductus arteriosus. The prognosis is excellent with surgery.

Valvular defects

Mitral/tricuspid valve dysplasia is due to malformation of the atrioventricular valves. Regurgitation of blood through the atrioventricular valve increases the workload for the atrium, leading to atrial enlargement and congestive heart failure. The prognosis is poor.

Aortic/pulmonic stenosis is a narrowing of the aorta/pulmonic valve, which obstructs the flow of blood leaving the ventricle. This leads to hypertrophy of the ventricle as the heart tries to maintain cardiac output. Clinical signs include syncope, exercise intolerance and heart failure. Pulmonic stenosis can be treated by surgery or by performing a balloon valvuloplasty.

Septal defects

A hole in the septum between the atria or ventricles allows blood to flow from the left to the right side of the heart, this leads to congestive heart failure. Ventricular septal defects are the most common congenital heart defect in cats. Treatment involves surgery to correct the defect.

Combined defects

Tetrology of Fallot causes congestive heart failure. It is made up of four components: pulmonic stenosis, ventricular septal defect, right ventricular hypertrophy and a dextraposed aorta. The prognosis is very poor.

Persistent right aortic arch

Persistent right aortic arch is a vascular ring anomaly. The oesophagus is trapped between the ligamentum arteriosus, aorta, pulmonary artery and heart base causing regurgitation of food. Affected animals are stunted and may have aspiration pneumonia. Treatment involves surgery to cut the ligamentum arteriosus.

Acquired heart disease

Endocardial disease

Endocardiosis refers to chronic degeneration of the heart valves, particularly the mitral valve. This leads to regurgitation of blood into the left atrium causing congestion and heart failure.

Bacterial endocarditis is due to bacterial infection of the heart lining and most commonly affects the aortic valve, causing leakage of blood back into the left ventricle. Clinical signs include lethargy, pyrexia, shifting lameness, anorexia and detection of a new heart murmur. Treatment involves antibiotics and symptomatic treatment of heart failure. The prognosis is poor due to permanent damage of the heart valves.

Myocardial disease

Dilated cardiomyopathy (DCM) is seen in large breeds such as Dobermann pinschers, Boxers, Great Danes and Irish Wolfhounds. It develops with heart enlargement, reduced contractility and congestive heart failure.

Hypertrophic cardiomyopathy is the most common form of heart disease in cats. Enlargement of the left ventricle leads to reduced myocardial relaxation and inadequate cardiac output, causing congestive heart failure. DCM may occur in cats as a result of taurine deficiency (e.g. feeding exclusively fish), but is uncommon now commercial diets are fed.

Restrictive cardiomyopathy leads to reduced myocardial relaxation and contractility resulting in congestive heart failure.

Pericardial disease

Pericardial effusion refers to the build up of fluid between the pericardium and the heart itself. This prevents the heart from expanding properly resulting in right-sided heart failure, with a pleural effusion and ascites. Pericardiocentesis should be performed and results in a rapid improvement. If the effusion recurs surgery to remove the pericardium may be necessary.

Diagnostic tests

In addition to taking a history and performing a full clinical examination the following diagnostic tests are available:

- Blood tests for haematology and biochemistry.
- Electrocardiogram (ECG).
- Thoracic radiographs (lateral and dorsoventral).
- Echocardiography.

Electrocardiogram   An ECG measures the electrical activity of the heart. It is used to diagnose arrhythmias and may be used in conjunction with other tests to detect chamber enlargement. A veterinary nurse should be able to record an ECG of diagnostic quality (see Table 17.14).

Echocardiography   This is ultrasound examination of the heart. A probe (the transducer) is placed in contact with the surface of the patient. A piezo-electric crystal in the probe emits high-frequency sound waves, which are eflected back by body tissue. The transducer detects the returning sound waves and converts them into an ultrasound image.

Two-dimensional echocardiography allows assessment of the heart for anatomical defects and the size of the chambers. M-mode allows myocardial function to be assessed and Doppler echocardiography enables the source of a heart murmur to be detected. Most ultrasound machines will perform two-dimensional and M-mode echocardiography, but Doppler is a more specialised technique. A veterinary nurse should be able to assist the veterinary surgeon with the ultrasound scan (see Table 17.15).

Acute heart failure

Animals with acute heart failure present with severe dyspnoea, cyanosis or pallor and cardiogenic shock. Animals are often distressed, have dilated pupils and will resist restraint. Severely dyspnoeic dogs are orthopnoeic and open-mouthed breathing is seen in cats. (Note: cats are obligatory nose breathers, so this is a very bad sign.) Clinical signs of cardiogenic shock include collapse, decreased awareness, tachycardia, weak peripheral pulses, cold extremities, pale mucous membrane and a prolonged capillary refill time.

Table 17.14 Procedure for an ECG

(1) Place the patient in right lateral recumbency, preferably on a rubber-topped table
(2) Attach the electrodes:
   Red – right fore
   Yellow – left fore
   Green – left hind
   Black – right hind
(3) Apply a conducting gel or alcohol to the electrodes
(4) Select the settings, 10 mm/mV and 25 mm/s are suitable for most patients
(5) Record the ECG (leads I, II, III, AVL, AVR and AVF)
(6) Label the ECG with date, settings, leads and case details

Tip: Remember where the electrodes go by thinking of traffic lights: start with the red on the right fore and work in a clockwise direction (red, yellow, green). The black electrode goes on the remaining limb, i.e. right hind

---

Table 17.15 Assisting the veterinary surgeon with cardiac ultrasound

(1) Clip the hair over the transducer positions (left parasternal, right parasternal and subcostal)
(2) Restrain animal in lateral recumbency and pull the forelimbs cranially
(3) Apply ultrasound gel to the probe
(4) After the procedure clean the probe and wipe the gel from the animal's coat

---

Initial treatment should be aimed at stabilising the patient rather than investigating the cause of cardiac failure. Most patients will resent restraint, so handling of patients should be kept to a minimum. Oxygen should be administered by the easiest least stressful method available. If possible an intravenous catheter should be placed, but do not stress the animal. Drugs used to treat pulmonary oedema include diuretics and vasodilators. Diuretics should be administered intravenously for rapid effect. Water should be provided ad lib. Nitroglycerine ointment is a venodilator, which can be administered topically, usually on the inside of the pinna. (N.B It is absorbed through the skin so gloves should be worn to prevent direct contact, otherwise hypotension may occur.) Poor cardiac output and tissue perfusion lead to hypothermia, so the animal should be kept warm.

Cardiac arrest may occur at any time so resuscitation equipment should be set up ready. Equipment required includes endotracheal tube, laryngoscope, ambu bag or circuit, oxygen supply, tie to secure tube and a cuff inflator. All personnel should be trained in and be proficient at performing cardiopulmonary resuscitation (see Table 17.16).

Nursing care

- **Do not stress** (this is of particular importance in cats).
- Administer oxygen.
- Cage rest.
- Keep warm.
- Monitor vital signs.
- Administer drugs as per veterinary surgeon's instructions.
- Perform cardiopulmonary resuscitation if cardiac arrest occurs.

Table 17.16 Procedure for performing CPR (cardiopulmonary resuscitation)

AIRWAY	Place an endotracheal tube
BREATHING	Attach to anaesthetic circuit or ambu bag
	Perform artificial ventilations at 10–20 breaths per minute
CIRCULATION	Perform cardiac massage at 60–120 compressions per minute

Anaemia

Anaemia describes a low circulating volume of red blood cells. Anaemia occurs in three ways: through haemorrhage, increased red cell destruction (haemolysis) or decreased production of red blood cells. Anaemia can be classified as regenerative or non-regenerative. Regenerative anaemia describes an increase in red cell production in response to cell loss due to haemorrhage or haemolysis. Non-regenerative anaemia describes an inappropriate response to a reduction in the number of red blood cells and severe cases are commonly associated with bone marrow disorders.

Anaemia can be described as chronic or acute. Chronic anaemia occurs gradually over time and causes include liver disease, nutritional disorders (e.g. iron deficiency), bone marrow disorders, viral infections (e.g. FELV, FIV), parasites (*Haemobartonella felis*) and immune-mediated disease. Acute anaemia occurs suddenly as a result of haemorrhage or haemolysis and may be due to trauma, surgery, clotting disorders, warfarin poisoning and haemangiosarcomas.

Clinical signs of anaemia are due to a decrease in oxygen-carrying capacity of the blood and include pallor of mucous membrane, lethargy, weakness, exercise intolerance, collapse, tachycardia and tachypnoea.

Diagnostic tests available:

- Blood tests for routine biochemistry and haematology (including reticulocyte and platelet counts). Cats should also be screened for FELV/FIV viruses and the blood parasite, *Haemobartonella felis*.
- Blood tests for clotting disorders including activated clotting time (ACT), prothrombin time (PT), activated partial thromboplastin time (APTT), von Willebrand's factor, buccal mucosal bleeding time and assays for clotting factors.
- Blood tests for immune-mediated disease including in-saline agglutination, Coombs and antinuclear antibody tests.
- Blood tests for iron deficiency, including serum iron and total iron binding capacity.
- Thoracic and abdominal radiographs.
- Bone marrow aspirate/biopsy in non-regenerative anaemia.

Treatment should be aimed at the underlying condition, e.g. give immunosuppressants for immune-mediated disease, Vitamin K for warfarin poisoning, tetracycline for *Haemobartonella felis*, chemotherapy for leukaemia or lymphoma and erythropoietin for renal disease.

However, if the packed cell volume falls to such a level that the red blood cells are unable to carry sufficient oxygen to tissues and clinical signs are evident, a blood transfusion is indicated. In chronic anaemia, compensatory mechanisms occur over time, enabling animals to tolerate a lower PCV than those with acute blood loss.

Nursing care

- Keep quiet.
- Avoid stress.
- Monitor vital signs
- Administer drugs as per the veterinary surgeon's instructions.
- Administer blood products and monitor for adverse reactions.
- Feed a diet high in iron and B vitamins.

Clotting disorders

Abnormal haemostasis is due to vessel wall defects, thrombocytopenia, platelet dysfunction or coagulation factor deficiencies. Haemorrhage may occur spontaneously or following surgery, trauma or loss of deciduous teeth.

The site of haemorrhage varies depending on the type of clotting disorder. Multifocal pinpoint/petechial haemorrhages on the skin or mucous membranes are seen with impaired clot formation. Melaena, haematemesis, epistaxis, haematuria and retinal/intraocular haemorrhage can be seen with thrombocytopenia or platelet dysfunction. Haematoma formation or bleeding into body cavities, including joints are associated with clotting factor deficiencies.

Diagnostic tests available include:

- Routine biochemistry and haematology (including platelet count).
- Activated clotting time (ACT).
- Prothrombin time (PT) and activated partial thromboplastin time (APTT).
- Buccal mucosal bleeding time.
- Von Willebrand's factor.
- Factor VIII.
- Other clotting factor assays.
- Fibrin degradation products (FDP).

Clotting disorders can be hereditary and may have a higher incidence in certain breeds, e.g. Von Willebrand's disease in Dobermann pinschers and Haemophilia A (Factor VIII deficiency) in German Shepherd dogs. Haemophilia A is sex-linked, affecting only male dogs, although females can be carriers of the disease. Immune-mediated thrombocytopenia (IMT) is an inherited disease causing destruction of platelets. Inherited defects are present at birth but clinical signs may not develop until later in life, e.g. at the time of neutering. Affected animals should not be used for breeding.

Some clotting disorders are acquired, i.e. develop over time and are usually seen in older animals with no previous history of bleeding episodes. Acquired disorders may be due to oestrogen toxicity, warfarin poisoning, liver disease or disseminated intravascular coagulation (DIC).

Plasma, platelet-rich plasma or whole blood may be required to stabilise patients with clotting disorders. Specific therapy involves administration of steroids for immune mediated thrombocytopenia, desmopressin (DDAVP) in Von Willebrand's disease, vitamin K with warfarin poisoning and heparin with DIC.

Nursing care

- Handle gently.
- Avoid stress/excitement.
- Monitor vital signs.
- Administer drugs following the veterinary surgeon's instructions.
- Administer blood products and monitor for adverse reactions.

N.B. Do **not** use the jugular vein for venipuncture in these patients. All blood samples should be taken from a peripheral vein and pressure applied to the venipuncture site for 5–10 minutes following blood sampling.

Diseases of the alimentary system

The alimentary system comprises the oesophagus, stomach, small intestine and colon. Dysfunction of these organs may lead to regurgitation, vomiting or diarrhoea. It is important to differentiate between regurgitation and vomiting. Regurgitation is seen with oesophageal disorders, vomiting with gastric disorders and diarrhoea is associated with intestinal disease. Vomiting and diarrhoea may occur together.

Regurgitation

Regurgitation is a passive process, where the head is lowered and undigested food is ejected from the mouth. There is no contraction of abdominal muscles. Causes include megaoesophagus, oesophagitis, oesophageal stricture, persistent right aortic arch and oesophageal foreign bodies. This may lead to aspiration pneumonia due to inhalation of food particles or saliva. Severity ranges from regurgitation of solid food to regurgitation of all ingested material and saliva.

Diagnostic tests available:

- pH of vomitus (to differentiate between regurgitation and vomiting).
- Blood tests for routine haematology and biochemistry. Specific tests to detect myaesthenia gravis, hypothyroidism and Addison's disease, in animals with megaoesophagus.
- Radiography.
- Barium swallow.
- Oesophagoscopy.

Treatment varies depending on the cause of regurgitation, e.g. removal of oesophageal foreign bodies, ballooning of oesophageal strictures, surgery in animals with a persistent right aortic arch and medical management of an underlying disease causing megaoesophagus.

Gravity-assisted feeding is used to control clinical signs. The consistency of food is determined by the severity of regurgitation. In some animals all that is required is to feed from a height, in others only liquid food may be tolerated. It may also be necessary to tilt a dog, keeping the head and forelimbs raised for 10 minutes post feeding and in severe cases when even water is regurgitated, a permanent feeding tube (gastrostomy tube) must be placed.

Nursing care

- Monitor vital signs.
- Offer food and water from a height.
- Observe for and record any regurgitation.
- Observe for signs of aspiration pneumonia (depression, coughing, pyrexia).
- Keep animal clean, bath and groom as necessary.
- Monitor hydration status.
- Administer intravenous fluids if dehydrated.
- Administer medications as directed by the veterinary surgeon.
- Monitor and record weight daily.

Vomiting

Vomiting is an active process, where stomach contents are forcefully ejected out of the mouth by contraction of the abdominal muscles. Vomiting can be classified as acute or chronic and causes include dietary indiscretion, viral, bacterial or parasitic infections, neoplasia, obstruction (e.g. foreign bodies, pyloric stenosis), drugs (e.g. steroids, nonsteroidal anti-inflammatory drugs), poisons, toxins and systemic disease (e.g. diseases of the liver, kidneys or pancreas, peritonitis, pyometra). Vomiting results in loss of water, sodium, chloride and potassium from the body leading to dehydration, electrolyte imbalances and metabolic alkalosis. Clinical signs associated with vomiting include restlessness, nausea, inappetence and abdominal pain.

Diagnostic tests available:

- Blood tests for haematology and biochemistry.
- Abdominal radiographs or ultrasound.
- Barium meal.
- Gastroscopy (see Table 17.17).
- Exploratory laporotomy.
- Biopsies for histopathology (taken via endoscopy or laparotomy).

Treatment is aimed at treating the underlying disease, controlling the clinical signs and correcting dehydration. Drugs include antiemetics to control severe vomiting, histamine blocking drugs to reduce gastric acid secretion, antacids to neutralise gastric acid and antibodies to treat specific bacterial infections. Surgery may be used to correct pyloric stenosis or remove a gastric foreign body. Fluid therapy

Table 17.17 Endoscopy	
	Guidelines for preparation
Upper GI endoscopy	Starve for 12–18 hours
Lower GI endoscopy	Starve for 36–48 hours Administer at least two warm water enemas to empty the colon Oral laxatives may be administered 12–18 hours prior to endoscopy

should be administered at a rate sufficient to replace any fluid deficit, provide maintenance requirements and replace ongoing losses. A 0.9% sodium chloride solution may be used to correct the metabolic alkalosis caused by vomiting.

Nursing care

- Starve animal for 24 hours, then feed small frequent meals.
- Feed a bland diet such as chicken and rice or a commercial prescription diet.
- Keep animal clean, bath and groom as necessary.
- Monitor vital signs.
- Monitor hydration status.
- Administer intravenous fluids if dehydrated.
- Observe and record any vomiting.
- Administer medications as directed by the veterinary surgeon.
- Isolate animal and barrier nurse if an infectious agent is suspected.
- Monitor and record weight daily.

Diarrhoea

Diarrhoea can be classified into small- or large-intestinal diarrhoea depending on frequency, volume and appearance of faeces. In general, animals with small-intestinal diarrhoea pass large volumes of soft to liquid faeces three to four times daily and those with large-intestinal diarrhoea pass small amounts of soft faeces (which may contain mucus or fresh blood) up to 10 times daily. Diarrhoea may be due to primary intestinal disease or secondary to metabolic disorders such as hyperthyroidism, liver disease, Addison's disease and pancreatitis. Diarrhoea results in loss of water, bicarbonate and potassium from the body leading to dehydration, electrolyte imbalances and metabolic acidosis. Fluid therapy should be used to correct dehydration, metabolic imbalances, electrolyte imbalances, provide maintenance requirements and replace ongoing losses.

Diagnostic tests available.

- Blood tests for haematology, biochemistry, trypsin-like immunoreactivity, folate and cobalamin.
- Faecal analysis for parasites, culture, *Giardia, Cryptosporidia* and an ELISA test for parvoviral antigen.
- Abdominal radiographs or ultrasound.
- Barium meal.
- Endoscopy of the upper or lower gastrointestinal tract (see Table 17.17). Fibre-optic or video endoscopes can be used to examine the oesophagus, stomach, proximal duodenum and colon. Mucosal biopsies are taken for histopathology.
- Exploratory laparotomy.
- Biopsies for histopathology (taken via endoscopy or laparotomy).

Acute diarrhoea can be mild or severe. In mild cases, the animal appears bright and is not dehydrated but in severe cases, the animal appears dull and depressed, is dehydrated and has other clinical signs such as pyrexia, abdominal pain and melaena.

Dietary causes of acute diarrhoea include sudden change of diet, scavenging and dietary intolerance or hypersensitivity. Other causes include intestinal obstruction, haemorrhagic gastroenteritis and viral, bacterial or parasitic infections. Obstruction of the intestine may be caused by intussusceptions, neoplasia or foreign bodies, items such as toys, stones and fish hooks are commonly seen in dogs, whereas linear foreign bodies, e.g. needle and thread are usually seen in cats. Viral infections include canine parvovirus, feline panleucopaenia, FELV and FIV and are more common in young or unvaccinated animals. Bacterial infections include *Salmonella, Campylobacter, Clostridium* and pathogenic *E. coli*. Intestinal parasites include *Toxocara, Giardia* and *Cryptosporidia*.

In mild cases, clinical signs usually resolve with starvation and dietary management alone, but severe cases require aggressive fluid therapy and investigation and treatment of the underlying disease. Treatment includes antibiotics for specific bacterial infections, anthelmintics for roundworm infections, metronidazole for giardiasis and surgery for intestinal obstruction. An exclusion diet should be fed if a food allergy is suspected (involves feeding a single source of protein that the animal has not been previously exposed to).

Chronic diarrhoea is due to maldigestion or malabsorption of food. Exocrine pancreatic insufficiency (EPI) is a maldigestive disease caused by a lack of digestive enzymes. Malabsorptive disorders include inflammatory bowel disease (IBD), lymphangiectasia and intestinal neoplasia.

Inflammatory bowel disease describes a group of disorders where there is infiltration of the intestinal mucosa by inflammatory cells. Types of IBD include lymphocytic–plasmacytic enteritis and eosinophilic enteritis. Other clinical signs associated with IBD include vomiting, inappetence and weight loss. Long-term corticosteroid therapy and dietary modification are used to treat IBD. Dietary therapy involves feeding a hypoallergenic diet that is low residue and highly digestible.

Lymphangiectasia is a lymphatic abnormality where there is obstruction to lymphatic drainage causing dilation and hypertension of intestinal lymphatic vessels. This results in leakage of lymph, which is high in protein, causing hypoproteinaemia. Clinical signs include diarrhoea and weight loss. Treatment involves feeding a diet that contains high-quality protein and is low in fat. Corticosteroids are used to reduce inflammation.

Neoplasia of the intestinal tract is usually malignant. The two most common types of intestinal neoplasia are lymphoma and adenocarcinoma. Clinical signs include vomiting, diarrhoea, weight loss, lethargy and inappetence. The cause of intestinal lymphoma is often unknown; however, feline leukaemia virus (FELV) can increase the risk of intestinal lymphoma in cats. Chemotherapy is used to treat animals with intestinal lymphoma. Treatment for intestinal adenocarcinoma involves surgical excision.

Malabsorptive disorders can cause mild to severe hypoproteinaemia. Peripheral oedema, ascites and respiratory problems may develop, as reduced osmotic pressure allows fluid to leak out of the circulation.

Acute colitis is associated with dietary indiscretion, which results in secondary bacterial infection and IBD. The cause of chronic colitis is unknown, although it is thought to be caused by an immune response to antigens in the colon. Colitis may be controlled by avoiding stress, feeding a high-fibre diet and administering medications such as steroids or sulphasalazine.

Nursing care

- Feed a diet which contains high-quality protein and is low in fat.
- Feed small frequent meals.
- Monitor vital signs.
- Observe for and record any diarrhoea.
- Take outside frequently to give the animal opportunity to defecate.
- Keep the animal clean, bath and groom as necessary.
- If diarrhoea is severe: bandage tail, clip around anus and apply a barrier cream such as sudocream or vaseline.
- Monitor hydration status.
- Administer intravenous fluids if dehydrated.
- Monitor and record weight daily.
- Administer medications as directed by the veterinary surgeon.
- Isolate animal and barrier nurse if an infectious agent is suspected.

Liver disease

Liver disease may be congenital (e.g. portosystemic shunt) or acquired. Causes of acquired disease include canine infectious hepatitis, toxins, drugs and neoplasia.

Clinical signs of liver disease include jaundice, depression, vomiting, diarrhoea, anorexia, weight loss, polydipsia, polyuria, ascites, abdominal pain and signs of hepatic encephalopathy.

Jaundice or icterus is the yellowing colouring of skin, sclerae and mucous membranes caused by a build-up of the bile pigment bilirubin. There are three types of jaundice: haemolytic (prehepatic), hepatocellular (intrahepatic) and obstructive (posthepatic). Haemolytic jaundice is caused by the excessive breakdown of red blood cells, hepatocellular jaundice occurs with liver disease and obstructive jaundice is seen with bile flow obstructions.

Diagnostic tests include:

- Blood tests including haematology, biochemistry, bile acids (see Table 17.18) and ammonia.
- Urine tests including specific gravity, dipstick and sediment.
- Abdominal ultrasound or radiography.
- Liver biopsy (a coagulation screen should be run first).

Antibiotics and lactulose are used to treat liver patients showing signs of hepatic encephalopathy. Antibiotics are used to kill ammonia-producing bacteria in the intestines, and lactulose (a synthetic disaccharide) reduces absorption of ammonia from the intestines. Congenital portosystemic shunts can be surgically ligated.

Nursing care

- Monitor vital signs.
- Feed a restricted protein diet.
- Administer medication as per the veterinary surgeon's instructions.
- **Barrier nurse if an infectious disease is suspected**.

Diseases of the pancreas

Pancreatitis

Pancreatitis is defined as inflammation of the pancreas and is caused by self-digestion of the pancreas by digestive enzymes. It may be acute or chronic. Clinical signs include depression, vomiting, severe abdominal pain. Collapse and shock may occur in severe cases. Pancreatitis is a serious condition that can be fatal.

Diagnostic tests available:

- Blood tests for haematology, biochemistry, amylase and lipase.
- Abdominal radiography.
- Abdominal ultrasound.

Treatment involves withholding food and water for at least 72 hours, until clinical signs have resolved, then gradual reintroduction of water and food. Intravenous fluid

---

Table 17.18 Procedure for a bile acid stimulation test

(1) Take a baseline blood sample into a plain or heparinised tube
(2) Feed
(3) Take a second blood sample 2 hours later

therapy is administered to treat shock and provide fluid requirements. Analgesia is administered to control pain.

Nursing care

- Monitor vital signs.
- Ensure nothing is given per os for at least 72 hours.
- Feed other patients away from the animal, so that it cannot smell their food.
- Administer intravenous fluids as per the veterinary surgeon's instructions.
- Administer analgesia and monitor for abdominal pain.
- Once clinical signs have resolved, offer small amounts of water and monitor for vomiting, pain, etc.
- If the animal tolerates water, introduce small frequent meals of a low-fat diet.

Exocrine pancreatic sufficiency

This is failure of the pancreas to produce sufficient digestive enzymes, leading to maldigestion and malabsorption of food. Pancreatic atrophy occurs. Clinical signs include diarrhoea, steatorrhoea, ravenous appetite, coprophagia and weight loss. German Shepherd dogs are most often affected.

Diagnostic tests include:

- Blood test for haematology, biochemistry and trypsin-like immunoreactivity (TLI).
- Faecal analysis.

Treatment involves dietary management and supplementation of food with pancreatic enzymes. The animal should be fed small frequent meals of a low-fat highly digestible diet. The enzyme replacement supplement should be mixed with the food.

Nursing care

- Feed a low-fat diet.
- Feed small frequent meals.
- Mix enzyme supplement with food.
- Monitor faecal consistency, amount and colour.
- Monitor weight.
- Monitor vital signs.
- Keep animal clean, bath and groom as necessary.
- Prevent faecal scalding.

Ascites

Ascites is the accumulation of abnormal fluid within the abdominal cavity. Animals with ascites often present with abdominal enlargement. A sample of fluid should be collected by abdominocentesis (see Table 17.19) and analysed to determine the type of fluid present.

Table 17.19 Abdominocentesis

Equipment	21 gauge needle 5 or 10 ml syringe Clippers Cotton wool and skin preparation solutions
Method	(1) Restrain the animal in lateral recumbency (2) Clip mid-ventral abdomen (3) Prepare the abdominocentesis site (4) Veterinary surgeon performs abdominocentesis (5) Send fluid for cytology and culture

The fluid can be classified as transudate, modified transudate, exudate, blood or chyle. Transudates are seen with hypoproteinaemia (e.g. protein-losing enteropathy, liver disease and glomerulonephritis). Modified transudates are seen with heart disease, neoplasia and venous obstructions. Exudates occur with urinary tract rupture, pancreatitis, feline infectious peritonitis and bacterial infection (e.g. intestinal perforation and abscesses). Haemorrhage occurs with trauma (e.g. ruptured spleen), neoplasia (e.g. haemangiosarcomas) and clotting disorders (e.g. warfarin poisoning, von Willebrand's disease and thrombocytopenia). Chyle is seen with lymphatic rupture due to neoplasia or trauma.

Renal disease

The kidneys regulate the composition of body fluids, restrict water loss and excrete nitrogenous waste products. They are responsible for the production of renin and erythropoetin and for vitamin D activation. Renal disease results in failure of these mechanisms. Renal failure may occur suddenly (acute) or gradually over a period of time (chronic).

Acute renal failure

Animals with acute renal failure have a sudden onset of clinical signs. Clinical signs include depression, vomiting, anorexia and polydipsia. Affected animals are usually anuric or oliguric, but can be polyuric.

Causes of acute renal failure include hypovolaemia (e.g. dehydration, haemorrhage), heart failure, toxins (e.g. ethylene glycol poisoning), infectious agents (e.g. leptospirosis) and obstruction to or rupture of the urinary tract.

Diagnostic tests available include:

- Blood tests for haematology and biochemistry.
- Urine sample for specific gravity, dipstick and sediment examination.
- Abdominal radiography.
- Abdominal ultrasound.

Treatment of acute renal failure involves supportive care and identification and correction of the underlying cause. Fluid therapy should be administered to correct dehydration and improve urine output. If oliguria persists, diuretics such as frusemide, dopamine and mannitol may be administered to improve urine production. Persistent vomiting may be controlled by administration of antiemetics. Antibiotics are used to treat leptospirosis or other infections. Peritoneal dialysis is used to remove nitrogenous waste products from the bloodstream, when administration of treatment fails to restore urine production.

Nursing care

- Administer fluid therapy.
- Monitor hydration status.
- Monitor and record bodyweight.
- Monitor vital signs.
- Monitor urine output (normal urine output = 1–2 ml/kg/ hour).
- Administer drugs as per the veterinary surgeon's instructions.
- Feed a low-protein, low-phosphorus diet.
- Encourage animal to eat.
- Monitor and record vomiting.
- Keep animal clean, groom and bath as necessary.
- Barrier nurse if an infectious cause is suspected.

Chronic renal failure

Chronic renal failure causes clinical signs such as polydipsia, polyuria, inappetence, weight loss, halitosis, vomiting and depression. Animals with chronic renal failure often have oral ulceration, poor coat condition, pale mucous membranes and uraemic breath. Affected animals may be hypothermic and hypertensive.

There are many causes of chronic renal failure including chronic interstitial nephritis, glomerulonephritis, pylonephritis, hydronephrosis, hypercalcaemia, leptospirosis, polycystic kidney disease and renal neoplasia.

Diagnostic tests available include:

- Blood tests for haematology and biochemistry.
- Urine sample for specific gravity, dipstick, sediment and culture.
- Abdominal radiography.
- Abdominal ultrasound.
- Renal biopsy.

Treatment of chronic renal failure involves supportive care and identification and correction of the underlying cause. Drugs used to treat patients with renal failure include antiemetics to control vomiting, antihypertensives to reduce blood pressure and antibiotics to treat leptospirosis or other infections.

Dietary management involves feeding a diet that is low in protein and phosphorus and high in B vitamins. The protein must be of high biological value (see Chapter 9 on nutrition). Water must be freely available at all times.

Nursing care

- Monitor vital signs.
- Provide water ad lib.
- Take outside frequently.
- Monitor and record any vomiting.
- Monitor hydration status.
- Administer fluid therapy to correct dehydration.
- Feed a low-protein, low-phosphorus diet.
- Encourage to eat if inappetent.
- Keep animal clean, groom and bath as necessary.

Nephrotic syndrome

Nephrotic syndrome is classified as end-stage kidney disease. Hypoalbuminaemia and proteinuria occur, leading to formation of oedema and ascites. Supportive care should be given. Plasma expanders or transfusions may be required.

Lower urinary tract disease

The lower urinary tract is made up of the ureters, bladder and urethra. Lower urinary tract disease is due to inflammation, obstruction or dysfunction of one or more of these organs.

Diagnostic tests available include:

- Blood tests for haematology and biochemistry.
- Urine sample for specific gravity, dipstick, sediment.
- Urine sample for culture and sensitivity (must be collected by cystocentesis).
- Abdominal ultrasound.
- Abdominal radiography.
- Intravenous excretory urography (IVU).
- Retrograde urethrogram.

Cystitis

Cystitis is defined as inflammation of the urinary bladder. Clinical signs are pollakiuria, tenesmus, haematuria and incontinence. A urine sample should be collected by cystocentesis and sent for urine specific gravity, dipstick, sediment and culture and sensitivity. Causes of cystitis include neoplasia, urolithiasis and bacterial infection. The bacteria responsible for urinary tract infections include *E. coli*, *Staphylococcus* spp., *Klebsiella* spp., *Proteus* spp., *Streptococcus* spp. and *Pseudomonas* spp. Treatment involves administration of a suitable antibiotic (dependent on the sensitivity results).

Nursing care

- Monitor vital signs.

- Ensure water is freely available and encourage animal to drink.
- Take outside frequently.
- Monitor urination (note volume, frequency, if straining or haematuria).
- Administer medications as per veterinary surgeon's instructions.

Canine urolithiasis

Urolithiasis is a condition where stones known as uroliths or calculi form within the urinary tract. These stones cause irritation and can get lodged in the kidney, ureter, bladder or urethra. Clinical signs of urolithiasis vary but may include pollakiuria, straining, haematuria, pain or urination, distended bladder, depression, anorexia, polydipsia and polyuria. Predisposing factors include urinary tract infection, high dietary intake of certain minerals, systemic disease (e.g. liver disease) and genetic disorders (e.g. urate calculi in Dalmatians).

Diet plays a major role in the control and management of some types of urinary calculi (i.e. struvite, urate or cystine). Specially formulated diets are used to change environmental conditions such as urine pH and mineral content, aiding dissolution of calculi and preventing their recurrence. Acidifying diets are used in the treatment of struvite and alkalinising diets in the treatment of urate or cystine calculi.

Where dissolution is not possible, calculi such as calcium oxalate, calcium phosphate or silica may be removed by cystotomy or urethrotomy (depending on the site of obstruction).

Nursing care

- Monitor vital signs.
- Ensure water is freely available and encourage animal to drink.
- Take outside frequently.
- Monitor urination (note volume, frequency, if straining or haematuria).
- Administer medications as per veterinary surgeon's instructions.

Feline lower urinary tract disease (FLUTD)

Feline lower urinary tract disease causes inflammation of the urinary bladder and urethra, producing clinical signs such as restlessness, stranguria, pollakiuria and haematuria. Young inactive cats that are obese and fed a dry diet are more at risk of developing the condition. It affects both male and female cats. FLUTD may be obstructive or non-obstructive. Cystic calculi may be present.

Cats with non-obstructive disease are able to urinate. The clinical signs are attributed to inflammation and the urinary bladder is thickened and empty on palpation. All female cats and some male cats fall into the category.

Obstructive disease is seen in male cats when the urethra becomes blocked by calculi or clumps of crystals and mucus (urethral plugs). The obstruction usually occurs at the tip of the penis where the urethra is narrowest. Affected cats will become distressed, frequently strain to urinate and constantly lick their genitalia. The bladder will become distended causing abdominal discomfort and renal failure will start to develop.

Urethral obstruction is a serious condition that requires urgent medical treatment if the animal's life is to be saved. Blood tests should be performed to assess metabolic status (particularly urea, creatinine and potassium levels). Intravenous fluids should be administered to correct dehydration and support renal function; a non-potassium-containing fluid such as 0.9% sodium chloride should be used. Cystocentesis should be performed to empty the bladder and a sample sent for analysis and culture. Once stable, the cat should be anaesthetised and retrograde urethral flushing performed to dislodge calculi. An indwelling Jackson cat catheter should then be placed. A buster collar should be used to prevent patient interference. The catheter should either be capped and the bladder drained every 4 hours or a urine collection system should be attached.

Dietary management of FLUTD involves feeding a diet that is low in magnesium, protein and ash. It should also have a relatively high sodium content and contain a urinary acidifier.

Nursing care

- Monitor vital signs.
- Monitor urine output.
- Feed an appropriate diet.
- Tempt to eat.
- Keep clean and dry, bath as necessary.
- Apply a barrier cream to prevent urine scald.
- Groom regularly.
- Care of indwelling urinary catheter (use an aseptic technique and prevent patient interference).
- Administer medications as per the veterinary surgeon's instructions.
- Administer fluid therapy as per the veterinary surgeon's instructions.

Incontinence

Incontinence is described as the involuntary passage of urine. Leakage of urine may be continuous or intermittent and may occur when the animal is recumbent or standing. Causes of incontinence include ectopic ureters, urethral sphincter mechanism incompetence, neurological disease, prostatic disease and neoplasia. Treatment is specific to the underlying cause, e.g. ureteral reimplantation with ectopic ureters, drugs to increase urethral tone or colposuspension surgery with urethral sphincter mechanism incompetence and castration with prostatic disease.

Nursing care

- Monitor vital signs.
- Monitor and record urinations.
- Keep clean and dry; bath and groom as necessary.
- Apply a barrier cream to prevent urine scald.
- Provide suitable bedding such as vet beds that allow drainage of urine away from the patient.

Endocrine disease

Endocrine glands secrete hormones into the circulation, where they are transported to the target organ. There are many types of hormones, each of which has a regulatory effect on metabolic processes. Endocrine disease is caused by dysfunction of one or more of these glands leading to under or over production of hormones. Diseases of the pituitary gland, thyroid gland, parathyroid gland, adrenal gland and endocrine pancreas will be discussed here (see Table 17.20).

Diabetes mellitus

Diabetes mellitus is caused by insufficient production of insulin by the pancreas, leading to hyperglycaemia. Predisposing factors include obesity and endocrine disease such as Cushing's disease or hypothyroidism. Clinical signs include polyuria, polydipsia, increased appetite, weight loss, lethargy and cataracts.

Diagnostic tests include:

- Blood tests for haematology and biochemistry.
- Urine sample for specific gravity, dipstick, sediment and culture.

Treatment involves administration of insulin by subcutaneous injection. There are various types of insulin available. Neutral insulin is short acting and has rapid onset of action. It can be used to stabilise ketoacidotic diabetics. Lente insulin has an intermediate duration of action and protamine zinc insulin (PZI) has a long duration of action. These can be used in long-term stabilisation of diabetics.

Insulin should be stored in a refrigerator. Opened bottles must be dated and discarded after 30 days. Insulin should be mixed gently before use. The correct size of insulin syringe must be used: most insulin preparations contain 100 IU/ml, but it should be noted that Caninsulin (Intervet) contains 40 IU/ml.

Initial stabilisation of a canine diabetic patient involves once- or twice-daily administration of an intermediate-acting insulin. A long-acting insulin may be preferable in cats. The patient should be fed twice daily, at the time of the insulin injection and again 6–8 hours later, coinciding with peak insulin activity. If the patient is receiving twice-daily insulin therapy, the two meals should be provided 12 hours apart, at the time of insulin administration. The patient should be fed a high-fibre diet, which has a low carbohydrate content and is consistent in composition. The type, amount and time of feeding should be the same each day, as should exercise.

It is important that owners monitor their pet's water and food intake as these are reliable indicators of how well the disease is controlled. Some treatment protocols also advocate home monitoring of the patient by measurement of urine glucose concentrations. This can be done shortly before administration of the morning insulin. The principle is that the dose of insulin should be increased in a stepwise fashion if there is persistent glucosuria. However, this method of monitoring can be misleading and lead to owners overdosing their pets with insulin without adequate veterinary guidance. If insulin is overdosed, hypoglycaemia occurs and the body responds by releasing hormones, such as cortisol, to increase blood glucose levels. This causes a rebound hyperglycaemia, known as Somogyi overswing. The hyperglycaemia and glucosuria associated with Somogyi overswing is detected in the morning urine test and may be misinterpreted as a need for an even higher insulin dose.

In unstable diabetics a serial blood glucose curve (blood glucose levels are measured every 2 hours over a 24-hour period) should be performed. This will identify problems such as insulin resistance, Somogyi overswing or insufficient duration of action of the insulin. Adjustment to the management regime can then be made, e.g. by reducing the insulin dose, administering twice-daily insulin or switching to a longer-acting insulin. If twice-daily insulin doses are given, the patient should be fed at the time of each injection.

Table 17.20		
Endocrine gland	**Hormone**	**Function**
Anterior pituitary	Thyroid stimulating hormone (TSH)	Stimulates thyroid gland to produce thyroxine
	Adrenocorticotropic hormone (ACTH)	Stimulates adrenal cortex to produce steroids
Posterior pituitary	Antidiuretic hormone (ADH)	Stimulates reabsorption of water by the kidneys
Thyroid	Thyroxine	Controls metabolic rate
Parathyroid	Parathormone (PTH)	Increases blood calcium levels
Adrenal cortex	Corticosteroids	Increases blood glucose levels
	Mineralocorticoids	Increasing sodium reabsorption in the kidneys
Pancreas	Insulin	Regulates blood sugar levels

If the patient does not eat its food, a half dose of the insulin should be given and the cause investigated. Patients undergoing anaesthesia should also be given a half dose of insulin (without food). They should be placed on a dextrose saline infusion and blood glucose levels should be monitored.

Insulin resistance is due to antagonism of insulin and may occur in pregnant or obese animals, or when other diseases such as Cushing's disease, hyperthyroidism, hypothyroidism, pancreatitis and bacterial infections occur concurrently with diabetes. The underlying cause should be identified and treated, and the insulin dose adjusted accordingly. Diabetic bitches should also be spayed because of insulin resistance during seasons.

Nursing care

- Assist veterinary surgeon with diagnostic test.
- Administer insulin as directed by the veterinary surgeon.
- Feed an appropriate diet at the times requested.
- Ensure water is freely available.
- Take outside frequently.
- Monitor blood glucose levels.
- Monitor urine for glucose and ketones.
- Monitor vital signs.
- Monitor clinical signs.
- Administer fluid therapy as directed by the veterinary surgeon.
- Administer medications as directed by the veterinary surgeon.

Complications associated with diabetes mellitus include hypoglycaemia, ketoacidosis, cataracts and bacterial infections (e.g. conjunctivitis and urinary tract infection).

Hypoglycaemia produces clinical signs such as restlessness, ataxia, muscle twitching and seizures. It is most likely to occur at the time of peak activity of the insulin, i.e. mid-afternoon if a once-daily dosing regime is used. Immediate action must be taken; this may involve feeding, rubbing sweet foods such as honey onto the gums or administration of intravenous dextrose. If left untreated, coma and death will result.

In addition to carbohydrate metabolism, insulin is also important for protein and fat metabolism. In cases where diabetes goes undiagnosed, or in unstable patients, excessive breakdown of fat occurs leading to a build-up of ketones. This leads to a condition known as diabetic ketoacidosis. Clinical signs include anorexia, dehydration, vomiting, depression and collapse. Affected animals are hyperglycaemic and have glucose and ketones in their urine. This is a serious condition that requires immediate action. Treatment involves fluid therapy with potassium supplementation to correct dehydration, acidosis and electrolyte imbalance and administration of soluble insulin to stabilise blood glucose levels. Blood glucose levels should be monitored hourly and glucose supplementation administered as necessary. Close monitoring of vital signs, serum potassium and phosphate levels and acid–base status is essential. Once stable, the patient may be switched to intermediate- or long-acting insulin.

Nursing care for a ketoacidotic diabetic

- Monitor vital signs.
- Monitor blood glucose levels hourly.
- Administer insulin injections as directed by the veterinary surgeon.
- Administer intravenous fluids as directed by the veterinary surgeon.
- Supplement intravenous fluids with potassium as directed by the veterinary surgeon.
- Administer intravenous dextrose as directed by the veterinary surgeon.
- Monitor the animal's response to treatment.

Hyperadrenocorticism (Cushing's disease)

Hyperadrenocorticism may be caused by excessive administration of steroids (iatrogenic), or overproduction of steroids by the adrenal cortex. The latter may be due to pituitary or adrenal neoplasia. Clinical signs include polydipsia, polyuria, polyphagia, abdominal distension, muscle atrophy and weakness, lethargy, skin changes and alopecia.

Diagnostic tests include:

- Blood tests for haematology and biochemistry.
- ACTH stimulation test.
- Low-dose dexamethasone screening test (LDDST).
- High-dose dexamethasone suppression test (HDDST).
- Endogenous ACTH assay.
- Abdominal ultrasound.
- Abdominal radiography.

Cushing's disease may be confirmed with an ACTH stimulation test and/or a LDDST. The HDDST and endogenous ACTH assay are used to determine whether the disease is adrenal or pituitary dependent. (See Table 17.21 for test protocols.)

Pituitary-dependent hyperadrenocorticism is the most common form of Cushing's disease (80% cases) and is due to a pituitary tumour – most are small and benign – overproducing ACTH. The negative feedback system fails and the pituitary continues producing ACTH despite the high cortisol levels. Adrenal-dependent hyperadrenocorticism is less common and is due to excessive production of steroids by the adrenal gland. Pituitary-dependent hyperadrenocorticism is normally treated medically with drugs such as mitotane or trilostane. Adrenal tumours may be surgically removed.

Nursing care

- Monitor vital signs.
- Assist veterinary surgeon with diagnostic tests.

Table 17.21 Lab test protocols	
ACTH stimulation test	(1) Take a baseline blood sample (plain/ heparinised tube) (2) Inject ACTH (Synacthen) intravenously (If < 15 kg give 0.5 ml and if > 15 kg give 1 ml) (3) Take a second blood sample after 30–60 minutes (plain/heparinised tube) (4) Label the tubes with the case details and the time that the samples were taken (5) Send for cortisol levels
LDDST	(1) Keep the patient quiet and do not perform any other investigation during the test (2) Take a baseline blood sample (plain/ heparinised tube) (3) Inject 0.01 mg/kg of dexamethasone intravenously (4) Take a second blood sample after 3 hours (plain/heparinised tube) (5) Take a third blood sample after 8 hours (plain/heparinised tube) (6) Label the tubes with the case details and the time that the samples were taken (7) Send for cortisol levels
HDDST	(1) Keep the patient quiet and do not perform any other investigations during the test (2) Take a baseline blood sample (plain/ heparinised tube) (3) Inject 0.1 mg/kg of dexamethasone intravenously (4) Take a second blood sample after 3 hours (plain/heparinised tube) (5) Take a third blood sample after 8 hours (plain/heparinised tube) (6) Label the tubes with the case details and the time that the samples were taken (7) Send for cortisol levels
Endogenous ACTH assay	(1) Take a blood sample into a chilled EDTA tube (2) Centrifuge immediately (3) Draw off plasma and freeze (4) Send the frozen sample to the laboratory for endogenous ACTH levels

- Ensure water is freely available.
- Take outside frequently.
- Administer medication following the veterinary surgeon's instructions.
- Monitor clinical signs.

Hypoadrenocorticism (Addison's disease)

Addison's disease is a reduction or failure of steroid secretion by the adrenal glands causing fluid and electrolyte imbalances, including hyponatraemia, hyperkalaemia and dehydration. Clinical signs include anorexia, lethargy, weakness, vomiting, diarrhoea, polydipsia, polyuria, hypotension, bradycardia and collapse. Causes include atrophy of the adrenal cortex, neoplasia and certain drugs (e.g. mitotane therapy or long-term steroid administration).

Diagnostic tests include:

- Blood tests for haematology and biochemistry.
- Sodium : potassium ratio.
- ACTH stimulation test.

Addison's disease may be chronic or acute. Treatment of both forms of the disease involves administration of glucocorticoids and mineralocorticoids. Chronic cases may have vague clinical signs making diagnosis difficult. Acute conditions (**Addisonian crisis**) are life threatening. Affected patients are hypovolaemic, collapsed and have severe bradycardia. Addisonian crises require urgent medical treatment including intravenous corticosteroids and aggressive fluid therapy with a non-potassium containing fluid.

Nursing care

- Monitor vital signs.
- Assist veterinary surgeon with diagnostic tests.
- Administer medication following the veterinary surgeon's instructions.
- Administer fluid therapy following the veterinary surgeon's instructions.
- Ensure water is freely available.
- Take outside frequently.
- Monitor clinical signs.

Hyperthyroidism

Patients with hyperthyroidism have an overactive thyroid gland leading to excess production of thyroxine. Clinical signs are associated with a high metabolic rate and include hyperactivity, tachycardia, weight loss, polyphagia, polydipsia, polyuria, diarrhoea and vomiting. Hyperthyroidism is common in older cats, but rare in dogs.

Diagnostic tests include:

- Blood tests for haematology and biochemistry.
- Total T4 levels.

Treatment involves administration of carbimazole, thyroidectomy or radioactive iodine treatment.

Nursing care

- Monitor vital signs.
- Assist veterinary surgeon with diagnostic tests.
- Ensure water is freely available.
- Feed an appropriate diet.
- Keep clean, bath and groom as necessary.
- Clean kennel as necessary.

- Administer medication following the veterinary surgeon's instructions.
- Post op nursing following thyroidectomy (see Chapter 19).
- Follow protocol for radioactive iodine treatment (only performed at specialist centres).
- Monitor clinical signs.

Hypothyroidism

Patients with hypothyroidism have an underactive thyroid gland, leading to reduced thyroxine production. Clinical signs are associated with a low metabolic rate and include obesity, lethargy, weakness, bradycardia and dermatological changes such as alopecia, seborrhoea and hyperpigmentation. Hypothyroidism is most common in middle-aged dogs and rare in cats.

Diagnostic tests:

- Blood tests for haematology and biochemistry.
- Thyroxine levels (total or free T4).
- Endogenous TSH assay.

Treatment involves daily oral administration of thyroxine.

Nursing care

- Monitor vital signs.
- Assist veterinary surgeon with diagnostic tests.
- Administer medications following the veterinary surgeon's instructions.
- Feed an appropriate diet.
- Monitor clinical signs.

Diabetes insipidus

Diabetes insipidus is caused by a failure of the kidneys to reabsorb water. There are two forms of diabetes insipidus: central and nephrogenic. Central diabetes insipidus is caused by a deficiency of ADH (antidiuretic hormone) and nephrogenic diabetes insipidus is due to a failure of the renal collecting ducts to respond to ADH. The principal clinical signs are polydipsia and polyuria, with affected animals passing large volumes of very dilute urine (SG < 1.008).

Diagnostic tests include:

- Blood tests for haematology and biochemistry.
- Urine specific gravity, dipstick and sediment.
- Water deprivation test (see Table 17.22).
- ADH response test (used if patient fails to respond normally to water deprivation test; see Table 17.22).

Intranasal DDAVP is used to treat central diabetes insipidus and thiazide diuretics may be used to treat the nephrogenic form.

Table 17.22 Water deprivation and ADH response tests	
Water deprivation test	(1) Catheterise and empty bladder. Measure urine specific gravity (2) Withhold all food and water (3) Every hour: empty bladder, measure urine specific gravity and weigh patient (4) Stop when urine SG reaches 1.030 or when the patient has lost 5% of its body weight
ADH response test	(1) Continue to withhold all food and water (2) Administer desmopressin (DDAVP – a synthetic ADH) (3) Empty bladder and measure the urine specific gravity every hour for four hours

N.B. Following these tests water must be reintroduced gradually; otherwise water toxicity may occur

Nursing care

- Monitor vital signs.
- Assist veterinary surgeon with diagnostic tests.
- Administer medication as per the veterinary surgeon's instructions.
- Ensure water is freely available (except during water deprivation or ADH response tests).
- Take outside frequently.

Hyperparathyroidism

Hyperparathyroidism is due to excessive parathyroid hormone secretion. Causes include neoplasia of the parathyroid gland (primary hyperparathyroidism), renal disease (renal secondary hyperparathyroidism) and nutritional deficiencies (nutritional secondary hyperparathyroidism).

Diagnostic tests include:

- Blood tests for haematology and biochemistry.
- PTH assay.
- Radiography.

Primary hyperparathyroidism

Primary hyperparathyroidism leads to hypercalcaemia. Clinical signs include polydipsia, polyuria, inappetence, lethargy and weakness. Parathyroid tumours may be surgically removed.

Nursing care

- Monitor vital signs.
- Assist veterinary surgeon with diagnostic tests.
- Monitor ionised calcium levels.
- Ensure water is freely available.
- Take outside regularly.

- Encourage patient to eat.
- Administer fluid therapy (use 0.9% sodium chloride).
- Post-operative care (see surgical nursing chapter).
- Administer medications as per the veterinary surgeon's instructions.

Secondary hyperparathyroidism

Secondary renal hyperparathyroidism may be seen in patients with severe chronic renal failure. Excessive calcium resorption from bone occurs, leading to renal osteodystrophy. Clinical signs include rubber jaw, skeletal pain and pathological fractures. Treatment is aimed at reducing phosphate levels by using phosphate binders and feeding a low-phosphorous diet.

Nutritional secondary hyperparathyroidism is caused by continuously feeding diets that contain excessive phosphate and insufficient calcium (e.g. red meat or offal) to young growing animals. This leads to reabsorption of calcium from bone, causing lameness, reluctance to move, skeletal pain, limb deformity and pathological fractures. Treatment involves feeding a balanced diet.

Nursing care

- Monitor vital signs.
- Assist veterinary surgeon with diagnostic tests.
- Feed an appropriate diet.
- Administer medications following the veterinary surgeon's instructions.
- Gentle handling of patient.
- Cage rest.
- Administer analgesia as required.

Diseases of the nervous system

Seizures

Seizures may be partial, affecting only part of the body, or generalised, affecting the entire body. During partial seizures the animal remains conscious and shows clinical signs such as vocalisation, jaw champing, disorientation, circling, twitching of facial muscles and localised muscle rigidity. The clinical signs associated with generalised seizures include convulsions, jaw champing, hypersalivation, vocalisation, loss of consciousness and involuntary urination and defecation. Seizures may be single, multiple (cluster seizures) or continuous (status epilepticus).

The owner of a seizuring animal may ring the veterinary surgery in a distressed state. The veterinary nurse should calm the owner and give first aid advice. The owner should be told to darken the room, remove any objects that may injure the pet and provide a quiet environment (e.g. turn off the radio/TV and remove other animals or people from the room). They should be told not to touch or restrain the seizuring animal, as it could result in injury to themselves or their pet. They should observe from a distance and once the seizure has finished bring the animal to the surgery.

Causes of seizures include epilepsy, hydrocephalus, head trauma, neoplasia, hypoxia, inflammation, bacterial/viral infections (e.g. canine distemper virus), toxins (e.g. lead poisoning) and metabolic disturbances (e.g. hypoglycaemia, hypocalcaemia, hepatic encephalopathy and uraemia).

Diagnostic tests available include:

- Blood tests for haematology and biochemistry.
- Cerebral spinal fluid (CSF) tap.
- Electroencephalography (EEG).
- Magnetic resonance imaging (MRI scan).
- Computed tomography (CT scan).

The underlying cause of the seizures should be identified so that, where possible, specific therapy can be administered. When seizures are prolonged (i.e. over 1 minute) or cluster seizures occur, anticonvulsant drug therapy is indicated. Seizures may be controlled by administration of diazepam. Diazepam is usually given intravenously but can be given per rectum if intravenous access is not possible. Repeat boluses can be given (up to a maximum of three doses) but if this fails to control the seizures, a diazepam infusion, intravenous phenobarbitone or pentobarbitone should be considered. Phenobarbitone is the most important drug in long-term management of epilepsy. Potassium bromide can be used in conjunction with phenobarbitone if the seizures are refractory.

Nursing care

- Observe and record seizures.
- Dim lights or put a towel over the front of the kennel.
- Pad the kennel with foam or bedding.
- Keep the room quiet by restricting access to personnel, talking quietly and moving barking dogs elsewhere.
- Place an intravenous catheter and keep it patent by flushing every 4 hours with heparinised saline.
- Administer medication as per the veterinary surgeon's instructions.
- Administer fluid therapy as per the veterinary surgeon's instructions.
- Keep airway clear.
- Administer oxygen as necessary.
- Monitor vital signs.
- Cool the patient if hyperthermic.

Unconsciousness

Unconsciousness is defined as a lack of awareness and lack of response to sensory stimuli. Brief loss of consciousness is called syncope. Coma is a state of deep, prolonged unconsciousness. Causes include metabolic disorders, toxins, seizures, airway obstruction, shock, head trauma and barbiturate overdose.

Nursing care

- Keep airway patent, remove airway foreign bodies and suction secretions.
- Intubate and administer oxygen.
- If patient is not breathing, perform IPPV at 10–20 breaths per minute.
- If no heart beat is detected, start cardiac massage at 60–120 beats per minute.
- Monitor vital signs.
- Administer fluid therapy following the veterinary surgeon's instructions.
- Administer drugs following the veterinary surgeon's instructions.
- Turn every 4 hours.
- Check bladder and express as necessary.
- Keep clean and dry, bed bath as necessary.

Spinal injuries

Compression of the spinal cord leads to clinical signs such as pain, ataxia, weakness and paralysis. Causes include intervertebral disc disease, wobbler syndrome, cauda equina syndrome, discospondylitis, spinal fractures or luxations, fibrocartilagenous embolism and neoplasia.

Sudden onset of paralysis should be treated as an emergency. The owner should be asked to bring the animal to the surgery. The patient's spine should be kept straight – this can be achieved by transporting the animal on a board.

The neurological assessment consists of:

- Localisation of pain.
- Examination of gait.
- Detection of proprioceptive deficits.
- Detection of muscle atrophy.
- Assessment of muscle atrophy.
- Assessment of muscle tone.
- Assessment of limb, anal and panniculus reflexes.
- Assessment of deep pain.
- Assessment of bladder function.

Diagnostic tests available include:

- Radiography.
- Myelography.
- MRI scan.
- CSF analysis.

Conservative management may be used in patients that do not require surgery, or if other considerations, such as financial constraints, preclude surgery.

Nursing care

- Cage rest.
- Provide soft bedding.
- Monitor urination and empty bladder if unable to urinate voluntarily.
- If recumbent, turn every 4 hours or support in sternal.

- Monitor vital signs.
- Perform physiotherapy.
- Keep clean, bath immediately if coat becomes soiled with urine or faeces.
- Monitor for pain and administer analgesia as necessary.
- Administer medications as per the veterinary surgeon's instructions.
- Monitor progress.

Complications that may affect recumbent spinal patients include pressure sores, urine scalding, faecal scalding, hypostatic pneumonia and urinary tract infections. See Chapter 16 on general nursing for information on how to prevent and treat these complications.

Diseases of the musculoskeletal system

The musculoskeletal system involves bone, joints and muscle.

Bone disease

Nutritional secondary hyperparathyroidism

See section on endocrine disease.

Rickets

This disease is seen in young growing animals that are fed a diet deficient in vitamin D. The affected animal is unable to absorb calcium from the intestines, leading to reduced bone mineralisation around the growth plates. Clinical signs include lameness, bowing of limbs and swollen joints. Radiographic examination shows enlargement of growth plates. Treatment involves feeding an appropriate diet for a young growing dog.

Nursing care

- Feed a balanced diet suitable for a growing puppy.
- Administer analgesics as necessary.
- Provide soft comfortable bedding.

Metaphyseal osteopathy

Metaphyseal osteopathy occurs in young growing dogs, particularly giant breeds. It is associated with abnormal metaphyseal bone formation, usually affecting long bones of the distal limbs. Clinical signs include swelling, pain, lameness, pyrexia, depression and anorexia. The cause of metaphyseal osteopathy is unknown. Treatment consists of pain relief and feeding an appropriate diet for a young growing dog.

Nursing care

- Feed a balanced diet suitable for a growing puppy.
- Administer analgesics as necessary.
- Provide soft comfortable bedding.

Hypertrophic osteodystrophy (Marie's disease, pulmonary osteopathy)

Hypertrophic osteodystrophy may occur secondary to thoracic or abdominal space-occupying lesions disease, such as tumours or abscesses. It leads to abnormal bone formation around the metaphysics of long bones. Clinical signs include pain, lameness and symmetrical swelling of the distal limbs.

Nursing care

- Monitor vital signs.
- Provide soft, comfortable bedding.
- Administer analgesics as necessary.
- Administer medications as per the veterinary surgeon's instructions.

Osteomyelitis

Osteomyelitis is inflammation, most commonly due to infection, of bone. Clinical signs include pain, swelling, pyrexia, depression and inappetence. A draining sinus tract may develop. Causes include bacterial or fungal infection (the latter is uncommon in the UK) and corrosion of surgical implants. Radiography reveals destruction of existing bone and new bone formation. Treatment includes administration of antibiotics (based on culture and sensitivity results), antifungals and removal of surgical implants or necrotic bone fragments (sequestra) that may be associated with the osteomyelitis.

Nursing care

- Monitor vital signs.
- Provide soft, comfortable bedding.
- Administer analgesia as necessary.
- Administer antibiotics as per the veterinary surgeon's instructions.
- Provide post-operative care.

Bone tumours

Bone tumours may be benign or malignant. Benign bone tumours include osteoma and chondroma. Malignant bone tumours include osteosarcoma, chondrosarcoma, fibrosarcoma, and haemangiosarcoma.

Primary osteosarcomas and haemangiosarcomas usually affect the long bones of the limbs causing pain, bone swelling and lameness. They frequently metastasise to the lungs and other organs. Chrondrosarcomas affect bones such as ribs and the nasal cavity and rarely metastasise. Fibrosarcomas usually affect the bones of the axial skeleton, including the skull and mandible.

Radiographic evaluation reveals bone destruction and new bone formation. A bone biopsy should be taken to differentiate the lesion from infection and determine the type of bone tumour. Thoracic and abdominal radiographs should be taken to check for metastasis. Surgical options include excision, amputation or limb salvage. The best results are achieved by combining surgery with chemotherapy.

Nursing care

- Monitor vital signs.
- Provide soft, comfortable bedding.
- Provide analgesia as necessary.
- Provide adequate nutrition.
- Provide post-operative care.
- Assist veterinary surgeon with administration of cytotoxic drugs.
- Administer medications as per the veterinary surgeon's instructions.

Joint disease

Arthritis

Arthritis is defined as inflammation of a joint. Polyarthritis is the inflammation of several joints. Causes include infectious agents and immune-mediated disease such as rheumatoid arthritis, systemic lupus erythematosus (SLE) and idiopathic polyarthritis.

Diagnostic tests available include:

- Blood tests for haematology, biochemistry, rheumatoid factor and antinuclear antibodies.
- Radiography.
- Joint tap (arthrocentesis) for cytology and culture.

Bacterial infectious arthritis (suppurative arthritis) causes acute lameness, normally of one joint, but sometimes of multiple joints in young animals. Clinical signs include heat, pain and swelling of the affected joint. A joint tap should be performed and a sample of synovial fluid sent for culture and sensitivity. Treatment involves administration of antibiotics and non-steroidal anti-inflammatory drugs.

Immune-mediated arthritis often affects multiple joints – this is termed polyarthritis. Polyarthritis may be of specific immune-mediated diseases (e.g. rheumatoid arthritis, SLE), may be secondary to other disease processes such as neoplasia or inflammatory bowel disease or may be a primary idiopathic process. Dogs with polyarthritis often present with shifting limb lameness, reluctance to move, pyrexia, inappetence and lethargy.

Diagnostic tests are aimed at characterising the arthritis (joint taps, radiographs) and identifying underlying causes – for example by measuring rheumatoid factor and antinuclear antibody and looking for concurrent diseases.

Many animals with polyarthritis will require lifelong immunosuppressive therapy with corticosteroids and sometimes other adjunctive treatments.

Nursing care

- Monitor vital signs.
- Provide soft, comfortable bedding.
- Encourage frequent walks of short duration.
- Diet if obese.
- Administer medications as per the veterinary surgeon's instructions.

Osteoarthritis (degenerative joint disease)

Osteoarthritis is a non-inflammatory process causing deterioration of articular cartilage and increased formation of new bone at joint surfaces. It usually occurs as a chronic sequel to previous joint damage. Causes include trauma (e.g. ruptured cruciate ligament), developmental disorders (e.g. hip dysplasia) and inflammatory arthritis. Clinical signs include pain, lameness and stiffness after rest. The clinical signs in many patients can be controlled with conservative measures alone – especially weight reduction and sensible exercise regimes. Exercise should be adjusted to a level that does not cause pain or discomfort – short, frequent exercise periods are normally advised. Anti-inflammatory drugs may be administered if these measures are ineffective. Non-steroidal drugs such as carprofen and meloxicam that are suitable for long-term use are most appropriate.

Nursing care

- Monitor vital signs.
- Diet if obese.
- Provide soft, comfortable bedding.
- Administer medications as per the veterinary surgeon's instructions.
- Take for frequent short walks.
- Monitor clinical signs.

Hypervitaminosis A

An excessive intake of vitamin A over a prolonged period of time may lead to hypervitaminosis A. It is most common in cats and is usually caused by feeding large quantities of liver or over supplementation of cod liver oil. Excessive quantities of vitamin A lead to new bone formation, which causes ankylosis of vertebrae and joints. The neck is often particu-

larly affected. Clinical signs include pain, lameness, postural changes and reluctance to move. The animal may find it difficult to eat or groom. Treatment involves feeding a balanced diet and providing analgesia.

Nursing care

- Monitor vital signs.
- Provide analgesia.
- Feed a balanced diet.
- Assist feeding: position the bowl so that cat can reach it or hand feed.
- Groom regularly.

Muscle disease

Muscle disease may be localised, affecting only one muscle group or more generalised, affecting many groups (polymyopathy). Skeletal muscle is most commonly affected. Clinical signs include muscle weakness and loss of function. Causes of muscle disease include infectious agents (e.g. *Toxoplasma gondii, Neospora caninum*), immune-mediated disease and endocrine disorders (e.g. hypothyroidism, Cushing's disease).

Diagnostic tests include:

- Blood tests for haematology, biochemistry, creatinine kinase, *Toxoplasma, Neospora*, acetylcholine receptor antibodies and specific endocrine function tests.
- Electromyogram (EMG).
- Muscle biopsy.

Treatment will depend on the underlying disease.

Nursing care

- Monitor vital signs.
- Assist walking if required.
- Provide soft, comfortable bedding.
- Turn every 4 hours if recumbent.
- Physiotherapy.
- Assist feeding if dysphagic.
- Feed liquid food from a height if regurgitating.
- Administer medications as per the veterinary surgeon's instructions.
- Monitor progress.

Diseases of the cutaneous system

Essential terminology to be familiar with when involved with an animal suffering a skin disease includes:

- **Alopecia** – the absence of hair from areas of skin where it is normally present. This might be partial or complete, focal or generalised, patchy or diffuse, reversible or nonreversible. It may present in congenital, inherited or acquired form and may be attributed to primary disease of the hair follicle or to secondary disease.

- **Pruritis** – a sensation within the skin that provokes the desire to scratch. The animal may be seen to be persistently licking, chewing or rubbing at itself. It may demonstrate changes in character and inflict self-trauma in attempts to remove hair. The skin may be seen to be reddened and inflamed (**erythema**) with evident damage (**excoriations**) and changes such as **lichenification** and **alopecia.**
- **Seborrhoea** – excessive secretion of sebum by the sebaceous glands within the skin, giving the skin an oily appearance.
- **Pyoderma** – a **pyogenic** (pus forming, e.g. infected) condition – most occur secondary to other skin conditions.

Ectoparasitic skin disease

Of all the ectoparasites to concern our domestic pets the flea is the biggest problem. It causes the majority of pruritis cases and with the off-host component to its life cycle can be the most difficult to manage/treat appropriately. See Chapter 15 for full details.

The diagnosis of ectoparasites usually depends on history and clinical signs along with successful identification of the particular organism, either by coat brushings or skin scrapings.

Hormonal alopecia

This is usually associated with hair loss to the flanks and/or ventral abdomen and usually occurs without pruritis, self-trauma or inflammation. In advanced cases it may involve the whole trunk of the body but hair will usually remain on the head and limbs. There is a specific group of hormonal diseases that tend to cause bilateral symmetrical alopecia and these are:

- Hypothyroidism (see 'Endocrine Disease').
- Hyperadrenocorticalism (see 'Endocrine Disease').
- Sertoli cell tumour.
- Canine ovarian imbalances.
- Feline symmetrical alopecia.

Sertoli cell tumour

This is the commonest occurring testicular tumour to induce alopecia in middle- to old-aged dogs. Dogs that are cryptorchid are 13 times more likely to develop this tumour.

Clinical signs are associated with the hyperoestrogen seen with the tumour:

- Bilateral non-pruritic alopecia of perineal area, inner surfaces of the hindlimbs, ventral abdomen and flanks.
- Gynaecomastia (enlarged mammary tissue).

- Pendulous prepuce.
- Attractiveness to other male dogs.
- Internal neoplastic testicle is frequently enlarged, while the normally positioned testicle is atrophied.
- Non-regenerative anaemia in advanced cases as the oestrogen affects the bone marrow.

Diagnosis is made upon evaluation of clinical history, signs and examination. Diagnostic tests may include plasma oestrogen assay testing.

Treatment is usually castration.

Canine ovarian imbalance

Although the aetiology of this condition is not fully understood, the hormone oestrogen plays a significant role, either as an oestrogen responsive dermatosis or dermatosis induced by hyperoestrogenism.

Hyperoestrogenism, or classified type I, is usually linked to cystic ovarian disease or ovarian tumours. Clinical signs are:

- Generalised bilateral symmetrical alopecia that commences in the perineal region.
- Vulval enlargement.
- Abnormal oestrous cycles.
- Seborrhoea (secondary).

Treatment is ovariohysterectomy with owners informed of possible lag period (up to 6 months) before cessation of signs.

Oestrogen responsive dermatosis, or classified type II, is a rare condition of the bitch occurring after ovariohysterectomy. Clinical signs are:

- Perineal alopecia, spreading to inner hindlimbs and ventral abdomen.
- Juvenile vulva and nipples.
- Soft and puppy-like coat in character.

Treatment involves hormone replacement such as oestrogen or testosterone.

Feline symmetrical alopecia

This is a rare condition that is not clearly understood; it is more commonly seen in neutered cats.

The alopecia is seen around the perineal area but soon spreads to involve the inner aspects of the hindlimbs and ventral abdomen – in some cases it becomes generalised.

Clinical examination and exclusion of other possible causes from the list of differentials leads to the diagnosis.

Treatments include:

- Thyroid hormone replacement.
- Megoestral acetate therapy.
- Testosterone therapy in males and females.

Pyoderma

This is associated with an underlying disease in the dog; the most common pathogen involved in canine pyoderma is *Staphylococcus intermedius*. Secondary opportunist bacteria such as *Proteus, Pseudomonas, Corynebacterium* may also be isolated, usually in association with the *Staphylococcus*.

Normally resident bacteria are thought to be important in the skin's normal defence mechanisms.

The severity of the infection is determined by the depth of the penetration – and this is how pyodermas are classified.

Pyoderma is rare in the cat.

Surface pyodermas

Acute moist dermatiti Frequently occurs where skin becomes damaged due to self-trauma. Occurs over face, feet, hindquarters and tail. The area will be wet due to serum exudates, painful with areas of hair loss and /or hair matting.

Treatment Remove underlying cause (ear infection, anal gland engorgement), clip hair from site, cleanse area with antibacterial products such as chlorhexidine. Use of Elizabethan collar will reduce likelihood of further trauma.

Skin fold dermatitis Common around the lip fold, vulval fold or tail fold, especially in Pekinese and Sharpei: this is a conformation-related condition. This is an infection of acute moist dermatitis within these areas, often with full extent obscured by anatomy.

Treatment: Chlorhexidine washes, followed by cosmetic surgery to correct anatomy.

Superficial pyodermas

Impetigo Otherwise known as juvenile pustular dermatitis (puppy pyoderma). Seen in young puppies, especially along ventral abdomen; clinical signs include multiple pustules and yellow scab.

Treatment Antibacterial shampoos with the addition of antibiotics if extensive.

Folliculitis Formation of pustules with hair protruding, sometimes the lesions are observed in a ring-like formation, especially along ventral abdomen, with overall 'out-of-condition' look to coat. Underlying disease is the cause of this condition.

Treatment Identify and treat underlying disease, give antibiotic medication.

Deep pyodermas

Interdigital pyoderma (pododermatitis) Seen in short-haired dogs; the paws become swollen and painful and may exude pus. Areas of alopecia will be seen with ulceration and fistulas in severe cases.

Treatment Surgical drainage of infected material, treatment of underlying cause, long-term antibiotic therapy.

Furunculosis Often associated with demodicosis, ringworm, hypothyroidism or general debility. Clinical signs will include pustules, discharging pus, fistulas, alopecia and pain. Lesions often found on nose, muzzle, flanks and anal region, but can extend to any part of the body.

Treatment Correct underlying disease and give long-term antibiotic therapy (systemic).

Feline pyoderma

This is associated with cat bites; bacteria such as *Pasteurella, Staphylococcus* and *Fusiformis* spp., which are found routinely in the cat's mouth, cause cellulitis when bite wounds penetrate deep within skin. Other clinical signs are pyrexia, anorexia, depression, pain and swelling at site of bite wound.

Treatment Systemic antibiotics with drainage at site.

Ringworm

This is also known as **dermatophytosis**, ringworm can infect skin, nails or hair. In the dog and cat two organisms of the fungal disease are important: *Microsporum* spp. and *Tricphyton* spp. (see Chapter 15).

Allergic dermatitis

Urticaria

An acute allergic reaction, causes vary widely and include certain drugs, vaccines, insect bites and stings.

Clinical signs These lesions appear suddenly as multiple swellings or wheals on the skin, with the hair becoming erect. They are likely to be pruritic and may last hours or days.

Diagnosis This is based on clinical signs and historical evidence.

Treatment Remove cause and administer corticosteroids.

Atopic dermatitis

Causes vary widely and are many – amongst the most common are house dust, house dust mites, fungi and pollens.

Clinical signs In **dogs**, signs are often first seen at around 1–3 years of age and may include general pruritis but especially around face, feet, axilla and ventral abdomen. Self-inflicted trauma may lead to secondary infection, alopecia and pigmentation of the skin. Some dogs develop ocular discharge and otitis externa.

In **cats**, similar clinical signs are presented but may also show miliary eczema, symmetrical alopecia, eosinophilic granuloma complex or facial pruritis.

Diagnosis   Intradermal skin testing with multiple allergens to determine causes:

(1)   To avoid drug interactions only xylazine and atropine sulphate should be used.
(2)   Lay the animal on its side and clip full flank coat.
(3)   Using a felt-tip marker pen label the site for each allergen test area.
(4)   Inject 0.05 ml of the allergen intradermally, together with a positive control (histamine) and a negative control (sterile diluent).

After 30 minutes, examination of the testing area will reveal positive or negative results. A positive is where the wheal is greater than half the difference of the diameter of the positive and negative control sites.

Treatment   Usually a lifelong-held allergy with suitable changes to environment required, along with management of symptoms by prescribing corticosteroids, antihistamines and essential fatty acid supplementation. In some cases a topical shampoo such as colloidal oatmeal, washed onto the animal every 3 days may be indicated.

Food hypersensitivity

Causes are individual to each animal but products such as beef, horse meat, milk, eggs and fish are commonly implicated with this condition (see Chapter 9, Nutrition).

Clinical signs   Associated with pruritic skin disease and/or gastrointestinal symptoms.

Diagnosis   Attempts are made to eliminate the cause of the irritation by feeding an elimination diet – one that is very digestible (therefore few waste products to potentially cause reaction) and contains a nutritional source not previously presented to the animal – thus no reaction should occur. Once all clinical signs have ceased, usually within a 6–8-week period, individual foodstuffs may be reintroduced to determine any role in the hypersensitivity. If no reaction occurs, these foods may be deemed suitable to be part of the animal's menu.

In some cases where severe disease has been suffered the owners of the animal may wish to remain on the elimination diet if this proves successful in eradicating the disease. Provided this diet is suitable for maintenance feeding and is palatable to the animal, this is a viable option.

Treatment   Avoidance of specific allergens identified to cause reaction at time of elimination diet trial. Long-term feeding of special clinical diet may be an option.

Contact dermatitis

Common causes of this condition include soaps, detergents, shampoos, topical drugs, plastic, rubber, nylon and other synthetic products.

Clinical signs   Lesions are found mostly on feet, ventral abdomen, neck and chin. These are likely to be pruritic, erythematous and often incur secondary infections following self-trauma. They may develop after just 4–6 weeks but often intolerance to the material may build up over time and this could take as long as many months or years.

Diagnosis   *Patch testing* – the suspected allergen is applied to a clipped area of skin and held in contact over a 48-hour period. The area is then examined for signs of reaction.

Contact elimination – the animal is withdrawn from its usual environment and hospitalised. If the clinical signs resolve, this leads to further evidence of contact dermatitis. Periodic reintroduction of single items from own environment may lead to identification of 'safe' items and ultimately the allergenic ones.

Treatment   Avoid contact with identified allergens.

Further reading

Barr, M. C., Olsen, C. W. and Scott, F. W. (2000) Feline viral diseases. In Ettinger, S. J. and Feldman, E. C. (eds), *Textbook of Veterinary Internal Medicine*, 5th edn, W. B. Saunders, London.

Breitschwerdt, E. B. (2000) The rickettsioses. In Ettinger, S. J. and Feldman, E. C. (eds), *Textbook of Veterinary Internal Medicine*, 5th edn, W. B. Saunders, London.

Greene, C. E. (2000) Bacterial diseases. In Ettinger, S. J. and Feldman, E. C. (eds) *Textbook of Veterinary Internal Medicine*, 5th edn, W. B. Saunders, London.

Simpson, J. (1998) Medical disorders and their nursing. In Lane, D. R. and Cooper, B. (eds), *Veterinary Nursing*, 2nd edn, Butterworth-Heinemann, Oxford.

Swango, L. J. (2000) Canine viral diseases. In Ettinger, S. J. and Feldman, E. C. (eds), *Textbook of Veterinary Internal Medicine*, 5th edn, W. B. Saunders, London.

Taboada, J. and Merchant, S. R. (2000) Protozoal and miscellaneous infections. In Ettinger, S. J. and Feldman, E. C. (eds), *Textbook of Veterinary Internal Medicine*, 5th edn, W. B. Saunders, London.

A further source of information on diseases affecting cats is:

The Feline Advisory Bureau, Taelselbury, High Street, Tisbury, Wiltshire SP3 6LD. (www.fabcats.org.)

18

Obstetric and paediatric nursing of the dog and cat

W. Adams and *G. C. W. England*

Learning objectives

After studying this chapter, students should be able to:

- State the criteria for successful breeding.
- Describe the diseases of the reproductive tract of the dog and cat.
- Explain the methods used to control reproduction.
- Identify the techniques used to determine pregnancy.
- Describe normal and abnormal pregnancy.
- Describe the care and management of the neonate.
- State the abnormalities that may occur during the neonatal period.

Introduction

Breeding of domestic pets may occur as a planned event by the experienced breeder or novice but enthusiastic owner. Commonly, however, pet animals become pregnant as a result of an unintentional mating of an oestrus female. The latter situation occurs most frequently because of a lack of education on behalf of the owner. This situation is lamentable, especially considering the thousands of unwanted pets that are destroyed by humane societies every year. It is a responsibility of the veterinary profession to educate owners of new pets so that they are fully aware of the reproductive physiology and the risks of pregnancy. In the majority of cases sterilisation of the puppy or kitten should be recommended.

Breeding should not be undertaken lightly; both the male and female should be carefully assessed and should be clinically sound, free from hereditary diseases, have excellent temperaments, be good examples of the breed and should be free from infectious disease. Many animals that are used at stud do not meet these criteria. Before breeding from a dog or cat the owner should give careful consideration to the quality of their animal as well as the availability of homes for the potential offspring.

There are both moral and legal responsibilities (under the Sale of Goods Act) for breeders of animals to ensure that the offspring are clinically healthy and have a sound temperament. There are many hereditary defects that should preclude animals from breeding and these are discussed in detail in other chapters of this text. In the case of cryptorch-

idism the affected male and both parents should be considered to be carriers and should not be used for breeding.

Control of hereditary disease

Three schemes created in collaboration with the Kennel Club and the British Veterinary Association aim to control the incidence of hereditary diseases in pedigree dogs.

(1) The BVA/Kennel Club/International Sheepdog Society Eye Scheme is designed for the control of specific known inherited conditions including: (i) generalised progressive retinal atrophy, (ii) persistent pupillary membrane, (iii) goniodysgenesis, (iv) total retinal dysplasia, (v) hereditary cataract, (vi) Collie eye anomaly, (vii) primary lens luxation, (viii) multifocal retinal dysplasia, (ix) persistent hyperplastic primary vitreous and (x) congenital hereditary cataract. There are also other conditions that are currently under investigation including coloboma, abnormal pigment deposition, multiocular defects and optic nerve hypoplasia. Dogs should be examined every 12 months to ensure that they remain clear from the hereditary condition. This is very important for certain diseases (such as hereditary cataracts and certain retinopathies) which are not evident at birth. However, in practice, examination generally ceases when the dog exceeds the age at which the disease is commonly identified. The examination is performed by an appointed eye panelist (lists are available from the BVA or the Kennel Club).

(2) The BVA/Kennel Club Hip Dysplasia Scheme is designed to help control hip dysplasia in pedigree dogs. Dogs are usually radiographed on one occasion after they reach 12 months of age. The radiographs are assessed on nine detailed points and are scored for abnormality; radiographically normal hips score zero (0:0) and the maximum score is 106 (this figure does not represent the worst possible hips, only the maximum score that can be achieved on this scoring system). Average values are calculated from all the scores recorded for a given breed and these are regularly published. In some breeds the average may not represent the true status of the breed, since some breeders refuse to have very bad hips submitted for scoring. However,

it is hoped that breeding from animals with scores less than the average will result in improved quality of hips in subsequent generations.

In the United States a different scheme is in operation. This scheme evaluates the degree of laxity of the hip joint, by taking two radiographs, one with the femoral head pushed into the joint and the other with it 'pulled' away from the joint. The distance that the femoral head moves is indicative of the degree of joint laxity. The system is often referred to as the 'Penn Hip' scheme, referring to the University of Pennsylvania where it was originated.

(3) The BVA/Kennel Club Elbow Dysplasia Scheme is designed to help control elbow disease in pedigree dogs. Three radiographs are taken of each elbow and a score awarded according to the presence of typical dysplasia or secondary osteoarthritits. Each elbow is scored 0 to 3, and the overall score is the higher of the two elbows (the scores are not summed as in the Hip Dysplasia Scheme). It is recommended that breeding should only occur of animals with overall elbow grades of 0 or 1.

Other schemes have been adopted by certain breed societies to monitor the level of specific diseases. Examples are the monitoring of cardiac disease in Boxers, and the assessment of Dobermann pinscher dogs for cervical spondylopathy. Certain breed societies have established codes of conduct, which aim to control the number of litters bred per bitch and the age of first mating. The Kennel Club will not register pups born from bitches over the age of 7 years.

The Governing Council of the Cat Fancy (GCCF) provides for the registration of cats and the production of certified certificates. In addition, it classifies breeds, licenses shows and publishes rules that control those functions. Whilst the GCCF publishes leaflets of general advice, it issues no specific guidelines regarding hereditary disease.

Assessment of animals for breeding

Potential breeders should take advice from many sources before breeding from any male or female animal. Animals should be screened for hereditary disease as discussed above. In addition the animals should be in good general health and should be of a suitable age for reproduction. In both the female and male this should be after their temperamental and conformational qualities can be properly assessed, whilst in the female it should be after the animal is skeletally mature.

In dogs in the UK, there are no bacterial venereal pathogens and therefore routine bacteriological swabbing for the prepuce or vagina is a waste of time. However, in the cat it is important to screen for feline leukaemia virus before embarking upon breeding.

The male

Male dogs and tomcats are sexually active throughout the year, although a minor seasonal effect may be noted in some countries. The testes are descended into the scrotum at birth in the cat, and they descend into the scrotum by 10 days after birth in the dog. Both pups and kittens may show sexual activity from several weeks of age; however, puberty does not occur until 6–12 months in the dog and 8–12 months in the cat. For both species, spermatogenesis (the production of spermatozoa) commences at approximately 5 months of age.

It is preferable not to use a male at stud until he is at least 12 months of age, since it is not possible to fully evaluate his qualities until this time, and even then the occurrence of certain hereditary diseases may not be apparent. It is advisable that the first mating attempts should be with an experienced female.

The fertile lifespan of a male varies considerably, and is probably related to the longevity of that particular breed. It is certain, however, that average seminal quality of male stud dogs is reduced from 7 years of age onwards.

Endocrinology

The interstitial (Leydig) cells are the source of testosterone production from the testes. **Luteinising hormone** (LH), a gonadotrophin hormone released from the pituitary gland, stimulates the production of this hormone. A second pituitary gonadotrophin called **follicle stimulating hormone** (FSH) appears to increase the process of sperm production (spermatogenesis) directly via the Sertoli cells. Testosterone has a negative feedback effect upon the release of FSH and LH, which is mediated by **gonadotrophin releasing hormone** (GnRH) (Fig. 18.1).

Control of reproduction in males

The majority of male dogs do not cause problems if they remain entire. However, there are situations where control of 'antisocial' behaviour may necessitate the control of male hormone release. The situation in the entire tomcat is rather different because the problems of territory marking, roaming and aggression are greater than the dog.

Exogenous hormones

Chemical control of reproductive function can be achieved in both species on a short-term basis with hormones that suppress the normal release of testosterone. The most commonly used agents include the progestogens (drugs with progesterone-like activity) which may be administered daily orally (e.g. megestrol acetate), or as a depot injection (e.g. proligestone or delmadinone acetate). These drugs do not produce infertility, only a reduced libido. No single drug

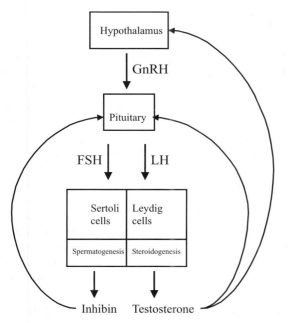

Fig. 18.1 Schematic representation of the endocrine control of testicular function in the male.

is commercially available as a male contraceptive agent; complicated drug regimes are required for this effect.

Surgical contraception

The most common method for the regulation of sexual activity is castration, which is not reversible. Castration before puberty may result in failure of development of the secondary sexual characteristics. In some males a change in metabolic rate may result in increased bodyweight. Castration after puberty and correct dietary control eliminate the majority of problems associated with castration.

Vasectomy is rarely performed in the dog or tom. It involves removal of part of the vas deferens, which prevents sperm being ejaculated. The procedure does not interfere with sexual behaviour, and since in many cases this is the primary aim, it has no advantages over castration.

Vaccination

As technology advances, it is becoming more likely that vaccines will be developed against components of the reproductive system. Currently, however, whilst some experimental vaccines are available for use in females in other species (directed against the zona pellucida), there are none available for use in the male dog or cat.

Diseases of the reproductive tract of the dog and tomcat

There are a variety of conditions that may affect the reproductive organs of both the tomcat and the male dog.

Endocrinological abnormalities

Primary abnormalities in the secretion of pituitary hormones may result in the poor development of gonadal tissue, a condition called **hypogonadism**. This is rare but has been reported in both species.

Diseases of the testes

An absence of the testes (**anorchia**) is very rare; in most cases the testes are retained within the abdomen. These undescended testes belong to the condition known as **cryptorchidism**, which literally means 'hidden testicle'. Often the condition is unilateral, with one testicle present within the scrotum and the other retained within the abdomen. These cases are often wrongly called monorchids; monorchidism refers to an animal with a single testicle. Some cryptorchid animals are bilaterally affected and no testes are seen within the scrotum. The treatment for all cryptorchids is removal of both testes, because of the high incidence of neoplasia within the abdominal testis, and the fact that the condition is likely to be inherited.

Inflammation of the testes (**orchitis**) is rare but may follow trauma (particularly in the tomcat) or ascending bacterial infection. In some countries (but not the UK) orchitis may be caused by the bacterium *Brucella canis* which is a venereal pathogen transmitted at coitus.

Testicular tumours are the second most common tumour affecting the male dog but are rare in the tomcat. There are three common tumour types: those affecting the Leydig cell (Leydig cell tumour), those affecting the Sertoli cells (Sertoli cell tumour), and those affecting the germ cells (seminoma). Some of these tumours may be endocrinologically active and secrete female hormones (oestrogens) which produce signs of feminisation.

Diseases of the accessory glands

The prostate gland in the male dog is the only accessory sex gland. The tomcat has both prostate and bulbourethral glands, although disease of either is rare.

Prostate abnormalities in the dog are common and include benign enlargement (**hyperplasia**), bacterial prostatitis, prostatic cysts and prostatic tumours. The clinical signs of these diseases may be similar and include difficulty urinating and defecating and the presence of blood within urine and/or semen.

Diseases of the penis and prepuce

It is common for there to be a purulent discharge from the prepuce of the male dog, which should be considered normal unless it is excessive. It is not seen in the tomcat.

Phimosis is a condition where there is inability to extrude the penis due to an abnormally small preputial orifice. This may occur either congenitally or as a result of trauma or inflammation, and may result in pain during erection. **Paraphimosis** is a failure to retract the penis into the prepuce and may also be due to a small preputial orifice. The penis becomes dry and necrotic and urethral obstruction may result. **Priapism** refers to the persistent enlargement of the penis in the absence of sexual excitement.

Lymphoid hyperplasia is a relatively common condition in the male dog, where the bulbus glandis is covered with multiple 2–3 mm diameter nodules. These are usually smooth and do not cause any significant disease, although they may be traumatised at the time of mating or semen collection.

Antisocial behaviour

In many cases behaviour which may be normal for a male animal is considered to be antisocial by man. These problems include territory marking, mounting inappropriate objects and aggression towards other males. These problems often necessitate treatment that may include behavioural modification therapy in conjunction with drugs that inhibit male hormone production such as progestogens. Castration may be required in certain cases.

Normal mating

The sexual behaviour of the tomcat and male dog is considerably different from each other and from other species. It is important therefore that the events of natural mating are understood so that abnormalities can be recognised whilst remembering that the modern mating environment is often artificial. On the day of mating, bitches and queens are frequently transported large distances, are introduced to the male briefly and then expected to mate immediately. This situation eliminates the normal courtship phase associated with proestrus behaviour and may result in mating problems. In addition many females are presented to the male at an inappropriate time, either because this is convenient for the owner or because of inexact assessment of the stage of the oestrus cycle. In these events, sexual behaviour of both the male and female may not be optimal.

Mating behaviour in the domestic dog

The dog and bitch will normally exhibit play behaviour when they are first introduced to each other. Generally the bitch should be taken to the designated area first. The dog can then be introduced. He should be restrained on a lead to ensure that the bitch is happy for the dog to be there and is receptive to him. Once this has been established, the dog can be allowed off his lead. This is when they will normally play for a few minutes (Fig. 18.2a). Very experienced studs may forgo this playtime and mount the bitch straight away, so it is important to establish the willingness of the bitch to be mated in the first instance. The bitch will normally settle and stand with her tail deviated to one side in order to allow mating to take place. This tail deviation is known as 'flagging'.

The dog may ejaculate a small volume of clear fluid either before mounting the bitch or whilst he is trying to gain intromission into the bitch. This fluid is the **first fraction** of the ejaculate and does not contain sperm. It originates from the prostate gland and probably flushes any urine or cellular debris from the urethra. The dog will continue to mount, thrust and dismount (Fig. 18.2b), until his position allows the penile tip to enter the vagina. This is known as **intromission** (Fig. 18.2c). The dog will now achieve a full erection. The dog appears to move much closer to the bitch and the thrusting movements increase rapidly. He will now ejaculate the **second fraction** of ejaculate, which is sperm rich. Once thrusting has subsided the dog will turn through 180 degrees and dismount the bitch whilst his penis remains within the vagina. The dog and bitch will now stand tail-to-tail, and this is called the **tie** (Fig. 18.2d). The tie is associated with the dog ejaculating the **third fraction** of ejaculate. This is again clear fluid and prostatic in origin and its purpose is to flush the sperm forwards through the cervix into the uterus. The tie lasts on average for 20 minutes but this varies considerably between dogs and can be as short as 5 minutes or over an hour in length.

Once the tie is over, the dog and bitch will separate. The bitch should be checked for any bleeding. There is normally a small amount of fluid that comes away when the tie ends. This is just the last portion of prostatic fluid and is normal. The fluid can sometimes be bloodstained depending on the bitch's discharge. Bitches with heavy discharge tend to have a heavier staining of this fluid. If this fluid is very heavily bloodstained, the bitch and the dog should be checked thoroughly. If all is normal, then the bitch is taken away from the area first. The dog will normally lick at himself to help the penis re-enter its sheath. At this time the dog should be checked to ensure that his penis has returned to its sheath correctly. Occasionally, during the mating process, small blood vessels in the dog's penis will burst, resulting in a small amount of bloody discharge. This should subside quickly.

Mating behaviour in the domestic tomcat

The period of sexual introduction and play is variable in the cat, depending upon the experience and aggression of the male. The normal sequence of events occurs rapidly compared with the dog. The male usually approaches the female from the side or back and grasps her neck in his mouth. Whilst maintaining this grasp he mounts the female and positions himself to align the genital regions. The queen normally lowers her chest and elevates the pelvic region whilst deviating her tail. Pelvic thrusting and ejaculation occur rapidly. During intromission the queen often emits a cry and attempts to end mating by rolling, turning and striking at the male. The female then exhibits a marked post-coital reaction consisting of violent rolling and excessive licking. She will not allow further mating at this time.

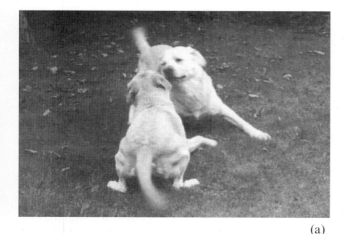

(a)

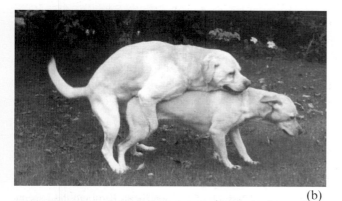

(b)

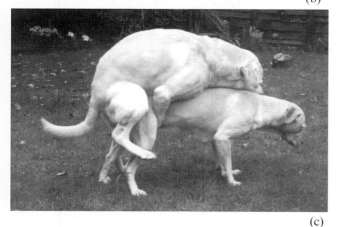

(c)

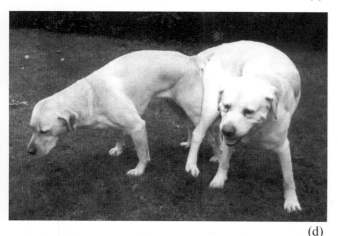

(d)

Fig. 18.2 (a) Playing prior to mating. (b) Mounting behaviour prior to intromission. Fig. 18.2 (Continued) (c) Intromission. (d) The 'tie'.

Problems at mating

The mating of dogs and bitches always seems a straightforward process, but often there can be problems. The most common difficulty is that the dog does not 'tie' with the bitch. This is not considered a satisfactory outcome, although it is quite possible that such matings will still result in the bitch conceiving if the dog has ejaculated. The most common reason for a mating with no tie is that there is a height difference between the dog and the bitch. The dog must be able to enter the bitch as straight as possible and if he is too short or too tall this could make it difficult. If the dog is too short, use a step to make him taller and vice versa. Sometimes the dog will not tie because he has had an unpleasant past experience that has reduced his confidence, often causing a failure to achieve a full erection. In these instances holding the dog and bitch together as soon as the dogs' thrusting has stopped may be helpful. This is known as a held tie, but this in itself can be very difficult to achieve. Normally, one either holds the dog and bitch together as soon as the dog loses his confidence. The dog should not be allowed to mate the bitch too many times without achieving a tie. It is better to try a few times and then rest the dog until the next day.

Often the bitch's position can be a problem; she may not elevate her vulva correctly or she may not deviate her tail very well, or she keeps moving her tail from side to side. In these instances, elevating the bitch's vulva to the correct position, or holding her tail out of the way can help the dog. These problems are commonly associated with inexperienced bitches. These bitches can be a little overwhelmed by the whole process and require much more support than an experienced bitch. They will often stand at first and then completely change their minds. In these cases, patience is a virtue and the bitch just requires a little more time to get used to the stud and the idea of being mated. These matings can sometimes take several hours to achieve, but the bitch should not be rushed and most certainly must not be forced to stand. This could result in putting her off the mating game altogether. Some bitches can be difficult if the stud dog is playing too much and leaping on the bitch. This is rectified by gentle restraint of the bitch, so as not to upset the stud. This is a more common problem with inexperienced stud dogs. Whenever possible, a new stud dog should always be put with an experienced bitch and vice versa.

In the cat, it is frequently very difficult to be present during a mating since this puts off all but the experienced males. In most cases it is necessary to be present as an observer. As with the bitch it is always best to have an experienced partner when a queen or tom is mated for the first time.

Assessment of fertility

Male fertility may be assessed by the evaluation of semen quality. Semen may be collected by stimulating the male dog to ejaculate by hand; artificial vaginas are no longer used for this purpose. Semen collection is more difficult in the tom-cat, and may require general anaesthesia and electroejaculation. A special artificial vagina may be used to collect from trained tomcats. Collection equipment should be warmed before use.

Semen, once collected, should be placed into a water bath at body temperature to prevent damage to the sperm. The second fraction of the dog ejaculate and the entire cat ejaculate should be used for evaluation.

(1) The volume should be measured and the colour recorded. Normally the semen is white and milky in colour, and up to 2.0 ml (of second fraction) for the dog and 0.1–0.5 ml in the tomcat.

(2) After gently mixing the sample, a drop should be placed upon a warmed microscope slide and a subjective assessment made of the percentage of sperm with vigorous forward progression.

(3) A small portion of the sample should be diluted with water to kill the sperm and therefore stop their movement. The spermatozoal concentration can then be measured using a haemocytometer counting chamber. The total sperm output should be calculated by multiplying this value with the volume of the sample.

(4) A portion of the sample should be stained to allow the differentiation of live and dead sperm and the assessment of spermatozoal morphology. A combination of the two stains **nigrosin** and **eosin** is suitable for this purpose. Normally four parts of the stain are mixed with one part of semen, and then a smear is immediately made onto a glass microscope slide. When examined under high magnification, nigrosin appears as a background stain. The eosin is a vital stain – it stains only sperm with a damaged membrane, i.e. dead sperm (Fig. 18.3). Using nigrosin and eosin, sperm are stained either pink (these are termed dead), or are unstained (these are termed live).

The semen characteristics of fertile dogs are given in Table 18.1.

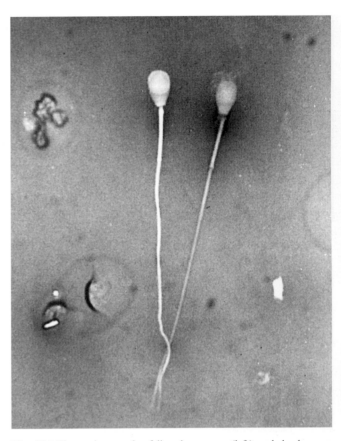

Fig. 18.3 Photomicrograph of live dog sperm (left) and dead sperm (right) with clamped acrosome

The domestic queen

Queens have multiple oestrous cycles each year. They are seasonally polyoestrus, and typically cycle from February to September. Ovulation is induced by coitus and the interval between each oestrous cycle varies depending upon whether the queen has ovulated, or fails to ovulate either because she is not mated or because there is insufficient hormone release at mating. Unmated queens return to oestrus at intervals of 14–21 days. Queens that ovulate but do not become pregnant generally return to oestrus after approximately 45 days.

The female

The domestic bitch

Bitches generally have one or two oestrous cycles per year. Each oestrus ends with spontaneous ovulation, which is followed by the luteal phase. A variable period of acyclicity (called **anoestrus**) follows the luteal phase. The bitch is **polytocous** (produces numerous offspring in each litter) and the oestrous periods are non-seasonal. The interval between each cycle can vary between 5 and 13 months, although the average is 7 months.

Puberty

The domestic bitch

In the bitch the onset of cyclical activity (puberty) is normally between 6 and 23 months of age, with most bitches having their first oestrus by the age of 12–14 months. Bitches that do not exhibit oestrous behaviour by the anticipated age are considered to have delayed puberty, but it should be remembered that many normal bitches will not cycle until they are 2 years old. The majority of bitches start to cycle about 6 months after they have reached adult height

Table 18.1 Characteristics of the second fraction of the ejaculate from 53 fertile dogs				
	Normal progressive motility (%)	Volume (ml)	Concentration ($\times 10^6$/ml)	Total sperm output ($\times 10^6$)
Mean	85.2	1.3	310.5	403.4
S.D.	6.2	0.4	82	120
Range	42–92	0.4–3.4	50–560	36–620

and weight, which may explain some of the variations exhibited between breeds.

The domestic queen

Female cats generally exhibit their first oestrus at 6–9 months of age, but this is dependent upon the photoperiod. Those that are born in the summer frequently commence cycling at the first spring; however, those that are born in the winter may not cycle until they are at least 12 months of age.

The oestrus cycle

The domestic bitch

The stages of the oestrous cycle in the bitch are **proestrus, oestrus, metoestrus (dioestrus)** and **anoestrus** (Fig. 18.4). The terms 'in season' or 'in heat' are used to indicate the stage of the cycle when the bitch is receptive to the male dog, i.e. oestrus.

During proestrus the bitch is receptive to the dog but will not allow mating. Oestrus commences when the bitch will accept the male, and it is during this stage that the eggs are released from the ovaries; a process known as ovulation. Ovulation in the bitch occurs spontaneously towards the end of oestrus. Each egg is contained within a fluid-filled structure called a **follicle**. After ovulation, the follicle develops into a solid structure called a **corpus luteum**. One corpus luteum forms from each follicle that has ovulated and the corpus luteum produces a hormone called **progesterone**.

In many species the phase of progesterone production (the **luteal** phase) is divided into two. The early luteal phase is termed metoestrus and the mature luteal phase is termed dioestrus. However, in the bitch the early luteal occurs during standing oestrus (i.e. when the bitch will stand to be mated), making this terminology difficult to adopt (since metoestrus would then be occurring during oestrus). In the bitch the terms metoestrus and dioestrus are therefore often used synonymously to reflect the luteal phase of the cycle after the end of standing oestrus. This phase is therefore characterised by the presence of the corpora lutea upon the ovaries and the presence of the hormone progesterone in the blood.

The bitch is unusual compared with other species in that the duration of metoestrus is similar whether the bitch is pregnant or not (Fig. 18.5). This explains why the condition known as **false** or **pseudopregnancy** is common in the bitch (see later). Metoestrus is followed by a period of quiescence termed anoestrus.

The hormonal changes of the oestrous cycle are shown in Fig. 18.6.

Late anoestrus   During late anoestrus two hormones are released from the pituitary gland: follicle stimulating hormone (FSH) and luteinising hormone (LH). These initiate the growth of follicles within the ovaries and cause the follicles to produce the hormone oestrogen.

Proestrus   Proestrus is characterised by increased plasma concentrations of oestrogen that cause swelling of the vulva and the development of a serosanginious vulval discharge. Oestrogens also induce the release of specific pheromones that are responsible for attracting male dogs.

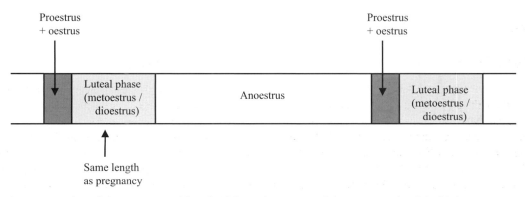

Fig. 18.4 Schematic representation of the sequence and length of the various stages of the oestrus cycle of the bitch.

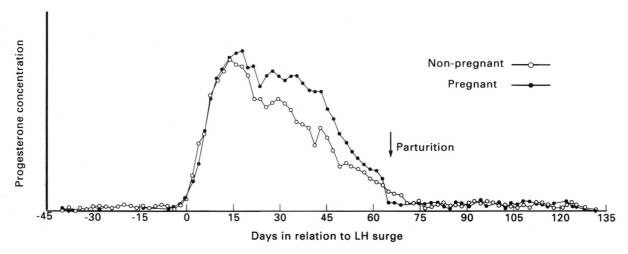

Fig. 18.5 Changes in plasma progesterone concentration in the pregnant and non-pregnant bitch

During proestrus the bitch will not allow mating but may show increased receptivity to the male. This period lasts for approximately 7 days. Oestrogens also cause thickening of the vaginal wall and an increase in the number of epithelial cell layers. During proestrus the elevated concentrations of oestrogen have a negative feedback effect upon the release of the gonadotrophin hormones from the pituitary gland, and the concentrations of FSH and LH are reduced compared with late anoestrus.

Oestrus   During oestrus the bitch demonstrates characteristic behaviour towards the male dog including deviation of the tail and presentation of the vulva and perineum. The bitch will stand to be mated. This period lasts for approximately 7 days. The onset of oestrus is related to a decline in the concentration of plasma oestrogen and at the same time the production of progesterone. The bitch is unusual in that progesterone is produced in low concentrations by luteinisation of the follicle, a process which occurs before ovulation. In many species progesterone is only produced after ovulation. It is this decline in

the concentration of oestrogen and the slight increase in the concentration of progesterone that is responsible for stimulating a surge of both FSH and LH. This surge is the trigger for ovulation that occurs approximately 2 days later. It can therefore be seen that the hormonal stimulus for ovulation occurs during oestrus (i.e. when the bitch will stand to be mated) and that the release of eggs also occurs during this period. After ovulation, corpora lutea form and produce greater amounts of progesterone. The end of standing oestrus is associated with relatively high concentrations of progesterone in the blood.

Metoestrus (dioestrus)   The period of metoestrus lasts whilst the corpora lutea continue to produce progesterone and is approximately 55 days in length. In the pregnant bitch the period of metoestrus is synonymous with pregnancy, for the birth of pups occurs when progesterone secretion is terminated. In the non-pregnant bitch the corpora lutea persist for a similar period of time.

Towards the end of metoestrus another hormone called **prolactin** is released from the pituitary gland. This is respon-

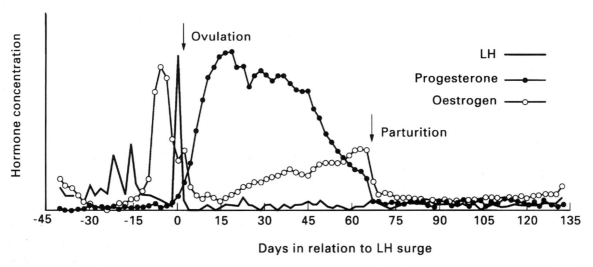

Fig. 18.6 Changes in plasma hormones during the oestrus cycle of the pregnant bitch

sible for the development of mammary tissue and the onset of lactation. Prolactin is produced in both the pregnant and the non-pregnant bitch, and is the reason why pseudopregnancy is a common event in the bitch.

Anoestrus Metoestrus is followed by a period of quiescence, during which time there is effectively no hormonal activity. In the non-pregnant bitch there is no sudden decline in the concentration of progesterone but values gradually reduce and the transition to anoestrus is smooth. The situation is slightly different during pregnancy because progesterone concentrations rapidly decline, and it is this event which stimulates the onset of parturition. The length of anoestrus varies considerably between bitches, but it is 4 months on average.

The domestic queen

The stages of the oestrous cycle in the queen are **anoestrus, proestrus, oestrus** and **interoestrus** (Fig. 18.7). The terms 'in season' or 'in heat' are used to indicate the stage of the cycle when the cat is receptive to the male, i.e. oestrus. During winter there is essentially no hormone activity; the queen is in anoestrus. In spring-time cyclical activity commences and in the unmated queen periods of sexual activity (proestrus and oestrus) are interrupted by periods of non-receptivity (interoestrus). If the queen is mated and ovulation is induced, the queen enters metoestrus or pregnancy.

Pregnancy follows a fertile mating; metoestrus (also called pseudopregnancy) follows a sterile mating. The duration of pseudopregnancy in the queen is shorter than that of pregnancy unlike the situation in the bitch.

Proestrus Follicular development occurs during this phase due to the release of LH and FSH. This causes the secretion of oestrogen that is responsible for the development of the signs of proestrus including attraction of the male and the changes in the vaginal epithelium similar to those seen in the bitch. Proestrus in the queen is often poorly recognised unless a male is present; however, during this stage the queen will not accept mating. Proestrus lasts between 2–3 days.

Oestrus The exact hormonal changes that cause the onset of standing oestrus are uncertain, although this may be associated with declining concentrations of oestrogen similar to that seen in the bitch.

The clinical signs of oestrus (also termed **calling**) include: persistent vocalisation, rolling and rubbing against inanimate objects. In the presence of the male the queen may show persistent treading of the hind feet, lateral deviation of the tail and lordosis of the spine. Oestrus lasts between 2 and 10 days.

Interoestrus In the absence of mating, or when mating does not result in ovulation, the signs of oestrus gradually decline and the queen enters a stage of non-receptivity. This period may last for between 3 and 14 days. After this time the queen returns to proestrus and oestrus.

Pregnancy Ovulation in the queen is caused by the release of LH, which is stimulated by mating. Each mating results in a surge of LH, however there appears to be a threshold value below which ovulation will not be induced. Multiple matings are therefore more likely to result in ovulation than are single matings.

Ovulation is followed by an increase in the plasma concentration of progesterone released from the newly formed corpora lutea. Peak progesterone concentrations are reached approximately 1 month after mating and are maintained for the duration of pregnancy that varies between 64 and 68 days. It is not uncommon for queens to have an absence of cyclical activity during lactation. This has been called **lactational anoestrus**.

Metoestrus (pseudopregnancy) Non-fertile matings result in ovulation without conception. Ovulation may also occur following stimulation of the vagina (e.g. following collection of a vaginal smear), stimulation of the perineum (which may be self-induced) or may occur spontaneously in some queens. Ovulation results in the formation of corpora lutea and the production of progesterone in a similar manner to early pregnancy. After approximately 40 days, progesterone concentrations decline and the queen returns to cyclical activity. Should pseudopregnancy occur late in the year (autumn) the queen may not return to cyclical activity but may enter anoestrus.

Determination of the optimum time for mating

The domestic bitch

The determination of the time of ovulation in the bitch is important because the bitch is monoestrous and the mean interoestrus interval is 31 weeks. The clinical signs of oestrus are not always reliable indicators of the time of ovulation; in

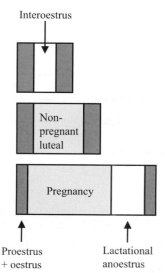

Fig. 18.7 Schematic representation of the sequence and length of the various stages of the oestrus cycle of the queen.

many bitches the behavioural signs do not correlate well with the changes in hormone concentration. There are, however, two natural methods which increase the likelihood of conception despite these potential problems. The first is the relatively long fertile period of eggs and the second is the relatively long survival of spermatozoa within the female reproductive tract.

There are several methods by which the optimum time for mating can be detected and these include clinical assessments, measurement of plasma hormone concentration and vaginal cytology.

Clinical assessments The clinical signs of oestrus do not correlate well with the underlying hormonal events. The 'average bitch' ovulates 12 days after the onset of proestrus and should be mated from day 14 onwards when oocytes have matured. However, in some bitches, ovulation may occur as early as day 5 or as late as day 30 after the onset of proestrus. These would be unlikely to become pregnant if mated on the 12th and 14th day, which is common breeding practice.

Studies on laboratory-kept dogs have shown that the LH surge often occurs around the same time as the onset of standing oestrus. Although there is some variation of this event, mating 4 days after the onset of standing oestrus may be a suitable time in many bitches.

One clinical assessment that may be useful in the bitch is the timing of vulval softening (Fig. 18.8). This often occurs during the LH surge when there is a switch from oestrogen dominance to progesterone dominance of the reproductive tract.

If only clinical assessments are available the combination of the onset of standing oestrus and the timing of distinct vulval softening may be useful in the prediction of the best mating time, since each event occurs on average 2 days before ovulation.

Measurement of plasma hormone concentration The three relevant plasma hormones are LH, oestrogen and progesterone. The measurement of plasma concentrations of LH would indicate impending ovulation; the fertile period is between 4 and 8 days after the LH surge. There is, however, no simple method by which plasma LH concentrations can be readily measured.

There is little value in the measurement of plasma oestrogen concentrations because the oestrogen plateau is not predicative of the timing of ovulation. Plasma progesterone concentrations are, however, very useful since this hormone is absent during proestrus and begins to increase coincidentally with the plasma surge of LH, thus detecting a rise in the concentration of plasma progesterone is predictive of ovulation. Progesterone can be easily measured in the practice laboratory within 30 minutes of sample collection using a commercial enzyme-linked immunosorbent assay test-kit. This method simply involves comparison of a colour change in the sample, with the colour change in low- and high-concentration progesterone controls.

Vaginal cytology The changes in the concentration of plasma hormone concentrations have a marked effect upon the vaginal mucosa.

When the bitch is not cycling, there are approximately two or three layers of cells lining the vagina. However, during oestrus, the vagina develops many cell layers in order to protect itself during mating. The cells within these layers differ from each other in their shape and size. When cells are collected from the vagina (the technique called a **vaginal smear**), only the cells on the surface of the vagina are removed. Different cell types are therefore collected at the various stages of the reproductive cycle. Staining of these cells and subsequent microscopic examination allows an assessment of the underlying hormone changes to be made. Cells can be collected either by aspirating vaginal fluid using a pipette, or using a cotton swab. Once collected cells are placed onto a glass microscope slide, spread into a thin film and stained so that they can be individually examined (Fig. 18.9).

During anoestrus the vaginal wall is only a few cells in thickness; these cells are small and spherical in shape.

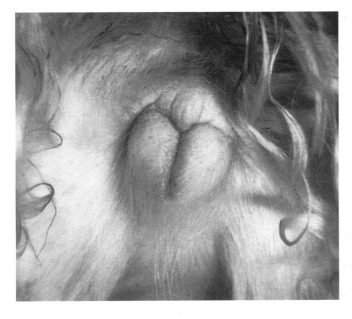

Fig 18.8 Photograph of swollen bitch's vulva, just before the LH surge.

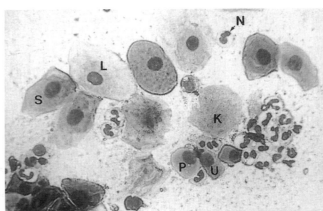

Fig. 18.9 Photomicrograph of the vaginal smear of a bitch in the luteal phase S = small intermediate epithelial cell, L = large intermediate epithelial cell, K = keratinised cell, N = neutrophil, U = uterine cell..

Because they are positioned close to the basement membrane they are called **parabasal cells**. The anoestrus vaginal smear is characterised by the presence of these cells. There are also normally a few white blood cells (**neutrophils**) which remove cell debris and bacteria.

During proestrus the vaginal mucosa increases in thickness under the influence of oestrogen. The mucosa may be up to five or six cells thick. The cells further away from the basement membrane are larger in diameter than those nearer to the membrane. These cells have a large area of cytoplasm surrounding the cell nucleus and are called **small intermediate cells**. When the surface cells are collected during proestrus they are therefore predominantly these small intermediate cells, although there will also be a small number of the parabasal cells present. White blood cells are also present during proestrus; however, numbers are reduced compared with anoestrus. This is because the increased thickness of the vaginal mucosa prevents movement of the white blood cells into the lumen of the vagina. Red blood cells are also present in the vaginal smear during proestrus. These cells originate from the uterus and pass into the vagina via the cervix.

During oestrus the vaginal mucosa continues to thicken and the number of cell layers increases. There may be up to 12 cell layers during oestrus. Surface cells are large and irregular in shape and are called **large intermediate cells**. Cells of this size may accumulate the material keratin and are then termed **keratinised**. The nucleus of these large keratinised cells often disappears. The cells are then called **anuclear** because of the absence of the nucleus. White blood cells are not found in the vaginal smear during oestrus because the thick vaginal wall does not allow them to penetrate. Red blood cells are present in large numbers during oestrus.

During metoestrus there is sloughing of much of the vaginal mucosal epithelium. This is caused by the increasing concentrations of the hormone progesterone. The number of cell layers is reduced and the surface cells are again the small intermediate epithelial cells or parabasal cells. Several of the epithelial cells may have vacuoles within the cytoplasm, giving the cell a 'foamy' appearance. Foam cells and epithelial cells with cytoplasmic inclusion bodies are characteristic of metoestrus. Because of the large amount of degenerate cellular material within the vaginal lumen there is a rapid influx of white blood cells as soon as the mucosa is thin enough to allow their penetration. Large numbers of white blood cells are therefore found in the metoestrus vaginal smear. Few red blood cells are present during metoestrus.

The bitch should first be mated when the percentage of anuclear cells is maximal (usually 80% or above) (Fig. 18.10). There are, however, variations from the normal; some bitches may have two peaks of anuclear cells and some have a low percentage of anuclear cells during the fertile period.

Other tests   A number of other tests have been evaluated in the past including the measurement of electrical resistance, pH and glucose concentration in the vagina; none of these methods is reliable.

However, examination of the vaginal wall using an endoscope (**vaginoscopy**) may be valuable for identifying the optimal time for breeding, as the vaginal wall undergoes specific changes around the time of ovulation.

The domestic queen

Unlike the bitch, in the queen ovulation is induced by coitus. After mating, assuming that a sufficient release of LH has occurred, follicles increase in size and ovulation follows 24–36 hours later. Mating is best planned during the peak of oestrus and vaginal cytology may be used to assess this time; however, collection of the smear may induce ovulation. Multiple copulations should be permitted to ensure an adequate release of LH and therefore ovulation.

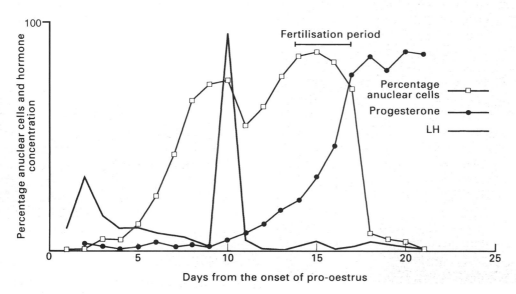

Fig. 18.10 Schematic representation of the changes in the percentage of anuclear cells during oestrus of the bitch.

Assisted reproduction

The domestic bitch

There are several techniques that may be used to assist reproduction in the bitch. These include the induction of oestrus (see later) and **artificial insemination**. Artificial insemination is the technique of collecting semen from a male animal, and placing it into the reproductive tract of the female.

Artificial insemination may involve the use of freshly collected semen, semen that has been diluted and chilled or semen which has been frozen and then thawed. Artificial insemination has several advantages over natural mating:

- It reduces the requirement to transport animals.
- It is an acceptable way of overcoming, to some extent, the quarantine restrictions that prevent the movement of animals from one country to another.
- It increases the genetic pool available to an individual breed within a country.
- It reduces the disease risk that is always present when unknown animals enter a kennel for mating. In some countries the use of artificial insemination may reduce the spread of infectious diseases.
- In certain circumstances, artificial insemination may be useful when natural mating is difficult (for example bitches which ovulate when they are not in standing oestrus or bitches that have hyperplasia of the vaginal floor).
- Semen may also be collected from male animals that are unable to achieve a natural mating due to age, debility, back pain or premature ejaculation.

The greatest area of interest is probably the storage of genetic material by freezing semen for insemination at a future date. This may be necessary in male animals that are likely to become infertile due to castration or to medical treatments with certain hormones. The more common reason is, however, the preservation of semen from superior animals for use in future generations.

Collected semen may be deposited easily into the vagina of the bitch using a long inseminating pipette that is gently introduced near to the cervix. When semen is placed in this position, spermatozoa must swim through the cervix, into the uterus and up the uterine horns. During a natural mating, contractions of the vagina and uterus help in transporting semen. These contractions generally do not occur during insemination, although some may be produced by stimulating the vagina. Vaginal insemination is therefore not ideal, but usually when fresh or chilled semen is used the spermatozoa will live long enough to fertilise the eggs. However, in the case of frozen semen the spermatozoa do not live for long after thawing and so vaginal inseminations are not very satisfactory.

The chance of pregnancy can be improved if the semen is placed directly into the uterus rather than into the vagina. It is very difficult to place a catheter through the bitch's cervix into the uterus (a technique that is simple in many other animals) because the vagina is long and narrow and because the cervical opening is small and at an angle to the vagina. A special insemination pipette has been developed for this purpose. Recently, some research workers have been able to catheterise the cervix using an endoscope. However, in certain countries the commonest way of performing uterine insemination is surgically via a laparotomy.

Because of the short lifespan of the preserved sperm, it is most important that inseminations are accurately timed in relation to ovulation. The ideal time is between 2 and 5 days after ovulation, and this is best assessed by using the measurement of plasma progesterone concentration and the study of vaginal cytology.

In the UK, pups that are the result of artificial insemination can only be registered if the Kennel Club has given prior permission. The permission of the Kennel Club is not required before semen is imported or exported. There are, however, specific regulations set by the Department for Environment Food and Rural Affairs in this country, and similar organisations in other countries, which aim to prevent the introduction of infectious diseases. Import regulations vary between countries but are particularly stringent for the UK. Import permit requirements usually include health certification before, and a set time period after semen collection, quarantine of semen until the second health examination and various serological tests.

The domestic queen

Whilst artificial insemination has been widely practised in the domestic cat as a research model for wild cats, the technique is not commonly used in this country. Techniques used in the cat are, however, further advanced than those in the dog, and include the induction of ovulation, *in vitro* fertilisation and embryo transfer.

Control of reproduction

There have been many methods employed to control the reproductive cycle of the bitch and queen. These involve surgical methods and medical control of cyclical activity. More recently, advances have been made in the induction of oestrus, and the termination of pregnancy.

The domestic bitch

Surgical neutering **Ovariohysterectomy** is the removal of both ovaries and the uterus to the level of the cervix. The term **spaying** is commonly used to describe this procedure. In some countries it is more common to remove only the ovaries (called **ovariectomy**). Either technique should be considered in any bitch not required for breeding. Both have several advantages including a reduction in the incidence of mammary tumours, elimination of the problems of false pregnancy and of pyometra as well the obvious advantages of absence of oestrous behaviour and inability to produce offspring. There are, however, several claimed adverse effects including an increased incidence of incontinence, changes in coat texture and a tendency to gain weight. Whilst little can be done regarding the former two conditions, the latter may easily be controlled by correct dietary management.

There is considerable discussion concerning the correct time to perform the procedure on a bitch. There is no doubt that surgery is technically easier and recovery is more rapid in young animals, and some veterinary surgeons perform surgery as early as 4 months of age. However, it has been suggested that when performed before puberty (the first oestrus) there is an increased tendency for underdevelopment of the secondary sexual characteristics and there may also be effects on the closure time of the animals' growth plates. Prepubertal neutering does significantly protect the female against the development of mammary tumours later in life. However, waiting until after the first oestrus suffers the risk of pregnancy and false pregnancy.

Medical inhibition of cyclical activity There are a variety of compounds that may be used to inhibit cyclical activity including progesterone or progesterone-like compounds (progestogens), testosterone or other male hormones (androgens) and gonadotrophin-releasing hormone agonists and antagonists. Drugs may either be administered during anoestrus to prevent the occurrence of an oestrus (the term **prevention** is used), or may be given during proestrus or oestrus to abolish the signs of that particular oestrus (the term **suppression** is used). The most commonly used compounds are the progestogens, which are formulated as depot injections or as oral tablets.

The depot injections may be used during anoestrus to prevent the occurrence of the next anticipated oestrus. The oral tablets may be used either during anoestrus for oestrus prevention, or during proestrus to suppress the signs of that oestrus. A normal oestrus often occurs between 4 and 6 months after the administration of these hormones.

These drugs are not recommended for use before the first oestrus or in an animal that is required for breeding. The side-effects of these drugs include increased appetite, weight gain, lethargy, mammary enlargement, coat and temperament changes and the risk of inducing pyometra.

The termination of pregnancy Unwanted matings are commonly seen in general practice. The term **misalliance** is often used to describe these cases. There are several treatment options should pregnancy termination be necessary. If the bitch is not required for breeding, an ovariohysterectomy may be performed early in metoestrus, approximately 2 weeks after the end of oestrus. Medical therapy using oestrogens on several occasions after mating is often successful in preventing conception but suffers the risk of induction of pyometra and the disadvantage that oestrus will be prolonged. In later pregnancy it is possible to use various drugs (e.g. prolactin inhibitors and/or prostaglandins) which lower the concentration of progesterone in the blood and therefore induce resorption or abortion. Recently progesterone-receptor antagonist have been licensed for use.

Induction of oestrus With the development of new drugs and new drug regimes it has become possible to induce an oestrous cycle in the bitch. In many cases the success rate in terms of the birth of live pups is poor and the administration of the drugs is complicated. However, these methods may be useful in those bitches which have longer than average interoestrus intervals, those which are slow to reach puberty and those which do not exhibit behavioural signs of oestrus.

The domestic queen

Surgical neutering The indications and potential adverse effects of ovariohysterectomy and ovariectomy in the cat are similar to those of the bitch. The procedure is usually performed when the queen is 5–6 months of age regardless of the onset of puberty; poor development of the external genitalia does not cause problems. In the UK the surgical procedure is frequently performed through a flank incision. This approach is, however, best avoided in oriental breeds where coat colour is a temperature-dependent effect, and clipping the coat may result in the growth of dark-coloured hairs.

Medical inhibition of cyclical activity The drugs available for use in the queen are similar to those described for the domestic bitch. Long-term drug therapy is, however, less commonly used because queens that are not wanted for breeding are usually surgically neutered.

Termination of pregnancy Treatment of an unwanted mating can be achieved by the administration of progestogens if the queen is still in oestrus. In most cases, however, pregnancy termination is performed 1 month after mating using similar drug regimes to those described in the bitch.

Induction of oestrus Various drugs may be used for the induction of oestrus and ovulation. In most cases, however, it is important to remember that the queen is a seasonal breeder, and that her cyclicity is governed by photoperiod.

Diseases of the reproductive tract

The domestic bitch

There are several abnormalities of the reproductive tract in the domestic bitch. These may be considered under general headings of endocrinological, ovarian, uterine or external genital abnormalities.

Endocrinological abnormalities The common endocrinological abnormalities of the bitch include:

- Delayed onset of puberty (cyclical activity is not present at 24 months of age).
- Prolonged anoestrus (failure of return to cyclical activity resulting in a prolonged interoestrus interval).

- Silent oestrous cycles (normal cyclical activity including ovulation but without the external signs of oestrus).
- Split oestrus (signs of proestrus but this does not terminate in ovulation and is followed 2–12 weeks later by a normal cycle).
- Ovulation failure (when bitches have apparently normal oestrous periods with an absence of ovulation – these bitches often return to oestrus with shorter than normal intervals).

One specific endocrinological condition frequently seen in the bitch is **pseudopregnancy** (false pregnancy, phantom pregnancy or pseudocyesis). The signs of the condition include anorexia, abdominal enlargement, nest making, nursing of inanimate objects, mammary development and lactation. False pregnancy should be considered normal in the bitch because the changes in plasma hormones are similar in both pregnant and non-pregnant individuals. It has been wrongly thought that pseudopregnancy is produced by either an overproduction of progesterone or abnormal persistence of the corpus luteum. The actual mechanism is related to the decline in plasma progesterone concentration during late metoestrus, which is associated with an increase in plasma concentrations of prolactin. In many cases therapy is not required because the signs will gradually decline. However, in certain cases it may be necessary to use hormonal therapy to reduce the plasma concentrations of prolactin.

Diseases of the ovary

There are few abnormalities of the ovary. An absence of ovarian development (**agenesis**) may occur; this usually affects one side only and may affect fertility. Ovarian cysts are rare and may be associated with signs of persistent oestrus; however, most cysts originate from the ovarian bursa and are not endocrinologically active. Ovarian tumours are also rare.

Occasionally bitches with both ovarian and testicular tissue are seen. These animals are termed **intersex** and may be recognised because of the appearance of their external genitalia. The vulva may be cranially positioned and an os clitoris may develop. The gonads may be found in a normal ovarian position or within the scrotum. These animals are usually sterile.

Diseases of the uterus

Developmental problems of the uterus include **aplasia** (abnormal development) or **agenesis** (failure of development); in these cases reproductive cyclicity will be normal but the bitch may fail to become pregnant. Intersex animals may have the presence of both uterine tissue and vasa defferentia.

The most common uterine disease of the bitch is **cystic endometrial hyperplasia** (CEH) which may develop into **pyometra**. Hyperplasia of the endometrium occurs in response to progesterone during normal metoestrus. In young animals the hyperplasia resolves at the end of the luteal phase. This is not the case in older bitches, and small cystic regions develop within the glandular tissue. The uterus in this state is probably more prone to infection than the normal uterus, and should bacteria enter during oestrus (when the cervix is open) they may proliferate. The accumulation of pus within the uterus (pyometra) leads to the bitch to becoming unwell. Clinical signs may include the presence of a malodorous vaginal discharge, lethargy, inappetence, pyrexia, vomiting, polydipsia and polyuria. In some cases the cervix is not open and a vaginal discharge is absent; these cases are called **closed pyometra**. In all cases of pyometra the treatment of choice is ovariohysterectomy following stabilisation of the patient using appropriate fluid therapy. Medical treatment (with combinations or prolactin inhibitors and prostaglandins) has been advocated and success rates appear to be quite reasonable, although in most cases the best option is surgery.

Treatment of bitches with progestogens for the prevention or suppression of oestrus, or oestrogens for the treatment of unwanted matings may predispose to the development of pyometra.

Diseases of the vagina and vestibule

Congenital abnormalities of the caudal reproductive tract include segmental aplasia and hymenal or vestibular constrictions.

Vaginitis (inflammation of the vagina) is sometimes seen in prepubertal bitches and usually resolves after the first oestrus. Specific infectious causes of vaginitis include **Brucella canis** (not present in the UK) and herpes virus. Many bacteria are found within the vagina as normal commensal organisms including beta-haemolytic streptococci that many dog breeders wrongly consider to be venereal pathogens. There is little value in routine bacteriological swabbing of the vagina before breeding, since usually only these commensal bacteria are isolated.

Diseases of the external genitalia

Congenital abnormalities such as vulval atresia and agenesis are rare. Clitoral hypertrophy may occur associated with intersexuality.

The domestic queen

Endocrinological abnormalities

Delayed puberty may be difficult to assess in the queen since the onset of cyclical activity is related to the season of the year at birth (see above). Delayed puberty and prolonged anoestrus has, however, been seen although they are rare.

The most common abnormality is ovulation failure that often results from insufficient reflex release of LH at mating. The majority of queens will ovulate if 4–12 matings are allowed in a 4-hour period.

Pseudopregnancy also occurs in the queen, although this condition is dissimilar to that seen in the bitch and usually follows a sterile mating (or occasionally spontaneous ovulation). After ovulation there is an increase in plasma progesterone, which does not occur in the absence of mating, and no return to oestrus for a further 35 to 40 days (Figs 18.4 and 18.7 and 18.11). The clinical signs are an absence of oestrus; treatment is not required.

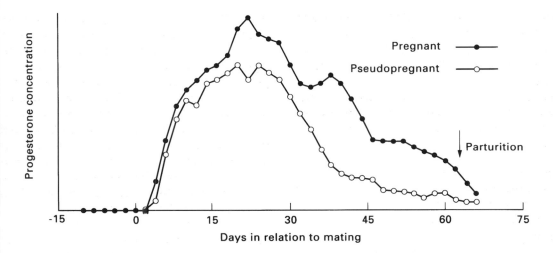

Fig. 18.11 Schematic representation of progesterone profiles in pregnant and pseudopregnant cats

Diseases of the ovary

Congenital diseases of the ovary such as ovarian agenesis and ovarian hypoplasia are rare. Ovarian cysts and neoplasms may develop similar to those seen in the bitch and are also rare.

Premature ovarian failure may be seen in queens aged 8 years and above; these animals stop cycling for an unknown reason.

Diseases of the uterus

The range of uterine abnormalities seen in the cat are similar to those of the bitch. Pyometra may be less common because in the absence of mating ovulation does not occur and the luteal phase is therefore absent. However, spontaneous ovulations or the common use of progestogens may cause the development of cystic endometrial hyperplasia and pyometra.

Diseases of the vagina, vestibule and external genitalia

Congenital abnormalities of the vagina, vestibule and external genitalia are rare but include: vaginal and vulval aplasia and defects associated with intersexuality. Vaginitis is uncommon.

Pregnancy

The domestic bitch

The length of pregnancy in the bitch is relatively consistent at 64, 65 or 66 days from the preovulatory LH surge. However, the apparent length of pregnancy, assessed from the time of mating, may vary between 56 and 72 days, since both early and late matings may be fertile:

- Early matings require sperm survival within the female reproductive tract until ovulation and egg maturation; such matings produce a long apparent pregnancy.
- Late matings occur when eggs are waiting to be fertilised for some time after ovulation; such matings produce a shorter pregnancy.

The clinical signs of pregnancy might include:

- Increased bodyweight and abdominal enlargement; however, these signs may not be obvious if the number of pups is small.
- A reduced food intake and a vaginal discharge are common approximately 1 month into the pregnancy. Enlargement and reddening of the mammary glands may be noted especially from 40 days after mating (these signs may, however, be present in bitches with pseudopregnancy).
- The production of milk (a variable finding: some bitches produce serous fluid from day 40 and milk from day 55 onwards, whilst in others this may not occur until just before parturition).

Certain physiological changes occur during pregnancy and include the development of a normochromic, normocytic anaemia and a reduction of the packed cell volume; these changes are normal.

Food intake does not increase during the first 30 days of pregnancy. After this time the absolute requirement for carbohydrate and protein increases. During the last half of pregnancy food consumption may be doubled. Provided that diet is well balanced and contains suitable amounts of vitamins and minerals it is not necessary to provide extra supplementation although it may be necessary to provide the food divided into two or three meals during the day. Supplementation with calcium and vitamin D should be avoided, since this does not prevent eclampsia and can be dangerous.

Regular exercise should be provided throughout pregnancy, limited by the amount the bitch is willing to undertake.

For the control of ascarid infections (*Toxocara*) it is necessary to administer medication during pregnancy to reduce or prevent perinatal transmission. Various drugs (benzimidazoles) and treatment regimes have been advocated for the treatment of pregnant bitches.

It is advisable to ensure that routine vaccination has been performed before mating. Vaccination during pregnancy is unlikely to be damaging to the fetus and therefore may be undertaken if necessary, but no live vaccine is licensed for this purpose.

Pregnancy diagnosis   As well as observation of the clinical signs already described (noting that mammary gland development, increased weight and abdominal enlargement may be present in pseudopregnancy as well as in pregnancy), there are several methods for pregnancy diagnosis in the bitch:

- **Abdominal palpation**. This is best performed approximately 1 month after mating when the conceptual swellings are approximately 2.0 cm in diameter. The technique can be highly accurate but may be difficult in obese or nervous animals, and may be inaccurate if the bitch was mated early such that pregnancy is not as advanced as anticipated. After day 35, individual conceptuses cannot easily be palpated and diagnosis becomes more difficult.
- **Identification of fetal heart beats**. In late pregnancy it is possible to auscultate the fetal heart beats using a stethoscope, or to record a fetal ECG. Both of these methods are diagnostic of pregnancy; fetal heart rate is more rapid than that of the dam.
- **Radiography**. From day 30 it is possible to detect uterine enlargement with good-quality radiographs. However, this is not diagnostic of pregnancy, since pyometra may have a similar appearance. Pregnancy diagnosis is not possible until after day 45 when mineralisation of the fetal skeleton is detectable radiographically. At this stage it is unlikely that there will be radiation damage to the fetus, however, sedation or anaesthesia of the dam may be required and is a potential risk. In late pregnancy the number of pups can be reliably estimated by counting the number of fetal skulls.
- **Hormone tests**. Plasma concentrations of progesterone are not useful for the detection of pregnancy in the bitch. Measurement of the hormone **relaxin** is diagnostic of pregnancy, and there is now a rapid ELISA test kit that can be run within the practice laboratory to measure this hormone. Alternatively a blood sample can be sent away to a commercial laboratory.
- **Acute phase proteins**. The rise in the concentration of acute phase proteins has been used as the basis of a commercial pregnancy test in the bitch. Concentrations of these proteins (including fibrinogen and C-reactive protein) increase from approximately 25 days onwards. The test is reliable, although these proteins are also released in inflammatory conditions such as pyometra.
- **Ultrasound examination**. Diagnostic B-mode ultrasound is now commonly used for pregnancy diagnosis (Fig. 18.12). The technique is non-invasive and without risk to the pups, dam or veterinary surgeon. The bitch can be examined in the standing position with minimal restraint.

    With ultrasound it is possible to diagnose pregnancy as early as 16 days after ovulation, although because in most cases this time is not known it is prudent to wait until 28 days after mating. At this time the fluid-filled conceptuses can easily be imaged, and embryonic tissue can be identi-

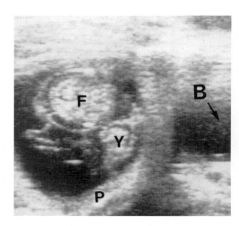

Fig. 18.12 Ultrasound image of a pregnant bitch. F = fetus, Y = yolk sac, B = bladder

fied. It is possible to assess the number of conceptuses, however, this can be inaccurate, especially when the litter size is large. Movement of the fetal heart can be seen ultrasonographically and this confirms fetal viability. It is possible to examine the bitch at any time after day 28 to diagnose pregnancy and to confirm fetal viability and growth. With later examinations it is less easy to estimate the number of pups.

The domestic queen

The average length of pregnancy in the queen is 65 days with a range of 64–68 days. The clinical signs of pregnancy include increased bodyweight and abdominal enlargement (these signs are often apparent in all but young queens) and mammary development which is obvious from approximately day 40. These changes are usually diagnostic for pregnancy, since pseudopregnancy is not common and is not usually associated with clinical signs.

During the second half of pregnancy there is an increase in food intake and in the requirement for both carbohydrate and protein. Provided that the diet is well balanced and contains suitable amounts of vitamins and minerals, it is not necessary to provide extra supplementation.

Many queens continue to be active during pregnancy; the amount of exercise is best limited by the individual cat. It is advisable to ensure that routine vaccination has been performed prior to mating.

Pregnancy diagnosis in the queen

- **Abdominal palpation**. Conceptual swellings can be palpated from approximately 21 days after mating. These are discrete until 30 days after mating but then become more difficult to palpate from this time onwards.
- **Identification of fetal heart beats**. In late pregnancy the fetal heart beats may be auscultated using a stethoscope; however, at this time it is usually possible to palpate the fetus in all but the most obese cats.
- **Radiography**. From day 30 it is possible to detect uterine enlargement with good-quality radiographs. Mineralisa-

tion of the fetal skeleton is detectable radiographically from 40 days after mating.

- **Hormone tests**. Plasma concentrations of progesterone are elevated in both pregnancy and pseudopregnancy, therefore measurement of this hormone is not diagnostic. Plasma relaxin concentrations are elevated from day 25; this hormone is diagnostic of pregnancy and can be measured as described for the bitch.
- **Ultrasound examination**. Diagnostic B-mode ultrasound may be used for pregnancy diagnosis in the cat. The pregnancy length can be assessed from mating time, unlike the bitch. Conceptuses can be imaged from 12 days after mating, and embryonic tissue can usually be seen from day 14. From this time onwards it is possible to identify pregnancy, confirm fetal viability and assess fetal growth. It is more difficult to assess the number of kittens in later pregnancy.

Abnormalities of pregnancy

A great concern for owners is the risk of **resorption** or **abortion** during pregnancy. To understand the differences in these processes it is necessary to define the stages of development:

- In general, the term **embryo** is used when the characteristics of the pup are not discernable.
- From approximately 35 days after ovulation the characteristics of the pup become obvious and the term **fetus** is used.
- **Resorption** refers to the resorption of the entire conceptus and occurs during the embryonic stage of development.
- **Abortion** refers to the expulsion of the fetus and the fetal membranes before term (i.e. before 58 days after ovulation).
- A **stillbirth** is the expulsion of the fetus and fetal membranes after day 58 (i.e. close to term).

The incidence of resorption or abortion of the entire litter is not known, although it is certain that up to 5% of bitches suffer isolated resorption of one or two conceptuses with continuation of the remaining pregnancy.

There are many potential causes of resorption/abortion, which include infectious agents, trauma, fetal defects and maternal environment. In the dog the infectious agents *Brucella canis* (not present in the UK), canine distemper virus, canine herpes virus and *Toxoplasma gondii* infection have all been implicated as causes of abortion and resorption. In the cat, feline herpesvirus I, feline panleukopaenia virus, feline leukaemia virus, feline infections peritonitis virus and *Toxoplasma gondii* infection may produce abortion, resorption or stillbirths.

In many cases embryonic death and pregnancy loss is best assessed using real-time diagnostic B-mode ultrasound. Resorption may be unrecognised by the owner unless it is associated with a period of illness. Abortion of fetal tissue may be obvious but may not be noticed should the dam eat the aborted material. In the face of an abortion there is little except supportive therapy that can be administered to the patient.

Pregnancy hypoglycaemia has been reported in the bitch and is associated with reduced blood glucose concentrations during late pregnancy. The clinical signs include weakness that may progress to coma.

The condition may be confused with hypocalcaemia, which occurs at a similar time (see later).

Parturition

Preparation for parturition

In the last few weeks of pregnancy, attempts should be made to encourage the bitch or queen to accept a nest in a suitable place. This ideally should be a warm, clean, draught- and damp-proof room, which can be heated. The room is best isolated from the main thoroughfare of the household, where the bitch or queen can rest quietly, into which a whelping or kittening bed can be placed. Ideally the bed should be large enough to allow the dam to stretch and have sufficient room for a large litter. The sides should be high enough to prevent the puppies or kittens escaping until they are approximately 4 weeks old.

In some cases, particularly with very hairy dogs, it might be useful to remove some of the hair from around the perineum and ventral abdomen, prior to the whelping. This will help the puppies gain access to the nipples and allows cleaning of the dam after parturition.

The environment in which the litter is to be born, and ultimately to be reared, is especially important. Hypothermia is a major cause of neonatal mortality and so the environmental temperature is critical. Neonates are unable to regulate their own temperature for the first week of life and therefore rely on the dam and other neonates to keep warm. A chilled neonate will not respond normally, move properly or be able to suck, which may then result in the dam neglecting it. It is therefore recommended that the whelping/kittening area must be able to be heated to 25–30°C for the first few days of the neonates' life. This temperature is often unbearable for the dam and so can be safely reduced to approximately 22°C after this time. It is most important that the litter is kept well away from any draughts that might chill them.

The room can easily be heated using a thermostatically controlled heater, or underfloor heating. A heat lamp can be suspended over the bed, but care must be taken to ensure that the neonates don't overheat. It is recommended that perhaps only half of the box is heated in order for the dam to move out of the heat if she wants to. Well-protected hot-water bottles or circulating water blankets also provide good alternatives.

The actual place where parturition and rearing are to take place are also important. Whilst it is important not to place the dam's whelping/kittening bed near a thoroughfare, it is beneficial for socialising the puppies/kittens, if noises from washing machines, radios and people talking can be heard.

The room should also be of a sufficient size to allow the growing puppies/kittens to play and where possible have access to an outside area, should the weather permit.

Useful equipment

A plentiful supply of newspaper is necessary for the whelping/kittening area, and plenty of bedding, that can easily be removed when soiled, should be available. Shredded paper can be used, but with care, since very small neonates may get caught up in it. If using a fabric bedding material, then at least three or four of these will be needed. A supply of blankets will suffice. A pair of weighing scales, clock and notepad are useful items to have to enable one to keep a record of times and weights of neonates being born. A thermometer should be kept in order to record the bitch's rectal temperature prior to whelping.

Sometimes dams can be clumsy at the time of whelping and if she is whelping a large litter, it may be useful to put some of the neonates out of harm's way in a small box within the nesting bed. It is important to ensure that the neonates are kept warm whilst away from their mother. This can be achieved by wrapping a hot-water bottle in some towels and placing it in the bottom of the box.

A supply of milk substitute can be offered to the bitch or queen during whelping/kittening. No food should be offered at this time just in case the dam gets in to difficulty and requires veterinary intervention.

There should be suitable equipment to facilitate the artificial rearing of the neonates if this is required.

Stages of parturition

In the last week of pregnancy it is prudent to record the bitch's rectal temperature at least twice daily. This is to detect the prepartum hypothermia that precedes the onset of parturition by 24–36 hours. This decline in body temperature is mediated by a sudden reduction in the plasma concentration of progesterone. The rectal temperature usually changes from approximately 39°C to below 37°C.

There are five stage of parturition:

(1) Stage of preparation.
(2) First stage of parturition (onset of contractions).
(3) Second stage parturition.
(4) Third stage parturition.
(5) Puerperium (after parturition).

The **stage of preparation** is associated with the decline in plasma progesterone concentration and hence the decrease in rectal temperature. At this time the vaginal and perineal tissue will relax and the dam may show some signs of impending parturition.

She may start to prepare her whelping nest, by shredding and ripping up the bedding. She will probably be more restless than usual. She may also show an increased mucus discharge from her vulva, which will probably be slightly more swollen. Some bitches may seek the company of others, while some will try to find solace in a quiet place on their own.

It is important to remember that some may show no signs of preparation at all. Few bitches will be happy with an audience for the whelping, so it is best if just one person stays with her at that time.

The **first stage of parturition** commences with the onset of uterine contractions and can be 1–12 hours in duration, although this is very variable between bitches. By this time milk is usually present within the mammary glands or should appear at this stage.

With the onset of contractions the bitch might become increasingly restless, pant and/or shiver and her nesting behaviour might become more frantic. Some bitches will refuse food at this time or may vomit their last meal. Most cats will seek seclusion at this time.

The uterine contractions will push the fetus against the cervix, which has begun to dilate, and this may result in the rupture of the allantochorion and allantoic fluid may then be produced from the vulva.

The **second stage of parturition** is characterised by an increase in uterine contractions initiation of abdominal contractions and propulsion of the fetus through the cervix into the vagina. Abdominal contractions begin when the first fetus enters the pelvic canal. These are normally quite noticeable. The bitch will appear to squeeze from her ribs towards the perineal area and then relax. The time of the first contractions should be recorded, in case there is any delay in the whelping. The time between the onset of straining and the birth of the first fetus is variable. It can be as short as 10 minutes or up to 30 minutes or longer, particularly in maiden bitches. If the bitch continues to have contractions for more than 2 hours without producing a puppy or her waters have broken and a puppy has not been produced, veterinary advice should be sought, as this could indicate **dystocia** (see below). Most bitches will be in lateral recumbency during whelping, but some bitches may prefer to stand. Delivery of the fetal head is often most difficult and may be associated with some pain, but once this is delivered the rest of the fetus is usually delivered rapidly.

A membrane, the **amnion**, surrounds the fetus. This is often seen at the vulva during straining. It may appear and then disappear with the contractions. This membrane may rupture spontaneously or be broken by the dam. The fetus may also be born within it. After delivery of the fetus, the dam will normally commence vigorous licking, removing the membranes and clearing fluid from around the neonate's face. If the dam fails to remove the membranes immediately after the birth, it must be done for her swiftly. Occasionally young or maiden bitches may need help and encouragement with the immediate licking and cleaning. This can be achieved using a clean soft towel. The neonate should be given a vigorous rub with a towel to stimulate it, help to clear the airways of any fluid and to dry it so as to avoid it being chilled. When rubbing a neonate it is best if it is held with its head lower than its bottom, to aid the drainage of fluid from its lungs, and not too high from the ground, in case it is dropped.

The birth of the fetus is usually followed by the passage of the **allantochorion** or **placenta** (afterbirth). Normally a bitch separates the puppy from the placenta by chewing through the cord and then eating the placenta when it is expelled. It is important to ensure the dam does not chew the umbilicus excessively as this can cause damage to the neonate. If the bitch does not sever the umbilicus, the placenta can be separated by tearing or cutting the cord using scissors. Care must be taken if the cord is torn. This can be achieved by holding the cord an inch or so away from the puppy's abdomen and tearing it with the other hand. A bitch should be given every opportunity to clean and fuss over the puppy, before it is removed for weighing and checking, etc. (see 'Examination'). Once all the procedures have been carried out, the puppy can be returned to the dam. The neonates are best left with their mother during the remainder of the delivery, as removing them might distress the bitch, inhibiting further straining. If the dam is young, inexperienced or particularly clumsy, it can be a good idea to put a few of the neonates in a warm box, once she has attended to them. This will keep them safer whilst the dam continues giving birth.

The **third stage of parturition** is the passage of the placenta. In the bitch and the queen the passage of the placenta occurs usually during the second stage of parturition, although, occasionally one or more fetuses are delivered without their placentae. These are expelled at a later stage or delivered with subsequent fetuses. It is a good idea to count the number of placenta passed as a larger number of fetuses compared with the number of placentae may indicate that the bitch has retained one or more.

After the bitch has finished whelping there is normally a dark-coloured vulval discharge present. This contains a green-coloured pigment that originates from the placenta. This discharge should normally decline after about a week.

The **puerperium** is the period after parturition during which the reproductive tract returns to its normal non-pregnant state. During this time the uterus starts its involution and it is common to see a mucoid vulval discharge that may last for up to 6 weeks.

Dystocia

The term **dystocia** literally means difficult birth; it is used to indicate any problem that interferes with normal birth. Dystocia is rare in the queen; however, problems are not uncommon in the bitch, especially in brachycephalic breeds such as the Bulldog and Boston terrier. The two main causes of dystocia are maternal factors and fetal factors.

Maternal dystocia

Maternal dystocia may be divided into two categories; poor straining efforts by the dam and obstruction of the birth canal.

Poor straining efforts of the dam Poor straining may be the result of nervousness or pain that inhibit normal parturition, but it is more commonly the result of poor myometrial contractions, a condition that has been termed **uterine inertia**. Inertia may be primary, in which case parturition does not commence, or may be secondary to some other factor occurring during parturition.

Primary uterine inertia is rare in the cat but is seen not uncommonly in young bitches with only one or two pups, or in older overweight bitches with large litters. The cause of the condition is unknown; however, it may relate to poor condition of the uterine musculature in fat or debilitated animals, overstretching of the uterus when the litter size is large, poor stimulus for parturition when there are only a few fetuses, or low plasma calcium concentrations.

The endocrinological events of parturition are usually normal; however, subsequent uterine contractions are not fully initiated and parturition does not follow. A green vulval discharge, which indicates placental separation, may be seen some days after the expected date of parturition. In some cases the owner may have observed initial weak uterine contractions or have noted the decline in body temperature. At this stage the administration of the hormone **oxytocin** may stimulate uterine contractions. Some cases may respond to the intravenous administration of **calcium borogluconate**. Repeated doses of oxytocin may be necessary but oxytocin should only be given when it is certain that there is no obstruction to the birth canal. However, it is not possible in the bitch to assess the patency of the cervix by digital palpation (the vagina of an average 20 kg bitch is 20 cm long). In certain cases, caesarean operation may be necessary.

Primary uterine inertia may be anticipated in some bitches because of a previous history of this problem or because of their age, physical condition or the number of pups. The best assessment of the bitch is to monitor the rectal temperature twice daily during the last 7–10 days of pregnancy.

Secondary uterine inertia is the cessation of uterine contractions after they have started. Most commonly this is the result of uterine exhaustion following obstructive dystocia but may occur spontaneously during second stage parturition, presumably because of factors similar to those seen with primary uterine inertia. If the cause of the dystocia can be relieved, the administration of oxytocin and calcium may be suitable treatments. In some cases, however, caesarean operation may be necessary.

Obstruction of the birth canal Obstruction may be the result of abnormalities of the birth canal, such as:

- **Deformity of the pelvic bones**. These may be congenital malformations, developmental abnormalities or the result of previous trauma, commonly following a road accident.
- **Soft tissue abnormalities within the pelvis** which press against the reproductive tract. They might include pelvic neoplasms, although these are rare in animals of breeding age. Abnormality of the reproductive tract itself (for example, torsion of the uterus or congenital vaginal or uterine constrictions).

Fetal dystocia

Fetal oversize   Oversize of the fetus relative to the birth canal may be the result of:

- **Breed conformation** (dystocia may be considered almost normal for certain breeds with exaggerated physical characteristics such as a large head size).
- **Actual fetal oversize**, when the litter size is small and large fetuses develop within the uterus.
- **Fetal abnormalities**, including fetal monsters, resulting in relative oversize and dystocia.

In the majority of these cases caesarean operation is necessary for the delivery of the fetuses, whether normal or abnormal.

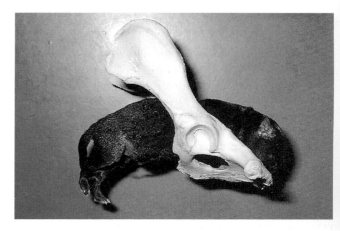

(a)

ORIENTATION OF THE FETUS

- The **presentation** of a fetus is a description of the direction of its long axis in relation to the long axis of the dam. Pups and kittens can only be delivered in longitudinal presentation (i.e. the long axis of the fetus is parallel to the long axis of the dam) but may have either anterior (fetal head delivered first) or posterior (fetus delivered backwards) presentation (see below).
- The **position** of a fetus is a description of its dorsal axis with respect to the dorsum of the dam; this describes the degree of rotation of the fetus. Most species are normally born in dorsal position (i.e. the back of the fetus is uppermost in the same orientaion as the dam).
- The **posture** of a fetus is a description of the orientation of the head and legs, which may be extended or flexed. For anterior presentation the head must be extended, and this occurs naturally during a posterior presentation.
- A **breech birth** refers to a fetus delivered in posterior longitudinal presentation, usually in dorsal position with the hind limbs flexed. This means that the fetus is presented 'bottom first' with its hind legs directed towards the dam's head (Fig. 18.13). A fetus delivered in posterior presentation with the legs extended is not a breech presentation.

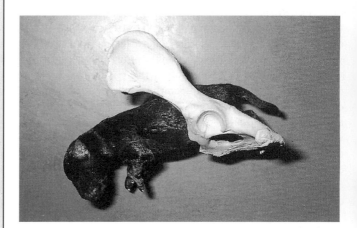

(b)

Abnormalities of fetal alignment   The normal presentation, position and posture of the fetus during delivery have been previously described. Variation from the normal disposition may result in dystocia. This may be corrected in certain cases by manipulation per vaginum; however, caesarean operation may be necessary.

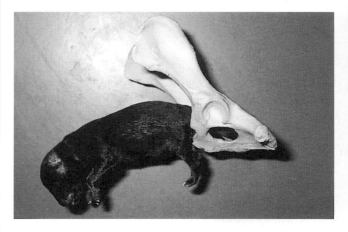

(c)

Fig 18.13. Presentations of a fetus. (a) normal anterior presentation (b) normal posterior presentation (c) breech presentation.

Recognition of dystocia

The normal events of parturition should be clearly understood so that recognition of dystocia can be achieved rapidly, thus allowing prompt intervention.

Collection of a relevant history is essential in the evaluation of a potential case of dystocia. This includes the estimation of the stage of pregnancy. Determining of the mating time is most helpful in establishing the stage of pregnancy of the cat, but this is not very useful in the bitch, where pregnancy length can vary between 56 and 72 days from mating. Regular monitoring of rectal temperature is therefore essential in the bitch. It should be established whether this has been done by the owner, and if so what changes were observed.

Of particular importance is the time-course of events from the onset of parturition, e.g. the onset of behavioural changes such as restlessness, nest making and panting. The time when straining first occurred and the character of the straining efforts may also be useful as an indicator of dystocia, as will the times that any fetuses were produced.

It is not possible to give definite guidelines regarding potential cases of dystocia but examination of the patient is warranted in certain situations:

(1) A bitch has exceeded 70 days from the last mating and has no signs of impending parturition.
(2) A cat has exceeded 65 days from the last mating and has no signs of impending parturition.
(3) The dam is unsettled and strains forcefully but infrequently.
(4) There are signs of straining which then cease.
(5) There is a black/green vulval discharge with no signs of parturition.
(6) There has been a decline in rectal temperature and parturition has not commenced within 48 hours.
(7) There has been ineffectual straining for 1 hour or more.
(8) Several fetuses have been produced, the last more than 2 hours ago, and the dam is restless.
(9) Several fetuses have been produced, the last more than 2 hours ago, and a larger litter is expected (may not be known by the owner).

Investigation of potential cases of dystocia

In most cases it is necessary to ensure that the animal is pregnant and/or that viable fetuses remain within the uterus. This can be achieved by transabdominal palpation, auscultation of fetal heart beats, real-time ultrasonography and radiography, as described earlier for pregnancy diagnosis.

Further investigation involves digital examination of the vagina to assess whether a fetus is present and to establish fetal alignment. This should only be performed after cleaning the vulval area thoroughly with an antiseptic solution and scrubbing the hands or wearing surgical gloves. A water-soluble lubricant should be applied to the fingers and the vestibule and vagina should be carefully examined. The presence of bone or soft tissue abnormalities of the pelvis should be noted. The presentation, position and posture of the fetus should be established before any further intervention is contemplated.

For normal presentations, delivery can be assisted using the thumb and forefinger placed in a cradle manner around the fetal head (anterior presentation) or pelvis (posterior presentation). Traction should only be applied during the straining effort of the bitch; however, pressure on the roof of the vagina with a finger may be applied with the finger to stimulate straining. Sterile gauze or similar fabric may help the nurse to grip the puppy or kitten when assisting delivery. Undue force should never be applied to the feet as these are easily damaged or deformed.

Caesarean operation

There are many reasons for performing a caesarean operation. In many cases this may be for the relief of dystocia, whilst occasionally it may be an elective procedure when there is concern over foeto-maternal disproportion.

Anaesthesia

It is important to remember that there are several marked physiological changes during pregnancy that may affect the requirements for anaesthesia. These physiological changes result in decreased minimum alveolar concentrations of anaesthetic gases, an increased oxygen requirement, and commonly hypoventilation and subsequent hypoxia and hypercarbia. In addition, in cases of dystocia the animal may be debilitated and may have recently been fed.

The general aims are to:

(1) Ensure adequate oxygenation (intubation and oxygen administration).
(2) Maintain blood volume and prevent hypotension (intravenous fluid therapy).
(3) Minimise depression of the fetus and dam during and after surgery (reduce the dose of anaesthetic agents used).

There are many anaesthetic regimes suitable for this procedure, they include the use of volatile agents for induction and maintenance of anaesthesia and the use of rapid acting intravenous induction agents (such as propofol) followed by maintenance of anaesthesia using a volatile inhalational anaesthetic.

Complications

There are several complications of caesarean operation in both species. These include:

(1) Anaesthetic risks in the dam and the neonate.
(2) Risks during surgery of uterine rupture and haemorrhage resulting in hypovolaemia.

(3)   Post-operative risks including wound infection and wound breakdown.
(4)   Interference with the wound by neonates trying to suck.
(5)   Problems in the dam of accepting the litter.

Some veterinary surgeons prefer to perform the operation via a flank incision to avoid the problem of wound interference when the neonates try to suck.

The problem of rejection of the litter by a young dam after a caesarean operation may be overcome by placing the offspring with the dam as soon as possible after surgery. The mother's milk should be squeezed on to the newborn's head if rejection is a problem. The dam should be carefully observed until she is able to coordinate sufficiently enough to not damage them and she must not be left unattended until successful sucking has been noted.

Post-parturient care

Care and management of the neonate

The first essential steps after birth are:

(1)   Establish a clear airway and stimulate respiration.
(2)   Cut the umbilicus.
(3)   Keep the neonate warm until active.
(4)   Encourage the neonate to suck.

It is essential that a clear airway is established as soon as a fetus has been born (or delivered via a caesarean operation). This involves removal of the surrounding fetal membranes and clearing of the mouth and nose of fetal fluid using either a dry towel or a small pipette. Gentle compression of the chest usually results in the establishment of respiratory effort. If this is not the case but the heart is beating, respiratory stimulation should continue by rubbing the thorax and removal of further fluid by gently swinging the neonate in a small arc (but this should be avoided unless absolutely necessary because of the risk of brain trauma).

In certain cases the administration of respiratory stimulant agents such as doxopram hydrochloride may be efficacious, as may the administration of oxygen. If respiration does not commence then artificial respiration can be attempted by blowing gently into the nose and mouth of the neonate. This should be done carefully to induce only slight lung expansion without overinflating the lungs. If the heart is not beating, external cardiac massage combined with artificial respiration may be attempted.

The umbilicus should be cut approximately 3 cm from the fetal abdomen; excessive bleeding can be prevented by the application of a ligature.

Once regular respiratory efforts are maintained the neonate may be placed into a prewarmed box or incubator until it is active when it may be returned to the dam and encouraged to suck. Sucking normally occurs immediately after birth and at intervals of 2–3 hours for the first few days.

Examination

Once the neonate has been born and the mother is sufficiently happy for you to remove it, it should be checked for abnormalities.

- The neonate's birth weight should be recorded. Normally the neonate will gain between 5–10% body weight per day and a failure to do so, may indicate poor health.
- The neonate should also be checked for congenital abnormalities, such as cleft palate or harelip.
- The umbilicus should also be checked for herniation. It should be clean and show no evidence of further bleeding. If the umbilicus is bleeding then this can be ligated, to prevent further blood loss.
- Respiration should be regular and even. The normal respiratory rate for a neonate is 15–40 breaths per minute. There should not be excessive noise. If there is excessive noise, this may indicate that the neonate still has fluid in its lungs and the appropriate action should be taken (see 'Second Stage Parturition').
- There should be no discharge from the eyes or ears. Any other birth defects can also be recorded now, as well as the neonate's colour and gender.
- The neonate's rectal temperature could also be taken and recorded at this time, but in reality this is unnecessary. The normal rectal temperature for the first week after birth should be 32–34°C.

Neonatal characteristic

Neonatal pups and kittens are unable to stand at birth. They should, however, be quite mobile, using their limbs to crawl. Neonates should be assessed for their general strength and the weakest should be carefully observed, since these do not feed adequately and may fail to thrive. Standing may be seen from 10 days from birth and most neonates should be able to walk at 3 weeks of age.

Pups and kittens are born with their eyes closed; separation of the upper and lower lids with opening of the eyes should occur by approximately 10–14 days after birth. The cornea at this stage may appear slightly cloudy, although this will disappear over the first 4 weeks. Many kittens are born with strabismus that persists until they are 8 weeks old.

Care of the litter

During the first few weeks of life the dam will take care of the needs of the litter. However, the litter should be checked regularly for signs of problems, ensuring that all of them are receiving an adequate supply of milk from the dam and that no one pup/kitten is missing out on feeding opportunities. There should be a plentiful supply of clean bedding available, so that the dam and her offspring are comfortable and not lying on soiled or wet bedding.

Normally the dam will lick the perineal region in order to stimulate the neonate to defecate or urinate and this should be performed for the first 2–3 weeks after birth. After this time the neonates will urinate and defecate voluntarily and therefore the amount of soiling in the whelping bed will increase and will require more frequent changing.

The litter should be weighed on a regular basis, usually weekly to ensure that all of the litter are gaining weight adequately. At 10–14 days the eyes of the puppies or kittens should open, and gradually they will be able to focus on objects. They will become stronger on their legs and begin to crawl around. At this time it is advisable to ensure that all the puppies are able to use their hind legs properly. Sometimes very large or fat puppies fail to get up on their hind legs properly and will haul themselves around on their front legs and bellies. If this becomes apparent then the pup should be checked to ensure there is nothing physically wrong with the legs. It should be encouraged to use its hind legs by placing a hand under the pup's bottom and pushing it on to its rear legs. This condition rarely persists due to the increased competition for food, but with a small litter it may become a problem.

Once weaning commences the dam may be less inclined to clean up their mess. The litter should be encouraged to soil away from the nest so that cleaning is more easily facilitated. This may hasten toilet training.

Care of the dam

Once the dam has finished whelping/kittening, she should be cleaned, paying particular attention to her perineum. This will make her feel more comfortable. She should also now be given the opportunity to exercise and urinate/defecate. Usually the dam will then settle with her litter during feeding. Soiled bedding should be changed for clean, fresh material.

The dam can now be offered some food. It must be remembered that depending on the amount of afterbirths she has eaten, if any, she may be prone to gastrointestinal upset. It is therefore recommended that for the first day or so she should be offered something nutritious but 'light'. Chicken, fish, rice and pasta are all suitable. The dam should be offered her diet in 5–6 small meals. This can be a pre-prepared diet specifically suitable for lactation or a well-balanced diet. The amount she receives should depend on the litter size. Obviously a bitch with a large litter will need significantly more food than one with only a small litter. The dam should, however, remain on 5–6 small meals per day for the first few weeks. It should also be remembered that the diet should not be altered too quickly as this may worsen any gastrointestinal upset.

Normally a veterinary surgeon should be called to examine the dam when parturition is finished in order to check her health and that of her newborn litter.

During the first 2 weeks, after the birth of the litter, the dam will spend much of her time with the litter and therefore it may be preferable to feed the dam close to the whelping/kittening bed. A readily accessible supply of fresh water should be close by. Once weaning begins, the dam should be encouraged to leave the nest for increasingly longer periods.

The dam should be encouraged to exercise during lactation, but where possible, this should be close to the house and where she will not come into contact with other animals, due to the risk of taking infection back to the litter.

Once weaning has begun and is well under way, the demands on the dam start to reduce and therefore her relevant food intake should also gradually begin to lessen. Obviously, if the dam has lost a great deal of weight through her efforts to feed the litter, then her food intake should remain high so she can replace some of the lost bodyweight. Once she has regained some weight her food intake can then be reduced.

The dam's general health should also be closely monitored throughout lactation. Common problems to look for are signs of **eclampsia** (see later), **mastitis** (see later), pyrexia, and a foul smelling vulval discharge. If any of these are observed, veterinary attention should be sought. The litter should also be closely monitored for fading pups/kittens.

Periparturient abnormalities

There are several conditions that may occur during late pregnancy or soon after parturition in both the domestic bitch and queen. Certain conditions are emergencies and prompt recognition of the clinical signs is essential to allow successful treatment.

Hypocalcaemia (eclampsia, puerperal tetany)

Low plasma concentrations of calcium are related to calcium loss in the milk and poor dietary calcium availability. The condition is most commonly seen during late pregnancy or early lactation. It is rare in the cat. The clinical signs include restlessness, panting, increased salivation and a stiff gait that may progress to muscle fasciculations, pyrexia and tachycardia. If untreated, tetany and death results. The slow administration of calcium borogluconate by intravenous injection produces a rapid resolution of the clinical signs. During administration cardiac rate and rhythm should be monitored. Calcium supplementation may then be given orally or by subcutaneous injection to prevent recurrence of the condition.

Placental retention

The retention of placental tissue is uncommon in both the bitch and the cat; however, it causes great concern for many owners. Placentae are normally delivered following each pup or kitten and may be quickly eaten by the dam. If a placenta is retained the clinical signs are a persistent green-coloured vulval discharge. This should be differentiated from the normal haemorrhagic discharge that may persist for 1 week after parturition (a mucoid discharge may be present for up to 6 weeks). If a retained placenta is diagnosed by either ultrasound examination or palpation, the administration of oxytocin is usually curative.

Post-partum metritis

Infection and inflammation of the uterus may occur following prolonged parturition, abortion, fetal and/or placental retention or obstetrical manipulation. The clinical signs commonly include a persistent purulent vulval discharge, lethargy and pyrexia. Treatment with broad-spectrum antimicrobial agents should be instituted immediately; fluid replacement therapy may be required.

Mastitis

Inflammation of the mammary gland is not common in the bitch or queen, although it may have disastrous results should the dam reject the litter because of pain on suckling. It is usually the result of bacterial infection following trauma (sucking). The mammary glands are tender, warm and firm upon palpation and the milk may be contaminated with blood and inflammatory cells so that it becomes yellow, pink or brown in colour. The dam may become lethargic and anorexic if the condition is not treated. Bathing and massaging the gland with warm water and gently removing the infected fluid may be helpful; however, antimicrobial agents are usually required. It should be remembered, however, that these agents will be excreted in the milk and ingested by the neonates.

Artificial rearing of neonates

In some circumstances it may be necessary to artificially rear some or all of the litter. Some instances are:

(1) Death of the dam.
(2) A large litter.
(3) A sick dam.
(4) A dam showing no interest in her litter.
(5) A dam with an inadequate milk supply.

Obviously, artificial rearing, where possible, is best avoided. In some cases it may be possible to foster the pups/kittens onto another dam, for example, a lactating bitch or queen that has just whelped/kittened and lost its litter, or one that has a pseudopregnancy at the time.

In the case of an excessively large litter, it may be possible to rotate some of the litter between artificial rearing and being reared by the dam. It has been suggested that just some neonates should be entirely artificially reared, rather than be rotated, although these authors do not advocate this method. In any case, the neonates should remain in the nest, with the dam, to ensure normal socialisation.

It is essential that all neonates should receive the colostrum from the dam to ensure an adequate uptake of immunoglobulins. If the dam has died, it may still be possible to express some colostrum from her, as long as it is not contaminated with drugs or toxins.

All the equipment for artificial rearing should be readily available and where possible should be included in the equipment acquired in preparation for parturition, so it is there if needed. There are several commercially available milk substitutes available for artificial rearing for both pups and kittens. It is important that the neonate receives the right formulation of milk. Cow or goat milk is not a suitable substitute, since their composition is very different from that of the bitch or queen. It is possible to make up a milk substitute, but this must have the appropriate lactose, fat and protein content and is time-consuming. It is better to make up a pre-prepared milk substitute. The milk should be warmed to body temperature (39°C) and be fed according to the manufacturer's instructions, bodyweight and age of the neonates.

Artificial rearing is both demanding and time-consuming, especially if rearing is done entirely without the dam. The neonates normally feed every 2–4 hours during the first 5 days of life, which then reduces to every 4 hours after day 5. Feeding can be achieved by using a commercial feeding kit, which contains a bottle and teat. This encourages normal suckling, but can be more time-consuming. The teat aperture should be large enough to prevent the neonate sucking in air but small enough so as to prevent excessive volumes of milk flowing through it. Feeding can also be achieved using a dropper bottle or syringe feeding. A 2 ml syringe should be adequate for the first few days. When using either of these methods, care must be taken not to rush the neonate, as this may result in it inhaling the milk rather than swallowing it, which may cause pneumonia.

In some cases it may be beneficial to feed the neonates by means of a stomach tube (orogastric tube) especially during the first few days of life, for rapid feeding or for particularly sick neonates. The procedure is relatively simple. A small 2 mm diameter piece of soft polythene tubing should be measured against the neonate's mouth and to the end of the level of the ninth rib. This length should be marked on the tube. The outside of the tube should be lubricated with a small volume of water on the outside.

The head is held in the normal position and the mouth is held just open using a finger and thumb; if the head is extended or flexed, passage of the tube into the trachea is more likely. The tube is directed gently over the tongue into the back of the throat. Swallowing greatly assists passage into the oesophagus; however, this is not essential. The tube can usually be seen on the left side of the neck as it passes down the oesophagus. There is little resistance as the tube is introduced into the stomach; the length of the tube is the best guide. Once in position, the syringe can be attached and its contents slowly injected into the stomach. The tube is then gently removed.

When artificial rearing has to take place entirely without the dam, the neonate is fully reliant upon you as its carer.

Neonates are unable to open their bladder or bowels voluntarily and normally the dam would stimulate the pup to urinate or defecate by stimulating their anogenital region. This would normally be done after feeding and in the absence of the dam this stimulation can be carried out by using a moistened piece of cotton wool. This should be performed every 2 hours.

Any spilt milk should be cleaned off the neonate, as during the early days this may result in chilling of the neonate. Once it is allowed to dry it will cause matting of the coat.

The orphans' only other need is to be kept warm and out of draughts. They should be maintained at an environmental temperature of 25°C.

Weaning

Weaning is a gradual process, which normally starts at about 2.5 weeks and will be complete by about 5 weeks. The neonates will still suck from their mother throughout the process, but once weaning has begun, the dam will normally spend increasingly more time away from her offspring. She should still be allowed frequent access to them during the day and will normally still spend the night with them.

Until the weaning process begins, the neonate is reliant on the dam for all of its nutritional needs, but once weaning has begun, each pup or kitten should be closely monitored for continued weight gain. Signs associated with undernutrition include crying, inactivity and poor weight gain.

Small quantities of food can be offered to the neonates on a finger, allowing the pup or kitten to lick or suck the finger. The range and volume of food can be increased as the neonates get used to feeding. The food offered can be of a proprietary brand specifically designed for weaning or cooked minced beef or rice pudding can be offered. Some pups/kittens will wean easily, taking solids and lapping straight away, whilst others may take longer. It is therefore especially important to treat each pup/kitten individually and be patient.

Neonates being weaned directly from the dam will gradually increase the amount of solid food being eaten and should be on 5–6 feeds per day by the age of 5 weeks. Neonates being hand reared will gradually have the volume of milk they receive reduced as the weaning process continues, in a similar manner as if being weaned from the dam.

Abnormalities of the neonatal period

A number of diseases may affect pups and kittens early in life. A certain percentage of neonates may die before weaning and it has been suggested that this can be as high as 15–20%. However, with good management systems (including the avoidance of hypothermia) the number of offspring lost should not be greater than 5%.

Fading puppy and kitten syndrome

The most common problem noted within the neonatal period is that of fading puppies or kittens. Most commonly, neonates die when less than 1 week of age. There are numerous factors associated with this loss; however, most commonly it is the inherent susceptibility of the newborn that results in its ultimate demise. Neonates have poor mechanisms of thermoregulation, fluid and energy balance, are immunologically incompetent and may have abnormal lung surfactant composition. When combined with poor management regimes and poor mothering behaviour of the dam, the risk of neonatal mortality can be high. Approximately 50% of neonatal deaths can be attributed to (i) infection, (ii) maternal and management-related deficiencies, (iii) low birthweight, and (iv) congenital abnormalities.

Neonatal septicaemia

The inherent vulnerability of the neonate puts it at risk for colonisation by a number of bacterial agents. This may result in a rapid death with very few initial clinical signs. However, in some circumstances, ill-health results in frequent crying, restlessness, and hypothermia, and this progresses to clinical signs of diarrhoea and/or dyspnoea with resultant dehydration or cyanosis, and ultimately death. In certain circumstances some neonates are more chronically affected and fail to grow as expected prior to the onset of obvious clinical disease. The majority of passive immunity follows from the intake of colostrum, and gut transfer occurs only during the first 48 hours of life. It is vital, therefore, to ensure an adequate intake of colostrum to protect against these organisms.

Regardless of the cause, rapid and aggressive treatment using intravenous fluid therapy, oral electrolytes, broad-spectrum antimicrobial agents and oxygen administration is essential. Despite such treatment the mortality rate can be high.

Neonatal viral infection

Viral infections are not common in the neonate, especially when vaccination programmes are practised in the adult. Maternally derived antibody frequently provides protection for several weeks.

Canine herpes virus may result in the birth of congenitally infected pups that are weak and die soon after birth.

In the queen, feline immunodeficiency virus and feline leukaemia virus can both infect kittens transplacentally as well as perinatally, and result in neonatal death after a few weeks of age. Neonatal deaths and the birth of kittens with cerebellar hypoplasia are not uncommon following infection with feline panleukopaenia virus during pregnancy. Feline infectious peritonitis virus has also been implicated in cases of upper respiratory tract disease and fading kitten syndrome.

Congenital abnormalities

Congenital abnormalities are those abnormalities that are present at birth. Common problems include cleft palate where there is failure of the normal fusion of the palatine arches. The defect may occur anywhere along the length of the hard or soft palate, although most commonly it arises caudal to the incisor ridge. The defect is common in certain breeds and it has been suggested that it is a trait inherited either in a recessive or polygenic manner. In most cases euthanasia of the neonate with this problem is advisable because of the problems of sucking and aspiration of milk.

There are many other congenital abnormalities that may affect each organ system, such as hernias, fetal monsters, hydrocephalus, microphthalmus, flat puppies (swimmers), congenital heart disease and atresia of the terminal rectum. A thorough clinical examination of each pup after birth should allow these abnormalities to be readily detected.

KEY POINTS

Understanding of normal reproductive physiology is important so that advice on the management of breeding, investigation of infertility and management of parturition can be sensible and appropriate.

- Reproductive physiology in the dog and cat differs significantly from other mammals.
- Advice on the control of breeding is essential to help prevent the later destruction of unwanted animals.
- The commonest cause of infertility is managemental and relates to a misunderstanding of the normal physiology of reproduction.
- Diagnosis of pregnancy is important to enable suitable management regimens to be established and also if the litter size is determined as a warning to the possibility of uterine inertia.
- Careful monitoring and nursing care during and after parturition is essential to facilitate survival of neonates.

Further reading

England, G. C. W. (1998) *Allen's Fertility and Obstetrics in the Dog*, 2nd edn, Blackwell Scientific Publications, Oxford.

Hoskins, J. D. (1995) *Veterinary Pediatrics: Dogs and Cats from Birth to Six Months*, 2nd edn, W. B. Saunders, Philadelphia.

Jackson, P. G. G. (1995) *Handbook of Veterinary Obstetrics*, W. B. Saunders, London.

Simpson, G. M., England, G. C. W. and Harvey, M. J. (1998) *Manual of Small Animal Reproduction and Neonatology*, BSAVA Publications, Cheltenham.

19

Surgical nursing

D. Anderson and *J. Smith*

Learning objectives

After studying this chapter, students should be able to:

- Describe the basic physiology and treatments of surgical diseases.
- Describe the physical signs of normal and delayed healing of tissues and wounds.
- Provide information to the owner on the post-operative nursing care required for surgical diseases.
- Discuss the common complications and nursing requirements of surgical diseases

---

Physiology of surgical nursing

Inflammation

Inflammation may be a normal **physiological** response to injury or irritant, or part of a **pathological** process causing disease. An inflammatory response will be present as part of the healing process, but then persist for longer than expected if disease develops. For example, the redness and swelling of the inflammation seen along the line of a surgical incision over the first 2–3 days post surgery are normal. If the animal licks at the sutures or the surgical incision becomes infected, the inflammation will persist and then would be considered

---

The **cardinal signs** of inflammation are:

- Redness.
- Swelling.
- Heat.
- Pain.
- Loss of normal function of the tissue.

---

part of a pathological response to continued injury.

These signs of inflammation have been recognised for 2000 years. The redness, heat and swelling are due to an increase in the blood flow to the tissue. Swelling occurs as white blood cells and protein-rich fluid leave the blood vessels and accumulate in the tissue. Pain is due to stimulation of the nerve endings in the tissue as a response to the increased pressure because of the swelling, as well as inflammatory mediators and toxins released by the cells in the area. This fluid is known as **inflammatory exudate** and is an important part of the inflammatory process.

Inflammatory exudate serves a number of functions:

- Dilution of irritant substances in the tissues.
- Delivery of immune cells to the tissues.
- Delivery of immunoglobulins and other immune response substances.
- Delivery of fibrinogen into the area to help with 'walling off' of the inflamed site.
- Initiation of the response to injury and start of the healing process.

However, the inflammatory response can also lead to loss of function either due to destruction of the tissue (e.g. destruction of cartilage in erosive arthritis) or just due to muscle spasm and pain.

Acute inflammation

Acute inflammation is the immediate and rapid response to injury. In ideal circumstances where the injury is self limiting, the inflammation should settle down very quickly, i.e. within 2–3 days.

There can be systemic signs of acute inflammation including:

- Fever.
- Increased pulse rate.
- Increased circulating white blood cells, particularly polymorphonuclear leucocytes (PMNL).

In most circumstances, the acute inflammation resolves quickly once the injury is repaired or the initiating factor is eliminated. However, where inflammation persists, it may become chronic, and pathological (Table 19.1).

Chronic inflammation

Chronic inflammation refers to the fact that the inflammatory response has gone on for longer than expected – maybe weeks or months. These changes in the tissue may become irreversible and affect the normal function of the tissue permanently. The main difference in the tissue is that instead of PMNL, a mononuclear cell population is seen together with proliferation of fibroblasts. There are three common situations where the inflammation persists and chronic inflammation results:

Outcome	Notes
Resolution	No significant tissue injury
Healing	Tissues are slowly regenerated or repaired
Abscessation	An accumulation of pus which persists in a walled off cavity
Degeneration	Damaged cells degenerate and are not repaired
Mineralisation	Calcified deposits are laid down in soft tissues in response to chronic inflammation
Necrosis	Cell death occurs and the affected tissue is sloughed. Particularly seen in the skin or intestinal epithelium in response to severe inflammation
Gangrene	Cell death is associated with loss of the local blood supply and putrefaction of the tissues by anaerobic bacteria

Table 19.1 Outcome of inflammation in tissues

- Persistent low grade infections, e.g. intracellular organisms or fungi.
- Prolonged exposure to foreign material, e.g. suture material.
- Autoimmune diseases – in these diseases, the inciting cause is the animal's own tissues and treatment aims to reduce the inflammatory response rather than remove the cause.

Inflammation of specific tissues

Inflammation of certain tissues has specific names (Table 19.2). The same basic processes occur, with production of fluid, swelling, oedema, increased blood supply and sometimes increased pain. For example, inflammation of the pancreas (pancreatitis) results in oedema and reddening of the pancreas with severe cranial abdominal pain. Peritonitis has been likened to an 'internal burn' as the peritoneum may become bright red, and produce large amounts of abdominal fluid.

Treatment of acute inflammation

The aims of treatment of inflammation are to remove the inciting cause and to prevent the development of chronic inflammation or long-term disease.

Removal of the inciting cause may be as simple as **lavage** (washing away) of debris or chemicals, or treatment of a bacterial infection with antibiotics. In the early stages, inflammation can sometimes be reduced by using **cold compresses** to reduce blood flow and thereby reduce swelling. Rapid treatment of burns (within 20 minutes) with cold water can reduce the extent of the injury by dissipating the heat and reducing the inflammatory response around the edge of the burn.

Sometimes, it is necessary to limit the inflammatory response, and drugs can be used. Drugs can reduce the inflammation and often have a secondary analgesic effect due to reduced stimulation of nerve endings and reduction of swelling. The commonly used drugs are corticosteroids and non-steroidal anti-inflammatories (**NSAIDs**). These two groups of drugs have potential toxic side effects; they should

never be used together and are only used under the direction of a veterinary surgeon.

Fluid accumulation

Fluid can accumulate in tissues or in body spaces as part of a pathological process or as a response to injury and often is part of the inflammatory response. Analysis of the fluid is necessary in order to make a diagnosis of the disease process causing the fluid to accumulate.

Types of body fluid

- **Exudate** is the term used to describe inflammatory fluid that contains white blood cells and proteinaceous debris.
- **Blood** may accumulate in body cavities after organ haemorrhage or in tissue planes.
- **Serosanguinous exudate** is fluid that has the appearance of blood, but on analysis has a lower packed cell volume (PCV) than blood and other inflammatory cells predominate.
- **Transudate** is fluid that has shifted across semi-permeable membranes and is largely acellular. It may accumulate due to loss of osmotic pressure (proteins in the circulating blood) or increased venous pressure.
- **Modified transudate.** When a transudate has been in the body cavity for a while, it causes irritation in its own right and some cells start to move into the transudate as part of the inflammatory response.
- **Physiological fluid in an inappropriate space (e.g. urine, bile, chyle, saliva).** The body produces some fluids that should always travel out through lined ducts; if there is a leak in the system, large volumes of these fluids may be identified in inappropriate spaces such as free urine or bile in the abdomen.

Fluid-filled mass

Fluid-filled masses are often identified as part of investigation of disease, and they are differentiated according to the type of fluid within:

Table 19.2 Surgical terminology

Terminology	Meaning
General terms	
Prognosis	The prognosis is an indication of whether the animal is likely to survive the procedure – or at least how long the disease is likely to be controlled. For example a poor prognosis suggests that the animal will die fairly soon despite treatment, whereas an excellent prognosis suggests that the disease may be cured
Post-operative morbidity	This refers to the degree of complications that the animal may be expected to suffer after the surgery. High morbidity would suggest that an animal will need a lot of nursing care (e.g. paraplegics), whereas low morbidity suggests that the animal is expected to make a rapid and full recovery
Emergency surgery	Surgery that is performed immediately as a life-saving procedure despite increased anaesthetic and recovery risks in the ill patient
Elective surgery	Surgery that is planned and can be performed at a time convenient to the veterinary surgeon or owner
Stay sutures	These are long lengths of suture material temporarily placed in tissue so as to hold the tissue without causing bruising during surgery. Usually, the ends are held together with artery forceps and these used as 'handles' to manipulate the tissue
Temporary openings	The suffix -**otomy** denotes a procedure for temporarily opening or dividing tissue during surgery. The tissue is then repaired to allow it to heal normally

Laparotomy or celiotomy	A temporary opening into the abdomen. These are the standard terms of abdominal surgery. These terms can be further defined by identifying the site of the incision:
	    midline (linea alba)
	    paramedian (slightly to one side of the midline)
	    parapreputial (to one side of the prepuce)
	    paracostal (caudal and parallel to the last rib)

Thoracotomy	A temporary opening into the thorax
Cystotomy	A temporary opening into the bladder
Urethrotomy	A temporary opening into the urethra
Nephrotomy	A temporary opening into the kidney
Hysterotomy	A temporary opening into the uterus (e.g. a caesarean)
Enterotomy	A temporary opening into the intestine
Gastrotomy	A temporary opening into the stomach
Tracheotomy	A temporary opening into the trachea
Rhinotomy	A temporary opening into the nasal cavity
Arthrotomy	A temporary opening into a joint space
Osteotomy	A temporary division of a bone
Tenotomy	A temporary division of a tendon
Myotomy	A temporary division of a muscle
Permanent openings	The suffix -**ostomy** denotes the creation of an opening or **stoma** which communicates with the outside through the skin. Usually a device is used to keep the stoma open, and then this is removed when the opening is allowed to close. Permanent stoma are sutured to the skin and allowed to heal open
Cystostomy	An opening in the bladder, to divert urine from the urethra, via a drain
Urethrostomy	A permanent opening in the urethra, to allow urination when there is an obstruction or stricture in the urethra distally
Jejunostomy	An opening in the jejunum, to allow feeding bypassing the stomach and duodenum via a special feeding tube
Gastrostomy	An opening in the stomach to allow decompression or feeding bypassing the oesophagus, via a tube
Pharyngostomy	An opening in the pharynx, to allow feeding via a tube, or placement of an endotracheal tube bypassing the mouth
Tracheostomy	An opening in the trachea, to allow the animal to breathe when there is an obstruction in the larynx or pharynx, or when it is important not to have the endotracheal tube in the mouth during surgery. The opening may be temporary via special tracheostomy tube, or it can be a permanent airway
Removal of structures	The suffix -**ectomy** denotes the surgical removal of all or part of a structure. Where part of a structure is removed, the remaining part must be sutured back together. The point at which the tissue is rejoined is called the **anastamosis**
Nephrectomy	Removal of a kidney
Cystectomy	Removal of part of the bladder wall
Enterectomy	Removal of a length of intestine
Colectomy	Removal of part or all of the colon
Pancreatectomy	Removal of part of the pancreas
Gastrectomy	Removal of part of the stomach
Splenectomy	Removal of part or all of the spleen
Cholecystectomy	Removal of the gall bladder
Ovariohysterectomy	Removal of the ovaries and uterus (spay)
Orchidectomy	Removal of the testes
Lung lobectomy	Removal of a long lobe
Tonsillectomy	Removal of the tonsils
Mastectomy	Removal of some or all of the mammary glands
Ostectomy	Removal of a section of bone
Inflammation of tissues	The suffix -**itis** indicates inflammation and or infection of that tissue. They may be chronic (long term) or acute (sudden in onset)
Uveitis	Inflammation of the iris of the eye

Table 19.2 (Continued)

Terminology	Meaning
Dermatitis	Inflammation of the skin. Specific terms may be used to describe the nature of the inflammation, e.g. pyoderma – an infected inflammation of the skin
Nephritis	Inflammation of the kidney, often called pyelonephritis to denote infection in the kidney
Cystitis	Inflammation of the bladder
Urethritis	Inflammation of the urethra
Metritis	Inflammation of the uterine lining. Pyometra denotes a concurrent infection of the inflamed uterus
Vaginitis	Inflammation of the vagina
Orchitis	Inflammation of the testes
Colitis	Inflammation of the colon – often referred to as 'irritable bowel'
Enteritis	Inflammation of the small intestines (i.e. diarrhoea)
Gastritis	Inflammation of the stomach (i.e. vomiting) Symptoms of vomiting and diarrhoea may be referred to as gastroenteritis
Pancreatitis	Inflammation of the pancreas
Hepatitis	Inflammation of the liver
Peritonitis	Inflammation of the abdominal lining
Pleuritis	Inflammation of the thoracic lining
Pneumonia	Inflammation of the lungs
Tracheitis	Inflammation of the trachea
Rhinitis	Inflammation of the nasal cavity
Gingivitis	Inflammation of the oral gingiva
Otitis	Inflammation of the ear. This may be the external ear canal (otitis externa) or the middle (otitis media) or inner ear (otitis interna)
Arthritis	Inflammation of a joint
Neuritis	Inflammation of a nerve or nerve roots
Conjunctivitis	Inflammation of the conjunctiva of the eye
Adenitis	Inflammation of a gland
Aspiration of fluid	The suffix **-centesis** denotes the aspiration of fluid or air from a body cavity. This may be necessary to collect fluid for analysis for diagnostic reasons, or it may be for therapeutic reasons
Cystocentesis	Aspiration of urine from the bladder. This may be to get a sterile sample of urine for analysis or to relieve pressure when the urethra is obstructed
Abdominocentesis	Aspiration of fluid from the abdominal cavity
Paracentesis	Sampling of abdominal fluid using a needle or catheter
Thoracocentesis	Aspiration of fluid or air from the thoracic cavity. Fluid or air are not normally present in the thorax, and this may be carried out as a life-saving procedure
Pericardiocentesis	Aspiration of fluid from the pericardial sac
Arthrocentesis	Aspiration of synovial fluid from a joint
Endoscopic procedures	The suffix **-oscopy** denotes examination via a specialised instrument. The endoscope may have an eyepiece or may be attached to a video screen for viewing more easily. The endoscope may only be used for viewing, or some will have attachments that allow removal of foreign bodies (forceps), biopsy samples, or even surgical procedures
Endoscopy	An examination of a body system using an endoscope. The endoscope may be flexible (fibre-optic) or a rigid tube with a light source and eyepiece. The instrument used may have special names: Bronchoscope (respiratory tract) Laryngoscope (larynx) Proctoscope (large bowel) Auroscope (ear) Ophthalmoscope (eye)
Cystoscopy	Endoscopic examination of the bladder
Proctoscopy	Endoscopic examination of the rectum and colon
Gastroscopy	Endoscopic examination of the stomach
Laparoscopy	Endoscopic examination of the abdominal cavity and minor surgical procedures, using instruments introduced via a separate opening
Oesophagoscopy	Endoscopic examination of the oesophagus
Bronchoscopy	Endoscopic examination of the bronchi
Thoracoscopy	Endoscopic examination of the thoracic cavity and minor surgical procedures, using instruments introduced via a separate opening
Tracheoscopy	Endoscopic examination of the trachea
Laryngoscopy	Endoscopic examination of the larynx
Rhinoscopy	Endoscopic examination of the nasal cavity. This may be carried out via the nares (normograde) or round the back of the soft palate (retrograde)
Otoscopy	Endoscopic examination of the ear
Arthroscopy	Endoscopic examination of a joint, and minor surgical procedures, using instruments introduced via a separate opening

- **Seroma** is probably the commonest fluid-filled mass encountered in surgical nursing. It is usually an accumulation of inflammatory exudate within the tissue underneath a surgical site. Some surgeries result in loss of normal tissue structure (**dead space**) and the spaces fill with fluid rapidly after the surgery. If measures are not taken to prevent this, then the fluid may take a long time to resolve or even need drainage.
- **Haematoma** is the term used for a 'blood blister' where a blood vessel bursts due to trauma or surgery and the blood accumulates in the surrounding tissues. It is important to differentiate between haematoma due to direct trauma (or surgery) and haematoma due to clotting defect or vessel wall abnormality.
- **Abscess** is an accumulation of inflammatory exudate that is full of dead and dying white cells (pus) in response to severe irritation or infection. It is usually walled off with a fibrous reaction (see below).
- **Physiological fluid leak.** Sometimes normal body fluids can leak into tissue planes and get walled off by the inflammatory response to form a persistent fluid-filled mass. A good example of this is the **salivary mucocoele** where saliva leaks from the salivary duct and forms a fluctuant subcutaneous mass.

Abscesses and cellulitis

Abscesses and cellulitis are a very common presentation of acute inflammatory disease in veterinary practice. When pyogenic organisms locate in a solid tissue they cause cell death and a strong inflammatory response. This leads to the formation of pus. If this is not localised, then it may diffusely distribute throughout the tissue and is known as cellulitis.

Abscesses are nearly always secondary to bacterial infection, and the pus is full of bacteria and dead bacteria inside white blood cells. However, an abscess can also be sterile when there are no bacteria involved but there is an accumulation of dead and dying cells and tissues within a fibrous capsule.

Within an abscess, there are often several stages of inflammation going on at the same time, with pus in the centre, an acute inflammatory response around this with PMNL reacting to the toxins produced in the pus and on the outside, a chronic inflammatory response with mononuclear cells and fibroblasts laying down a fibrous capsule. Sometimes the toxins produced by the abscess are not contained and they cause a **toxaemia** which makes the animal systemically ill. The toxaemia can be life threatening, causing pain, fever, vomiting, shock or even heart or kidney failure. Once the pus is discharged from the abscess, the systemic signs resolve and recovery is usually very rapid.

Abscesses that occur superficially, for example cat bite abscesses in the skin, often rupture spontaneously, releasing the pus through a hole in the overlying skin. Some abscesses occur internally, e.g. prostate, liver or peritoneal. If these abscesses rupture and release the pus generally throughout the abdomen, the consequences could be fatal.

Treatment of abscesses and cellulitis

Cellulitis is too diffuse to be treated except with systemic antibiotics, analgesics and anti-inflammatories, but abscesses can often be drained and this provides immediate relief from symptoms. Once the abscess is drained, the cavity collapses and the fibrous tissue granulates in and the hole heals over rapidly. If the diagnosis is not certain, a small needle and syringe can be used to aspirate some fluid from the abscess for analysis prior to treatment. Treatment of abscesses is most effective if done under general anaesthetic, but at the very least, sedation and analgesics should be administered prior to treatment, as abscesses can be extremely painful.

TREATMENT OF ABSCESSES
- Hot compresses can be applied to very superficial abscesses. The principle is to soften the overlying skin and encourage rupture of the abscess through the surface. The use of poultices containing boric acid is not to be recommended as they irritate the surrounding skin.
- Surgical drainage is a much quicker and more reliable way of treating abscesses. A hole is made in the skin at the most superficial point of the abscess using a scalpel blade. The pus is allowed to drain and the cavity lavaged with sterile fluids. The drainage hole should be encouraged to stay open for a few days either using a drain (see later) or by daily bathing with lavage of the cavity.
- Resection of abscesses: very deep abscesses or internal abscesses are not suitable for treatment by simple lancing. Deep abscesses may be dissected out around the fibrous capsule and removed in one piece. Internal abscesses may be either resected (e.g. a lung lobe abscess) or they may be suctioned out under sterile conditions and the omentum used as a natural drain (e.g. prostatic abscesses).
- Rabbits are a special case as they can get recurrent abscesses in the submandibular and cheek area. These are filled with a particularly thick type of pus that is very difficult to drain and remove. It is important to adequately open up the abscess in order to allow treatments for some days afterwards. Compounds that debride the inside of the cavity such as hydrogels or debriding solutions are often used to continue the cleaning process inside the cavity while it granulates. Sometimes the abscess is related to tooth root disease and this must also be treated in order to prevent recurrence. In some cases, there are multiple abscesses and it may be necessary to resect them.

Wound healing

Generally, acute inflammation of tissue is followed by healing. There are some basic processes that are common to all tissues:

- Removal of dead and foreign material.
- Clearance of the inflammatory response.
- Regeneration of lost tissue components if possible.
- Replacement of lost tissue components by connective tissue.

The different outcomes of the healing process depends on the type of tissue and the degree of damage, there may be **resolution**, **regeneration** or **organisation**.

Resolution

Where there is no tissue destruction and the inflammatory process is very mild, the tissue can return to its original state prior to the injury, e.g. a superficial graze.

Regeneration

The damaged tissue is completely replaced by proliferation of the remaining cells. This depends on the type of tissue, as regeneration can only occur if the lost cells can be replaced and if the connective tissue and vascular supply are still intact. Cells are classified in this context, into three basic groups:

- **Labile cells**. These cells can divide and proliferate throughout life. They are highly capable of regeneration, e.g. epithelial cells, blood cells and lymphoid tissue.
- **Stable cells**. These cells do not normally divide, but can do so in response to certain stimuli, and may divide following injury to the tissue, e.g. cells in the liver, kidney, endocrine glands, bone and fibrous tissue.
- **Permanent cells**. These cells only divide during fetal growth and are incapable of regeneration, e.g neurons, cardiac muscle cells and to some extent, skeletal muscle cells.

Organisation

Where the cells cannot repair the damage by regeneration, then the tissue heals by the formation of scar tissue, which is organised fibrous tissue with a large number of collagen fibres. Often this means that the tissue will lose its normal function, or be more susceptible to recurrent damage, e.g. scar tissue in skin (see later).

Most tissues heal by a combination of these processes, with some parts capable of regeneration and others forming scar tissue.

Skin is a good example of tissue that heals in the dermis by the formation of scar tissue (organisation) and by regeneration in the epidermis.

Normal wound healing in skin

The normal process of healing follows a predictable pattern that can be used to determine the progress of any healing tissue. There is always overlap between the phases as they progress from one predominant cell type to another, and they are not distinct.

- **Inflammatory phase**. After injury, there is an initial inflammatory phase triggered by activation of the platelets and fibrin in the blood clot, that in turn attracts neutrophils to the damaged tissue. The neutrophils will clear up bacteria, necrotic tissue and foreign material. They also release inflammatory mediators that attract macrophages into the tissue. Once the macrophages arrive, the final debridement process begins and the tissue starts to proliferate to repair the damage. The wound will look exudative, swollen and red during this phase.
- **Proliferative phase**. The proliferative phase is triggered by the macrophages, and involves fibroblasts that lay down the matrix of the tissue, endothelial cells that lay down new blood vessels and epithelial cells that migrate over the top of the wound to reconstitute the epidermis. This phase is the most crucial part of wound healing as it demonstrates that it is progressing normally. The classic appearance of this phase is the development of **granulation tissue**. Granulation tissue is bright red, very vascular and has a granular surface due to the capillary loops growing into the tissue. It is highly resistant to infection and is a sign that the wound is clear of bacterial infection. During the formation of granulation tissue, the wound starts to contract and this process alone can close a wound by up to 30% of its area. Gradually, the granulation tissue is replaced by collagen fibres and scar tissue is laid down.
- **Remodelling phase**. Once the proliferation and repair of the tissue is complete, the scar will remodel and strengthen over a period of days to weeks as the hair regrows and the fibroblasts rearrange the matrix of the tissue according to the tensions during normal function.

In a clean surgical wound in skin, the inflammatory phase should only last 24–48 hours, then a thin layer of granulation tissue develops between the edges of the surgical wound. By the time the sutures are removed at 7–10 days, the remodelling phase is well under way.

In larger skin wounds, the inflammatory phase may last longer due to infection or foreign material and the granulation tissue may not start to develop until at least 3–5 days. Depending on how large the wound is, the proliferative phase (granulation, contraction and re-epithelialisation) may take days to weeks to be completed.

Normal wound healing in other tissues

All tissues follow the same basic healing pattern as skin, with inflammatory, proliferative and remodelling phases.

Tendon and muscle injuries are often associated with trauma and other tissues may be simultaneously damaged, prolonging the healing process. The basic pattern is as for skin, but the remodelling phase is much more important as tendons and muscles have to retain function as well as strength. Muscle should heal quickly but may have to be immobilised to allow development of strength in the scar. Tendons take a very long time to develop strength and have to be supported and only gradually reintroduced to weight bearing otherwise they may stretch or rupture.

The gastrointestinal, urinary and reproductive tract tissues heal more rapidly than skin, with the fibrin clot helping to seal the wound initially, but the main support comes from the sutures for the first 3 days. The epithelium can regenerate and starts to close the wound almost immediately, with fibroblast proliferation giving the wound strength by 3 or 4 days after wounding. The urinary bladder heals the fastest and the colon the slowest. Normal healing in the gut depends on good nutrition and a good blood supply. Nutrition for the surgical wound comes from the lumen and feeding the patient will also stimulate blood supply to the gut and accelerate healing. This simple concept emphasises the importance of post-operative nursing and feeding of the patient.

Factors that affect normal wound healing (Table 19.3)

Normal wound healing in companion animals is fairly efficient. Most wounds are delayed in healing either because the animal has another undiagnosed disease or because the management of the patient is poor. Sometimes treatments affect the rate of healing and these may have to be modified until the wound is healed.

Summary

Inflammatory processes may be a normal part of the healing process but they can also be part of the pathology. Prolonged inflammation is usually a sign that the healing process is delayed. Responses to inflammation can aid in the diagnosis of the disease process. Some tissues can heal by regeneration, but others may have to heal by the formation of scar tissue.

Wounds

Classification of wounds

Wounds may be classified according to aetiology, depth of skin loss, contamination or infection, extent of soft tissue or bony involvement, duration since wounding and site. For example: 'An abrasive, full thickness, infected injury to the distal hindlimb with shear and fracture of the lateral metatarsal bone and loss of ligaments'.

It is important to know how the wound was incurred in order to determine the extent of the injuries and the expected progression of the wound. Some types of injuries affect the way in which the tissues heal and their susceptibility to infection.

Aetiology

There are 10 basic groups of aetiology of wounds:

- Surgical.
- Surgical wound dehiscence.
- Laceration.
- Puncture.
- Abrasion/shear.
- Degloving/ischaemic/skin slough.
- Burns – chemical, cold and heat, electrical.
- Ballistic/gunshot
- Crush injury
- Chronic fistulae/sinuses.

These general groups are distinguished by the degree of tissue trauma, contamination and associated injuries. Identifying the cause of injury helps in determining appropriate wound management and also in the expected healing time. Wounds that are heavily contaminated or with large amounts of tissue loss will have longer inflammatory phases and longer healing times.

Table 19.3 Causes of delayed wound healing	
Factors affecting healing	**Clinical examples**
Systemic diseases	Hypothyroidism, hyperadrenocorticism (Cushing's), protein-losing disease, renal or hepatic disease, diabetes mellitus, malnutrition, cachexia, cancer, severe cardiovascular disease
Wound management	Choice of wound dressing (primary layer), bandage technique, inadequate bandage protection, infrequent dressing changes, patient interference with the wound
Surgical factors	Prolonged anaesthetic time, wound infection, overly tight sutures, tension on the suture line, choice of suture material, poor surgical techniques, contamination of instrumentation or surgical site during surgery, inadequate closure or drainage of dead space. Foreign material left in the wound, including suture material may delay healing by increasing the inflammatory response
Therapy	Corticosteroids, antimetabolite chemotherapeutic drugs, radiotherapy

Degree of contamination

The only truly clean wound is a surgical wound; all other types of wounds can be considered contaminated or infected. The optimal time for treatment of an open wound is within the first 6 hours. This is known as the 'golden period' and the wound is considered as contaminated, but not infected:

- 0–6 hours – little bacterial multiplication.
- 6–12 hours – bacteria beginning to divide.
- Over 12 hours – bacterial invasion of tissues.

Viability and vascular supply to the tissue

Wounds may also be more susceptible to infection if there is associated tissue damage. Tissue that is devitalised (or necrotic) due to laceration or compression of blood vessels, is more likely to become infected. Surgical wounds are more at risk of infection if a tourniquet has been used and cardiovascular disease may also delay healing due to poor blood supply to the limbs. Shock can also result in vasoconstriction and if this circulation is not regained, then there may be reduced blood supply (and therefore increased risk of delayed healing or infection) to wounds in any area of the body.

Different types of tissue have a greater or lesser ability to resist infection. Well-vascularised areas of skin have good bacterial defences, and should heal well and resist infection. Tissue may become devitalised due to poor handling or desiccation during surgical debridement, which then increases the risk of infection or delayed healing.

Foreign material

All foreign material has to be removed before the wound will be able to heal, but the immune system can cope better with less irritant particles, such as sand, than with clay soil particles or organic debris.

> **CLOSURE OF WOUNDS**
> - **Primary closure (first intention healing).** Wounds that are closed surgically heal rapidly with a very short healing phase because there is little foreign material or bacteria.
> - **Delayed primary closure.** Some wounds that are contaminated are best cleaned and managed as an open wound for 1–3 days in order to ensure that there is no residual infection. These wounds are then closed surgically once the earliest signs of granulation tissue formation are seen.
> - **Secondary closure.** Wounds that are heavily contaminated, or where the surrounding skin is thought to be damaged, may be managed as an open wound for several days until it is possible to close the wound surgically. These wounds will
> have well-established granulation tissue filling the wound and it may be necessary to excise some of the granulation tissue in order to close the wound.
> - **Second intention healing.** In some instances, it is not possible or unnecessary to close the wound surgically, and it is dressed and bandaged until the wound heals. In these cases, the wound heals by **granulation**, **contraction** and **epithelialisation**. Large wounds may take weeks or months to close in this way, and during this time, the wound has to be regularly rebandaged. It is often more cost-effective and better for the patient to attempt secondary closure using a reconstructive technique than continue with second intention healing.

Management of primary closure wounds

This group of wounds covers all surgical incisions that are sutured, and will be the commonest wound management area that veterinary nurses have to provide advice on. Prevention of complications associated with surgical wounds relies on meticulous management in four main areas:

- Pre-operative preparation of the patient.
- Systemic or local wound factors that may affect wound healing (see above).
- Surgical technique and wound closure (see later).
- Post-operative management.

Pre-operative management of the patient

The general principle behind pre-operative management is that the patient should be as as healthy as possible at the time of the surgery in order to reduce post-operative risks. Therefore **elective procedures** may be delayed if, on the day of admission, the animal has another incidental condition (e.g. diarrhoea). Patients that have concurrent injuries should be stabilised as much as possible prior to surgery, particularly if a long operation is necessary. However, longer stays in hospital before operations also increases the risk of wound infection and breakdown. The specific reasons for this are not known, but it is probably due to increased stress during hospitalisation and the colonisation of the patient's skin with micro-organisms other than its normal skin commensals.

Skin preparation and patient preparation are important in reducing the bacterial load and therefore also the risk of inflammation and infection post surgically (see Chapter 21).

Prior to surgery, the number of micro-organisms on the skin should be reduced as much as possible. Very dirty animals (e.g. farm dogs) may benefit from a general bath with non-medicated soap to remove dust and dirt which might contaminate the wound – as well as the operating theatre! However with 'normal' levels of contamination, bathing makes no difference unless antiseptic solutions such as 4% w/v chlorhexidine are used. Generally, it is not necessary to bathe pre-op, and standard skin preparation is adequate.

Clean wounds do not generally become infected post-operatively. The risks of infection can be determined by classifying the type of surgery and using an appropriate antibiotic protocol peri-operatively (see later).

Hair removal

Ideally the hair is removed prior to anaesthesia after the pre-medication has been administered so as not to prolong anaesthetic time. This also allows for loose hairs to fall off prior to skin preparation. The clipping should always be done outside theatre so that the contaminated hair can be removed from the vicinity of the surgery. Depilatories and shaving have been shown to increase the wound infection rates, and so clipping is the recommended technique for the removal of hair. Coarse hair is clipped with a No. 10 blade first and all clips are completed with a No. 40 blade. The blade is held gently against the skin and run in the opposite direction to the lie of the hair. Lubricants and coolants are applied regularly to prevent overheating of the blade and it is important to ensure that the blade is sharp and has no missing teeth. Poor technique results in nicks in the skin, dermatitis and increased risk of post- surgical wound infection. A vacuum cleaner is often used to remove the loose hair from the patient and the table.

A minimum of 15 cm either side of the proposed incision site should be clipped. For reconstructive procedures, the whole side of the animal may need to be clipped. For surgery on the limbs, the whole circumference and up to or beyond the adjacent joint should be clipped.

Small exotic species of animal will have much thinner skin than dogs and cats, and extra care must be taken during hair removal. Although a No. 40 clipper blade is often used, variable high-speed clippers specifically designed for animals with fine hair are much better. These clippers make hair removal easier and cause less accidental cutting and burning of the skin. Preparation of avian skin requires feathers to be plucked rather than clipped, in order to ensure regrowth of the feather.

Skin preparation

The patient's skin can never be made completely sterile. The aim of pre-operative preparation is to reduce the bacterial count without damaging the skin's natural barriers to infection. First a **surgical scrub** solution is used which has antiseptic and detergent properties to degrease and kill bacteria on the skin surface. Second a **surgical antiseptic** solution is applied to leave some residual activity to kill bacteria that may migrate out of the hair follicles or sebaceous glands

during the surgery. For procedures that require particularly high standards of surgical asepsis for prolonged periods (e.g. specialist orthopaedic surgery), an adhesive impermeable transparent drape may be applied after the skin has been prepared. The surgeon then incises through the drape, which remains stuck to the edges of the skin incision, thereby protecting the surgical site from contamination during the operation.

Post-operative management of surgical wounds

When an animal is discharged, the owner should be given instructions for wound care, potential problems and when to seek advice. It is a good idea to explain the procedure that has been performed and to show the owner the wound before the animal goes home. Some surgeries will require specific instructions such as limited exercise, special diet, care of a bandage or physiotherapy. It is advisable that the owner is given *written instructions* on post-operative care so that there can be no misunderstanding at a later date if there is a complication associated with poor home care.

Immediate peri-operative care

At the end of the surgery, blood stains and clots should be gently wiped away using sterile fluid such as saline. Avoid wetting the surgical incision if possible. Agents such as hydrogen peroxide solutions may be used to help clean the fur, but should not be used on the peri-surgical skin as it may cause a dermatitis.

The main principles of managing a clean surgical wound are:

- Dressing the wound.
- Observation of the wound and patient.
- Prevention of self-mutilation.
- Suture removal.

Dressing surgical wounds

Surgical wounds are dressed if necessary for various reasons:

- To protect the wound from contamination or trauma.
- To protect the wound from self-mutilation.
- To absorb exudate from the wound.
- To limit movement of the wound to reduce pain, or tension on the sutures.
- To limit swelling of the surgical site.

Some surgical wounds do not require a dressing. Simple dressings consist of a non-adherent primary layer with a thin absorbent pad held in place by an adhesive tape. After 24 hours, this dressing can be removed as the wound will have formed a fibrin seal which is resistant to bacterial contamination. A commercial example of this kind of dressing is

Primapore (Smith & Nephew) which has a strip of non-adherent dressing with an adhesive edge to hold it to the skin. Spray-on dressings can also be used to seal the wound in the first 24 hours with a waterproof and gas permeable polymer layer.

In some cases, additional padding is required and a thick cover of absorbent material such as cotton wool or gamgee may be used which is held in place by tertiary dressings. Pressure bandages (e.g. Robert Jones) should always have substantial padding to prevent focal pressure points. All bandages should be replaced 24 hours after surgery to prevent the development of pressure injuries secondary to swelling under the dressing.

Wounds that are expected to exude heavily may need to be dressed more than once daily in order to ensure that the absorptive capacity of the dressing is not exceeded and the healthy tissues are kept dry and clean.

Monitoring of post-surgical wounds

Veterinary nurses are well placed to detect early signs of wound complications by careful observation of the surgical wound. If a dressing has been placed on the wound it may not be possible to directly observe the wound, but the skin surrounding the wound and the dressing itself can be observed.

The factors to pay particular attention to are:

- **Exudate** – note the amount, colour and type (serous or purulent). If exudate continues to leak through a dressing, the dressing must be changed to observe the wound.
- **Erythema** (reddening) – note whether this is limited to the vicinity of the sutures or whether it extends further. Has the erythematous area increased or decreased in size since the surgery?
- **Oedema** – note how severe the oedema is and whether it is increasing or reducing.
- **Haematoma** – note how severe the haematoma is and whether it is increasing or reducing.
- **Pain** – note the severity of the pain (a subjective score of 1–10 is sometimes helpful) and whether the pain is continuous, intermittent, only present when the wound is handled, or if there is no pain.
- **Odour** – Note if there is a foul odour from the wound.

In addition to monitoring the wound, good post-surgical wound care also involves monitoring the patient for any signs of systemic illness which may be associated with wound complications. Both subjective and objective assessments should be performed:

- **Subjective assessment** – note whether the animal is bright, alert and responsive or whether there has been a change in demeanour since before the surgery. Also note progressive changes in demeanour throughout the post-operative recovery phase.

- **Objective assessment** – daily monitoring of temperature, pulse and respiration rates, a note of appetite, defecation and urination should consitute the minimum daily assessment of hospitalised patients in the post-operative phase. In some cases, a more detailed clinical examination including other factors such as water intake, neurological reflexes or blood parameters may be necessary.

Prevention of self-mutilation

Self-mutilation at the surgical incision often leads to wound dehiscence. Some tendency to lick the wound post-operatively is seen in almost all animals, but persistent licking or chewing at the wound may be an indicator of wound complications. Animals may also lick or chew at the wound because of concern at the foreign material on the skin (the sutures) or due to generalised skin disease causing pruritus.

Dressings will help reduce self-mutilation, but a determined animal or young animals will soon destroy most bandages. Bitter sprays are available to protect either the bandage or the surgical site, but they are not as effective as preventing access to the wound altogether. The Elizabethan collar is one of the most useful and commonly employed devices to prevent self-mutilation. They are available as opaque or clear plastic and are placed around the neck secured by a collar or harness. They must be large enough to prevent the nose from reaching over the edge of the collar and accessing the wound. Scratching with the hind feet can be prevented using well-padded bandages on the feet, and other devices available include neck braces or body braces that prevent the animal turning round to reach the wound. Basket muzzles are helpful to prevent animals from destroying bandages, but they must be carefully fitted to ensure that the animal can pant and drink water through the muzzle. Owners should be warned that other pets may interfere with the wound by grooming or playing.

Exotic species may require some ingenuity to prevent them interfering with sutures. One alternative is to use subcuticular sutures so that there are no skin sutures to irritate the fine skin. Elizabethan collars may be made out of light card or plastic and splints can be made out of syringe cases or ice-lolly sticks. Care should be taken to ensure that the collar does not irritate the skin around the neck, and some species, e.g. rabbits, may 'freeze' on application of an Elizabethan collar and refuse to eat or drink. As it is important that herbivores eat as soon as possible after surgery, an 'anti-scratch collar' may be more appropriate in these situations (Hoyt). It may be difficult to protect a laparotomy wound in cavies or rodents where the surgical site is in constant contact with the floor. These animals should be housed separately until the wound is healed and the bedding changed to a non-powdery source such as shredded paper. The bedding must be completely changed daily to ensure minimal contamination of the wound with urine or faeces.

Removal of sutures

Sutures approximate the wound edges and this allows rapid first intention healing with minimal scarring. Sutures are removed as soon as the skin is healed and in most cases, this will be in 7–10 days. However, in some young animals, healing may be quicker, and in older animals, the sutures may be left in for a few extra days. Subcuticular sutures may be used to appose the skin edges using absorbable suture material where the surgeon does not wish to use skin sutures. In these cases, the wound should still be checked 7–10 days later to ensure that the wound has healed normally.

Reptiles are a special case, in that the sutures may remain in place until the next **ecdysis** (moult), as then the epidermis is more active and healing may be considered complete.

Complications of surgical wounds

The main complication of surgical wounds is **dehiscence** (the breakdown of a wound along all or part of its length).

FACTORS THAT INCREASE THE RISK OF WOUND DEHISCENCE
- Poor post-operative care of the wound.
- Infection of the wound.
- Seroma formation.
- Poor pre-operative preparation of the patient.
- Poor surgical technique.
- Poor suture technique or inappropriate suture materials.
- Decreased blood supply to the wound.
- Poor general health of the patient.

Infection is by far the commonest cause of dehiscence and may be caused either by the poor post-operative care or by the surgical preparation and technique.

Other complications of wound healing include:

- **sinus** formation – this is a late infective complication. It is usually a small blind ending tract lined with granulation tissue leading to an abscess cavity. Sinuses in surgical wounds are often focused around suture material or other foreign material inadvertently left in the wound at the time of surgery. Suture sinuses are often seen surrounding skin sutures if they are left in place for too long. They resolve on removal of the foreign material.
- **fistula** – this is an abnormal tract that forms between two epithelialised surfaces, or connects an epithelial surface to the skin. It can be a complication of wound healing, for example in anal or oronasal surgery. Occasionally it is seen as a congenital abnormality (e.g. rectovaginal fistula). Fistulae have to be surgically repaired.
- **incisional hernia** – this is a late complication of abdominal surgery where there is dehiscence of the incision in the

muscle layers, while the skin repair remains intact. Abdominal contents may herniate out and lie in the space between the muscles or under the skin. It should be repaired as a matter of urgency in case the skin ruptures and the abdominal contents become contaminated.

Management of contaminated or infected wounds

Initial assessment

First aid measures are important in the initial assessment of the injury:

- Take brief details on the duration and site of the injury.
- Assess bleeding and determine if arterial or venous.
- Arrest bleeding using a bandage or tourniquet if necessary.
- Cover the wound with a sterile dressing to prevent further contamination in the hospital.
- Assess the animal's general state of health; look for signs of shock.
- Assess the animal for other life threatening injuries.
- Provide antibiotic cover and analgesia, as directed by a veterinary surgeon and treat shock if necessary.
- Take a more detailed full history from the owner.

The history helps to determine the origin of the wound and the likely concurrent injuries. It will also determine whether the wound is classified as infected or contaminated.

Principles of management

The first stage is **decontamination** as far as possible, given the state of the wound and the condition of the patient. This also means prevention of further contamination in the hospital or by the animal. The second stage is **debridement** of necrotic or devitalised tissue and removal of any foreign debris. The final result should be control of infection and establishment of a healthy wound bed enabling closure of the skin deficit.

One of the important first steps is to clip and clean the surrounding undamaged skin. This not only helps to clean the wound, but also helps to assess the extent of the wound and viability of the skin. Ideally, the wound should be protected from further contamination, and so if possible, it may be closed using towel clips or a continuous suture. This is not always possible, so most wounds are packed with sterile swabs or filled with a water-soluble jelly (KY®, Johnson & Johnson) during clipping and cleaning. The jelly can then be washed away with any hair or dirt from the adjacent skin later on. The clipper blades must be properly disinfected and without chips that might cause dermatitis on nearby skin. Hair at the edges may be trimmed with scissors wetted with saline, or dipped in mineral oil. Thorough and wide removal of hair is important in keeping the wound clean during the next phases of management.

Lavage and debridement of wounds

The principles of wound lavage are to wash debris out of the wound, dilute the bacteria, and finally not to cause any further damage. It is therefore important to use large volumes of fluids and also not to lavage too vigorously. This may be achieved by using a 20 ml syringe with an 18 gauge needle or catheter attached to a giving set on a bag of fluids.

Gross contamination or necrotic tissue may be washed away with gentle tap water lavage using a hand shower. After this, the wound should be treated in a sterile manner to prevent further contamination. Not all solutions are suitable for wound lavage; substances added to a lavage solution may damage the host cells and delay healing (see Table 19.4). Although it is tempting to use antiseptic solutions for infected wounds, they do not stay in the wound for long and may delay wound healing. In general it is best just to use large volumes of sterile isotonic fluids to lavage wounds (see box). If antiseptic solutions are used, it is important to use the solution, rather than the surgical scrub, as the latter contains detergents which irritate the wound.

WOUND LAVAGE PROCEDURE
(1) Select at least a 1000 ml bag of sterile isotonic fluids.
(2) Attach a giving set with a three-way tap on the end.
(3) Attach a 20 ml syringe and an 18 gauge needle or catheter onto the three-way tap.
(4) Lavage the wound over a bowl or tray to catch the fluid using the 20 ml syringe to spray the wound surface.
(5) Keep refilling the syringe from the fluid bag until all the fluids have been used to clean the wound or the wound fluid runs clear.
(6) Carefully dry the healthy skin adjacent to the wound and cover the wound with sterile dressings.

Debridement of wounds is the next crucial step in wound management. Debridement involves removal of all infected, necrotic or contaminated tissue from the wound. This may be done in three ways:

- Surgical debridement.
- Primary layer dressings.
- Enzymatic debridement.

Surgical debridement
This is the best way to remove grossly contaminated tissue. The wound should be draped and prepared as for surgery and a scalpel is used to cut away necrotic or dirty tissue. The instruments and gloves/drapes may be exchanged for sterile ones as the debridement progresses and the wound becomes cleaner. Surgical exploration of the wound also enables visualisation of local anatomical structures, and to determine the extent of the wound.

Debridement dressings
These are used in the initial stages until it is clear that there is no residual infection or necrotic material. Debridement dressings should not be left on the wound for more than 24 hours and in some instances may need changes twice daily. There are three main dressing types available for debridement (see section on primary layer bandaging):

- Adherent dressings.
- Hydrogels.
- Hydrocolloids.

Other techniques
Commercial enzyme preparations can be applied to the wound to break down and allow removal of necrotic debris but they are stopped once the granulation tissue is established. Maggots have been used to debride wounds, allowing rapid establishment of healthy granulation tissue. Sterile maggots are produced commercially and are available at the correct larval stage for clinical use. They must be removed from the wound before they start to invade healthy tissue.

Table 19.4 Suitability of solutions for wound lavage

Solution	Concentration	Indications
Sterile saline	0.9%	Any wound – no tissue damage; no antibacterial action other than dilution
Lactated Ringer's solution	As supplied	As above
Chlorhexidine (Hibitane 4%)	0.5%	Contaminated or infected wounds – *S. aureus* often resistant. Toxic to fibroblasts. Residual activity good
Povidone–iodine (Pevidine solution: BK)	1%	Contaminated or infected wounds. Inactivated by debris, pus or blood. Broad spectrum, poor residual activity. Toxic to host cells
Hypochlorite (Dakin's solution)	0.125%	Toxic to cells. Irritant for 4–5 days after use *Not recommended*
Hydrogen peroxide	1–3%	No bactericidal activity. Very toxic to all cell types *Not recommended*
Cetrimide/chlorhexidine (Savlon)		Very toxic to cells. Irritant *Not recommended*

Antiseptics or antibiotics should not be a substitute for good surgical debridement. Debridement is the single most important step in the management of a wound and is often performed inadequately.

Management of secondary closure wounds

Principles of wound dressings

Wound dressings are usually applied to the wound in three layers; the primary, secondary and tertiary layers. The general construction of the dressing depends on the location of the wound and the function of the dressing.

Wound dressing functions:

- Absorption of exudate.
- Analgesia.
- Protection of the wound.
- Prevention of infection.
- Promote wound healing.

All dressings should be closely monitored by both the owner and the nursing staff for signs of complications. Poorly managed dressings will cause delayed wound healing and may cause further damage; dressings that have been applied too tightly to the limb can cause damage ranging from areas of skin loss to loss of the whole limb or even death.

REASONS TO REMOVE THE DRESSING
- Persistent chewing at the dressing.
- Foul smell from the dressing.
- Soiling or wetting of the dressing while on a walk or with urine.
- 'Strike-through' of exudate from the wound to the outside of the dressing.
- Slippage of the dressing from its original placement.

Primary layer

The primary layer is the material that is placed in contact with the wound itself. The principle behind the primary layer is that it should at least do no harm to the wound and at best, improve the rate of healing of the wound. There are numerous products available for wound dressings sold to a relatively poorly informed veterinary and veterinary nursing profession. It is important to realise that there is no perfect wound dressing, and by understanding the way in which the different classes of dressings work, the veterinary nurse should be better equipped to use these dressings appropriately.

Wound dressings should be considered according to their function, and knowledge of the normal process of wound healing enables the veterinary nurse to choose the appropriate dressing at different stages of healing.

The aim of the primary layer will include some or all of the following at different stages:

- Debridement of necrotic tissue – this may require rehydration, lysis of fibrin attachments and physical removal from the wound.
- Absorption of fluid away from wound – if the fluid is allowed to remain on the wound surface it can macerate the tissues or provide a reservoir for infection.
- Stimulation of granulation tissue – some dressings will actively promote and speed up the formation of granulation tissue.
- Promotion of epithelialisation – epithelialisation can only occur across healthy granulation tissue and is faster in a moist warm environment.

Categories of primary layer dressings

Wound dressings can be described according to their basic characteristics, although some dressings may fall into more than one category, or dressings may be designed so that they have more than one general function:

- Adherent or nonadherent.
- Absorbent or non-absorbent.
- Passive, interactive or bioactive (passive have no action on the wound, interactive respond to the wound environment in some way and bioactive have a biological effect on the wound).
- Occlusive, semi- or non-occlusive (this refers to the degree of permeability to gas or vapour of the dressing).

Adherent and non-adherent dressings Saline-soaked gauze swabs are often used as passive adherent dressings in the early stages of wound management for debridement of necrotic tissue. These are cheap to apply and very effective, but they may be painful to remove and can damage healthy tissue. They are often referred to as **wet-to-dry** dressings.

Passive non-adherent dressings are typically used over surgical wounds, skin grafts or granulation tissue. Perforated polyurethane membrane and paraffin gauze are commonly seen examples. These do not interact with the wound in any way, but prevent the secondary layers from sticking to the wound.

Absorbent dressings Sometimes, the secondary layer of the dressing is used to absorb exudate, but some primary layer dressings are specifically designed to absorb fluid and prevent it accumulating at the wound surface causing maceration of the tissues. Foam dressings usually have a semi-permeable membrane backing that allows absorption of fluid and some controlled evaporation so that the wound environment remains moist without being too wet. These passive dressings can be useful for exudative granulating wounds as they allow epithelialisation in a moist environment.

Wounds that are producing copious amounts of fluid can be dressed with ordinary disposable baby nappies. These can be weighed to calculate how much fluid the animal is losing.

Complex dressings   **Alginate** dressings are bioactive and interactive. They are sheets of a protein derived from seaweed, which release sodium or calcium when in contact with body fluids. This results in the stimulation of haemostasis and inflammation. They are used to stimulate the formation of granulation tissue and for haemostasis in low level bleeding. Once they are wet, they form a gel which keeps the surface of the wound moist. The disadvantage is that sometimes they cause the formation of excessive granulation tissue.

Hydrogel dressings are interactive, consisting of insoluble hydrophilic polymers. They are provided either as a sheet with a semi-permeable backing or as a gel. The hydrogel can rehydrate necrotic tissue, absorb exudate and reduce oedema. Where it is in gel form, a second primary layer must be put over the gel to prevent it from drying out and often the foam dressings are used for this purpose. It is useful where parts of the wound are granulating well and other parts require further debridement as the gel will not harm healthy granulation tissue. The disadvantage is that the debridement process is very slow, and the combination of dressings may be expensive.

Hydrocolloids are bioactive and interactive suspension of polymers in an adhesive matrix. They are usually provided as a sheet with an occlusive backing which prevents dehydration of the wound. They can both rehydrate and debride necrotic wounds and will stimulate the formation of granulation tissue. Because they are adhesive, they may prevent contraction of the granulating wound by sticking to the edges and sometimes cause exuberant granulation tissue. They should not be used in infected wounds, and need to be changed regularly, so may be expensive.

Topical wound treatments

- **Aloe vera ointment** actively stimulates the development of granulation tissue, but only if the very pure products are used.
- **Silver sulphadiazine ointment** (Flamazine®, Smith & Nephew) is a topical broad-spectrum antibiotic, with prolonged activity, and is the agent of choice for prevention of sepsis from burns.
- **Zinc bacitracin ointments** may enhance epithelialisation.
- **Malic, benzoic and salicylic acid solution** (Dermiso®, Smithkline Beecham) – this product has a very low pH and is a debriding agent, it is toxic to granulation tissue and should not be left in the wound.

Secondary bandage layer

The secondary layer of a dressing is used either to hold the primary layer in place, to provide padding to the wound underneath, absorb exudate or to distribute the pressure of the bandage evenly. The secondary layer is most commonly an **orthopaedic wool** which is available as rolls of viscose or polyester fleece in different widths. The bandage is applied evenly in a spiral with overlapping layers of 50% of the width of the material. If the bandage is required to distribute pressure (see Robert Jones bandage) then more substantial material such as rolls of cotton wool are used. For heavy levels of exudate, cotton wadding such as gamgee may be incorporated into the secondary layer. The secondary layer is then stabilised using a conforming stretch bandage. This layer is again applied evenly with 50% overlap of width, only slightly compressing the wool layer underneath. It is important not to overstretch the bandage during application, particularly over narrow points in the limb as pressure points may arise.

Tertiary bandage layer

The tertiary layer is primarily to protect the main functional layers of the bandage from soiling or mutilation by the animal. This outer layer is usually an elastic cohesive or adhesive bandage, applied in a spiral with 50% overlap of width. It is important that this layer is applied with even pressure as the layers cannot slide over one another to relieve pressure points when the animal moves around in the bandage. At the top of the bandage, this layer must not extend over the top of the secondary layer padding as it will cause chafing of the skin. Finally, adhesive bandages should not be used to stick the bandage to the bare skin or fur as an attempt to help keep the bandage in place. The bottom of the bandage may be covered with an elastic adhesive bandage to increase wear. In order to keep the bottom of the bandage dry, empty intravenous fluid bags or commercially available canvas boots may be used to protect a foot temporarily, but they should not be left on permanently.

Reconstructive surgery

General principles

Major reconstructive procedures are used when there is inadequate skin or other tissue available to close the deficit created by the surgery or trauma. Usually the surgical procedure is planned in advance, so that the patient can be prepared and positioned appropriately. The general principles behind reconstructive surgery include:

- The patient should be haemodynamically stable prior to surgery.
- The patient should be prepared for a long period of anaesthesia.
- A very wide area of skin should be clipped and surgically prepared to allow for moving skin around into the wound.
- The skin must be handled gently to prevent bruising that might damage its blood supply.

> Reconstructive procedures require good wound management in advance of the surgical procedure. Often the success of the surgery relies on the elimination of infection and foreign or necrotic material prior to surgery.

When an incision is made in the skin, or a skin deficit occurs after trauma, the elastic recoil of the skin makes the edges gape apart. When the skin edges are advanced to close the large wound, there may be too much tension on the edges, causing delayed healing or dehiscence. The skin of the dog and cat generally is extremely mobile and can be manipulated to close skin deficits, but by taking into consideration the tension lines prior to surgery, sometimes the problems associated with the recoil of the skin edges can be avoided.

Suturing skin

Sutures are used to appose the tissues together so that they heal more quickly. Sutures in the skin should *appose* the tissues and not cause eversion or inversion of the skin edges. Generally, absorbable sutures are used in deep tissues where they are not accessible for removal and non-absorbable sutures, which cause less tissue reaction, are used in the skin and then removed about 7–10 days after the surgery. Sutures should not be placed too tightly, particularly in the skin, which swells slightly in the first 2–3 days after surgery. Tight sutures may either tear out as the skin swells, or cause itchiness which encourages the animal to interfere with them. Finally, sutures that are placed too tightly may also constrict the vessels at the wound edge and delay wound healing.

Strategies to combat tension may be employed in most simple wounds, either as a single procedure or in combination. **Subcuticular sutures** are used to hold the dermis together so that the skin sutures do not have to be too tight. **Walking sutures** can be used which advance skin towards the centre of the wound, taking the tension off the main incision line. **Vertical mattress sutures** can also be used as tension relieving sutures to take the pressure off the incision line for a few days and then they are removed before the incision sutures.

Sutures and tissue responses to sutures

There are many different types of suture materials, all developed to perform different tasks in different surgical situations.

Suture materials are divided into two main groups: the natural materials and the synthetic materials. Within these categories, suture materials may be (i) **braided** or **monofilament** and (ii) **absorbable** or **non-absorbable**.

Suture materials are manufactured in different sizes. The metric gauge is the actual suture diameter in millimetres multiplied by 10. However, often suture sizes are referred to by the United States Pharmacopeia sizing which has a different figure for the same suture: e.g. 2 metric is the same gauge as 3-0 USP.

Suture can be purchased in individual sterile packets, which has a needle attached to the end of the material by a method known as **swaging**. This is the ideal way to use suture material as then it is known to be reliably sterile, the needle sharp and the material undamaged. Some suture materials are provided on a reel in surgical spirit, where the suture material is pulled off and a length cut as needed. This is a much less reliable way of storing suture materials and should be avoided for internal use. Finally, suture materials can be purchased as lengths which are then threaded onto resterilisable needles. This causes more tissue trauma due to drag through the tissues where the suture material is doubled over through the eye of the needle. The needle is also more likely to become blunt.

When choosing a suture material, the veterinary surgeon or nurse needs to know the following information (Table 19.5):

- How secure is the knot? Monofilament materials have high **memory** (i.e. they are very springy) and therefore the knots are less secure than braided materials.
- How strong is the material? Often braided materials are stronger than monofilament materials of an equivalent size.
- How long does the material last in the tissues? This may depend on the mechanism by which the suture material is broken down in specific tissues, but some materials are designed to be long lasting, e.g. polydioxanone.

Table 19.5 Suture materials

Physical characteristics	Natural	Synthetic
Braided, absorbable	Catgut	Polyglycolic acid, polyglactin 910
Monofilament, absorbable		Poliglecaprone 25, polydioxanone, polyglyconate
Braided, non-absorbable	Silk, linen, cotton	Caprolactam, polyester
Monofilament, non-absorbable		Nylon, fishing line, polypropylene, stainless steel

- How much **drag** is there when the material is drawn through tissues? Generally, the braided materials drag through the tissues more than monofilament and are more likely to cause damage.

Tissues treat all suture materials as foreign material and mount an inflammatory response. Therefore it is a good surgical principle to use the minimum of suture material possible to achieve closure of the wound, and to use the smallest gauge of suture material that will be strong enough.

Generally, the natural materials cause much more inflammation and are less reliable than the synthetic materials.

Primary closure of large skin deficits; skin reconstruction

Large skin defects may not be amenable to simple closure and special surgical techniques have to be used. These techniques often involve moving flaps of skin around and it is important that the blood vessels supplying the flap are carefully protected from damage during the surgery. Very fine rat-toothed forceps, **stay sutures** or specialist skin hooks may be used to handle the skin. The vessels should also be prevented from going into spasm during the surgery – hypotension, hypothermia, shock, dehydration, pain will all decrease blood flow to the skin and risk damage to the skin flap. These cases need very careful peri- and post-operative nursing.

RECONSTRUCTIVE SURGERY
(1) Clip and prepare very wide areas of skin surrounding the surgical site.
(2) Protect the drapes from 'strike through' that might compromise aseptic technique.
(3) Watch for hypothermia and dehydration during surgery.
(4) Count the swabs and estimate blood loss.
(5) Provide soft bedding, good post-operative analgesia and close observation to improve circulation to the skin.

Some oncologic surgeries will entail removal of part of the abdominal or thoracic wall and in these cases, a synthetic mesh made of absorbable or non-absorbable material may be used to close the defect. These meshes are expensive and can result in the development of sinus tracts if aseptic technique is not good enough.

Random skin flaps

Incisions are made running away from the skin defect to create a flap of skin that is then undermined so that it can be advanced to cover the defect. These flaps rely on the network of blood vessels in the dermis to supply the skin edges at the end of the flap. They have to have a wide base to ensure that enough vessels run into the flap to keep it alive and can only be moved into adjacent areas as far as the tension will allow.

Axial pattern flaps

These are specialist skin flaps that are defined and named by the specific artery and vein that supply that area of skin. The skin is elevated according to anatomic landmarks and the artery and vein identified underneath. The flap of skin can then be moved as far as the vessels will allow. This flap is very reliable as it has a well-defined blood supply and can be used over wounds that have poor blood supply.

Free skin grafts

Skin grafts are pieces of skin removed from a donor site and then sutured in place onto a wound. They are usually used for wounds on the limbs which are difficult to repair using skin flaps. The skin graft is very susceptible to failure as it has to rely on the wound bed for nutrition from the first day and has no independent blood supply. If the blood supply fails to grow into the skin graft within 3–4 days, then the graft will fail.

Skin grafts may be harvested as **split thickness grafts**, which include only the epidermis and superficial dermis, or **full thickness grafts** (FTSG) which include the whole of the epidermis and dermis. In animals, we usually use full thickness pieces of skin, as this also transfers the hair follicles and then the final result is more cosmetic and hard wearing. If it is difficult to harvest a large piece of skin from the flank, then **punch grafts** or **stamp or strip grafts** may be taken and embedded into the wound allowing the surface to re-epithelialise by growing out from the islands of little skin grafts. Punch grafts are usually taken with a skin biopsy punch and pushed into little holes in the granulation tissue. Stamp or strip grafts are small squares or strips of skin laid onto the granulation tissue with gaps between the grafts. These tend to have very sparse hair regrowth in between the grafts and are quite fragile. Usually FTSG are **meshed** by making little stab incisions in the skin to allow it to conform better to the surface of the wound and also to allow drainage of fluid out from underneath the graft.

MANAGEMENT OF FREE SKIN GRAFTS
(1) A well-padded bandage (Robert Jones) must be kept on for the first 5–7 days to immobilise the limb.
(2) Bandage changes must be done carefully so that the graft does not move.
(3) Aseptic wound management to prevent infection.
(4) A non-adherent primary dressing layer is essential.

Post-operatively, grafts are dressed with a non-adherent dressing such as paraffin gauze or silicone mesh and heavily bandaged (e.g. with a Robert Jones bandage) to prevent movement of the graft site. The dressing is changed as infrequently as possible in order to minimise disruption of the fragile process of graft healing over the first 7 days.

Free skin grafts fail due to inadequate preparation of the wound bed (e.g. chronic avascular granulation tissue), infection of the graft, failure to immobilise the graft or adherence of the primary dressing to the graft. They may also fail if serum or haemorrhage accumulates underneath the graft and lifts it off the wound surface so that the blood vessels cannot grow into the graft quickly enough.

Complications associated with reconstructive surgery

Many reconstructive procedures are long surgeries with large areas of tissue exposed for some time. Patients may dehydrate and become hypotensive more rapidly than expected and also become hypothermic resulting in longer recovery times and poor skin circulation. If the surgical technique is poor, these skin flaps have a high risk of failure. If the circulation fails in the skin flap, it rapidly becomes ischaemic and over the first 3–4 days is cold to the touch, finally becoming hard and blackened as the skin dies.

Drains

> **INDICATIONS FOR DRAINS**
> Drains are used in three circumstances:
> - Where there is a need to perform repeated lavage of a space.
> - Where there is a need for repeated aspiration of fluid (or air) from a space.
> - Where the surgeon wants to prevent the accumulation of fluid in a space (e.g. seroma).

Passive versus active drains

Passive drains rely on gravity and capillary action, whereas active drains have a suction apparatus on one end – either intermittent or continuous.

The commonest passive drain is the **Penrose drain** which is a soft latex tube usually placed in the dead space created at surgery to allow drainage of fluid after surgery. One end of the drain is anchored in the wound with an absorbable suture and the other is anchored at the skin. The end of the drain should always exit through the skin through a separate incision site to the surgical incision so that it does not interfere with wound healing. As it relies on gravity, the drain should exit at the lowest possible point, and to increase drainage, a larger drain or several drains may be placed (drainage volume depends on surface area for the capillary action).

Active drains are usually rigid walled and may have a radio-opaque marker down the side so that their position can be checked. The most common use is the thoracic drain where a drain is placed through the skin, under a skin tunnel and then between the ribs into the thorax. The end of the drain is securely closed with clamps and bungs. The drain may be used to aspirate air or fluid out of the chest or to introduce treatment into the chest cavity (e.g. in pyothorax). The drain can be attached to a syringe for intermittent suction or to a suction device that continuously drains the chest. These drains have to be very carefully bandaged in as the animal could die if it chews the end of the tube and the chest communicated with the outside directly.

Active drains are also used underneath surgical wounds, attached to suction devices that are little vacuum tubes. The continuous gentle suction applied to the dead space is a very effective way of preventing the formation of a seroma.

Closed versus open drains

The thoracic drain is always a closed drain and the system is sealed from the outside. Active drains are closed as they collect the fluid in a reservoir bottle or tube. Passive drains will always be open as they allow the fluids to drip out onto the patient or the floor.

When a passive drain is used, there is a potential risk of bacterial contamination of the wound as bacteria may migrate up the sides and lumen of the tube. In addition, there is increased nursing involved in keeping the skin clean and dry underneath the wound and preventing the fur from becoming matted with exudate. The skin may be protected either by using a thin layer of barrier cream under the end of the drain or using a commercial synthetic spray that makes a breathable but waterproof barrier on the skin to help prevent maceration Cavilon (3M, Arnolds). Where possible the drain should be bandaged in place with a sterile dressing to absorb the fluid from the end of the drain. This has to be changed regularly to ensure that the skin does not become macerated. Active drains still have some risk of bacterial contamination as there will be some migration of bacteria up the sides of the tube, but the risk is smaller, particularly as they can often be bandaged into place using antiseptic ointments and sterile dressings.

Care and management of drains

All drains should be handled in an aseptic manner, and the animal treated with broad-spectrum antibiotics until they are removed. The animal must be prevented from interfering with the drain and the drain must be protected from the animal's urine or faeces. Drains are removed by cutting the skin suture and then are pulled quickly out with light pressure over the hole to help it to seal. Thoracic drains should have a purse-string suture pre-placed in the skin ready to close the skin on removal. Most other drains are removed and the hole allowed to granulate over.

Summary

Wounds heal in a predictable manner which can be manipulated by the veterinary surgeon or veterinary nurse to accelerate – or delay – the recovery of the animal. Classification of wounds is important in order to make a rational plan of approach to management of a case. Wounds allowed to heal by second intention should be assessed closely at each bandage change in order to determine what stage of healing the tissues have reached and to apply the appropriate dressing. Recon-structive surgery is the technique of choice where possible.

Fracture management

Initial assessment and management

It is essential that the patient is adequately restrained before examining or treating with first aid. However placid an animal is under normal circumstances, it will often attempt to bite when in a lot of pain. A muzzle is often required.

Fractures may be accompanied by other injuries and some of these can be life threatening. More often than not, the fracture is of lesser priority and its repair (depending on its nature) can be left for several days until the patient is in a stable condition. It is important to prioritise these injuries and the most life threatening is dealt with first. Once these issues are dealt with, a full and careful examination can be carried out by the veterinary surgeon, analgesics administered and the limb temporarily supported with splints and bandages. (See Chapter 4, First Aid.)

When the veterinary surgeon has established that there is a fracture, *two orthogonal radiographic views* must be taken in order to make a specific diagnosis.

Physiology of fractures

A fracture is a complete or incomplete break of bone continuity, with or without displacement of the resulting fragments.

Fracture healing

Indirect fracture healing (previously called secondary healing)

Local events immediately after fracture are the same as in other tissues: haemorrhage, formation of a clot, and acute inflammation. The clot is gradually replaced by granulation tissue and blood vessels grow into the organising clot from periosteal blood vessels and blood vessels in the medullary canal of the bone. Fibrous tissue is produced by fibroblasts in the organising clot around the fracture and forms a cuff around the bone ends. This fibrous tissue is important as it stabilises the fracture and allows cartilage to develop. This large cuff of stabilising tissue is known as **callus**. Callus is composed of fibrous tissue, cartilage and immature bone and it envelops the ends of the bone.

The cartilage is then slowly replaced by bone in endochondral fashion. Cells called **chondroclasts** resorb cartilage and new bone is formed when **osteoblasts** line the surfaces and secrete a mineralised matrix. As this process progresses, the callus gradually contains more cartilage and bone and less fibrous tissue. As the callus becomes stiffer, the fracture becomes more stable until eventually the callus rigidly unites the bone ends and this is the point of **clinical union**. Callus is not always good news; sometimes the callus formed may be disorganised and excessive and can interfere with the normal movements of muscle and tendons.

There is then a long remodelling phase where the callus is replaced by mature bone. **Osteoclasts** are responsible for bone resorption in the remodelling phase, they remove the mineral part of the callus and degrade the collagenous and non-collagenous proteins. Simultaneously, mature bone is laid down by osteoblasts, thus re-creating the original bony structure.

Haversian remodelling is a process of bone resorption and formation within the cortex and is the final step in restoration of the normal compact bone structure. The surface of the cortices is smoothed out and the bone's strength restored in response to normal weight bearing.

Direct fracture healing (previously called primary healing)

Direct fracture healing occurs when the bone edges are so close together that callus formation does not occur and the bone forms without the interim stage of fibrous tissue and cartilage. In cases where callus formation is detrimental to the return of function, e.g. joint surfaces, direct fracture healing is preferable and this usually requires surgical intervention as soon as possible after the trauma. The fragments must be held in rigid anatomical alignment (i.e. with plates, screws and/or wires or a combination), and this allows Haversian systems to cross a minute fracture gap and repair the cortical bone directly with little or no callus formation.

The rate of fracture healing

Provided there are no complications, clinical union is usually achieved in 12–16 weeks in adult dogs and cats. Remodelling may continue for many months or even years, after clinical union has occurred. The rate of fracture healing is assessed by clinical examination to detect the increase in rigidity and the firm swelling associated with union by callus formation. Radiographs are taken to assess the degree of callus formation and the extent of mineralisation within the callus. Many factors influence the rate at which fractures heal and it is important to be aware of these when contemplating fracture repair.

- Fractures in immature animals heal more quickly than in adult animals.
- Fractures in geriatric animals heal more slowly.
- Fractures in debilitated animals heal more slowly. Debilitation may be due to poor nutrition or systemic illness such as hormonal disorder or kidney failure.
- **Osteomyelitis** interferes with healing and is one of the most common causes of poor fracture healing after surgical repair. Healing can progress normally once the infection is overcome.
- Fractures of cancellous bone heal more quickly than fractures in cortical bone.
- Fractures in bones that have a good blood supply heal more quickly than those in areas with a poor blood supply. For example the pelvis and scapula are covered by large muscle masses which have a good blood supply and these bones heal well. The distal one-third of the radius and ulna has little muscle cover and a poor blood supply, therefore fractures at this site heal poorly, especially in very small breeds of dog.
- Oblique fractures heal more quickly than transverse fractures because there is a larger area of contact to promote tissue regrowth.
- Poor reduction or fixation of a fracture will result in a slow rate of healing.

Complications associated with fracture healing

- **Nonunion** – complete failure of the fractured ends of the bone to unite.
- **Delayed union** – fracture healing progresses slowly. Clinical union is not achieved within the expected time.
- **Mal-union** – fracture heals in an abnormal position. Untreated fractures and those not treated properly often heal in an abnormal position.
- **Shortened limb** – limb shortening occurs if there is healing with inadequate reduction of overriding fracture fragments. Limb function may be severely compromised.
- **Osteomyelitis** – inflammation of the bone. Bacterial osteomyelitis is commonly caused by inadequate asepsis during surgery. It is more likely to occur if there is also damage to the local blood supply. This is recognised by heat, pain and swelling of the affected part, systemic illness, inappetence and fever.
- **Fracture disease** – this is a syndrome of muscle wastage and inability to flex joints in a limb after fracture repair. One or more joints in the affected limb may be held rigid due to scar formation within the joints or within muscles surrounding the fracture site. Fracture disease is more common after fixation by external coaptation or when there is inadequate reduction.

- **Sequestrum** – a necrotic piece of bone not incorporated successfully in the fracture repair.
- **Implant failure** – this can occur through poor choice of implants or technique, stress applied through the implant through overactive behaviour of the patient, or failure of the implant itself. This will result in a sudden deterioration, with instability and pain returning at the fracture site.

Classification of fractures

Modern classification of fractures provides information for both treatment and prognosis: the bone involved, type of displacement, direction of the fracture line and the number and type of fragments.

(1) **Open versus closed**:

- A **closed** fracture describes a fracture with no break in the skin.
- An **open** fracture has a wound that has penetrated the skin and the fracture ends are open to the outside environment. This type carries a bigger risk of infection and is often contaminated, e.g. a road traffic accident where the limb has been dragged along the road.

(2) **Anatomical description**

- **Articular** – involving the joint.
- **Diaphyseal** – a fracture in the midshaft, or diaphysis of the bone.
- **Metaphyseal** – a fracture of the area between the midshaft and the end of a long bone (epiphysis).
- **Physeal** – a fracture through the growth plate of an immature animal.
- **Epiphyseal** – a fracture of the epiphysis.
- **Condylar** – a fracture of the epiphysis when condyles are involved, for example the distal humerus or femur.

Other common sites of fractures include the pelvis, the mandibles and the ribs.

(3) **Type of displacement**:

- **Greenstick** – an incomplete (i.e. only one cortex) fracture of a bone of an immature animal.
- **Fissure** – a fine crack which may displace during surgery or when stressed.
- **Depressed** – especially fractures of the skull where fragments may be pushed into the underlying cavity.
- **Compression** – often refers to fracture of a vertebral body where a compressive force has resulted in the shortening of a vertebra by a crushing effect.
- **Impacted** – cortical fragments are forced into cancellous bone.
- **Avulsion** – a fracture in which a bony prominence has been torn away from the rest of the bone, usually by the pull of a muscle. For example, fracture of the olecranon or avulsion of the tibial crest.

(4) **Direction of fracture line**:

- **Transverse** – fracture line is at 90° to the axis of the bone.
- **Oblique** – fracture line is at an angle of at least 30°.
- **Spiral** – fracture line curves around the bone.
- **Longitudinal, Y or T** – refers to the appearance of the fracture lines on the bone.

(5) **Number or types of fracture**:

- **Simple** – one fracture line creating two fragments.
- **Comminuted** – more than one fracture line creating more than two fragments.
- **Wedge** – a multifragmented fracture with some contact between the main fragments after reduction.
- **Segmental** – one or more large complete fragments of the shaft of a long bone.
- **Irregular** – a diaphyseal fracture with no specific pattern.
- **Multiple** – more than one fracture in the same or different bones.

Some fractures are further classified to provide more detail about the appearance. Epiphyseal or growth plate fractures are classified by the Salter–Harris system ranging from Type I to Type VI. Accessory carpal bone and central tarsal bone fractures are important fractures in racing greyhounds and are each classified Type I to Type V.

Diagnosis of fractures

Clinical signs

Owners may have witnessed what happened to their pet and can give the veterinary surgeon vital information. A good clinical history may then give the veterinary surgeon a good indication of the nature of the injuries.

The first signs, as with any injury can be attributed to acute inflammation. The major clinical signs seen with fractures are:

- Pain localised to the affected bone.
- Local swelling and heat.
- Bruising at the fracture site leading to discoloration of the overlying soft tissues.
- Marked loss of function.
- Visible or palpable deformity of the affected bone.
- Abnormal mobility at the fracture site.
- Crepitus when the injured part is moved.

Radiography

General anaesthesia is usually necessary to obtain good quality radiographs. At least two views are essential to enable the veterinary surgeon to make a proper diagnosis and a plan for repair. Radiographs of the normal contralateral limb are useful in planning reconstruction of a severe fracture, e.g. comminuted or multiple fractures. Although it may be obvious that a limb is fractured, a good-quality radiograph will confirm details like hairline fractures, small fissures/chips or alterations in bone density, which could alter the treatment plan.

The principles of fracture repair

The primary aim of fracture fixation is to restore the functional anatomy of the fractured bone. This is achieved by:

- Restoring the continuity of the bone.
- Restoring the length of the bone.
- Restoring the functional shape of the bone.
- Maintaining essential soft tissue function.

Essential soft tissues include the blood vessels supplying the bone, muscles acting on the bone and the nerves supplying the muscles. Any techniques for fracture repair must be sympathetic to these tissues because without them there is no chance of restoring function to the injured limb. Many techniques exist for successfully restoring bone continuity length and shape. However, the same basic principles apply to all the techniques:

- **Reduction** – The fracture fragments should be brought together in the correct anatomical alignment. This may be done 'closed', by traction and manipulation of the limb or 'open', by performing surgery at which time the fracture is visualised and the individual fragments manipulated back into position.
- **Fixation** – The fragments should be immobilised in the correct alignment until clinical union occurs. The fragments may also be compressed together to narrow the fracture gap.
- **Blood supply** – the blood supply to the bone fragments must be preserved. Fractures will only heal if there is an adequate blood supply.

Stabilisation of fractures

After reduction of a fracture the bones must be held in position until healing occurs. In some cases, such as greenstick fractures and some pelvic fractures, immobilisation may be unnecessary and simple restriction of activity will suffice.

INDICATIONS FOR IMMOBILISATION AT THE FRACTURE SITE
- To relieve pain.
- To prevent displacement of the fragment (loss of reduction).
- To prevent movement that might cause delayed union or non-union.

Fracture fixation techniques are broadly classified into three groups:

- **External coaptation**, using casts or splints.
- **Internal fixation** using pins, plates, screws and other devices.
- **External – internal fixation** using 'external fixators'.

There are a number of ways to repair fractures and there are a number of factors to be taken into account before deciding on the technique for repair. For example a young dog's fractures will heal more quickly than an older dog, and a fracture in a small breed, such as a Chihuahua, presents different problems than the same fracture in a Great Dane.

FACTORS AFFECTING FRACTURE REPAIR
- Classification of the fracture.
- Age of the patient.
- Size of the patient.
- Temperament of patient.
- Presence of any underlying disease.
- Cost to owner.
- Expectations of owner (i.e. working animal versus pet).

Casts and support bandages

The aim of external coaptation is to limit motion at a fracture site by immobilising the joints above and below the fracture. If the joints above and below the fracture cannot be immobilised then external coaptation is not suitable.

Methods of external coaptation fall into three main groups: casts, splints and extension splints.

Advantages of external coaptation techniques

- Technically simpler than some internal fixation techniques.
- They are economical.
- They are non-invasive.

Disadvantages of external coaptation techniques

- They have limited applications; for example casts are most useful for fractures below the stifle in the hindlimb and below the elbow in the forelimb.
- They do not provide sufficient stability for many fractures, particularly comminuted or severely oblique fractures.

- They are at risk of causing pressure sores.
- Slower healing of fracture and greater callus formation.
- They restrict activity of joints and muscles in the limb and are therefore prone to causing fracture disease.

Types of fracture suitable for casting

Relatively stable fractures are ideal: greenstick fractures or simple oblique or spiral fractures that are stable after manual reduction. Where one bone is fractured close to an intact bone which provides a splint-like mechanism, a cast can be used, e.g. a fractured radius with an intact ulna. Casts are also used for post-operative support of arthrodeses, internal fixations or tendon repair.

There are various types of casting materials available, which all attempt to conform to the ideal requirements of a cast.

CASTS – IDEAL REQUIREMENTS
The ideal casting material:
- Easy to apply.
- Conformable.
- Reaches maximum strength quickly.

The ideal finished cast:
- Hard wearing.
- Radiolucent to enable monitoring of fracture healing without removal of the cast.
- Strong and lightweight but not too bulky.
- Easy to remove.
- Water resistant, but 'breathable'.
- Economical.

- **Polypropylene impregnated with resin** (e.g. Dynacast Optima, Smith & Nephew) – easy to apply, radiolucent, strong lightweight and hard wearing.
- **Fibreglass impregnated with resin** (e.g. Vetcast Plus, 3M) – easy to apply, strong and lightweight but less hard wearing than a polypropylene cast. Causes slightly reduced radiographic detail. Some newer products can be immersed in water and then dried with a hairdryer.
- **Thermoplastic polymer mesh** (e.g. Hexcelite, Hexcel UK) and **thermoplastic sheets** (e.g. Turbocast, Transthermo Systems) – easy to apply, radiolucent although the mesh creates a distracting pattern on the radiograph. Hard wearing. Expensive to purchase but can be re-used making it more economical.
- **Plaster of Paris** – conformable but messy to apply. Makes a heavy, bulky and weak cast. Slow to reach maximum strength and loses strength when in contact with water. Radio-opaque and has to be removed to monitor fracture healing. Cheap to purchase.

Application of a cast

The casting material must be applied in close proximity to the bone to be able to give good support to the fracture. There is a fine line between using too much padding and too little. Too much will allow the fractured ends to move within the cast or cause the cast to slip. Too little padding causes pressure sores. The cast must contain at least one joint above the fracture and one below.

The manufacturer's instructions should be followed closely for preparation of the casting material.

(1) Collect all the materials needed before applying the cast:

- Gloves.
- Stockinette.
- Synthetic cast padding such as Soffban (Smith & Nephew).
- Enough rolls of casting material of appropriate size.
- A bowl of water at the temperature recommended by the manufacturer.

(2) Open or surgical wounds are dressed appropriately.
(3) Stockinette is rolled up the limb, taking care to prevent any creases.
(4) Cast padding is carefully and evenly wound onto the limb with 50% overlap at each turn, paying special attention to any bony prominence. Do not overpad these parts, instead use ring 'donuts'. Donuts can be made by cutting holes in small pads made out of cast padding; these are usually placed on the accessory carpal bone and olecranon of the front limb or the calcaneus of the hindlimb. This prevents pressure ulceration on these structures.
(5) One roll of casting material is prepared by immersing in the bowl of water and squeezing several times to allow the water to penetrate into the roll.
(6) Excess water is squeezed out and the roll of casting material is applied to the limb in the same manner as the padding but with even tension. The casting material starts to set within minutes (depending on the type used) therefore it is important to work quickly.
(7) Each roll is wetted individually just before application. Depending on the type of casting material used and the size of the patient, usually 2–3 layers are applied with 4–6 layers for larger dogs.
(8) The pads and nails of the middle two toes are left exposed at the bottom of the cast.
(9) A 1–2 cm length of padding is left exposed at the top and bottom of the cast.
(10) Once the cast has hardened the stockinette and padding at each end are turned down over the edge of the cast and secured with tape.
(11) A cast can be made stronger by applying splints made out of several lengths of casting material laid longitudinally down the compression side of the cast.

Splints

Zimmer and gutter splints can be used as a fixation technique in some fractures, particularly those occurring below the carpus or hock in cats and small dogs. Splints can also be made from casting material (except plaster of Paris). A cast is applied as before, and then an oscillating saw is used to cut the length of the cast on the medial and lateral sides. The limb is dressed and bandaged appropriately and the two halves of the cast are reapplied to the limb and secured with an adhesive bandage.

Post-operative care of casts and splints

- Owners should be given *written* instructions of how to look after the cast and what to look out for if things start to go wrong.
- When the patient is taken outside, the bottom of the cast should be covered with a plastic bag (old drip bags are useful for this) and secured with tape – never elastic bands as these may easily be forgotten and cause problems later on.
- Casts may have to be reapplied if the animal chews extensively or damages the cast. Growing animals will need a new cast every week to allow normal growth of the limb.
- Give medication as prescribed.
- Check cast daily and any of the following signs should be reported to the veterinary surgeon immediately:

  - Swelling of the limb or toes.
  - Chafing at the edges of the cast.
  - Staining of the cast with a discharge.
  - A foul smell coming from the cast.
  - Slipping of the cast from its original position.
  - Chewing or other signs of discomfort.
  - Collapse or bending of the cast (especially plaster of Paris).
  - General illness – depression, lethargy, lack of appetite.

Complications of casts

- Limb swelling – if the cast is too tight, it restricts the lymphatic and venous drainage which results in oedema of the lower limb. This is usually seen within 1 hour of applying the cast and needs urgent attention.
- Pressure sores – usually seen if the cast is poorly padded or is slightly loose and sliding on the skin.
- Cast loosening – if the cast was put on when the limb was swollen, the cast may loosen once the swelling subsides.
- Prolonged immobilisation of the limb may cause any of the following complications:

  - Joint stiffness and fibrosis.
  - Cartilage degeneration.
  - Muscle atrophy.
  - Osteoporosis of disuse.

- Joint laxity – rapidly growing young large-breed dogs are particularly at risk.
- Delayed union, mal-union and non-union may be seen with poor case selection, poor cast selection, poor casting technique or frequent reapplication of the cast and movement of the fracture site.
- Refracture on removal of the cast – provided the limb had good callus formation (clinical union) on the radiograph at the time of cast removal, this should not happen.

Removal of the cast

Generally limbs remain in a cast for 4–6 weeks. Radiographs are taken to establish the degree of healing and callus formation. The patient should be sedated or anaesthetised. An oscillating saw is the most suitable tool for removing casts. Two cuts are made in the cast and the line of cut is carefully chosen to avoid bony prominences. The saw should never come into contact with the skin. The saw moves in an arc of 5°–6° and only cuts the solid casting material; the padding underneath catches on the blade and is not cut. The oscillating blade can become hot while cutting the cast and the saw should be rotated to use a cooler part of the blade. The padding underneath can then be removed with scissors. Plaster shears can also be used; they are inserted at the distal end of the cast and the cut is advanced proximally in small regular steps.

Internal fixation

Internal fixation uses pins, plates, screws and wire to repair fractures.

Advantages of internal fixation

- Suitable for fractures in any bone.
- Versatile and can handle the full range of fracture types.
- Allows accurate reduction and rigid fixation.
- Allows the limb to return to full function early, encouraging fracture healing and minimising the risk of fracture disease.

Disadvantages of internal fixation

- Relatively expensive and time-consuming.
- Some internal fixation techniques are technically demanding.
- There is capital expenditure on the equipment.
- The risks of surgery (wound healing problems, infection) are inherently greater in an open reduction and fixation than in closed reduction and fixation.
- Open fractures with extensive soft tissue injury may not be suitable.

Implants and techniques used in internal fixation

Intramedullary pins These are called Steinman pins; they are stainless steel rods with a sharp trocar point at each end, and it is possible to have one end threaded. They come in different widths ranging from 1.6 to 8 mm in diameter and are placed into the medulla of the bone that is fractured. They are inserted with a Jacobs chuck or power drill.

- **Advantages:** cheap to purchase, quick to use, require minimal surgical exposure, easier to implant and remove than bone plates.
- **Disadvantages**: less stable fixation, slower return to function, secondary bone union (i.e. slower healing), more after care required, not suitable for unstable fractures.

Post-operative management of intramedullary pins:

- Two radiographic views are required to assess repair.
- Provide clients with written instructions outlining convalescent period and dates for follow-up examinations.
- Give medication (analgesics and maybe antibiotics) as directed.
- Exercise restrictions; lead exercise only to allow patient to urinate and defecate. Cats should be restricted to a cage or a section of a room.
- Avoid stairs and prevent animal jumping on or off furniture.
- Sutures are usually removed after 10 days.
- At the first check, evaluate for limb function and assess joints adjacent to the fracture for range of motion. The point where pin emerges from bone is examined for swelling or evidence of pin migration. Regular checks to monitor bone healing and watch for pin migration.
- The pin is usually removed under anaesthetic once clinical union is achieved.

Interlocking nails These are solid rods of 4, 4.7, 6, or 8 mm in diameter with holes through which screws are inserted. The nails are placed in the medulla and the screws fix the rod within the bone. Diaphyseal fractures are suitable for this method of repair and it gives a more reliable fixation than an intramedullary pin. It requires expensive equipment and technical expertise to insert. Equipment and implants are available in this country but few referral centres have this system.

Arthrodesis wires and K wires These are smaller pins in widths of 0.9 to 2 mm in diameter. Arthrodesis wires have trocar points at each end and K-wires have a flattened bayonet point at one end and trocar point at the other. These pins can be used as intramedullary pins in very small bones, as an aid in stabilising a fragment while primary fixation is taking place or to create a tension band wire. They are also used in various types of fractures in small dogs and cats but not for midshaft fractures of long bones.

Cerclage wire   This is malleable monofilament stainless steel wire. It is often used to supplement the use of intramedullary pins, external skeletal fixators and bone plates. It compresses large fragments by encircling the bone and the fragment and then is twisted with wire twisters, pliers or special tighteners. It is also used to create a tension band wire (see below).

Tension-band wire   This is used to fix an avulsed fracture. It uses two different directional forces to create compression of the fracture. A K-wire or pin is placed into the fragment and main bone and a wire is placed in a figure-of-eight pattern around the end of the pin. It is anchored through a predrilled hole to a solid part of the bone on the opposite side to the ligament or muscle that pulled off the fragment.

Venables and Sherman plates   A Venables plate is a rectangular bone plate with round holes. The number of holes varies from 4 to 8. The plate is secured to the bone, bridging the fracture with Sherman self-tapping screws. A Sherman plate is similar to the Venables plate but narrows between the holes making it lighter and not as strong. Sherman screws are also used to attach the plate to the bone. **Self-tapping screws (Sherman)** differ from tapped screws by their slotted heads and two notches at the tip of the screw. They are available in two widths (7/64 and 9/64) and various different lengths.

After the plate has been contoured (bent to fit the bone), it is held in position with **bone-holding forceps**. Each hole is drilled with the correct-size drill bit to include both near and far cortices. The hole is then measured with a depth gauge and the correct length screw selected. The screw is driven into the hole with a screwdriver. They cut their own thread as they are screwed into the hole. (For this reason they cannot be taken out and replaced in the same hole because they would strip the thread as it was replaced and not be secure.) Screws are not inserted into holes that cross the fracture line, these holes are best left empty or a lag screw (see later) placed prior to placing the plate.

ASIF/AO systems   ASIF stands for the Association for the Study of Internal Fixation, and is used in North America to name the patent and copyright of the system of orthopaedic equipment used for internal fixation. However, the European designation for the same equipment is AO which stands for Arbeitsgemeinschaft für Osteosynthesefragen.

There is a wide variety of different plates and equipment for repairing every conceivable type of fracture. The most commonly used plate in veterinary practice is the **dynamic compression plate (DCP)**. It is a strong plate with oval shaped holes. These are available in different widths named by the size of screw they take, and lengths or number of holes. A 2.0 mm plate takes 2.0 mm screws, a 2.7 mm plate takes 2.7 mm screws, 3.5 mm and 4.5 mm plates come in narrow or broad widths and take 3.5 and 4.5 mm screws respectively.

The DCP can serve various functions depending on how it is applied to the fractured bone. It can be used as a **compression** plate, as a **neutralisation** plate, or as a **buttress** plate. A compression plate is used in simple transverse diaphyseal fractures to compress the ends of the bone together. A neutralisation plate is used in oblique, spiral and comminuted fractures where compression is not possible, and the fracture has been reconstructed with wires or screws but the repair needs additional support. A buttress plate is used to help stabilise the fracture site and to bridge a fracture that is not reconstructable. The defect at the fracture site is usually filled with a **cancellous bone graft**.

Pre-tapped screws (AO type)   These screws are identified by the hexagonal head, which needs a special type of screwdriver to be able to place them. They are available in different widths and lengths, and some larger screws are **cortical** or **cancellous**. Table 19.6 is a guide to the sizes and drill bits to use.

Technique   A drill bit is selected to drill a hole the size of the core of the screw; for example, if a 3.5 mm cortical screw was to be used, a 2.5 mm drill bit will be selected. The hole is then measured with the depth gauge and the correct length of screw is selected. The hole is then 'tapped' to create a thread for the screw. A **tap** is a special device designed to cut the thread in the bone. It is especially important to use the correct tap for the screw being inserted. The tap designed for the 4.0 mm cancellous screw cannot be used for the 3.5 mm cortical screw even though both screws are of similar widths because the thread has a different pitch. The screw is finally driven into the hole using the hexagonal head screwdriver.

Lag screw technique   A lag screw is not a type of screw but a technique. It is used to stabilise and compress fragments in a fracture. The fracture is reduced and held in place using bone-holding forceps. A hole is drilled the same width as the screw (the gliding hole), in the fragment, and the far cortex is then drilled with a drill bit the same size as the core of the screw. The far cortex is tapped, but the near cortex (in the fragment) is not. When

Table 19.6 Sizes of AO-type screws and corresponding drill bits

Size of screw (mm)	Drill bit for core (mm)	Drill bit for gliding hole (mm)	Tap (mm)
1.5[a]	1.1	1.5	1.5
2.0[a]	1.5	2.0	2.0
2.7[a]	2.0	2.7	2.7
3.5[a]	2.5	3.5	3.5
4.0[b]	2.0	4.0	4.0
4.5[a]	3.2	4.5	4.5
6.5[b]	3.2	6.5	6.5

[a] *Cortical;* [b] *cancellous*

the screw is driven into the hole, it does not grip the fragment but just grips the far cortex; this has the effect of compressing the fragment into place.

Post-operative care after internal fixation

- Two radiographic views are required to assess the repair immediately post-operatively.
- Analgesia and nursing during recovery aims to enable a smooth and peaceful recovery of consciousness.
- Early recovery of appetite and adequate nutrition is important.
- Long anaesthetic times and blood loss during reconstruction of the fracture may necessitate continuation of intravenous fluids into the recovery period.
- Assisted walking may be necessary to allow the animal an opportunity to urinate and defecate while limiting the use of the fractured limb.
- Daily monitoring of temperature, pulse and respiratory rates during hospitalisation.
- Give medication and analgesia as directed in the days following the surgery.
- Sutures are usually removed after 10 days.
- Clients should be provided with written instructions outlining the convalescent period and dates for follow-up examinations and re-radiography. These should be on a regular basis as directed by the veterinary surgeon. The owners should be instructed on how to recognise possible complications and how to seek veterinary advice if these occur.
- Exercise restrictions – cage rest is outdated with modern methods of rigid immobilisation. It is considered to be beneficial to fracture healing and well-being of the patient to give short controlled bouts of lead exercise: 10–15 minutes (on a lead) a couple of times a day for the first 3–4 weeks is usually sufficient. Swimming is also of great benefit once any wounds have healed, but must be controlled in the early stages of healing to prevent overenthusiastic movements.

Complications associated with internal fixation

The most common complications are osteomyelitis and infection associated with the implants, and implant failure. Both are often due to poor technique or poor choice of implants. In some cases, the post-operative care in the home environment is not sufficiently rigorous to protect the implants from failure.

External skeletal fixation (ESF)

External skeletal fixation stabilises fractures using pins that are inserted through a small stab incision in the skin and then into the bone. They usually travel through both cor-tices and are then fixed on the outside of the limb with bars and clamps or acrylic resin. Different types of frame can be made according to the requirements of the fracture. A simple frame would consist of one bar and three or four pins exiting from the bone. A more complex frame could consist of multiple pins and three or more bars in three different planes.

Pins come in different sizes (2 mm, 3 mm, 4 mm, and 5 mm). Pins may be smooth with a trocar end or have threaded ends. End-threaded pins have either a negative thread, where the thread is cut out of the pin and the overall diameter of the pin remains the same, or a positive thread where a thread is wound onto the pin and the overall diameter of the pin is slightly larger. Pins are also available with a positive thread in the middle of the pin rather than the end. The advantage of a threaded pin is that it is less likely to loosen or be pulled out than a smooth pin. Pins are placed in both cortices of the bone but do not necessarily exit both sides. The centrally threaded pins are designed to exit both sides of the limb. Clamps and bars are available to fit each size of pin.

EXTERNAL SKELETAL FIXATION
Advantages:
- Minimal instrumentation required.
- Clamps and bars are re-usable.
- Minimal disruption of soft tissues.
- Minimal foreign body at fracture site.
- Open wound management easy.
- Easy to combine with other implants.
- Rigidity and alignment easily adjustable.
- Assessment of fracture healing easy.
- Easy to remove.

Disadvantages:
- Soft tissue problems possible.
- Application technique requires practice.
- Premature pin loosening common.
- Difficult to apply to proximal limb.
- Can be difficult to get good radiographs of the limb.

APEF system

The acrylic pin external fixator (APEF) system uses corrugated tubing which is filled with **polymethylmethacrylate**, a type of bone cement. All the pins are placed in the bone and the corrugated tubing is fixed onto the ends of the pins. The cement is mixed and poured into the tubing. The tubing is then held in alignment until the cement has hardened. The hardening process is a chemical reaction between the liquid and powder components and intense heat is generated. It is important to protect the soft tissues (and fingers!) from this heat. Heat can also be conducted down the pins and cause necrosis of the bone. Sterile swabs soaked in cool sterile saline can be placed on the tissues to help protect them; saline can also be dribbled from a syringe onto the pins. The cement takes up to 10 minutes to set. Mandibular fractures are particularly suitable for this system; the acrylic can be formed around the pins and the shape of the jaw into a 'bumper bar'.

Bone grafts

Bone grafts can be harvested from either **cortical** or **cancellous** bone. They are used to supplement fracture repair and accelerate healing across a wide fracture gap during reconstruction. The term **autograft** refers to bone taken from a site and used elsewhere in the same dog. An **allograft** refers to bone taken from one patient and transferred into another patient of the same species.

Cortical bone grafts consist of a whole segment of solid bone or else chips of cortical bone either in a fracture or taken from a non-essential site. These bone grafts are very robust and can even be taken from a different dog for use in **limb salvage** although this is a very specialised technique. It takes a long time for the cortical graft to become fully incorporated in the repair.

Cancellous bone is harvested from inside the medulla of long bones and typically, the commonest sites used are the proximal humerus or the ilium. A drill is used to make a hole in the cortical bone and the cancellous bone is scraped out from the inside of the bone using a curette. Cancellous bone is very sensitive as it contains live cells. It should be handled in a sterile manner and stored in a blood soaked swab on the trolley until used. Cancellous bone grafts are an essential part of repair of complex fractures as they contribute cells and growth factors involved in bone healing.

Types of fracture suitable for external fixation

- Long bone fractures.
- Comminuted fractures.
- Open and infected fractures.
- Delayed unions and non-union.
- Mandibular fractures.

Post-operative care of external fixators

- Open wounds should be treated and dressed appropriately.
- The limb should have a compressive bandage applied for 2–3 days (changed daily) to minimise swelling. This bandage should go between the limb and the bars/acrylic and in between the pins, and should include the toes.
- The ends of the pins protruding from the clamps or tubing should be covered with self-adhesive tape to prevent damage to furniture and owners.

- Air should be allowed to circulate between the skin and pins.
- Cats should be confined to cage rest.
- Exercise should be limited to lead exercise only, taking care to avoid fences/objects that are likely to catch the frame.
- Owners should be told to expect a small amount of scab formation at the site of the pin, this is normal and does not need cleaning on a daily basis. However, excess exudate does need to be cleaned and should be seen by the veterinary surgeon.
- Generally external fixators are well tolerated by the patient but an Elizabethan collar can be put on to prevent the patient interfering with the frame.
- Written instructions should be given to the owner regarding medication, post-op checks and radiographs.

Complications of external fixation

- Swelling of the soft tissues impinging on the clamps or acrylic bars.
- Excessive exudate from the pin site caused by movement of the skin and soft tissues.
- Loosening of pins, but in some cases individual pins can be removed without losing the stability of the frame.

Luxations and subluxations

A **luxation** (also called a dislocation) is a displacement of articular surfaces from the normal position within a joint. The joint surfaces no longer touch each other. A **subluxation** is a partial dislocation of the joint surfaces.

Luxations and subluxations may be classified into two types: congenital and acquired.

- **Congenital** luxations or subluxations are anatomical abnormalities present at birth, which may or may not be inherited. The most common congenital luxation is that of the patella. In most cases a surgical procedure can replace the patella in its normal position. However, some congenital luxations are so severe that they cannot be corrected. Some small dogs and cats may be able to cope with the permanently luxated joint, but in larger breeds severe congenital luxation may cause great disability.
- **Acquired** luxations and subluxations result from some form of trauma, such as a road traffic accident. The ligaments keeping the joint in its normal position are damaged and the joint is forced out of alignment. Acquired luxations most commonly occur in the hip and elbow joints. Also affected but less commonly are phalangeal joints, the hock and shoulder joints.

First aid treatment for dislocations should follow that for fractures. The presenting signs and the trauma suffered are often similar.

Clinical signs and diagnosis of joint luxation

The signs shown by the patient can mimic those of a fracture and it can be difficult to differentiate between them. Pain, deformity, loss of motion, non-weight bearing and crepitus are common signs to both. Sometimes typical stance positions are characteristic of an animal with a dislocation. Radiography is essential to confirm the diagnosis and also the presence or absence of other conditions, e.g. small fractures.

Treatment of joint luxation

Treatment of luxations requires the return of the joint to its normal anatomical position and repair of the damaged ligaments. Like fracture reduction, reduction of luxations may be achieved in several ways:

- **Closed reduction** is reduction of the joint by manipulation of the limb. This is the method that should be attempted first. Closed reduction should be attempted as soon as possible after injury as the longer the delay the less chance there is of successful reduction of the joint. Most joints are impossible to reduce under sedation, causing unnecessary pain and suffering to the patient, and reduction should be carried out under general anaesthetic. The joint should be re-radiographed afterwards to check that the reduction has been successful.
- **Open reduction** involves a surgical approach to the joint; the luxated bones are visualised and manipulated back into the joint. Some form of stabilisation technique is usually required.

Postoperative care is similar after both open and closed reductions except that open luxations require the added precautions taken following surgery. The main post-operative aim is to avoid forces that could cause a recurrence of the luxation.

- Once the joint is reduced it must be immobilised. After a hip dislocation the hindlimb is supported in an **Ehmer** sling; similarly, after a shoulder dislocation the forelimb can be supported in a **Velpeau** sling. These slings are kept on for 5–7 days.
- Exercise should be restricted for 3–4 weeks and then slowly increased.

Complications

- Re-luxation is the most common complication, especially if activity is not sufficiently restricted or if there is other pathology in the joint, such as a fracture.
- Joint infection is a risk, especially if an open reduction has been performed.
- There may be injury to surrounding soft tissues, associated either with the original trauma or with the reduction of the joint. These injuries may not be obvious at first. They include damage to nerves in the region of the joint.

Oncologic surgery

Oncology is the study of cancer and its related diseases. A **neoplasm** or tumour, is an abnormal uncontrolled growth of cells which develop faster than the surrounding normal tissues. Most tumours arise as the animal ages and typically they are found in dogs or cats over 8–10 years of age. However, there are some very aggressive tumours which occur in dogs or cats as young as a few months old. Some breeds of animal are specifically susceptible to certain tumours and may develop more than one tumour at the same time (e.g. Boxers, mast cell tumours; Flat Coated Retrievers, sarcomas). Many owners will be very concerned by the possibility that their animal has cancer, and they must be reassured that many tumours are benign and, if removed completely, will not grow again.

> Neoplasia is extremely common in small-animal practice and all unexplained lumps on an animal should be investigated with the possibility of neoplasia in mind.

Neoplasia

Tumours may arise from any body tissue and the name of the neoplasm is derived from its tissue of origin. Very aggressive tumours may lose all their identifying characteristics because they are growing so fast, and in these cases, it may not be possible for the pathologist to identify the original tissue of origin. It is important to know the tissue of origin, because this enables the veterinary surgeon to predict how the tumour will behave and also what treatment is most appropriate. Neoplasms may be **benign** or **malignant** and this description indicates whether the tumour is likely to spread to other organs or tissues in the animal and result in its death.

The terminology used in oncology is very specific and often describes both the type of tumour and how it behaves.

Benign tumours usually grow quite slowly and are discrete and encapsulated. They are often freely mobile relative to neighbouring tissues and the suffix '-oma' is used to indicate the tumour is benign (although there are a few exceptions):

- **Lipoma** – a benign tumour of adipose (fat) cells, very common in the subcutaneous tissues of older overweight animals.
- **Papilloma** – a benign wart-like tumour of epithelial cells, most often seen on the skin of cats and dogs (e.g. at the lip margins, eyelid and ear) but they also occur in the bladder and rectum.
- **Melanoma** – a benign pigmented skin tumour of melanocytes. Some melanomas, however, are highly malignant particularly if they arise in the mucous membranes of the mouth (**malignant melanoma**).
- **Fibroma** – a benign tumour of fibrous tissue, present as firm superficial tumours of the skin, and may be difficult to differentiate from other more malignant skin tumours.

- **Adenoma** – a benign tumour of glandular tissue, may be quite common in older dogs (e.g. anal adenoma).

Malignant tumours may grow quickly or slowly. They may not have a definite capsule and may be closely attached to neighbouring tissue. Some malignant tumours will spread (**metastasise**) very readily to other organs such as the lungs, liver, spleen and bones. Metastasis may occur via various routes:

- In the circulation after invasion of blood vessels.
- In the lymphatic system to the draining lymph node and beyond.
- By direct contact of tumour cells with neighbouring organs by direct invasion (**extension**) or by exfoliation of tumour cells into a cavity such as the abdomen (**transplantation**).

Malignant tumours are also classified according to the tissue from which they arise:

- **Carcinoma** is a malignant tumour arising from epithelial cells:

    - **Squamous cell carcinoma** arises from squamous epithelium such as the oral cavity.
    - **Transitional cell carcinoma** arises from the transitional epithelium characteristic of the bladder epithelium.
    - **Adenocarcinoma** is a malignant tumour of glandular tissue in epithelia.

- **Sarcoma** is a malignant tumour arising from mesenchymal tissues (mainly connective tissues):

    - **Lymphosarcoma** is a tumour of the lymphoid tissues, common in dogs, and may be seen in association with feline leukaemia virus in cats.
    - **Fibrosarcoma** arises from fibroblasts, and may be found in any connective tissue.
    - **Osteosarcoma** is a malignant tumour of osteoblasts and is usually in the limb bones. In the dog, they are commonly found in the distal radius or ulna, proximal humerus, distal femur or proximal tibia.

When the tumour is examined histopathologically, it can be further graded to determine its degree of malignancy by assessing its rate of proliferation and degree of differentiation of the cells.

Preparation for oncologic surgery

Many forms of neoplasia are amenable to surgery; however, in order to plan treatment and advise the owner, a specific diagnosis of the type of tumour is necessary. This entails taking a **biopsy** from the tumour and submitting it for histopathology. Benign tumours may be completely cured by **excisional surgery** and there are a number of treatments available for malignant tumours that will extend the lifespan of the animal while maintaining its quality of life.

Many animals are older and will require some investigation to establish whether there is evidence of other disease before the surgery is carried out. The dog also should be radiographed or scanned to check whether the neoplasia has spread to other sites. Finally, many patients may be cachexic, malnourished or suffering from **paraneoplastic disease** that makes them increased surgical risks. Attention to nutrition, planning for post-surgical care and nursing is important for successful oncologic surgery.

All animals should have a right and left lateral chest X-ray taken to check for metastases.

Paraneoplastic disease

Tumours can cause other signs of illness apart from the physical effects of the mass itself. Some tumours secrete biologically active hormones that may cause generalised non-specific ill-health, or they may cause well-defined syndromes of disease. Sometimes the paraneoplastic syndrome is more acutely life threatening than the tumour itself.

Some examples include:

- Anal adenocarcinoma and lymphosarcoma can cause **hypercalcaemia** which causes polydypsia, polyuria and renal failure.
- Insulinomas secrete active insulin which causes episodes of acute **hypoglycaemia.**
- Mast-cell tumours can secrete histamine causing generalised or local acute inflammatory responses.
- Thyroid adenomas secrete excess thyroxine, causing tachycardia, weight loss and hyperactivity.

Tumours can also cause pyrexias, **cachexia** and generalised poor nutrition due to other substances released into the circulation.

Biopsy

There are different ways of obtaining tissue for diagnostic purposes:

- **Fine-needle aspirate biopsy** – this is the commonest and most useful method of diagnosis of tumours. It is also used to assess draining lymph nodes for evidence of metastasis. A fine gauge hypodermic needle is inserted into the tumour to aspirate a few cells for cytological analysis. The skin is clipped and surgically prepared in a small patch immediately overlying the tumour. The tumour is then fixed in one hand and the other hand used to introduce the needle into the centre of the tumour. Sometimes ultrasound guidance is used to direct needles into intra-abdominal or intra-thoracic tumours. The needle is then redirected in several directions to obtain cores of cells, and withdrawn. An air-filled syringe is then attached to the needle and the contents of the needle blown onto a clean glass slide. The cells are then gently spread into a smear and air dried for cytology.

FINE-NEEDLE ASPIRATE BIOPSY

(1) Clip and prep a small area of skin over the mass.

(2) Prepare several clean glass slides, labelled with the patient's identity.

(3) Use a 23 gauge needle and a 5 ml syringe.

(4) Fix the mass still with one hand and introduce the needle into the mass. Redirect the tip of the needle in several different directions inside the mass and then withdraw it.

(5) Fill the syringe with air and attach it to the needle so that any tissue in the tip of the needle can be expelled onto a slide. Do this several times onto different slides.

(6) Use a clean slide to gently make a smear of each sample on the slides.

(7) Air dry the slides and submit for cytology.

- **Bone marrow biopsy** – aspirates are also used to sample bone marrow, using a special bone marrow biopsy needle. Usually the sample is taken from the wing of the ilium under sedation with local anaesthesia, or general anaesthesia. The overlying skin is prepared as for surgery and a small skin incision is made over the bone. The bone marrow biopsy needle is driven through the cortex of the bone with the stylet in place. Once in the medullary cavity, the stylet is removed and a syringe used to aspirate bone marrow. The samples are then dripped onto slides tilted at 60° to the vertical so that they run down the slide forming a smear. These are air dried and submitted for cytology.

- **Needle core biopsy** – a small cylinder of tissue is obtained using a specialised instrument such as a **Tru-Cut needle**. There is a central notched obturator, with an outer sleeve or cannula with an attached handle. General or local anaesthesia of the overlying skin is necessary. A stab incision is made in the skin to allow the loaded instrument to be introduced through the soft tissues, and ultrasound guidance may be used to direct the instrument into the centre of the tumour. Once the obturator is in the tumour, the sleeve is pushed sharply over the notch in the obturator, cutting a tiny cylinder of tissue out. The closed instrument is withdrawn and a hypodermic needle used to gently dislodge the biopsy from the opened obturator.

- **Punch biopsy** – punch biopsies are taken using small circular cutters, from superficial lesions in the skin. The biopsy site may be closed using a single interrupted suture.

- **Trephine biopsy** – trephine biopsies are taken from bony tumours, using a **trephine** or a **Jamshidi needle**. A core of bone/tumour a few millimetres in diameter is obtained and pushed out of the trephine or needle using a stylet.

- **Incisional biopsy** – incisional biopsy is used for tumours that are big enough to remove a piece of tissue from without affecting the ultimate surgical treatment. Usually a wedge of tissue is taken from a part of the tumour that appears to be actively growing and then the wedge is repaired with sutures. This is the most reliable way to obtain a diagnosis.

- **Excisional biopsy** – this is usually used for small tumours that are easy to remove with a margin of normal tissue, particularly if they are suspected to be benign. It involves the complete removal of the tumour at the first surgery.

Principles of oncologic surgery

The mainstay of any cancer therapy is to maintain the animal's quality of life, and side-effects of treatment must be balanced by the clinical improvement – or cure. Most tumours are treated with surgical excision, and usually the aim is to remove the entire tumour. However, sometimes it is the mass of the tumour that is causing the animal discomfort and **debulking surgery** may be used to remove as much of the tumour as possible in order to improve the animal's quality of life until it regrows.

Benign well-encapsulated tumours may be cured by simple excision of the tumour. However, many tumours require a **surgical margin** around the tumour in order to ensure that the tumour is entirely removed. Fibrosarcomas are a good example of tumours that are very invasive and require very wide margins of excision in order to attempt to cure the tumour. This may in turn require complex reconstructive surgery to repair the defect made where the tumour was removed. Intra-operatively techniques may be used to reduce the risk of spreading the tumour into normal tissues. For example, the surgeon may change gloves, instruments or drapes prior to closure.

In some areas, a 'clean' surgical margin may not be possible and further types of therapy for the cancer may be indicated after the surgery. Some tumours are so malignant, that post-operative chemotherapy or radiotherapy may be suggested even if the tumour appears to have been completely removed.

Palliative Surgery may be used to remove a tumour to improve the animals quality of life although it does not alter the prognosis.

Submission of tissue for histopathology

All tissue removed from an animal should be submitted for histopathology or stored in formalin in case of recurrence.

Ideally all tissue removed from the animal should be submitted to the pathologist with a detailed history in order to maximise the information available with which to analyse the tumour. However, large tumours may be difficult to submit by post, and representative samples may have to be taken from the mass. In this case, the main bulk of the tumour should be kept until the pathologist's report is complete in case more tissue is requested. Very bony samples have to be decalcified prior to cutting and this may result in a delay of up to 3 weeks prior to the report being received by the veterinary practice.

Where the tumour is malignant or locally invasive, the pathologist should be requested to assess the margins of the tumour in order to determine whether excision has been complete. Sometimes the surgeon may orientate the tumour by placing a marker suture at the cranial/caudal ends, or the edges of the mass can be painted with different colours of Indian ink, which are allowed to dry before fixation.

Tissue should be fixed in 10% neutral buffered formalin in a volume ratio of 1 part specimen to 10 parts of formalin solution. Tissue thicker than 1 cm may need to be incised to allow more rapid access of the formalin to the deeper parts of the tissue so that adequate fixation occurs. Once the tissue has been fixed for 2–3 days, it can be posted with a ratio of tissue-to-formalin of 1:1. Formalin is a carcinogen and health and safety regulations must be observed during handling of the solution and preparing packages for posting. (See Chapter 13, Clinical Pathology and Laboratory Diagnostic Aids.)

Other treatments

- **Cryosurgery** is where tumour tissue is destroyed by freeze–thaw cycles that cause the cells to rupture due to ice crystal formation. This is not very selective and normal cells are also killed.
- **Chemotherapy** is the use of cytotoxic drugs to kill tumour cells selectively; it is only used for specific tumour types.
- **Radiotherapy** is used in specialist centres to kill dividing tumour cells.
- **Hyperthermia** is also a specialist technique that uses local application of heat via needles introduced into the tumour to try and kill the dividing tumour cells.
- **Photodynamic therapy** is a specialist technique using photosensitising chemicals and light to kill tumour cells.
- Often treatments may be combined with surgery and **adjunctive therapy** in the form of analgesics, antibiotics, anti-inflammatories, specialist nutritional requirements and nursing management may be an important part of managing these patients.

Post-operative management and advice

Ongoing nursing and monitoring of cancer patients is often necessary. Radiographs may be repeated at 4–6 month intervals to check for the development of metastases.

Oncologic surgery carries with it the stigma of the dreaded word 'cancer' and many owners will continue to be concerned about the outcome long after the surgical wound has healed. Some animals have a very good quality of life for a considerable period of time even if the treatment has not been curative, and owners may need reassurance that the animal is not suffering. Some tumours carry a poor prognosis despite surgery and owners may need extra time and advice on how to observe their animal for recur-

rence and quality of life. It can be very distressing for owners to think that the animal will die from the condition and be waiting for it to happen, and all staff should be aware of the condition. Discussion about what to look for and how they might want to manage the final euthanasia may be best carried out before the animal is terminally ill. (See Chapter 26, Managing Animal Death.)

Surgery and diseases of specific body systems

This section covers the main surgical diseases in the different body systems, and outlines the surgery and nursing implications of disease or potential surgical complications.

Nearly all surgical procedures are carried out under general anaesthetic and much of the post-operative nursing involves monitoring of the recovery from anaesthesia, and assessment and provision of analgesia. However, some surgical procedures also require post-operative monitoring for specific complications such as haemorrhage, infection, suture dehiscence or respiratory difficulties.

Surgical intervention in different areas of the body can be classified in terms of their potential for infection. Areas that can be prepared for aseptic surgery are a different risk to those that are clearly infected and impossible to make aseptic.

SURGICAL CLASSIFICATIONS

I **Clean** surgery – a surgical wound made under aseptic conditions that does not enter any contaminated viscus, and there is no break in sterile technique.

II **Clean-contaminated** surgery – a surgical wound made under aseptic conditions which enters the oropharynx, respiratory, alimentary or urogenital tracts, but there is no other source of contamination.

III **Contaminated** surgery – there is a major spill of contaminated material at surgery, or a break in sterile technique, or entry into a viscous with a high bacterial load (e.g. the colon or rectum).

IV **Infected** surgery – the surgical site is known to be already infected.

These classifications of surgical procedures enable the surgical team to assess the risk of post-operative infection and treat appropriately. For example, category I does not require antibiotics post-operatively, and category IV may be treated with antibiotics both before, during and after surgery (Table 19.7). The most effective way to use antibiotics during surgery is to give an intravenous preparation before the first incision. **Antibiotics given after the surgery has been completed will make no difference to the incidence of infection.**

<table>
<tr><td>

REDUCING RISK OF INFECTION

During surgery, the risks of infection can be reduced by other means too:

- Thorough lavage of contaminated tissue using sterile fluids.
- The surgeon may change gloves or re-scrub after handling infected or contaminated tissue prior to closing the unaffected tissue.
- The instruments may be changed for fresh sterile instruments.
- Suture material should be discarded if used in contaminated areas and fresh material supplied for closure of clean areas.
- The drapes may be covered with fresh sterile drapes prior to closure.

These techniques are commonly used after surgery on the gastrointestinal tract.

</td></tr>
</table>

The eye

Ophthalmic surgery is one of the most meticulous areas of small animal surgery, where preparation, technique and post-operative care can have an enormous impact on outcome. General anaesthesia is required for all but the most minor procedures. Specialised instruments, theatre equipment and facilities for magnification may be necessary for some ophthalmic surgery.

General principles and preparation for eye surgery

The conjunctival sac is filled with a gel or lubricant and the fur is clipped very carefully from a small area surrounding the eye. The first stage is to clean gross contamination or exudate off the eye and eyelids using gauze swabs soaked in sterile saline. Skin preparation is then completed using diluted povidone–iodine solution (note that surgical scrub solutions are *not* used in eye preparation) in preference to chlorhexidine solutions. The corneal and conjunctival surfaces should then

Table 19.7 Surgical procedures and risks of infection

Classification of risks	Examples of surgical procedures
I Clean surgery	Neutering; uncomplicated hernias
II Clean contaminated surgery	Lung lobectomy; gastrotomy; tracheotomy
III Contaminated surgery	Abdominal surgery where the gut contents spilled accidentally; oral surgery; wounds less than 4 hours old; lower bowel surgery
IV Infected surgery	Aural surgery; abscesses; old wounds; removal of necrotic tissue

be irrigated with sterile balanced salt solutions or saline and a drop of broad-spectrum antibiotic solution may be instilled onto the surface prior to surgery. Alcohol solutions should not be used near the eye surface. During surgery, Lacrilube® (Allergan) may be used to keep the eye lubricated while the eyelids are held open for the surgery.

Post-operatively, the eye is usually protected using an Elizabethan collar, and sometimes it is necessary to bandage the front paws. Bandages are difficult to keep secure over the eye and limit post-operative monitoring and treatments. Inflammation of the eye in the post-operative phase is often detrimental, particularly where specialist surgery has been performed on structures within the eye. In this regard, ocular surgery is unusual as corticosteroids may be used in the post-operative phase to reduce inflammation despite the delay in wound healing. Post-operative treatments may include topical ointments or drops for administration of antibiotics, steroids or cycloplegics (reduce pupil spasm). In general, ointments can be applied less frequently than drops and may be easier for the owner to administer.

Analgesia is important and will make administration of treatments easier. Owners may need special advice and instruction on how to administer treatments safely.

Surgical conditions of the cornea and conjunctiva

Conjunctivitis ?twb = 0.5w > This is inflammation of the conjunctival membrane characterised by reddening of the conjunctiva. Usually the animal also shows increased tear production and overflow (**epiphora**). If the eye is very sore, the animal may hold the eyelids closed and be very reluctant to allow examination of the eye (**blepharospasm**). It is not a surgical disease in its own right, but is often a symptom of other conditions in the eye. In cats and rabbits it can be a primary infection.

Keratitis and ulceration Keratitis is inflammation of the cornea, which may be accompanied by ulceration. The inflamed cornea has a cloudy appearance due to the oedema. Using the dye **fluorescin** in the eye allows ulceration to be visualised, and is important in diagnosis and monitoring of the healing of the ulcer. Where ointments containing corticosteroids are to be used to treat the keratitis it is extremely important to ensure that there is no ulceration present as the corticosteroid will prevent the ulcer from healing.

Ulcers may be secondary to penetration of the conjunctiva by a foreign body or due to keratitis or exposure of the surface of the eye and drying out of the conjunctiva. Severe ulcers may cause erosion of the cornea and ultimately result in rupture of the eye.

Ulcers are treated using techniques to protect the surface of the eye while the ulcer heals by second intention. Small ulcers may be treated with removal of the initiating cause and antibiotic ointment. Large ulcers may require surgical treatment. Traditionally, the third eyelid used to be sutured across the front of the eye to cover the ulcer. However, newer techniques such as conjunctival flaps and corneal contact lenses provide better visualisation of the ulcer to monitor healing and make it easier to apply treatments.

Keratitis can also be caused by the instillation of irritant chemicals onto the surface of the eye. This may be accidental, malicious or iatrogenic, and requires *emergency treatment* to prevent permanent scarring to the cornea. The eye should be irrigated with copious amounts of water or sterile saline to wash as much of the chemical out as possible. The eye should then be closely monitored for ulceration and treated appropriately.

Foreign bodies   Presentation with acute severe conjunctivitis may indicate the presence of a foreign body such as a grass seed trapped behind the eyelids. Careful examination of the inner surfaces of both eyelids and the third eyelid is necessary to identify and remove the foreign material. In calm animals, it may be possible to do this after application of local anaesthetic drops, but many animals will require sedation or general anaesthesia, as it can be very painful. After removal, the eye should be checked for ulceration.

Surgical conditions of the eyelids

Entropion   This is inversion of the eyelid margin such that the eyelashes rub on the cornea. There is often secondary conjunctivitis and keratitis. Entropion is treated by surgery to return the eyelid margin to its normal position.

Ectropion   This is eversion of the eyelid margin. In most cases, ectropion does not require surgical intervention, but in some dogs, it prevents normal lubrication of the eye and gives rise to a chronic exposure keratitis. Certain breeds of dog may have both ectropion and entropion at different points along the eyelid margin.

Distichiasis   This is the most common of a group of disorders characterised by abnormal growth of hairs at the eyelid margin so that the hairs rub the surface of the cornea. In many cases, the hairs do not cause a clinical problem, but in some cases, they cause a chronic keratitis requiring treatment. There are several surgical treatments described to remove the offending hairs and the follicle permanently.

Tumours   Tumours on the margin of the eyelid are very common in older dogs. They cause irritation by rubbing on the surface of the cornea and some are malignant. They are treated by excising a wedge of the eyelid margin containing the tumour.

Surgical conditions of the globe

Eyeball prolapse   Complete **prolapse** of the eyeball out of its socket (**proptosis** of the globe) can occur particularly in brachycephalic dogs. *First aid treatment is important* if there is to be any chance of saving the eye. The eye must be kept moist using KY jelly (Johnson & Johnson) or Lacrilube® (Allergan), supported by sterile saline soaked swabs. Definitive surgery to replace the eye in the socket must be carried out as soon as possible.

Lens luxation   The lens is usually held in place by ligaments behind the pupil, but if these fail, it can luxate either into the anterior chamber of the eye or caudally. This is usually a spontaneous event often in Terrier breeds, but can also be seen as a result of trauma. It requires emergency treatment to remove the lens as it will lead to the development of glaucoma and blindness.

Glaucoma   This is an acute elevation in the pressure within the eye which can result in *permanent blindness* within 24 hours if not treated. There are several causes of glaucoma, but the commonest are **anterior uveitis** and lens luxation. The eye is extremely painful, the sclera engorged and the pupil is usually dilated. Emergency medical treatment includes analgesia and intravenous hypertonic fluids (mannitol) to try to draw fluid out of the eye. Surgical treatments are available in specialist centres.

Cataracts   A cataract is the opacification of the fibres or capsule of the lens of the eye, ultimately resulting in blindness. It should be distinguished from ageing changes in the lens that result in an apparent blue colour of the lens, but that the animal can still see through. Cataracts may be a primary disease or secondary to other conditions such as diabetes mellitus. They may be left untreated or they can be surgically removed by specialist ophthalmic surgeons. Removal of the lens enables the animal to recognise objects and people as the lens is not as important in focusing as it is in people. This restores quality of life to the older animal.

Ocular trauma   The eye may be penetrated by foreign bodies or lacerated by claws or teeth during fights with other animals. All these conditions may potentially result in loss of the eye and should be examined and treated as an *emergency*.

Retina   Most retinal diseases are not amenable to surgery, but the retina is an important site of disease in the eye. Of particular importance are a group of inherited diseases of the retina known as **progressive retinal atrophy** which are known to occur in certain breeds.

Skin

Skin biopsy

Skin biopsies are indicated for diagnosis of skin disease. Minimal preparation of the skin surface should be performed in order not to disrupt surface cells that may aid the pathologist in making a diagnosis. The sample is taken using either a **skin biopsy punch** or just with a scalpel blade. Several biopsies should be taken from representative sites and the incisions closed with simple interrupted sutures. In severely diseased skin, there may be delayed wound healing.

Skin tumours

Skin masses should ideally be histologically identified prior to removal. The best way to identify the tumour is using a **fine-needle aspirate biopsy**. Surgery should be performed in the normal aseptic way and the skin closed with sutures. It is important to be aware that some small skin tumours may require tissue margins *in three dimensions* and therefore some fat and muscle may need to be removed along with the overlying skin.

Surgical management of local pyoderma

Some chronic local skin infections are related to long-term skin disease such as atopy (allergic skin disease) and are then exacerbated by the animal's anatomical skin folds. If the skin folds are not due to obesity, then it may be appropriate to resect the skin folds in order to prevent the recurrence of painful pyoderma. The common examples are vulval folds, screwtail folds and lip folds. Certain breeds such as the brachycephalics and spaniels are more likely to suffer from these conditions. Patients with allergic skin disease are most likely to interfere with their sutures as they are always itchy.

Urine/faecal scalding and pressure sores

Recumbent or incontinent patients are prone to soiling with urine or faeces and it is a *failure of nursing management* which then results in the development of pressure sores or 'scald' (**dermatitis**). The skin and fur must be kept clean and dry at all times. In some cases, this may involve several baths per day or clipping away fur to enable exposure of the skin so that it can be checked easily. Traditional treatments are to protect the skin with a thin layer of vaseline or similar oil-based cream, so that the urine does not irritate the skin surface. However, these do not allow the skin to breathe and although they will prevent the skin from becoming worse, they will not help treat any dermatitis. Commercial spray-on products are available (e.g. Cavilon™) which provide a semi-permeable membrane under which the skin can heal while it is protected from the urine/faeces. The skin can also be covered with self-adhesive semi-permeable membranes.

Prevention of pressure sores is much easier than cure. Padded bedding will help prevent the development of pressure points in recumbent, obese or bony patients, and the use of 'Vetbed' material or incontinence pads will help keep the skin dry, by wicking moisture away from the surface. Paralysed patients should be turned every 2–4 hours and all pressure points protected. Physiotherapy will help encourage the blood supply to the skin and reduce the risk.

Anal sacs

The anal sacs are situated on either side of the anus and contain anal glands which produce a creamy coloured pungent exudate. The sacs are normally emptied on top of the faeces at the time of each defecation, and should not swell up or cause irritation. If anal sacs become impacted they fill with fluid which then becomes secondarily infected, or they can eventually rupture and spill irritant infected contents into the tissues around the anus. This is often the case with animals with chronic **anal furunculosis**. Anal furunculosis is a deep-seated infection with sinus tracts in the skin around the anus and under the tail. It is very painful and usually associated with colitis, dietary intolerance and auto-immune disease.

The classic clinical sign of anal gland irritation is persistent chewing at the rump or tail and/or rubbing the perineum on the ground, particularly after defecation. Anal gland disease may be secondary to a number of non-surgical diseases such as flea allergic dermatitis, atopy, obesity or diarrhoea. In some cases, it is necessary to remove chronically diseased anal sacs to prevent recurrence of infection.

Interdigital disease

Interdigital disease may be part of generalised skin disease, but some breeds are particularly predisposed to development of interdigital cysts or interdigital foreign bodies such as grass seeds. Dogs with long fur between the toes are particularly at risk of grass seeds becoming embedded in the thin interdigital skin. This causes painful swellings or abscesses; sometimes it is possible to identify the end of the grass seed in the swelling and it is removed with forceps. However, if the seed has migrated into the leg, the sinus tract must be surgically explored. Surgical exploration is often easier if done with a tourniquet on the leg during the surgery. During the summer and autumn months, owners should be advised to check between and under the toes daily, or else keep the fur trimmed very short.

Aural surgery

The most common conditions of the ear are usually related to generalised skin disease. Recurrent shaking of the head and scratching at the ears can result in an aural haematoma, and persistent dermatitis may result in otitis externa.

Aural haematoma This is the most common injury of the pinna. It is secondary to self-induced trauma and there is nearly always underlying otitis externa. A blood vessel bursts, usually on the underside of the pinna and forms a large haematoma. They are painful and if not treated, cause the pinna to scar in a deformed shrivelled shape. Generally they are treated surgically. The haematoma is drained and cleaned out, allowing the skin to flatten again against the cartilage. Recurrence is then prevented by suturing the skin to the cartilage to close the dead space, with the knots tied on the outer surface of the pinna. Buttons, quills or X-ray film have all been used to help flatten the skin and prevent the sutures from pulling out.

Post-operatively it is important to treat any underlying skin or ear disease and to prevent the patient from scratching at the ear again. This is either with an Elizabethan collar or with a figure-of-eight head bandage.

Otitis externa　This is extremely common in both dogs and cats. There are many causes and these have to be investigated prior to treatment:

- Foreign bodies in the ear canal (e.g. grass seeds).
- Ear mites (*Otodectes*).
- As an extension of generalised skin disease (e.g. atopy).
- Poor ear conformation, especially in the floppy-eared breeds or very hairy breeds.
- Polyps or tumours.
- Bacterial or yeast infection of the ears – this is usually secondary to one of the above.

Animals usually present with head shaking, scratching at the ears, aural pain and there may be bleeding or discharge out of the ear canals.

It may be necessary to clean the ears with saline before they can be examined. They are often extremely painful and this procedure should be done with analgesia or under anaesthetic.

Tumours in the ear, or where cases of otitis externa have become very severe, are treated surgically:

- **Lateral wall resection**: the lateral wall of the vertical canal is removed so as to open up the ear to the air and allow better drainage and access for cleaning. This is only suitable for ears that have no disease on the medial wall of the vertical canal or in the horizontal canal.
- **Vertical canal ablation**: the vertical canal is completely removed and the horizontal canal opening is sutured to the skin. This is only for ears where the disease is confined to the vertical canal.
- **Total ear canal ablation**: this procedure is most commonly used and is usually for severe long-term otitis externa. Often the infection has ruptured the tympanic membrane and there is otitis media too. The middle ear (tympanic bulla) is accessed at the time of surgery by enlarging the bony opening (**bulla osteotomy**) and the middle ear is scraped and lavaged clean. The whole of the vertical and horizontal ear canal are removed and the tissue and skin sutured closed over the top. This procedure is more challenging than the others but often is the only solution as it removes all the diseased tissue.

Ear surgery is regarded as infected and antibiotics are usually given both before, during and after the surgery. Post-operatively, the patients need analgesia, and the ear must be protected from self-inflicted injury. An Elizabethan collar may be used, or a head bandage, or the pinnae may be bandaged together to stop them flapping against the wound. There is often a discharge of blood or exudate from the wound for several days and this must be gently cleaned away using sterile saline. The sutures may have to stay in slightly longer than usual, but small areas of dehiscence are allowed to heal by second intention.

Otitis media　In the dog, this is often an extension of otitis externa, but in the cat, it may occur as a primary disease as an ascending infection via the eustachian tube. Access to the middle ear is either via a total ear canal ablation as described above if there is external disease or via a ventral approach (**ventral bulla osteotomy**). The animal is placed in dorsal recumbency and the dissection made directly over the tympanic bulla. A small drill is then used to make a hole in the bulla to allow drainage and lavage.

Otitis interna　Inflammation of the inner ear structures causes loss of balance, vomiting, head tilts, nystagmus and disorientation (**vestibular syndrome**). If this is secondary to severe middle ear disease, then surgical management of the middle ear disease may be necessary to resolve in the otitis interna.

Mammary tumours

Mammary neoplasia is the commonest tumour in the bitch, and the second most common tumour in all dogs. It is less common in the cat, although it is seen in breeding queens, particularly Siamese, or cats that have been treated for oestrus suppression or skin disease using megoestrol acetate (Ovarid)®.

In bitches, the most commonly affected glands are the two caudal pairs while in queens, cranial glands are most often affected. About 50% of mammary tumours in the bitch are benign, but in cases with multiple masses, they may all be different tumour types. In cats, over 80% of mammary masses are malignant, and carcinomas tend to be particularly aggressive, most having metastasised by the time of presentation.

Fine-needle aspirate biopsies are rarely helpful except to differentiate mammary tumours from mastitis or hypertrophy. The type of tumour is rarely confirmed prior to surgery as it does not change the management of the disease.

Surgery is the treatment of choice for mammary tumours. In the bitch, the type of surgery has little effect on the survival time, and as many tumours are benign, radical surgery is generally unnecessary. Surgery involves either removing just the gland affected (**mammectomy**), or the gland and an adjacent gland (**local mastectomy**) or all the glands on the affected side (**radical mastectomy** or '**mammary strip**'). In the cat, the tumours are often aggressive and radical surgery is more important.

All mammary gland surgery is prone to dehiscence and ideally a drain should be used and post-operative antibiotic therapy. Surgery on both sides is simultaneously usually avoided to reduce the risk of wound complications.

Although in humans there are many other treatments used alongside surgery for mammary tumours, in dogs and cats there are currently no other treatments that are known to make a difference to survival after removal of malignant mammary tumours.

Gastrointestinal tract

Many diseases affecting the GI tract have serious adverse effects on the fluid and electrolyte status of the patient.

These deficits should be identified and stabilised prior to anaesthesia and surgery. Long periods of anorexia or vomiting and diarrhoea will cause the animal to be dehydrated and in a negative energy balance and therefore a poor candidate for surgery. Steps must be taken to replenish nutritional deficits and to maintain nutrition to minimise the effects of surgery on the patient. This may mean placement of feeding tubes prior to, or during the surgical procedure to help nurse the patient post-operatively. For example, an anorexic cat is likely to recover much more quickly if feeding tubes are placed at the time of surgery, than if hand feeding or 'tempting' food is relied upon in the early post-operative stages.

Oral surgery
Dental disease and management

- **Periodontal disease** is disease of the tissues and structures that surround the teeth.
- **Dental plaque** is a film-like deposit on the surface of the tooth consisting of a mixture of salivary deposits, bacteria and food particles.
- **Dental calculus** is mineralised, stone-like concretion of accumulated dental plaque.
- **Gingivitis** is a reddening of the gums around the teeth, signifying inflammation.
- **Dental caries** is erosion of the tooth enamel and dentine which may extend into the tooth pulp.

Periodontal disease associated with the build up of dental plaque and calculus is the most common dental condition encountered in small-animal practice. The animal presents with **halitosis**, gingival bleeding or ulceration, gingivitis and sometimes lip ulceration. Very severely affected animals may have tooth root abscesses, osteomyelitis or even septicaemia. Cats can present with just a gingivitis and erosive **neck lesions** of the teeth that cause them to fracture.

Veterinary dentistry is a speciality in its own right, and specialists can crown teeth, fill root canals, treat dental caries and repair fractures. The bulk of veterinary dentistry in general practice involves basic dental hygiene and removal of calculus and plaque. Owners should be encouraged to help prevent the build up of dental plaque by regularly brushing their animals' teeth, using either 0.2% chlorhexidine solution or a proprietary veterinary toothpaste. Ideally, the owner should be shown how to do this when the animal is young, to ensure compliance.

Specialised instruments are used to remove scale manually prior to using electronic scalers. **Dental scalers** may be ultrasonic or sonic, and release the plaque by vibration from high frequency sound waves. A continuous spray helps keep the scaler tip and the tooth surface cool, but operator technique is also important in preventing damage to the tooth surface (see box). The tip of the scaler must be used as flat as possible to the tooth and never at an angle less than 45°, and never with any pressure applied. Polishing the teeth after scaling is essential to smooth

---

DENTAL SCALING
(1) General anaesthesia is essential, and allows a full and detailed examination of the mouth.
(2) A cuffed endotracheal tube should be used and the table tipped slightly head-down. The back of the pharynx should be packed with a roll of bandage or swabs (counted in and out!).
(3) The operator should wear a mask and eye protection and sterile surgery should not be done in the vicinity for at least 1 hour after dental work.
(4) Dental calculus is removed manually using a **supragingival scaler** to pull the calculus off the tooth away from the gingiva.
(5) The scaler tip is held as flat as possible to the tooth surface and continuously moved in light overlapping strokes, applying no pressure.
(6) Each tooth should only be scaled for 15 seconds and then rested to allow the heat to dissipate.
(7) A **subgingival curette** is used to clean underneath the gingiva alongside the teeth.
(8) The teeth are polished to smooth out the scaled surface using a **prophylaxis cup** and **prophylaxis paste** with fluoride.
(9) The mouth is cleaned of debris and wiped dry and the pharyngeal pack removed prior to recovery from anaesthesia.

---

out the scaled tooth surface so that the plaque and calculus do not rapidly adhere and reaccumulate. A slow-speed electronic rotator handpiece is used together with a small soft rubber cup filled with **prophylaxis paste**. The cup rotates on the tooth and polishes the surface with the paste acting as a lubricant to prevent build up of heat. The cup should be applied quite firmly so that the edges flare out to polish underneath the gingival edge. Finally, the gingival recesses may be gently flushed with a dilute antiseptic solution (0.2% chlorhexidine) to remove debris, calculus or prophy paste.

Dental extractions are commonly necessary, but essentially are an indication of the failure of dental management for the patient. Teeth should be removed if there is evidence of tooth root infection, exposure of the pulp cavity, fractures, neck lesions (in cats), or advanced dental caries or periodontal disease. If there is any doubt as to whether a tooth is in good health, radiography using high-detail dental non-screen film will help to assess the tooth root. Occasionally young animals present with retained deciduous teeth which are causing periodontal disease by trapping food material and debris between them and the permanent teeth. These are removed as described below, but it is important to be very careful and ensure that no leverage or damage occurs to the permanent teeth.

Dental extraction should be carried out carefully and gently, taking time to systematically loosen the attachments. Use of excessive force will increase the risk of fistulas, haemorrhage, tooth root fracture and even fracture of the jaw.

DENTAL EXTRACTION
(1) Prepare the patient and operator as for dental scaling.
(2) Assess all the teeth and radiograph if necessary.
(3) The soft tissue attachment between the gingiva and the tooth is cut using a sharp **dental luxator** or a number 11 scalpel blade.
(4) The tooth is loosened using a dental **root elevator**.
(5) The tooth is then cut to separate the roots, or the overlying bone elevated as necessary (see text).
(6) The tooth is thoroughly loosened using a dental luxator to cut the periodontal ligaments and then a root elevator to lever the root and loosen it.
(7) Dental **extraction forceps** are used to remove the tooth only once it is properly loosened, gently rotating it to pull it out.
(8) The tooth roots are examined to ensure that all the root has been removed and none is remaining in the socket.

The most common complication of dental extraction is incomplete removal of a tooth root which may result in pain and/or abscessation. More rarely, the alveolar socket may haemorrhage. In normal animals, this should stop with gentle pressure, but persistent bleeding is suggestive of a bleeding disorder or other disease.

INDICATIONS FOR ANTIBIOTICS
Antibiotics are used in the following circumstances:
• The animal also has renal, hepatic or cardiac disease.
• Where it was not possible to remove all the diseased teeth.
• Where there is associated oral ulceration or septicaemia.
• Where there is osteomyelitis.
• The animal has orthopaedic implants that may become infected.

The first step is to cut the periodontal ligaments all the way down the tooth root. The **dental luxator** is used for this, it is a sharp instrument and is made of soft metal, so it is not used for leverage or applying any force to the tooth. Next, the tooth is gently rocked using the **root elevator** to loosen the root until the tooth can be lifted out with the forceps.

Multi-rooted teeth cannot be removed in a single piece as the roots flare and point in different directions. The crown of the tooth is therefore cut into sections to split the roots into single items which can then be removed one by one. Ideally, an oscillating saw is used for this, but a hacksaw blade may be used to manually cut the tooth, although this will cause much more soft tissue damage. Teeth with very large deep roots (e.g. the canine) have to be elevated by removal of some of the mucoperiosteum and bone overlying the root. This is then repaired surgically after the tooth has been removed.

Great care should be taken when removing teeth from cats and small breed dogs particularly in the rostral part of the jaw where the canine tooth roots are long. Even gentle extraction methods can result in mandibular fracture or the development of oronasal fistulas.

As a general rule, although the oral cavity is contaminated, antibiotics should not be used routinely for all dental procedures. A single intravenous dose of a bactericidal antibiotic (e.g. ampicillin) at the time of the dental work should be sufficient to treat the transient bacteraemia.

Oral tumours   These are generally seen in older dogs and cats. Tumours may arise on any structure of the oro-pharynx (tongue, gingiva, lips, palate, tonsils, etc.), and the prognosis depends very much upon both the site of the tumour and the type of tumour. As owners generally do not inspect their pet's mouth regularly, these tumours may be large before they are presented for treatment. The first sign of a tumour may be halitosis, loss or displacement of teeth or facial swelling, and the tumour may only be identified at the time of dental examination by the veterinary surgeon.

Surgical resection carries the best prognosis for all oral tumours in the dog and cat. Where tumours are on the mandible or maxilla, bone and teeth may have to be removed along with the tumour in order to get adequate margins. The defect is then closed using flaps of mucosa from the lips and sutured with absorbable suture material. Post-operative nursing focuses on analgesia and ensuring that the patient can eat and drink easily. Food should be soft and formed, but not dry/abrasive (which might tear the sutures) or too sloppy (which might seep between the sutures). Tumours of the tonsils or palate often carry a worse prognosis, particularly in cats.

Oronasal fistulas   These may be secondary to trauma, dental extraction or tumour resection. All fistulas should be repaired surgically, to prevent food material impacting in the nasal cavity and causing a rhinitis. Pre-op preparation involves using saline and then dilute chlorhexidine or povidone–iodine solution to flush out debris accumulated in the cavity and nasal passages. Post-operatively, the defect should heal rapidly and may be kept clean with gentle oral lavage using chlorhexidine solutions.

Cleft palate   Puppies should always be checked for cleft palate at the time of birth, but it can also be traumatic in origin. Some clefts are simply repaired using advancement flaps, and others require more advanced techniques, depending on the degree of involvement of the soft and hard palate. Protection of the suture line in the mouth is difficult and restriction of food intake or use of feeding tubes are counterproductive. The animal should be given soft formed food that will not get stuck in the suture line and is easy to swallow.

Foreign bodies and penetrating injuries For-eign bodies such as sticks, bones, fish hooks or grass seeds may lodge in the soft tissues of the mouth and pharynx. All cause pain associated with the mouth, difficulty in swallowing and drooling.

The mouth can be opened in the conscious animal by using ropes behind the canine teeth of the upper and lower jaws, but the examination will be more effective under general anaesthesia. Penetrating injuries of the oeso-phagus and pharynx caused by sticks thrown for dogs by the owners can be potentially life threatening and should be surgically explored as an emergency.

Oesophageal surgery

Oesophageal foreign bodies Partial obstruction of the oesophagus with bones is common in Terrier breeds and results in regurgitation of food and sometimes fluids. In cases where there is complete obstruction, dehydration is extremely rapid and hypovolaemia may be life threatening. *These cases are always emergencies.* The foreign body is usually retrieved by extraction via the mouth through a rigid endoscope, but occasionally bones may have to be pushed down into the stomach. Digestible foreign bodies (such as bones) are not removed from the stomach but plas-tic toys or balls have to be removed via a gastrotomy. Post-operatively, the patient is treated with drugs to reduce gastric acidity in case of gastric reflux, which will exacerbate oesophagitis. The oesophagus is also assessed for tears and inflammation, using the endoscope. Small tears or bruising may be treated with nil by mouth and food and water via a gastrostomy tube for 3–5 days. Severe full thickness tears may have to be explored via a thoracotomy to prevent development of sepsis, and the prognosis is very poor.

Oesophageal stricture This condition may arise as a result of trauma secondary to an oesophageal foreign body, but is also known to arise as a consequence of gen-eral anaesthesia. The animal presents 2–4 weeks after the initiating cause with a history of regurgitating all solid food. It is difficult to treat successfully and therapy relies on stretching the stricture endoscopically and using steroid therapy to reduce the rate of recurrence of scar tissue. An-imals may manage on a liquidised diet.

Gastric surgery

Foreign body The cardinal sign of a gastric foreign body is persistent or intermittent vomiting. Diagnosis may be confirmed by radiography, contrast radiography or gas-troscopy. Some foreign bodies may be retrieved endoscopi-cally, but many will require surgical removal. The stomach is accessed via a cranial midline laparotomy and pulled out of the abdomen as far as possible. The rest of the ab-dominal organs are packed off with sterile moist towels or swabs to protect them from contamination. The incision is usually made in an avascular area of the body of the sto-mach. The whole stomach should be inspected for other foreign bodies and mucosal damage prior to closure with a synthetic absorbable suture material.

Pyloric obstruction This can be due to a foreign body, but more often it is due to pyloric thickening, either due to hypertrophy of the muscle or to neoplasia. These diseases are often known as **gastric outflow diseases**, and congenital forms are more common in specific breeds such as brachycephalic dogs or Siamese cats. Once the diagnosis is confirmed, surgery is performed to either widen the pylorus (**pyloroplasty**) or to remove the pylorus altogether (**pyloric resection**).

Immediately post-operatively, small amounts of water are made available to the patient and then small quantities of a liquidised low-fat diet are offered 24 hours later. It is impor-tant to stimulate normal gastric motility without inducing vomiting, and some cases may have a gastrostomy tube placed at the time of surgery to help decompress the sto-mach post-operatively for a few days.

Gastric dilatation/volvulus This is a peracute ra-pidly fatal syndrome resulting from accumulation of food and gas in the stomach. The stomach dilates initially and this precipitates rotation of the stomach around its axis re-sulting in occlusion of the oesophagus and the venous drainage. Severe hypovolaemic and toxic shock starts dur-ing the dilatation phase and escalates once rotation occurs. If not treated promptly, death results from the shock, gas-tric wall necrosis, ventricular dysrhythmias and DIC (**dis-seminated intravascular coagulation**). The specific aetiology is poorly understood, but usually the dogs are deep chested, often middle to older aged, and the condition may be associated with a nervous temperament. Pre-operatively, nursing involves aggressive management of the shock and attempts to deflate the stomach either by passage of a stomach tube or by percutaneous needle gas-trostomy. (See Chapter 14, First Aid.)

Confirmation of rotation of the stomach is obtained with a right lateral abdominal radiograph and indicates that surgical derotation is necessary.

GASTRIC DILATATION/VOLVULUS
(1) Treat for shock with rapid administration of large volumes of intravenous fluids.
(2) Intravenous antibiotics.
(3) Decompression of the stomach via passage of a stomach tube.
(4) Right lateral radiograph to confirm volvulus.
(5) ECG – treat if necessary for ventricular dysrhythmias.
(6) Surgery for decompression, derotation and assessment of stomach wall viability.

Usually a gastrostomy tube is placed at the time of sur-gery to allow decompression of the stomach if there is reduced gastric motility post-op, and may be used for feeding if the animal is moribund. In order to prevent recurrence of the rotation, a **gastropexy** may be carried out where the pylorus is anchored to the body wall with sutures, although this does not prevent the recurrence of dilation. Post-operative nursing continues treatment of fluid and electrolyte losses and in particular monitoring and treating ventricular dysrhythmias.

Gastric neoplasia　Gastric neoplasms are often aggressive and may be very advanced before diagnosis. Clinical signs include haematemesis, weight loss and gastric pain. Some neoplasms can be resected if they are on the greater curvature of the stomach.

Tube gastrostomy　This is a useful tool for nutritional support and/or decompression of the stomach. The tube is anchored in the stomach and exits through the body wall, where it is sutured to the skin and bandaged in place. The tube can be placed without surgery using an endoscope to push the end of the tube through the skin (per endoscopic gastrostomy tube or **PEG tube**) or it is placed via a laparotomy. A **dePezzer** (mushroom tipped) catheter is usually used, although a **Foley catheter** may also be substituted. It is important to protect the tube from self-mutilation, particularly if it was placed endoscopically, as it is less secure in the stomach wall than if sutured. Tubes are removed by pushing a probe into the end of the mushroom tip to straighten out the tip and allow it to be pulled through the abdominal wall. They should not be removed too early (< 3 days) before a seal has formed around the hole in the gastric wall. The resultant wound in the body wall may leak gastric contents for 1–2 days, but is kept clean with skin antiseptics and allowed to granulate closed.

Small intestine

Surgery on the small intestine (duodenum, jejunum and ileum) is common in small animal practice. The intestines are lifted out of the abdomen during surgery so that other organs are not contaminated if gut contents spill. They should be kept moist using sterile saline-soaked swabs or towels, but this will mean that waterproof surgical drapes are necessary. Heat loss is rapid when the intestines are removed from the abdomen and it is necessary to provide a heating pad or warmed fluids.

Biopsy　Intestinal biopsy is usually indicated when investigations of gastrointestinal signs such as persistent or recurrent vomiting or diarrhoea, have been unrewarding. It is not possible to biopsy the jejunum or ileum via endoscopy and these have to be accessed via a laparotomy. Animals presented for intestinal biopsy may be poor candidates for surgery. Healing may be delayed due to hypoproteinaemia or cachexia. Small samples of intestine are taken from several sites all the way down the gastrointestinal tract and submitted in separate containers, each labelled with the site of the biopsy. All the biopsy sites are sutured closed and wrapped with omentum.

Post-operatively, the animal is encouraged to eat and drink as soon as possible in order to encourage rapid healing of the biopsy sites.

Enterotomy; foreign body removal　Foreign bodies in the cat small intestine are often **linear foreign bodies**, i.e. they are string, wool or thread and needle. The material may be lodged behind the back of the tongue or trapped at the pylorus and travel all the way down the GI tract into the small intestine. Smooth muscle contraction of the gut wall then concertinas the gut up the linear material and eventually either blocks the lumen or cuts through the wall of the intestine. Dogs more commonly ingest balls or plastic toys which pass to a point along the jejunum and then become lodged.

Sometimes the foreign body can be palpated through the abdominal wall, but often X-rays are necessary to make the diagnosis. The animal is stabilised and the foreign body removed via a laparotomy.

Usually the foreign body can be removed via a scalpel incision in the gut wall and then the hole is closed with synthetic absorbable sutures. Sometimes, the gut is very inflamed and appears necrotic, in which case an enterectomy may be necessary.

Enterectomy　Enterectomy is indicated where the gut is necrotic or there is a tumour in the wall. A section of the gut is removed and then the ends are sutured together to form an **anastamosis**. The affected section of gut is separated off using Doyen **bowel clamps** or just an assistant's fingers to prevent leakage from the remaining bowel, and then cut with a scalpel to remove it. Once it is removed, the cut ends are held close together while the surgeon sutures the edges using synthetic absorbable suture material. Often the anastamosis is then wrapped in omentum to help seal the surgical site. Post-operatively, healing is enhanced if the animal is encouraged to eat as soon as possible.

Intussusception　This is a condition where the small intestine invaginates into itself (like a telescope closing up). It is very rare in the cat, but usually seen in young dogs, often secondary to an episode of diarrhoea. The invaginated portion of intestine is called the **intussusceptum** and the outer part is the **intussuscipiens**. The blood supply to the intussusceptum is compromised and it often becomes necrotic. Symptoms are similar to intestinal obstruction and the diagnosis is usually made by X-ray. Surgery to reduce the intussusception is necessary and if the intussusceptum is necrotic it is resected. Sometimes the disease recurs and the intestines may be sutured to each other to prevent this (**enteropexy**).

Volvulus　Mesenteric volvulus is rarely reported in the dog and cat, although it is relatively common in horses. In all species it is rapidly fatal due to endotoxic and hypovolaemic shock secondary to death of most of the small intestine.

Large intestine

Surgery of the large intestine carries greater risk than higher up the GI tract as there is an increased bacterial load and a slower rate of healing. Enemas near the time of surgery are detrimental to surgical asepsis as the slurry is more likely to spill and contaminate the abdomen. Pre-operative oral antibiotics with anaerobic activity may help to reduce the bacterial load, but peri-operative antibiotics are essential and should be continued post-operatively. Hospital feeding should be careful not to induce a dietary enteritis – i.e. easily digested protein sources may be better than high-protein diets that may cause a nutritional diarrhoea. Often constipation or tenesmus are a symptom of the disease and dietary fibre supplements, faecal modifiers such as Isogel or Peridale (GSL) are used to increase faecal mass and increase peristalsis. Paraffin pastes or liquids are less suitable as they only lubricate the faeces and do not alter the water content or soften impacted faeces.

Biopsy

Biopsy of the rectum and distal colon can be achieved using rigid **proctoscopy**, although these biopsies are only partial thickness. Full-thickness biopsies are taken via laparotomy, and carry an increased risk compared to small intestinal biopsies. Strict aseptic technique, packing off the uncontaminated viscera and thorough lavage of the abdomen at the end of the procedure are important.

Colectomy

Removal of the colon is most often indicated for the treatment of chronic constipation in cats. Cats present with multiple episodes of complete obstipation requiring enemas and evacuation each time. Eventually, the episodes become more frequent and the colon loses all function. It is important to check that the cat does not have an obstruction to defecation in the pelvic canal by rectal examination and radiography of the pelvis. Surgery involves careful identification and ligation of the vessels supplying the colon, and resection and reanastomosis of the colon ends. Animals that are severely affected may require the ileo-caeco colic valve to be removed as well. The animal is prepared for surgery with antibiotics, but an enema is not performed as it is easier to prevent contamination of the abdomen during surgery if the faeces are dry and hard and can be removed within the colon.

These animals are often inappetent post-operatively, and early nutritional support is important to healing in the colon. Dehiscence of the anastamosis is often fatal.

Rectal polyps/tumours

Rectal polyps (papillomas) cause faecal tenesmus, bleeding and discomfort and are often treated initially as a colitis. Removal of the polyps is indicated because they are a pre-malignant change of the rectal mucosa. They can be removed by using a 'pull out' technique where the rectum is everted through the anus to allow removal of the polyp. The defect should be sutured using monofilament absorbable material and post-operative care is directed at reducing post-op straining using analgesics, anti-inflammatories, local anaesthetic gel and dietary fibre. Where the tumour is identified as malignant or has invasive characteristics, a wider excision is carried out to remove the full thickness of the rectal wall.

Rectal prolapse

This is eversion of the wall of the rectum through the anus. It is usually secondary to chronic straining and may be associated with a rectal tumour. Successful management requires treatment of the primary disease as well as reduction of the prolapse itself. The prolapse should be protected from self-mutilation and kept moist and lubricated, using lignocaine gel. Once the rectum is reduced, it is maintained using a loose temporary purse string suture around the anus. This may have to be loosened intermittently to allow defecation. Again, dietary faecal modifiers should be given to make the faeces soft and bulky.

Imperforate anus

This is a congenital condition where the anus fails to unite with the rectum, thus creating complete obstruction to the normal passage of faeces from the moment of birth. Sometimes it is possible to correct surgically.

Peritoneum

The peritoneum is the lining of the abdominal cavity and functions to help with healing of the intestinal tract and to protect it from infection if it becomes contaminated. Peritonitis occurs if there is contamination or irritation that results in an inflammatory response. Peritonitis can be due to surgical contamination, urine leakage from the bladder, intestinal content leakage due to perforation of any part of the GI tract, penetrating abdominal injury or leakage from the biliary or pancreatic systems. Initially, if there is no infection, peritonitis develops in response to the

---

CONTAMINATION OF THE ABDOMEN AT SURGERY

(1) Thorough abdominal lavage using sterile isotonic fluids (Hartmanns or saline) at body temperature.

(2) Repeated lavage until the fluids come out clear.

(3) All lavage fluid must be removed from the abdomen as remaining fluid reduces the ability of the immune system to clear remaining bacteria.

(4) Use omentum to cover any potential sites of leakage.

(5) Change the surgeon's gloves, instruments and redrape with sterile drapes over the top of the contaminated drapes (preferably with waterproof drapes).

(6) Give a second dose of intravenous antibiotics. Do not use topical antibiotics or antiseptics in the abdomen.

irritant nature of the fluid (e.g. urine or bile), and clinical signs may take a few days to develop. However, if the fluid is septic, or where there is leakage from the GI tract the peritonitis becomes infected and this rapidly leads to severe illness, with septicaemia, shock and cardiovascular collapse within a few hours.

It is important for nurses to recognise peritonitis as part of post-operative monitoring of a patient particularly after surgery on the GI tract. An animal may show some, or all, of the following clinical signs:

- Pyrexia.
- Anorexia.
- Depression.
- Tachycardia.
- Vomiting.
- Ascites.
- Abdominal pain.

The mainstay of treatment is to surgically explore the abdomen and find the source of contamination. In mild cases, or where there is no infection, thorough lavage of the abdomen may be sufficient. Where there is infection, the abdomen is best treated with **open peritoneal drainage**.

Abdominal lavage involves pouring large volumes of warmed sterile isotonic fluids into the abdomen via a laparotomy and using suction to remove them until they come out clear. It is important to remove all the contaminated fluid to be effective and waterproof surgical drapes should be used.

Open peritoneal drainage is a technique whereby the abdomen is not fully closed after the lavage and the abdomen is dressed with sterile dressings and a thick absorbent bandage (or disposable nappies). This dressing is changed using sterile technique 2–3 times per day while the infection drains from the abdomen. At each dressing change, the abdomen may be lavaged again through the open wound. Nursing of these patients is very complex and involves close monitoring of blood albumin and electrolyte levels, hydration and care of the bandage.

Respiratory tract

Respiratory distress is potentially life threatening in any species and the veterinary nurse must be able to recognise respiratory difficulties quickly in order to respond with potentially life-saving first aid.

Respiratory difficulty arises from inadequate oxygen delivery to the tissues which causes **hypoxia**. There are a number of ways this can come about:

- Obstruction to the passage of air into the respiratory tract, e.g. laryngeal paralysis, tracheal collapse, foreign body.
- Inefficient oxygen exchange at the air–tissue interface, e.g. pulmonary oedema, pneumonia.
- Inadequate blood supply to the alveoli, despite normal delivery of gases (**ventilation perfusion mismatch**), e.g. pulmonary thromboembolism, right-sided heart failure.

- Inadequate oxygen-carrying capacity, e.g. severe anaemia, carbon monoxide poisoning.
- Inadequate blood delivery to the tissues, e.g. hypovolaemia, circulatory collapse.

The clinical signs of respiratory distress will develop from an initial increase in respiratory rate, and effort to visible cyanosis of the mucous membranes, loss of consciousness and death:

- Increased respiratory rate at rest.
- Increased respiratory effort (there may be visible 'heaving' of the ribs).
- Exercise intolerance.
- Open mouth breathing (particularly cats).
- Cyanosis of the tongue and gingiva.
- Collapse.

First aid treatment is essential even for only mildly affected patients. Animals that show any signs of respiratory difficulty may suddenly decompensate when they are stressed during examination, and become profoundly hypoxic.

RESPIRATORY DISTRESS
- **Do not stress**.
- Keep patient away from other animals.
- Monitor continuously.
- Provide oxygen supplementation.
- Sedate if necessary.
- Keep the patient cool (this prevents panting and improves ventilation).
- Be prepared for emergency tracheostomy, CPR or endotracheal intubation for ventilation.

Nasal disease

Nasal disease in the dog and cat have a different pattern of disease, with the cat being predominantly affected by infectious agents causing acute or chronic rhinitis. Diagnosis of nasal disease can be very challenging and relies mainly on radiography, rhinoscopy, biopsy and in some cases MRI or CT scanning.

Rhinoscopy and biopsy Rhinoscopy is used to visualise the nasal turbinates to take biopsies or look for a foreign body. Ideally a small rigid endoscope is used, but sometimes an auroscope is used or a small flexible endoscope to look behind the soft palate at the choanae.

Biopsy of the nose in most instances relies on radiographic diagnosis of a lesion and then a blind biopsy using biopsy forceps measured against the radiograph. In some cases, the biopsy may be taken using the rhinoscope to guide the biopsy forceps. Biopsy of inflamed turbinates bleeds profusely, and the pharynx must be packed. Usually pressure over the external nares is sufficient to arrest bleeding, but in severe cases, adrenaline diluted to 1:100 000 may be sprayed up the nares to assist vasoconstriction of superficial vessels. Successful biopsy of nasal tumours often results in little haemorrhage.

Rhinotomy   Occasionally, it is necessary to open the nasal cavity to take biopsies, remove foreign bodies or remove a benign tumour. This is done via an incision on the bridge of the nose and the nasal cavity accessed through the nasal bones. Post-operative complications can include **emphysema** of the head and neck due to air leaking out through the rhinotomy incision.

Nasal aspergillosis   This is a fungal infection of the nasal cavity usually seen in younger doliocephalic breeds of dog. It causes a purulent nasal discharge and often causes **epistaxis**, which can be very severe. Diagnosis is made sometimes on biopsy or rhinoscopy, but it is more usually diagnosed with a blood test for the aspergillus antibodies. Treatment usually involves flushing the nasal cavity with an antifungal via tubes implanted in through the frontal sinus. The flushing has to be done conscious so that there is no risk of the dog aspirating the drug into the lungs.

Nasal neoplasia   Nasal tumours tend to affect older doliocephalic dogs and are most often carcinomas. In the cat, the Siamese may be more at risk and adenocarcinoma is the most common diagnosis, but lymphoma is also seen. The diagnosis is made by radiography and biopsy of the abnormal region seen on the radiograph. Surgical treatment is not usually an option, and nasal tumours are treated with a course of radiotherapy.

Stenotic nares (BAOS)   Brachycephalic airway obstruction syndrome (**BAOS**) is a syndrome affecting brachycephalic breeds with deformed airways, resulting in difficulty breathing. The commonest breeds affected are the Bulldogs, Pekingese and Pugs; occasionally Persian cats may be affected. The animal presents with noisy breathing which results from a combination of obstructions to the upper airway:

- Stenotic nares.
- Overlong soft palate.
- Tonsillar hypertrophy.
- Pharyngeal hypertrophy.

Some of these dogs may also have collapsed larynx and a narrow trachea.

Severely affected animals may have exercise intolerance and episodes of cyanosis and **syncope**. Animals may present as an emergency in hot weather when they may be suffering from heat stroke, dehydration, cyanosis and severe stress. Nursing requires oxygen supplementation, cooling, sedation and if necessary an emergency tracheostomy.

Surgical treatment depends on the most severely affected part of the airway, the stenotic nares can be widened and the tonsils and part of the soft palate resected to improve upper airway flow.

Laryngeal surgery

Surgery on the larynx is a complex procedure and can potentially result in severe difficulty during recovery due to mucosal swelling. The animal must be closely observed for signs of respiratory distress and facilities available for oxygen supplementation or emergency tracheostomy if necessary.

Laryngeal paralysis   This typically occurs in the older medium-sized breeds of dog. It is rarely seen in the cat. The disease results from paralysis of the recurrent laryngeal nerve which then means that the dog cannot abduct its arytenoid cartilages to open the airway on inspiration. The clinical signs range from increased noise on breathing when excited, panting or exercising, to cyanosis and collapse. These dogs often present in the summer when they are panting more to lose heat and the paralysed larynx becomes oedematous and swollen, thereby further reducing airflow. They may collapse and be brought into the practice cyanotic and struggling to breathe. In hot weather they may also have heat stroke.

In an acute situation, the animal may have to be anaesthetised so that the airway can be intubated and oxygen administered. Prior to recovery, the appropriate surgery is to 'tie back' the arytenoid cartilage so that it no longer obstructs the airway. If this is not possible, then it would be necessary to place a tracheostomy tube to bypass the larynx and allow the dog to breathe until surgery is possible.

Some breeds of dog are predisposed to laryngeal collapse which is not amenable to laryngeal tieback and is treated with a permanent tracheostomy. The diagnosis is made on laryngoscopy. These dogs sometimes respond to weight loss and medical management.

Laryngeal tumours   These are rare, but also cause respiratory obstruction. Complete resection of the larynx is not very successful and unless the tumour is sensitive to chemotherapy, there is little treatment possible.

Trachea

The trachea is a rigid cartilaginous structure that prevents collapse of the airway when the animal creates negative pressure on inspiration.

Collapsing trachea   This is most often seen in toy or miniature breeds of dog, most notably the Yorkshire Terrier. The tracheal rings are not rigid and when the dog is excited or exercising, the trachea flattens and causes a harsh honking cough. Severely affected dogs may become cyanotic during coughing episodes or even syncopal. Some dogs respond to medical management of weight loss, anti-inflammatories, antitussives and use of a harness rather than a collar. Dogs that are severely affected may require surgery to place rings around the outside of the trachea to provide a rigid support for the airway. There are other techniques that place the support on the inside of the trachea. The surgery is very complex and the post-operative period very risky as the surgery can make the tracheal irritation worse.

Avulsion of the trachea   Typically this is seen in the cat after a road traffic accident. The trachea is torn apart usually quite distal within the thorax. The cat may initially appear normal, but becomes tachypnoeic over the first few days after the accident and may develop emphysema over the neck and shoulders. Surgical repair is urgent and involves a thoracotomy to re-anastamose the ends of the trachea. The surgery is technically difficult and the anaesthetic complicated by the fact that the cat requires IPPV during the surgery through a sterile endotracheal tube placed by the surgeon through the incision into the distal trachea. Post-operatively, a chest drain is placed to monitor for pneumothorax and the cat is closely monitored for signs of leakage from the anastamosis.

Tracheostomy   This may be temporary or permanent. It may be used for administration of anaesthetic gases during oral surgery or as a means of bypassing an obstructed upper airway. Most often it is used as a life-saving procedure in an emergency situation to bypass an obstructed upper airway.

EMERGENCY TRACHEOSTOMY
Procedure
(1) Make sure that the oxygen delivery tube will fit the tracheostomy tube.
(2) Clip and surgically prepare the ventral aspect of the neck.
(3) Have a sterile surgical kit ready, together with the appropriate-sized tracheostomy tube, and suture material to open up the tracheal incision.
(4) Suction may be necessary for the lower airway.
(5) Prepare for post-operative monitoring.

Management of a tracheostomy tube
(1) Constant monitoring for at least the first 12–24 hours.
(2) Regular suction of the tracheostomy tube every hour.
(3) Humidify the trachea by instilling 5–10 ml sterile saline into the tube every hour.
(4) Change the tracheostomy tube for a fresh sterile one every 2–6 hours depending on the quantity of exudate.

Emergency airway
If an animal is very close to death and the materials are not immediately available, oxygen can be administered via a wide-gauge hypodermic needle or catheter pushed quickly through the ventral midline of the neck between the tracheal rings. This can then be used to administer oxygen via a narrow tube or urinary catheter.

Usually the airway is not completely blocked and administration of oxygen with a face mask provides some relief while the animal is prepared for tracheostomy. However, where the animal is unconscious or severely cyanotic, the veterinary nurse should be prepared to perform the tracheostomy using only local anaesthetic or no anaesthetic and no surgical preparation if the animal is likely to die with any delay. If airway obstruction is anticipated, for example after surgery on the upper airway, the ventral aspect of the neck may be prepared in readiness for an emergency tracheostomy.

Foreign body/neoplasia   Rarely an animal presents with obstruction of the trachea. If this is a foreign body, it may be removed under anaesthesia using endoscopic forceps. Small tumours can be removed by resection of some of the tracheal rings and re-anastamosing the trachea.

Lungs

Principles of thoracotomy   The thorax can be approached by either entering the cavity between the ribs (lateral or **intercostal thoracotomy**) or by splitting the sternum and approaching the thorax from the ventral aspect (**sternal thoracotomy** or sternotomy). If more access is required, a rib can be resected.

The intercostal thoracotomy is the commonest approach and allows the surgeon access to the lungs, heart, oesophagus and pleural cavity on one side only. The advantage of a sternotomy is that both sides of the chest can be explored at the same procedure. Sternotomy in large dogs requires the facilities to saw through the sternum. During the thoracotomy, the animal must be on IPPV continuously, and it should be monitored for heat loss and dehydration.

Following thoracotomy, great care is taken to close the incision with an airtight seal. A chest drain is used to remove the pleural air during closure and also post-operatively to monitor air or fluid leaks within the chest. A sterile drain is placed through a skin tunnel between the ribs and the other end is linked to a water seal which allows continual aspiration of air or it may be occluded and drained intermittently (see 'Drains', above).

Analgesia is very important after thoracotomy, and it is important to get large dogs up and moving around as soon as possible to reduce the risk of **thromboembolism**.

Lung lobectomy   Lung lobes are removed via an intercostal thoracotomy as this gives the best access to the arteries, veins and bronchus. The vessels and bronchus may be ligated and oversewn manually or a lung lobectomy stapling device can be used to perform the procedure in one step. After the lung lobe has been removed, the bronchus is checked for air leaks by filling the chest with warm sterile saline, inflating the lungs, and looking for bubbles.

Pyothorax   This is an infection of the pleura in the thoracic cavity. It is commonly seen in cats probably secondary to cat bites and dogs, probably due to migrating grass seeds. The animal presents with difficulty breathing due to large volumes of pus in the thoracic cavity. Mostly these are treated by placing thoracic drains in both sides of the chest and draining and lavaging the chest twice daily with sterile fluids and antibiotics. Persistent cases may require a thoracotomy to open up the chest cavity and debride infected tissue or look for the foreign body.

Cardiovascular system

Heart

Persistent ductus arteriosus (PDA)   This occurs
when the ductus arteriosus fails to close at birth, and blood bypasses the lungs and left side of the heart, travelling from the pulmonary artery directly into the aorta. It creates a characteristic **heart murmur** that should be easily detected at the first vaccination check. If the condition is left untreated, then the dog will eventually die from heart failure. The treatment is surgery via a left lateral thoracotomy to tie off the PDA.

Vascular ring anomaly   Congenital defects of the
heart and great vessels sometimes occur and result in entrapment of the oesophagus between the ligamentum arteriosum (the remnants of the closed ductus arteriosum) and the other vessels. The commonest is a **persistent right aortic arch** (PRAA) when the aorta is found on the right side instead of the left and the ductus crosses the oesophagus and makes a constriction that prevents the normal passage of food on swallowing. The treatment is ligation and separation of the ductus from the surface of the oesophagus via a left-sided thoracotomy.

Arteries and veins

Vascular access – 'cut-down'   Intravenous treat-
ments are usually given via an intravenous catheter placed in the cephalic vein. However, in patients that are very collapsed, dehydrated or in severe shock it can be very difficult to identify the superficial veins in order to place the catheter. If it is not possible to place a jugular catheter instead, a **'cut-down'** technique may be used to access a vein. The area over the vein is clipped and prepared surgically and a tourniquet placed above the vein to increase visibility. An incision is made directly over the vein, and careful dissection down through the tissue planes used to identify the vessel. The catheter is then placed routinely, flushed with heparin–saline and usually sutured in place. The skin is then sutured over the surgical site, and the wound dressed.

Aortic thromboembolism   This is a serious emer-
gency condition, usually seen in the cat, when a blood clot (**embolism**) breaks off and travels down the aorta to block the iliac arteries at the end of the aorta. This completely blocks the blood flow to one or both hindlimbs. The hindlimbs are cold, stiff, very painful and there is no palpable femoral pulse. Occasionally the condition is responsive to medical management and surgical removal of the thromboembolism has been reported, but is only rarely successful. The disease is usually secondary to heart disease and the prognosis is poor.

Emergency vessel occlusion   Vessels may be la-
cerated or ruptured during the course of surgery or as a result of severe trauma. If the event occurs during surgery, small arteries (< 2 mm) and veins (< 4 mm) can be sealed using electrodiathermy, or may stop bleeding with a few minutes of direct pressure. Large vessels are ligated or double ligated, using absorbable synthetic suture material with good knot security. There are also commercial staples available to seal arteries and veins during surgery.

Traumatic haemorrhage may have to be stemmed prior to identifying the specific vessel. If the bleeding is clearly arterial (pumping), surgical exploration and ligation of the artery is a priority. However, the bleeding may be profuse and non-specific. Initially direct hand-held pressure on the wound using a sterile pack of absorbent material may be sufficient to slow the bleeding. If the bleeding continues to be profuse, other options are a tourniquet above the site of bleeding on a limb, application of a very heavily padded bandage or immediate surgical exploration under anaesthesia. It is very important to time the duration of a tourniquet to prevent ischaemic necrosis and also important to remove the bandage as soon as possible, otherwise high pressures underneath the bandage may result in the same effect. Weighing the material used to absorb the blood before and after use will help to estimate blood loss.

Major arteries may be repaired if necessary and blood flow can be temporarily stopped during the repair using bulldog clips or a **Rommel tourniquet**. Very fine gauge polypropylene suture material is usually used to repair arteries or veins, as it causes very little tissue reaction.

Endocrine system

Thyroid

Thyroidectomy – dog   In the dog, thyroidectomy is
usually carried out as treatment for thyroid carcinoma. Small tumours may be easy to remove, but they can be very vascular and may be attached to vital structures in the neck.

Thyroidectomy – cat   **Hyperthyroidism** is a com-
mon condition of the older cat due to a thyroid adenoma (a benign tumour) which secretes excess thyroid hormone. It results typically in restlessness, weight loss, polyphagia and tachycardia. Some cats may also have concurrent kidney disease and heart failure. The thyroid gland may be palpated in the neck, or it may be diagnosed from a blood sample. Initially, the cat is usually stabilised using

an orally administered antithyroid drug (neomercazole), but ultimately, surgery is a curative treatment, removing the affected thyroid gland or glands. The main risk associated with surgery is damage to the **parathyroid glands** which are closely attached to the cranial end of the thyroid gland. This results in loss of control of calcium metabolism and **hypocalcaemia** develops in the first 2–3 days after surgery. If the damage is severe, the cat may need calcium supplementation intravenously and then orally for weeks until the parathyroid glands recover.

Adrenal glands

The adrenal glands in the dog and cat are sometimes removed as a treatment for Cushing's disease (**hyperadrenocorticism**) or **phaeochromocytoma**, where the adrenal gland is the primary source of the problem. Surgery involves deep dissection in the region of the dorsal abdominal vena cava, and there can be severe haemorrhage. The patients may have delayed wound healing due to the medical condition and should be closely monitored for wound dehiscence. Sudden hormonal changes in the post-operative period can also destabilise a patient and they should be closely monitored for electrolyte abnormalities, hypotension and vomiting/diarrhoea.

Adrenal tumours are the most common tumour in the ferret and they are often removed successfully.

Pancreas

The pancreas is a lobulated gland that is closely associated with the stomach and duodenum. The commonest disease is a sterile inflammation (**pancreatitis**), which causes severe abdominal pain and vomiting. This is not a surgical disease and surgical exploration will make the symptoms worse. Other conditions include pancreatic abscesses, damage due to abdominal trauma and pancreatic tumours.

Pancreatectomy
Abscesses and tumours may be removed by a partial pancreatectomy. If the lesion is in the body of the pancreas or involves the blood supply to the duodenum, it is generally considered inoperable. The commonest tumour of the pancreas is an **insulinoma** which is a tumour that secretes excess insulin and causes hypoglycaemia. After the surgery, the animal has to be carefully managed to ensure that acute pancreatitis does not occur. No food or water is given by mouth for the first 48 hours, and hydration is maintained with intravenous fluids and electrolytes. Monitoring of the glucose levels is critical in post-operative management of insulinoma patients and they may need a glucose drip. When the animal is fed, it should initially be given small quantities of a low-fat diet.

Pancreatic biopsy
In some patients with chronic low-grade pancreatitis, it is difficult to diagnose the disease without a biopsy. Ideally, this is done via **laparoscopy** ('key-hole' surgery) to reduce the risk of a flare-up of the

disease. Otherwise, a small piece of pancreas is removed via laparotomy and the patient managed as above.

Liver

Liver disease can potentially result in a number of medical conditions that would adversely affect the success of surgery. Many patients may have low albumin levels, vitamin K and increased susceptibility to sedatives or anaesthetic drugs. Animals with suspected liver disease should always have blood clotting times tested prior to surgery, and they may need a transfusion of fresh frozen plasma. However, the liver also has remarkable powers of regeneration and can compensate for removal or damage to liver lobes.

Biopsy

The purpose of performing a liver biopsy is to achieve a specific diagnosis. It can either be done by laparoscopy, or via a laparotomy incision. Usually, just a small piece of the edge of a liver lobe is removed, and normal clotting stops the bleeding spontaneously. Occasionally a Tru-Cut needle may be used with ultrasound guidance to obtain the biopsy.

Lobectomy

A whole liver lobe may need to be removed if it is diseased or damaged. The blood supply to the liver may be temporarily shut off using a small tourniquet during the surgery. Post-operatively, the animal must be monitored closely for haemorrhage into the abdominal cavity as this is the commonest complication of the surgery.

Portosystemic shunt

Portosystemic shunt (PSS) is a congenital or acquired vascular anomaly that redirects blood flow in the portal vein so that it bypasses the liver. The clinical signs include poor growth, abnormal behaviour a few hours after feeding (**hepatic encephalopathy**), seizures, urate calculi in the urinary tract and hypoglycaemia. The disease is usually diagnosed with blood tests and ultrasound scans of the liver. More detailed investigations such as a **portovenogram** (contrast material injected into a mesenteric vein), contrast fluoroscopy or ultrasound may be necessary. Small breeds of dog are most commonly affected with congenital shunts which are usually single large vessels draining into the abdominal vena cava (**extrahepatic shunts**). Large breeds of dog are usually affected with **intrahepatic shunts**. Acquired shunts are seen in older dogs or cats and are related to the development of veins that bypass the liver secondary to chronic liver disease that obstructs the normal flow of blood in the portal vein.

Only congenital PSS is treated surgically. The patient is usually stabilised with medical management first and then the shunt is tied off with silk via a laparotomy, in either one or more surgical procedures. Some referral centres use constrictor devices to slowly occlude the shunt to allow the liver more time to adapt to the increased blood flow. Post-operative complications include abdominal pain, hypoglycaemia, diarrhoea, vomiting, hypotension, hypothermia, prolonged recovery time due to poor metabolism of anaesthetic drugs, seizures and shock.

Cholecystectomy

Cholangitis or cholecystitis (infection or inflammation of the biliary ducts and gall bladder), cholelithiasis (stones in the gall bladder) may be treated by removal of the gall bladder. The surgery is carried out through a cranial midline laparotomy and the gall bladder ligated and removed. The bile continues to drain into the duodenum through the bile duct and the only difference is that it does not collect in the gall bladder between meals. Post-operatively the animal should be treated with antibiotics, but abdominal drains are not necessary.

Spleen

The spleen is a large vascular organ in the abdomen on the left side next to the stomach. Although in humans, removal of the spleen can result in the development of septicaemia, this has not been reported in dogs and cats and total splenectomy is not usually associated with any long-term problems.

Splenectomy

The indications for removal of the spleen include neoplasia, splenic torsion, trauma and haemorrhage. Haemangiosarcoma is the most common primary tumour of the spleen and some tumours will be metastases from elsewhere. However, up to half of splenic tumours may be benign or even just haematomas, so splenectomy can carry a good prognosis.

Sometimes patients present with acute haemorrhage from the spleen and splenectomy is performed as an emergency procedure. More often, the bleeding is intermittent and the spleen is removed as an elective procedure to prevent a haemorrhagic crisis. If the haemorrhage has been severe, the animal may require a blood transfusion prior to surgery, and if the haemorrhage is due to trauma and *not* neoplasia, an **autotransfusion** of blood can be carried out. At the time of the laparotomy, the blood is suctioned via sterile apparatus out of the abdomen, mixed with the appropriate volume of anticoagulant, filtered and transfused into a peripheral vein. If there is any likelihood of neoplastic disease, autotransfusion should not be carried out.

The most common post-operative complication is haemorrhage as a result of displacement of a ligature in the abdomen. The patient needs to be closely monitored for signs of intra-abdominal bleeding.

Urinary tract

All surgery on the urinary tract runs the potential risk of acute renal failure if kidney function is affected and urine production stops post-operatively. Urine production should be maintained at a minimum of 2 ml/kg/hour using intravenous fluid therapy during the post-operative period. Urine needs to be collected and measured in order to calculate these figures, and diuretics or other treatments given if urine output is inadequate. Blood samples can also be analysed for urea, creatinine and electrolyte (potassium) levels which also indicate renal function.

Kidney

The kidneys are **retroperitoneal**, which means that they lie outside the peritoneal cavity of the abdomen. They receive 25% of total cardiac output and are one of the vital organs of the body. Surgical handling or trauma that might disrupt the blood supply or cause the artery to spasm could potentially be life threatening.

Ureteronephrectomy
A kidney may be removed if there is severe trauma, neoplasia, **hydronephrosis** (enlargement of the kidney secondary to back pressure from the bladder), or severe **pyelonephritis** (infection). It is essential to be sure that the other kidney is functioning normally prior to this procedure, otherwise the animal may go into renal failure post-operatively. The kidney is removed together with its ureter which is traced all the way down to the bladder and the arteries and veins ligated. Post-operatively, intravenous fluids should be maintained until normal urine flow has been monitored and recorded.

Nephrotomy
Calculi can occasionally form in the kidney. These are very painful and result in severe secondary infections of the kidney which may cause permanent damage. They are removed by a nephrotomy into the renal pelvis when the calculus is removed and the incision repaired. Post-operative intravenous fluid therapy is important to ensure good urine production, and close monitoring of blood urea and creatinine to check for evidence of urine leakage.

Renal biopsy
The kidney can be biopsied, but this is only done after extensive investigation of the renal disease, as it carries considerable risks of haemorrhage and damage to renal function. Ideally, the biopsy is taken through a surgical incision, but sometimes it is done percutaneously using a **Tru-Cut needle** with ultrasound guidance. Post-operatively, pressure is used to stop bleeding and urine output monitored with intravenous fluids and urinalysis.

Ureter

The ureters travel in the retroperitoneal space from the kidney to the bladder. They can be imaged using intravenous excretory urography or ultrasound examination, but are not seen on plain radiographs.

Avulsion of the ureter   Rarely, the ureter may be torn secondary to abdominal trauma. This causes urine leakage into the retroperitoneal space causing cellulitis with electrolyte abnormalities. In some cases the damage can be repaired surgically, but often ureteronephrectomy is necessary. It is important to stabilise the animal with respect to renal and electrolyte parameters prior to anaesthesia.

Ectopic ureters   This is a congenital condition where one or both ureters implant distal to the bladder so that urine flows directly into the urethra. This results in a constant urinary incontinence, usually in a young dog. Golden Retrievers, Poodles and Labradors are most commonly affected. The condition is diagnosed using excretory urography and ultrasound. The ureters are often enlarged and abnormal due to ascending infections. In some cases, the ascending infection results in severe pyelonephritis and a ureteronephrectomy is carried out. Where the ureter and kidney are healthy, it is possible to reimplant the ureter surgically into the bladder. Surgery on the ureter can result in spasm that causes the kidney to stop producing urine on that side for up to 48 hours. Ideally, therefore, if both ureters need surgery, one side should be done at a time. As in renal surgery, urine production is carefully monitored post-operatively. In some cases, the incontinence may persist due to other bladder abnormalities.

Ureteric entrapment   The ureters run down to the bladder and in the female pass the uterine body and cervix. At this position they are at risk of entrapment in the ligature during routine ovariohysterectomy. This is life threatening, particularly if both ureters are involved. If the ligature is removed within 7 days, little damage is done to the kidney and it should completely recover.

Bladder

Surgery on the bladder is common in veterinary practice. It lies in the caudal abdomen and can be accessed via a midline laparotomy. The bladder should be emptied prior to surgery, either using a catheter via the urethra or using a small-gauge needle and syringe at surgery. The bladder wall is delicate and prone to oedema and bruising with rough handling, so it is usually held during surgery using stay sutures or fine forceps. Urine continues to collect in the bladder during surgery, so it is important to protect the other abdominal organs from contamination with the urine during the cystotomy.

Cystotomy and cystectomy   The commonest indications for cystotomy are to remove calculi (stones) or tumours. Usually, the incision in the bladder wall is made in the ventral aspect and more stay sutures may be placed lateral to the incision to help open up the bladder for inspection. Sometimes the calculi are located well down the bladder neck and it may be necessary to place a urethral catheter and flush them into the bladder with sterile saline. For removal of neoplasms, the full thickness of the bladder wall is cut away with a margin around the tumour, and the bladder reconstructed. The incision is closed in two layers using a synthetic absorbable suture material. Post-operatively, the animal should be given the opportunity to empty the bladder as frequently as possible and monitored for normal urination and evidence of urine leakage (uraemia, hypothermia, abdominal pain) for 3–4 days.

Bladder rupture   This occurs either secondary to blunt abdominal trauma or to prolonged urethral obstruction causing severe back pressure and accumulation of urine. Occasionally bladder rupture occurs when attempting to manually express the bladder in paralysed patients. The condition may be diagnosed from the history, absence of urine in the bladder or using diagnostic imaging techniques. The immediate concern is the **uroperitoneum** and the metabolic consequences of the absorption of urine from the peritoneum. There may be uraemia, electrolyte imbalances, dehydration and shock, which may have to be treated prior to surgery. At surgery, the abdomen should be lavaged with sterile saline to remove urine and contaminants, and the bladder is repaired. Post-operatively, blood urea levels and urine production should be closely monitored.

Tube cystostomy (urinary diversion)   This is the placement of a drain through the abdominal wall in order to drain the bladder, bypassing the urethra. This may be used as a temporary measure prior to urethral surgery or after bladder or urethral surgery to divert urine flow. It can also be used for diversion of urine in patients with urethral obstruction due to tumours, or paralysis of the bladder. A **Foley catheter** is drawn into the abdomen through a stab incision lateral to the midline. The tip is placed into the bladder and the balloon inflated with sterile saline, and the catheter secured with sutures and omentum. The catheter is then secured to the outside of the body wall with sutures or zinc oxide butterfly tapes. In the hospital, this should be attached to a closed urine collection system to prevent the risk of ascending infections. In long-term use, the bladder is emptied at least four times daily by removing a bung from the end and attaching a syringe. When the drain is removed, the tip should be submitted for culture and then appropriate antibiotics used to treat any associated infection. Use of antibiotics while the drain is in place will not prevent infection and only increases the likelihood of resistant strains developing.

Urethra

Surgery on the urethra is most often done secondary to damage caused by calculi. Pre-operatively, the systemic consequences of urethral obstruction may need to be addressed prior to anaesthesia and often a urinary catheter is passed before surgery to make identification of the urethra easier.

Urethral obstruction Blockage of the urethra in any species results in accumulation of urine in the bladder which if not relieved causes back pressure on the kidneys and then bladder rupture. The urine spills into the abdomen and causes uraemia and death. The clinical signs may be severe abdominal pain with persistent straining to urinate.

> Animals straining to urinate should be checked as an emergency to assess the bladder.

The cat is usually more severely affected than the dog, which may only have partial obstruction.

The urethra in the female is short and wide and unlikely to obstruct except secondary to neoplastic growth. In the male dog and cat, the urethra is narrower, particularly at the tip in the male cat and at the level of the os penis in the male dog. This anatomical characteristic makes it prone to obstruction by **urinary calculi** (stones). The type of stone that blocks the urethra depends on the disease and it should be submitted for analysis in order to determine the most appropriate prophylactic treatment for the future.

Male cats also develop obstruction of the urethra secondary to feline lower urinary tract disease (**FLUTD**) and in these cases, the obstruction is not always due to a calculus, but can be a mucoid plug.

The priority is to stabilise the animal with intravenous fluids and to decompress the bladder. If a urinary catheter cannot be passed, then it may be necessary to empty the bladder by cystocentesis. Once the pressure is reduced, it may then be possible to pass a catheter or to flush the urolith or plug back into the bladder with sterile saline (**retropulsion**). If it is not possible to remove the calculus this way then urethrotomy is necessary.

KEY POINTS

Cystocentesis
(1) Sedation is only necessary in very fractious animals, although analgesia should be provided.
(2) The distended bladder is identified as a hard mass in the caudal abdomen.
(3) A small area of skin on the ventrolateral abdomen directly over the bladder is clipped and surgically prepped.
(4) A 20 gauge needle of the appropriate length for the size of animal is selected and attached to a 20 ml syringe via a three-way tap.
(5) Sterile gloves are put on or a short hand scrub performed.
(6) The bladder is gently held still with one hand and the needle introduced into the bladder through the prepared area of skin.

---

(7) The urine is drawn off and the three-way tap used to expel the urine into a bowl, this is repeated until the bladder feels empty.
(8) The volume of urine is recorded.

Urethrostomy In some circumstances, either the cause of the urethral obstruction cannot be treated (e.g. calcium oxalate crystals) or the tip of the urethra is so damaged that it is prone to recurrent obstruction. In these cases, it may be necessary to create a new opening for urination through a wider part of the urethra. In the dog this is done at the level of the scrotum. In an intact male dog, castration and scrotal ablation is performed and then an incision into the urethra at that level sutured to the skin edges (**scrotal urethrostomy**). In the male cat, the penis is amputated and the urethra opened out and sutured to the skin edges (**perineal urethrostomy**). A urinary catheter should not be placed after surgery, and it is extremely important that the animal does not lick at the site at any stage during the healing process. Initially, there may be considerable bleeding associated with urination and it may be easier to hospitalise the patient until this has reduced. Nursing involves keeping the site clean and free of urine or blood, and preventing urine scald until the animal learns how to reposition during urination.

Urethral rupture The urethra is exposed to damage in the male dog as it runs down the perineum and inguinal area, and in all animals as it runs through the pelvic canal. The most common cause of rupture is trauma to the pelvic area and it is often seen secondary to pelvic fractures. The urine leaks out of the urethra and can cause severe inflammation of the pelvic tissues. Reabsorption of the urine then causes changes in the blood biochemistry such as uraemia, and hyperkalaemia, which cause systemic illness. If the tear is small, the urethra may be treated with placement of a soft silicone indwelling urinary catheter, allowing it to heal by second intention. Larger tears or complete ruptures (avulsion) should be repaired surgically once the animal is stabilised for the anaesthetic. Urine is then diverted through a cystostomy tube until the site is healed.

Urethral neoplasia This is more common in the bitch than the dog and is occasionally seen in the cat. It usually presents with acute obstruction to urination, although there may be a history of cystitis. Surgery can be performed to try to remove the urethra and reconstruct it using part of the vagina, but the prognosis is very poor.

Urinary incontinence Incontinence is most common in the bitch. It has to be investigated in order to determine the primary cause (causes):

- Ectopic ureters.
- Pelvic bladder.
- Short bladder neck.
- Urinary tract infection.
- Urinary sphincter mechanism incompetence (USMI).

Ectopic ureters is the only condition that has to be treated surgically. The other conditions often present in a slightly older bitch or in the young bitch after spaying. They may respond to medical management, but occasionally surgery is necessary to try to reposition the bladder neck to increase the pressure around the sphincter, and thereby increase the holding capacity of the bladder and reduce incontinence. This is specialist surgery and post-operative care involves carefully monitoring for urinary tract infections and ensuring that there is no retention of urine.

Incontinence in the male dog is usually secondary to prostatic disease. Castration may make the incontinence worse and it is very difficult to treat successfully either with drugs or surgery.

Genital tract

Testes

The testes are the reproductive organ producing spermatozoa in male animals. They should normally descend after birth into the scrotum and remain externally located.

Elective castration (orchidectomy) Castration may be carried out for therapeutic reasons (treatment of orchitis, perineal hernia, anal adenoma, testicular tumours or prostatitis), social reasons or as part of a neutering programme. Occasionally, castration is recommended to control behavioural abnormalities or difficulties such as roaming, excessive libido or aggression. Castration in the tomcat is usually carried out to prevent territorial spraying.

Castration in the cat is usually carried out via an incision in the scrotum, the testis pulled out gently and then either ligated with suture material or the vas deferens and vascular bundle tied in a knot to secure haemostasis. The vascular bundle is released into the scrotum and the procedure repeated on the other side. The cat is observed post-operatively for signs of haemorrhage, and then discharged with instructions to use a litter tray with shredded newspaper for 2–3 days. The wounds in the scrotum are not sutured, but allowed to heal by second intention.

Castration in the dog can be carried out either through a pre-scrotal mid-line incision or via scrotal ablation. Pre-scrotal castration involves pushing the testes forwards into the single incision and then the arteries and veins are ligated before removal of each testis. The skin incision is sutured closed, and the scrotum is left in place. Scrotal ablation involves removal of the scrotum and then the testes are removed with ligation as described above directly through the scrotal area. The skin is sutured closed. Pre-scrotal ablation is quicker but leaves an unsightly scrotal sac behind and risks seroma or haematoma formation in the scrotum. Scrotal ablation takes longer, but has fewer complications associated with the healing of the surgical site.

Post-operatively, it is important that the owner is warned not to let the dog lick the sutures and that the dog is monitored for signs of ventral abdominal or scrotal swelling or bruising that might indicate ligature slippage.

Retained testes (cryptorchidism) Failure of one or both testes to descend is an inherited condition, is more common in small breed dogs, and is very rare in the cat. Both the retained testis and the descended testis are at risk of the development of neoplasia and they should be removed. Owners should be encouraged not to breed from affected animals.

The retained testis may be found at any point from the kidney down through the inguinal canal to just above the scrotal sac. The path is carefully surgically explored to locate the testicle and then it is removed in the standard way. The removed testis should be submitted for analysis to confirm that the correct tissue was removed.

Testicular neoplasia These tumours are relatively common, and are usually seen in older dogs. There are three main tumour types:

- Sertoli cell tumour (SCT).
- Seminoma (SEM).
- Interstitial cell tumour (ICT).

Sertoli cell tumours are more likely to metastasise than the other types to the lymph nodes, lung or liver. Sometimes SCT or SEM can cause a paraneoplastic syndrome associated with the production of hormones. Usually a **feminisation syndrome** is seen which causes hair loss, **gynaecomastia** (enlarged mammary glands), prostatitis, atrophy of the unaffected testis, a pendulous prepuce and may be attractive to other male dogs. More severely affected dogs may also have bone marrow suppression, causing changes such as anaemia.

Treatment with castration should carry a good prognosis.

Prostate

The prostate gland completely regresses after castration, and should not develop disease later in life. Uncastrated dogs may develop prostatic disease secondary to the influence of the hormone testosterone. Symptoms may include infertility, impotence, incontinence, dysuria, haematuria, caudal abdominal pain and faecal tenesmus. The prostate can be examined by caudal palpation of the abdomen or rectal examination. Ultrasonography and radiography is also useful. Samples of the prostate gland can be taken by needle aspirates through the abdomen, alongside the rectum or via a urinary catheter. Ejaculation samples will also give some information about the fluid that the prostate is secreting.

Benign prostatic hyperplasia (BPH) This occurs in the older male dog, when the prostate becomes acutely enlarged and very painful. It may be secondarily infected. Castration may be indicated to prevent recurrence. Antitestosterone drugs can also be used (delmadinone acetate).

Prostatic cysts and abscesses If BPH persists, the prostate may develop cysts or abscesses, which can become enormous. Prostatic abscesses may be life threatening, presenting with toxaemia and systemic disease similar to pyometra in the bitch. Cysts and abscesses should be operated on before they rupture causing peritonitis. The approach is through a midline laparotomy, the abscess or cyst is drained and lavaged with sterile fluids until clean, and then packed with omentum before routine closure.

Prostatic neoplasia

Cancer can develop in the prostate gland of older dogs, castrated or entire. The gland is very painful and has similar signs to other prostatic diseases. Prostatic carcinoma rapidly spreads to the adjacent lymph nodes and sometimes the vertebral bodies. The prognosis is poor and prostatectomy is unsuccessful at achieving a cure and results in complete urinary incontinence.

Penis

Amputation

Penile amputation is indicated where there is severe trauma to the penis or if there is neoplastic disease. The penis is extremely vascular, and the procedure should be done under a tourniquet. Usually the whole of the os penis is removed and the urethra is reconstructed at the end of the inguinal part of the penis.

Mucosal eversion

Occasionally, hypersexed dogs may present with mucosal eversion of the tip of the urethra on the end of the penis. The mucosa is very vascular and bleeds because of the trauma. Castration may help, but usually the mucosa has to be resected from the end of the penis. Again it helps to use a tourniquet during surgery and then absorbable fine gauge suture material is used to resuture the mucosa at the end of the urethra. Post-operatively, there may be some bleeding and wadding may be used inside the prepuce to help provide gentle pressure to stop this.

Ovaries and uterus

Elective ovariohysterectomy (spay)

In the United Kingdom, female companion animals are usually neutered (removal of the uterus and ovaries) to prevent unwanted litters and prevent oestrus activity. Bitches are also neutered to decrease the risk of development of mammary tumours, the best effect of this is seen if the bitch is neutered before the first season. Bitches, rabbits and ferrets are also neutered to prevent the development of pyometra (uterine infection) later in life.

The ovaries are identified and the arteries tied off before cutting the ovarian ligament. Then a ligature is placed around the uterine stump as close to the cervix as possible, to tie off the uterine arteries, before removal of the whole of the genital tract. The most important part of the procedure is to ensure that the ovaries are removed intact and no remnants are left behind that might secrete hormones. In some countries, only the ovaries are removed (**ovariectomy**); this is a shorter procedure and there is no documented increased risk of uterine disease. Bitches and exotic pets are usually operated on from the midline, but in the UK

cats are usually operated on from the left flank approach lying in lateral recumbency. There is some suggestion that spaying increases the likelihood of urinary incontinence in some breeds of dog, although this is not certain and only likely if there is already an underlying bladder abnormality.

Post-operative analgesia and observation are important. The wound should be observed for signs of bleeding or bruising, and the recovery monitored. Any post-operative spay that has a prolonged recovery from anaesthesia should be assessed for the possibility of intra-abdominal haemorrhage. Pale mucous membranes, generalised weakness, a rapid thready pulse, hypothermia, bleeding from the laparotomy wound or vagina are all symptoms that should be investigated. Post-operative instructions relate to wound care and restricted activity to prevent dehiscence of the abdominal repair.

Pyometra

This is the accumulation of pus in the uterus, which may be infected or sterile. It occurs most commonly in middle- to older-aged animals which have never had a litter. It is potentially life threatening and often presents as an emergency. Affected animals may be depressed and polydipsic and may have a history of abnormal or more frequent oestrus. They may have a fever and often vomit. If the cervix is open (**open pyometra**), there is a vaginal discharge and they may be less ill than when the cervix is closed (**closed pyometra**) and all the pus is retained in the uterus.

The animal may be in severe toxaemic shock, and they often require intensive fluid therapy before they are fit for anaesthesia. Ovariohysterectomy is needed as a life-saving procedure as soon as the animal is stable enough for surgery. Intensive nursing is required in the post-operative phase to ensure that recovery from the toxaemia and renal function is complete after the removal of the infected uterus. Fluid therapy should continue until renal function and urine output is normal.

Caesarean section

This is necessary when a bitch or queen presents with dystocia. The caesarean may be necessary if the animal is not able to progress with normal birth (e.g. hypocalcaemia, uterine inertia) and not responding to medical management, or sometimes the fetus becomes stuck or dies in the birth canal and caesarean is carried out to save the remaining litter.

Any attempts to assist the animal to deliver the fetuses per vagina must be carried out under strict aseptic conditions to reduce the risk of post-delivery infections. Generally, the decision is made based on the possibility of live offspring and the duration of the labour so far.

Usually caesarean section is carried out under general anaesthetic, although where the facilities are available, epidural anaesthesia is the technique of choice. Preparation for the caesarean section focuses around the provision of enough personnel to resuscitate the pups/kittens (see Chapter 18 on neonatal care). Most veterinary surgeons use a midline approach to the abdomen despite the possibility of interference with the sutures by the young. Preparation of the abdomen for aseptic surgery must be thorough, but avoid using antiseptics that might cause dermatitis around the mammary glands. The incision is closed routinely, although some surgeons may use a subcuticular closure so as not to have skin sutures in the region where the offspring will be suckling.

Post-operative care involves close monitoring of the recovery from anaesthesia, and prevention of hypothermia. Regular post-operative checks are necessary to ensure that the dam is suckling and caring for the litter, despite the stress of hospitalisation and surgery. Many cases will be discharged to their home environment as soon as possible after recovery and monitored with home visits. It is particularly important that the owner is given advice on nutrition of the dam post-operatively and frequent small meals offered in the early stages post-operatively. Often they will develop a transient diarrhoea due to hormonal influences as well as eating placentae. The litter and bedding must be kept as clean as possible to prevent post-operative sepsis.

In some circumstances, an ovariohysterectomy will be performed at the same time as the caesarean section. This is not ideal but is sometimes indicated where there is uterine rupture or risk of recurrent unwanted pregnancy (strays).

Neoplasia   Older animals may develop tumours of the ovaries or uterus. They can be very aggressive, but some are benign. Ovariohysterectomy is indicated.

Vagina

The vagina is usually only affected by disease in the entire bitch or queen and rarely causes problems after neutering.

Hyperplasia   Vaginal hyperplasia is seen most often in brachycephalic breeds. The vaginal mucosa has an exaggerated hyperplastic response to the oestrogens secreted during oestrus, and excessive folds of vaginal mucosa protrude through the vulva. It often has the appearance of a tumour, but it regresses at the end of oestrus. The exposed mucosa must be kept clean and lubricated with KY® jelly. Treatment is to prevent recurrence by ovariohysterectomy.

Prolapse   Vaginal prolapse is less common than hyperplasia, but occurs in the same breeds. Mild prolapses may not require treatment other than protection of the exposed mucosa. Spontaneous regression should occur during the dioestrus period.

Neoplasia   Neoplasia of the vulva and vagina are seen occasionally. Most large fibrous tumours identified in the wall of the vagina are leiomyomas, and are infiltrative hard nodules usually in the dorsal vaginal wall. The tumours are removed using an **episiotomy** to access the vaginal lumen from the perineum, and the bitch is also neutered. The urethra should be catheterised during surgery, so that the urethral orifice can be identified during the resection. Neoplasms of the vulva tend to be more aggressive carcinomas or mast-cell tumours and require complex surgery for removal and reconstruction.

Hernias and ruptures

A **hernia** is an abnormal protrusion of an organ or organs through a physiological opening in the lining of the cavity in which it is normally enclosed. A **rupture** is a pathological tear in the lining of the cavity through which enclosed organs may protrude.

Most hernias and ruptures affect the abdominal cavity, but a few occur elsewhere. An example outside the abdomen includes herniation of the occipital or temporal lobes of the brain under the bony tentorium cerebelli as a complication of space-occupying lesion of the cranium.

The openings through which a hernia may occur are either a normal opening which has enlarged to allow organs through (e.g. inguinal canal), or an opening which should have closed during normal development (e.g. umbilicus). Hernias and ruptures share some characteristics in terms of the risks associated with the protrusion of viscera; however, as hernias are physiological, they are usually lined by an outpouching of the cavity lining, e.g. the peritoneum. Ruptures are not lined and the cavity lining is ruptured along with the body wall.

Hernias and ruptures are further described:

- **Reducible**. The contents of the hernia or rupture can be replaced in the original anatomical location by gentle pressure on the swelling to push the viscera back through the defect itself.
- **Irreducible** or **incarcerated**. The contents of the hernia or rupture cannot be replaced usually because of the formation of adhesions in chronic cases.
- **Strangulated**. The contents of a hernia or rupture can become devitalised due to entrapment of the blood vessels passing through the defect. Strangulation is life threatening and a serious emergency.

Umbilical hernia

This is a congenital condition where the umbilicus fails to close over properly and fat and/or abdominal contents protrude through under the skin. Small hernias are of no consequence as they usually do not increase in size as the puppy grows. Large hernias should be repaired due to the risk of incarceration of small intestine or other abdominal organs.

Inguinal hernia

Aetiology (male and female)   Herniation occurs through the inguinal canal which is a physiological opening in the muscle of the caudal abdominal wall. It is more common in females than males, particularly in elderly overweight small-breed dogs. In the bitch a swelling may be seen in the groin extending towards the vulva. The hernia may contain fat in the broad ligament, uterus, intestines or bladder. If the bitch is pregnant, the gravid uterus can become strangulated. In male dogs, fat or intestine may herniate into the scrotal sac and can become strangulated because of the small opening.

Management The hernia should be scanned or X-rayed to determine what structures are in the hernia and the owner warned about the possibility of strangulation. All hernias should be surgically corrected and the inguinal canal narrowed to prevent recurrence. Ideally the animal should also be neutered.

Perineal hernia

Aetiology Perineal hernia occurs almost exclusively in older male dogs. It is associated with degeneration of the muscles of the pelvic diaphragm (coccygeus and levator ani). Affected dogs have difficulty defecating and have an obvious swelling on one or both sides of the anus. The swelling is associated with impaction of faeces in the rectum as well as herniated abdominal contents. An important complication of perineal hernia is retroflexion and incarceration of the bladder and prostate. This can result in acute urethral obstruction and is an emergency.

Management There are a number of surgical techniques described for hernia repair that involve apposing the remains of the atrophied muscles using a monofilament long-lasting suture material (e.g. PDS or polypropylene). Some techniques also involve transferring muscle flaps to help support the hernia repair and these techniques are usually more successful. All dogs are castrated to help prevent recurrence.

PRE- AND POST-OPERATIVE NURSING FOR PERINEAL HERNIA

Pre-operatively, the animal should be assessed for bladder position and the possibility that the bladder could be **retroflexed** into the hernia, obstructing the urethra. If there is doubt, the hernia may be X-rayed or the urethra catheterised in order to empty the bladder. Sometimes the bladder has to be emptied by cystocentesis before it can be catheterised or reduced. The surgical site is considered contaminated and peri- and post-operative antibiotic cover is required. Before the surgical preparation, the rectal sacculation is manually emptied of faeces and a purse string suture is placed to prevent faecal material contaminating the surgical site during surgery. Enemas are not used as they may result in a loose slurry that could easily spill into the surgical site. Post-operatively, the purse string is removed and faecal modifiers (Sterculia, Isogel) given in the food to prevent straining against the hernia repair and also to improve rectal function. Bilateral hernia repairs sometimes develop rectal prolapse and which requires a loose purse string suture around the anus for a few days until the anus regains normal tone.

Diaphragm

Aetiology (congenital, traumatic) Diaphragmatic rupture is most commonly associated with trauma such as a road traffic accident, causing a sudden increase in abdominal pressure when the glottis is closed. The diaphragm tears either around the edge (**circumferential**) or across from the centre to the edge (**radial**). The loss of a functional diaphragm makes breathing more difficult and this is coupled with herniation of abdominal contents such as intestine, liver, spleen or stomach into the pleural space. The trauma may also have caused pulmonary contusion (bruising of the lungs) which adds to the animal's respiratory distress. Some cases are missed at the time of the original trauma and may present months later with dyspnoea when more abdominal contents herniate through into the chest.

Congenital defects in the diaphragm are also seen, the commonest of which is the **pericardial–peritoneal diaphragmatic hernia**. In this condition, the ventral portion of the diaphragm is absent and abdominal contents herniate into the mediastinum (not the pleural space). Often the animal also has a large umbilical hernia.

Management All diaphragmatic hernias are repaired surgically. Congenital defects are repaired as elective procedures, but ruptures may need to be operated on as an emergency if the stomach is in the chest and it begins to dilate. Ideally the animal should be stabilised after the accident to improve the anaesthetic risk, but in some cases, the dyspnoea is so severe that surgery is necessary. The tear is sutured closed using long-lasting absorbable suture material. Chronic cases may be difficult to reduce due to adhesions to the pleura, and also due to contraction of the abdominal muscles, the abdomen may be difficult to close, once all the abdominal contents are returned. A chest drain may be necessary, particularly in chronic cases where there may be a pleural effusion.

PRE- AND POST-OPERATIVE NURSING FOR DIAPHRAGMATIC RUPTURE

Pre-operative nursing focuses on provision of supplementary oxygen, reducing stress on handling, analgesia and treatment of shock. The nurse should be prepared to provide IPPV during the anaesthesia and monitor for sudden changes in blood pressure when the abdominal viscera are moved back into the abdomen. A catheter may be used to aspirate air out of the thorax as the rupture is closed or a chest drain may be used. Post-operatively, the animal should be watched carefully for signs of discomfort associated with increased abdominal pressure and evidence of continuing difficulty with oxygenation due to pulmonary contusions. Some cats may be inappetent after surgery due to liver damage.

Prepubic tendon or abdominal wall rupture

Aetiology This condition is usually seen as a consequence of abdominal wall trauma, most commonly a road accident, but also due to a blunt blow such as a kick. There may also be other injuries associated with the trauma. Usually there is an extensive area of severe bruising over the rupture and the associated subcutaneous swelling.

Management The rupture is repaired surgically using long-lasting absorbable materials such as PDS. Very macerated muscle tissue may not repair easily and a synthetic mesh might be necessary to replace devitalised muscle. Where the prepubic attachment is ruptured, wire sutures may be used to reattach the ventral abdominal wall to the pubic bone.

PRE- AND POST-OPERATIVE NURSING FOR PREPUBIC TENDON OR ABDOMINAL WALL RUPTURE
The animal should be stabilised and given analgesia prior to surgical repair. If the bladder is in the rupture, urine production should be closely monitored or the animal catheterised to ensure that the bladder neck is not entrapped. Analgesia is important as the abdominal wall is often very bruised. Anti-inflammatories may help with resolution of bruising, as well as padded bedding and cage rest. Faecal modifiers should be given to assist with defecation so that the animal does not strain and put pressure on the abdominal repair. Animals that require a mesh implant should be closely monitored for signs of infection or sinus tracts associated with the implant. Post-operative exercise is restricted and the animal prevented from jumping up or stretching the abdomen.

Musculoskeletal

Tendon and muscle repair

Tendon and muscle damage is usually secondary to trauma, unless a **myotomy** or **tenotomy** has been performed as part of a surgical approach to a joint.

Muscle damage is usually repaired as soon as possible after injury using absorbable monofilament material. Trauma to muscle often results in very macerated fragile tissue and it can be difficult to reappose successfully. Normal healthy muscle heals quickly after a myotomy as it has a good blood supply.

Tendons heal very slowly and have to be supported to ensure that they do not stretch and lose function. Orthopaedic implants may be used to protect the tendon until it has fully repaired and remodelled.

Limb amputation

Amputation is an unfortunate but not infrequent surgical procedure in all of the companion animals. It is a very difficult concept for many owners to come to terms with and they may need special counselling and advice. Most dogs cope with amputation much better than the owner will expect and may even be walking and running within hours of anaesthetic recovery.

Amputation may be recommended for the following reasons:

- Curative removal of a benign tumour (e.g. haemangiopericytoma).
- Palliative removal of a malignant, but very painful tumour (e.g. osteosarcoma).
- Injury to the distal limb that is beyond repair (e.g. shear injury).
- Nerve root avulsion resulting in permanent paralysis of the limb.
- Economic reasons if the complex fracture or soft tissue injury is too expensive for repair.

The most important aspect of assessment of a patient for amputation is establishing that the other three limbs are fit and free of arthritic or other disease. On admission it is very important to check and state on the consent form exactly which limb should be amputated. Obese patients or very large breeds may not be suitable candidates for amputation as they will have difficulty shifting the centre of gravity over to the remaining legs and may be less agile.

POST-OPERATIVE NURSING FOR AMPUTATION
Post-operative nursing is important to help these patients to their feet as soon as possible so that they can quickly adapt to a new gait. Walking must be assisted if the floor is slippery or else rubber mats may be laid down to give the dog confidence. Surgery may be prolonged and there can be considerable blood loss from the cut muscle ends if diathermy is not available, so intravenous fluids are important to ensure a rapid recovery. Prevention of seroma formation at the site of the amputation can be achieved by bandaging or use of a drain.

Arthrotomy

Some surgical conditions of the joints require surgery inside the joint itself (**arthrotomy**). The commonest indications for joint surgery in the dog and cat are dislocations, ligamentous injuries (in particular cruciate ligament rupture), osteochondrosis (abnormal development of cartilage in the joint), penetrating wounds of the joint and fractures involving the joint surface. The elbow, stifle and hip are the most commonly affected joints.

Strict asepsis is extremely important as post-operative infection in the joint is devastating. Equally important is careful haemostasis and meticulous repair of the surgical approach through the joint capsule. The joint is usually flushed out with sterile saline at the end of the surgery, and the repair made using monofilament suture materials. Joint surgery can be very painful and good analgesia is important; some surgeons may use local anaesthetic into the joint. Seroma formation is a common post-operative complication and some veterinary surgeons will put a pressure bandage on the joint to prevent this, and to immobilise the joint for a few days. However, it is difficult to immobilise the elbow and stifle and often bandages are ineffective. Exercise is usually limited to a strict regime and it is important that the owner is given clear written instructions.

In some specialist centres, joint surgery may be carried out using **arthroscopy**. This enables access to the inside of the joint without the disadvantages and post-operative complications of the surgical approach. The arthroscope must be sterile and specialist instruments are used that are introduced into the joint via a separate hole. The joint is kept clear during surgery with a continuous high-pressure sterile fluid lavage. A sterile sleeve is used to cover the cable from the arthroscope to the viewing screen.

Arthrodesis

Arthrodesis is the surgical fusion of a joint to prevent its movement, and is used when there is intractable joint pain, chronic instability of the joint or an irreparable joint fracture. The principle is that the joint surfaces are obliterated using curettes or power driven burrs or saws, and then the joint is fused in a normal standing position, using plates or screws to compress the surfaces together. The joint is often supported with a cast post-operatively until the arthrodesis has fully healed and can support the animal's weight. Again strict asepsis is essential to the success of the procedure. Sometimes the surgery is done under tourniquet (e.g. carpal arthrodesis) to reduce blood loss and improve visibility during surgery.

Fractures

Fractures are often the result of traumatic incidents, but in small-breed dogs, they can occur if the dog jumps down from a height – e.g. out of the owner's arms or off the sofa. Some fractures are pathological and are associated with bone disease or neoplasia.

In most instances, fractures are repaired surgically, although this depends on the type of fracture (see earlier). It is important that two good-quality radiographs are obtained of the fracture prior to surgery in order to plan the repair. Immediately post-operatively, two views are taken to assess the success of the repair and to determine the position of any implants.

MAIN PRINCIPLES FOR NURSING THE FRACTURE PATIENT

- Assessment and treatment of concurrent injuries.
- Provision of analgesia.
- Assisted walking to ensure that the animal does not slip over when taken out.
- Provision of adequate dry bedding so that the animal remains dry and clean.
- Monitoring for pressure sores.
- Monitoring the temperature, pulse and respiration rate as indicators of pain, infection or distress.
- Observation of the surgical wound for signs of post-operative infection.
- Detailed communication with the owner over the exercise regime and prevention of excessive use of the limb during the healing process.
- Regular radiography of the repaired fracture to monitor healing.

Specialist orthopaedic surgery

Some orthopaedic surgery is only done in referral centres, such as the tibial plateau levelling osteotomy (a treatment for cruciate rupture), total hip replacement (for chronic hip arthritis due to hip dysplasia) or very complex fractures. These procedures require detailed assessment of the animal and the surgery is done under very strict aseptic conditions. The equipment is expensive and the nursing staff must be experienced in the use and care of these instruments.

For example, when a total hip replacement is carried out, the animal is assessed for skin disease that may increase the risk of bacterial contamination at the time of surgery, obesity, gastrointestinal disease that might cause a diarrhoea during hospitalisation, as well as its orthopaedic disease.

During surgery, the surgeons may wear two pairs of gloves, use adhesive waterproof disposable drapes, and personnel in theatre are limited to reduce aerosol contamination. Often a culture swab is taken from the surgical wound just before closure to check for any contamination in the surgical wound during surgery.

Spinal surgery

Neurosurgical procedures require certain specialised equipment and skills and are usually carried out in referral centres. Diagnosis of spinal injuries or diseases are carried out using a combination of clinical examination and neurological tests and radiographs, contrast radiography (myelography) and advanced imaging techniques (e.g. MRI or CT). Samples of spinal fluid may be taken for analysis either from between the skull and first cervical vertebra (**cisternal puncture**) or from between the lumbar vertebrae (**lumbar puncture**).

Spinal cord injury arises from any pressure on the cord within the vertebral canal. The resulting inflammatory response can result in continued injury to the nerves even after the cause of the pressure has been relieved. Recovery from spinal injuries is very slow and requires a committed and caring nursing staff.

Recumbent animals are at high risk of a number of complications that can be alleviated or prevented by good nursing.

NURSING SPINAL INJURIES
(1) Ensure that the bladder is emptied regularly.
(2) Check for pressure sores three times daily.
(3) Turn the patient regularly – at last every 2 hours.
(4) Monitor conscious or unconscious defecation and urination.
(5) Monitor neurological reflexes and record improvements.
(6) Maintain adequate nutrition.
(7) Physiotherapy of all joints to prevent stiffness and cartilage degeneration.
(8) Keep the skin clean and dry.
(9) Provide regular assisted walks and attention; move the patient into a place where it can watch general activity.

Spinal patients are at risk from the following:

- Pneumonia.
- Pressure sores.
- Dermatitis due to urine or faecal skin soiling.
- Limb oedema.
- Muscle wasting.
- Urinary tract infection.

Most dedicated owners can manage small to medium-sized recumbent patients at home once the animal is urinary continent, but will need detailed written guidelines on nursing care. Regular visits help to monitor the animal's progress and to provide support to the owners that they are doing everything correctly.

Fractures

Spinal fractures are usually the result of trauma, and the radiograph may not accurately reflect the degree of spinal cord damage done at the time of impact if the spinal muscles have pulled the bones back into alignment. If a spinal fracture is suspected, the patient should not be sedated or anaesthetised for radiography, as the muscles may be holding the bones in place and preventing further spinal cord damage. Some fractures are managed with cage rest if the spinal cord injury is not severe. In other cases, the vertebrae have to be stabilised using pins, plates or external fixation.

Disc disease

The intervertebral discs can cause severe spinal cord injury if they dislodge and erupt into the spinal canal, hitting the ventral aspect of the spinal cord. This classically occurs in the small-breed dogs such as Dachshunds, Pekingese and Jack Russell Terriers which have a defect in the cartilage component of the disc (Type 1). These disc protrusions can occur very suddenly and result in acute paralysis of the patient. Another disc disease syndrome is seen in ageing larger-breed dogs, which causes slow compression of the spinal cord and results in chronic nerve pain (Type 2).

Both types of disc disease are alleviated by surgery to open up the spinal canal (**laminectomy**) and to remove the fragments of disc pressing on the spinal cord. This is very specialised surgery and careful assessment of the patient is necessary to determine which part of the spinal canal is affected. Post-operatively, the patient may be slightly worse before the neurological symptoms improve and will require prolonged nursing care. Acute cases of paraplegia should be operated on as soon as possible to reduce the damage to the spinal cord.

Neoplasia

Tumours are occasionally diagnosed causing neurological symptoms secondary to slow compression of the spinal cord as they grow within the confined space of the spinal canal. Surgical removal of benign tumours of the meninges via a laminectomy can be successful, but tumours arising from the vertebrae themselves are usually inoperable.

KEY POINTS
- Good surgical nursing requires that the nurse understands the normal physiological processes of tissue damage and repair.
- In order to be able to nurse an animal effectively both before and after the surgery, the nurse needs to understand the disease and the surgical options that are available to help treat the animal.
- Halstead's principles are the mainstay of good surgical technique and provide a good basis on which to start nursing a patient:
    Strict aseptic technique.
    Gentle tissue handling.
    Preservation of the blood supply.
    Removal of necrotic tissue.
    Accurate haemostasis.
    Closure or drainage of dead space.
    Anatomic approximation of tissues without tension.
- Some surgeries have very specific potential post-operative complications and the nurse should be aware of these in order to monitor for them or try to prevent them.
- An appreciation of the potential surgery for a condition enables the veterinary nurse to prepare the patient and theatre appropriately.

Further reading

Anderson, D. M. (1997) Practical approach to reconstruction of wounds in small animal practice. Part 1. *In Practice*, vol. 19, pp. 463–471.

Anderson, D. M. (1997) Practical approach to reconstruction of wounds in small animal practice. Part 2. *In Practice*, vol. 19, pp. 537–545.

Anderson, D. M. (1999) Nursing patients undergoing skin reconstruction. *Veterinary Nursing*, vol. 14, pp. 52–61.

Anderson, D. M. and White, R. A. S. (2000) Ischemic bandage injuries: a retrospective study in nine dogs and two cats. A review and discussion of the literature. *Veterinary Surgery*, Nov–Dec, pp. 488–498.

Aspinall, V. (2003) *Clinical Procedures in Veterinary Nursing*, Butterworth-Heinemann, Oxford.

Bennett, R. A. (1998) Soft tissue surgery in reptiles. In Bojrab, M. J., Ellison, G. W. and Slocum, B. *Current Techniques in Small Animal Surgery*, 4th edn, Williams & Wilkins, Baltimore.

Bistner, S. I. and Ford, R. B. (2000) *Handbook of Veterinary Procedures and Emergency Treatment*, 7th edn, W. B. Saunders, Philadelphia.

Coughlan, A. R. and Miller, A. (eds) (1998) *BSAVA Manual of Small Animal Fracture Repair and Management*. British Small Animal Veterinary Association, Cheltenham, p. 348.

Ellison, G. W. (1993) Visceral healing and repair disorders. In Bojrab, M. J. (ed.) *Disease Mechanisms in Small Animal Surgery*, 2nd edn, Lea & Febiger, Philadelphia.

Flecknell, P. (1988) Developments in the veterinary care of rabbits and rodents. *In Practice*, vol. 20, pp. 286–295.

Harari, J. (ed.) (1993) *Surgical Complications and Wound Healing in the Small Animal Practice*, W. B. Saunders, Philadelphia.

Hotson Moore, A. and Simpson, G. (eds) (1999) *Manual of Advanced Veterinary Nursing*, British Small Animal Veterinary Association, Cheltenham.

Hoyt, R. F. (1998) Abdominal surgery in pet rabbits. In Bojrab, M. J., Ellison, G. W. and Slocum, B. (eds) *Current Techniques in Small Animal Surgery*, 4th edn, Williams & Wilkins, Baltimore.

Jeffery, N. D. (1995) Postoperative care and physical therapy. In *Handbook of Small Animal Spinal Surgery*, W. B. Saunders, London.

Langley-Hobbs, S. J., Abercomby, R. H. and Pead, M. J. (1996) Comparison and assessment of casting materials for use in small animals. *Veterinary Record*, pp. 258–262.

Lee, A. H., Swaim, S. F. and Henderson, R. A. (1986) Surgical drainage. *The Compendium of Continuing Education*, vol. 8, pp. 94–103.

Moore, M. and Simpson, G. (eds) (1999) *Manual of Veterinary Nursing*, British Small Animal Veterinary Association, Cheltenham.

Morgan, D. A. (2000) *Formulary of Wound Management Products*. In Morgan, D. A. (ed.), 9th edn, *Guides for Health Care Staff*. Euromed Communications Ltd., Haslemere, Surrey.

Morris, J. and Dobson, J. (2001) *Small Animal Oncology*, Blackwell Sciences, Oxford.

Perren, S. M. (1993) Primary bone healing. In Bojrab, M. J. (ed.), *Disease Mechanisms in Small Animal Surgery*, 2nd edn, Lea & Febiger, Philadelphia.

Piermattei, D. L. and Flo, G. L. (1997) Immobilization (fixation). In *Handbook of Small Animal Orthopedics and Fracture Repair*, W. B. Saunders, Philadelphia.

Piermattei, D. L. and Flo, G. L. (1997) Fractures: classification, diagnosis and treatment. In *Handbook of Small Animal Orthopedics and Fracture Repair*, W. B. Saunders, Philadelphia.

Piermattei, D. L. and Flo, G. L. (1997) Delayed union and nonunion. In *Handbook of Small Animal Orthopedics and Fracture Repair*, W. B. Saunders, Philadelphia.

Pope, E. R. (1993) Skin healing. In Bojrab, M. J. (ed.), *Disease Mechanisms in Small Animal Surgery*, 2nd edn, Lea & Febiger, Philadelphia.

Seim, H. B. and Creed, J. E. (1998) Restraint techniques for prevention of self trauma. In Bojrab, M. J., Ellison, G. W. and Slocum, B. (eds), *Current Techniques in Small Animal Surgery*, 4th edn, Williams & Wilkins, Baltimore.

Smeak, D. D. (1998) Selection and use of currently available suture materials and needs. In Bojrab, M. J., Ellison, G. W. and Slocum, B. (eds), *Current Techniques in Small Animal Surgery*, 4th edn, Williams & Wilkins, Baltimore.

Villiers, E. and Dunn, J. (1998) Collection and preparation of smears for cytological evaluation. *In Practice*, vol. 20, pp. 370–377.

Williams, J., McHugh, D. and White, R. A. S. (1992) Use of drains in small animal surgery. *In Practice*, vol. 14, pp. 73–81.

20

High-dependence nursing

E. Leece and *N. Hill*

Learning objectives

After studying this chapter, students should be able to:

- Describe the nursing skills necessary for the care of small animal patients requiring a more intensive nursing protocol than routine in-patients, including:
  - Monitoring and support of the different organ systems.
  - Pain control.
  - Fluid therapy.
  - Nutrition.

Introduction

High dependency nursing is defined as one-to-one nursing, and can range from the following:

- Managing a paraplegic patient.
- Administering hourly ophthalmic drops to a patient with a deep corneal ulcer.
- Calculating the intake and output of a patient with acute renal failure.
- Managing an intensive care case (Fig. 20.1).

These patients require a lot of nursing skill, time and effort. Time and staffing is of paramount importance and the following should be provided:

- Adequate skilled staff.
- 24-hour nursing care.
- Dedicated monitoring equipment.
- Communication.
- Record keeping.
- Time!

Adequate skilled staff and a combined team approach are required to ensure good patient care is not overlooked.

Twenty-four-hour care is often needed for these patients. This involves working shifts, nights and weekends. A good stable nursing team and dedicated approach is required.

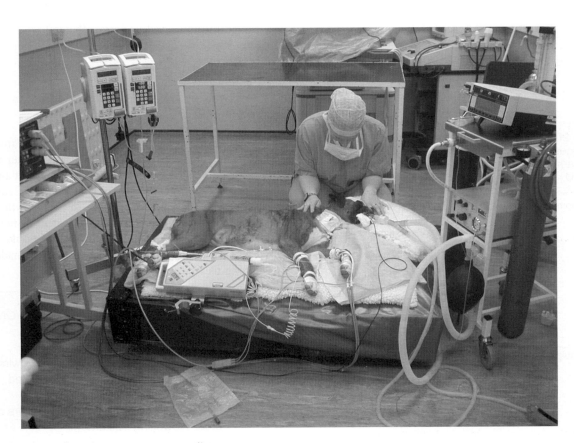

Fig. 20.1 Managing an intensive care case on a ventilator.

Table 20.1 lists some of the basic equipment required for the management and monitoring of a high-dependency case along with some of the desired equipment for intensive care.

Communication is not only important between nurses and veterinary surgeons, but also between staff and the owners. Some patients may be presented in a critical state, or the patient may be undergoing major surgery. It is not just these patients, but all patients that need communication with the owners.

On admission of the patient, the owners should be made aware of the following:
(1) What the patient is coming in for and which tests are going to be performed.
(2) Risks of any anaesthesia.
(3) Approximate length of stay and estimate of costs.
(4) Ongoing updates on the patient and the cost of treatment so far.
(5) For all high-risk patients, resuscitation should be discussed with the owners with particular attention being paid to the patient's condition and long-term prognosis. The option of resuscitation versus no resuscitation should be presented to the owner along with whether closed or open chest resuscitation should be performed if these facilities are available at the clinic.

Table 20.1 The basic equipment required for the management and monitoring of a high-dependency case and also some of the desired equipment for an ICU

Basic equipment required	Heat lamps, pads and/or incubator
	Thermometer
	Intravenous catheters and fluid delivery systems
	Urinary catheters
	Oxygen delivery systems
	ECG/blood pressure monitor
	PCV/TP/BUN
	Refractometer
	CPR equipment (crash trolley or box)
	24-hour nursing
Desired equipment	Haematology and biochemistry
	Electrolyte analyser
	Blood gas analyser
	Pulse oximeter
	Capnograph

PCV = packed cell volume; TP = total serum protein; BUN = blood urea nitrogen; CPR = cardiopulmonary resuscitation

Record keeping is a crucial part of high-dependency nursing. It allows for monitoring both physiological trends and the patient's response to therapy as well as enabling an accurate record of treatments and nursing care. The record should allow for continuity in patient care between nursing staff. Case notes should include a plan for the monitoring and treatment of critical cases and these may need to be changed and updated several times per day. Obviously the type of clinical record depends on the type of patient and may range from a simple card system for a patient receiving physiotherapy to a full intensive care record such as the one shown in Fig. 20.2 for the critical care patient.

Nosocomial infection

Nosocomial infections are infections acquired by a patient as a result of their stay in hospital. Critical care patients are at higher risk of infection, with urinary tract and wound infections being more prevalent than more serious chest infections or bacteraemia.

Nosocomial infections have a multifactorial aetiology:

(1) Patient factors:

   - Disease process can lower the threshold to infection.
   - Endogenous and exogenous immunosuppression (e.g. corticosteroids, chemotherapy).
   - Malnutrition.
   - Invasive monitoring and supportive techniques (e.g. intravenous and urinary catheters).

(2) Hospital factors:

   - Poor hygiene
   - Transfer by staff between patients.
   - Overuse of antibiotics.

Prevention of nosocomial infections is imperative in the critical care setting. This will be discussed further throughout the chapter. It is important to remember that antibiotics may prevent and treat systemic infection by susceptible organisms but they may predispose to overgrowth by resistant micro-organisms, making the treatment of nosocomial infections extremely difficult. Antibiotics should only be used when necessary and not to cover up any inadequacies in nursing technique.

PREVENTION OF NOSOCOMIAL INFECTION
- Disinfection of kennels between patients.
- Barrier nursing.
- Reduce risk of infection through the following:
   (a) Wound management, changing soiled bandages.
   (b) Management of intravenous catheters and other indwelling equipment.

RESUSCITATION: DNR / closed chest / open chest

Date:	Case no:	Name:	Age:	Sex:
Clinician:	Anaesthetist:	Start ICU	End ICU	
Admission weight:	Today's weight:	Blood volume:		

Reason for ICU: (case summary, anticipated problems)

Phone nos:

Anaes:	Clinician:	Owner:

PLAN 0-12 hrs

1	
2	
3	
4	
5	
6	

PLAN 12-24 hrs

1	
2	
3	
4	
5	
6	

Catheter incl. urinary (position,size,date)	F: flushed	D: dressed

Fig. 20.2 Example of an ICU record running over a 24-hour period.

Instructions / medications	DATE: / / TIME:																					
	1																					
	2																					
	3																					
	4																					
	5																					
	6																					
	7																					
	8																					
	9																					
	10																					
	11																					

| Vital signs | Resp: o   Pulse ●   BP >\|<   ETCO₂ Δ | 200 180 160 140 120 100 80 60 40 20 | | | | | | | | | | | | | | | | | | | | |

Monitoring	SpO₂ / ABG																					
	Vent. *IPPV, normal, dyspnoea, tachypnoea*																					
	CRT																					
	Mucous membrane colour																					
	CVP																					
	Pulse quality *strong, fair, poor, weak*																					
	Mentation *excited, alert, sleep, depressed, coma*																					
	PLR, pupil size *normal, dilated, ppt, anisc.*																					

INS	Nutrition: BER: IER:																					
	FLUID 1 rate ml/hr / amount																					
	FLUID 2 rate ml/hr / amount																					
	FLUID 3 rate ml/hr / amount																					
	TOTAL INS ml/hr / Total amt																					

OUTS	URINE OUTPUT ml/hr / amount																					
	USG																					
	DRAIN ml/hr / Type: amount																					
	OTHER *emesis, diarrhoea etc.*																					

| | Comments, blood results etc | | | | | | | | | | | | | | | | | | | | | |

Fig. 20.2 (Continued)

	TIME
	1
	2
	3
	4
	5
	6
	7
	8
	9
	10
	11

Instructionss / medications

Vital signs

200 180 160 140 120 100 80 60 40 20

Resp: o   Pulse •   BP > | < $ETCO_2$ Δ

SpO2 / ABG	
Vent. *IPPV, normal, dyspnoea, tachypnoea*	
CRT	
Mucous membrane colour	
CVP	
Pulse quality *strong, fair, poor, weak*	
Mentation *excited, alert, sleep, depressed, coma*	
PLR, pupil size *normal, dilated, pinpoint, anisc.*	

Monitoring

Nutrition: BER: IER:	
FLUID 1	
FLUID 2	
FLUID 3	
TOTAL INS	

INS

URINE OUTPUT	
USG	
DRAIN type	
OTHER *emesis, diarrhoea etc.*	

OUTS

Comments, blood results etc	

Fig. 20.2 (Continued)

Date:	Case no:	Sheet no:

Fig. 20.2 (Continued)

Barrier nursing

Isolation is required if a patient has a known infection or disease, or shows signs that could be transmitted to other patients. In the critically ill patient it is important to reduce the risk of infection because often these patients are immunosuppressed and much more susceptible to infection (Fig. 20.3). More information on barrier nursing may be found in Chapter 16, General Nursing.

Patients with a suspected or known infection should be placed in a kennel away from the rest of the in-patients.

- Ideally the patient should be placed into an isolation ward.
- The ward should be a self-contained unit with its own entrance separate from that of the hospital.
- The room should have its own equipment for use in that room only:

  (a) Bedding.
  (b) Feed bowls.
  (c) Clinical waste.
  (d) Litter trays and litter.
  (e) Monitoring equipment.
  (f) Gloves, gowns, masks, shoe covers, and a change of clothing.
  (g) Disinfectants.
  (h) Foot bath.

- There should be good ventilation, separate from that of the main ward.
- One nurse should be allocated to the patient and should not come into contact with other patients.

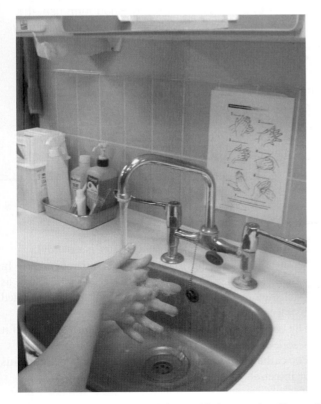

Fig. 20.3 Hands should be washed thoroughly between handling each patient.

Reducing the risk of infection

Good wound management

Any wound, whether it is clean or contaminated, should be treated like a clean wound.

- Sterile gloves should be worn.
- Any swabs, cotton buds or instruments entering the wound should be sterile.
- Irrigation solution used to flush the wounds should be sterile.
- Any bandaging materials used should be sterile.
- Dressings should be changed regularly or if soiled or wet.
- Prevent self-trauma by the patient by using an Elizabethan collar and providing adequate pain relief.

Proper care of indwelling catheters and drains

Intravenous (IV) catheter selection:

- The choice of catheter, gauge, length and site should be considered when catheterising a patient.
- A correctly placed catheter of suitable gauge and length, which is well maintained, can increase the indwelling time.
- For long-term catheterisation, the choice of catheter type is important. Silicone or polyurethane catheters are minimally reactive and are therefore less thrombogenic, whereas polyvinyl chloride, polyethylene and polypropylene are the most reactive.
- If large volumes of fluids are to be administered, a larger gauge catheter will be required.
- If central venous pressure is to be monitored, the length of the catheter is important. The tip of the catheter needs to reach the vena cava within the thoracic cavity close to its entry point to the right atrium.
- If an overlong catheter is used in the cephalic or saphenous vein, positional occlusion could be a problem for running intravenous fluids.
- More information on types of intravenous catheters can be found in Chapter 22, Fluid and Shock Therapy.

EQUIPMENT REQUIRED FOR INTRAVENOUS CATHETER PLACEMENT (FIG. 20.4)
- Clippers.
- Lint-free swabs soaked in chlorhexidine scrub solution.
- Lint-free swabs soaked in spirit.
- Catheter of suitable gauge and length.
- Tape to secure the catheter to the patient.
- Bung with injection port or extension set.
- Heparinised saline.
- Occlusive dressing.
- Bandaging equipment.

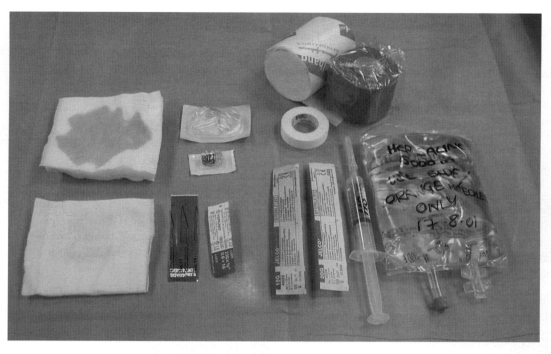

Fig. 20.4 Equipment required for intravenous catheterisation of a peripheral vein.

Catheter placement (Fig. 20.5):

(1) Ensure you have all the equipment ready before starting.
(2) Restrain the patient on a non-slip surface.
(3) Clip an area over the vessel and any long hairs.
(4) Wash hands thoroughly.
(5) Aseptically prepare the skin using an antimicrobial solution.
(6) Spray or wipe off any excess antimicrobial solution on the skin, with the spirit solution.
(7) Allow the spirit solution to evaporate first, then pinch the skin over the vessel with the thumb and forefinger and make a small incision in the skin using a no.11 scalpel blade or a needle.
(8) Insert the catheter into the vessel.
(9) Once there is a flashback of blood in the hub of the stylet one can run the catheter off the stylet into the vessel.
(10) Attach a bung or extension set to the catheter.
(11) Tape in the catheter by placing 1 cm of the first piece of tape sticky side up underneath the hub of the catheter. Bring the tape over the hub of the catheter and around the limb. Place a tab on the end of the tape for easy removal.
(12) Place the centre of a second piece of tape sticky side up on the underneath of the bung or extension set. Criss-cross the tape over the top of the bung or extension set and around the limb.
(13) Flush the apparatus with heparinised saline.
(14) Bandage in place with some cast padding (Velband®, Softban®) initially, then use an adhesive dressing (Co-flex®, Vetrap®).
(15) The bung or extension set should be left exteriorised from the dressing. This enables drugs to be administered or blood samples to be taken.

USEFUL TIPS FOR PLACEMENT OF LONG-TERM CATHETERS

• When a small incision is made in the skin prior to catheter placement, this allows the catheter to be smoothly placed into the vessel and prevents burring of the catheter. Although not necessary prior to placing a catheter for short-term use, it is advisable prior to placing a catheter which will stay in more than 24 hours.
• An occlusive dressing should be applied for long-term use or in immunocompromised patients (Fig. 20.6).
• A T-port extension set minimises handling of the catheter at its point of entry through the skin and so minimises the risk of transferring infection.

Basic catheter maintenance:

• Continuous assessment of the catheter is essential.
• Monitor for swelling above or below the bandage. In some cases, often in cats or short-legged breeds such as Dachshunds, the bandage may need to be extended distally to include the toes of the patient.
• The bandage should be changed at least once daily or if it is soiled or wet.
• The catheter site should be observed for signs of phlebitis or infection:

(1) Redness.
(2) Swelling.

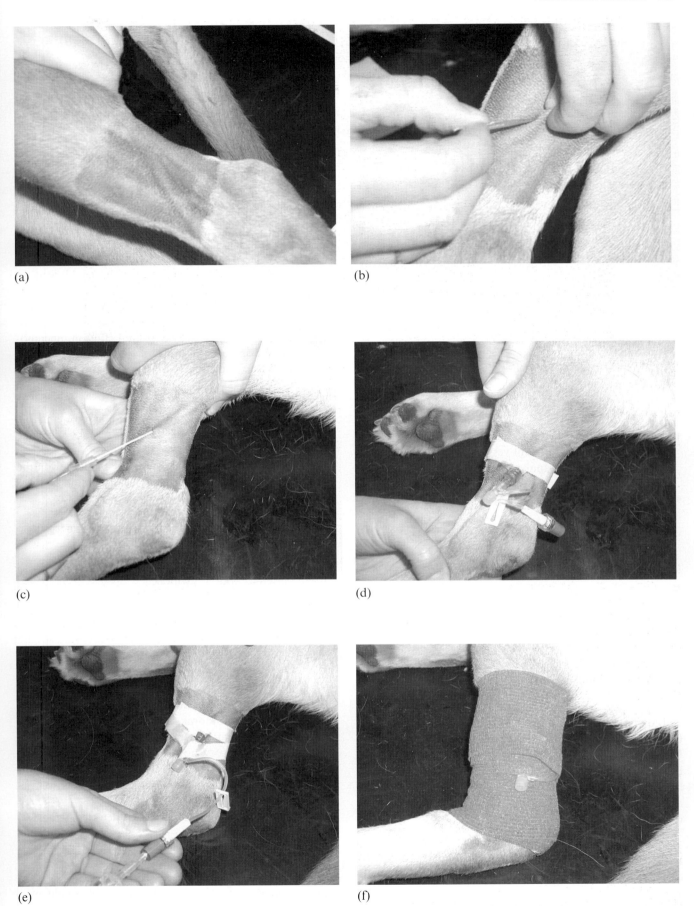

Fig. 20.5 Saphenous catheter placement in the dog. (a) Saphenous vein being raised by an assistant. (b) Scalpel blade being used to make a small incision in the skin. (c) Insertion of an over the needle catheter. (d) Attachment of T-port extension set to catheter and secured with tape. (e) Flushing catheter with heparinised saline. (f) Limb bandaged with T-port exposed for access.

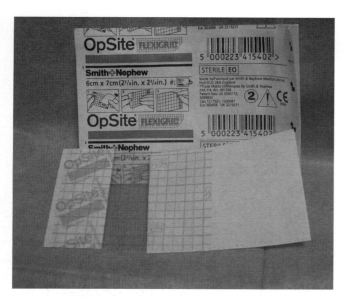

Fig. 20.6 An occlusive dressing should be applied to a long-term catheter.

(3) Heat.
(4) Discomfort.

- If this occurs the catheter should be removed and another catheter placed in a different vessel (the tip of the catheter can be sent away for analysis to determine the cause and type of infection).
- The catheter should be flushed every 6 hours when not in use.

Patient monitoring in high-dependence nursing

The ability to monitor the different organ systems is imperative to high-dependency nursing and can be applied to a variety of situations. In the severely ill patient, all organ systems should be monitored. It is necessary to be able to use equipment available and to interpret results obtained and apply them to the patient. The nursing and veterinary team can then provide supportive measures necessary. Monitoring applied to each of the body systems listed below will be described along with a brief discussion on how the common abnormalities detected can be treated, although these are covered in greater detail in other chapters.

- Respiratory system.
- Circulatory system.
- Thermoregulatory system.
- Gastrointestinal system.
- Urinary system.
- Neurological system.
- Musculoskeletal system.

Respiratory system (pulmonary system)

The function of the respiratory system is to oxygenate blood and remove carbon dioxide. This requires normally functioning lungs to allow gas exchange along with normal minute ventilation, which is controlled by respiratory rate and tidal volume.

(1) Respiratory rate:

- Normal values vary widely.
- The respiratory rate does not tell you about tidal volume.

(2) Respiratory depth and rhythm:

- Marked variations in depth or rhythm can signify a problem which, if left untreated, could lead to respiratory failure.
- Excessive abdominal effort may be an indication that the patient is trying to compensate for a problem such as lung disease, pleural effusion, pneumothorax, or upper respiratory tract obstruction, and should be immediately investigated further.

(3) Mucous membrane colour:

- Ashen or cyanotic colours indicate hypoxaemia.
- Cyanosis will not be seen in severely anaemic patient.
- Cyanosis may occur if there is low blood flow in the capillary bed (alpha-2-agonist sedation, severe shock).

> **NOTE**
> Ambient lighting can, in certain circumstances, cause membranes to appear cyanotic.

(4) Auscultation:

- Both sides of the chest should be auscultated for air flow.
- Decreased air movement may indicate lung pathology, pneumothorax or pleural effusion.
- If there is upper respiratory tract obstruction, then a harsh inspiratory noise may be auscultated at the level of the trachea with the stethoscope placed on the ventral aspect of the patient's neck as well as being heard over the lung fields.
- Abnormal lung noises may be detected (crackles, wheezes).

> **NOTE**
> Veterinary attention should be sought if abnormalities are detected and may be further investigated by thoracic imaging.

(5) Pulse oximetry:

- Pulse oximeters measure haemoglobin oxygen saturation and therefore the ability of the lungs to deliver oxygen to the blood.
- Probes may be placed on the tongue, the lips or on unpigmented foot pads in cats.
- Displays oxygen saturation and pulse rate.
- Rely on good cardiovascular stability to work properly (poor performance with vasoconstriction or low blood pressure).
- Probes need to be moved on a regular basis to prevent sluggish blood flow beneath the clip and therefore lower readings.
- When receiving oxygen-enriched air, pulse oximetry is not a good indicator of hypoventilation.
- If hypoxaemia is detected then measures should be taken to provide an enriched oxygen environment and the cause determined.

> *TIP*
> Normal oxygen saturation > 93%. Oxygen therapy should be implemented if the reading falls below this value.

(6) Blood gas readings:

- Arterial blood samples may be taken and the levels of oxygen and carbon dioxide measured accurately using a blood gas machine.
- Expensive equipment, may only be available in large hospitals.
- Arterial catheters (Fig. 20.7) may be placed to enable repeated samples to be taken (as well as direct blood pressure monitoring). These must be maintained aseptically, ideally glued in place to minimise movement, flushed every 2 hours, clearly marked as arterial so that no drugs are inadvertently injected.

(7) Capnography:

- Requires a specialised piece of monitoring equipment that can only be used in intubated patients (Fig. 20.8).
- Measures expired carbon dioxide levels (normal end tidal CO_2 35–40 mmHg).
- High levels indicate hypoventilation.

Oxygen therapy

Oxygen therapy should be instituted in the event of hypoxaemia, respiratory failure or severe anaemia (haemoglobin < 5 g/dl or PCV < 10%). Higher levels of inspired oxygen can be supplied to the patient in a variety of ways depending on how long the patient is likely to require enriched oxygen and what the patient will tolerate. Many hypoxaemic patients, especially cats, are extremely distressed and do not tolerate handling and restraint. Persistent attempts to restrain

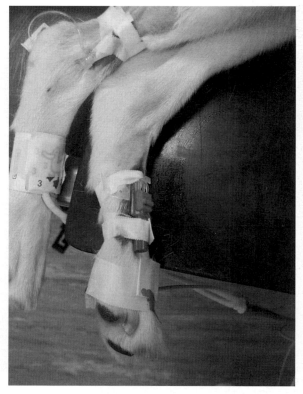

Fig. 20.7 Arterial catheter placed in the metatarsal artery of the hindlimb.

these patients may result in excessive struggling, leading to a respiratory crisis. It is imperative to try to stabilise these patients by providing oxygen and allowing the patient to calm down before examination is performed. The methods of providing an oxygen-enriched environment are listed below and a more detailed description of their use can be found in Chapter 17 on medical nursing.

- **Face mask**
- **Nasal catheters** are well tolerated in dogs (Fig. 20.9) or **nasal prongs** may be used in larger dogs (Fig. 20.10).

> *PLACEMENT OF NASAL CATHETERS*
> - Use a soft rubber tube (feeding tubes or proper nasal tubes).
> - Measure the distance from the tip of the nose to the level of the medial canthus of the eye, mark the tube.
> - Spray the nasal cavity with local anaesthetic.
> - Lubricate tubing.
> - Guide the tube into the nose ventrally and medially in short, smooth movements, allow the patient to relax before advancing the tubing further.
> - Insert up to the mark made earlier.
> - Secure the tubing in place with butterfly tape attached to skin with superglue, sutures or staples and secure at the back of the head to a collar.
> - Attach to oxygen supply and turn the flowmeter on slowly to prevent an unpleasant burst of cold air into the nasal cavity.

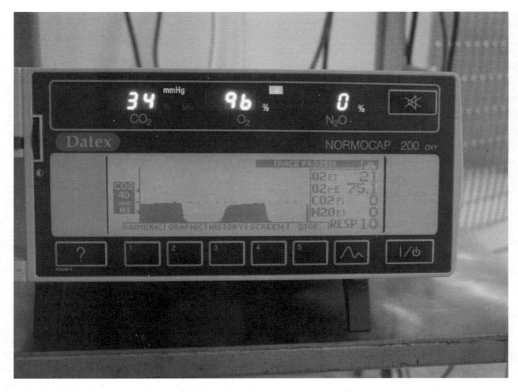

Fig. 20.8 Capnograph demonstrates a trace of expired carbon dioxide, end tidal carbon dioxide and inspired oxygen.

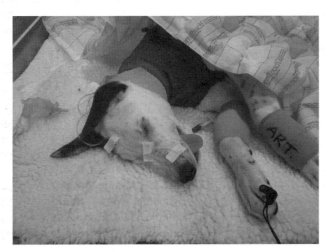

Fig. 20.9 Nasal catheter for oxygen insufflation.

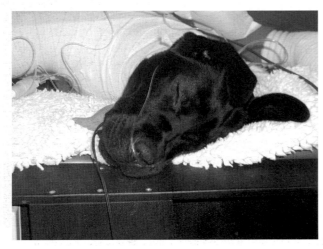

Fig. 20.10 Nasal prongs in place.

- **Oxygen collars.**
- **Oxygen cages.**

Pulmonary support

This chapter will briefly cover basic pulmonary support, nursing care for patients undergoing ventilation and management of chest drains and tracheostomy tubes. Pulmonary support involves the treatment and support of respiratory function, specific to the patient's presenting problem.

(1) Turning – this prevents hypostatic congestion in the lungs of recumbent patients.

(2) Nebulisation and coupage – nebulisation is the formation of mini-droplets of water or saline in the inspired gases. These droplets can be carried down to the smaller airways in order to hydrate and mobilise secretions.

The easiest method of nebulisation is to bubble the flow of oxygen through a canister containing sterile water or saline. A fine spray of small droplets can be visualised in the gases. A simple facemask can be used to deliver these to the patient for 10 minutes prior to coupage.

(3) Humidification of inspired gases – this may be achieved by nebulisation or, if the patient is intubated, by the use of a heat and humidity exchanger placed at the end of the endotracheal tube (Fig. 20.11).

(4) Coupage should be used following nebulisation to aid in mobilisation of secretions and encourage coughing. Coupage should not be performed in cases where rib

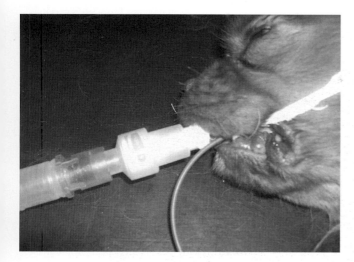

Fig. 20.11 Heat and humidity exchanger in use.

fractures are present or when there is active bleeding in the chest.
(5) Artificial ventilation (IPPV – intermittent positive pressure ventilation).

LONG-TERM VENTILATION
Mechanical ventilation assists or controls the patient's breathing by forcing a mixture of air and oxygen into the lungs via an endotracheal tube. The technique requires specialised staff and equipment and may be used in trauma patients, in central nervous system disorders and other forms of pulmonary disease. Descriptions of the different ventilatory modes are beyond the scope of this chapter, however, a few simple points should be noted for the nursing care of a ventilated animal.
Ventilated patients require the following specialist care from nursing staff:
- Sedation or general anaesthesia.
- Regular turning every four hours.
- Humidification of inspired gases.
- Moistening of the mouth.
- Replacement of endotracheal tubes (red rubber tubes every 6 hours, silicone tubes every 24 hours), suctioning of tubes.
- Lubrication of eyes.
- Inspired gases made of a mixture of air and some oxygen.
- 24-hour nursing and constant supervision.

Care of chest drains

The use and care of chest drains are discussed in relation to high-dependency nursing, although more details can be found in Chapter 17 on medical nursing. Indications for a chest drain:

- Intrathoracic surgery for post-operative drainage of air and fluid, for example lung lobectomy or ruptured diaphragm.
- Pyothorax.
- Pneumothorax.
- Pleural effusions.
- Chylothorax.
- Haemothorax.

Types of chest drains Different types of chest tubes are available and some come with a trocar or stylet. Tubes should be flexible, non-collapsible and easily sterilised. These include red rubber, PVC and silicone. Unless continuous drainage is performed, the tubes must remain closed in between drainage to prevent aspiration of air through the tube and the development of a pneumothorax. The tubes must be sealed by one of the following:

- Three-way tap and gate clamp.
- Heimlich valve.
- Underwater seal.

Aspiration of the chest tube may be performed intermittently with a syringe and three-way tap or continuously by means of suction. Intermittent drainage is adequate for most cases, although continuous drainage may be required if the rate of air or fluid accumulation is likely to be rapid. The frequency of drainage is governed by the amount of fluid or air accumulated.

- Three-way tap/gate clamp – a three-way tap and clamp are often used together (Fig. 20.12). The three-way tap is attached to the drain with a spigot to create a closed system. The end of the drain is then bent over and the clamp applied. The three-way tap is then left in the position that is off to the patient. This system allows intermittent drainage of the chest and is ideal for any size patient.
- Heimlich valve – this is a clear plastic device comprising a one-way rubber flutter valve. It is connected directly to the drain. Air or fluid is expelled from the chest during expiration. This system can be intermittently drained by

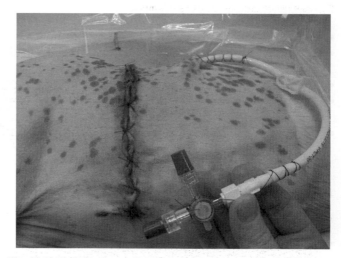

Fig. 20.12 Use of a three-way tap and clamp to create a closed system.

syringe or connected to a suction machine for continuous drainage. The Heimlich valve has a tendency to block and requires regular changing. This valve may be used in patients weighing above 15 kg.

- Underwater seal system – this comprises a sterile bottle with sterile saline/water to the depth of a few centimetres. The bottle has a bung, into which two tubes are inserted, one of which is submerged 2 cm into the saline/water, the other remaining above the fluid. The fluid creates a back-pressure and seals the pleural cavity from the atmosphere. This system can provide intermittent or continuous drainage.

Technique for intermittent drainage:

(1) Gather equipment.
(2) Sterile gloves, syringe and container/kidney dish.
(3) Ensure the patient is comfortable.
(4) Before commencing drainage, ensure the clamp is on and the three-way tap is off to the patient.
(5) Connect the syringe to the three-way tap.
(6) Unscrew or unclip the clamp.
(7) Close the three-way tap to the atmosphere (the three-way tap will now be open to the patient and syringe, allowing drainage).
(8) Gently withdraw the plunger of the syringe to aspirate the air or fluid.
(9) Once the syringe is full, close the three-way tap off to the patient and expel the contents of the syringe into a suitable container.
(10) Continue until a vacuum is felt in the syringe.
(11) Close the three-way tap off to the patient and close the clamp.

> **TIP**
> Patients with a chest drain should ideally never be left unattended.

Nursing management of chest drains:

- Chest drains should be bandaged lightly in place to prevent dislodgement or damage by the patient (Fig. 20.13).
- Bandages should be changed daily unless soiled or wet.
- The point of insertion should be kept covered and checked regularly.
- The point of insertion should be cleaned daily.
- The presence of an indwelling chest drain will cause 2 ml/kg of fluid to be produced per day.
- Intermittent drainage should be carried out at regular intervals dependent on the amount of fluid produced.

Care of tracheostomy tubes

Indications for placement of tracheostomy tubes:

- To allow for delivery of oxygen and volatile anaesthetic agents during certain upper airway or intranasal procedures.

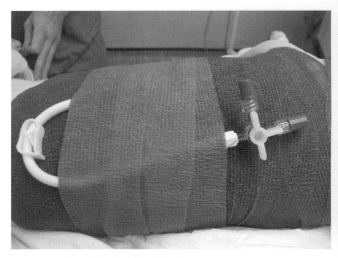

Fig. 20.13 Chest drain bandaged in place.

- To relieve upper airway obstruction (e.g. laryngeal paralysis).
- Facilitate the removal of lower airway secretions.
- To allow manual/mechanical ventilation.

Types of tracheostomy tubes:

- Silicone and nylon are non-irritant materials used for tracheostomy tubes.
- Metal tubes are seldom used today.
- Single or double lumen tubes available.
- Double lumen tubes may not be suitable for small dogs or cats.
- Cuffed or uncuffed.

> **TIP**
> Cuffed tubes predispose the patient to pressure necrosis and post-intubation stenosis.

Nursing care of tracheostomy tubes:

> The objective of regular management is to prevent the build-up of secretions that may block the tube and to provide aseptic wound care and humidify inspired air.

- Observe the patient continually for early detection of occlusion.
- Any sign of distress, dyspnoea, coughing or pawing at the site could indicate an obstruction.
- Regular checks from every 15 min to every 2 hours are often needed.
- Humidify inspired air, by use of a humidity exchange filter (artificial nose), nebulisers or by instilling 0.5–3 ml

of sterile saline every 1–2 hours into the tracheostomy tube.

- Clean the tracheostomy site and adjacent skin every time the tube is cleaned.
- Use sterile saline on cotton buds or gauze swabs.
- Antiseptic solutions may be used, but need to be kept away from the incision and wound area because they will irritate the tracheal mucosa.
- The tube can be removed and a new one replaced. The tube can be placed back into the trachea easily by pulling the tracheostomy open using the traction sutures placed at the time of the surgery.
- Regular suctioning helps prevent accumulation of secretions.
- Frequency of suctioning depends on the patient.
- Cats often need more frequent suctioning.

Suction technique:

(1) Restrain the patient gently in a stress-free environment.
(2) Pre-oxygenate the patient.
(3) Use a sterile pliable suction catheter or soft urethral catheter.
(4) Introduce the catheter aseptically into the trachea.
(5) Intermittent and light suction is applied to the catheter.
(6) Allow the patient to have a few breaths in-between suctioning.
(7) Each suction attempt should take no longer than 15 seconds.

TIP
Do not suction too soon after the patient has been fed as it can initiate gagging and vomiting.

If a tube is obstructed, action must be taken immediately:

- Extend the patient's head and check the tube is not obstructed externally by skin folds or bedding.
- Attempt to suction the tube unless the patient is cyanotic.
- Remove the tracheostomy tube and replace with another tube, either a fresh tracheostomy tube if available or an endotracheal tube of suitable size.
- Ventilate with 100% oxygen.

Transtracheal catheterisation

This may be performed in an emergency situation when there is an upper airway obstruction. A large-bore needle is placed percutaneously into the trachea between the tracheal rings distal to the obstruction and attached to a source of high-flow oxygen. This technique may be performed to stabilise a patient and provide oxygen for a few minutes until a tracheostomy can be performed.

Cardiovascular system

The function of the cardiovascular system is to pump oxygenated blood around the body to supply tissues and organs with oxygen and nutrients and to remove waste products. Monitoring is important in a variety of cases that may require high-dependency nursing such as trauma, haemorrhage, shock, cardiac arrhythmias, and electrolyte imbalances. There are a number of easy ways to assess cardiovascular function; however, it is better to use a technique that assesses blood pressure and perfusion in the peripheral tissues. Some techniques are described in further detail in Chapter 17.

(1) Auscultation:

- Used to assess heart rate, rhythm and the presence of any cardiac murmurs.
- Auscultation does not give any information on the cardiovascular system as a whole.

(2) Electrocardiogram:

- Used to assess heart rate and rhythm via detection of the electrical rhythm.
- Does not tell you how well the heart is actually contracting.
- Useful for monitoring arrhythmias and response to therapy.
- Crocodile clips attached to the skin may be used but for more prolonged use adhesive pads should be applied to the foot pads (Fig. 20.14).

(3) Mucous membranes:

- Mucous membrane colour can give some information about the cardiovascular status of the patient.
- Pale mucous membranes may be an indication of anaemia or vasoconstriction, which may be a result of sympathetic stimulation, e.g. pain, fear, shock, dehydration.
- An ashen colour is an indicator of poor perfusion.
- A brick-red colour may be a result of endotoxaemia.

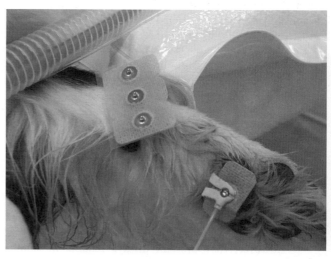

Fig. 20.14 Adhesive ECG pads in use.

- Capillary refill time should be less than 2 seconds in the healthy patient. Prolonged refill times are indicative of poor perfusion.
- Mucous membranes should be moist to the touch.

(4) Peripheral pulses:

- Palpation of peripheral pulses is an invaluable tool in cardiovascular monitoring.
- Peripheral pulses should be palpated if possible, such as the dorsal metatarsal artery, since this gives an indication of good peripheral blood flow. Palpation at these sites takes practice but should be possible. The femoral pulse can also be palpated.
- In cases of low blood pressure and hypovolaemia, the peripheral pulses are lost before the femoral pulses due to vasoconstriction.
- When feeling the pulse, it is actually the difference between the systolic and diastolic blood pressures that can be appreciated and is not an indication of the blood pressure itself.
- It is important to try to occlude the artery as this gives an indication of actual blood pressure. Although very subjective, if a pulse is easy to occlude it can mean poor blood pressure and warrants further investigation.

(5) Arterial blood pressure: it is important to monitor this in critical patients since organ perfusion relies heavily on a mean arterial blood pressure above 60 mmHg. Blood pressure may be monitored invasively or non-invasively. Invasive monitoring is by means of an arterial catheter attached to a manometer or an electrical transducer giving a reading of the arterial waveform. More commonly non-invasive monitoring is carried out by the following techniques:

(a) *Doppler blood pressure monitoring (Fig. 20.15)*:

- This is the cheapest and most reliable method of measuring blood pressure indirectly.
- A piezoelectric crystal is taped in place over a peripheral artery so that a pulse can be detected audibly on an amplifier.
- An occlusive cuff is placed around the limb proximally to the crystal and attached to a manometer.
- The cuff is then inflated to a pressure that occludes the artery, therefore the sound of the pulse is lost.
- The cuff is slowly deflated until blood flow can be audibly detected once more and the corresponding pressure read on the manometer. This is the systolic blood pressure.
- The cuff is then fully deflated between readings.

(b) *Oscillometric measurements (Fig. 20.16)*:

- This is a fully automated method and is easy to use; however, they are not always reliable in smaller patients or when arrhythmias are present.

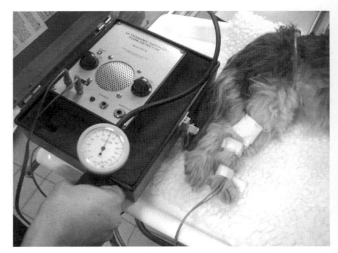

Fig. 20.15 Doppler blood pressure monitor: amplifier, crystal and cuff.

- A cuff of appropriate size is placed over a peripheral artery (the cuff width must be approximately 40% of the circumference of the limb).
- The machine inflates the cuff to occlude the artery, then allows the cuff to deflate.
- As the cuff deflates, the machine detects changes in oscillations in pressure in the cuff as a result of blood flow and from these changes can determine systolic, mean and diastolic pressure.

NORMAL VALUES FOR BLOOD PRESSURE
Systolic > 80 mmHg
Mean > 60 mmHg

---

(6) Central venous pressure (CVP) – this is a guide to right ventricular filling pressure and so is a balance between intravascular volume, cardiac function and venous

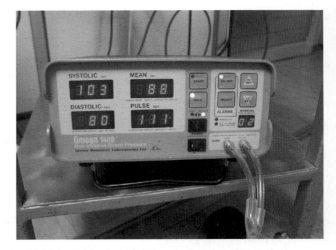

Fig. 20.16 Oscillometric blood pressure monitor.

compliance. Trends in CVP may be important in rehydration fluid therapy, cardiac problems when the pumping system may be failing (congestive heart failure or pericardial tamponade) and fluid therapy in oliguric renal failure, when excessive fluid administration is not eliminated by the kidneys.

- Decreased CVP is most commonly caused by hypovolaemia leading to decreased venous return to the heart.
- Raised CVP may be due to fluid overload, poor cardiac contractility, and pericardial tamponade.
- Further interpretation of CVP readings is beyond the scope of this chapter and more information can be found in Chapter 22 on fluid therapy.

Measurement of CVP:

- CVP is measured using a long catheter, which is normally inserted via the jugular vein so that its tip lies in the vena cava within the thoracic cavity close to the right atrium.
- The patient should be restrained in lateral recumbency and the neck placed on a sandbag.
- The length of catheter required should be measured (from the point of entry to the heart base).
- The area over the jugular vein should be clipped and prepped, and a suitable drape placed over the site.
- Sterile gloves should be worn during this procedure.
- A small incision should be made through the skin overlying the vein prior to catheter placement.
- The catheter may be introduced into the vein using a variety of techniques. The two most commonly used techniques in veterinary practice are the peel away catheter and the Seldinger technique.
- The **peel away technique** involves placing a specially made short introduction catheter into the vein over a needle, removing the needle and then sliding the jugular catheter through the preplaced catheter. Once in position the introduction catheter is peeled away leaving the jugular line in place.
- The **Seldinger technique** again utilises an introduction catheter or needle, which is inserted into the vein. A guidewire is then introduced into the vein and the catheter removed. A special dilator is then passed over the wire to dilate the entrance through the vessel wall. Once this is removed, the jugular catheter can be fed over the guidewire into the vein and the guidewire then removed.
- The catheters can then be sutured in place and an occlusive dressing applied.
- Some jugular catheters are multi-lumen catheters which enable fluids and drugs to be given through separate lines, whilst still having a dedicated lumen for CVP monitoring.
- The catheter can be connected up to a transducer or manometer. However, expensive equipment is not required and an alternative technique is described in Chapter 22 on fluid therapy and shock.

(7) Cardiac output – this can be measured using a variety of techniques; however, this level of monitoring is rarely employed in veterinary patients.

Thermoregulatory system

Regular monitoring of body temperature may be important in certain patients which are suspected to be at risk of infection or where thermoregulatory control may be impaired, for example postoperatively. Measuring the difference between rectal temperature and toe web temperature (measured by placing the thermometer in between the foot pads) can be a useful indicator of peripheral perfusion. The normal difference is usually less than 3°C and may be elevated in shock or with vasoconstriction.

Gastrointestinal system

It is important to monitor gastrointestinal function in all critical care patients, regardless of presenting signs. The following parameters should be noted:

- Changes in appetite.
- Amount and consistency of motions.
- Amount of vomiting.
- The patient should be weighed daily.
- Presence of abdominal pain.

It is important to maintain nutrition in ill patients and if a patient refuses to eat this should be addressed. A patient should not be allowed to go for more than 3 days without nutrition. Estimates of the amount of fluid lost through vomiting and diarrhoea should be calculated and added to the daily fluid therapy plan. PCV, TP and electrolytes should be monitored in any patient with vomiting or diarrhoea, since electrolytes will be lost from the body and dehydration may occur.

Urinary system

The normal patient produces 1–2 ml/kg/hr of urine. Urine output may be decreased for a variety of reasons including decreased renal perfusion (dehydration, shock), renal failure, pain and opiate analgesia. Urine output should be monitored (Fig. 20.17a) in patients presented in severe shock and can be a good guide to successful fluid resuscitation, animals undergoing spinal surgery or trauma patients who may not be able to empty their bladder voluntarily, and in patients with marked renal failure. Urine specific gravity should be serially measured in patients undergoing fluid therapy to monitor the degree of concentration of the urine; as the patient becomes rehydrated the urine should become less concentrated. In many intensive care patients the daily fluid intake can be matched to the urine output and other known losses. Urine output can be measured by catching urine produced, by cystocentesis or by urinary catheterisation. Daily cathe-

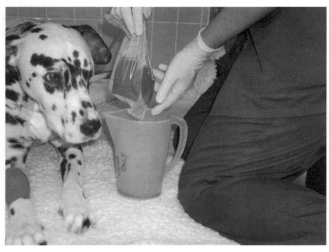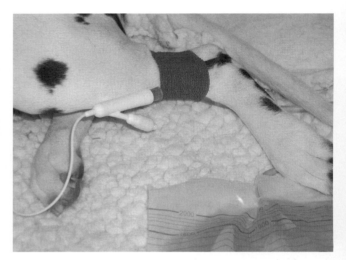

Fig. 20.17 (a) Monitoring urine output includes measuring volume per kg per hour and specific gravity. (b) Urinary catheter taped to hindlimb to prevent any further trauma to the urethra from excessive pulling.

terisation of the bladder can be performed as long as it is well tolerated and performed in an atraumatic and aseptic manner (Fig. 20.17b).

INDICATIONS FOR INDWELLING URINARY CATHETERS
- Monitor urine output, e.g. acute renal failure, critically ill patients.
- Recumbent patients where there is a risk of urine scald.
- Repeated catheterisation is not tolerated.
- Difficulty expressing bladder manually.

Traditionally, urinary catheterisation has been linked with nosocomial infection and urethral trauma; however, if the following points are observed then there is no reason why indwelling catheters should not be used as long as they are not used indiscriminately.

- Catheters are placed aseptically and good nursing care taken in their daily maintenance.
- A closed system is maintained at all times.
- In feline patients atraumatic catheters made from silicone are now available for indwelling use.
- Indwelling catheters should be removed once they are no longer required.
- A urine dipstick should be performed daily to check for developing infection; if this happens then the catheter should be removed.
- The bladder should be palpated daily to make sure that there is no discomfort.
- Blood will be seen in the urine bag during the first 24–48 hours after placement, this is normal and the catheter should not be removed at this time.

MAINTENANCE OF AN INDWELLING CATHETER
- Flush the prepuce or vulva once daily (dilute pevidine solution).
- Ensure a closed system at all times.
- Flush with sterile saline once daily.
- Urine dipstick once daily to check for infection.
- During the first 24–48 hours of placing the catheter, blood will be seen in the urine bag, this should clear within a few hours and is not a reason to remove the catheter.

Neurological system

Monitoring patients with neurological dysfunction can be challenging during high-dependency nursing and the amount of time spent doing so will vary between cases, for example:

- An epileptic being monitored for seizures will only need intravenous catheter care to maintain intravenous access during a seizure and must be in a cage that can be seen by a nurse at all times.
- A patient that has spinal paresis or has undergone surgery will need time-consuming nursing care if recumbent, i.e. physiotherapy, pain monitoring and repeated checks on bladder size and function.
- Patients exhibiting signs consistent with raised intracranial pressure, such as head trauma or brain tumour, will need the following parameters intensively monitored:

    (a) Changes in mentation, especially increased depression or decreased response to stimulus.
    (b) Pupil size (should be equal).
    (c) Pupillary light responses (changes should be noted).
    (d) Respiratory pattern.

(e) Gag reflex and other cranial nerve signs.
(f) Deep pain responses.
(g) Proprioceptive reflexes.

Musculoskeletal system

Attention to the musculoskeletal system is important in recumbent animals. Patients should be encouraged to stand and walk if able to do so and physiotherapy should be implemented unless contraindicated.

Physiotherapy

Physiotherapy is the use of physical and therapeutic techniques to help alleviate pain and suffering, overcome or prevent disabilities and aid in the treatment of muscle, nerve, joint and bone disease. The body has an amazing ability to repair itself, but unfortunately, disease, concurrent problems, poor nutrition, inactivity or inappropriate activity can inhibit or slow the process. Physiotherapy can play a very important role in:

* Improving quality of repair post injury or trauma.
* Improving the well-being and quality of life of the patient whilst function is being returned.
* In some cases, speeding the rate of recovery.

Physiotherapy, by various means, aims to:

* Improve the circulation of the compromised area.
* Transport oxygen and nutrients, to assist the body to repair.
* Maintain and regain flexibility of all parts of the body and full range of movement of all joints.

Conditions suitable for physiotherapy:

(1) Neurological disorders:

* Rehabilitation post spinal surgery.
* Wobbler syndrome (CSM).
* Paresis/paralysis.
* CDRM (canine degenerative reticulomyopathy).
* Peripheral nerve lesions.
* Fibrocartilaginous emboli.

(2) Orthopaedic disorders:

* Hip dysplasia.
* Hip replacements.
* Arthritis.
* Congenital deformities.
* Cruciate ligament injuries.
* Joint, muscle, tendon, ligament sprain or injury.

(3) Wound healing:

* Non-healing wounds.
* Decubitus ulcers.

TIP
Always seek veterinary advice prior to performing any forms of physiotherapy.

The different forms of physiotherapy are summarised in Table 20.2.

Massage   This can be used on the whole body. Massage enhances the circulatory, muscular and nervous systems (Table 20.3). It is relaxing and in most cases helps prevent or relieve stress. Massage is easily applied and easily learnt, although can be time consuming.

MASSAGE TECHNIQUES

* Stroking – used to familiarise yourself with the patient. Gently stroke the patient all over the body in one direction.
* Efflurage – similar to stroking, although more pressure is applied and has more of an effect on musculature and the circulation. Firm long strokes are used in one direction, preferably towards the heart. This helps promote venous return.
* Petrissage – used on the muscular areas of the patient (Fig. 20.18). Using hands and fingers, gently squeeze and knead the muscles. A knowledge of the muscular system is required. Begin at the distal limb, working proximally through the muscle groups. This warm up period is used prior to passive joint movements. It helps break down adhesions and areas of muscle tension and spasm. Work across the muscle fibres. Petrissage can also be used on other muscle groups and not just on the appendages. Do not forget about the muscles around the spine, neck and ribs.

Remember: Begin gently and increase pressure slowly.

Table 20.2 The forms of physiotherapy	
Physical therapy	Massage
	Passive joint movement
	Active exercise
	Hydrotherapy
	Coupage
Electrotherapy	Ultrasound
	Laser
	Muscle stimulation
	TENS
Others	Contrast bathing
	Application of heat
	Application of cold

Table 20.3 Indications and contraindications of massage	
Indications	**Contraindications**
To increase circulation of body fluids, facilitating the transport of nutrients and oxygen to tissues and waste products away from tissues	Shock and dehydration
To enhance muscle tone and relieve spasm	Hyperthermia
To maintain strength and flexibility of the muscular system	Acute trauma, sprain or painful condition
To reduce oedema	Malignancy
To improve the emotional bond with patient	Inflammation

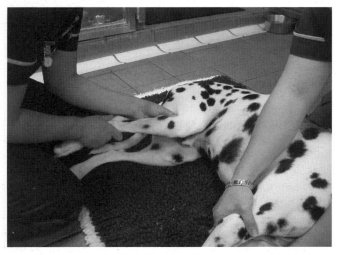

Fig. 20.18 Petrissage.

Passive joint movement (PJM)
This involves movement of the patient's limbs and joints to:

- Help maintain flexibility and good range of movement in joints.
- Improve muscle tone and strength.
- Help improve or eliminate stiffness.

Passive joint movement may be beneficial for many patients, but particularly in patients where movement is severely compromised.

TECHNIQUE FOR PERFORMING PASSIVE JOINT MOVEMENT (FIG. 20.19)
(1) Ensure the patient is comfortable. Lateral recumbency is preferred.
(2) Support the limb (sandbags and bedding may be used).
(3) Begin at the distal limb and move each joint through its range of movement. This is done slowly and is performed by flexing and extending the joint. Initially the joint is moved through mid-range of movement and progressively to full range of movement, depending on the patient and its condition.

---

(4) Support above and below the joint.
(5) The joints above and below the joint you are working on must be supported and no excessive force should be used. Work progressing proximally and then move the limb as a whole. Ensure the limb is supported.
(6) The patient can then be turned for work on the opposite side.
(7) Finish with efflurage.

Remember:
- Muscles need to be prepared and warm prior to PJM.
- Your patient needs to be relaxed and comfortable before you begin.
- Select a suitable environment: quiet, peaceful and no draughts.
- Consider your mood, temperament and time!
- If patient seems uncomfortable or in pain, stop and seek veterinary advice.

Assisted active exercise
This can be used in several ways.

- If the patient is small enough, one person can assist the patient to stand.
- For larger patients, two or even three people are sometimes needed. Simply supporting the patient's weight with your arms and hands does this.
- Towels may be used as a sling, crossed under the chest or supporting the abdomen. Purpose-built slings (Fig. 20.20), mechanical hoists (Fig. 20.21) and carts may also be used.

TECHNIQUES FOR ASSISTED ACTIVE EXERCISE
Once you have assisted the patient to get up and stand, aided or unaided, encourage the patient to walk or take a few steps. Stimulating the patient in several ways can do this:
- Simply take the patient outside for fresh air, to sniff around on the grass.
- Use the patient's favourite food.
- Other patients in runs next to where the patient is.

Help the patient bear weight on affected limb(s). This can be performed as follows:
(1) Lift the unaffected limb so the patient has to bear weight on the affected limb.
(2) Support the fore or hindquarters with both hands and gently rock the patient from side to side, back and forth. This can aid in improving muscle tone and strength, and help the coordination and balance of the patient.

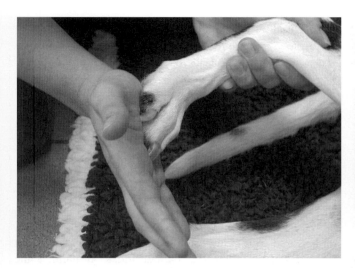

Fig. 20.19 Passive joint movements of the distal phalanges.

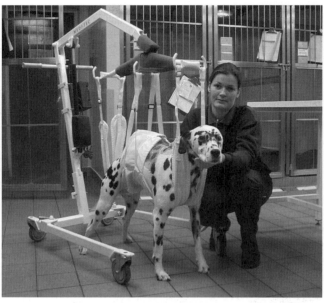

Fig. 20.21 Use of mechanical hoist to support a paraplegic patient.

Hydrotherapy (Fig. 20.22) Swimming is an excellent all-round exercise that allows the patient to use its limbs in a non-weight-bearing environment. This can encourage the use of full range of movement of joints and help build up muscle around areas, which are normally painful in the weight-bearing position. It is also good for cardiovascular fitness, but one should ensure the patient is fit enough to cope with the swimming.

Coupage This is the percussion of the thorax with cupped hands and loose wrists. This aids in the loosening and expulsion of secretions. In a recumbent patient that is unable to move or change position, coupage may be beneficial. Pooling of secretions may occur on one side of the patient's chest if it is allowed to stay in one position for too long. (For further reading see Chapter 17.) Nebulisation may be used in conjunction with coupage to aid the removal of bronchial secretions. This is useful in patients with pulmonary disease.

Electrotherapy There are three types:

- Ultrasound – high-frequency sound waves are used to treat muscle, tendon and soft tissue injury.
- Laser treatment – may be used to increase tissue healing, reduce pain and inflammation. It is also used for the healing of open wounds.

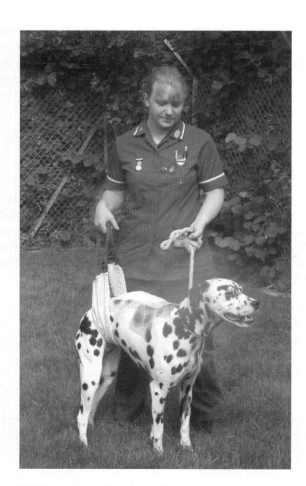

Fig. 20.20 Assisted exercise using a sling.

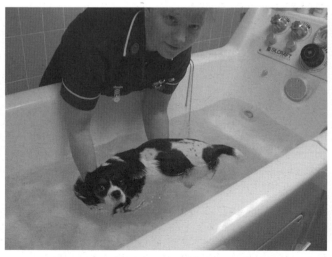

Fig. 20.22 Hydrotherapy used as part of a rehabilitation programme post spinal surgery.

- Muscle stimulation – the use of electrical pulses to produce muscle contraction. It is useful for patients where exercise is restricted, can aid in strengthening the muscles and aid in the recovery of peripheral nerve lesions.

Transcutaneous electrical nerve stimulation (TENS)　The TENS machine helps to achieve pain relief by use of a low-intensity stimulation of sensory nerve endings underneath the skin.

Other therapies　The application of **heat** can help relieve muscle tension and spasms, reduce oedema and help relieve pain. Using the following can do this:

- Hot-water bottles.
- Heated intravenous fluids.
- Warm water in disposable gloves.
- Heat pads.
- Microwavable pads.

> *TIP*
> Use a small towel to wrap around the application.

The application of **cold** can aid in reducing oedema, bruising and also help relieve pain. Using the following can do this:

- Intravenous fluids that have been kept in the refrigerator.
- A bag of frozen vegetables.
- Cold running water.

> Take care not to apply direct heat or cold onto the patient!

Contrast bathing is the application of heat and cold together. This promotes good circulation. Use heat initially, then cold. Alternate every 2–3 min. This can be used 48 hours post injury.

Pain management in high-dependence nursing

One critical area of high-dependency nursing is the recognition and basic management of pain. Patients may be in pain for a variety of reasons such as post-operative pain, trauma, pancreatitis, etc. It is important to recognise pain and provide analgesia. Inadequate analgesia in intensive care can result in the following:

- Psychological stress, depression and sometimes aggression.
- Insomnia.
- Poor nutritional intake.
- Prolonged recumbency.

- Increased stress response to the illness.
- Cardiovascular and respiratory compromise (tachycardia, vasoconstriction, tachypnoea, hypoventilation).

Inadequate analgesia can lead to slower recoveries for the patients as well as presenting a welfare problem.

Managing pain

Pain can be assessed by looking at behavioural responses of the patient in conjunction with physiological changes. There will be similarities in pain perception between humans and animals and so it is important to treat for anticipated pain regardless of whether the patient looks in pain. Some patients may look comfortable but display signs of pain when handled and so it is vital to have contact with the patient and to gently palpate around any wounds to ensure that the animal is comfortable. If in doubt as to whether a patient is in pain, analgesia should be provided regardless and the patient's response assessed.

Non-pharmacological analgesia

As well as providing the patient with analgesic drugs, it is important to ensure that the patient is comfortable by providing adequate bedding, comfortable ambient temperature and peace and quiet. A distended bladder will also cause great discomfort to a patient, so urinary output and bladder size should be checked. Adjunctive therapy such as acupuncture and physiotherapy may also be utilised for a variety of conditions.

Analgesic agents

More information can be found on analgesic agents in Chapter 23, Anaesthesia and Analgesia. Ideally a multimodal approach to analgesia should be used, combining opiates for severe or acute pain, NSAIDs to control inflammation and more long-term pain and local techniques where applicable:

- Opiates (pure and partial agonists).
- NSAIDs.
- Local anaesthetics.
- Alpha-2-agonists.
- Ketamine.

> It is important to remember that some of the drugs mentioned in this section are not licensed for veterinary use.

Opiates

Opiates tend to be reserved for acute or moderate to severe pain. They are often used in the first 24–48 hours after an operation or trauma. At clinical dose rates, opiates can be used safely in the majority of circumstances. Pure agonists (morphine, methadone, and pethidine) can be titrated to effect and if an overdose occurs then their actions can be reversed using naloxone. The duration of action of opiates may vary between patients and can depend on the initial dose used. In general if a patient appears sedated a repeat dose should not be administered. Table 20.4 summarises some of the types of opiate available in veterinary patients.

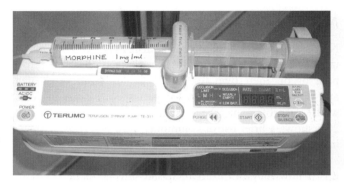

Fig. 20.23 Morphine diluted 1:10 administered continuously via syringe driver.

Continuous analgesia Dosing every few hours can lead to peaks and troughs in plasma concentrations of analgesic agents and so some drugs such as morphine can be used as continuous intravenous infusions and the infusion rate adjusted according to the patient (Fig. 20.23).

Transdermal fentanyl patches are increasingly used in veterinary practice and are especially effective in cats in severe pain, since they minimise the number of injections and therefore the amount of handling required. They consist of a permeable membrane that allows the slow release of fentanyl, which is absorbed across the skin (Fig. 20.24). The skin should be clipped and cleaned with water prior to application and the patch placed in an area that the animal cannot reach (on the back of the neck in dogs or lateral thorax in cats). The dose used is 2.5–5 µg/kg/hr. It can take up to 8 hours to reach therapeutic plasma levels; however, the patches will provide analgesia for up to 3 days. Patients should not be placed on heated pads as this can increase the rate of absorption and may lead to overdose.

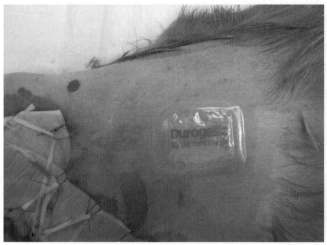

Fig. 20.24 Providing analgesia by use of a fentanyl patch.

Table 20.4 Examples of opiate analgesia used in intensive care cases

Drug	Dose rate and route	Dosing interval	Adverse effects
Morphine	Dogs: 0.1–1 mg/kg SC, IM, slow IV Cats: 0.1–0.5 mg/kg SC, IM, slow IV (IV infusion 0.1–0.3 mg/kg/hr)	1–4 hours	Sedation Vomiting (therefore do not use in patients with suspected raised intraocular or intracranial pressure)
Methadone	0.1–0.5 mg/kg SC, IM	2–5 hours	No vomiting
Pethidine	3–10 mg/kg IM, SC	1–2 hours	Can be painful on injection **Should not be administered IV**
Buprenorphine	0.006–0.2 mg/kg IM, SC	6–8 hours	Slow onset of action Partial agonist
Butorphanol	Dogs: 0.1–0.4 mg/kg IM, SC Cats: 0.4–0.8 mg/kg IM, SC	1–2 hours 2–4 hours	Poor analgesia Partial agonist
Fentanyl	1–5 µg/kg IV	30 min	Potent analgesia Can cause severe respiratory depression and bradycardia Normally used intraoperatively Can be given by infusion
Fentanyl patches	2.5–5 µg/kg/hr transdermal	3 days	See 'Continuous Analgesia'

SC = subcutaneous; IM = intramuscular; IV = intravenous

NSAIDs

Non-steroidal anti-inflammatory drugs (NSAIDs) may be used as an adjunct to opiates for acute or post-operative pain or on their own for mild, chronic pain. Carprofen and meloxicam are licensed for peri-operative use in dogs, whilst carprofen may be used for cats and exotics. Table 20.5 shows a brief list of commonly used NSAIDs in veterinary patients.

NSAIDs act by inhibition of prostaglandin synthesis and this is how they can exert their side-effects, namely gastrointestinal ulceration and renal failure in the face of hypotension. Carprofen is a very weak prostaglandin inhibitor and should therefore be associated with fewer side-effects.

Alpha-2-agonists

Alpha-2-agonists can provide good short-term sedation and analgesia, even at low doses, and can potentially be employed to provide analgesia in some cases.

Ketamine

Ketamine has been used to provide analgesia in subanaesthetic doses, although there is still the risk of encountering side-effects such as muscle tremors. The authors normally reserves this drug for severe breakthrough pain.

Local anaesthetics

Using a local technique directly blocks transmission of pain signals in the sensory nerve fibres. This is an ideal way of providing analgesia since it prevents the pain signals from entering the spinal cord which can initiate a wind-up process in the CNS and make adequate provision of analgesia more difficult. Lidocaine is a short-acting local anaesthetic agent which is sometimes used and can be combined with adrenaline to prolong its duration of action; however, bupivicaine has a much longer duration of action (6–8 hours) and is the drug of choice in pain management. Examples of local anaesthetic techniques used in high-dependency nursing include intercostal nerve blockade and intrapleural anal-gesia following thoracotomies or thoracic trauma and epidural analgesia, which will be discussed in more detail.

Intercostal nerve block　Local anaesthetic is injected around two intercostal nerves cranial and two caudal to a lateral thoracic wall incision, maximum 2 mg/kg 0.5% bupivicaine, approximately 0.5 ml/nerve.

Intrapleural infiltration　This technique can be employed when there is a chest drain in place and is used for post-thoracotomy pain and following trauma. The local anaesthetic diffuses to the intercostal nerves. 1.5–2 mg/kg diluted to 1 ml/kg is administered via the chest drain every 6 hours.

Epidural analgesia　Lumbosacral epidural anaesthesia is an easy and effective technique for providing pain relief distal to the umbilicus in dogs. Indications include abdominal surgery, straining, and hindlimb analgesia. Since the spinal cord normally terminates at L6, there is little risk of entering the subarachnoid space. In cats the cord finishes slightly more caudally and so care should be taken when placing lumbosacral epidurals. The technique is quite simple once experienced and the patient is normally sedated or anaesthetised.

Contraindications to placement of epidurals:

- Skin disease.
- Bleeding disorders.
- Neurological disease.
- Bacteraemia.
- Anatomical abnormalities.

Drugs used in epidural anaesthesia include local anaesthetics, opiates and less commonly alpha-2-agonists.

- Local anaesthetics – these drugs cause sensory blockade followed by motor blockade at higher doses. Bupivicaine can be used on its own to produce analgesia for approximately 6 hours. The volume of agent injected governs the spread of the block cranially. If the blockade spreads too far cranially, the respiratory musculature could become paralysed. Vasodilation in the area of analgesia is caused by blockade of sympathetic innervation to blood vessels could potentially result in hypotension and so patients should be placed on intravenous fluid therapy.

Table 20.5 Commonly used NSAIDs			
Drug	**Dose**	**Dosing interval**	**Adverse actions**
Carprofen	4 mg/kg SC cats 4 mg/kg SC, IV, PO dogs	Repeat injection after 24 hours 24 hours then 2 mg/kg PO twice daily	Gastrointestinal irritation
Meloxicam	0.2 mg/kg SC in dogs followed by 0.1 mg/kg PO once daily	24 hours	Gastrointestinal irritation
Ketoprofen	2 mg/kg SC dogs and cats then 1 mg/kg PO once daily	24 hours then 1 mg/kg once a day	Gastrointestinal irritation avoid in hypotension Can be used for 5 days

SC = subcutaneous; IV = intravenous; PO = per os

Fluid therapy in high-dependence nursing

TECHNIQUE FOR PLACEMENT OF EPIDURAL INJECTION

- Restrain dog in lateral recumbency or in sternal recumbency with the hindlimbs pulled forward.
- Clip and prepare the skin, wear sterile gloves and use a sterile drape.
- Palpate the iliac prominences and draw a line between them. In the midline the dorsal spinous process of L7 should be palpated in this region. Moving caudally the lumbosacral space can be felt followed by the sacrum.
- Once happy with the position of the lumbosacral space, a spinal needle can be introduced in the midline perpendicular to the skin.
- The needle should be advanced until a popping sensation is detected as the needle passes through the interarcuate ligament.
- The stylet is then removed and the needle aspirated to check for the presence of CSF or blood.
- The presence of the needle in the epidural space is verified by testing for loss of resistance. Either a small amount of air or saline is injected, if resistance is detected then the needle should be repositioned and tested again.
- The drugs may then be injected slowly and the needle removed.

A typical dose used for abdominal and hindlimb analgesia is bupivicaine 1 ml/5 kg 0.5% solution up to a maximum of 6 ml/dog.

More commonly, local anaesthetics are combined with morphine, enabling a lower dose of bupivicaine to be used resulting in less motor blockade and providing prolonged analgesia.

- Opiates – preservative-free morphine may also be injected into the epidural space either alone or in combination with bupivicaine at a dose of 0.1 mg/kg. Morphine will produce prolonged analgesia (up to 24 hours) with no motor blockade.
- Alpha-2-agents – these are commonly used in the epidural space in large animal patients to provide profound and prolonged analgesia. Medetomidine has been used in small animal patients; however, systemic absorption leads to sedation and cardiopulmonary effects.

Epidural catheters Placement of a silicone catheter into the epidural space via lumbosacral puncture can be utilised in veterinary patients to provide long-term analgesia. Placement of the catheter in the epidural space can be verified radiologically and the catheter advanced cranially depending on the level that analgesia is required. The catheter must be securely positioned and maintained in a sterile fashion to minimise the risk of infection. A bacterial filter is also fitted to the injection port of the catheter.

Fluid therapy in high-dependence nursing

Fluid therapy is a vital part of high-dependency nursing. Nurses should have a basic understanding of the physiology involved, administration of fluid therapy and how to monitor a patient's response. The following section will give an overview of general fluid therapy in the intensive care setting; for more information the reader is referred to Chapter 22 on fluid therapy.

Physiology of fluids

Total body water makes up approximately 60% of the bodyweight in healthy patients. This fluid is distributed throughout the body in various compartments as described in Chapter 22. Fluid distribution between these areas is affected by a variety of homeostatic mechanisms including sodium concentrations and protein concentrations in different areas of the body. It is important to understand how changes in these levels can affect distribution, and the goal of fluid therapy is to maintain homeostasis.

Total circulating blood volume

Intravascular fluid within the blood vessels makes up 5% of bodyweight; when red cell volume is added to this it represents total circulating blood volume which is approximately 8–10% bodyweight (50–55 ml/kg in cats and 80–90 ml/kg in dogs).

TOTAL CIRCULATING BLOOD VOLUME
Cats: 50–55 ml/kg
Dogs: 80–90 ml/kg

Assessment of fluid requirements

Fluid therapy should be directed at the requirements specific to each individual patient such as volume deficits and electrolyte imbalances. The calculation of fluid deficits is covered in Chapter 22 and working out a fluid therapy plan should include the following:

(1) Correcting fluid deficit:

- Determine fluid loss.
- Usually replace with a fluid solution that is similar in composition to that lost, usually isotonic (Fig. 20.25).
- Goal is to increase intravascular fluid content initially.

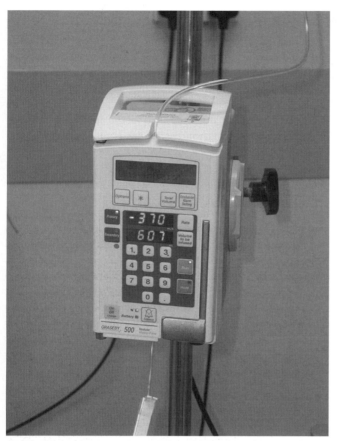

Fig. 20.25 Fluid pumps and syringe drivers deliver accurate volumes of fluids or drugs to the patient.

(2)   Maintenance requirements:

  • Maintenance requirements describes the fluids lost through normal physiological processes, i.e. respiratory tract, urinary tract and gastrointestinal tract.
  • In the normal patient, maintenance is approximately 2 ml/kg/hr or 50 ml/kg/day.
  • Remember if a patient is panting, pyrexic or is polyuric due to the disease or drug therapy, this should be taken into consideration.
  • Maintenance losses are normally hypotonic and so a relatively hypotonic solution should be used.
  • If a patient is not eating then potassium should be added to the maintenance fluid at 20 mEq/l (see section on potassium supplementation).

(3)   Ongoing losses:

  • Daily losses associated with the disease process are included here such as vomiting, diarrhoea, pleural effusions.

NURSING
In the critical care setting keep a record of the daily outputs of the patient (urinary, vomiting, etc.) so that fluid therapy can be matched to cover these losses.

Types of intravenous fluids

Crystalloids

A crystalloid is a fluid containing solutes such as ions or glucose and are described in greater detail elsewhere. They are generally used as replacement and maintenance fluids. The ion concentrations govern the distribution of the fluid once it is in the body. Crystalloids can be classed according to their ion concentrations relative to plasma:

  • Hypertonic.
  • Isotonic.
  • Hypotonic.

Potassium supplementation
Serum potassium may be decreased in a variety of conditions requiring intensive nursing. Hypokalaemia results in muscle weakness, ileus, and arrhythmias. Hypokalaemia should be suspected if the patient has poor nutritional intake is dehydrated or has ongoing abnormal losses (e.g. diarrhoea) and the extent of the hypokalaemia estimated according to the duration of the problem. Potassium can be easily measured using electrolyte machines and this facility should be available in any intensive care unit. Potassium may be added to the crystalloid under veterinary supervision using Table 20.6 as a guide, and the bag must be clearly labelled.

Potassium should not be administered faster than 0.5 mEq/kg/hr due to potential cardiac effects.

Mild hypokalaemia should correct itself if the patient is eating and drinking adequately, although potassium may also be supplemented orally.

Colloids

The word colloid refers to a high-molecular-weight substance, the molecules of which are too large to pass through normal capillary walls; therefore the substance remains in the intravascular space. The molecules' size and positive charge attracts water to them, holding it in the intravascular space. Albumin normally performs this role in the blood; however, in certain disease states protein levels can fall, e.g. liver disease, protein losing enteropathies or due to dilution with excessive crystalloid administration.

INDICATIONS FOR SYNTHETIC COLLOID ADMINISTRATION
  • Haemorrhage.
  • Intravascular space resuscitation.
  • Total protein < 3.5 g/dl.
  • Albumin < 2 g/dl.
If albumin falls below 1 g/dl then plasma should be administered instead of synthetic colloids.

Table 20.6 Guidelines for potassium supplementation to intravenous fluids

Estimated potassium level	Actual potassium measurements (mEq/l)	Guideline for potassium chloride (KCl) mEq added to 500 ml NaCl 0.9%
Increased	>5.5	0
Normal	3.5–5.5	5
Mild decrease	3.0–3.5	15
Moderate decrease	2.5–3.0	20
Severe decrease	2.0–2.5	30
	<2.0	40

Blood and blood products

> **INDICATIONS FOR USE OF BLOOD PRODUCTS (FIG. 20.26)**
> - PCV <20%, Hb <8 g/dl.
> - Severe haemorrhage (>30% total circulating blood volume in healthy patient).
> - Anaemia associated with thrombocytopaenia.
> - Anaemia associated with coagulopathies.
> - Disseminated intravascular coagulation (DIC).

For further information on transfusion medicine see Chapter 22; however, an important aspect of high-dependency nursing concerns the monitoring of patients during blood administration to detect transfusion reactions. Ideally pre-emptive measures should be taken to minimise the risk of a transfusion reaction:

- Crossmatching.
- Administration of an antihistamine, such as chlorpheniramine 0.4 mg/kg IV, SC, prior to administration.
- Start the infusion slowly 1–2 ml/kg/hr and check for evidence of reaction before increasing the infusion rate.
- Monitor the patient regularly, especially in the initial period of the transfusion.
- Electrolyte abnormalities may occur following large transfusions, particularly hypocalcaemia. Cardiac arrhythmias may also be seen in these cases and ECG monitoring may be useful.

> **MONITORING DURING TRANSFUSION**
> - Rectal temperature.
> - Respiratory rate.
> - Pulse rate +/− blood pressure.
> - Urticaria, pruritis.
> - Vomiting.
> - Also monitor signs of blood volume overload.

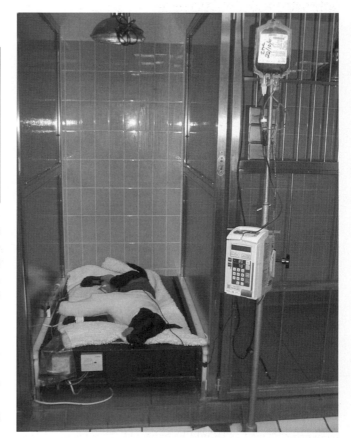

Fig. 20.26 Patient receiving whole blood due to severe haemorrhage at surgery.

Oxygen-carrying fluids

Oxyglobin® is an ultrapurified polymerised haemoglobin solution of bovine origin, which is available on the veterinary market. Oxyglobin is a volume expander (a synthetic colloid) and provides extra oxygen-carrying capacity as it circulates in the plasma and can be used as an alternative to whole blood. It is indicated in anaemia, haemolytic anaemia, haemorrhage caused by trauma and surgery. The small molecular size of Oxyglobin means that is extremely effective in improving oxygen delivery to tissues but it also means that it is eliminated from the body quickly (12 hours). It can interfere with some laboratory tests, particularly PCV, after transfusion and so haemoglobin should be measured. Remember that Oxyglobin® contains no clotting factors and so there is a risk of coagulopathies with large infusions.

The recommended infusion rates for oxyglobin are 3–10 ml/kg/hr in dogs with a total amount of 30 ml/kg and 3–5 ml/kg/hr in cats. Again the patients should be monitored for transfusion reactions and for signs of circulatory volume overload.

Monitoring response to fluid therapy

Monitoring the patient's response to fluid therapy is discussed in Chapter 22. In high-dependency nursing it is important to recognise and record this response using the following as a guide:

- Improved mental status of the patient.
- Decreased heart rate and increased pulse quality and blood pressure.
- Improved mucous membrane colour and capillary refill time.
- Increased central venous pressure (CVP) if monitored.
- Increased urine production.
- Decreasing urine specific gravity.
- Decreasing measured values such as PCV and urea.

Nutrition in high-dependency nursing

Importance of nutrition

If a critically ill patient is deprived of protein-rich nutrition, then the patient will enter a state of negative energy balance. A patient in ICU will therefore develop complications of acute malnutrition, such as impaired immune responses, poor wound healing, muscle weakness and organ failure much faster than in any normal patient. Any critically ill patient that has not eaten for 3 days is an indication for nutritional support, along with any patient that is not recovering as well as should be expected. There is no clinical test to determine nutritional status and so it is important in high dependency nursing to provide optimum nutritional support. Refer to Chapter 16 on general nursing for more information on nutrition in the critically ill patient.

ENTERAL VERSUS TOTAL PARENTERAL NUTRITION (TPN)
Enteral nutrition uses the gastrointestinal tract for administration of nutrition, whereas TPN bypasses the guts and nutrition is provided intravenously. Enteral nutrition should be used whenever the intestinal tract is functional since it preserves normal gut function and flora as well as being cheaper and less hazardous than parenteral nutrition.

Total parenteral nutrition (TPN)

- Parenteral nutrition is only indicated when the gut is not working mechanically or it is not able to digest the food presented to it. Ideally nasogastric, oesophagostomy or gastrotomy tubes should be used if at all possible (Figs 20.27, 20.28). Table 20.7 lists the complications arising from enteral feeding and what nursing action should be taken.
- Parenteral nutrition is expensive and associated with much higher risk compared to enteral nutrition.
- It is administered into a large vein (jugular) to prevent thrombophlebitis.
- The catheter should only be used for nutrition. If a multiple-lumen catheter is available, one lumen should be the dedicated nutrition line.
- Risk of sepsis is minimised with proper nursing care of the intravenous catheter.
- Commercial solutions are available.

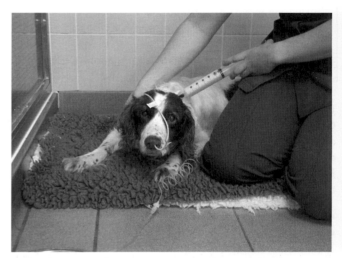

Fig. 20.27 Nasogastric tubes and gastrotomy tubes are well tolerated in dogs.

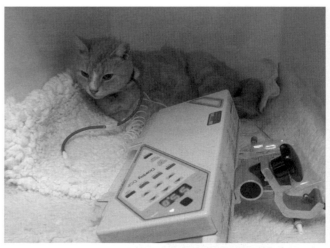

Fig. 20.28 Oesophagostomy tubes are extremely well tolerated in cats for long periods of time.

Table 20.7 Complications of enteral feeding	
Complication	**Treatment**
Vomiting	Stop feeding for 2 hours then feed slower with smaller volumes
Diarrhoea	Use correct food product
Tube ejection	Remove and replace
Blockage	Flush before and after each feed Do not crush tablets up and administer via tube
Infection	Wound management

ASSESSMENT OF NUTRITION
- Return to normal attitude and appetite.
- Improved recovery rates.
- Wounds heal quickly.

Table 20.8 Complications in the recumbent patient	
Possible complications	**Prevention/treatment**
Infection	Aseptic catheter, drain and wound management Antibiotics when necessary
Decubitus ulcers	Padded bedding Frequent turning
Scalding/soiling	Absorbent bedding Clip and clean coat Barrier creams
Lung atelectasis	Frequent turning
Hypostatic pneumonia	Frequent turning Nebulisation and coupage Maintenance sternal where possible
Myopathy/neuropathy	Soft, padded bedding Frequent turning Physiotherapy
Muscle atrophy	Physiotherapy HBV protein diet
Aspiration pneumonia	Nebulisation and coupage Postural drainage Feed in upright position (orally or via tubes) Antibiotics

Recumbency in high-dependence nursing

Many of the patients requiring high-dependency nursing involve managing the recumbent patient. The patient may be recumbent for many different reasons. The nursing involvement and management of these cases are discussed in Chapter 16. There are many points to consider when caring for a recumbent patient. These patients may already have a severe disease or have undergone major surgery, so complications need to be anticipated and prevented where possible. A summary of complications is shown in Table 20.8.

Attention needs to be directed towards not only the physical complications but to the mental state of the patient. The patient may be scared, frustrated and may not understand why it cannot get up and walk. These patients require a lot of nursing time and encouragement. They need to be stimulated several times during the 24 hour period. Even if they cannot walk, this does not mean they cannot be taken outside. Simply taking them outside for a sniff about and some fresh air 3–4 times per day can prevent them becoming apathetic and lazy.

STIMULATION OF THE RECUMBENT PATIENT
- Kennel the patient near activity and do not isolate the patient.
- Take outside at least 3 times a day. Encourage them to bear weight and place their feet for them. Once strong enough, some patients can be left in a mechanical hoist for a small part of the day.
- Feed small meals frequently. May need to hand feed if cannot reach food/water on own.
- Give them toys to play with if allowed.
- Physiotherapy is often indicated in recumbency. May help to form a bond with patient.
- Most patients enjoy swimming.
- *STIMULATION, TLC and TIME!*

KEY POINTS
- High-dependency nursing requires highly trained staff that can dedicate time to individual patients.
- The nursing team should work closely with the veterinary surgeon involved, along with the owners, to provide optimal patient care.
- The correct management of indwelling catheters and drains will help to minimise the risk of nosocomial infections in intensive care.
- A thorough working knowledge of monitoring equipment used for critically ill patients is necessary, along with the knowledge required to interpret and act on results obtained.
- Nurses need to be able to recognise and treat pain in all patients and minimise psychological stress during hospitalisation.
- The veterinary nurse must be aware of fluid and nutritional requirements of all in-patients.

21

Theatre practice

D. McHugh

Learning objectives

After studying this chapter, students should be able to:

- Explain the principles of surgical asepsis.
- Describe the role of the veterinary nurse in the establishment and maintenance of asepsis in the operating theatre.
- Describe the different methods of sterilisation available and discuss their suitability and use for a range of surgical instruments and equipment used in veterinary surgery.
- Describe the care and maintenance of surgical instruments/packs and equipment.
- Recognise a range of surgical instruments used in all types of veterinary surgery.
- Describe the preparation of a patient for surgery, intra-operative and immediate post-operative care of a patient.
- Explain the role of a veterinary nurse in the operating theatre as both a scrubbed and circulating nurse.
- Describe the ideal properties of suture materials and discuss the advantages and disadvantages of different types.
- Recognise different suture patterns commonly used in veterinary surgery.

The veterinary nurse is usually given the responsibility for running the operating theatre. This involves maintenance of hygiene in the theatre; care and maintenance of instruments and equipment, preparation of theatre, the patient and the surgical team, and assistance as both scrubbed and circulating nurse.

DEFINITIONS

Sepsis – the presence of pathogens or their toxic products in the blood or tissues of the patient. More commonly known as **infection**.

Asepsis – freedom from infection, i.e. exclusion of micro-organisms and spores.

Antisepsis – prevention of sepsis by destruction or inhibition of micro-organisms using an agent that may be safely applied to living tissue.

Sterilisation – the destruction of all micro-organisms and spores.

Disinfection – the removal of micro-organisms but not necessarily spores.

Disinfectant – an agent that destroys micro-organisms, generally chemical agents applied to inanimate objects.

The most important factor in successful theatre practice is the establishment and maintenance of a good **aseptic technique**, i.e. all the steps taken to prevent contact with micro-organisms.

Factors influencing the development of infection

Infection of a clean surgical wound is always a matter of great concern. Obviously it is far better to prevent infection than to try and treat it. The use of antibiotics should not be relied upon to protect patients from the consequences of poor asepsis.

It has been established that most surgical wound infections occur at the time of surgery, not during the post-operative period. Poor aseptic technique will undoubtedly affect the success of any surgery and in the long term the success and reputation of the practice. Strict theatre discipline is essential if high standards are to be maintained. There has to be a specific protocol that is adhered to rigidly and that everyone involved with surgery respects. This will include correct theatre attire, scrubbing-up procedures, patient preparations, draping techniques, sterilisation, organisation of surgical lists, cleaning protocol and conduct during surgery.

Sources of contamination in the operating theatre include:

- Operating room.
- Equipment.
- Personnel.
- Patient.

Operating room and environment

Many micro-organisms are airborne and any movement within the operating theatre will disperse them. Good ventilation is necessary as hot, humid conditions are a great threat to asepsis. Cleaning procedures should be performed first because micro-organisms from contaminated sites will remain in the air. The operating room itself must be easily cleaned and should contain as little furniture and shelving as possible.

Equipment and instruments

All equipment and instruments used in the operative site must be sterile. There must be a new set of instruments for each operation.

Personnel

The more people present in theatre, the greater the likelihood of infection. All theatre personnel should wear theatre clothing, caps, masks, scrub suits and antistatic footwear. These are only worn in the designated theatre area. In addition, those who are in the surgical team should prepare their hands aseptically and wear sterile gowns and gloves.

The patient

The patient is probably the greatest source of contamination, especially as animals are covered in hair. The source of micro-organisms may be endogenous or exogenous.

> **Endogenous** – those that originate from within the body of the patient.
> **Exogenous** – those that are found on the outside, i.e. the skin and coat. This term is also used with reference to environmental sources of micro-organisms (e.g. air, equipment, etc.).

It does not necessarily follow that introduction of micro-organisms will result in an infected wound. Micro-organisms can and will enter any wound that has been exposed to air but whether infection follows depends on several variable factors, including the balance between the **virulence** (disease-producing ability) of the organism and the **resistance of the patient**. Other factors that influence wound infection include:

- **Duration of surgery** – bacterial contamination increases the longer the wound is open. Infection rate doubles for every hour of operative time.
- **Surgical technique** – excessive trauma to tissues and damage to vascular supply may increase the likelihood of infection.
- **Impaired host resistance** – this may increase the risk of infection if it is due to drugs, nutrition or underlying disease.
- **Contamination of the wound** – surgical wounds are classified with respect to their potential for contamination and infection.

> *CLASSIFICATION OF SURGICAL WOUNDS*
> **Clean** – where there is no break in asepsis. The respiratory, gastrointestinal and urinary tracts are not entered and there is no break in aseptic technique.
> **Clean-contaminated** – where a contaminated area is entered but without spillage or spread of contamination (i.e. ingesta, urine, mucus). Minor break in asepsis.
> **Contaminated** – where there is spillage from a viscus or severe inflammation is encountered, but no infection present. Open fresh traumatic wounds.
> **Dirty** – infected where there is pus present or viscus perforation spilling pus. Traumatic wound containing devitalised tissue or foreign bodies.

Sterilisation

Sterilisation can be divided into two types (Table 21.1).

Heat sterilisation

Steam under pressure (autoclave systems)

Steam under pressure is the most widely used and efficient method of sterilisation. It is also the most economical, although the initial outlay may be large. Items which may be sterilised in the autoclave include:

- Instruments.
- Drapes.
- Gowns.
- Swabs.
- Most rubber articles.
- Glassware.
- Some plastic goods.

Heat-sensitive items which may be damaged in the autoclave include fibre-optic equipment, lenses and plastics (especially those designed to be disposable, such as catheters).

The three main types of autoclave are the vertical pressure cooker, the horizontal or vertical downward displacement autoclave and the vacuum-assisted autoclave.

Vertical pressure cooker This is a very simple machine which operates by boiling water in a closed container like a household pressure cooker. It usually has an air vent at the top which is closed once the air has been evacuated, and pressure (15 p.s.i.) is allowed to build up. As the air vent is at the top, the main disadvantage of this type of autoclave is the danger that some air will be trapped underneath the steam. The temperature in this area will be lower and sterility cannot be guaranteed. It is also manually operated and there is room for human error in the sterilising cycle.

Table 21.1 Heat and cold sterilisation	
Heat sterilisation	Autoclave (steam under pressure)
	vertical
	horizontal
	vacuum-assisted
	Dry heat
	hot-air oven
	high-vacuum oven
	convection oven
Cold sterilisation	Ethylene oxide
	Commercial solutions:
	commercial
	alcohol based
	Gamma irradiation

Horizontal or vertical downward displacement autoclave This type is larger and usually fully automatic. It uses an electrically operated boiler that is incorporated in the autoclave as a source of steam. Air is driven out more efficiently by downward displacement. There is an air outlet at the bottom and a steam outlet at the top.

Most of these machines are designed for loose instrument sterilisation only, rather than packs, as they have insufficient penetrating ability and drying cycles: packs may seem to be dry but they remain damp, allowing entry of micro-organisms during the storage period.

There is usually a choice of programmes on this type of autoclave with temperatures of 112, 121, 126 or 134°C.

Vacuum-assisted autoclave (porous load) This type of autoclave works on the same principle as the other two but uses a high-vacuum pump to evacuate air rapidly from the chamber at the beginning of the cycle. Steam penetration after evacuation is almost instantaneous and sterilisation occurs very quickly. A second vacuum cycle rapidly withdraws moisture after sterilisation and dries the load. It is suitable for all types of instruments, drapes and equipment and there is a choice of cycles using different temperatures and pressures.

Vacuum-assisted autoclaves are fully automatic, with fail-safe mechanisms (usually warning lights and alarms) which indicate whether the load is non-sterile or has been sterilised effectively. They are generally much larger and more sophisticated than other types and are invariably connected to a central boiler to supply steam. The cost of purchase and maintenance are higher, but the machine's efficiency and reliability in sterilisation far outweigh those of the smaller types.

Principles of sterilisation using steam under pressure

Although autoclaves vary in size and type the basic principle of function remains the same. When water boils at 100°C it is converted to steam and the temperature remains the same however long it is heated. Many bacteria, spores and viruses are resistant to heat, and remain unchanged even if exposed to such a temperature for a long time. By increasing the pressure, the temperature of the steam is raised and resistant micro-organisms and spores will be killed by coagulation of cell proteins. It is the increased temperature, not the increased pressure, that leads to this destruction of micro-organisms. The higher the temperature, the shorter the time needed to achieve sterilisation (Table 21.2).

The autoclaving process The central sterilising chamber of the autoclave is surrounded by a steam jacket. The pressure in the jacket is raised (depending on the cycle). Steam then enters the chamber and as it does so air is displaced downwards, because steam is lighter. When all the air is evacuated, exhaust vents are closed and steam continues to enter until the desired pressure is reached.

Table 21.2 Autoclave temperature, pressure and time combinations		
Temperature (°C)	Pressure (p.s.i. [kg/cm^2])	Time (min)
121	15 [1.2]	15
126	20 [1.4]	10
134	30 [2]	$3\frac{1}{2}$

It should be noted that this is only the sterilising time. The length of the whole cycle will vary from 15 to 45 minutes

The more sophisticated types of autoclave have a vacuum prior to introduction of steam to displace air from materials to be sterilised. If any air remains in the chamber the temperature will be lower than steam at that pressure and sterility cannot be guaranteed.

Once the air has been evacuated, steam that has entered the chamber begins to condense on the colder surfaces in the chamber, i.e. instruments, etc. The steam produces heat which penetrates to the innermost layer of the pack. The moisture increases the penetrability of the heat. After the given amount of time the steam is exhausted. As the temperature drops, the pressure returns to normal. In vacuum-assisted autoclaves the instruments are then heat dried: filtered air replaces the exhausted steam. On modern machines the door cannot be opened until the end of this stage.

Effective sterilisation also depends on correct loading of packs into the autoclave. There should be adequate space between them to allow steam to circulate freely. Care should be taken to avoid overloading and blocking of the inlet and exhaust valves. Before packing for sterilisation, instruments must be free of grease and protein material to allow effective penetration of steam.

Maintenance of the autoclave All types of autoclave should be serviced by a qualified engineer to ensure that they remain in good working order and remain electrically safe. Vacuum-assisted autoclaves with a separate boiler should be serviced every 3 months to comply with Health and Safety regulations. Thermocouple testing is recommended at least annually to ensure effective sterilisation is taking place.

Monitoring efficacy of sterilisation in the autoclave **Chemical indicator strips** show colour changes when the correct temperature, pressure and time have been reached. A strip is placed inside each pack. It is important that the appropriate strip is used for each different pressure/time/temperature cycle, otherwise a false result may be given.

Browne's tubes work on the same principle, i.e. a colour change. Small glass tubes are partly filled with an orange-brown liquid which changes to green when certain temperatures have been maintained for a required period of time. Tubes are available which change at 121, 126 or 134°C. It is essential to ensure that the correct type of tube is selected for any particular temperature cycle. Browne's tubes are also available for hot-air ovens.

Bowie–Dick indicator tape is commonly used to seal instrument and drape packs. It is a beige-coloured tape which is impregnated with chemical stripes that change to dark brown when a certain temperature is reached (121°C). As with ethylene oxide indicator tape, it is not reliable as an indicator of sterility as it does not ensure that the temperature was maintained for the required time.

Spore tests are strips of paper impregnated with dried spores (usually *Bacillus stearothermophilius*). A strip is included in the load; on completion of the cycle it is placed in the culture medium provided and incubated at the appropriate temperature for up to 72 hours. If the sterilisation process has been successful, the spores will be killed and there will be no growth.

Spore systems are more accurate than chemical indicators but the delay in obtaining results is a major disadvantage. A combination of both systems is recommended: chemical indicators should be included in each pack and spore strips should be used at regular intervals.

Vacuum-assisted autoclaves will usually have visible temperature and pressure **gauges** on the front. Some systems have a paper **recording chart** which indicates the efficiency of sterilisation.

Thermocouples (electrical leads with temperature-sensitive tips) are placed in various parts of the sterilising chamber with the leads passed out through an aperture to a recording device outside. The temperature within the chamber can be constantly recorded throughout a cycle to check that required temperatures are received and held for the specified time.

Dry heat

Dry heat kills micro-organisms by causing oxidative destruction of bacterial protoplasm. Micro-organisms are much more resistant to dry heat than when heated in the presence of moisture and so higher temperatures are required (150–180°C). Dry heat below 140°C cannot destroy bacterial spores in less than 4–5 hours.

The range of equipment sterilised in this way is restricted: fabrics, rubber goods and plastic cannot withstand these high, dry temperatures and are easily damaged.

There are certain items for which dry heat sterilisation is the method of choice. These include glass syringes, cutting instruments, ophthalmic instruments, drill bits, glassware, powders and oils.

Hot-air ovens   These are heated by electrical elements (Table 21.3). They are usually small but are economical in terms of purchase and running costs. They have been largely superseded by the autoclave, which is more efficient and suitable for most types of material.

A long cooling period is needed before the items may be used. The door should be fitted with a safety device to prevent it being opened before the oven is cool. It is important to ensure that the oven is not overloaded and that items are placed so that air can flow freely.

Table 21.3 Temperature and time ratios recommended for hot-air ovens

Item	Temperature (°C)	Time (min)
Glassware	180	60
Non-cutting instruments Powders, oils	160	120
Sharp-cutting instruments	150	180

Spore strip tests and Browne's tubes are available which are designed specifically for testing sterility in hot-air ovens.

MOIST HEAT (BOILING)
Boiling is no longer considered as a method of sterilisation. It cannot be guaranteed to kill all micro-organisms and spores, because the maximum temperature of 100°C is insufficient to kill resistant spores.

Cold sterilisation

Ethylene oxide

Ethylene oxide is a highly penetrating and effective method of sterilisation. However, concerns have been expressed about its use in veterinary practice as it is toxic, irritant to tissue and a very inflammable gas. Its use is currently permitted and the danger to operators should be negligible as long as the manufacturer's recommendations are followed. COSHH Regulations may, however, make its use impractical in some veterinary practices. Ethylene oxide inactivates the DNA of the cells, thereby preventing cell reproduction. The technique is effective against vegetative bacteria, fungi, viruses and spores. Several factors influence the ability of ethylene oxide to destroy micro-organisms, including temperature, pressure, concentration, humidity and time of exposure. As the temperature increases, the ability of ethylene oxide to penetrate increases and the duration of the cycle shortens. However, the only system available in the UK operates at room temperature for a period of 12 hours.

Use of the ethylene oxide steriliser   The steriliser consists of a plastic container which is fitted with a ventilation system to prevent gas entering the work area. It should be located in a clean, well-ventilated area (e.g. fume cupboard) away from working areas. The temperature of the room must be at least 20°C (68°F) during the cycle.

Individually packed items to be sterilised are placed in a polythene liner bag. A gas ampoule containing ethylene oxide liquid is placed within the liner bag which is then sealed with a metal twist tie and placed in the steriliser unit. The top of the glass vial is snapped from outside the liner bag to release the sterilant gas. The door to the steriliser unit is closed and locked, the ventilator turned on and the items left to sterilise. The sterilisation process is frequently performed overnight. At the end of the 12-hour period a pump is switched on to aerate the container. The door may be opened after 2 hours and the load removed.

The items should then be left for a further 24 hours in a well-ventilated room to allow the ethylene oxide to dissipate.

Items which may be sterilised using ethylene oxide

Ethylene oxide is effective for the sterilisation of many different types of equipment but its use is limited by the size of the container, the duration of the cycle and concerns about toxicity. Its use therefore tends to be restricted to items which are damaged by heat:

- Fibre-optic equipment.
- Plastic catheters, trays, etc.
- Anaesthetic tubing, etc.
- Plastic syringes.
- Optical instruments.
- High-speed drills/burrs.
- Battery-operated drills.

Some commercially available products are now sterilised by this method, e.g. syringes, synthetic absorbable suture materials and catheters.

> Avoid sterilising equipment made of polyvinylchloride (PVC) by this method as it may react with the gas.

Preparation of materials for sterilisation

Materials to be sterilised by ethylene oxide must be cleaned and dried. The presence of protein and grease will slow the sterilisation process. Water on instruments at the time of exposure may react with the gas and reduce its effectiveness.

Occlusive bungs, caps or stylets must be removed from instruments so that gas can penetrate freely. Syringes should be packaged disassembled.

Ethylene oxide penetrates materials more readily than steam so a wider variety of packaging materials may be used when preparing items for sterilisation and storage. However, nylon film designed for autoclaving should not be used as it has been shown that there is poor penetration by ethylene oxide.

Testing efficiency of ethylene oxide sterilisation

Indicator tape with yellow stripes which turn red when exposed to ethylene oxide may be used as an indicator of exposure to the gas, but they do not guarantee sterility as they give no indication that exposure was for the correct length of time. In fact, the colour change will occur after a very short period.

Chemical indicator strips which undergo a colour change when exposed to ethylene oxide for the correct time may be placed in the centre of a pack or load to test the penetration efficiency.

Spore strips placed into a load are added to a culture medium on completion of the cycle and are incubated for 72 hours. This is a useful test of the efficiency of the system but is obviously not suitable as an immediate indicator of sterility.

Commercially produced solutions

There are a number of chemical disinfectant solutions produced commercially. Some are ready for use, others require dilution (usually with purified water) prior to use.

Until recently a solution containing gluteraldehyde has been the most widely used product for chemical disinfection. Although it is still readily available, COSHH regulations may prevent its use in veterinary (and medical) practice.

Chemical solutions

This method should really only be considered as a means of **disinfection**, although some manufacturers guarantee sterilisation following prolonged immersion (usually 24 hours).

It remains a useful method for surgical equipment which may not be sterilised by any other means. It has gained particular popularity for the disinfection of endoscopic and arthroscopy equipment.

Care should be taken to use the specific concentrations and time stipulated by the manufacturer. Before immersion, check with the manufacturer that the equipment will not be damaged by wet disinfection. The chemical solution and the article to be disinfected should be placed in a tray or bowl, preferably with a lid to prevent evaporation and contamination by airborne micro-organisms. Following immersion in chemical solutions, instruments should be rinsed in sterile water before use. Chemical solutions should be discarded after use and a fresh solution made up each time.

Alcohol-based solutions

A variety of these have been used, e.g. ethyl alcohol and isopropyl alcohol. They work by denaturation and coagulation of proteins.

Irradiation

This form of sterilisation is a form of gamma irradiation and can only be carried out under controlled conditions.

Many pre-packaged items are sterilised by this method, including suture materials and surgical gloves.

Packing supplies for sterilisation

Various materials and containers are available for packing supplies for sterilisation, each having advantages and disadvantages. Choice will depend on several factors:

- Size of autoclave/gas steriliser.
- The packaging material must be resistant to damage when handled and not damage the equipment to be sterilised.
- Steam or gas must be able to penetrate the wrapping for sterilisation to occur and must be easily exhausted from the pack once sterilisation is complete.
- Micro-organisms must not be able to penetrate from the outer surface of the wrap to the inner.
- Cost.
- Personal preference.
- Time taken to achieve sterility.

Materials and containers

Nylon film   Nylon film designed specifically for use in the autoclave is available in a variety of sizes. It has the advantages of being reusable and transparent so that items can be easily seen. Its main disadvantage is that it becomes brittle after repeated use, resulting in development of tiny unseen holes and therefore contamination of the pack. It may also be difficult to remove sterile items from packs without contaminating them on the edges of the bag. The packs are often sealed using Bowie–Dick tape.

Seal-and-peel pouches   Disposable bags, consisting of a paper back and clear plasticised front with a fold-over seal, are available in a wide variety of sizes. They may be used with ethylene oxide or the autoclave. The risk of contamination during opening is small. Double wrapping decreases the risk of damage to the instrument during storage or when opening the pack. They are most suitable for individual instruments.

Paper   Paper-based sheets are used for packing instruments. The most suitable type consists of a crepe-like paper which is slightly elastic, conforming and is water-repellent. It is therefore ideal as an outer layer for packs. Although it is frequently re-used, it is intended to be disposable. It is available in large sheets which can be cut to the appropriate size.

Textile   Textile sheets, usually linen or cotton/polyester combination, are used to wrap surgical equipment for sterilisation. They are conforming, strong and reusable but have the major disadvantage of being permeable to moisture. Usually a double layer of linen is covered by a waterproof paper-based wrap for surgical packs.

Drums   Metal drums with steam vents in the side, which are closed after sterilisation can be used for instruments, gowns and drapes. Their main disadvantage is that they are frequently multi-use, so that there is a degree of environmental contamination each time the lid is opened.

There is also a risk of contamination of items touching the edge or outside of the drum when they are removed. Initial outlay is relatively high but they will last for years.

Boxes and cartons   A variety of cardboard boxes and cartons are available for use in the autoclave. They are useful for gown or drape packs and for specialised kits (e.g. orthopaedic kits). They are relatively inexpensive and may be re-used.

Care and sterilisation of equipment

Gowns and drapes

After use, surgical gowns and drapes should be washed, dried and inspected for damage. Gowns should then be folded correctly so that the outside surface of the gown is on the inside (Figs 21.1 and 21.2). This is so that the surgical team can put on gowns in an aseptic fashion (described later). Plain drapes may be folded concertina style (Fig. 21.3) or so that two corners are on the top surface (Fig. 21.4). Fenestrated drapes are usually folded concertina style.

Sterilisation   Both gowns and drapes may be sterilised by ethylene oxide but this method is often uneconomical in a large practice owing to the small size of the steriliser, duration of the cycle (12 hours) and the airing time of 24 hours. Autoclaving is a quicker, more efficient method but it is essential that the machine has a porous load cycle to ensure complete penetration and drying of the load. A hot air oven is unsuitable as it will lead to charring of the material.

Gowns and drapes may be sterilised in drums, boxes, bags or packs. A handtowel is usually placed with the gown when packing for sterilisation. Drapes are sometimes incorporated into the instrument pack.

Disposable sterile gowns and drapes are now widely used and are to be recommended (see 'Draping the Patient').

Swabs

Swabs may be purchased sterile or non-sterile. Each pack should have a consistent number which is known to all surgery staff, usually packs of 5. Swabs may be incorporated into the instrument pack, supplied in drums or packed individually in packets.

Sterilisation   Swabs should be sterilised in the same way as gowns and drapes.

Urinary catheters

Although designed for single use, most urinary catheters may be resterilised once. The exception to this is the Foley catheter, which will usually be unfit for re-use. After use,

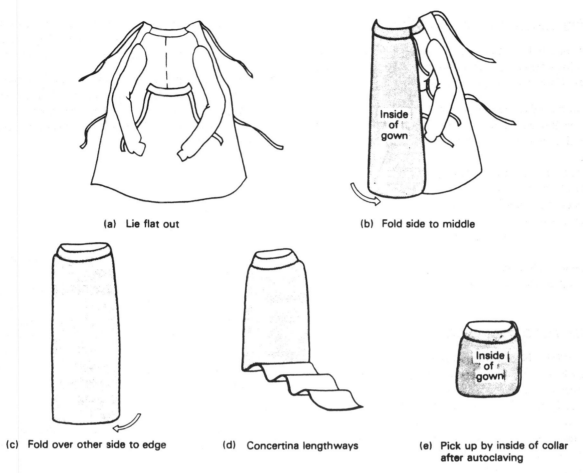

(a) Lie flat out   (b) Fold side to middle

(c) Fold over other side to edge   (d) Concertina lengthways   (e) Pick up by inside of collar after autoclaving

Fig. 21.1 Folding a gown.

catheters should be washed, rinsed and then dried. They should be packed, without coiling if possible, in appropriate bags.

Sterilisation Many brands of catheter may be sterilised by autoclaving but some will be damaged by heat. Ethylene oxide can be successfully used for all types of catheter. It is essential to ensure that they are aired for the recommended time before use.

Syringes

Plastic syringes are designed to be disposable. To ensure sterility after storage they must be packed individually. It is therefore rarely economical to resterilise small syringes but it may be profitable to resterilise 30 and 50 ml syringes. They should be disassembled, washed thoroughly and dried prior to sterilisation.

Sterilisation Most plastic syringes can be autoclaved safely but some brands will be damaged. Ethylene oxide may be used effectively to sterilise syringes. The plungers should be removed from the barrel prior to this. Glass syringes may be sterilised using a hot-air oven, autoclave or ethylene oxide.

Liquids

It is usual to purchase liquids pre-sterilised, although more sophisticated autoclaves have a cycle for the sterilisation of fluids. The risk of breakage of glass bottles is high and it is probably more economical to purchase fluids which have been commercially prepared.

Power tools

Air drills, saws and mechanical burrs are usually autoclavable but individual manufacturer's instructions should always be followed. Autoclaving can in some cases lead to jamming of the motor. Ethylene oxide can be used for all air-driven tools. Battery drills frequently have a plastic casing which would melt in an autoclave but they can be sterilised by using ethylene oxide.

Storage after sterilisation

There should be a separate area for storage of sterile packs. It should be dust free, dry and well ventilated. Ideally all packs should be kept in closed cupboards. They should be handled as little as possible to minimise risk of damage, and

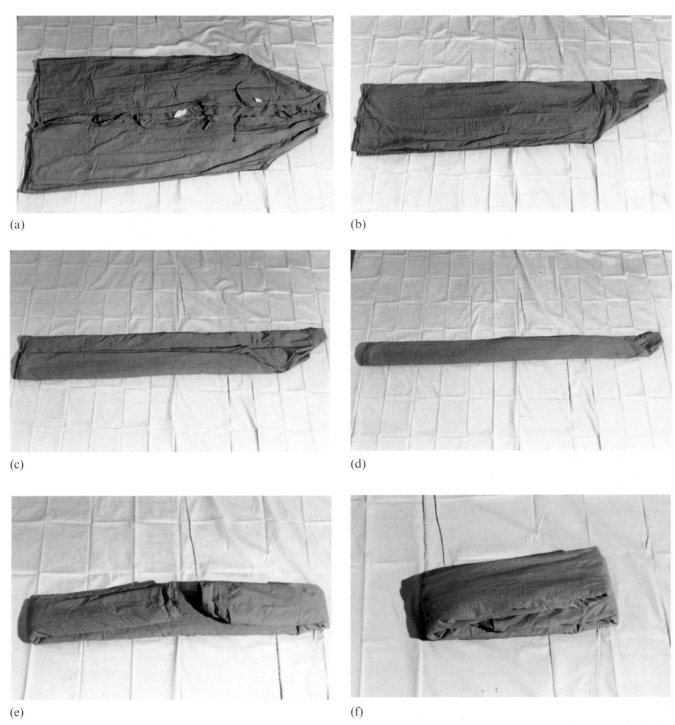

(a)

(b)

(c)

(d)

(e)

(f)

Fig. 21.2 Alternative method of folding a gown. (a) The gown is folded inside out, (b) folded in half lengthways, (c) folded in half lengthways again, (d) and again in half lengthways; (e) the top and bottom edges are folded to the middle; (f) the gown is then folded in half again.

packed loosely on shelves so that bags are not damaged. The length of time for which packs may be safely stored after sterilisation is the subject of much debate, with recommendations varying from a few weeks to 6 months. A sealed pack should remain sterile for a limitless period but it may become contaminated by excessive handling, resulting in damage to the pack, or moisture. It is therefore recommended that unused packs should be repacked and resterilised after 6–8 weeks.

The operating theatre

The design and layout of the operating theatre will rarely be within the control of the veterinary nurse. It is important, however, to have some knowledge of ideal requirements and desirable features in order to appreciate differing standards or aseptic techniques and to try and make the best of existing facilities. The operating theatre suite should ideally consist of:

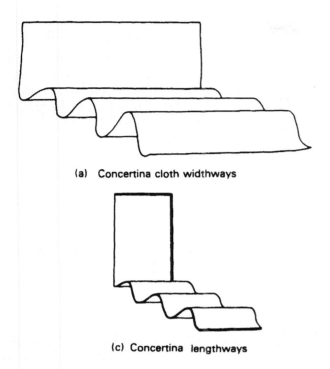

(a) Concertina cloth widthways

(c) Concertina lengthways

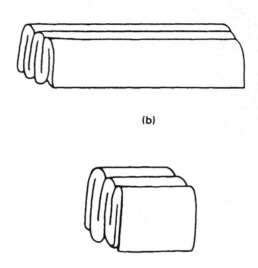

(b)

(d) Pack cloths in autoclave drum or autoclave bags sealed with indicating tape

Fig. 21.3 Folding surgical drapes.

- The operating theatre.
- Anaesthetic preparation area.
- Area for washing and sterilising equipment.
- Sterile storage area.
- Scrubbing-up area.
- Changing rooms.
- Recovery room.

The operating theatre

Many practices have just one operating theatre which is used for all surgery. Larger hospitals may have theatres which are used specifically for particular types of surgery, e.g. orthopaedic work, general surgery and 'dirty' surgery (e.g. dental work). The size of the theatre will depend on the purpose for which it is intended. If it is to be used for simple, routine surgery it can be quite compact. However, if it is to be used for orthopaedic surgery a large amount of surgical equipment may be needed. If the theatre is too small, working conditions will be compromised and it may be difficult to maintain a high standard of asepsis. It has to be large enough to accommodate the patient, anaesthetic equipment, surgical instrument trolley, other equipment and personnel.

There are several other requirements that are essential, or at least desirable:

- The operating theatre should be an end room, not a thoroughfare to other rooms.
- It must be easily cleaned. Walls and floors must be made of impervious, non-staining materials, floors should be

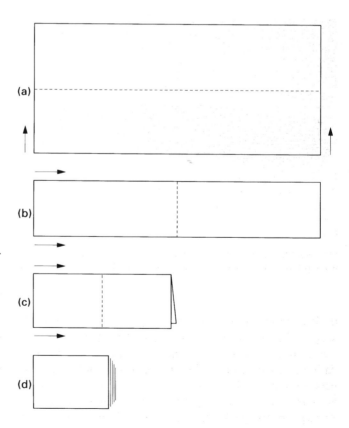

Fig. 21.4 Folding a plain drape corner to corner. (a) The drape is folded in half widthways; (b)–(d) it is then folded in half lengthways three times so that there are two corners at the top.

non-slip and hard wearing. The use of drains should be avoided where possible but should not pose a problem if maintained properly. Walls and ceiling should be painted with a light-coloured 'waterproof' paint. The corners and edges of all walls should be coved to facilitate easy cleaning.

- There should be as little shelving and furniture as possible as it will harbour dust.
- Good lighting is essential. Advantage should be taken of natural daylight. Ideally lighting should be concealed within the ceiling with additional side lights on the wall and an overhead theatre light.
- There should be a good supply of electric sockets (in waterproof casing), preferably recessed into the wall. Heating is an important consideration since anaesthetised animals are unable to control their own body temperature. The ambient temperature should be between 15 and 20°C. Fan heaters cause air and dust movement and should be avoided. Modern wall-mounted radiators are the most realistic method of heating. Panel heating within the walls is ideal, but expensive.
- A system of air-conditioning and ventilation is necessary, and may become mandatory under COSHH Regulations.
- A scavenging system for anaesthetic waste gas will also be necessary.
- An X-ray viewer, preferably flush with the wall, is an important fixture in operating theatres.
- An air supply for power tools may be needed. This should ideally be piped into the theatre from cylinders housed outside the theatre. Anaesthetic gases can be delivered in the same way.
- All equipment, including the operating table, must be easily cleaned.
- A wall clock is needed for anaesthetic monitoring and timing of surgery.
- A dry-wipe board is useful for recording details such as swab numbers, suture details, blood loss, etc.
- The rooms should have double swing doors which should normally be kept closed.
- There should be no clear-glass window to the outside, as this will be distracting. Windows should not open, as this will be a threat to asepsis.
- The operating table should be adjustable to facilitate positioning of the patient and to suit the height of the surgeon. The base of the table may be static or maintained on wheels for easy moving. There is usually a hydraulically operated pump to adjust the height, and some electrically operated pumps are also available.

Anaesthetic preparation area

There should be a separate area where the induction of anaesthesia pre-operative procedures (e.g. clipping, catheterisation of the bladder and preparation of the surgical site) can be carried out. It should lead directly into the operating theatre.

Area for washing and sterilising equipment

There needs to be a room where dirty instruments are washed, packed and sterilised. It should be situated close to the operating theatre but away from the sterile storage area. It should include a washing machine and tumble drier (specifically for theatre wear, gowns and drapes), sterilisation facilities and possibly an ultrasonic instrument cleaner.

Sterile storage area

Sterile supplies should be stored in closed cupboards away from the instrument washing area, but adjacent to theatre. Here instrument trolleys can be laid out prior to surgery. Entry should be directly into the theatre.

Scrubbing-up area

There should be a separate scrub room within the theatre suite but outside the theatre itself. This should lead directly into the sterile preparation area and theatre. Swing doors which can be foot operated should separate the rooms.

Changing rooms

Changing rooms for personnel should be situated at the entrance to theatre. It is a good idea to have a red line delineating the sterile area and appropriate notices displayed to indicate these areas. Footwear for use in theatre should be placed at the entrance to theatre beyond the red line. This barrier should be adhered to at all times to ensure a high level of asepsis. The layout of rooms within the theatre suite is important for the sake of asepsis. There should be a one-way traffic system, so that the surgical team and sterile supplies enter through one door and unscrubbed personnel enter and leave through a separate doorway.

Recovery room

A room where the patient can recover following surgery may be situated near the operating theatre suite. It should be quiet and warm and contain essential equipment to deal with any post-operative emergencies which could occur.

Maintenance and cleaning of the operating theatre

A routine cleaning programme in the operating area is essential if a high standard of asepsis is to be maintained:

- At the beginning of each day, all the surfaces and all the furniture and equipment in the theatre suite should be damp-dusted using a dilute solution of disinfectant. A dry duster would simply move dust around the room.

- In-between cases, the operating table should be wiped clean.
- At the end of the day, the floors in all rooms of the theatre suite should be vacuumed to remove debris and loose hair. They should then be either wet-vacuumed or washed using disinfectant. All waste material should be removed. Surfaces, equipment, lights and scrub sinks should all be washed down with disinfectant.
- Once a week there should be a more thorough cleaning session where all equipment is removed from the room and the floors and walls are scrubbed. A disinfectant with detergent properties which will remove organic matter and which is active against a wide range of bacteria, including *Pseudomonas* spp., should be used. After removing any excess solution, allow the disinfectant to dry on the surface rather than rinsing it off, for longer residual activity. All equipment should be meticulously wiped over.
- Cleaning utensils should be designated specifically for use in the theatre suite. They should be rinsed and allowed to dry after use. Buckets should always be emptied and rinsed out. Autoclavable mops are available and should be used whenever possible. Failing this, cloths and mop heads should be washed daily in a washing machine. All utensils should be stored away from the sterile area.
- It is a good idea to take a selection of swabs for bacterial culture from a variety of sites in the operating theatre from time to time to ensure efficacy of your cleaning regime and to alert you to any potential problems. There should be no growth of bacteria from sterilised equipment and most other sites, e.g. sinks, operating tables, trolleys, drains, positioning aids, surfaces, lights.

Preparation of the surgical team

If good surgical asepsis is to be achieved, all those involved in the surgery should change from their ordinary clothes into correct theatre attire before entering the operating theatre suite.

Theatre wear, which should be worn only within the suite, usually consists of a simple two-piece **scrub suit**. A clean suit should be worn each day, or it should be changed more frequently if it becomes soiled. Theatre **footwear** should be antistatic and traditionally has consisted of white clogs or wellingtons. These have the advantage of being easy to clean. Canvas shoes are sometimes worn but have the disadvantage of being difficult to clean on a daily basis and should be covered by waterproof overshoes. All footwear should be wiped over with a disinfectant at the end of the day. Plastic overshoes are available which fit over normal shoes, but they are not recommended since they wear through in a very short time.

Various different styles of **headwear** are available to accommodate longer hairstyles and beards. These are usually disposable and paper-based.

The purpose of **masks** is to filter expired air from the nose and mouth and to prevent transmission of micro-organisms from surgical team to patient. Masks are effective filters

for relatively short periods only and so should ideally be changed between operations.

Scrubbing up

Pre-operative scrubbing up is a systematic washing and scrubbing of the hands, arms and elbows which is performed by all members of the surgical team before each operation. As it is not possible to sterilise the skin, the aim of the scrubbing-up routine is to destroy as many micro-organisms from the surface of the arms and hands as possible, prior to donning a sterile surgical gown and gloves. Many different scrub routines have been described and no single technique is necessarily better than another. It is recommended that one of the tried and tested regimes is adopted and adhered to strictly. For example:

(1) Remove watch and jewellery.
(2) Finger nails should be cut short and any nail varnish removed.
(3) Adjust the water supply (which should be elbow or foot operated) to a suitable temperature and flow. Once the scrubbing-up routine has started, the hands should not touch the taps, sink or scrub dispenser. If they are inadvertently touched, the last stage of the procedure should be repeated.
(4) Wash the hands thoroughly using a plain soap. At this stage, clean the nails using a nail pick.
(5) Once the hands have been washed, wash the arms up to and including the elbows. Always keep the hands higher than the elbows so that water drains down towards the unscrubbed upper arms rather than the other way round (which would lead to recontamination). The purpose of this stage of the procedure is to remove organic matter and grease from the skin.
(6) Rinse the hands and then the arms by allowing water to wash away the soap from the hands towards the elbows.
(7) Repeat this procedure using a surgical scrub solution, e.g. povidone–iodine or chlorhexidine (Table 21.4). Use only sufficient water to produce a lather, as bactericidal properties of the scrub solution are dependent on contact time with the skin. Excessive amounts of water will rinse away the scrub solution before it has achieved its aim.
(8) Rinse off the scrub solution as in stage (6).
(9) Take a sterile scrubbing brush and systematically scrub the hands. Scrub the palms of the hand, wrist and four surfaces of each finger and thumb (back, front and both sides) and the nails. Either rinse the brush and use it on the other hand or discard it and take a second brush. It is not recommended that the backs of the hands and arms are scrubbed as this may lead to excoriation, which predisposes to infection.
(10) The final stage is a repeat of stage (7). Wash the hands and arms in surgical scrub but this time the scrubbing process is not extended to include the elbow, so that there is no danger that a previously unscrubbed area is touched.

Table 21.4 Ideal properties of surgical scrub solutions	
Wide spectrum of antimicrobial activity	
Ability to decrease microbial count quickly	
Quick application	
Long residual lethal effect against micro-organisms	
Remain active and effective in the presence of organic matter	
Safe to use without skin irritation or sensitisation	
Economical	
Practical for veterinary use	
Commonly used agents	
Povidone–iodine	Iodine combined with a detergent
	Broad-spectrum antimicrobial activity – bactericidal, viricidal and fungicidal
	May cause severe skin reactions and irritation in some individuals
	Efficacy impaired by organic matter
Chlorhexidine	Effective against many bacteria, including *E. coli* and *Pseudomonas* spp.
	Viricidal, fungicidal and sporicidal properties
	Effective level of activity in the presence of organic material
	Longer residual activity than povidone–iodine
	Relatively low toxicity to tissue
Triclosan	A newer agent, claimed to be antibacterial against both Gram-positive and Gram-negative bacteria

(11) Rinse the hands and arms as before.

(12) Take a sterile handtowel, holding it at arm's length. Use a different quarter to dry each hand and each arm. Then discard the handtowel.

The scrubbing procedure should take between 5 and 10 minutes.

Check the clock as you start and as you begin the final stage to ensure that you have not rushed the procedure.

Putting on a surgical gown

There are two different types of gown: back-tie and side-tie. The technique for putting on the gown is similar for both, with slight variation:

(1) The sterile gown (folded inside out) is taken from its sterile pack, held at the shoulders and allowed to fall open (Fig. 21.5a).

(2) One hand should be slipped into each sleeve (Fig. 21.5b). No attempt should be made to try and pull the sleeves over the shoulder or to readjust the gown as this will lead to contamination of the hands or outside of the gown. An unscrubbed assistant should pull the back of the gown over the shoulders (touching only the inside surface of the gown) and secure the ties at the back.

(3) With the hands retained within the sleeves, the waist ties should be picked up and held out to the sides (Fig. 21.5c).

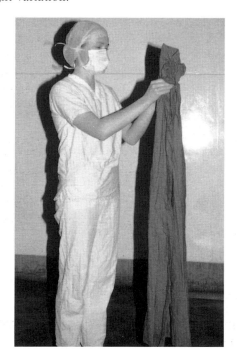

(a)

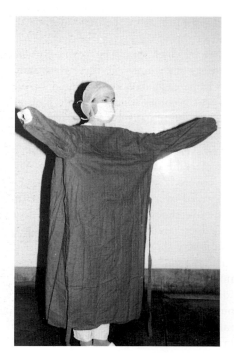

(b)

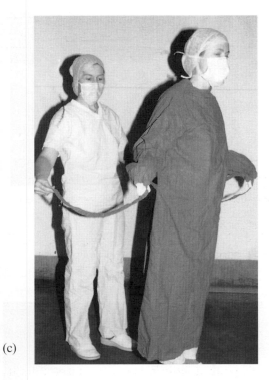

(c)

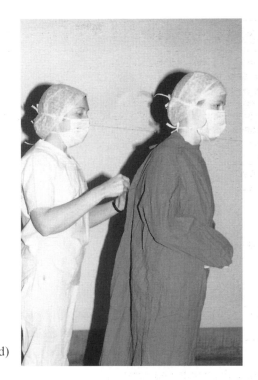

(d)

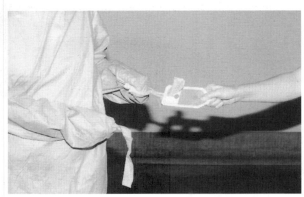

(e)

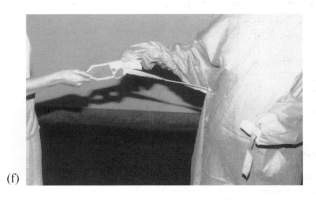

(f)

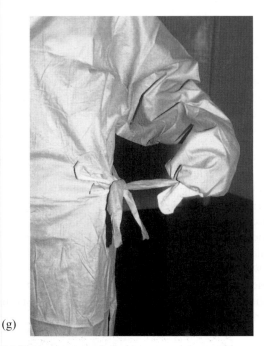

(g)

Fig. 21.5 Putting on a surgical gown.

In the case of **back-tying** gowns, the unscrubbed assistant will then take the ends of the waist ties and secure them at the back (Fig. 21.5d). The back of the gown is now unsterile and must not come into contact with sterile equipment, drapes and gowns.

In the case of the **side-tying** gown, the unscrubbed assistant takes hold of the paper tape on the longer waist tape and takes the tie around the back to the opposite side (Fig. 21.5e). The scrubbed person then pulls the tape, so that the paper tape comes away (Fig. 21.5f). The gown is tied at the waist by the scrubbed person (Fig. 21.5g). This type of gown provides an all-round sterile field.

Putting on surgical gloves

Three methods are available: closed gloving, open gloving and the plunge method.

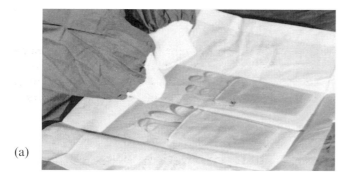

(a)

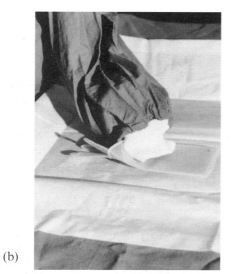

(b)

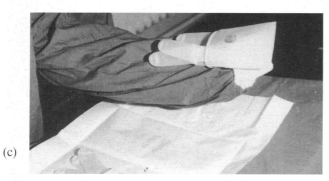

(c)

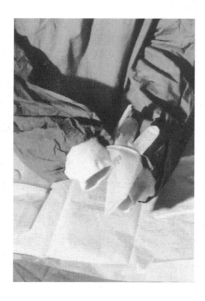

(d)

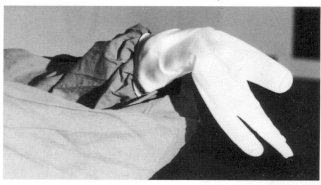

(e)

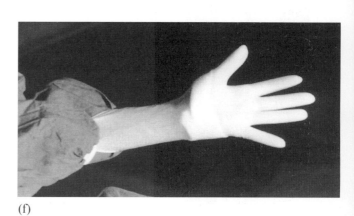

(f)

Fig. 21.6 Closed gloving technique.

Closed gloving

The hands are kept inside the sleeves while gloving takes place. This technique (Fig. 21.6) has the advantage that it minimises the chances of contaminating the gloves, since the outside of the gloves do not contact the skin.

(1) Hands remain within the sleeves of the gown. The glove packet is turned so that the fingers point towards the body. (The right glove will now be on the left and vice versa.)
(2) The glove is picked up at the rim of the cuff of the glove.
(3) The hand is turned over so that the glove lies on the palm surface with fingers of the glove still pointing towards the body.
(4) The rim is picked up with the opposite hand.
(5) It is then pulled over the fingers and over the dorsal surface of the wrist.
(6) The glove is then pulled on as the fingers are pushed forwards.

Open gloving

The hands are extended out of the sleeves while gowning. This technique (Fig. 21.7) has the disadvantage that the gloves are relatively easily contaminated by skin contact.

(1) The glove pack is opened by an assistant.
(2) With the left hand, pick up the right glove by the turned down cuff, holding only the inner surface of the glove.
(3) Pull on to the right hand. Do not unfold the cuff at this stage.
(4) Place the gloved fingers of the right hand under the cuff of the left glove and pull on to the left hand holding only the outer surface of this glove.
(5) The rim of the left glove is hooked over the thumb whilst the cuff of the gown is adjusted.
(6) Pull the cuff of the left glove over the cuff of the gown using the fingers of the right hand.
(7) Repeat for the right hand.

Plunge method

With this method (Fig. 21.8) the sterile glove is held open by a scrubbed assistant and the hand inserted. There is a risk of contaminating both personnel involved. This technique is not commonly employed in veterinary operating theatres.

Pre-operative preparation of the patient

Surgical cases may be categorised as follows:

- **Elective and non-urgent** – the patient is usually healthy and often young (e.g. ovariohysterectomy, castration, corrective osteotomy).
- **Necessary or urgent** – not immediately life-threatening but require prompt attention (fracture repair, airway, gastrointestinal surgery).
- **Emergency surgery** – life-threatening conditions (e.g. abdominal crisis), often traumatic (e.g. chest injury).

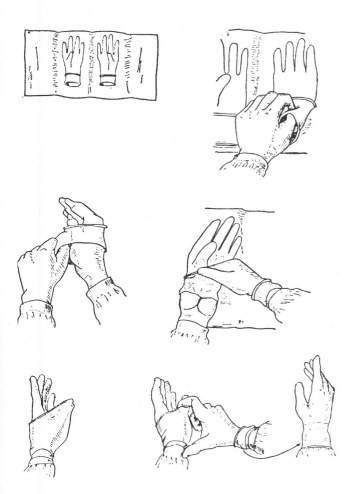

Fig. 21.7 Open gloving.

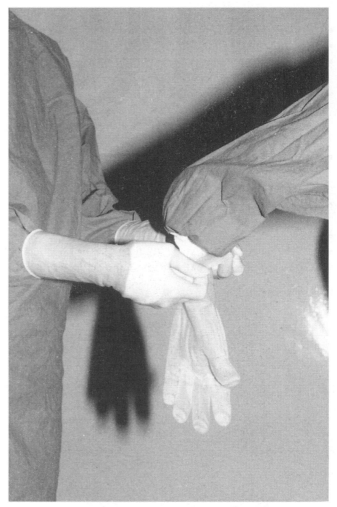

Fig. 21.8 The plunge method of gloving.

The time between admission and surgery will depend on various factors. In the simplest elective procedures, the patient is admitted on the morning of surgery and returns home later that day. Pre-operative preparations in these cases are minimal. In others there may be a delay before surgery is performed. Reasons for this may include:

- **Investigative procedures**, e.g. diagnostic tests, radiographic and ultrasonographic studies, etc.
- **Fluid therapy or transfusion** – to improve the patient's physiological status before surgery.
- **Presence of other injuries** which require treatment before surgery may be undertaken (e.g. thoracic trauma associated with a limb fracture).
- **To allow reduction of swelling/debridement of wounds** – bandaging of fracture site, application of wound dressings, etc.
- **Stabilisation** of patient with concurrent metabolic disturbance (e.g. diabetes mellitus, renal disease, Cushing's syndrome).

Admission of the patient (see also Chapter 3)

On admission of the patient:

- All relevant details must be recorded on the case records.
- Check the reason for admission.
- Where relevant, identify the site (draw a diagram if necessary).
- Ensure that the owner understands what is to be done and how the patient will look when discharged (e.g. it will have a clipped area and may be wearing a bandage, cast, Elizabethan collar, etc.).
- Ensure that the patient is in good general health or that symptoms have not changed since last seen by a veterinary surgeon.
- Always ensure that you have a contact telephone number and that an anaesthetic consent form is signed.
- The patient should then be weighed.
- It is sensible at this stage to fit a plastic identicollar containing the patient's name/number, weight, and

reason for admission to minimise the risk of mistakes occurring.

Pre-operative procedures

Starvation

Food is usually withheld for 12 hours prior to surgery. This is primarily to prevent regurgitation of food under general anaesthesia or during recovery. A full stomach could also interfere with the surgical procedure.

Clipping

Clipping the surgical site is necessary for most procedures (except intraoral). It may be carried out pre-anaesthesia or under general anaesthesia (Table 21.5). Certain considerations should be borne in mind when clipping:

- Clip a large area around the surgical site. Ensure that the clipping is neat. (This is what the owner will notice.)
- Ensure that clipper blades are in good order. Tears in the skin will cause irritation, which may encourage postoperative licking and scratching at the site.
- When clipping around a wound, K-Y jelly placed in the wound and on the coat at the edges of the wound will help to prevent hair entering the wound.
- Clean clipper blades in between cases. It may be necessary to sterilise them after clipping contaminated sites, e.g. abscesses.
- Clipping should be performed away from the operating theatre to minimise contamination by hair.
- Do not allow clipper blades to become too hot during use as this may cause inflammation or excoriation which is not apparent until the post-operative period. Have a second pair of blades ready so that you can swap them during procedures.
- Some surgeons advocate shaving of the skin after clipping but this may lead to severe excoriation of the skin, which encourages post-operative licking, scratching and soreness.

	Advantages	Disadvantages
Table 21.5 Clipping: advantages and disadvantages		
Under general anaesthesia	Often takes less time Fewer people required to restrain animal Desirable with fractious animals or painful/inaccessible sites	Decreases asepsis: small loose hairs are extremely difficult to remove even with a vacuum cleaner Increases anaesthetic time
Pre-anaesthesia	Shorter anaesthetic time Improves asepsis: loose hairs generally shed before surgery Can give initial skin preparation Improves operating theatre efficiency (more operations can be performed)	Patient may be un-cooperative Requires two or more people Clipping more than 12 hours before surgery may increase skin bacteria

Bathing

Ideally all patients should be bathed before surgery to decrease the risk of contamination but this is not always feasible. It should be considered in elective orthopaedic procedures such as total hip replacement.

Administration of an enema (see also Chapter 16)

For some surgery (e.g. rectal/colonic) it is desirable to give an evacuant enema prior to surgery. A soap-and-water enema is simplest. The patient may need bathing afterwards to remove faecal contaminants from the skin.

Preparation immediately before surgery

Some form of **premedicant** drug is usually given by intramuscular or subcutaneous injection, 15 minutes to 1 hour before induction of anaesthesia.

Antibiotic drugs are often given at the same time as the premedicant drugs to ensure effective antibiotic blood levels at the time of surgery. **Eye drops** are often applied immediately prior to ophthalmic surgery. **Catheterisation of the bladder** may be required for the following reasons:

- Monitor urine output during and after surgery.
- Minimise risk of soiling during surgery.
- Facilitate access to abdominal organs.
- Prevent risk of bladder perforation or rupture during surgery.

Other possible preparations are described in Table 21.6.

Preparation of the skin

The skin and coat are two of the greatest sources of wound contamination as it is not possible to remove all bacteria from the skin. The aim is to significantly reduce the number present without damaging the skin itself. Common skin bacteria include species of *Staphylococcus, Bacillus* and occasionally *Streptococcus*.

As antiseptic and detergent properties are required in skin-cleansing agents, surgical scrub solutions such as chlorhexidine and povidone–iodine are ideal. An antiseptic solution (which may be water- or alcohol-based) is then usually applied to give residual bacterial activity.

Initial skin preparation should be done in the preparation room. There are several different techniques which are used commonly and one that is recommended is as follows:

(1) Surgical gloves should be worn to prevent contamination of the patient's skin from the nurse's hands. It is not necessary for the gloves to be sterile during the initial preparation.
(2) Using lint-free swabs, wash the site using a surgical scrub solution and a little warm water, beginning at the proposed incision site and working outwards. Once the edges of the clipped area are reached, discard the swab and take a new one.
(3) Continue this procedure until the area is clean, i.e. there is no discoloration on a white swab.
(4) A small amount of a 70% alcohol solution can then be sprayed over the site to remove any remaining detergent. It should not be used on open wounds or mucous membranes.
(5) Move the patient into theatre and position for surgery. For limb surgery, a tape is applied over the foot and attached to a drip stand to allow preparation around all sides of the limb.
(6) As the site is likely to have been contaminated to some extent in the transition to the theatre, the skin is given another wash in the manner previously described. This time, however, use sterile gloves, water and swabs.
(7) The final stage of preparation is carried out by the scrubbed surgical team with an antiseptic solution using sterile swabs on sterile Rampley sponge-holding forceps, which are then discarded.

> Care should be taken to avoid soaking the coat as this will increase the risk of 'strike through' from the drapes and may make the patient hypothermic.

Table 21.6 Other preparations immediately before surgery

(1) Purse-string suture around anus to prevent contamination by faecal material during surgery in the peri-anal region. The nurse should ensure that it is removed at the end of surgery.
(2) Application of Esmarch's rubber bandage and tourniquet for a bloodless operating field during surgery on distal limbs.
(3) Introduction of a throat pack to prevent aspiration of blood, mucus, etc., during oral or nasal surgery. Usually a dampened conforming bandage is used for this purpose.
(4) Cover any additional wounds not associated with the surgery to prevent risk of further contamination.
(5) Application of a foot bandage to cover any unclipped areas where the surgery involves a limb.

Preparation of eyes and mucous membranes

The solutions commonly used for preparation of the skin are likely to be irritant and cause damage to mucous membranes and in particular the eye. Dilute solutions of povidone–iodine (0.1–0.2%) are commonly used to irrigate the eye and may also be used on oral and other mucous membranes. Chlorhexidine solutions are shown to be more irritant to the surface of the cornea. Alcohol-based solutions should not be used on this sensitive tissue.

Some surgeons do not advocate clipping around the eye for intraocular surgery but use adhesive drapes to protect the eye from the hair and skin. Others prefer to clip a minimal amount of hair around the eye. Application of petroleum or K-Y jelly to the hair prior to clipping with a narrow fine blade will help to prevent hair being introduced into the eye. The skin around the eye is extremely thin and sensitive, and so it is important that the clippers are in good order and great care is taken when clipping. The eye should then be irrigated several times with physiological saline before irrigating with a povidone–iodine solution, as described. The skin should also be prepared with the povidone–iodine solution.

Positioning the patient for surgery

Most surgeons have individual preferences with regard to positioning of the patient for surgery, although there are some standard positions for specific operations. The veterinary nurse needs to be familiar with positioning for different surgical techniques and individual variations. When there is any doubt, the nurse should check well in advance of surgery.

Some operating tables have adjustable sides and tilting facilities which assist positioning of the patient. If not, the use of additional restraining aids such as troughs, sandbags and tapes will be necessary. Care should be taken to avoid placing heavy sandbags over the limbs or tying tapes tightly, which may occlude blood supply to the area.

Draping the patient

The reason for draping the patient is to maintain asepsis by preventing contamination of the surgical site by hair and the immediate environment. Drapes must therefore cover the entire patient and operating table, leaving only the surgical site exposed. Drapes may be disposable or re-usable. The relative advantages of each type are shown in Table 21.7.

- **Disposable drapes** are usually paper based. Many different types are available and cost tends to reflect the quality. Most of these are designed for the medical market but many are suitable for veterinary use. They are usually water-resilient and may be purchased pre-sterilised. One disadvantage is that cheap varieties tend to be non-conforming and may tear easily.
- **Re-usable drapes** are usually linen or cotton/polyester mixes. They may be custom made to suit practice needs.

Draping systems

Plain drapes   Four rectangular drapes are used to create a 'window' (**fenestration**) for the surgical site (Fig. 21.9). The fenestration created can be of any size. The first drape should be placed between the surgeon and the nearest side of the table. Then a drape is placed over the opposite side of the patient (i.e. furthest from the surgeon). Drapes are then placed over both ends. They are then secured in place using towel clips.

Fenestrated drapes   Fenestrated drapes achieve the same effect as the plain drapes in leaving a surgery

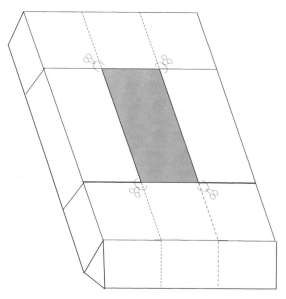

Fig. 21.9 Draping the surgical site with plain drapes, placed longitudinally on both sides of the operating table. Plain drapes are then placed over each end and secured by towel clips.

Table 21.7 Drapes: advantages and disadvantages		
	Advantages	**Disadvantages**
Disposable	Labour saving Less laundry Pre-sterilised Usually very water repellent Always in perfect condition	Expensive Cheaper brands can be less conforming Large stock needed
Re-usable drapes	Cheaper	Porous – all fluids leak through leading to a break in asepsis Time-consuming – washing and folding Danger of threads detaching and gaining access to wounds After repeated use quality becomes poor

window, but the window is already formed in a single ready-made drape. Fenestrated drapes can be large enough to cover the entire animal and table top. A selection of different-sized fenestrations are needed, however, to cater for all the different surgical sites.

Adhesive 'barrier' drapes Sterile clear adhesive plastic sheets are sometimes placed over the surgical site. Standard drapes are then applied in the usual way. The skin incision is made through the adhesive material.

Draping limbs There are various ways of draping limbs for surgery (Fig. 21.10). The surgeon's individual preference will govern the choice of method. Commonly, the lower limb is tied to a drip stand, using tape. A sterile drape is placed on the table top underneath the limb. Then either a sterile drape or stockinette is secured to the lower limb and the suspending tape is cut. The surgical site is then draped in a routine fashion.

Sub-draping Additional towels are sometimes used to protect the incision site from contamination. They are applied to each side of the incision by towel clips. The towel is then folded back over the towel clips.

Surgical assistance

The theatre nurse has two main roles (Table 21.8):

- Scrubbed nurse.
- Circulating nurse.

Guidelines for the scrubbed nurse

The role of the scrubbed nurse is an extremely important one and requires rigid adherence to a set of rules. It is very easy to make mistakes if corners are cut or changes made. Knowledge of the procedure to be performed is important so that the needs of the surgeon can be anticipated:

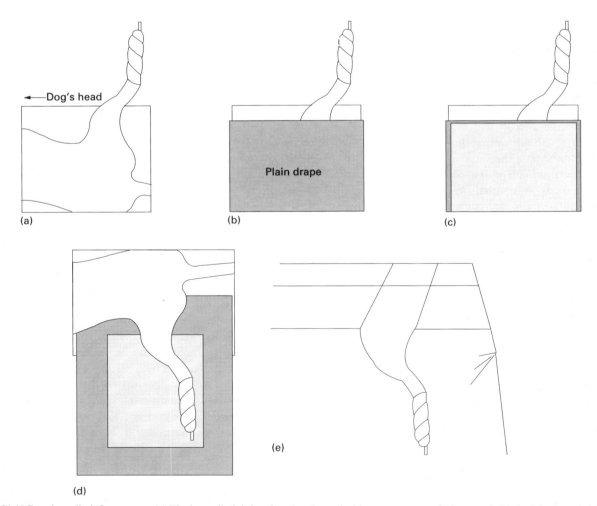

Fig. 21.10 Draping a limb for surgery. (a) The lower limb is bandaged and attached by tape to a transfusion stand. (b) A plain drape is laid over the body and the opposite limb of the patient. (c) A smaller plain drape is laid on top of this. (d) The tape is then cut and the limb lowered on to the inner drape. (e) The drape is carefully wrapped around the limb and secured with a towel clip; plain drapes or a fenestrated drape are then applied over the surgical site.

Table 21.8 Duties of a circulating nurse and of the scrubbed nurse

Duties of a circulating nurse:

(1) Help prepare theatre, instruments and equipment for surgery.
(2) Tie the surgical team into gowns.
(3) Help position the patient on the table.
(4) Preparation of the surgical site.
(5) Connect apparatus (diathermy, suction, airlines, etc.).
(6) Open packs of sutures/instruments, etc.
(7) Count swabs, sutures, etc., with the scrubbed nurse.
(8) Be in theatre at all times when surgery is in progress.
(9) Assist the anaesthetist.
(10) Prepare post-operative dressings.
(11) Help move patient to recovery.
(12) Help clear theatre at the end of surgery.

Duties of the scrubbed nurse:

(1) Prepare the instrument trolley.
(2) Assist in draping the patient and connecting equipment, e.g. suction
(3) Pass instruments, swabs, etc., to the surgeon.
(4) Assist with surgery: retract tissue, cut sutures, etc.
(5) Be responsible for all equipment, swabs, sutures, needles, etc.
(6) Keep instrument trolley tidy.

(1) It is essential to know exactly what instruments and equipment are on the trolley at the start and throughout surgery.
(2) All swabs, sutures, needles, etc., must be counted before surgery begins and again before the wound is closed, to prevent any items being accidentally left within a wound cavity.
(3) The nurse should watch the operation carefully in order to anticipate the surgeon's needs.
(4) Instruments should be passed to the surgeon so that they are ready to be used, i.e. not upside down.
(5) Instruments should be returned to the same place on the trolley each time so that the nurse knows exactly where they are. They should not be left around the surgical site, because they are likely to fall on the floor and because they will not be immediately to hand when needed.
(6) Instruments should be wiped over with a dry swab when they are returned to the trolley.
(7) Only one swab should be given to the surgeon at any time and the nurse must keep a constant check on the number of swabs.
(8) Swabs should be applied firmly to a bleeding site, without wiping across the tissue, which may both damage the tissue and disturb a clot.
(9) All tissues should be handled gently to avoid trauma. Viscera in particular should be handled very carefully.
(10) One of the nurse's roles may be to irrigate the tissues with warmed saline to prevent desiccation, particularly during long operations.
(11) On completion of surgery ensure that all instruments, needles and swabs are returned to the trolley and that needles, blades and glassware are safely disposed of.

GENERAL RULES FOR MAINTENANCE OF ASEPSIS

(1) Correct theatre attire to be worn at all times.
(2) There should be a minimum number of people present and movement should be kept to a minimum.
(3) There should be a new set of sterile instruments for each operation, even when dealing with a contaminated site.
(4) Plan to perform 'clean' operations first, i.e. orthopaedic operations (especially when implants are used), and contaminated surgery to be carried out last (i.e. aural and oral).
(5) Wherever possible there should be a room for 'dirty' procedures.
(6) Adopt an efficient sterilisation programme.
(7) Ensure that the theatre is maintained at an ambient temperature and the ventilation is good. Hot, humid conditions will encourage the growth of pathogens, in particular *Pseudomonas* spp.
(8) Wherever possible, clip and bath the patient before taking it to theatre.
(9) The surgical team must ensure that they do not touch any non-sterile surfaces during surgery. Any break in asepsis must be reported and rectified.
(10) Ensure that any contaminated instruments or equipment are not returned to the sterile trolley.
(11) Keep a record book of all operations so that if any sepsis problems arise the cause can be detected.
(12) Maintain a strict cleaning protocol.

Preparing an instrument trolley

Instrument trolleys should be prepared immediately prior to use. The longer that instruments are exposed to air, the greater the chance of contamination from the environment or personnel. If there is a delay once the trolley has been laid out, then a sterile drape should be placed over the top.

Trolleys can be laid up by a scrubbed nurse or by using sterile Cheatle forceps. The top of the metal instrument trolley will not be sterile and it is important to cover this with a waterproof, sterile drape first to prevent bacterial strike-through from the trolley if it becomes wet.

Instrument sets may be packed in trays complete with drapes, swabs, blades, etc. In these cases the outer wrappings of the set can be unfolded to cover the base of the trolley.

Where instruments are taken from multi-use containers the trolley should be covered by a waterproof drape followed by two layers of linen cloth. Swabs, drapes and instruments are then added.

Hazards in the operating theatre

The avoidance of accidents to patients and staff in the operating theatre is of the utmost importance. The Health and Safety at Work Act and the COSHH Regulations are designed to ensure safety in the workplace, including the operating theatre. (Refer to Chapter 5.)

Equipment

With the increasing use of new and sophisticated equipment, the risk of accidents has also increased. It is very important that all nursing staff are instructed in the use and maintenance of all new equipment. It is also important that all equipment is serviced regularly and tested for electrical safety to minimise risks.

Pollution from anaesthetic gases

All staff should be aware of the dangers associated with inhaling anaesthetic gases. An anaesthetic gas scavenging system must be fitted or absorptive filters used to minimise exposure to gases.

In the operating theatre, nursing staff will be exposed to various chemicals. Protective clothing, masks and gloves should be worn where appropriate.

Care of the patient during surgery

It is important to remember that underneath the drapes is a live patient! Care must be taken by the surgical team to avoid leaning on the animal's chest, which may compromise breathing in a small patient. Careful positioning of towel clips is important to avoid delicate structures such as the eye, which cannot be seen once drapes have been placed. Attention should be paid to the conservation of heat, especially in the small or very young. The use of heated water beds, insulation (e.g. bubble-wrap) and warmed intravenous and irrigation fluids should be encouraged. Careful positioning of the animal on the table is also important to avoid post-operative complications.

Immediate post-operative care

Recovery from anaesthesia

The patient should not be left unattended until it is conscious and sitting up. The endotracheal tube is usually removed just before the cough reflex returns. The animal should be watched closely to ensure that an adequate airway is maintained once the tube has been removed, especially in brachycephalic breeds or following airway surgery. A source of oxygen and a means of ventilation should be available during this time in case any problems arise. Colour of the mucous membranes, presence or absence of respiratory noise and effort will be indicators of effective ventilation by the animal. The ability to maintain body temperature is lost under anaesthesia, so steps should be taken to prevent hypothermia.

Haemorrhage

During recovery the patient should be observed for signs of external haemorrhage (which is usually obvious) or internal haemorrhage (signs of shock).

Recognition of pain

It is important to be able to recognise when an animal is in pain (see Chapter 3). The nurse should obtain instructions from the veterinary surgeon regarding post-operative analgesia.

Application of dressings of casts

Many orthopaedic and some soft-tissue cases will require post-operative bandages or casts. This should be done before the animal regains consciousness. Take care not to apply too tightly (especially head and ear dressings).

Comfort

Make sure that the animal has comfortable bedding, especially orthopaedic patients. Turn the animal regularly if it is disinclined or unable to do so by itself. Give opportunities for the animal to urinate, or empty the bladder manually if necessary. Do not forget to offer food and drink if this is allowed, especially in young and old patients.

Instrumentation

The cost of good-quality surgical instruments is extremely high but they will last for years if handled correctly, whereas cheaper instruments of poor quality will require early replacement.

- **Stainless steel** is the material of choice for most surgical instruments. It combines high resistance to corrosion with great strength and it has an attractive surface finish.
- **Tungsten carbide** inserts are often added to the tips of stainless steel instruments that are used for cutting or gripping, such as scissors and needle-holders. They are very hard and resistant to wear but tend to be expensive. Instruments with tungsten carbide inserts are often identified by their gold-coloured handles.
- **Chromium-plated carbon steel** surgical instruments are commonly used in veterinary practice because they are lower in price. However, they will rust, pit and blister

when in contact with chemicals and saline and they tend to blunt quickly.

Care and maintenance of surgical instruments

Surgical instruments should be handled carefully at all times. They should not be dropped into trays and sinks or onto trolleys. Special care should be taken of sharp edges and pointed instruments.

Care of new instruments

Most new instruments are supplied dry without lubrication. Before use, therefore, it is recommended that they should be carefully washed and dried and their moving parts should be lubricated with a proprietary instrument lubricant.

Cleaning after use

To comply with Health and Safety Legislation, the veterinary nurse must wear protective clothing (i.e. a plastic apron and rubber gloves) when dealing with surgical instruments.

Sharp items such as needles, glass vials and scalpel blades should be safely disposed of before removing other disposable items such as suture packets, swabs, etc. from the instrument trolley. Any specialised or delicate equipment should be separated from the general instruments and cleaned separately. Large instruments such as some orthopaedic instruments should be washed separately from general instruments as they may cause damage to them or be damaged themselves.

Instruments should be cleaned as soon as possible on completion of surgery to prevent blood, tissue debris or saline drying on them, as this will lead to pitting of the surface and subsequent corrosion. Initial soaking or rinsing in cold water is extremely effective for this. Hot water should not be used as this causes coagulation of proteins (e.g. blood). Alternatively, instruments may be soaked in a chemical cleaning solution specifically manufactured for instrument cleaning.

Where indicated, instruments should be dismantled and ratchets or joints opened before immersion.

Instruments should then be cleaned under cool or warm running water, using a hand brush with fairly stiff bristles. Particular attention should be paid to joints, ratchets, serrations, etc. Abrasive chemical agents should never be used as they may damage the surface of the instrument. Ordinary soap should also be avoided as it causes an insoluble alkali film to form on the surface, thus trapping bacteria and protecting them from sterilisation.

After washing, instruments should be rinsed thoroughly – preferably in distilled or deionised water – and then dried prior to packing, as water collecting in trapped areas may lead to corrosion.

After cleaning, each instrument should be inspected for distortion, misalignment, sharpness and incorrect assembly. Pivot movements, joints and ratchets should also be checked for correct function.

Ultrasonic cleaners

Bench-top ultrasonic cleaners suitable for veterinary use are readily available and are relatively inexpensive (Fig. 21.11). They are extremely effective at removing debris from areas inaccessible to brushes (e.g. box joints). They work by the production of sinusoidal energy waves with a vibration frequency in excess of 20 000/second. This produces minute bubbles within the cleaning solution. These form on the surface of instruments and as they implode, energy is released and breaks the bonds which hold debris on the surface.

Following an initial rinsing or soaking in cold water to remove excess blood and debris the instruments are placed in the wire mesh basket of the ultrasonic cleaner. The unit is filled approximately half full with water to which a specific ultrasonic cleaning detergent has been added. The basket is placed in the solution, the lid replaced and the unit switched

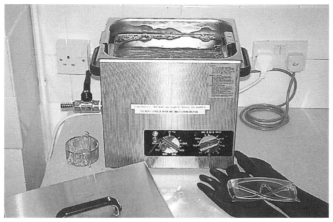
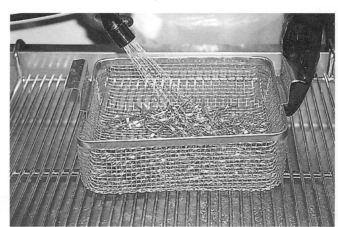

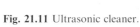
Fig. 21.11 Ultrasonic cleaner.

on. Usually a period of approximately 15 minutes is sufficient. On completion of the cycle, the basket is removed and the instruments rinsed individually under running water. They are then dried as already described.

All instruments should be dried after washing, as water collecting in trapped areas may lead to corrosion. After cleaning, each instrument should be inspected for distortion, misalignment and incorrect assembly. Pivot movements should be checked.

Lubrication

Lubrication of instruments on a regular basis is recommended, particularly after using an ultrasonic cleaner. It is important to use lubricants which are recommended by the manufacturer. Mineral oils and grease must be avoided as they leave a film on the surface under which bacterial spores may be trapped, preventing adequate penetration during sterilisation. Antimicrobial water-soluble lubricants (instrument milk) are available: instruments are dipped into the solution for a short period and then removed and allowed to dry. They do not need to be rinsed.

Cleaning of compressed air machines

Compressed air machines should never be immersed in water or put in ultrasonic cleaners. The machine should have detachable parts (drills, saw blades, etc.) which can be cleaned in a standard fashion as already described. The main handpiece should be detached from the air hose and cleaned according to the manufacturer's recommendations. For metal air drills and oscillating saws it is usually possible to wash the outside of the body of the handset under running tap water, taking care to avoid water getting into the air hose attachment and internal mechanism of the handpiece. With more delicate air- or battery-powered tools where this is not recommended, cleaning will usually involve wiping over the instrument thoroughly with a disinfectant cleaning solution, paying particular attention to triggers and couplings (Fig. 21.12). Use of a small brush such as a nailbrush may be necessary to remove debris. The air hose should be wiped over with a damp cloth in a similar fashion

and at the same time inspected to check that there is no damage to the outer sheath. The handpiece and hose attachments should be lubricated according to manufacturer's instructions. The machine should then be assembled and attached to the air supply and run for approximately 30 seconds to allow oil to circulate and ensure patency of the equipment prior to packing and resterilisation.

General surgical instruments

There is a wide variety of different surgical instruments available. It is not expected that the veterinary nurse should be familiar with them all but a broad knowledge of general instruments can be gained by reference to manuals and catalogues to learn the names and appearance of the more common ones.

Scalpel

The scalpel is the best instrument for dividing tissue with minimal trauma. Usually scalpel blades with interchangeable disposable blades are used (Fig. 21.13). A size 3 handle is commonly used for small animal surgery with blade sizes 10, 11, 12 and 15. A size 4 handle is used for large animal surgery with blade sizes 20, 21 and 22. The primary advantage of disposable blades is consistent sharpness. A scalpel with a blade and handle as a disposable package is available, as is a small, rounded (Beaver) handle with smaller disposable blades which has gained popularity with ophthalmic surgeons.

Dissecting forceps

These are commonly referred to as thumb forceps (Fig. 21.14) and are designed to hold tissue. They have a spring action and the jaws are opposed by holding the metal blades

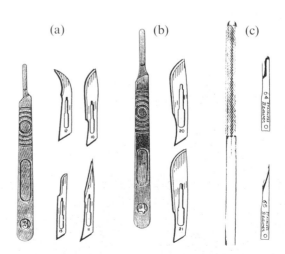

Fig. 21.13 Scalpel handles and blades. (a) Size 3 handle and sizes 10, 11, 12 and 15 blades. (b) Size 4 handle and sizes 21 and 20 blades. (c) Beaver handle with two different blades.

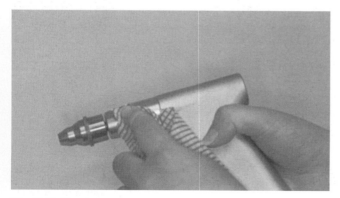

Fig. 21.12 Cleaning equipment.

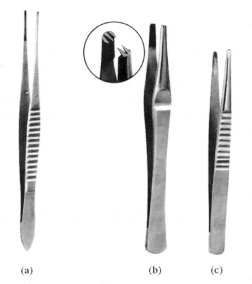

Fig. 21.14 Dissecting forceps. (a) Fine toothed. (b) Heavy-duty toothed. (c) Plain dressing forceps.

together. They may have plain or toothed ends. Generally, forceps with plain ends are used for handling delicate tissues such as viscera, whilst toothed forceps are used for denser tissues. Dissecting forceps should be held like a pencil.

Scissors

Operating scissors are available in various lengths and shapes (Fig. 21.15). Mayo dissecting scissors are commonly used for routine surgery; the finer, long-handled

Metzenbaum scissors tend to be used for more delicate work. Special suture scissors (e.g. Carless scissors) should be used for cutting sutures to prevent unnecessary blunting of dissecting scissors. For removal of sutures, Pains scissors are used. These are small and curved with the cutting surface of one blade hollowed out to fit under the suture easily. Scissors should be held with the ring finger and thumb inserted in the ring of the scissor and the index finger placed on the shaft to guide the scissors.

Haemostatic or artery forceps

Artery forceps (Fig. 21.16) are designed to clamp blood vessels and thus stop bleeding. They come in several different lengths and shapes. Most have transverse striations to facilitate holding tissue. There are many different patterns of artery forceps. Some of those commonly used include the Spencer Wells, Dunhill, Crile, Cairns and Kelly. Mosquito forceps are very small artery forceps for finer blood vessels, the most common type being the Halstead forceps. Like scissors, artery forceps should be held with the ring finger and thumb using the index finger to steady the forceps.

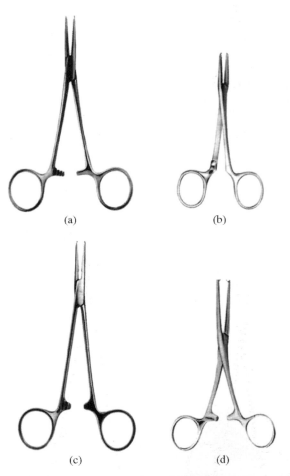

Fig. 21.16 Artery forceps. (a) Cairns, with a fine, slightly curved blade. (b) Spencer Wells, with a short, stubby blade. (c) Crile's, similar to Spencer Wells but longer and finer. (d) Kocher's, with a toothed end and long serrated jaw.

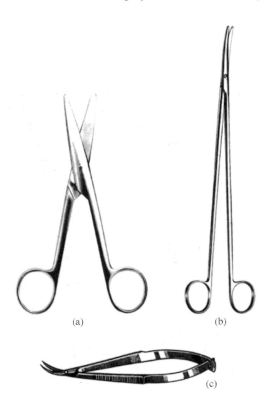

Fig. 21.15 Surgical scissors. (a) Mayo. (b) Metzenbaum. (c) Corneal.

Sponge-holding forceps

These are designed to hold sponges or swabs for skin preparation prior to surgery (Fig. 21.17b).

Tissue forceps

Allis tissue forceps and Babcock's forceps are the most commonly used type of tissue forceps (Fig. 21.18). They are designed to grasp tissue with minimal trauma but neither should be used to grasp and hold viscera; more specialised forceps such as Duvall's should be used for this.

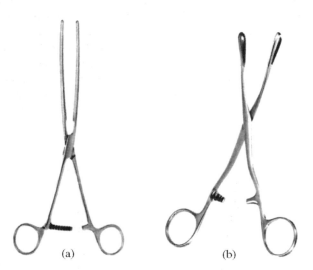

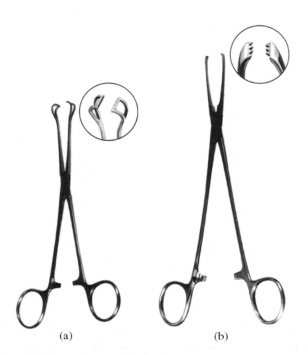

Fig. 21.17 (a) Doyen's bowel clamps. (b) Rampley's sponge-holding forceps.

Fig. 21.18 Tissue forceps. (a) Babcock's. (b) Allis.

Towel clips

These are used to attach drapes to the patient and instruments to the operating site (Fig. 21.19). Backhaus and Mayo forceps have a ringed handle and curved, pointed, tong-like tips. Gray's cross-action forceps, commonly used in veterinary surgery, have a strong spring-clip attachment.

Needle-holders

Needle-holders are forceps that are specifically designed for holding suture needles during suturing and for knot tying (Fig. 21.20).

Gillies needle-holders are very commonly used in veterinary surgery. They have a scissor action as well for cutting the suture ends. Their major disadvantage is that they have no ratchet, so that the needle has to be held in place by gripping the blades tightly.

Olsen–Hegar needle-holders also have a cutting edge but have the advantage of a ratchet to hold the needle securely in place. The disadvantage of the scissor edge is that the suture material may be inadvertently cut. Mayo–Hegar needle-holders resemble a pair of long-handled artery forceps. They have a ratchet but no scissor action. This is one of the most popular types of needle-holder.

McPhail's needle-holders traditionally have copper inserts in the tips, although those with tungsten carbide inserts are of superior quality. The handles have a spring ratchet so that by squeezing them together the jaws open and release the needle.

Retractors

These are used to facilitate exposure of the operating field (Fig. 21.21). They may be hand-held or self-retaining. Hand-held retractors include Langenbeck, Senn and Czerny; muscle and joint retractors include Gelpi, West's and Travers; examples of abdominal wall retractors are Gossett and Balfour; and Finochietto retractors are used for the chest.

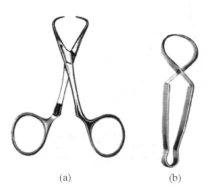

Fig. 21.19 Towel clips. (a) Backhaus. (b) Cross-action.

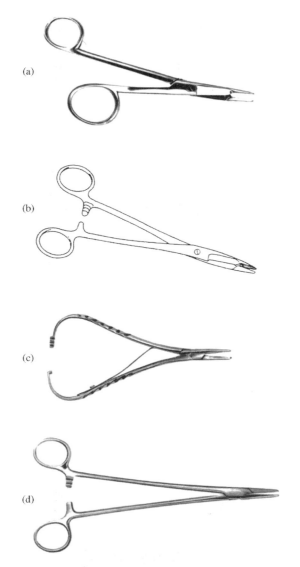

Fig. 21.20 Needle-holders. (a) Gillies. (b) Olsen–Hegar. (c) McPhail's. (d) Mayo–Hegar.

Orthopaedic instruments

See also Chapter 19, p. 503.

Osteotomes, chisels and gouges

These are used to cut or shape bone or cartilage (Fig. 21.22). They are available in a wide variety of sizes. The cutting edge of the osteotome is tapered on both sides, whereas the chisel is tapered on one side only. The gouge has a U-shaped edge to remove larger pieces of cartilage or soft bone.

Curettes

These have an oval-shaped cup. They scoop the surface of dense tissue to remove loose or degenerate tissue (e.g. car-tilage flaps, necrotic bone). The cup has a sharp cutting edge and is available in various sizes (Fig. 21.22).

Periosteal elevators

These are used to lift periosteum and soft tissue from the surface of bone (Fig. 21.23).

Bone-holding forceps

These are designed to grip bone fragments during reduction and alignment in fracture repair (Fig. 21.24).

Bone cutters and rongeurs

Bone rongeurs (Fig. 21.25a) are used to cut out small pieces of dense tissue such as bone or cartilage. Bone cutters (Fig. 21.25b) are designed to cut larger pieces of bone.

Bone rasps

Bone rasps may be used to remove sharp edges following arthroplasty procedures.

Retractors

Standard retractors are commonly used in orthopaedic surgery but in addition hand-held Hohmann retractors are often used for retracting muscle, tendons and ligaments (Fig. 21.26).

Drills, saws and burrs

Hand, battery and air drills are commonly used in orthopaedic surgery (Fig. 21.27). Hand drills are useful around delicate structures and when only minimal drilling is required but for most major surgery a battery-operated or air drill should be a prerequisite. These allow more speed and precision than hand drills. Battery drills tend to be slower and more cumbersome than most of the compact air drills available but they are suitable for most veterinary procedures and are less expensive. They should be recharged after each use.

Oscillating saws and mechanical burrs are either air or electrically driven. Great care should be taken when connecting attachments and during use. The power supply should not be applied until the couplings are assembled.

Wire forceps

Various wire-cutting and twisting forceps are available for applying cerclage wires and for stabilising bones with wire.

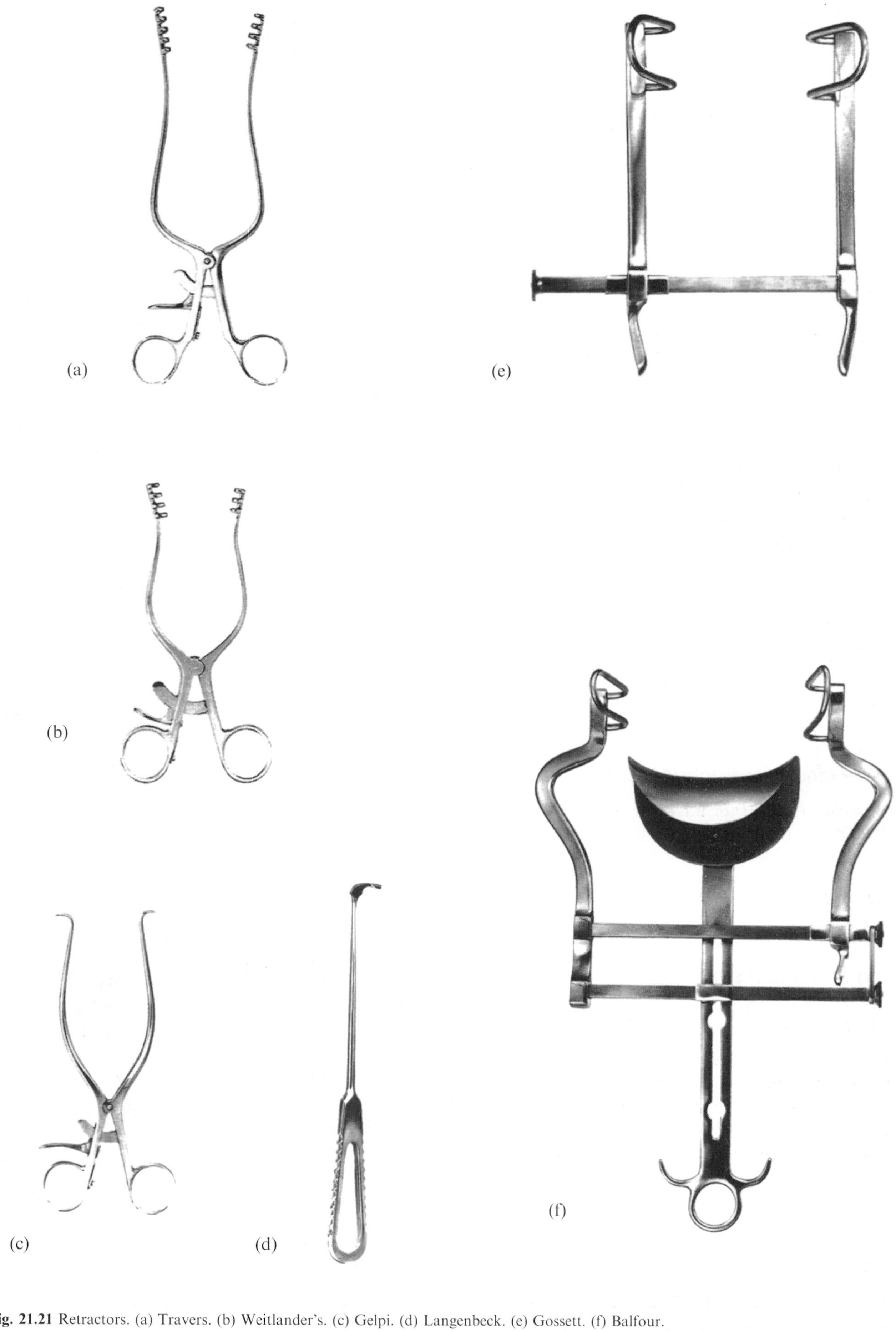

Fig. 21.21 Retractors. (a) Travers. (b) Weitlander's. (c) Gelpi. (d) Langenbeck. (e) Gossett. (f) Balfour.

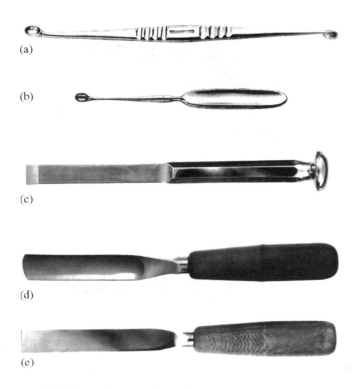

(a)

(b)

(c)

(d)

(e)

Fig. 21.22 Some basic orthopaedic instruments. (a) Volkmann's scoop. (b) Curette. (c) Chisel. (d) Gouge. (e) Osteotome.

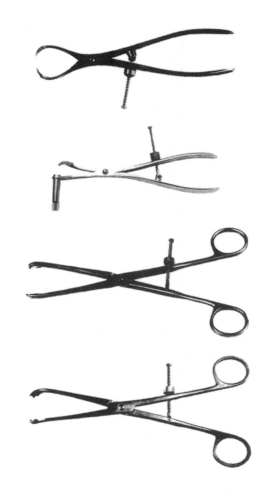

Gigli wire and handles

These are used in osteotomy techniques to saw through bone with a cheese-wire effect.

Instrumentation for fracture repair

The instruments required for fracture repair depend on the technique which is to be used. Materials used to repair fractures internally include Steinmann pins, orthopaedic wire, bone plates, screws and external fixator apparatus (see Fig. 21.28 and Table 21.9).

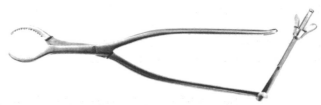

Fig. 21.24 Bone-holding forceps: self-centring forceps with speedlock fastening.

Packing a surgical set

Instrument sets are often packed together with swabs, drapes, suction tubing, etc. They are usually wrapped so that, when unfolded, the layers of wrapping will cover the base of the instrument trolley. A metal or plastic tray is usually lined with a towel or linen sheet. The instruments should then be laid out in a specific order. This is usually the

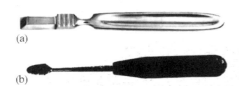

(a)

(b)

Fig. 21.23 Periosteal elevators. (a) Farabeuf's rugine. (b) Straight periosteal elevator.

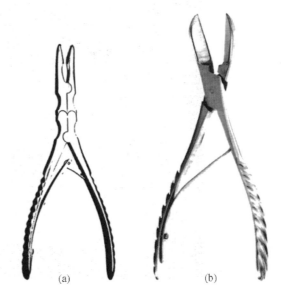

(a)   (b)

Fig. 21.25 (a) Bone rongeurs. (b) Bone-cutting forceps.

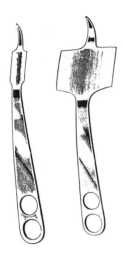

Fig. 21.26 Hohmann retractors.

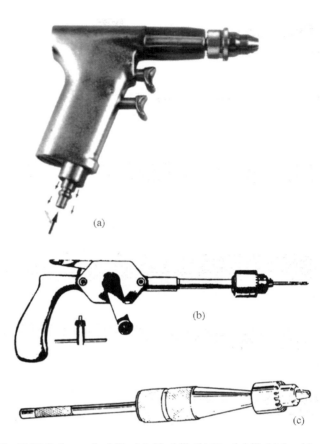

Fig. 21.27 Orthopaedic drills. (a) Air drill. (b) Hand drill. (c) Jacob's chuck.

order in which they are likely to be used (Fig. 21.29). Swabs, drapes, etc., are then added. A water-resistant paper wrap is then laid over the top of the trolley, followed by two layers of linen sheet. The tray is placed on this and the pack is then wrapped (Fig. 21.30). The set is secured with Bowie–Dick tape and tied with string. It should then be labelled and dated prior to sterilisation. Sharp or pointed instruments can be protected by application of autoclavable plastic tips.

Instrument sets

Instrument sets are made up to suit individual requirements and they vary from one practice to another. Some practices have sets for specific procedures (e.g. bitch spay set). Others have a standard instrument set that is used for all opera-tions, to which other instruments will be added depending on the procedure (Table 21.10). Often a smaller set will be available for minor procedures such as a cat spay. It is important that each of the standard instrument sets should

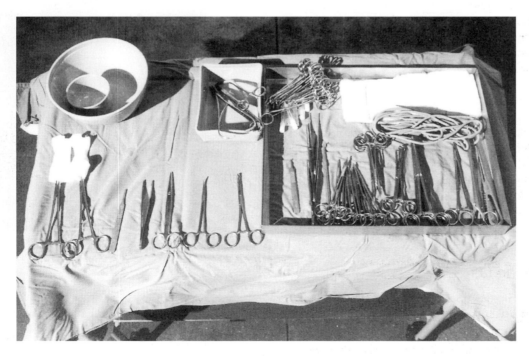

Fig. 21.28 Instruments laid out ready for use.

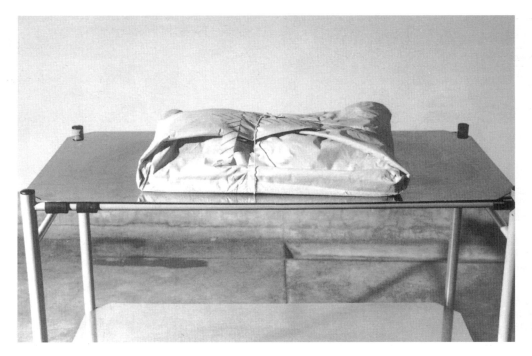

Fig. 21.29 Instrument set packed and ready for use.

Table 21.9 Drill and bone tap combinations for ASIF screws commonly used in veterinary surgery			
Screw dia. (mm)	Drill (mm) Gliding hole	Drill (mm) (Pilot hole)	Tap (mm)
5.5	5.5	4.0	5.5
4.5	4.5	3.2	4.5
3.5	3.5	2.5	3.5
2.7	2.7	2.0	2.7
2.0	2.0	1.5	2.0

contain the same number and type so that the surgical team always know what instruments they will have and so that it is easy to check that all are present at the end of the procedure. Instrument sets can be colour-coded by application of a piece of instrument identification adhesive tape. Table 21.10 lists suggested contents for various instrument sets required for surgical procedures but these are only guidelines.

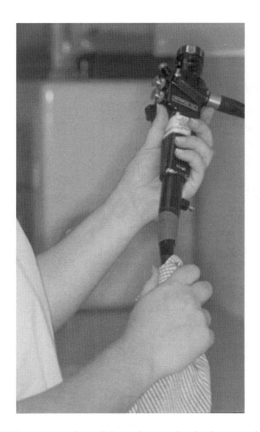

Fig. 21.30 The outer surface of the endoscope is wiped over and inspected for damage

Suction apparatus

A suction unit in the operating theatre is important for several reasons. It may be used for aspiration of the oropharynx and nasopharynx during or after surgery. It may be used for thoracocentesis following surgery or for suction of fluids and blood during the surgical procedure. Various suction machines are available and a size suitable for individual requirements should be chosen. It is sensible to choose a unit with two bottles so that there is always a spare when one bottle becomes full.

Table 21.10 Instrument sets for various surgical procedures: some suggested contents	

Standard instrument set	No. of pairs
Scalpel handle no. 3	1
Dissecting forceps –	
rat-toothed fine	1
rat-toothed heavy duty	1
fine plain	1
Mayo scissors – straight	1
Metzenbaum scissors	1
Artery forceps	10
Mosquito forceps	5
Allis tissue forceps	4
Suture scissors	1
Needle-holders	1
Langenbeck retractors	2
Gelpi retractor	1
Probe	1
Backhaus towel-holding forceps	10
Gallipot	1
Receiver	1
Suture tray	1
Suction tubing and tip	1
Electrocautery and handle	1
Swabs (X-ray detectable)	10
Scalpel blades sizes 10 and 15	2

Additional instruments for particular types of surgery

Abdominal surgery	Self-retaining retractors (e.g. Gossett)
	Doyen's bowel clamps (Fig. 21.17a)
	Long dissecting forceps
	Long artery forceps (e.g. Roberts)
	Towels to pack abdomen
Thoracic surgery	Rib cutters
	Finochietto rib retractors
	Periosteal elevator
	Chest drain
	Suture wire
	Oscillating saw if sternotomy approach
	Lobectomy clamps
	Long-handled artery forceps (e.g. Roberts)
	Rib raspatory
Orthopaedic surgery	General
	Osteotome
	Gigli wire and handles
	Chisel
	Periosteal elevator
	Curette
	Hand drill
	Gouge
	Mallet
	Hohmann retractor
	Putti rasp
	Hacksaw
	Lister's bone cutting forceps
	Bone rongeurs
	Power tools:
	Battery drill
	Air drill
	Mechanical burr
	Oscillating saw
	Implants:
	Stainless steel wire
	Intramedullary pins
	Kirschner wires
	Rush pins
	Staples
	Screws
	Plates

	In addition to general orthopaedic instruments:
	Bone pinning:
	Jacob's chuck and key
	Pin cutters
	Steinmann pin
	Wire fixation:
	Stainless steel wire
	Wire-holding forceps
	Wire-cutting forceps
	Bone staples:
	Bone staples
	Staple introducer
	Staple remover
	External fixator:
	Steinmann pins
	Kirschner Ehmer rods
	Kirschner Ehmer nuts
	Pin cutter
	Drill or Jacob's chuck
	Bone plating or screw fixation:
	Venables/Sherman bone plates
	Sherman screws
	Drill bit
	Air/hand drill
	Depth gauge
	Screw driver
	Plate bender
	ASIF technique (Fig. 21.28)
	(Association for the Study of Internal Fixation)
	Dynamic compression plates and screws
	Bone drills: standard and overdrill
	Bone tap and handle
	Drill guide – neutral and loaded
	Tap sleeve
	Drill insert
	Depth gauge
	Countersink
	Screwdriver
	Plate bender or irons
Ophthalmic instruments	No. 3 scalpel handle
	Scalpel blade sizes 11, 15 or Beaver handle and blades
	Fine dissecting forceps
	Fine scissors
	Corneal scissors
	Capsule forceps
	Vectis
	Iris repositor
	Castroviejo needle-holders
	Eyelid speculum
	Irrigating cannula
	Distichiasis forceps
Dental instruments	Mouth gag
	Dental scalers
	Dental elevators
	Dental chisels
	Dental forceps
	Ultrasonic descaler

Diathermy

Diathermy is a useful method of coagulation of blood vessels or cutting of tissues during surgery by means of high frequency alternating electrical current which produces heat within the tissues at the point of application.

Advantages of diathermy:

- Allows rapid control of haemorrhage and minimises blood loss – particularly important in very small patients, e.g. toy breeds and cats where even small amounts of blood loss may be life threatening.
- Allows clear visualisation of surgical field.
- Helps minimise surgery time.
- Reduces amount of foreign material in form of ligatures that need to be left in the surgical site.

The nature of the waveform of the applied current used in diathermy can vary the effect from curing to coagulation.

- Continuous waveforms are employed for cutting tissue.
- Interrupted waveforms are used for pure coagulation.

Diathermy unit

There are several different types of diathermy machines available for surgical use. Most units require the patient to be 'earthed' or 'grounded'. A ground or earth wire transfers the electrical current to a harmless place such as the ground. This 'earth' wire usually takes the form of a plate which is placed under the patient and is connected to the diathermy unit by a cable. If the patient is not sufficiently earthed, the electricity will pass along the line of least resistance which may be the patient or the surgeon. This may lead to serious burning or electric shock to the patient or surgeon. The earth plate may be disposable or re-usable. Some form of coupling gel, e.g. obstetrical lubricant spread on the earth plate is usually necessary in animals, since they are covered in hair, to provide a good contact between the plate and the patient. A diathermy probe, forceps or scissors are attached to one end of an insulated diathermy lead. The other end of the lead attaches to the diathermy unit. The lead and forceps must be sterilised for use during surgery. Current is usually activated by depression of a footpedal connected to the machine. Coagulation is achieved by applying the probe or forceps directly onto the bleeding vessel or by touching a pair of artery forceps clamping the vessel. Alcohol and other flammable materials should not be used with diathermy because of the risk of fire.

Care of the diathermy unit

After use the diathermy earth plate, if of the re-usable type, should be washed to remove coupling gel, hair, blood, etc. The cable and lead should be washed, inspected for patency and resterilised. The unit should be serviced and maintained by a qualified engineer.

Cryosurgery

Cryosurgery is a technique used to destroy living tissue by the controlled application of extreme cold. The aim is to kill cells in a diseased target while producing minimal damage to normal surrounding tissue.

By the application of a refrigerant, usually liquid nitrogen, to the tissues the temperature is reduced so that intracellular and extracellular water begins to freeze with the formation of ice crystals. This eventually leads to cell denaturation and death. A rapid freeze followed by a slow thaw is recommended and usually 2–3 freeze–thaw cycles are necessary to achieve maximal effect. As most veterinary practice requirements for liquid nitrogen are relatively low, it is usually possible to approach a local hospital or research facility to obtain small amounts of the refrigerant as required.

Precautions

Liquid nitrogen is a harmful substance. To comply with COSHH regulations, a standard operating procedure (SOP) should be employed to prevent possible accidents when handling the substance. All persons involved in using liquid nitrogen should be trained and aware of the SOP.

- Liquid nitrogen should be transported only in containers provided by the supplier of the liquid nitrogen or manufacturer of the cryosurgical equipment. These are insulated metal vessels of varying sizes.
- Wear protective eye goggles, apron and insulated gloves when handling the refrigerant and equipment.
- Avoid splashing liquid nitrogen on clothes, floors and equipment as it will splash and disperse over a wide area.
- Avoid skin contact with refrigerant and probes whilst in use.
- Care needed when filling cryosurgical unit. A metal funnel should be used to pour liquid nitrogen from reservoir vessel into unit.

Cryosurgical units

In veterinary practice small thermos-sized units are normally used. These are easy to handle and manipulate. The liquid nitrogen may be applied via a probe which adheres to the tissue surface or from a more diffuse pulsating spray.

PREPARATION OF THE SITE
- Clip hair around the site to allow effective contact of the liquid nitrogen with the lesion.
- The site should have a basic skin preparation with a surgical scrub solution.
- Protect surrounding healthy tissue with, e.g. polystyrene pieces. This is particularly important when using a spray around delicate structures such as the eye.

Care of equipment following use

- Once the probe/spray attachment has thawed, they should be washed using an instrument disinfectant.
- Any remaining liquid nitrogen should be poured back into the reservoir vessel.
- Probes may be autoclaved if desired.

POST-OPERATIVE CARE FOLLOWING CRYOSURGERY
- Initially there may be erythema and oedema which should be monitored carefully in the immediate post-operative period.
- A slough will then follow which may be moist. This should be cleaned once or twice a day. If there is any discharge, it is a good idea to apply petroleum jelly to the skin around the lesion to prevent excoriation.
- Owners should be warned beforehand that following cryosurgery the affected area may be unsightly and there may be a copious, foul-smelling discharge. They should also be told that following cryosurgery the skin may be unpigmented, resulting in white hair formation.

Endoscopes

There are two types of fibre-optic endoscopes in common use in veterinary practice:

- **Flexible** – used for diagnostic examination of body tracts, e.g. upper respiratory tract, bronchi, urinary tract, oesophagus, stomach, rectum and colon.
- **Rigid** – used for diagnostic evaluation of trachea and bronchi, oesophagus, nasal cavities. Used for evaluation of joints (arthroscopy) and abdominal cavity (laparoscopy).

In small-animal practice the flexible endoscope is more commonly used. Many instruments are obtained second-hand from the medical field and whilst this is an excellent source of good-quality, inexpensive endoscopes, caution should be employed when purchasing such instruments as it may prove difficult to obtain spare parts for older models when repairs are necessary.

The fragile fibre-optic bundles contained within the endoscope have two main functions:

- They transmit light (from a remote source) through the instrument, to illuminate the tissues under inspection.
- They carry the image back to the observer's eyepiece.

These fibre-optic strands are easily damaged by twisting and bending. The more fibres that are damaged, the less light will be transmitted. A second-hand instrument will almost certainly have some damaged fibres. A separate light source is needed to provide illumination. This may be purchased with the endoscope or separately. Relatively inexpensive, portable light sources are readily available. These will usually incorporate an air pump for insufflation and a water bottle for flushing and washing the lens during use.

---

(1) With immersible endoscopes a leak test should be performed after use to ensure that it is safe to soak the instrument when cleaning. A leak test kit and instructions will usually be provided by the manufacturer at the time of purchase. If there is evidence of fluid leakage within the endoscope, it should not be immersed and should be sent for repair immediately otherwise the instrument may be permanently damaged. If the leak test is satisfactory, the endoscope may be safely immersed.

(2) The outer surface of the endoscope is then wiped over with an instrument disinfectant, e.g. Meddis (Medichem). At this stage the instrument should be inspected for external damage. See Fig. 21.30.

(3) The biopsy channel should be flushed with the disinfectant solution and then a flexible wire brush introduced to clean the channel. It should then be flushed again. See Fig. 21.31.

(4) The endoscope is attached to its power source and the distal tip of the endoscope is placed in disinfectant solution and fluid aspirated by depression of the suction button. This should then be flushed with distilled water.

(5) The water and air buttons should be pressed to blow all water out of the system.

(6) If the flush channel is blocked, the tip of the endoscope should be gently brushed with a soft toothbrush to try and dislodge debris from this tiny orifice.

(7) Thorough drying of the endoscope is recommended. The instrument should ideally be hung up so that the tubing can hang straight down to allow drainage of any remaining fluid.

(8) Once dry, the endoscope may be packed in its case or preferably hung in a cabinet so that the cable may remain straight.

(9) Flexible endoscopes may be safely sterilised by ethylene oxide if desired. This is to be recommended, especially when used frequently or where there is a risk of infection. It is important to coil the fibre-optic cable in large loops when packing the steriliser unit to prevent risk of damaging the light fibres in the endoscope.

Care of endoscopes

Endoscopes should be cleaned as soon as possible after use, otherwise blood, mucus, etc. will become dried on and may block the air and fluid channels. All modern flexible endoscopes are designed so that the whole instrument can be immersed to allow thorough cleaning. In most older endoscopes, however, although the tubing is immersible, the handset is not and the internal mechanism will be irreparably damaged if it is soaked. It is very important therefore to follow the manufacturer's recommendations with regard to cleaning.

Rigid endoscopes are as easily damaged as flexible ones and they must be handled with care. Sterilisation by ethylene oxide is recommended, but where several procedures are to be performed in one day it will only be possible to use cold chemical disinfection. Although arthroscopy and laparoscopy are performed more extensively in equine practice, these techniques are becoming more common in small-animal practice. Frequently a video camera is attached to the endoscope so that a remote and enlarged image is produced on a TV monitor. (Flexible videoendoscopes are also available and used in small-animal practice.) This equipment is expensive and requires careful maintenance by a qualified engineer.

No single suture material in the wide range available possesses all of these ideal characteristics. Selection tends to depend on the surgeon's teaching and preferences. Table 21.11 gives the terms used to describe the characteristics of suture materials.

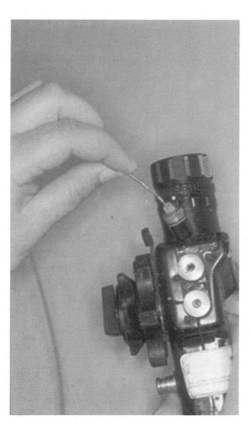

Fig. 21.31 Cleaning the biopsy channel.

Suture materials

The ideal suture material should:
- Be suitable for **use in any situation.**
- Be **readily available** and **inexpensive.**
- Be **readily sterilised** by steam or ethylene oxide.
- Show **high initial tensile strength**, combined with **small diameter material.**
- Have a **good knot security** – it should **tie easily**, with no tendency to slip or loosen, and the **knot should hold securely without fraying.**
- Produce **minimal tissue reaction** – it should be **inert** (i.e. not cause pain or swelling or delay healing), **non-allergenic, non-carcinogenic and non-electrolytic.**
- Show good **handling characteristics** – it should be easy to handle when wet or dry and pass through tissue without friction or cutting.
- **Not create an environment for bacterial growth**, i.e. not show capillary or wicking of fluids (ideally monofilament).
- **Be absorbed** after its function has been served.

Classification of sutures

Suture materials are either absorbable or non-absorbable. They may be further classified as natural or synthetic, and as monofilament or multifilament. Examples of each category are shown in Table 21.12.

Common suture materials

Absorbable sutures

These materials are degraded within the tissues and lose their tensile strength by 60 days. The natural fibres (i.e. catgut) are removed by phagocytosis, which tends to produce some degree of tissue reaction. The synthetic absorbable materials are hydrolysed and tend to produce minimal tissue reaction. In general, absorbable suture materials are used when closing internal tissue layers or organs which do not require long-term support.

Catgut   Catgut is a derivation of the word 'kid-gut'. It is made from the submucosa of sheep small intestine or the serosa of cattle intestines. 'Plain catgut' is untreated; 'chromic catgut' is tanned with chromic salts to slow its absorption, increase its strength and decrease the tissue reaction (Table 21.13). Catgut is absorbed by phagocytosis and enzyme degradation. The rate of absorption is influenced by infection, blood supply and tissue pH.

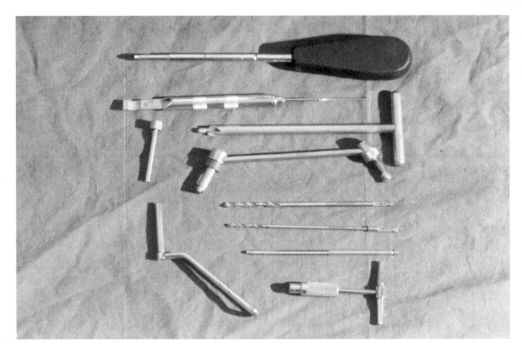

Fig. 21.32 ASIF (Association for the study of internal fixation). Instruments for internal fixation.

- It loses its initial tensile strength very rapidly.
- It always causes a mild to severe inflammatory reaction.
- In contaminated sites it may act as a nidus for infection.
- It handles well; the knots are secure when dry but may loosen as it swells when it becomes wet.
- It also tends to break if pulled sharply during knot tying.
- For many years chromic and plain catgut have been used in both human and veterinary surgery. **However, following a recent EC ruling they have been withdrawn from manufacture and sale**.

Polyglactin 910   This material is a copolymer of lactide and glycolide and is absorbed by hydrolysis. It is available in dyed and undyed preparations, the latter causing less tissue reaction; it is coated to improve its handling characteristics and it is braided.

- It has a higher initial tensile strength than catgut.
- It loses 50% of its strength in 14 days and is totally absorbed in 60–90 days.
- There is considerable tissue drag and careful placement of knots is necessary.

Table 21.11 Characteristics of suture materials: terminology

Tensile strength	The breaking strength per unit area of tissue
Knot security	Related to the surface frictional characteristics of the material Every suture is weakest where it is tied. Often the strongest sutures have the poorest knot security
Tissue reaction	The response of the tissue to the suture material involved
Tissue drag	The degree of frictional force developed as the material is pulled through the tissue
Capillarity	The extent to which tissue fluid is attracted along the suture material. Materials with high capillarity act as a wick and encourage fluids to move along them. Such materials should not be used in the presence of sepsis
Memory	The tendency of the material to return to its original shape. A material with high memory tends to unkink during knot tying, i.e. knot security is poor with materials possessing high memory
Chatter	The lack of smoothness as a throw of a knot is tightened down
Stiffness and elongation	The less force required to stretch a suture, the more it will elongate before it ruptures
Sterilisation characteristics	The ability of the material to undergo sterilisation without deteriorating. Autoclaving is satisfactory for the nylon materials. Repeated autoclaving will, however, weaken them. The natural products and synthetic absorbable materials should not be steam sterilised. Ethylene oxide sterilisation is safe for all sutures provided the packs are sufficiently aerated

Table 21.12 Examples of suture categories		
	Natural fibres	**Synthetic**
Absorbable sutures	Multifilament:	Monofilament
	Catgut: plain	Polydioxanone [PDS II][a]
	chromic	Polyglyconate [Maxon]
		Multifilament
		Polyglecaprone 25 [Monocryl]
		Polyglactin 910 [Vicryl][a]
		Polyglycolic acid [Dexon][b]
Non-absorbable sutures	Multifilament	Multifilament
	Silk	Braided polyamide [Nuralon][a]
	Linen [Supramid]	Polyester [Mersilene][a]
		Coated polyester [Ethibond][a]
		Monofilament
		Polyamide [Ethilon][a]
		Polypropylene [Prolene][a]
		Polybutylester [Novafil][b]
		Polyethylene [Dermalene][a]
		Stainless steel

[a] *Trademark Ethicon*
[b] *Trademark Davis & Geck Ltd*

Polyglycolic acid

This is an inert, non-antigenic, non-pyrogenic polyester made from hydroxyacetic acid and it is braided. It is absorbed by hydrolysis; the hydrolysed breakdown products have been found to be bacteriostatic experimentally, therefore its use has been advocated in infected sites.

- It loses approximately 30% of its strength in 7 days and 80% in 14 days.
- Tissue drag is considerable even in the coated formulation.
- It has poor knot security.

Polydioxanone

This is a monofilament absorbable suture which is absorbed by hydrolysis.

- It loses only 30% of its strength in 2 weeks and is minimally absorbed at 90 days.
- Tissue reaction is minimal.
- As it is monofilament, tissue drag is reduced.
- It is ideal in infected sites and where an absorbable material is required for a long period of time.
- Its main disadvantage is its springiness.

Polyglyconate

This is also a synthetic monofilament absorbable suture which is very similar to polydioxanone. It is slightly less springy and therefore easier to handle than polydioxanone.

Table 12.13 Catgut: approximate absorption times		
Plain gut	3–7 days	Severe tissue reaction
Mild treatment	14 days	
Medium treatment	21 days	Most commonly used
Prolonged treatment	40 days	

Polyglecaprone 25

This is a new synthetic monofilament absorbable suture that is similar to both polydioxanone and polyglyconate, though duration of tensile strength is shorter.

- Less springy than polydioxanone and polyglyconate.
- Tissue reaction minimal.
- Tissue drag minimal.
- Broken down by hydrolysis.
- Main disadvantage is that at 14 days only 30% original strength maintained.

Non-absorbable sutures

These maintain their strength for longer than 60 days. The material is neither hydrolysed nor phagocytosed: it becomes encapsulated within fibrous tissue. Non-absorbable sutures are used where prolonged mechanical support is required. The main indications for use are:

- In skin closure, where sutures are generally removed after 10 days.
- Within slow-healing tissues.

Silk

This is available as braided or twisted strands. It is obtained from threads spun by the silkworm larvae. It may be coated with silicone or wax to minimise the capillarity which may promote infection.

Silk has good handling characteristics, excellent knot security and good tensile strength. It is relatively inexpensive. Its main uses include cardiovascular and thoracic surgery, genital mucosa, and adjacent to eyes. It should not be used in infected sites, oral mucosa or hollow organs where it may act as a nidus for infection.

Linen

This is twisted from long strands of flax. It is easily sterilised, handles well and has excellent knot security. It does show capillary properties, however, and has been shown to contribute to sinus formation. It has been largely superseded since the advent of the synthetic absorbable materials.

Polypropylene

This is an inert, non-absorbable, monofilament material. It has high tensile strength but tends to stretch and will snap if crushed by needle-holders. The knot security is varied and a bulky knot may be formed. It is very springy but shows little tissue drag. It becomes encapsulated in a thin fibrous covering.

Polyamide

This may be either monofilament or braided. The monofilament form causes little tissue reaction, has little tissue drag and is non-capillary. Its handling characteristics are not good and knot security can be poor. It loses approximately 15% of its tensile strength each year. It can be used on fascia and muscle, but the buried ends can be irritant in serous or synovial cavities. The braided form is usually sheathed in an attempt to decrease capillarity but its use as a buried suture is not recommended. It shows more tissue drag than the monofilament variety, although it handles better.

Polyesters   Various braided polyesters are available. They are easy to handle and retain their tensile strength well. Some are coated with silicone, Teflon or polybutylate to reduce tissue drag. They tend to have poor knot-tying quality and some have shown signs of capillarity.

Stainless steel   This is available in monofilament or braided varieties. It is very strong, inert and non-capillary. It is relatively difficult to handle as the wire lacks elasticity and knots may be difficult to tie, but knot security is good. It is useful in slow-healing tissues such as bone, tendon and joint capsules, and in contaminated sites. It has become less popular in recent years as newer materials have become available.

Alternatives to sutures

Staples

Metal clips or staples for use in skin and other tissues have gained popularity in the field of veterinary surgery over the last few years. Staples designed for skin closure are packed in a gun-like applicator for rapid insertion. These instruments are intended to be disposable, although they may be safely sterilised by ethylene oxide.

The main advantage of staples is speed of insertion. They are inert and well tolerated. Re-usable staple-removing forceps are available to remove metal skin staples.

Stapling machines have also been designed for gastrointestinal anastomosis. Although designed for the human market, they are suitable for veterinary applications and are gaining popularity. They may permit resection of areas of bowel that are inaccessible to routine suturing, particularly in the equine abdomen. Their major disadvantage is cost, but their ease of use and the shortened surgery time have much to recommend them.

Metal clips are also available for use as ligatures. They come in various sizes with re-usable applicators. They are simple and quick to use.

Tissue glue

There are cyanoacrylate monomers which polymerise on contact with moisture in the wound. They have been found useful by some surgeons.

Adhesive tapes

Designed for use in humans, these have been of limited use in animals as they do not adhere well to moist skin.

Suture selection

The veterinary surgeon will normally select the suture material but the veterinary nurse should have some idea of which materials may be used in different tissues (Table 21.14) and

the sizes that will be required (Table 21.15). When selecting suture sizes, small-diameter materials should be chosen. These cause less tissue reaction, form smaller knots, knot more easily and are less likely to tie too tight (because they will break). If sutures are tied too tight, they will cut through friable tissue.

Packaging of suture materials

Individual packets   Most suture materials are purchased in pre-sterilised individual packets. This guarantees a sterile suture (unless the packet is damaged) and a needle in perfect condition where one is attached. The only disadvantage is that of cost. Synthetic absorbable suture materials are only available packaged in this way.

Cassettes   Multi-use cassettes are frequently used in veterinary practice for packaging catgut, nylon and stainless steel sutures. The disadvantage of these is the likelihood of contamination of cassettes during use – they often become damaged. It is also easy to contaminate the material as it is cut from the reel and transferred to the instrument trolley. Their use is to be discouraged.

Suture needles

Suture needles are designed to pass through tissue easily. They must be sharp enough to penetrate tissues with minimal resistance, rigid enough to prevent excessive bending and yet flexible enough to bend before breaking. They should be made from corrosion-resistant stainless steel.

Table 21.14 Suture materials suitable for different tissues

Skin	Monofilament nylon or polypropylene Metal staples Avoid materials with capillary action
Subcutis	Fine synthetic absorbable material with minimal tissue reaction, e.g. polydioxanone, polyglactin, polyglycolic acid
Muscle	Synthetic absorbable, non-absorbable, e.g. nylon
Fascia	Synthetic non-absorbable if prolonged suture strength required
Hollow viscus	Synthetic absorbable or polypropylene In bladder: monofilament synthetic
Tendon	Nylon, polypropylene, stainless steel
Blood vessels	Polypropylene: least thrombogenic is silk
Eyes	Synthetic absorbable, e.g. polyglactin, polydioxanone
Nerves	Nylon or polypropylene: minimal tissue reaction

Table 21.15 Sizes of suture material		
	USP – non-absorbable	
Metric	**Synthetic absorbable**	**Catgut**
0.2	10/0	
0.3	9/0	
0.4	8/0	
0.5	7/0	8/0
0.7	6/0	7/0
1	5/0	6/0
1.5	4/0	5/0
2	3/0	4/0
3	2/0	3/0
3.5	0	2/0
4	1	0
5	2	1
6	3 and 4	2
7	5	3
8	6	4

Sutures come in either metric or USP (US Pharmacopeia) sizes

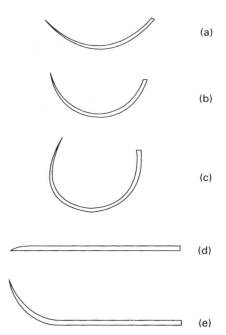

Fig. 21.33 Suture needle shapes: (a) $\frac{3}{8}$ circle, (b) $\frac{1}{2}$ circle, (c) $\frac{5}{8}$ circle, (d) straight and (e) $\frac{1}{2}$ curved.

Swaged needles

Swaged or atraumatic needles are attached to the suture material, i.e. they do not require threading. The advantage of this is that a needle in perfect condition is available with each strand and tissue trauma is minimised by the passage of material and needle of a comparative size. All of the pre-packed suture materials are available with a variety of different needle shapes and sizes.

Eyed needles

This type of needle requires threading. The primary indication for its use is economy of suitable material or use of speciality needles, e.g. for large-animal work. The disadvantages are increased tissue trauma due to the eye size, loss of sharpness of the needle tip, bending and corrosion following repeated use. The needle shape refers to both the longitudinal shape of the shaft and the cross-sectional shape.

Longitudinal shape

Of the great variety of different sizes and shapes that are available, some of those used in veterinary surgery are shown in Fig. 21.33.

Cross-sectional shape

Round-bodied   These are designed to separate tissue fibres rather than cut them, and are used for soft tissue or in situations where easy splitting of tissue fibres is possible.

Modified point   The **taper-cut** needle has a cutting tip on the point of the needle and a round body. This provides increased penetration of the needle without increased tissue trauma.

The **trocar-point** needle has a strong cutting head and a robust round body. This is useful in dense tissue.

Cutting needles   These are required wherever dense or tough tissue needs to be sutured. The cross-sectional appearance of the needle is usually a triangular cutting edge which extends at least half-way along the shaft. The reverse cutting needle has the cutting edge on the outside of the needle curvature to improve strength and resistance to bending.

Micropoint needles   These are very fine needles with a sharp cutting edge. They are designed for ophthalmic and microsurgery.

Selection of needles

The use of swaged needles is to be encouraged – their advantages far outweigh those of eyed needles. Other needles should be as close as possible in diameter to that of the suture. A large needle tract invites bacteria and foreign substances to enter the wound, thus delaying healing. The needle should be of the appropriate shape and size to enable the veterinary surgeon to close the wound accurately and precisely.

The smaller and deeper the wound, the greater the curve should be. Straight needles are designed to be hand held and tend to be used in the skin. Half-curved cutting needles have been commonly used in veterinary surgery but have little to recommend their use. The tissue type will determine the necessary point of the needle. Generally speaking:

- Round-bodied needles are used for viscera, subcutaneous and friable tissue.
- Taper-tip needles are used for easily penetrated tissue, i.e. for denser tissue.
- Cutting needles are generally used in the skin.

Suture patterns

Veterinary nurses maintained on the list held by the RCVS are now legally allowed to perform minor acts of surgery, including the suturing of wounds, and it is important that they should be familiar with basic suturing techniques. The veterinary surgeon should give practical instruction and reference should be made to surgical technique textbooks.

Suture patterns (Fig. 21.34) may be interrupted or closed, and may be further classified as apposing, everting or inverting:

- **Apposing** sutures bring the tissues in direct apposition.
- **Everting** sutures tend to turn the edges of the wound outwards.
- **Inverting** sutures turn the tissue inwards (e.g. towards the lumen of a viscus).

Surgical knots

- A surgical knot has three main components:
- The **loop** is the part of the suture material within the opposed or ligated tissue.
- The **knot** is composed of a number of **throws**, each throw being the linking of two strands of tissue around each other.
- The **ears** are the cut ends of the suture which prevent the knot coming untied.

Knots can be tied by hand or by an instrument. Hand ties may be single- or two-handed.

The basic surgical knot is the reef knot or square knot. A surgeon's knot has an initial double throw instead of a single throw. This reduces the risk of the first throw loosening before the second throw is placed.

Hand-tying helps to prevent slippage of the first throw, since tension can be kept on both ends of the suture throughout the procedure. However, it tends to be wasteful on suture material.

The knots of skin sutures should be pulled to one side of the incision and the suture loop should be loose. Sutures which are too tight compromise the vascular supply, enhance infection and delay healing. They are also uncomfortable and encourage the patient to interfere with the wound.

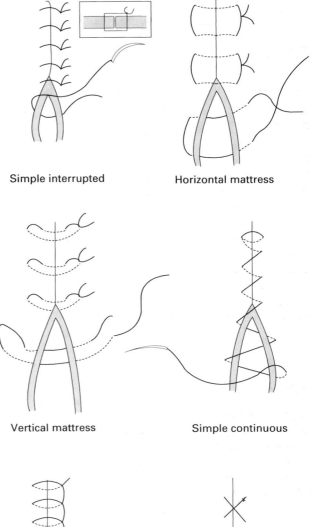

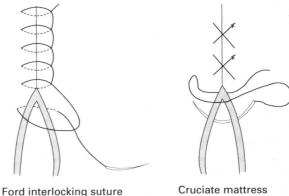

Simple interrupted   Horizontal mattress

Vertical mattress   Simple continuous

Ford interlocking suture   Cruciate mattress

Fig. 21.34 Common suture patterns used in the skin.

Suture material should not be crushed in the jaws of needle-holders. When tying knots, only the end of the suture material should be grasped. Needle-holders should not be clamped on to the eye of swaged needles as this will cause damage or breakage of the needle.

Interrupted sutures

The main advantage of the interrupted suture is its ability to maintain strength and tissue apposition if part of the suture line fails. Each suture is individually tied and cut distal to the knot. Its main disadvantage is the amount of suture material used and left within the tissue and the time required to suture.

Continuous sutures

These are neither knotted nor cut, except at each end of the suture line. The advantages of the continuous suture line are ease of application, use of minimal amount of suture material and ease of removal. The main disadvantage is that slippage of either the beginning or end knot is likely to cause failure of the entire suture line.

Common suture patterns

Skin Common suture patterns used in the skin (Fig. 21.34) include:

- Simple interrupted.
- Simple continuous.
- Ford interlocking.
- Interrupted vertical mattress.
- Interrupted horizontal mattress.
- Cruciate mattress.

Skin sutures should be placed at least 5 mm from the skin edge and be placed squarely across the wound. The skin should be handled gently with fine rat-toothed forceps. The wound edges should be apposed or slightly everted with no gaping or overlapping.

Muscle and fascia

- Simple interrupted.
- Simple continuous.
- Ford interlocking.
- Cruciate mattress.
- Horizontal mattress.
- Vertical mattress.
- Mayo mattress.

Hollow organ closure

- Simple interrupted.
- Parker–Kerr.

- Purse-string.
- Connell.
- Cushing.
- Lembert.
- Gambee.
- Halstead.

KEY POINTS
- Establishment and maintenance of a high level of asepsis should be the highest priority in the operating theatre – iatrogenic infections should not occur.
- A strict routine of work within the operating theatre is essential for efficient running of the theatre.
- Pre-operative planning is important – clean operations should be performed first and contaminated surgeries last.
- Surgical instruments and equipment should be regularly inspected to maintain them in good working order.

Acknowledgements

K. A. Wiggins (1999) Care and maintenance of surgical equipment. In D. R. Lane and B. Cooper, *Veterinary Nursing*, 2nd edn, pp. 559–567, Butterworth-Heinemann, Oxford.

Further reading

College of Animal Welfare (1997) *Veterinary Surgical Instruments*, Butterworth-Heinemann, Oxford.
Knecht, C. D., Allen, A. R., Williams, D. J. and Johnson, J. H. (1987) *Fundamental Techniques in Veterinary Surgery*, 3rd edn, W. B. Saunders, Philadelphia.
McCurnin, D. M. (1990) *Clinical Textbook for Veterinary Technicians*, 2nd edn, W. B. Saunders, Philadelphia.
Tracey, D. *Small Animal Surgical Nursing*, Mosby, St Louis.

22

Fluid therapy and shock

E. Welsh and *W. Busby*

Learning objectives

After studying this chapter, students should be able to:

- Define terms used to describe the concentration and movement of fluids.
- Explain the routes by which dogs and cats gain and lose water from the body and how the body regulates body water.
- Describe the distribution of water within the body and the differences in composition between intracellular and extracellular fluid.
- Discuss the different methods used to assess dehydration and calculate maintenance and replacement fluid requirements for dogs and cats.
- Discuss the advantages and disadvantages of different routes for fluid replacement therapy and describe one method used to place an over-the-needle intravenous catheter and to prime an administration set.
- Describe the different methods used to monitor patients receiving intravenous fluids.
- Define shock, describing common clinical signs associated with the syndrome and explain why fluid therapy plays an important role in treatment.

Introduction

Many medical and surgical conditions and interventions cause disturbances of fluid, electrolyte and acid–base balance within the body, and knowledge of the homeostatic mechanisms that normally govern these physiological processes is essential if disturbances within this system are to be identified, and rectified, in a logical and effective manner. This chapter will review the physiology of body fluid, electrolyte and acid–base balance and examine how to determine if fluid therapy is required, what the most appropriate fluids and routes of administration are, and how to assess patients' responses to treatment.

Units and definitions

It is important to be familiar with the various methods of measurement of fluids and electrolytes within the body, and to understand the units that describe them. Table 22.1 gives some important terms that will be used and their definitions.

IMPORTANT ELEMENTAL AND MOLECULAR SYMBOLS			
• Carbon:	C	• Potassium:	K
• Chlorine:	Cl	• Sodium:	Na
• Hydrogen:	H	• Bicarbonate:	HCO_3
• Nitrogen:	N	• Phosphate:	HPO_4
• Oxygen:	O	• Sulphate:	HSO_4
• Phosphorus:	P		

Table 22.1 Important terms and definitions

Term	Definition	Example
Solution	A solute dissolved in a solvent	Saline solution comprises a solute (sodium chloride) dissolved in a solvent (water). In the body, water is the main solvent
Electrolyte	A substance that yields ions when dissolved (dissociated) in water	Sodium chloride yields sodium and chloride ions in solution
Ion	A small water-soluble particle of atomic or molecular size which carries one or more positive or negative charges	Sodium chloride (NaCl) is an electrolyte that in solution in water dissociates into sodium ions and chloride ions. The sodium ion loses 1 electron (Na^+), while in contrast, the chloride ion gains 1 electron (Cl^-). Both sodium and chloride ions are referred to an **univalent** ions, whereas ions that lose or gain 2 electrons are referred to as **divalent** ions, e.g. Ca^{2+}
Cations	Ions carrying one or more positive charges	Sodium (Na^+), Calcium (Ca^{2+})
Anions	Ions carrying one or more negative charges	Chloride (Cl^-), Phosphate (PO_4^{2-}) *Mnemonic:* **Anion = a negative ion**

Frequently, the strength of biological solutions is measured in terms of their molecular, electrostatic or osmotic composition.

Molecular composition is described by the **molar concentration** measured in the number of moles per litre. However, since biological fluids are very dilute, it is more convenient to measure concentrations in millimoles per litre, that is one thousandth of a mole (1 millimole = 1/1000 mole). Molar concentration is determined as follows:

$$\text{Molar concentration (mmol/l)} = \frac{\text{Concentration (g\%)} \times 10\,000}{\text{Molecular weight}}$$

e.g. a 0.9% solution of sodium chloride (molecular weight 58.5) contains approximately 154 mmol/l.

The **equivalence** system is an older system of measurement that is still often used in physiology and in clinical practice, as it gives an indication of the ionic composition of a fluid. It is related to the molecular weight and the valence (see Table 22.1).

$$\text{Equivalent weight} = \frac{\text{Molecular weight}}{\text{valence}}$$

When the valence is 1 (univalent), the equivalent concentration in milliequivalents per litre (mEq/l) is the same as the molar concentration in millimoles per litre. Where the valence is 2 (divalent), the equivalent concentration is twice the molar concentration. In a solution, the sum of the equivalent weights of the cations must be balanced by the anions to ensure electroneutrality.

The **concentration of a solution** is measured by the mass of solute that is dissolved in a volume of solvent. The gram per cent (gram % or g/dl) unit describes the number of grams of solute in 100 ml of solvent. Therefore, a 1% solution has 1 g of solute in 100 ml of solvent (or 10 g per litre).

Osmosis is the process by which pure solvent (water) moves from a region of low solute concentration to a region of high solute concentration when separated by a **semi-permeable membrane**, to equalise or at least minimise, the difference in concentrations. Semi-permeable membranes are very common in the body and are effectively permeable to solvents but not to solutes. Osmosis is a specialised form of diffusion.

The **osmotic pressure** of a solution is the pressure needed to prevent osmosis from happening and it is proportional to the **number of particles** (not the size of the particles), both ions and undissociated molecules (e.g. protein), in the solution.

In general, isotonic solutions (Table 22.2) are used for parenteral administration, although hypertonic solutions are occasionally given intravenously. When fluids are administered to an animal, by whatever route, they initially enter the extracellular fluid (ECF), see below. If hypertonic solutions are added to the ECF, water will be drawn out of the cells into the ECF, causing cells to shrink in size and resulting in cellular dehydration. Conversely, if hypotonic solutions are added to the ECF, water may move into the cells, resulting in cellular swelling and possible lysis of the cells.

Protein molecules contribute to the osmotic pressure of certain body fluids, because they cannot diffuse freely across semi-permeable or cell membranes due to their large size. In contrast, both water and salts can move freely across biological membranes by osmosis and diffusion. Consequently, there is a steady osmotic pressure exerted by the protein that is referred to as the **effective osmotic pressure** (also called the colloid osmotic pressure or oncotic pressure). The osmotic pressure exerted by the blood proteins, primarily albumin, maintains the difference between the osmotic pressure of the plasma and the interstitial fluid. This difference is important in maintaining an adequate volume of fluid within the blood vessels. Similarly, non-diffusible proteins within the cells contribute to the effective intracellular osmotic pressure.

Body water

On average, the water content of the adult body is 60% by weight, ranging from 50–70% in normal healthy animals. The water content of the body varies with:

- **Age**. The water content of the body of young animals may be as much as 70–80%, while in older animals it may be as little as 50–55% of bodyweight. Such details highlight the importance of prompt and adequate fluid therapy in neonatal and young animals suffering from excessive fluid losses, especially as their kidneys are less efficient at producing concentrated urine.
- **Nutritional status**. The body water content is affected by the proportion of fat to lean tissue in the body since fatty tissue contains a much smaller amount of water than does other organs and soft tissues. To avoid the danger of over hydration, fluid therapy in obese animals should

Table 22.2 Terms relating to osmotic pressure of solutions		
Term	**Definition**	**Example**
Isotonic	An isotonic solution exerts equal osmotic pressure to body fluid	0.9% NaCl (normal saline)
Hypertonic	A hypertonic solution exerts greater osmotic pressure to body fluid	Hypertonic saline (7.5% NaCl) 10% dextrose
Hypotonic	A hypotonic solution exerts lower osmotic pressure to body fluid	Sterile water 0.45% NaCl

be based on the requirement of their ideal bodyweight, as they will have a slightly lower requirement than that calculated from their actual bodyweight.

Body water distribution

Almost two-thirds of the total body water is located inside the cells of the tissues (**intracellular fluid**; ICF), while the remaining one-third is located outside the cells (**extracellular fluid**; ECF). The ECF may be further divided into **intravascular fluid** (IVF), which is the water contained within the blood vessels, **interstitial fluid** (ISF) which is present in the spaces between the cells (also within dense connective tissue, bone, cartilage) and **transcellular fluids** (TCF) which are specialised fluids formed by active secretory mechanisms but comprising only a very small proportion of the ECF, e.g. cerebrospinal fluid, gastrointestinal secretions, etc. The distribution of body water into its principal compartments is shown in Fig. 22.1.

The composition of body fluids

The intracellular fluid and the extracellular fluid differ both in composition and function, although the interstitial fluid and the intravascular fluid are similar in composition (Tables 22.3 and 22.4). Transcellular fluid composition reflects its specialised function and may bear no resemblance to any other body fluid.

Plasma contains sodium (Na^+) as the main cation, with smaller amounts of potassium (K^+), calcium (Ca^{2+}) and magnesium (Mg^{2+}). Chloride (Cl^-) and bicarbonate (HCO_3^-) are the main anions with small amounts of phosphate (PO_4^{2-}) and protein. In all body fluids the number of positive charges must equal the number of negative charges so that an electrical gradient does not exist.

Normal blood capillaries have only a limited permeability and the large protein molecules cannot pass easily through this barrier. Therefore, ISF is an **ultrafiltrate** of plasma and contains everything found in plasma except proteins.

The intracellular fluid has potassium (K^+) and magnesium (Mg^{2+}) as its main cations and relatively small amounts of sodium. The major anions are phosphate (PO_4^{2-}) and protein. There is also some bicarbonate (HCO_3^-) and chloride (Cl^-) in the ICF.

Sodium is sometimes referred to as the 'osmotic skeleton' of the ECF, maintaining the volume of the ECF against the osmotic pull of the ICF. Protein, primarily albumin, acts in a similar manner within the blood vessels. Blood pressure (also known as hydrostatic pressure) tends to force fluid out of the arteriole end of capillaries and into the ISF, while the protein within the plasma acts to pull this fluid back into the capillaries at the venule end. Excess fluid in the interstitium is transported back into the intravascular space via the lymphatic system.

Table 22.3 The main cations and anions of body fluids		
Fluid compartment	Main cations	Main anions
Extracellular fluid (ECF)	Sodium, calcium	Chloride, bicarbonate
Interstitial fluid (ISF)	Sodium, calcium	Chloride, bicarbonate
Intravascular fluid (IVF or plasma water)	Sodium, calcium	Chloride, bicarbonate
Intracellular fluid	Potassium, magnesium	Phosphate, protein

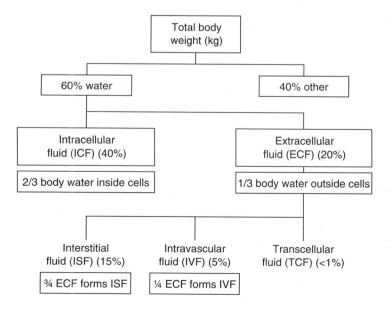

Fig. 22.1 The distribution of body water into its principal compartments.

Table 22.4 The approximate composition of intravascular fluid, interstitial fluid and intracellular fluid (mmol/l)

	Intravascular fluid	Interstitial fluid	Intracellular fluid
Cations			
Sodium	138	130	10
Potassium	4	4	110
Calcium	2.5	1.5	—
Magnesium	1	1	15
Anions			
Chloride	102	110	10
Bicarbonate	27	27	10
Protein	17	—	50
Phosphate	1	1	26

Body water and electrolyte balance

Dogs and cats require the following nutrients (in varying quantities) in order to live:

- Water.
- Protein.
- Carbohydrate.
- Fat.
- Vitamins.
- Minerals.

Water is often neglected as an essential nutritional requirement because of the ready availability of it in the UK! However, the majority of the bodyweight in dogs and cats is attributable to water.

Some functions of water in the body

- Solvent.
- Transport (of solutes, cells and gases).
- Temperature regulation.
- Digestion (many substances are digested by hydrolysis which requires water).

Body water and electrolyte balance

The water content within the body is a balance of the amount of water that is acquired by the body with the amount of water that is lost by the body. The normal healthy animal is able to match efficiently the intake and output of water and principal electrolytes.

Water is acquired and lost in a number of different ways.

Water intake The main methods by which animals gain fluids normally are:

- **Drinking water or other fluids**. Dogs and cats drink when they are thirsty. Thirst is controlled by the hypothalamus within the brain and is under voluntary control. Receptors within the mouth and throat are activated when they become dry and stimulate the sensation of thirst through activation of the thirst centre within the hypothalamus. In addition, osmoreceptors within the hypothalamus itself detect changes in the tonicity (concentration) of the blood leading to thirst and the release of angiotensin following hypovolaemia has a similar effect.
- **Eating**. Most moist or wet diets have significant water content. Dry diets may contain as little as 6–10% water.
- **Metabolism**. Metabolism of food within the body releases water as a by-product (providing 10–20% total fluid intake). Hydrogen within foods (protein, fat and carbohydrate) combines with oxygen to produce water. The amount of water produced depends on the type of food and how completely metabolised the food is (e.g. oxidation of fat produces more water than carbohydrate which in turn produces more water than protein).
- **Therapeutic**. Animals are occasionally administered fluid parenterally.

The majority of fluid is acquired through drinking and eating. Metabolic water contributes only a small amount.

Water loss The main methods by which dogs and cats lose water from the body normally are

- **Urination**. The normal kidney is able to regulate water loss. Fluid and electrolytes are lost.
- **Defecation**. The amount of fluid lost in faeces is surprisingly small. This is because the normal gastrointestinal tract has very efficient mechanisms for reabsorption of water. Fluid and electrolytes are lost.
- **Respiration**. Water is lost from the respiratory tract by evaporation. This happens normally during breathing and panting because air is humidified as it passes along the tracheobronchial tree and nasal passages. Fluid is lost.
- **Sweating**. Although sweating can cause significant water loss in some species, this is not the case in dogs and cats that sweat from the footpads only. The amount of fluid lost via this route is influenced by ambient temperature, humidity, activity and fever. Fluid and electrolytes are lost.

The fluid lost from the body by urination is sometimes referred to as **sensible** fluid loss. Because we do not see the water lost by other means (respiration and sweating), this is referred to as **insensible** or **inevitable** fluid loss.

In many situations an animal's ability to control body fluid balance will be compromised. Water intake may be abnormally increased or decreased by:

- Change in diet.
- Metabolic disorders.
- Anaesthesia (pre-operative fasting/general anaesthesia/recovery).
- Systemic illness.
- Mechanical difficulty (fractured jaw).
- Water deprivation.

Similarly, fluid loss may be different from normal because of:

- Altered urine production (e.g. renal disease).
- Altered faecal losses (e.g. diarrhoea an additional 4 ml/kg per stool or up to 200 ml/kg per day in severe cases).
- Vomiting (e.g. an additional 4 ml/kg per incident).
- Increased respiratory losses (e.g. excessive panting due to respiratory disease).
- Transudates, modified transudates and exudates (pyometra, burns, open wounds, peritonitis).
- Surgery (increased evaporative fluid losses from surgical sites).
- Blood loss.
- Lactation.

Therefore to maintain a normal water balance in a healthy dog or cat, a total of approximately 50 ml/kg/day of fluid is required (range 40–60 ml/kg/day) (Table 22.5).

As already mentioned, the inevitable water losses from the respiratory tract and skin cannot be regulated; however, within the body the **kidneys** play an important role in the regulation of not only water and electrolytes, but also of acid–base balance. At times of reduced intake or increased loss of water the osmotic concentration of the body fluids increases and the volume of the ECF, more specifically the intravascular fluid, is depleted. This has two effects on the animal. Firstly, the animal will become thirsty because of stimulation of thirst centres within the hypothalamus. Secondly, the increase in plasma osmotic concentration will be detected by **osmoreceptors** (cells which are sensitive to osmotic changes in the intravascular fluid) that stimulate the release of a hormone that is stored in the posterior pituitary, **antidiuretic hormone** (ADH). Release of ADH promotes the reabsorption of water from the renal tubules and this will increase the concentration of the urine that is voided. Conversely, if the osmotic concentration of the plasma is reduced, less ADH will be released and less water will be reabsorbed within the kidney, the urine becoming more dilute. In addition, a reduction in intravascular fluid will be detected directly by the kidneys as a reduction in renal perfusion. This stimulates the release of a kidney hormone, **renin**, generating **angiotensin** in the blood. In turn, angiotensin stimulates the release of **aldosterone** from the adrenal cortex. Aldosterone acts on the kidney to increase the reabsorption of sodium within the distal convoluted tubule, and thence water, resulting in more concentrated urine (see Fig. 22.2).

Urine specific gravity (USG) measures the solute concentration in urine and assesses the ability of the renal tubules to concentrate or dilute the glomerular filtrate. Urine specific gravity is a measurement of the density of urine compared to pure water. The number of molecules in urine, as well as their molecular weight and size influence the USG, therefore it only approximates solute concentration. Urine specific gravity may be measured by a refractometer, urinometer or dipstick.

The specific gravity of distilled water is 1.000. In dogs a urine specific gravity of greater than 1.030 and in cats a urine specific gravity of greater than 1.035 indicates adequate renal tubular concentrating ability.

Table 22.5 Fluid loss

Source of fluid loss	Volume of fluid loss (average) (ml/kg/24 hours)
Respiratory/cutaneous losses	20
Urinary loss (normal range)	20
Faecal loss (normal faeces)	10
Total	**50**

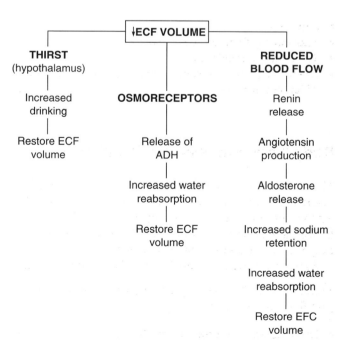

Fig. 22.2 Mechanisms involved in the restoration of extracellular fluid volume.

Urine specific gravity is affected by:

- Antidiuretic hormone and aldosterone concentrations.
- Temperature (USG decreases with increasing temperatures).
- Urinary concentrations of glucose.
- Urinary concentrations of protein.
- Urinary concentrations of sodium chloride and other crystalloids.
- Urinary concentrations of blood urea nitrogen (BUN).
- Drug administration (corticosteroids).
- Systemic illness (e.g. diabetes insipidus, Addison's disease, hepatopathy, etc.).

USG: TERMS AND DEFINITIONS
- **Isosthenuria**. Urine specific gravity and osmolality are the same as the glomerular filtrate/plasma (1.008–1.015). If the animal is azotaemic or dehydrated, isosthenuria is abnormal and indicates altered renal function.
- **Hyposthenuria**. Decreased urine specific gravity and osmolality, USG<1.015.
- **Hypersthenuria**. Urine specific gravity >1.015.

The management of water balance is probably more important than the regulation of electrolyte status. However, electrolytes too are delicately balanced within the body, and the balance of sodium, potassium, chloride and bicarbonate is the most important. Conditions that cause an increased loss of water may also cause loss of electrolytes. In the normal animal the daily requirement for sodium is approximately 1 mmol/kg/day and for potassium 2 mmol/kg/day.

Recording the daily intake and loss of fluid in veterinary patients is an important part of patient care, especially in those animals suffering from water and electrolyte imbalances. Recording methods will range from simply monitoring the drinking and urinary habits of elective surgical patients to accurate observations of volumes of fluid consumed orally and administered parenterally, measurement of urine and faecal output and recording of abnormal losses. Water balance ideally should be recorded on a chart detailing route of administration, type and volume of fluid given with details of fluid losses also provided. Each page would represent a 24-hour period and a glance at the chart would then be a useful guide to both the nurses and clinicians of each animal's fluid status (Fig. 22.3).

Disturbances of water and/or electrolyte balance

Many medical conditions and surgical interventions can disrupt the body's water and/or electrolyte status. Such conditions arise through altered intake or output of water and/or electrolytes. **Dehydration** is the term used to describe a reduction in the total body water and the signs and symptoms associated with such a loss. Dehydration can be caused by a loss of water only, which is known as **primary water depletion.** Primary water depletion is common where water intake is reduced or absent because of continued inevitable water losses, e.g. during excessive panting or when an animal is deprived of drinking water. In addition, certain disease states can cause a primary water depletion, e.g. diabetes insipidus. More commonly, water losses are accompanied by electrolyte losses, especially sodium, which is the main cation of the ECF, and this is referred to as **mixed water/electrolyte depletion**. The losses that are incurred during vomiting and diarrhoea include water, sodium, chloride and bicarbonate depletion. If diarrhoea is prolonged, potassium is also lost. In haemorrhage, protein, haemoglobin, platelets and clotting factors are lost in addition to water and electrolytes.

In conditions where urinary output has failed, e.g. blocked urethra, ruptured urinary bladder and acute renal failure, metabolites and electrolytes that are normally excreted in the urine accumulate within the body. In addition, insensible losses lead to water depletion. Therefore, the fluid imbalance that is present is very complicated and relates mainly to water loss, elevated serum potassium levels and acidosis.

A list of the common diseases and the principal fluid disorders they cause are given in Table 22.6.

Assessing fluid requirements

It is important to assess the degree of dehydration and the state of the circulation prior to initiating fluid therapy. There are a number of clinical and laboratory methods which may be used to establish the amount of fluid which is required by an individual animal.

History

A good history enables an accurate assessment of fluid deficits to be made. Questions about food and water consumption (anorexia, polydipsia), any gastrointestinal losses (vomiting, diarrhoea), urinary losses (polyuria, oliguria), abnormal discharges (open pyometra) and traumatic losses (blood loss, burns) should be sought from the owner.

Physical examination

Clinical signs are a useful, but not always accurate, means of assessing dehydration. Signs such as loss of skin elasticity and sunken eye do not start to appear until the

FLUID THERAPY MONITORING CHART

OWNERS NAME	ANIMALS NAME		
ADDRESS	BREED		
CONTACT TEL.	SEX	AGE	WEIGHT

DATE   VET NAME

REASON FOR ADMISSION   FLUID FOR INITIAL INFUSION

MAINTENANCE REQUIREMENT   _____

DEFICIT (dehydration/losses)   _____

TOTAL REQUIREMENT   _____   TO BE INFUSED OVER _____ HOURS

DRIP FACTOR: 20 drops/ml or 60 drops/ml or Blood at 15 drops/ml. (Circle as appropriate)

CALCULATION: total requirement (mls) × DRIP FACTOR (drops/ml) divided by time of infusion in minutes

Time	Bag size	Fluid type	Due to finish	Drip rate	Fluid total	MONITORING & COMMENTS				OUTPUT			
						Patient weight	T	P	R	COMMENTS	V+	D+	Urine	Discharges

Fig. 22.3 Example of a fluid therapy monitoring chart.

animal is approximately 5% dehydrated, and animals 15% dehydrated animals are moribund. It is important to remember when assessing the elasticity of the skin that in cachectic animals it is generally reduced, even when they are not dehydrated, while fat animals will lose their skin elasticity when more severely dehydrated than an animal of normal weight. Intermediate changes are described in Table 22.7.

EXAMPLE

10% dehydration in a 20 kg dog represents the following fluid deficit:

- 10% × 20 kg × 10 = 2000 ml. It is important to realise that the percentage loss is relative to bodyweight not body water.
- Using Table 22.8 (see italics). 100 ml per kg bodyweight = 100 ml × 20 kg = 2000 ml.

Table 22.6 Causes of the principal fluid abnormalities

(1) **Primary water depletion**
   Prolonged inappetence (fractured jaw, head or neck injury, etc.)
   Water unavailable (forgetful/neglectful owners)
   Unconsciousness (coma)
   Fever or excessive panting
   Diabetes insipidus

(2) **Water and electrolyte depletion**
   Vomiting
   Diarrhoea
   'Third space' losses (intestinal obstruction, peritonitis)
   Pyometra
   Wound drainage

(3) **Whole blood loss**
   Internal haemorrhage
   External haemorrhage
   Surgical losses

(4) **Potassium depletion**
   Prolonged inappetance (starvation)
   Vomiting
   Prolonged diarrhoea
   Prolonged diuretic therapy

(5) **Potassium accumulation**
   Ruptured urinary bladder
   Urethral obstruction
   Acute renal failure
   Addison's disease

Laboratory analyses

There are some simple laboratory tests that can be helpful in estimating losses.

Packed cell volume (PCV)

The PCV is an inexpensive but revealing parameter. For each 1% increase in the PCV, a fluid loss of approximately

Table 22.7 Clinical signs associated with dehydration	
Percentage dehydration	Clinical signs
< 5	No detectable clinical signs Increasing urine concentration
5–6	Subtle loss of skin elasticity (skin tent)
6–8	Marked loss of skin elasticity Slightly prolonged capillary refill time Slightly sunken eyes Dry mucous membranes
10–12	Tented skin stands in place Prolonged capillary refill time (> 2 seconds) Sunken eyes/protrusion of third eyelid Dry mucous membranes Early signs of shock (see later)
12–15	Signs of shock (see later) Moribund Death imminent

Table 22.8 Dehydration and fluid deficit	
Dehydration (%)	Fluid deficit (ml per kg bodyweight)
5 ($\leq$ = mild)	50
8 (≤ 8 = moderate)	80
10 (≤ 10 = marked)	*100*
12 (≥ 10 = shock)	120

10 ml/kg bodyweight has occurred. Rarely will the normal PCV of the patient be known, and therefore an estimate of 45% is made in dogs and 35% in cats.

Example If a 20 kg dog was found to have a PCV of 55%, the deficit should be calculated thus:

$$20\,kg \times 10\,ml/kg/\% \times (55\text{–}45\%) = 2000\,ml$$

The equation is unreliable where pre-existing anaemia is present unless the PCV prior to fluid loss is known. Similarly, acute blood cannot be evaluated by the PCV unless compensation has taken place or fluid has already been administered to replace the loss.

Haemoglobin

Dehydration will also result in an increase in the haemoglobin concentration of the blood and again care must be taken when interpreting results from an anaemic animal.

Total plasma protein (TPP)

Dehydration will cause a rise in TPP, but care must be taken because a dehydrated hypoproteinaemic animal may present with an apparently normal TPP. It is useful to assess both the TPP and PCV in an animal that has been diagnosed clinically as dehydrated because only rarely will pre-existing disease result in an elevation of both these parameters.

Blood urea and creatinine

Blood urea and creatinine levels will rise in the dehydrated animal (pre-renal azotaemia), but it is important to consider the possibility of renal disease that can also result in an elevation in these two parameters. Consequently, these parameters should be interpreted in the light of the urine specific gravity.

Plasma electrolytes

Estimation of the plasma electrolyte level (e.g. Na^+, K^+, Cl^-), is possible but is frequently of limited value as recorded values are not always an accurate reflection of the total body content of the individual ion. However, determination of serum potassium concentration is of value because a marked deficit of this ion can result in severe muscle weakness and cardiac disturbances, and equally an excess of this ion can also result in fatal cardiac dysrythmias.

Acid–base estimations

For details of assessment of acid–base balance see later.

Clinical assessment

These measurements can be used to estimate fluid deficits, but are more frequently used to monitor progress of fluid therapy and response to treatment in intensive care patients.

Bodyweight

Bodyweight is easily measured and acute losses may be due to fluid loss or catabolism (expected daily weight loss in an anorexic animal is 0.5–0.1% bodyweight). Acute increases in bodyweight are nearly always caused by increased fluid content.

Central venous pressure (CVP)

The CVP is a useful means of estimating the need for fluids in any situation but especially in congestive cardiac failure or where circulatory overload may be a problem (acute renal failure). Following severe, acute haemorrhage and in shock, CVP is invaluable in determining the adequacy of replacement fluid therapy.

The CVP is a measurement of the pressure in the right atrium, i.e. the chamber of the heart to which all the venous blood is returned. A long catheter is placed aseptically in a jugular vein, and advanced until the tip of the catheter lies within the chest. Ideally, the catheter should lie in the right atrium itself, but it is often located within the cranial vena cava that will reflect changes in the right atrial pressure. The catheter is connected to a water manometer and the CVP is measured in centimetres of water (cm H_2O).

Urinary output

Measuring urinary output is a useful means of assessing the adequacy of fluid replacement. As already discussed, urine output is low during dehydration (**oliguria**), and the return of normal urine output signifies that replacement is adequate. Urine output can be monitored casually by observation, but placing an indwelling urinary catheter allows accurate measurement of output. Normal urine output is 1–2 ml/kg/hour. A urine output of less than 0.5 ml/kg/hour is defined as oliguria. If fluid therapy fails to improve the urine output in an oliguric animal, the possibility of acute renal failure should be considered.

Acid–base balance

In a similar way to water and electrolyte balance, the acid–base balance is a closely guarded parameter which can be upset at times of disease. Within the body hydrogen ions are produced as a result of normal metabolic activity, and the body's acid–base status is a measure of the hydrogen ion concentration within its tissues. Hydrogen ions are measured according to the pH scale. The **pH** is defined as the negative logarithm (to the base 10) of the hydrogen ion concentration. The pH scale has a range of 1–14 and a pH of 7 is regarded as neutral, while pH of greater than 7 are alkaline and pH less than 7 are acidic.

In the normal animal, blood is slightly alkaline – it has a normal range of **pH 7.35–7.45**. When the pH of the blood falls below 7.35 a state of **acidaemia** is said to exist, whereas when the pH of the blood greater than 7.45 a state of **alkalaemia** is said to exist.

Acidosis and **alkalosis** describe abnormal processes and conditions that cause acidaemia or alkalaemia respectively if there are no secondary (or compensatory) changes in response to these processes and conditions. Acidosis and alkalosis can exist without producing acidaemia/alkalaemia because of the body's secondary compensatory mechanisms. Acidosis and alkalosis may be either **metabolic** or **respiratory** depending on their origin.

It is essential for proper cellular function that the blood pH is kept within the normal range. Large changes in pH may result in the animal becoming depressed and may ultimately lead to its death. Therefore the body has efficient mechanisms for dealing with the hydrogen ions that are produced within the body to prevent dramatic fluctuations of pH. There are three principal means of dealing with hydrogen ions, and these systems work in sequence to try and limit the effects of changes in hydrogen ion concentration. **Buffers** are the first to respond to alterations in the pH, followed by a **respiratory response** and finally a **renal response**.

Buffering

Buffers are able to react with acids and bases and reduce the extent of the pH change that they would normally produce. In the body, buffers act by trapping H^+ ions rather than eliminating them from the body. Buffers are required to keep pH within narrow limits until the H^+ ions can be delivered to either the lungs or to the kidneys, where they can be removed from the body. In general, buffers are weak acids or proteins. Because weak acids do not dissociate completely in water (unlike strong acids such as hydrochloric acid, HCl) they restrict the number of H^+ ions in solution, whereas proteins (such as haemoglobin) act as anions and have many sites to which cations such as H^+ ions may bind. Most buffering that occurs within the body occurs within cells, and proteins are among the most important intracellular buffers. Extracellular buffers include bicarbonate (HCO_3^-) and phosphate (HPO_4^{2-}).

$$H^+ + HCO_3^- \longleftrightarrow H_2CO_3 \longleftrightarrow CO_2 + H_2O$$

$$\text{Carbonic acid} \quad \text{Carbonic anhydrase}$$

$$H^+ + HPO_4^{2-} \longleftrightarrow H_2PO_4^-$$

The reaction which converts bicarbonate (HCO_3^-) to carbonic acid (H_2CO_3) does not become saturated in the same way as the phosphate reaction because the action of the enzyme carbonic anhydrase upon the carbonic acid results in the formation of carbon dioxide and water, both of which can be expelled from the body (or in the case of water incorporated in the body water).

Respiratory system

The respiratory system controls the level of carbon dioxide within the body. Carbon dioxide is in equilibrium with carbonic acid in solution in the body fluids. Increasing respiration will remove carbon dioxide from the body and therefore reduce acidity. Decreasing respiration will retain carbon dioxide and therefore, increase acidity.

It has already been noted that the reaction which converts bicarbonate (HCO_3^-) to carbonic acid (H_2CO_3) does not become saturated because of a build-up of water and carbon dioxide (see above); however, the reaction may be limited by the amount of available bicarbonate.

Renal system

Bicarbonate can be generated within the cells of the kidney by a reversal of the reaction that results in the formation of water and carbon dioxide.

$$CO_2 + H_2O \longleftrightarrow H_2CO_3 \longleftrightarrow H^+ + HCO_3^-$$

The bicarbonate that is generated enters the ECF pool, while the H^+ ions that are generated are excreted.

The pH of the body fluids is dependent upon the concentration of carbon dioxide and bicarbonate ions within the body.

$$pH = \frac{[HCO_3^-]}{pCO_2}$$

Therefore, the pH will fall if there is an increase in the concentration of carbon dioxide within the body, a fall of bicarbonate ions within the body or if H^+ ions are added to the system. Conversely, reducing the concentration of bicarbonate ions within the body, adding bicarbonate ions to the system or removing H^+ ions will cause an increase in the pH.

Acid–base abnormalities

To estimate acid–base balance an arterial blood sample is required, although venous blood samples can provide useful information if an arterial sample cannot be taken. In dogs and cats, arterial blood is generally taken from either the femoral artery, or a superficial branch of the femoral artery. The anticoagulant that is used is heparin, and the sample should be drawn anaerobically. If the arterial blood is not analysed immediately, it should be stored on ice, or at 4°C, until analysis. Analysis of the blood will give the pH of the sample, the bicarbonate ion concentration and the carbon dioxide tension (a measure of the amount of carbon dioxide within the sample), and from this information the clinician will be able to establish what deficits are present.

Acid–base abnormalities are not uncommon during disease and Table 22.9 shows the four major disturbances that can occur and the situations in which they are likely to arise. **Respiratory acidosis** arises through inadequate ventilation, or a failure of the respiratory system to respond to increased levels of carbon dioxide that are characteristic of rebreathing or increased production. Buffers will lessen the pH disturbance but renal compensation will only occur when the condition becomes long standing. **Respiratory alkalosis** occurs much less frequently than respiratory acidosis in veterinary practice.

Metabolic acidosis arises when acid metabolites are retained within the body or when the loss of buffer is marked. Respiratory compensation is rapid but incomplete, and ultimately the kidneys must restore balance, either by excreting hydrogen ions, retaining bicarbonate, or both. **Metabolic alkalosis** again occurs much less frequently.

The treatment of the various acid–base abnormalities should be directed at the source of the problem initially. Respiratory acidosis and alkalosis require therapy aimed at correcting the ventilatory disturbance. Metabolic acidosis can be ameliorated by providing extra buffer in the form of sodium bicarbonate (usually 1–2 mEq/kg IV is adequate). Often, reduced renal perfusion is the cause of a metabolic

Table 22.9 Causes of acid–base abnormalities	
Metabolic acidosis	
Accumulation of H^+	Shock
	Ruptured bladder/blocked urethra
	Diabetic keto-acidosis
	Aspirin/ethylene glycol poisoning
Loss of base (bicarbonate)	Chronic renal failure
	Chronic diarrhoea
Metabolic alkalosis	
Loss of H^+	Prepyloric vomiting
Accumulation of base (bicarbonate)	Overadministration of sodium bicarbonate
Respiratory acidosis	
Impaired ventilation	General anaesthesia
	CNS injuries (cerebral oedema)
	Severe lung damage
	Certain nerve/muscle diseases
Inspired carbon dioxide	Anaesthetic equipment
Increased carbon dioxide production	Malignant hyperthermia
Respiratory alkalosis	
Overventilation	Mechanical/manual ventilation
	Apprehensive/pain/fear

acidosis and using fluid therapy to restore renal perfusion will be sufficient to correct the abnormality.

Objectives of fluid therapy

The purpose of fluid therapy is to replace deficits from previous losses, improve and maintain renal function, supply maintenance requirements and provide for ongoing losses.

The most important initial treatment is to restore an adequate circulating volume, as severely dehydrated animals may be showing signs of shock (see later). After this, the remaining deficit can be replaced more slowly. In general, existing deficits should be replaced within the first 24 hours after admission. Thereafter, it is important to remember that while the animal is undergoing treatment, provision must be made to replace the continued inevitable and urinary losses as well as any continuing abnormal losses, e.g. diarrhoea.

Routes of administration of fluids

Oral fluid administration

If an animal is willing to drink, is not vomiting and does not have an intestinal obstruction, the oral route of fluid administration is a simple, cheap and painless method to treat an animal with mild dehydration. In addition, it is an ideal route by which to supply daily maintenance fluid requirements after initial deficits have been replaced. Moreover, the animal does not need to be hospitalised, allowing the owner to take the animal home.

The intestine acts as a barrier for selective absorption of water and electrolytes, providing a wide margin of safety. However, there are a number of disadvantages and if an animal is severely dehydrated, the oral route is not the route of choice. Although administering fluid orally does not require absolute sterility, only a limited range of fluids can be given (it is inappropriate for whole blood or plasma expanders such as dextrans), and it can be time consuming.

Where prehension is limited or impossible, oral therapy is not ruled out and fluid may be administered either by naso-oesophageal tube, pharyngostomy tube, oesophagostomy tube or gastrostomy tube. A **naso-oesophageal tube**, lubricated with a local anaesthetic gel, may be passed via the nostril to the distal oesophagus, and fluids given directly into the stomach. A **pharyngostomy tube** must be placed under anaesthesia via an incision in the skin of the neck. The tube is introduced via the pharynx into the oesophagus, allowing fluid and food to be administered. A **gastrostomy tube** again must be positioned under general anaesthesia, and is placed directly into the stomach via an incision in the left flank. Again, fluid and food may be administered through this tube. **Oesophagostomy tubes** are becoming more popular and are simpler to place than gastrostomy

tubes. In general, enteral feeding tubes are well tolerated by animals.

Isotonic or hypotonic fluids are recommended for oral administration to prevent the movement of water out of the ECF and into the bowel. A solution containing 120 mmol/l sodium chloride in 2% glucose will produce enhanced absorption of sodium and increased uptake of water. This can be prepared by mixing a teaspoonful of salt and a dessertspoon of glucose in 2 pints of water. There are many commercially available oral rehydration solutions available, and in general they use a similar principle to that described although some include glycine to further promote electrolyte and water absorption.

> *PRACTICAL TIP*
> The gastric capacity of the dog and cat is as follows:
> - Dog: 90 ml/kg.
> - Cat:
>   0.5–1.0 kg: 100 ml/kg.
>   1.0–1.5 kg: 70 ml/kg.
>   1.5–4.0 kg: 60 ml/kg.
>   4.0–6.0 kg: 45 ml/kg.

Subcutaneous administration (hypodermoclysis)

Subcutaneous administration of fluids is practical in small animals, where the animal is only mildly dehydrated and fluids cannot be administered orally. Because absorption from this route tends to be slow, especially where peripheral vasoconstriction is present, it is unsuitable for severely dehydrated animals. Only sterile isotonic electrolyte solutions, e.g. Hartmann's, should be administered subcutaneously, and only small volumes should be given at one time (10–20 ml/kg per site). Complete absorption of the fluid may take 6–8 hours. If fluid is not completely absorbed within this time an alternative route of fluid administration should be selected (e.g. intravenous). Repeated administration can be painful, and in addition there is a risk of skin infection or skin slough.

Intraperitoneal administration

The intraperitoneal route of fluid administration shares many of the advantages and disadvantages of the subcutaneous route, and should only be used where the animal is mildly dehydrated and fluids cannot be administered orally. It is best suited to neonatal dogs and cats and small mammals where intravenous access may be difficult. Hypotonic or isotonic electrolyte solutions may be administered intraperitoneally and the large adsorptive capacity of the peritoneum makes it a more efficient route of administration, but absorption is reduced during shock. Because of the risk of infection it is important that all manipulations are carried out aseptically, and great care must be taken not to puncture any of the abdominal organs.

To administer fluids intraperitoneally the animal is held almost vertically with its hindlimbs on the ground, and a second person aseptically introduces a short needle or catheter into the abdomen, just behind the umbilicus and in a cranial direction.

Intravenous fluid therapy

> ### INTRAVENOUS FLUID THERAPY
> Advantages:
> - Rapid administration of fluids intravascularly.
> - Large volumes of fluid may be administered.
> - Hypertonic solutions may be administered.
> - Plasma expanders may be administered.
> - Blood products may be administered.
>
> Disadvantages:
> - Risk of side-effects (phlebitis, thrombophlebitis, bacteraemia, thrombosis).
> - Specialised equipment necessary.
> - Training in technique required.
> - Risk of overhydration.
> - Patient interference.

A number of veins may be used to administer fluids intravenously:

- Cephalic and accessory cephalic.
- Lateral saphenous.
- Medial saphenous (particularly useful in cats).
- External jugular.
- Auricular (particularly useful in rabbits).

There are a number of different ways of administering fluids intravenously:

- **Needles** are inexpensive but are unsuitable for intravenous fluid administration. They are dislodged easily, and the sharp point will not only irritate the wall of the vein, but can penetrate the other side of the vein, thus delivering the fluid perivenously (extravasation).
- **Butterfly needles** (scalp vein sets) are safer because they can be secured to the limb more easily and are less likely to become dislodged. However, the sharp point of the needle may still irritate the wall of the vein. They are not suitable for long-term fluid administration.
- **Over-the-needle catheters** or cannulae are extremely useful in peripheral veins although they can also be used in the jugular vein of small dogs and cats. They can be secured to the limb and are less likely to become dislodged than needles. Moreover, the smooth tip of the catheter is less likely to cause phlebitis than needles or butterfly needles.

- **Through-the-needle catheters** or cannulae are longer and therefore, more appropriate for use in the external jugular vein. They are the only catheters suitable for monitoring central venous pressure.

Equipment required for placing an over-the-needle intravenous catheter:

- Hand-washing facilities: hands should be washed before commencing skin preparation and again before placement of the catheter.
- Assistant to restrain animal and raise vein as appropriate.
- Disposable gloves: gloves should be worn during skin preparation, discarded, and replaced following hand washing prior to catheter placement.
- Electric clippers: hair should be clipped liberally from the site of catheter placement ensuring that the barrel of the catheter will not contact contaminated hair or skin during insertion. In addition, fenestrated drapes may be used to limit contamination during placement of jugular catheters.
- Chlorhexidine- or povidone–iodine based surgical scrub.
- Sterile water or spirit (70%).
- Cotton wool or surgical swabs: the skin should be cleansed and prepared in a similar manner to a surgical site.
- Sterile No. 11 scalpel blade or hypodermic needle: to minimise the chances of catheter tip flaring during insertion, a small full thickness skin incision may be created directly over the point of catheter insertion.
- Suitable intravenous catheter: Fluid flows most rapidly through short, large-gauge catheters. Before catheter placement, the catheter may be primed with either sterile saline or heparinised saline. In any case the catheter plug or stopper should remain in place during catheterisation. Ensure that the bevel tip of the stylet extends beyond the end of the catheter. Just as when performing an intravenous injection the bevel of the stylet should be facing upwards as it is passed through the skin and into the lumen of the vein. Avoid touching the barrel of the catheter or the site of insertion directly. When the stylet enters the lumen of the vein, blood will appear in the clear flashback chamber (hub) at the distal end of the catheter. At this time the stylet is held steady as the catheter is advanced off the stylet and into the vein. There should be no resistance to this movement. Do not be tempted to pull the catheter back onto the stylet as this may cause the tip of the catheter to be sheared off and create a catheter embolus. Discard any catheters that develop flared or otherwise damaged tips. Because the tip of the stylet remains within the lumen of the catheter distally, blood spillage should be minimal.

  Over-the-needle catheters should be replaced at least every 48–72 hours. If long-term fluid administration is anticipated, a through-the-needle jugular catheter may be preferable.
- Syringe containing sterile saline for intravenous injection or heparinised saline: sterile saline or heparinised saline may be used both to confirm correct placement of the catheter and to flush the catheter following placement. Indwelling catheters used for intermittent drug adminis-

tration or blood sampling should be flushed through with heparinised saline (2–10 IU/ml) two to four times daily to maintain patency.

- Injection cap, three way tap, T-piece connector or primed administration set: Following insertion of the catheter, one of the above is placed to prevent blood flowing out of the catheter. Various other pieces of equipment are useful when intravenous fluids are being administered. Simple stylets are available that may be used to maintain patency of indwelling catheters when they are not in use, and are designed to remove the requirement for periodic heparinisation. These devices should be swabbed with alcohol (which is allowed to dry) before needle introduction or syringe attachment.
- Tape.
- Bandaging materials: once secured, the catheter and attachments are protected from patient interference by applying a soft dressing. It is important that the dressing is not constrictive. Bandages should be changed at least daily or more frequently if soiled by saliva, faeces, urine, vomit and discharges or if they otherwise become wet. At each bandage change, the site of insertion of the catheter should be inspected for signs of inflammation or infection. If unattended, many patients in addition may need Elizabethan collars or similar devices to limit patient interference with the catheter site.

Animals receiving fluid therapy will almost certainly have their physiological responses (temperature, pulse and respiration) monitored on a regular basis. In any event, patients with indwelling intravenous catheters similarly require twice daily evaluation. In the event of unexpected pyrexia, consider catheter related sepsis.

Indwelling intravenous catheters may be used for a number of other purposes in addition to fluid administration. These include:

- Drug administration.
- Blood sampling.
- Central venous pressure measurement.
- Administration of total peripheral or parenteral nutrition.

Equipment required for priming a fluid administration set:

- Hand-washing facilities: hands should be washed before commencing procedure.
- Gloves should be worn.
- Fluid for infusion (e.g. Hartmann's 500 ml or 1000 ml as appropriate): Check that the fluid bag selected contains the appropriate fluid, is still within the manufacturer's 'use by' date, is contained within sealed outer packaging and that the fluid within the bag is clear with no obvious contamination. Remove the fluid bag (or collapsible bottle) from the outer packaging and hang from the drip stand. Fluid may be warmed prior to administration.
- Fluid administration set: There are three main types of drip set (giving set or administration set) available. A normal administration set gives approximately 20 drops/ml. For smaller patients, a mini-drip fluid administration set (paediatric set) giving 60 drops/ml is useful

because it allows more accurate administration of small volumes. A burette often is incorporated into this type of set. This is useful when only small volumes of fluid are required, helping to prevent accidental overhydration. When blood is to be administered, a special blood administration set is required, which incorporates a nylon net filter to remove any aggregated red blood cells or other coagulation debris. A blood administration set gives approximately 15 drops/ml. Giving sets are supplied in sterile packaging and the number of drops per millilitre which they deliver will be written on the packaging and should be checked prior to calculating the drip rate.

A variety of automated infusion pumps and syringe drivers are available, which can be used to deliver a set amount of fluid over a defined period of time. These devices are usually fitted with an alarm system that will alert the nurse or clinician when the fluid line is obstructed, or when the fluid bag or syringe is empty. If infusion devices are used, it is important to remember that they are not a substitute for careful patient monitoring. In addition to infusion pumps and syringe drivers, drip rate counters may be purchased.

Select an appropriate fluid administration set, e.g. 60 drops/ml for smaller patients, filter administration set for blood products, and remove from the outer packaging. Position the roller clamp as required and place to the closed position. Prepare the fluid bag or bottle by removing the rip tab covering the port through which the stylet of the administration set is placed. Remove the cover from the administration set stylet and without touching the stylet with either your hands, or to the outside of the fluid bag, insert the stylet into the appropriate port on the fluid bag or bottle. Squeeze the drip chamber to allow fluid to flow into it and half fill it. The top drip chamber in filter administration sets should be filled completely, the second lower chamber being filled halfway. Without removing the protective cover from the patient end of the administration set, adjust the roller clamp and allow fluid to flow gently down the tubing until it reaches the patient end, ensuring that no bubbles are present. Close the roller clamp. The administration set is now primed and ready to use.

- Drip stand: extension tubing is available to lengthen the administration line and several extension sets may be used in sequence if required. A number of devices are also available to minimise kinking of the administration line tubing.

EXAMPLE

A 3 kg cat requires a total of 60 ml of fluid. The fluid is to be administered at 5 ml/kg/hour intravenously. A paediatric giving set that delivers 60 drops/ml is available. What flow rate (drops per minute) will be required?

$$\frac{60 \text{ drops/ml} \times 5 \text{ ml} \times 3 \text{ kg}}{60 \text{ minutes}} = 15 \text{ drops per minute} = 1 \text{ drop per 4 seconds}$$

Other methods of fluid administration

Rectal administration

This route of administration should not be used if an animal is suffering from diarrhoea, and is not suitable in severely dehydrated patients. Both isotonic and hypotonic fluids may be administered via this route, and sterility of fluid and equipment is not essential. It is important that the fluid is instilled into the colon and not into the rectum or an enema will result.

Intraosseous administration

Where it is difficult to place indwelling intravenous catheters, e.g. puppies, kittens, birds, adults with collapsed veins, intraosseous needles may be used. Fluid generally is administered by gravity flow into the medullary cavity of the chosen bone. The risk of severe infection must be considered.

A number of bone sites are suitable for placement of intraosseous needles including:

- Intertrochanteric fossa of the femur.
- Tibial crest.
- Greater tubercle of the humerus.
- Ilium.

Solutions commonly used in fluid therapy

Whole blood

RCVS guidelines do not allow the storage of whole blood or blood products, and blood collected from donor animals is generally used within a short period of time after collection. Blood for transfusion should be collected only from fit, healthy adult animals (cats should be FeLV, FIV and Haemobartonella negative), which have not previously been transfused. Approximately 10 ml/kg of blood may be collected from a donor dog, and a total of 30–40 ml from a cat. Animals should not be bled more than once in every 3–4 weeks. It is important that strict asepsis is observed when collecting the blood. Blood from a donor animal may be collected in commercially available collection sets containing an anticoagulant (either acid citrate dextrose (ACD) or citrate phosphate dextrose (CPD)) to prevent the blood from clotting. However, if the blood is to be used immediately, heparin or EDTA may be used as an anticoagulant. In cats, blood is generally collected into a syringe containing anticoagulant (0.14 ml CPD/ ml blood or heparin 2 IU/ml blood).

Blood is collected from the jugular vein in both dogs and cats, either by gravity flow or slow aspiration. As blood collects in the collection bag it must be agitated gently to prevent clotting. The volume of blood collected may be estimated by weighing the blood collection bag (1 gram = 1 ml).

Commercially available blood collection units contain sufficient anticoagulant for 450 ml of blood, and blood may be stored in these bags in the refrigerator until required. When ACD is used as the anticoagulant the blood may be stored at 4°C for a period of 3 weeks, whereas when CPD is used the blood may be stored for 4 weeks (see RCVS guidelines). Blood in which EDTA or heparin has been used as the anticoagulant should not be stored. When blood has been stored in the refrigerator, it should be warmed gently to a temperature of 37°C (and not greater than 40°C), prior to transfusion (see RCVS guidelines). Blood which has been stored in this manner is useful for replacement of red blood cells; however, where platelets are required, e.g. clotting abnormalities, blood must be given to the recipient immediately after collection.

Before infusion into the recipient animal, cross-matching and/or blood typing will have been carried out to ensure the blood is compatible for transfusion (Table 22.10). Although initial transfusion reactions are unusual, the A antigen is the most important factor in canine blood typing and ideally donor dogs should be A negative (DEA 1.1 negative). Most cats are type A, and there is < 40% chance of an incompatible reaction occurring if the blood is not typed prior to transfusion. Blood samples can be taken from both the donor and recipient animals for cross-matching to ensure compatibility before obtaining a large volume of blood from the donor. In-house blood typing kits are now available.

Indications for transfusion

- Haemorrhage – acute/chronic/internal/external.
- Anaemia – acute and chronic.
- Specific deficiencies – platelets, clotting factors.

Table 22.10 Blood cross-matching			
Cross-match type	**Donor**	**Recipient**	**Significance of agglutination or haemolysis**
Major cross-match	Red blood cells	Serum	Immediate transfusion reaction likely Delayed transfusion reaction possible
Minor cross-match	Serum	Red blood cells	Immediate transfusion reaction possible

Dangers associated with transfusion

- **Transfusion reactions** (Table 22.11). Transfusion reactions occur when incompatible blood is administered to an animal. The reaction is immune mediated and cross-matching or blood typing of donor and recipient blood can prevent this happening.
- **Pyrogenic reactions.** Fever due to pyrogens or bacteria in the blood or transfusion equipment. It is also possible to transfer viral and other agents, especially in cats.
- **Acidosis** (Metabolic.) After administration of stored blood.
- **Overadministration.** Causes circulatory overload (overhydration).
- **Air emboli.** This occurs infrequently when plastic blood collection bags are used, but is possible when blood is withdrawn using a syringe.
- **Citrate toxicity.** Hypocalcaemia.
- **Hypothermia.** Blood for transfusion should be administered at 37°C. Failure to do so may cause hypothermia in the recipient.

Blood products

- **Plasma.** If fresh blood can be obtained from donors, plasma may be extracted for immediate use. Blood should be centrifuged immediately after collection, and the plasma separated from the red blood cells. Remember to maintain sterility when transferring and decanting the plasma. Plasma is a useful replacement fluid in hypovolaemic animals and is suitable for animals that are hypoproteinaemic. Because plasma does not contain any red blood cells there is less risk of incompatibility reactions occurring.
- **Packed red blood cells.** Separated red cells (for example following the collection of plasma) can be given to animals that require red cell replacement. The red cells should be resuspended in an isotonic replacement fluid which does not contain calcium, e.g. 0.9 % NaCl, because calcium reacts with the citrate used to prevent clotting.

Plasma replacement fluids/colloids

When whole blood or plasma are unavailable, commercial plasma replacement fluids (colloids/plasma substitutes/plasma volume expanders) may be used. These fluids contain large molecules that will remain within the circulation, thus increasing the plasma's effective osmotic pressure and expanding plasma volume. These fluids may be used where there has been haemorrhage (although they will not replace red blood cells), or where the plasma volume is reduced for other reasons, e.g. fluid and electrolyte depletion.

- **Gelatins** (Haemaccel®; Gelofusin®). The gelatin solutions are derived from collagen and are isotonic with plasma. They are non-antigenic, and do not interfere with cross-matching tests for blood. The solutions will remain in the circulation for about 6 hours and the kidneys rapidly excrete them.
- **Dextrans.** These are solutions containing high-molecular-weight (MW) glucose polymers in either 0.9% NaCl or 5% dextrose. The solutions are hypertonic. The solutions are classified by the MW of the glucose polymer, e.g. dextran 70 (6% solution) has a molecular weight of 70 000 and dextran 40 (10% solution) a MW of 40 000. They remain in the circulation for times ranging from 2 to 24 hours depending on their MW. Unfortunately, these solutions tend to interfere with the red cells, some solutions promoting clumping of cells and others producing haemolysis. In addition, they interfere with the interpretation of cross-matching reactions. The raised plasma osmotic pressure caused by the dextrans will tend to draw water from the cells and ISF space into the blood vessels.

Table 22.11 Transfusion reactions

Reaction type	Timing	Clinical signs	Cause	Treatment	Prevention
Immediate immune-mediated haemolytic	Immediate (minutes – hours)	Pyrexia, salivation, vomiting, tachycardia, tachypnoea, muscle tremors, hypotension, prostration and haemoglobinuria	Recipient serum contains antibodies to donor red blood cells	Stop transfusion immediately. Fluid therapy to support vascular system	Cross-matching or blood typing
Immediate immune-mediated non-haemolytic	Immediate (minutes – hours)	Urticaria, pruritus, erythema, hypotension, bronchoconstriction, i.e. anaphylactic shock	Hypersensitivity reaction	Stop transfusion immediately. Antihistamines. Corticosteroids. Fluid therapy to support vascular system	Pre-treatment of recipient with antihistamines and corticosteroids has been used
Delayed immune-mediated	3 days to 3 weeks post-transfusion	Pyrexia, anorexia, jaundice	Recipient mounts immune response to donor red blood cells producing antibodies	No specific treatment	Blood typing

Therefore, crystalloids (see below) should be administered at the same time as dextrans to avoid cellular dehydration.

- **Starch (hydroxyethylstarch, HES).** HES (Hespan 6%®) is derived from amylopectin. Hespan 6% contains hetastarch, has high MW (450 000) and a duration of action of 24 hours.

Recently, a colloid has become available on the UK market that has the ability to carry oxygen. Oxyglobin® is a haemoglobin-based oxygen-carrier. It is compatible with all blood types and has a similar effect on intravascular blood volume as other colloids.

Crystalloids

In contrast to plasma volume expanders, crystalloids are non-colloidal substances that pass readily through cell membranes. This means that they will not remain within the ECF compartment but will equilibrate with the ICF compartment, and if renal function is normal, will be excreted in the urine. The most commonly used solutions in general practices are:

- **0.9% sodium chloride (NaCl).** Useful for replacing water and electrolyte losses, especially in vomiting, urinary obstruction, hepatopathy and Addison's disease. This is an acidifying solution.
- **5% dextrose (glucose) in water.** The dextrose in the solution is rapidly metabolised, and therefore, these solutions effectively provide free water that can be used to replace primary water deficits.
- **0.18% sodium chloride in 4% dextrose (also called glucose or dextrose saline).** Used to replace primary water deficits, and to replace the inevitable losses of sodium and water occurring on a daily basis (maintenance requirements). Potassium will also be required during long-term administration.
- **Hartmann's solution (also called lactated Ringer's).** Useful for replacing water and electrolyte losses, especially where the losses are post-gastric, e.g. diarrhoea or intestinal foreign body. Contains lactate that is metabolised by the liver to form bicarbonate, i.e. it is alkalinising.
- **Ringer's solution (also called compound sodium chloride solution).** Used to replace water and electrolyte losses especially where the losses are pre-pyloric, e.g. gastric vomiting. Contains potassium chloride and calcium chloride in addition to sodium chloride.
- **Potassium chloride (KCl)** can be used when potassium supplementation is needed. Ten millilitres of 10% KCl contains 13.4 mmol. If supplementary potassium is added to a crystalloid solution, it is important that the bag is clearly labelled to avoid possible overadministration (relative or absolute).
- **Sodium bicarbonate 8.4%** should be available to treat severe acidosis. This solution may be used intravenously as an injection but frequently it is added to intravenous infusions. However, do not add bicarbonate to any fluids that contain calcium (see Table 22.12), as a precipitate will be formed. Once again, if sodium bicarbonate is added to a crystalloid solution, it is important that the bag is clearly labelled to avoid possible overadministration (relative or absolute).

Table 22.12 summarises the principal constituents and some of the major indications for these fluids.

Volume and rate of fluid infusion

Replacement volume can be calculated from the history, clinical signs and simple laboratory tests as described earlier. Usually, this volume can be replaced within the first 24 hours of treatment, with half of the replacement being made in the first 6–8 hours. The animal also has maintenance requirements for fluids that must be met in addition to replacing existing deficits, and approximately 50 ml/kg/day of 0.18% NaCl with 4% dextrose (supplemented with additional potassium chloride) should be given to replace normal losses. It is important that potassium should not be administered at a rate greater than 0.5 mmol/kg/hour.

Table 22.12 The principal constituents and some of the major indications for commonly used intravenous fluids							
Solution		Na^+	K^+	Ca^{2+}	Cl^-	**Others**	**Indications**
Haemaccel	Isotonic	143	5	3	154	Gelatins	Restore circulating volume
Dextrans	Hypertonic	154	—	—	154	—	Restore circulating
	Hypertonic	—	—	—	—	5% dextrose	volume
0.9% NaCl	Isotonic	154	—	—	154	—	Replace ECF. Gastric losses from vomiting
Hartmann's solution (Ringer's lactate)	Isotonic	131	5	2	111	Lactate	Replace ECF. Especially from diarrhoea and post-gastric losses
Ringer's solution	Isotonic	147	4	2.5	156	—	Replace ECF. Gastric losses from vomiting
5% dextrose	Isotonic	—	—	—	—	5% dextrose	Primary water deficit replacement
0.18% NaCl + 4% dextrose	Isotonic	30	—	—	30	4% dextrose	Maintenance requirements. Primary water deficit replacement. Neonatal ECF replacement

Fluid requirement = losses + maintenance + ongoing
losses

The rate of fluid replacement often poses problems. A number of factors govern how fast fluids can be given:

- Rate of loss.
- Health of patient (cardiac and renal disease are of particular note).
- Type of fluid administered.
- Response by the patient to therapy.

During active severe haemorrhage and shock, fluids have to be administered rapidly (see 'Treatment of shock').

Overzealous fluid administration may result in the circulatory system becoming overloaded, or the body overhydrated. This is particularly a problem in smaller cats and dogs. Typically, excess of a colloid leads to circulatory overload with right-sided heart failure (indicated by an elevated CVP (see later)), and ultimately congestive cardiac failure. Too much crystalloid, on the other hand, will initially stimulate diuresis (via inhibition of ADH release), but as the electrolyte solution moves from the circulation into the remainder of the extracellular space, signs of oedema may develop, i.e. fluid will accumulate in the ISF space. Most seriously, pulmonary oedema may develop which will initially impair oxygenation; however, ultimately it can result in the death of the patient.

CLINICAL SIGNS ASSOCIATED WITH
OVERHYDRATION
- Serous nasal discharge.
- Restlessness.
- Chemosis.
- Respiratory distress caused by pulmonary congestion and oedema.

Overinfusion is most likely to occur with:

- **Reduced cardiac output**, e.g. congestive heart failure.
- **Renal/urinary conditions**, e.g. acute renal failure, ruptured bladder, where urine output is prevented.
- **Inadequate monitoring**. This is especially true of smaller patients.
- **Fluid administration to normovolaemic animals**, e. g. blood given in chronic anaemia.

Monitoring during fluid therapy

Monitoring during fluid administration should include:

- **Cardiovascular system**. Pulse (rate, rhythm, strength), mucous membrane colour, capillary refill time, jugular distension. In addition CVP, direct or indirect arterial blood pressure, chest auscultation (cardiac arrhythmias, pulmonary oedema).
- **Respiratory system**. Respiratory rate and depth, chest auscultation (pulmonary oedema). In addition arterial blood-gas analysis.
- **Temperature**. Core body and peripheral.
- **Urine output**. 1–2 ml/kg/hr.
- **Catheter site**. Check for signs of inflammation, extravasation, sepsis.
- **Administration set**. Check for kinking. Devices are available to minimise kinking of administration set tubing as it turns corners.
- **Bandages**. Check for soiling and comfort. Check for distal limb oedema and patient interference or self-mutilation.
- **General**. Check for peripheral oedema; check body-weight; skin turgor. Check fluid flowing!

Shock

Definition

Cells within the body require oxygen and nutrients to function normally (aerobic metabolism). Shock is an imbalance between the delivery of oxygen and nutrients to cells and utilisation of oxygen and nutrients by cells. When insufficient oxygen is supplied, cells change from aerobic to anaerobic metabolism. Anaerobic metabolism is an inefficient method of producing energy for cellular function and in addition results in the production of lactic acid. Lactic acid alters the acid–base balance within the body.

Shock may occur as a consequence of any syndrome, disease state or injury, that causes a critical decrease in effective blood flow with altered cell metabolism with or without cell death.

Classification of shock

- Hypovolaemic.
- Distributive.
- Cardiogenic.

Aetiology of shock

The following description of different forms of shock tends to suggest that each form occurs independently of the other. This is not the case. Many shocked animals will have components of more than one, or all forms of shock.

Hypovolaemic shock

Hypovolaemic shock represents absolute fluid loss and may occur following:

- Haemorrhage:

  - External.
  - Internal (chest, abdomen, osseofascial).
- Plasma loss.
- Third space losses (pyometra, peritonitis, ileus).
- Fluid depletion:

  - mixed water and electrolyte losses (vomiting and diarrhoea).
  - water losses (deprivation, diuresis).

Distributive shock

Distributive shock represents relative fluid loss. Distributive shock was previously referred to as vasogenic or vasculogenic shock. This form of shock occurs mainly following the release of naturally occurring vasoactive chemicals within the body. The primary changes are increased capillary permeability and increased vascular capacitance (that is there is an increased amount of blood within the venous system). There are a number of causes of distributive shock including:

- Endotoxaemia (**endotoxic shock**). Endotoxins are formed from the cell walls of principally Gram-negative bacteria, and act to release endogenous vasoactive substances. An initial rise in cardiac output may occur, but it does not compensate for the disturbance of the distribution of blood to the tissues and the increased vascular permeability.
- Anaphylaxis (**anaphylactic shock**).
- Neurogenic causes (**neurogenic shock**), e.g. vasomotor paralysis following spinal cord injury or overdose of general anaesthetic agents.
- Trauma.

Administration of drugs that have an effect on the capacity of the blood vessels, e.g. acetylpromazine, can induce distributive shock after absolute or relative overdose.

Cardiogenic shock

This is generally regarded as failure of the heart as an effective pump. However, shock may occur following obstructive problems:

- Cardiomyopathy.
- Valvular abnormalities.
- Arrythmias.
- Obstructive shock:

  - Pericardial tamponade.
  - Intracardiac neoplasia.
  - Aortic/pulmonary thromboembolism.

Pathophysiology of shock

The pathophysiology of hypovolaemic shock can be used as an example of the pathophysiological changes that occur in shock in general.

Initially, in response to falling blood volume a number of compensatory responses are triggered. These include:

- **Stimulation of the sympathetic nervous system**: Loss of blood, or effective circulating volume, reduces the venous return to the right side of the heart, and the output from the left side of the heart falls (cardiac output falls). Pressure-sensitive baroreceptors in the aorta and carotid artery detect the drop in blood pressure (hypotension) secondary to the fall in cardiac output. Centres within the medulla of the brain initiate compensatory mechanisms to restore blood pressure to normal. These compensatory mechanisms involve the sympathetic nervous system and stimulation of the adrenal medulla. Adrenaline and noradrenaline are released and cause the blood vessels of the skin, intestine, kidneys and muscles to constrict, i.e. there is an increase in peripheral vasoconstriction (increase in total peripheral resistance). This causes a direct increase in blood pressure and promotes increased venous return to the heart. At this stage, blood flow to the vital organs (heart, lungs and brain) is maintained. In association with these changes the heart rate increases and there is an increase in the force of contraction of the myocardium (heart muscle).
- **Endocrine influences**: release of the hormones aldosterone and ADH promote salt and water retention by the kidneys.
- **Extracellular fluid shift**: capillary hydrostatic pressure is reduced and water moves from the interstitial fluid space into the vascular space as the effective osmotic pressure of the plasma proteins predominates.

These early responses occur to compensate for the fall in vascular volume and aim to restore vascular volume, blood pressure and improve oxygen delivery to the tissues. If volume depletion is severe, then the mechanisms which are normally life saving can lead to the animal's death. Prolonged vasoconstriction and low perfusion cause continued tissue hypoxia, anaerobic metabolism and acidosis. Consequently, the peripheral vessels dilate and become engorged with blood. Moreover, cells in the capillary wall become non-functional and fluid is lost from the capillaries into the ISF space. Both of these mechanisms act to reduce the blood returning to the heart even further. The blood soon becomes viscous and slow moving, platelets may start to aggregate, and ultimately the blood will clot within the vessels. This effectively blocks the capillaries. If it is widespread, all the clotting factors will be used up resulting in a bleeding state known as disseminated intravascular coagulation (DIC).

The tissues most susceptible to hypoxia include:

- **Myocardium**: the heart is depressed by hypoxia, acidosis and the presence of the toxins.
- **Kidneys**: when blood flow to the kidneys is reduced urine output falls. Hypoxia causes the renal tubules to become damaged.
- **Gastrointestinal tract**: mucosal damage allows the invasion of bacteria, and bacterial toxins are absorbed.
- **Liver**.

In the lungs, although there is an initial increase in ventilation, eventually, microthrombi and other factors cause the lung to become very inefficient. Eventually, a state of multiple organ failure develops and the animal dies.

Clinical signs of shock

Hypovolaemic, cardiogenic and late distributive shock all share common clinical signs.

- Weak rapid pulse.
- Increased heart rate (tachycardia) with quiet heart sounds (due to poor cardiac filling).
- Pale mucous membranes (due to vasoconstriction).
- Prolonged capillary refill time (≥ 2 seconds) (due to vasoconstriction).
- Increased ventilation (due to metabolic acidosis/pain).
- Slow jugular refill and collapsed peripheral veins.
- Hypothermia and cold extremities (due to reduced metabolic rate and vasoconstriction).
- Depressed level of consciousness (due to reduced blood flow to brain).
- Muscle weakness (due to hypoxia, vasoconstriction, etc.).
- Reduced renal output (oliguria, anuria) (due to reduced blood flow to kidneys).
- Low CVP and low mean arterial blood pressure.
- Elevated PCV, Hb, TP, urea and creatinine (a blood sample should be obtained prior to fluid administration).

Treatment of shock

Fluid replacement

Adequate volume replacement is the single most important measure in the treatment of shock. However, fluids should be administered with care in cardiogenic shock, which is primarily a failure of the heart to pump fluid effectively around the body, rather than volume depletion.

After clinical assessment of the animal, at least one intravenous catheter should be inserted. If the peripheral veins are collapsed and difficult to catheterise, a jugular catheter may be used or fluids administered intraosseously.

To facilitate administration of large volumes of fluid over a short period of time, large gauge catheters are required, or more than one intravenous line should be established.

All fluids are given to effect, and the volumes required might be very large because of vasodilation or because of contraction of the ISF, which also must be replaced. Frequently, fluid replacement will be the only treatment required to promote recovery. Because fluid administration rates in shock are initially very high (Table 22.13), it is essential that the animal be monitored closely to avoid over hydration. Fluid rates are adjusted according to the patient's response.

Oxygen

It is important to ensure that shocked animals have a patent airway and are breathing efficiently. Because one of the problems in shocked patients is poor delivery of oxygen to tissues, the patient must be adequately oxygenated and administration of supplemental oxygen is a sensible measure. This may be achieved in a number of ways (flow-by, face-mask, nasal oxygen, incubator, tracheotomy tube, endotracheal tube, etc.).

Antibiotics

Antibiotics should be administered in all cases of shock either prophylactically or therapeutically. Intravenous broad-spectrum bactericidal agents should be used.

Glucocorticoids

There is much controversy over the use of steroids in shock. The administration of glucocorticoids tends to cause an improvement in the clinical state of the patient but will not necessarily decrease mortality. The greatest advantage will be seen if steroids are administered early in the course of shock and at high doses. Both methylprednisolone sodium succinate and dexamethasone sodium phosphate are suitable agents and are administered intravenously.

Table 22.13 Rates of fluid infusion for shock

Solution	Rate of fluid infusion (ml/kg)	
	Dog	Cat
Isotonic crystalloid[a]	60–90	40–60
Colloid	10–20	8–12
Hypertonic saline (7%)	4–7	2–4

[a] 5% dextrose and 0.18% NaCl/4% dextrose are not suitable for treatment of shock

Antiprostaglandins

The release of endogenous inflammatory mediators during shock can exacerbate the condition. Administration of drugs that help to block this reaction, e.g. non-steroidal anti-inflammatory drugs (NSAIDs) would therefore appear logical. Unfortunately, administration of these agents will also block production of prostaglandins essential to maintain renal blood flow and gastric mucosal integrity. Concurrent administration of NSAIDs and glucocorticoids is contraindicated.

Sympathomimetics

Where fluid therapy alone fails to improve cellular blood supply and oxygenation, the use of sympathomimetic drugs should be considered, e.g. dopamine, dobutamine, isoprenaline. These agents are useful in cardiogenic shock and in advanced shock where myocardial depression is present. They are administered as infusions because of their short half-lives within the circulation. Dopamine also will act to increase renal blood flow.

Sodium bicarbonate

Metabolic acidosis is common in shock mainly as a result of excess production of lactic acid. In general administration of intravenous fluids to improve perfusion will allow excess lactate to be metabolised.

If facilities are available to measure arterial blood gases and the blood pH falls to 7.2 administration of sodium bicarbonate may be considered.

General measures

If there is an obvious source of blood loss this should be stemmed if possible. Frequently, animals that are in shock will be, or will become, hypothermic. Although it is inadvisable to warm a hypothermic animal rapidly because vasodilation will occur, further loss of body heat can be prevented by ensuring a reasonable ambient temperature, avoiding draughts, lying the animal on an insulated surface, covering the animal and warming fluids to body temperature prior to administration.

Monitoring during shock

The same monitoring procedures that are used in fluid therapy also apply to animals that are in shock. Perhaps one of the most useful parameters that can be monitored is the CVP. This gives the nurse and the clinician an indication of the adequacy of fluid replacement and also serves as a useful indicator of the continuing fluid requirements of the animal.

KEY POINTS

- Many medical and surgical conditions and interventions cause disturbances of fluid, electrolyte and acid–base balance within the body, and knowledge of the homeostatic mechanisms that normally govern these physiological processes is essential if disturbances within this system are to be identified, and rectified, in a logical and effective manner.
- On average, the water content of the adult body is 60% by weight.
- Almost two-thirds of the total body water is located inside the cells of the tissues, while the remaining one-third is located outside the cells.
- To maintain a normal water balance in a healthy dog or cat, a total of approximately 50 ml/kg/day of fluid is required (range 40–60 ml/kg/day).
- Dehydration is the term used to describe a reduction in the total body water and the signs and symptoms associated with such a loss.
- There are a number of clinical and laboratory methods which may be used to establish the amount of fluid which is required by an individual dehydrated animal.
- Acid–base status is a measure of the hydrogen ion concentration within its tissues.
- The purpose of fluid therapy is to replace deficits from previous losses, improve and maintain renal function, supply maintenance requirements and provide for ongoing losses.
- Shock is an imbalance between the delivery of oxygen and nutrients to cells and utilisation of oxygen and nutrients by cells.

Further reading

Cannon, M. (2000) Fluid therapy for cats 1. Providing fluids to the feline patient. *In Practice*, vol. 22, pp. 242–251.

Cannon, M. (2000) Fluid therapy for cats 2. Restoring fluid and electrolyte balance. *In Practice*, vol. 22, pp. 317–326.

College of Animal Welfare (2000) *300 Questions and Answers in Anatomy and Physiology*, Butterworth-Heinemann, Oxford.

Hansen, B. D. (2001) Intravenous catheters. *Waltham Focus*, vol. 11, pp. 4–10.

Haskins, S. C. (1988) A simple fluid therapy planning guide. *Seminars in Veterinary Medicine and Surgery*, vol. 3, pp. 227–236.

Knottenbelt, C. and Mackin, A. (1998) Blood transfusions in the dog and cat. *In Practice*, vol. 20, pp. 110–113 and 191–199.

Rudloff, E. and Kirby, R. (2001) Resuscitation from hypovolaemic shock. *Waltham Focus*, vol. 11, pp. 11–22.

23

Anaesthesia and analgesia

D. C. Brodbelt

Learning objectives

After studying this chapter, students should be able to:

- Describe the necessary steps required to evaluate a patient for general anaesthesia.
- Discuss a suitable premedication plan for an individual patient.
- Discuss a potential analgesia plan to include pre-, peri- and post-operative analgesia.
- Describe local anaesthetic techniques.
- Discuss the administration and maintenance of general anaesthesia, including individual intravenous and inhalational agents.
- Check the anaesthetic machine prior to anaesthesia and to prepare for an anaesthetic.
- Discuss the potential risks of general anaesthesia.
- Assist the veterinary surgeon in the event of a cardio-pulmonary arrest during anaesthesia.
- Explain the veterinary nurse's role in anaesthesia and analgesia.

Introduction

Anaesthesia is the reversible production of a state of unconsciousness necessary to perform surgery or undertake diagnostic tests. It relies on the provision of analgesia, muscle relaxation and narcosis/unconsciousness: the 'triad' of anaesthesia. Safe and effective anaesthesia addresses these three components individually and by using a combination of anaesthetic agents satisfies these requirements whilst avoiding significant depression of normal physiological function. This is termed 'balanced' anaesthesia and provides good patient stability and reduces the potential for peri-operative complications. It is commonly employed in practice when a patient is premedicated with a sedative and analgesic, providing analgesia during and after surgery, and then maintained with an inhalation agent to provide narcosis.

The veterinary nurse is integrally involved in the provision of anaesthesia and analgesia of the patient presenting for surgery and diagnostic procedures. A solid understanding of each individual patient's requirements and the likely effects of the anaesthetic administered are important aspects of the nurse's duties when involved in an anaesthetic. Careful monitoring of the patient from admission, through the anaesthetic and until discharge is a task often delegated to the nurse by the veterinary surgeon, and the provision of good analgesia is an area the veterinary nurse can make a large impact and benefit the patient. In a survey of practitioners' views on analgesia, veterinary surgeons were most often likely to delegate the assessment and administration of analgesics to the veterinary nurse (Capner et al., 1999; Lascelles et al., 1999).

Safe anaesthesia requires a good knowledge of the underlying anatomy and physiology of the patient and an appreciation of the pharmacological effects of the anaesthetic given. The reader is recommended to review these subjects in Chapter 2 (Anatomy and Physiology) and other standard texts (see Further reading).

Pre-operative assessment and preparation

A thorough pre-operative examination is essential to identify higher-risk patients and allows appropriate preparation prior to anaesthesia. In those cases which are poor anaesthetic candidates (ASA classes 3–5), particular attention to preparation is required to minimise the risk of untoward events. Other considerations that affect the degree of preparation include the type of surgery; prolonged and/or invasive procedures require more preparation than superficial operations. Whether the procedure is elective or an emergency indicates how much preparation is possible. Emergency cases requiring immediate surgery may receive only cursory preparation. Elective procedures may be postponed without compromising the animal.

THE AMERICAN SOCIETY OF ANESTHESIOLOGISTS (ASA) RISK ASSESSMENT

Patients are classified into five categories:

Class 1   Normal, healthy patient.

Class 2   Patient with mild systemic disease.

Class 3   Patient with severe systemic disease that is not incapacitating.

Class 4   Patient with severe systemic disease that is a constant threat to life.

Class 5   Moribund patient not expected to survive 24 hours with or without surgery.

Pre-operative examination

The animal's medical condition is primarily determined by taking a good history, and performing a comprehensive clinical examination. When necessary, further tests may be required. Those systems of particular concern include nervous, cardiovascular, respiratory, renal and hepatic systems.

History

Much valuable information can be gained from questioning the owner. Questions relating to general health status include recent weight loss, behavioural changes, and signs of pain. Information pertaining to cardiovascular and pulmonary function can be gleaned by questioning the animal's response to exercise, presence of coughing and general demeanour when at rest. Excessive drinking may alert to endocrine, liver and renal problems and may lead to the performance of further tests prior to anaesthesia. Vomiting, diarrhoea, and inappetence prior to presentation may also alert the nurse to systemic disease. Reproductive status (neutered/in season) and the presence of discharges may be relevant (e.g. vaginal discharge). Other background information that may be of value includes:

- Duration of ownership.
- Previous medical history.
- Previous anaesthetic history.
- Vaccination status.
- Current medication, including 'over-the-counter' products. The dose, dosing frequency and duration of treatment should be established. Drugs of particular concern are listed in Table 23.1.

Physical examination

This concentrates on the organ systems affected principally by anaesthesia:

- Central nervous system status involves particular attention to the patient's state of mind and the presence of depressed function.
- Cardiovascular function is assessed with inspection of exercise tolerance, mucous membrane colour and capillary refill time, palpation of peripheral pulse rate and quality, and auscultation of cardiac murmurs and dysrhythmias. Pale mucous membranes suggest hypovolae-

Table 23.1 Drugs potentially affecting anaesthesia

Antibiotics

Glucocorticoids

Non-steroidal anti-inflammatory drugs

Organophosphorus compounds, flea collars, parasiticides

Anticonvulsants

Digoxin, beta-blockers, calcium channel blockers and ACE-inhibitors

Frusemide and other diuretics

Endocrine supplements, e.g. thyroxine

Antihistamines

Antitussives/bronchodilators

Antidepressants, e.g. selegiline

mia or anaemia, whilst cyanotic membranes indicate a sluggish circulation or poor oxygenation of arterial blood. Cool extremities can be seen during shock and reduced peripheral perfusion. Right-sided cardiovascular dysfunction is associated with pronounced jugular pulses, and peripheral oedema.

- Respiratory system examination includes observation of respiratory rate and pattern, auscultation and percussion of the chest. Auscultation of rales and crepitus suggest airway secretion and respiratory disease. Reduced sounds are associated with lung consolidation. Chest percussion with low resonance supports the presence of consolidation, whilst high resonance is consistent with pneumothorax.

> **PRACTICAL NURSING TIP**
> A good assessment of the patient's cardiovascular fitness for anaesthesia is its response to a short lead walk. If the animal becomes distressed, dyspnoeic or collapses after minimal exercise then the patient is at a significant risk for anaesthesia, whereas an animal that is unremarkable and remains undistressed should be fit for anaesthesia.

Further tests

Haematology and biochemistry

A blood sample should be examined if the history or physical examination raises the suspicion of anaemia, hypoproteinaemia, coagulation disorders, liver or renal pathology. Metabolic and electrolyte disorders, including hypo- and hyperkalaemia, can be detected. Liver function tests and liver enzymes can alert to liver pathology, whilst serum urea and creatinine are useful indicators of renal status. Urinalysis (especially urine specific gravity) is valuable in investigating renal function if particular concern exists.

Radiography

Animals involved in road traffic accidents, those with neoplastic disease and those with signs of cardiovascular or pulmonary disease should undergo radiographic examination of the thorax and abdomen. Presenting polydipsia and polyuria with or without a vaginal discharge in an unneutered bitch may warrant abdominal radiography to rule out pyometra.

Ultrasonography

Allows thorough investigation of cardiac function and abdominal pathology.

Electrocardiography

Abnormal pulse rhythms require further investigation.

Significance of clinical findings

Central nervous system disease

Behaviour better indicates an animal's suitability for surgery than age: a tail-wagging, active 15-year-old is a better risk than the depressed, small, inactive 8-month-old with a porto-systemic shunt. Depression increases patient sensitivity to anaesthetics and may indicate the presence of intracranial pathology (tumours, meningitis), systemic disease (pyrexia, hyperkalaemia, toxaemia) or cardiovascular problems.

Epileptic animals are more sensitive to anaesthetics if anticonvulsant therapy has only recently begun. In time, liver enzyme induction occurs and accelerates the metabolism of some anaesthetics, making the patient more resistant to anaesthetics.

Cardiovascular and respiratory disease

Signs of cardiac and respiratory disease (including exercise intolerance) are always important. When disease is present, the fundamental goal of preparation is to optimise the factors contributing to oxygen delivery to the tissues, i.e. cardiac output, haemoglobin content and pulmonary function.

Cardiac disease is not a contraindication to anaesthesia if the effects on cardiac function and blood flow are appreciated and drugs selected accordingly. In general, 'stress', pain and volume losses are less well tolerated by animals with cardiovascular disease. Drugs used for treating cardiac disease (e.g. digoxin, beta-blockers) may interact with anaesthetics. Cases with congestive heart failure may require cage rest, and institution of medical therapy. Pre-existing arrhythmias may require treatment.

Respiratory disease predisposes the animal to hypoxia and hypercapnia. It may contribute to secondary right ventricular changes (cor pulmonale) or polycythaemia. A common form of restrictive respiratory disease is morbid obesity. Restricted airways (e.g. nasal discharge, brachiocephalic canine anatomy) require careful attention for maintenance of an airway.

Causes of respiratory embarrassment (e.g. pneumothorax, gastric tympany) must be relieved pre-operatively. Pleural effusions should be drained pre-operatively. Excessive alveolar transudate may be cleared with diuretics, ACE inhibitors and drugs that improve cardiac contractility and function.

Liver and renal disease

Liver disease may prolong anaesthesia as most drugs administered undergo some hepatic metabolism. Consideration of anaesthetics with least reliance on hepatic function may be appropriate in such circumstances. Secondary problems include coagulation defects, hypoproteinaemia and hypoglycaemia (see below).

Patients with pre-existing renal disease are intolerant of renal hypoperfusion during anaesthesia. Significant cardiovascular depression and reduced kidney perfusion during anaesthesia can cause renal ischaemia and lead to subsequent renal failure. This is a particular concern in geriatric patients already in early chronic renal failure and can result in acute renal decompensation. Elderly patients (and those in renal failure) should be given fluids during anaesthesia and cardiovascular stability maintained.

Unstable blood glucose levels

Diabetes mellitus causes hyperglycaemia with diuresis, fluid loss and keto-acidosis. Severe hypoglycaemia resulting from an insulinoma or liver disease causes considerable neuronal damage if brain glucose supply is curtailed. Glucose levels must be controlled with soluble insulin or dextrose solutions pre-operatively.

Hypoalbuminaemia

This can indicate liver or renal disease and has two consequences. First, the albumin-bound fraction of drugs highly bound to plasma proteins (e.g. thiopentone) is lowered and so more free drug is available, potentially leading to overdose if a standard dose is administered. Second, plasma oncotic pressure may be lowered, promoting oedema and increased diffusion distance for gases in the lung and resulting in hypoxia if severe enough.

Coagulation problems

Clotting failure may be genetic (von Willebrand's disease in Dobermanns) or indicate liver failure. Fresh blood transfusion may be required pre-operatively.

Electrolyte and pH abnormalities

High potassium levels resulting from Addison's disease or renal failure must be lowered pre-operatively, while low serum potassium should be raised. High potassium levels are lowered with sodium bicarbonate solutions, calcium gluconate, insulin–glucose solutions, or cation-exchange resins. In extreme cases, peritoneal dialysis may be required. Potassium is raised by infusing solutions at rates not greater than 0.5 mmol/kg/hour. Extremes of pH are ameliorated by treating the underlying cause.

Hypovolaemia and dehydration

In dehydrated and hypovolaemic animals, tissue perfusion may become compromised during anaesthesia. Animals with chronic fluid loss (e.g. those with chronic vomiting and diarrhoea) may have electrolyte and/or pH disturbances.

Animals with renal failure cannot concentrate urine and become dehydrated if access to water is restricted. Dogs and cats with chronic renal failure, or any disease characterised by polyuria and polydipsia, must not have water withheld pre-operatively; if necessary, parenteral fluids may be given.

When reduced, circulating blood volume must be restored pre-operatively with appropriate fluids. Oral, intravenous, intraperitoneal, intraosseous or subcutaneous routes may be used, depending on the cause, fluid type and the time available.

Anaemia and polycythaemia

Low haemoglobin levels (below 8 g/dl) caused by blood loss or renal disease must be resolved before surgery; oxygen flux may become inadequate when compensatory changes (increased cardiac output and modest hyperventilation) are depressed by anaesthetics. In elective cases, low haemoglobin levels may be raised by treating the underlying cause; otherwise blood transfusion, preferably with 'packed' cells, may be required.

High haemoglobin levels can also be deleterious. Haematocrit values in excess of 55% make blood hyperviscous, causing it to 'sludge' in capillaries. They may also indicate that the animal is dehydrated or suffering from chronic hypoxia. High haematocrits (in normovolaemic patients) are lowered by the process of normovolaemic haemodilution. This involves the withdrawal of whole blood and simultaneous replacement with plasma or fluids.

Pyrexia

Pyrexia increases metabolic rate; there are rises in the consumption of oxygen and glucose and in the production of carbon dioxide. The cause of pyrexia should be sought because, while there is little problem anaesthetising animals with superficial abscesses, there is considerable risk when pyrexia results from endocarditis or meningitis. Pyrexia is treated with antibiotics if the cause is infectious.

Current medication

Pre-existing medical therapy and peri-operative medication may affect subsequently administered sedatives and anaesthetics. An understanding of the impact of these concurrent therapies is important to avoid unnecessary side-effects. Generally, however, most medications are continued through the peri-operative period. Individual considerations include:

- Aminoglycoside antibiotics, e.g. gentamicin, may induce neuromuscular blockade, which when combined with inhalation anaesthesia may result in significant ventilation depression. Further, at high doses these antibiotics can cause renal failure and may be better avoided in patients with pre-existing renal failure.
- Barbiturates given to control epilepsy should be maintained peri-operatively. Theoretically, enzyme induction may increase anaesthetic requirements, though clinically this is rarely seen.
- Cardiovascular therapy including the use of ACE inhibitors, beta-blockers, and calcium channel blockers is also best maintained. However, caution should be applied when administering anaesthetic agents and premedicants that decrease blood pressure (i.e. many drugs) and attention to maintenance of cardiovascular function during anaesthesia is particularly important. Digoxin therapy may induce intra-operative arrhythmias, though if cardiovascular function is stable it is best continued.
- Corticosteroids administered chronically prior to anaesthesia may inhibit the normal stress response to surgery and parenteral supplementation should be considered.
- Non-steroidal anti-inflammatory drugs must be used with caution in the peri-operative period because of their effects on renal autoregulation. In general these are best reserved for post-operative therapy.

Any 'emergency' case

There are cases where surgical delay is unacceptable:

- Thoracic visceral damage.
- Airway obstruction.
- Uncontrollable haemorrhage.
- Obstetric emergencies in which neonates are at risk.

In emergencies, preparation may be limited to catheterising a vein, administering fluids and enriching inspired breath with oxygen.

Final details

Before admitting normal animals for surgery, owners must:

- Be informed of the risks and possible outcomes.
- Have signed an anaesthetic consent form.
- Be asked to withhold food the night before (water can be given).

A full stomach reduces lung volume, limits breathing and predisposes to vomiting; this may result in fatal aspiration pneumonia. If an animal scheduled for surgery has received a large meal pre-operatively, the best option is to delay surgery to allow adequate emptying of the stomach (i.e. at least 6 hours).

KEY POINTS
- Clinical examination includes attention to patient history, physical examination findings and results of further tests.
- Careful patient evaluation identifies particular risks including cardiovascular and respiratory compromise, CNS depression, reduced liver and renal function and metabolic imbalances.
- Higher-risk patients require more pre-operative preparation.
- Adequate preparation avoids unnecessary anaesthetic complications.

Sedation and premedication

Sedatives and tranquillisers can be used on their own to allow minor procedures to be performed or as premedication in preparation for general anaesthesia. Many procedures require restraint only.

- *SOME PROPERTIES OF AN IDEAL SEDATIVE*
- Production of stoical indifference to the surroundings.
- Recumbency if required.
- Analgesia.
- No side-effects.
- The presence of a specific reversal agent.

Effective sedation and chemical restraint require a quiet environment without disturbance of the animal, adequate time to allow full effect, and calm, firm and sensible handling.

Practical nursing tip *For good effective sedation keep the animal in a quiet area of the practice, away from disturbances and allow adequate time for the sedative to work before handling the animal.*

Potential cardiovascular and respiratory depression can occur with the use of chemical restraint. Sedation is not always safer than general anaesthesia as often no oxygen is supplied, facility for intermittent positive pressure ventilation is not available and monitoring of the patient is frequently minimal. In debilitated patients that require more than just light sedation, a general anaesthetic with careful monitoring and intra-operative care may be more appropriate than heavy sedation.

THE OBJECTIVES OF PREMEDICATION
- To calm the patient and reduce anxiety prior to induction of anaesthesia.
- To provide sedation.
- To aid a 'smooth' induction and recovery.
- To reduce induction and maintenance agent requirements.
- To provide analgesia.
- To reduce associated side-effects of the anaesthetic to be given.
- To reduce adverse effects of surgery.

Premedication is given before anaesthesia to smooth subsequent events. Long-acting drugs like acepromazine smooth recovery after induction with barbiturates and other drugs. Similarly, analgesics smooth recovery after painful procedures. In providing 'background' narcosis,

premedication and analgesics lower the requirement for maintenance agents and consequently the incidence of associated side-effects. The premedication given should always be specific to the individual patient and procedure to be undertaken; some patients require greater sedation than others prior to anaesthesia. A good premedication will render the animal calm and tranquil, allowing a smooth, stress-free induction of anaesthesia (see Fig. 23.1).

Disadvantages of premedication include the potential for drug interactions and side-effects, prolongation of recovery, and the need to allow sufficient time for the drugs to have full effect. Not all animals require pre-anaesthetic medication, e.g. those already depressed by toxaemia, shock or head trauma. After haemorrhage or in shocked animals, normal doses produce more profound effects.

The route by which pre-anaesthetic medication is given influences time to peak effect, duration of action and the incidence of side-effects (Table 23.2).

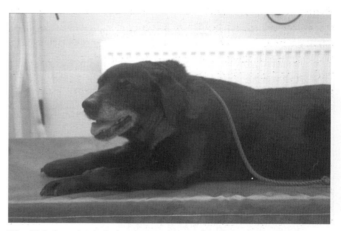

Fig. 23.1 A geriatric Labrador retriever, after light premedication, calmly awaits induction of anaesthesia.

Table 23.2 Comparison of drug administration routes	
Convenience	SC > IP > IM > IV
Pain on injection	IM > IP + IV > SC
Restraint needed	IV > IP > IM > SC
Animal tolerance	SC > IP > IM > IV
Onset of action	IV > IM > SC > IP
Duration of action	IP + SC > IM > IV
Predictability	IV > IM > SC > IP
Relative dose required	IP + SC > IM > IV
Technical ease	SC > IM > IP > IV

SC, subcutaneous; IP, intraperitoneal; IM, intramuscular; IV, intravenous

Phenothiazines – acepromazine

Phenothiazines are antagonists at central dopamine receptors. They are used routinely to premedicate animals prior to anaesthesia. Acepromazine (ACP, Vericore) the most commonly used phenothiazine in the UK, is available for small animals as a 2 mg/ml solution, and is administered at doses of 0.01–0.05 mg/kg intramuscularly or intravenously. It remains a popular and useful drug despite important side-effects. At normal doses the drug is safe and produces moderate sedation. Increasing the dose above this stated dose-range does not increase the degree of sedation but extends the duration of action and increases the severity of adverse reactions. The addition of an opioid potentiates sedation (i.e. neuroleptanalgesia, see below) and can be more effective with less side-effects than an increased dose.

PHENOTHIAZINES
Advantages
- Synergism: improve sedative effects of opioids.
- Antiarrhythmic: exert antiarrhythmic activity.
- Antiemetic: offset the emetic effects of some opioids.
- Spasmolytic: reduce discomfort when 'colic' results from gastrointestinal spasm.
- Antihistamine: useful with some histamine-releasing opioids.

Disadvantages
- Hypotension: this results from vascular smooth muscle relaxation. Problems occur when high doses are used or when normal doses are used in hypotensive or hypovolaemic animals. Acute decompensation and hypotension may result.
- Syncope: some breed-lines of Boxers collapse after low doses.
- Unpredictability: aggressive dogs are often resistant.
- Long-acting: dose-dependent duration of action; clinical sedation lasts 4–6 hours.
- Slow onset: peak effect does not occur for 10–20 minutes after IV and for 30 minutes after IM administration.
- No analgesia.
- Hypothermia: cutaneous vasodilatation and thermoregulatory depression cause heat loss.
- Poor muscle relaxation: no relaxant effects but reduces hypertonicity with ketamine.
- Penile prolapse may be seen in horses.
- Reduces threshold to seizures in epileptics.

Butyrophenones

These behave like phenothiazines though produce unpredictable results. Hypotension can be a concern at higher doses and they should be avoided in hypovolaemic patients. There are no butyrophenones with market authorisation for sole use in small animals, but fluanisone (Hypnorm, Janssen) and droperidol are available combined with opioids.

Neuroleptanalgesia

Phenothiazines and butyrophenones combined with opioids create a neuroleptanalgesic combination. The two components are synergistic; lower doses of each are needed, which lowers the incidence and severity of side-effects. Commercially available mixtures are convenient but effects can be sub-optimal:

- Hypnorm (fentanyl 0.315 mg, fluanisone 10 mg/ml).
- Small Animal Immobilon (etorphine 74 µg, methotrimeprazine 18 mg/ml).

Neuroleptanalgesics may be 'home-made': doses and drugs are modified to suit the individual case, e.g. acepromazine and buprenorphine. This form of neuroleptanalgesia is most commonly used in practice and can provide consistent and effective sedation.

NEUROLEPTANALGESIA
Advantages
- Lower incidence of side-effects.
- Increased degree of sedation.
- Increased predictability.
- Stable cardiopulmonary performance.
Disadvantages
- Animals remain sensitive to, and are aroused by, certain stimuli (e.g. noise).
- Only opioid antagonism is possible. The neuroleptic is not antagonised and is the longer-acting component.
- Behavioural changes are alleged to have occurred after neuroleptanalgesia in dogs.

Alpha-2-adrenoceptor agonists

Alpha-2 adrenoceptor agonists stimulate prejunctional alpha-2 receptors within the CNS, inhibiting release of noradrenaline, resulting in sedation. They are potent sedatives that provide analgesia, muscle relaxation and anxiolysis. However, they cause significant cardiopulmonary depression and should be used with caution in debilitated patients. They have specific antagonists, so their effects can be readily reversed.

Xylazine (0.5–2 mg/kg; Rompun, Bayer) and medetomidine (5–40 µg/kg (dog), 20–80 µg/kg (cat); Domitor, Pfizer) are alpha-2-adrenoceptor agonists with market authorisation in companion animals. Medetomidine is more potent, more specific to the alpha-2 receptor and longer acting than xylazine. The lower end of the dose range for both drugs in both species is to be recommended as cardiopulmonary depression is dose-dependent, increasing with increasing dose. Where heavier sedation is required the addition of an opioid (e.g. butorphanol) increases sedation without increasing cardiopulmonary depression.

Atipamezole (Antisedan, Pfizer) is an alpha-2 antagonist and is used to antagonise the effects of medetomidine in companion animals; the antagonist dose is the same volume as agonist injected in dogs and half the volume in cats (50–100 µg/kg im). Its use is desirable because the prolonged effect of medetomidine predisposes recipients to hypothermia, hypostatic lung congestion and prolonged recovery. After painful procedures, antagonism may expose the animal, acutely, to discomfort and appropriate analgesia must be administered.

ALPHA-2-ADRENOCEPTOR AGONISTS

Advantages

- Profound dose-dependent sedation.
- Duration of action is also dose-dependent.
- Marked drug-sparing effect: doses of induction and maintenance agents are considerably reduced. A greater lag time elapses before effects of induction agents are seen. Circulation time is prolonged, accelerating the uptake of volatile anaesthetics.
- Muscle relaxation: relaxant effects offset muscle rigidity seen with ketamine.
- Visceral analgesia.
- Specific reversal agent.

Disadvantages

- Cardiovascular depression: dose-dependent and profound cardiovascular effects occur; hypertension then hypotension, reduced cardiac output and bradycardia. Anticholinergic pretreatment, which counteracts bradycardia is controversial; though heart rate is restored, systemic vascular resistance remains elevated resulting in increased myocardial work. In dogs, xylazine sensitises the myocardium to adrenaline-induced arrhythmias during halothane anaesthesia.
- Respiratory depression: breathing is periodic with apnoeic pauses and mucous membranes turn grey. Muscle relaxation of redundant oropharyngeal tissue in brachycephalics may cause respiratory obstruction.
- Emesis: vomiting occurs in dogs and cats after xylazine and, to a lesser extent, after medetomidine.
- Diuresis: ADH inhibition and insulin suppression, contribute to this effect.

- Gut motility: this is reduced and barium meal interpretation may be confused.
- Thermoregulation: thermoregulation is impaired, generally resulting in hypothermia.
- Personal risk: The data sheet instructs that gloves should be worn when handling medetomidine.

Benzodiazepines

Benzodiazepines potentiate the inhibitory activity of the neurotransmitter gamma aminobutyric acid (GABA). They produce anxiolysis, muscle relaxation, sedation, hypnosis, and amnesia and have powerful anticonvulsant effects. Paradoxically, intravenous diazepam can cause marked stimulation in non-debilitated dogs. Diazepam as its water-insoluble formulation (Valium, Roche) causes pain on injection and thrombophlebitis. It is also available as a water-soluble emulsion (Diazmuls, Dumex) which is nonpainful on injection. Midazolam (Hypnovel, Roche) is water-soluble and also does not cause these problems. It is short-acting; is approximately twice as potent and is more effective after intramuscular injection than diazepam. Doses of 0.1–0.2 mg/kg of both drugs are routinely used.

Flumazenil

Flumazenil is a benzodiazepine antagonist used to treat overdosage in people and accelerate recovery in outpatient anaesthesia. In animals the cost often precludes its use.

BENZODIAZEPINES

Advantages

- Sedation: good sedation can be achieved in the debilitated patient.
- Safety: the drugs have high therapeutic indices and minimal cardiopulmonary effects.
- Drug-sparing effect: they prolong and enhance effects of other anaesthetics. Anaesthetic doses are lowered and predicted excitement (e.g. recovery after methohexitone) is prevented.
- Muscle relaxation: diazepam or midazolam are used with ketamine in cats to provide heavy sedation and eliminate excitation/convulsions and associated muscle hypertonicity of ketamine administration.
- Appetite stimulant in cats.

Disadvantages

- Unpredictable: in healthy animals, benzodiazepines often stimulate rather than depress but become increasingly effective as the animal's health status deteriorates.
- Formulation: diazepam causes pain on injection and thrombophlebitis.

Anticholinergic drugs

The routine use of anticholinergics for anaesthetic premedication is controversial. In previous times, the widespread use of diethyl ether anaesthesia in humans justified this practice; diethyl ether promotes oropharyngeal secretion, bronchosecretion and bronchoconstriction. Modern volatile anaesthetics do not produce excessive secretions and most cause bronchodilatation. In modern practice, anticholinergics are best administered when required. Uses include to

- Decrease salivation and bronchial secretion.
- Treat vagally induced bradycardia.
- Block the effects of certain drugs administered, e.g. anticholinesterases.

Atropine crosses the blood–brain barrier and the blood–placental barrier. The former can cause visual disturbances which can be disturbing, particularly for cats. It is given at 0.02–0.04 mg/kg intravenously, intramuscularly or subcutaneously. Glycopyrrolate (dose 0.01–0.02 mg/kg, Robinul, Anpharm) has a slower onset time, a longer duration of action and a greater antisialogogue effect than atropine. Tachyarrhythmias are said to be less likely and cardiovascular stability is better preserved. Glycopyrrolate does not cross the blood–brain barrier avoiding visual disturbance and may be a more appropriate agent in the cat.

ANTICHOLINERGICS

Advantages
- Bronchodilation, reduces total airway resistance.
- Rapidly controls intra-operative vagally mediated bradycardia.
- Protects against adverse vagal effects of anticholinesterases during antagonism of neuromuscular block.

Disadvantages
- Increases metabolic rate.
- Increases heart rate, increases myocardial oxygen consumption.
- Arrhythmogenic, causing bradyarrhythmias and/or tachyarrhythmias.
- Causes gastrointestinal ileus.
- Pupil dilatation and visual disturbance.

Pain and analgesia

Analgesia is a state of reduced sensibility to pain. Painful stimuli reach the brain in similar ways to other sensations but are amenable to interruption by a greater range of drugs. The perception of pain requires conscious awareness,

---

KEY POINTS
- For effective sedation and premedication a quiet environment, adequate time to allow full effect and careful patient handling are required.
- Sedation may be appropriate for simple procedures.
- Neuroleptanalgesia can produce more consistent sedation, with less cardiopulmonary depression, than a high dose of a single agent.
- Where general anaesthesia is required premedication is often valuable, smoothing anaesthesia and reducing complications.
- Phenothiazines, alpha-2-adrenoceptor agonists, benzodiazepines and anticholinergics are appropriate for premedication under different circumstances.

---

whilst nociception is the transmission of impulses to lower levels within the central nervous system in response to noxious stimuli. An animal's response to pain depends on the level of the central nervous system to which the pain message ascends (Fig. 23.2):

- Spinal responses include, for example, reflex limb withdrawal.
- Medullary responses include increased heart rate, blood pressure and respiratory rate.

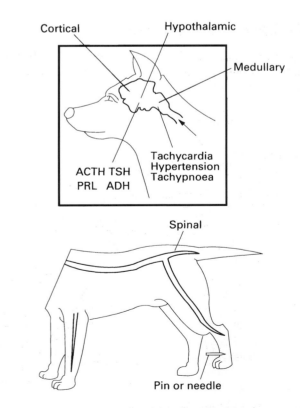

Fig. 23.2 Responses to pain.

- Hypothalamic responses take several forms. The hypothalamus initiates catecholamine release from the adrenal medulla and nerve endings of the sympathetic nervous system. This further increases heart rate and blood pressure. Less obviously, the hypothalamus secretes releasing factors which cause the pituitary gland to release 'stress' hormones such as adrenocorticotropic hormone (ACTH). Other pituitary hormones like thyroid stimulating hormone (TSH), antidiuretic hormone (ADH) and prolactin (PRL) are also released.
- Cortical responses are the most complex: they include activity like vocalisation and voluntary acts such as attempting to escape or to bite at the noxious stimulus.

Analgesics

Analgesics interrupt the ascending pain pathway at various levels (Fig. 23.3) and suppress the sensation of pain. Some, like the opioids, act at several points along this path. Blocking pain at a number of sites with the use of more than one type of analgesic can produce more effective analgesia; this is termed 'balanced analgesia'. Several drug groups suppress pain. These include:

- Alpha-2 adrenoceptor agonists.
- Benzodiazepines.
- General anaesthetics.
- Glucocorticoids.
- Local anaesthetics.
- Non-steroidal anti-inflammatory drugs (NSAIDs).
- Opioids.

Peripheral nerve endings

Glucocorticoids and NSAIDs reduce the production of pain-sensitising chemicals released from damaged tissues that stimulate nerve endings. Topical local anaesthetics block nerve endings.

Peripheral nerves

Local anaesthetics block nerve impulses in peripheral nerves. Local anaesthesia is frequently neglected as a method of pain relief but can produce very effective analgesia. Local anaesthetics are discussed later.

Spinal cord

Pain can be suppressed in the cord by the extradural injection of several drug types:

- Local anaesthetics block all nerve fibre types producing anaesthesia, analgesia and muscle relaxation.
- Opioids diminish sensitivity to pain but do not eliminate all sensation, proprioception or muscle function. Animals are therefore free from pain but can walk.
- Benzodiazepines, *N*-methyl-D-aspartate (NMDA) receptor antagonists and alpha-2 agonists have analgesic effects at the spinal level although they are less frequently used.
- Combinations of drugs that are compatible *in vitro* may be injected in order to capitalise on desirable properties of each, e.g. lignocaine or bupivacaine with morphine.

Brain

Opioids, alpha-2-adrenoceptor agonists and general anaesthetics cause analgesia through effects on the brain. Consciousness need not be lost for analgesia to be present.

Administration of analgesic drugs prior to tissue trauma is suggested to reduce post-operative analgesic requirements. This concept is called pre-emptive analgesia and, although work in the human literature remains equivocal (Richmond et al., 1993; Woolf and Chong, 1993), the general consensus is that analgesia given prior to surgery combined with adequate post-operative pain relief is the most effective. For example, premedication with the opioid buprenorphine and NSAID carprofen, followed by a local block prior to surgery and continued with regular dosing of an opioid post-operatively, will provide excellent analgesia and encourage a rapid recovery.

Opioid analgesics

Opioids are often included in premedication:

- To relieve pre-operative pain and therefore anxiety.
- To contribute to sedation.
- To provide analgesia during maintenance and on recovery.

While the properties of individual opioids differ, there are common advantages and disadvantages.

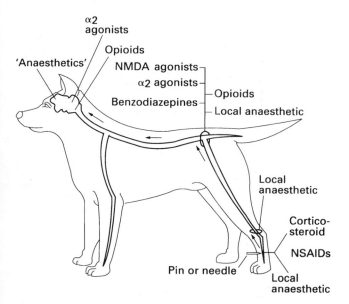

Fig. 23.3 Pain pathways and analgesia.

OPIOIDS

Advantages

- Profound, drug and dose-dependent analgesia.
- Benign cardiovascular effects: with some exceptions, opioids slow heart rate. In high doses, bradycardia and bradyarrhythmias may occur. Cardiac output is usually maintained.
- Anaesthetic-sparing effect: opioids reduce dose requirements of induction and maintenance agents.
- Sedation: some opioids produce sedation.
- Positive ventilatory effects: by reducing chest-wall pain after thoracotomy or trauma, opioids improve ventilation. This frequently offsets any respiratory depression seen.

Disadvantages

- Dysphoria: in pain-free animals, opioids may stimulate rather than sedate and cause excitation on overdosage (particularly cats). At normal analgesic doses, opioids in pain-free animals do not cause marked stimulation. Stimulation is also unlikely when neuroleptics are given concurrently.
- Respiratory depression: this is a greater problem in primates than companion animals, though some respiratory depression can be seen. Intra-operative alfentanil and fentanyl often depress breathing, mandating ventilatory support.
- Antitussive effects: opioids suppress the coughing reflex, which may be useful in animals requiring analgesia and prolonged intubation. However, accumulated bronchial secretion may impair respiration.
- Gastrointestinal effects: some opioids (e.g. morphine) cause vomiting in dogs. Opioids can induce constipation with prolonged use. With the exception of pethidine, opioids cause increased pressure in the biliary tree; they should be used with caution in pancreatitis and obstructive jaundice.
- Urinary retention: opioids cause urinary retention which may be of significance in cases of pre-existing bladder dysfunction.

Individual properties

Opioids have slightly different properties (Table 23.3) and their use in any situation is governed by several factors.

Potency   Although drugs vary in analgesic potency, this is of little relevance as 'weaker' opioids like pethidine are given at greater doses. The quality of analgesia is more important. Pure agonists (morphine, fentanyl) should be chosen if severe pain is anticipated.

Pharmacodynamic effect   The central nervous, autonomic, cardiopulmonary and gastrointestinal effects of individual drugs may render them useful or hazardous under different circumstances.

Pharmacokinetic factors   Onset time, duration of action and elimination pathways may be important considerations in choosing specific opioids.

Others   Personal preference, cost and controlled drug status may also influence choice.

Drug legislation

Because of their abuse potential, most opioids are controlled drugs (CD), i.e. their use is controlled by the Misuse of Drugs Act 1971.

Controlled drugs are 'scheduled' according to the degree of control applied to their use. Schedule 1 agents (e.g. LSD) are stringently controlled but unused in veterinary practice. Schedule 2 drugs like morphine, etorphine (Immobilon), fentanyl, alfentanil and pethidine are regulated in terms of:

- Special prescription requirements.
- Requisition requirements.
- Record keeping: acquisition and prescription must be recorded in a controlled drugs register (CDR).
- Safe custody. Schedule 2 drugs must be kept in a locked receptacle.
- Destruction of expired stocks.

Schedule 3 drugs include pentazocine and buprenorphine. These are subject to prescription and requisition requirements but transactions do not have to be recorded in the CDR. With the exception of buprenorphine, they do not have to be kept in a locked receptacle.

Table 23.3 Comparison of selected features of opioid analgesics

Drug	Controlled?	Potency	Efficacy	Duration (hours)
Morphine	Yes (Schedule 2)	1	++++	3–4
Pethidine	Yes (Schedule 2)	0.1	+++	1–2
Papaveretum	Yes (Schedule 2)	0.5	++++	3–4
Methadone	Yes (Schedule 2)	1	++++	3–4
Butorphanol	No	1	++	3–4
Buprenorphine	Yes (Schedule 3)	30	+++	6–8

Pure agonists (mu-agonists)

Opioids bind to specific opioid receptors in the CNS to produce analgesia. Mu receptor agonists bind to mu receptors to exert their analgesic effects. This group of analgesics is excellent for treating moderate to severe pain as their action is dose-dependent, with higher doses or repeated doses increasing the analgesic effect.

- Morphine: dose 0.1–0.5 mg/kg intramuscularly (dog), 0.1–0.2 mg/kg (cat). It is the gold standard analgesic, producing some sedation and lasting approximately 4 hours. However, it can cause vomiting and constipation, and at higher doses morphine can cause excitement in cats. When given intravenously it causes some histamine release.
- Methadone: dose as for morphine. It is said to produce less vomiting, sedation, excitement and histamine release compared to morphine and can hence be given intravenously.
- Papaveretum: dose 0.2–1.0 mg/kg intramuscularly. It is associated with less vomiting than morphine and greater synergy with acepromazine, producing greater sedation.
- Pethidine: dose 1–5 mg/kg intramuscularly. It rarely causes vomiting, or excitement in cats, and uniquely is spasmolytic on the intestines. It can be used in cases of pancreatitis and biliary obstruction. It causes histamine release if given intravenously, leading to significant hypotension.

Partial agonists/mixed agonist–antagonists

These agents are weak agonists at the mu receptor (partial agonists) or antagonists at the mu receptor and agonists at kappa opioid receptors (mixed agonist–antagonist), giving analgesia of moderate efficacy though variable consistency. They have a bell shaped dose–response curve meaning that at higher doses less analgesia may result. This is of significance if the animal is in severe pain as further doses of these drugs may not adequately treat the pain. As a group they are best reserved for procedures anticipated to result in mild to moderate pain only.

- Buprenorphine: dose 6–10 μg/kg (IM, IV). It is a partial agonist and has a relatively slow onset of action (45 minutes) but has a relatively long duration of action (6–8 hours). Tight mu receptor binding underlies the duration of action and also makes subsequent pure agonists (and vice versa) less effective. This is a useful agent for procedures producing mild to moderate pain.
- Butorphanol: dose 0.1–0.5 mg/kg (cats lower end of range). It is a mixed agonist–antagonist and analgesia is of an inconsistent nature though better for visceral than somatic pain. It has antitussant properties and provides good sedation when combined with a sedative.

Antagonists

Opioid antagonists may be beneficial to reverse some aspects of opioid activity. In veterinary medicine, naloxone is occasionally used to reverse sedation and respiratory depression, though analgesia is also reversed. Partial agonists such as buprenorphine can be used to reverse the fentanyl component of Hypnorm (Janssen Animal Health) to speed recovery without compromising analgesia.

Non-steroidal anti-inflammatory drugs (NSAIDs)

NSAIDs act peripherally as a group inhibiting cyclooxygenase and hence reducing the level of prostaglandins in the tissues. This reduction in prostaglandins reduces inflammation around the injured tissue. Direct analgesia is also said to occur though its mechanism is unclear. Pre-operative administration of some of the newer agents (carprofen and meloxicam) prior to tissue trauma can reduce tissue inflammation more effectively (i.e. pre-emptive analgesia).

However, due to prostaglandin inhibition, certain side-effects can occur:

- *Gastric irritation*: manifest as vomiting, diarrhoea and gastric haemorrhage. Prostaglandins inhibit gastric acid secretion, stimulate mucus production, maintain blood flow to the gastric mucosa and are involved in mucosal repair. Hence reduction in prostaglandins can compromise the gastric mucosa leading to ulceration.
- *Renal compromise*: prostaglandins modulate renal haemodynamics and are involved in autoregulation of blood flow to the kidneys. They are especially important in states of decreased renal perfusion, e.g. hypotension during anaesthesia, and under such circumstances, NSAIDs administration can lead to renal insufficiency. As a group they are not recommended pre-operatively.
- *Blood dyscrasias and platelet dysfunction*: thromboxane, and prostaglandins are involved in induction of aggregation of platelets. Thus NSAIDs prolong bleeding time.

NSAIDs used in veterinary practice include:

- Aspirin: dose 10–20 mg/kg (dog), 10 mg/kg (cat) per os. The duration of action is 12–24 hours (longer in the cat). Inhibition of platelet aggregation, gastric irritation, aplastic anaemia and hepatoxicity are notable side-effects.
- Paracetamol: dose 25–30 mg/kg (dog). Not safe in cats. The duration of action is 4–6 hours. It inhibits CNS cyclo-oxygenase and is a less effective analgesic than aspirin.
- Phenylbutazone: dose 10 mg/kg (dog). Duration of action is 6–12 hours. It produces moderate gastric irritation and sodium and water retention, so caution in renal and cardiac disease.

- Flunixin: dose 1 mg/kg (dog) (cats 1 mg/kg, not licensed). It has a 4-hour half-life but is found in tissue exudate for up to 24 hours. It is a good analgesic and antiendotoxic drug. Gastrointestinal toxicity and renal papillary necrosis have been recorded.
- Ketoprofen: dose is 1–2 mg/kg. It is a potent cyclo-oxygenase inhibitor and provides good analgesia.
- Tolfenamic acid: dose 4 mg/kg; the half-life is 6.5 hours. Though providing good analgesia it is associated with greater side-effects than some of the 'newer' NSAIDs.
- Carprofen: dose 2–4 mg/kg (SC, IV, PO). The duration of action is 12–24 hours. Carprofen produces poor inhibition of cyclo-oxygenase, thus is prostaglandin sparing. Less renal toxicity and gastric irritation are reported, but it has greater anti-inflammatory potency than phenylbutazone. It is recommended for administration pre-operatively prior to tissue trauma.
- Meloxicam: dose 0.2 mg/kg (SC) and is licensed for pre-operative administration in the dog. It provides good analgesia (18–24 hours after a single dose), and has been used for some time for chronic pain therapy.

Other agents used for analgesia

Alpha-2 adrenoceptor agonists provide good analgesia especially for visceral pain but these actions are reversed if an antagonist is subsequently administered (e.g. atipamezole). They can be administered epidurally and have been used in combination with local anaesthetics and opioids by this route.

Inhalation anaesthetics, including methoxyflurane and nitrous oxide, provide analgesia (see later).

Dissociative anaesthetics (e.g. ketamine) provide good analgesia for somatic pain. At subanaesthetic doses they can be used to reduce 'wind-up' and hypersensitisation of the CNS to painful stimuli.

The role of benzodiazepines as analgesics is controversial, though they have been found to provide analgesia in man when administered spinally and epidurally.

Supportive therapy

Good patient nursing is essential for post-operative comfort. Bandaging and support of injured areas, e.g. Robert Jones bandage, stabilises wounds and reduces pain on movement. Warmth, comfortable bedding, an empty bladder, food and water post-operatively and attentive care can significantly improve patient welfare.

Practical nursing tip *The provision of comfortable bedding, bandaging of the wound (where appropriate), a warm environment in which to recover and plenty of TLC are central to good pain relief in animals recovering from surgery.*

KEY POINTS
- Analgesia reduces post-operative morbidity and speeds recovery.
- NSAIDs, local analgesics and opioids are particularly useful.
- Balanced analgesia involves the concurrent administration of more than one type of analgesic to increase effective analgesia without increasing side-effects.
- Pre-emptive analgesia, administering the analgesic prior to surgical trauma, can produce better analgesia on recovery.
- Good nursing and supportive therapy are essential for effective analgesia.

Local anaesthesia

Local anaesthetics produce reversible block of nerve impulse conduction. Uses include:

- Superficial surgery: some minor procedures may be performed in the conscious animal using local anaesthetics alone (e.g. skin infiltration for wart removal). More invasive procedures may require moderate sedation (e.g. intravenous regional anaesthesia for toe amputation).
- Adjunct to surgical anaesthesia: local techniques may be superimposed on light general anaesthesia for major surgery. The local technique usually does not affect cardiopulmonary function, making the combined technique useful in high-risk cases. Animals also recover consciousness rapidly and, importantly, the surgical site remains pain-free.
- Facilitate procedures: topical anaesthetics facilitate intravenous and urethral catheterisation, endotracheal intubation and ophthalmic examination.
- Diagnosis: local anaesthetics are used to assist lameness diagnosis in horses.
- Antiarrhythmics: lignocaine is used to treat certain types of cardiac arrhythmia.

LOCAL ANAESTHESIA
Advantages
- Lower equipment requirement.
- Techniques are inexpensive.
- Excellent anaesthesia and muscle relaxation.
- Consciousness is retained when used alone; there is no loss of protective reflexes.
- There is little cardiopulmonary depression; techniques are relatively safe in ill animals.
- Some techniques allow titration: the degree, duration and anatomic 'level' of block can be varied.

Disadvantages
- Not all procedures can be performed with local anaesthetic techniques.
- Some techniques are difficult to perform and subsequent block may be incomplete.
- Some techniques are painful to perform; animals may require sedation.
- Active animals may require physical or chemical restraint for surgery.
- Overdosage and toxicity is possible with some drugs.
- Some techniques (e.g. extradural anaesthesia) can produce untoward cardiovascular effects.
- Some local anaesthetics have a short duration of action.

Mechanism of action

Nerve fibres carrying different sensations (e.g. touch, cold and pain) vary in response to local anaesthetics. Because pain fibres are among the most sensitive, it is possible for local anaesthetics to eliminate pain but allow touch and other sensations to persist. When this occurs, the drug behaves as a local analgesic. If all sensation is lost, the drug is an anaesthetic. Motor fibres are most resistant to local anaesthetics but are usually blocked, resulting in muscle relaxation.

Toxicity

Toxic central nervous signs – convulsions or coma – are seen if high levels of local anaesthetic are absorbed. Local anaesthetics can also induce cardiovascular side-effects. Lignocaine can be used to control ventricular arrhythmias, but at toxic doses electrical activity is suppressed and cardiac arrest may occur.

Toxicity depends on the route of injection (caution inadvertent intravenous injection), the total amount injected, the characteristics of the individual agent and whether a vasoconstrictor has been used. Overdosing is avoided by using low concentrations (the minimum dose required to produce effect), by using regional rather than local techniques (where appropriate) and by adding vasoconstrictors to the injected solution.

Pharmacokinetics

The speed of onset of a local anaesthetic block depends upon the agent diffusing into the nerve cell (usually the axon), where it has its effect. Factors influencing this include the proximity of the injection site to the site of action, the lipid solubility, concentration and volume of the agent used, and the use of potentiating drugs.

The duration of action of a local anaesthetic depends upon the lipid solubility of the agent used, the pH of the tissues, the pharmacological properties of agent, the blood flow at the site of action and the use of potentiating drugs.

Vasoconstrictors may be added to prolong the duration of block. The commonest vasoconstrictor used is adrenaline, added to local anaesthetic solutions at 1:100 000 concentration (0.01 mg/ml). This slows drug absorption from the injection site and prolongs block. Solutions containing adrenaline must not be overused in areas with poor or superficial blood flow; vasoconstriction may cause subsequent tissue ischaemia.

The state of the tissues into which local anaesthetic is injected also has an effect upon the action of the drug. For example, if local anaesthetic is injected into inflamed tissue it will have a reduced action. This is because inflamed tissue is more acidic than normal and so the agent will be more ionised and less able to diffuse through the tissue.

Local anaesthetic drugs

Lignocaine

This is the most commonly used local anaesthetic in veterinary practice. It is available as a gel, topical cream, a spray and in injectable forms. Injections are usually 1% or 2% solutions with or without adrenaline. The drug has a rapid (less than 5 minutes) onset of action. It spreads rapidly through tissues and produces almost complete block of 50–90 minutes. Adding adrenaline retards absorption (and toxicity) and prolongs the duration of block. Lignocaine can cause tissue irritation after injection.

Bupivacaine

This is about four times as potent as lignocaine and so is available in lower concentrations (0.25, 0.5 or 0.75%). It has a slower onset of action (up to 20 minutes) but may last from 4 to 6 hours. It does not irritate tissue but may cause cardiac arrest if inadvertent intravascular injection is made.

Mepivacaine

This drug is favoured for conduction blocks in the equine limb as it is less irritant than lignocaine. Its duration of action is similar to that of lignocaine.

Ropivacaine

This is a homologue of bupivacaine with similar clinical effects but much reduced cardiotoxicity. It is used in human anaesthesia.

Types of local anaesthesia

A number of different types of block can be performed.

Local block

Desensitisation is produced only at or near the site of application. Applications include:

- Surface or topical: anaesthetic is applied to skin/mucous membranes to give loss of sensation at the site of application, e.g. EMLA cream can be applied to the ear margin in rabbits to allow pain free catheterisation of the auricular vein.
- Intradermal: anaesthetic is injected into the skin to form a desensitised weal.
- Infiltration: a primary injection of local anaesthetic is made at the surgical site, using as small a needle as possible (23–25 s.w.g.). The next injection is made through this site and the process repeated until the surgical area is 'infiltrated' with local anaesthetic. Liberal infiltration must be avoided as overdosage is possible, especially in small animals and birds. Irritant drugs like lignocaine and those containing vasoconstrictors may interfere with wound healing.
- Intrasynovial: local anaesthetics injected into painful joints and synovial sheaths relieve pain but the effects are not long-acting.

Regional block

Anaesthetic is used to produce desensitisation remote from the site of injection.

- Perineural: this involves drug injection in proximity to identifiable nerves, as opposed to nerve endings. The technique requires knowledge of topographical anatomy. Injection is made using sterile needles and syringes. For example, the intercostal nerves (behind each rib) are often blocked with bupivacaine after thoracotomy. This relieves post-operative chest-wall pain, allowing adequate ventilation.
- Intravenous regional anaesthesia (IVRA): this is used for surgical procedures on limb extremities (e.g. digit removal). The limb is first exsanguinated using an Esmarch's bandage, which is then left in place as a tourniquet. Local anaesthetic (e.g. 2–5 ml lignocaine without adrenaline) is then injected into any vein distal to the tourniquet. Surgery may begin after 15 minutes. Anaesthesia persists until the tourniquet is removed.
- Spinal and epidural block: anaesthetic is injected within the bony confines of the spinal canal (see below).

Epidural anaesthesia

In this method, drug is injected into the space between the dura mater (the thick fibrous outermost covering of the spinal cord) and the periosteum lining the spinal canal. Here, the drug blocks the nerves as they leave the cord. A large spinal needle is used and usually injection is made into the L7–S1 interspace. The technique is useful for pain relief

and muscle relaxation during pelvic-limb orthopaedic procedures in dogs, and less commonly in cats. In current practice, the technique is usually performed on heavily sedated or anaesthetised animals. Lignocaine or bupivacaine combined with an opioid (e.g. preservative-free morphine) are commonly used. The main advantage of epidural opioids is prolonged and profound analgesia.

Spinal anaesthesia

This technique is rarely used in clinical veterinary anaesthesia. It involves a midline injection at the L5–L6 interspace or, at a higher level, into the CSF-filled space below the arachnoid mater, lying below the dura. Lower doses produce the same effects of extradural injection but there is a slightly greater risk of overdosage.

KEY POINTS
- Local anaesthesia can be used on its own for certain simple procedures.
- As an adjunct to general anaesthesia it can produce excellent analgesia, reduce the general anaesthetic requirements and provide balanced anaesthesia.
- Commonly used drugs include lignocaine, bupivacaine and mepivacaine.
- Local blocks include surface desensitisation and dermal injection.
- Regional blocks include IVRA, spinal and epidural blocks.

Injectable anaesthesia

General anaesthesia can be induced and maintained with injectable anaesthetics. The intramuscular and intravenous routes are most often used but occasionally, particularly in small mammals, the intraperitoneal route may be used. Recently, maintenance of anaesthesia via the intravenous route has received more interest. Total intravenous anaesthesia (TIVA) can provide a good alternative to gaseous anaesthesia, providing good cardiovascular stability without the potential pollution hazards of the inhalation agents (see later). Whichever route is used, the provision of a patent airway and a supply of oxygen are always to be recommended. If the intravenous route is to be used the placement of an intravenous catheter is to be recommended, particularly for prolonged and complicated procedures (Fig. 23.4).

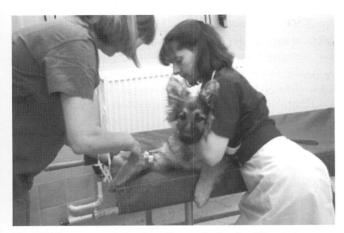

Fig. 23.4 Intravenous induction of anaesthesia after IV catheter placement.

INJECTABLE ANAESTHETICS

Advantages
- Convenient; simple to inject.
- Inexpensive – less equipment needed.
- Intravenous injection usually causes a rapid loss of consciousness.
- No airway irritation.
- No explosion/pollution hazard.
- Rapid recovery after a single dose.
- Some drugs can be antagonised.
- Endotracheal intubation is not always necessary.
- Rapid deepening of anaesthesia is possible.
- Respiratory function does not influence drug behaviour.

Disadvantages
- Stressful restraint may be required.
- Technical skill required for intravenous injection and catheterisation.
- Myositis and pain may result from injection.
- Perivascular injection may cause irritation with certain drugs.
- Effects may be slow to be reversed; for drugs without antagonists, recovery depends on cardiovascular, hepatic and renal function.
- Anaesthesia is readily deepened, but not lightened.
- Wide dose-range requirements.
- Self-administration is hazardous with some drugs.
- Repeated doses may cause drug accumulation and prolonged recovery.
- Injectable drugs have varying side-effects.
- Airway protection and supply of oxygen are often neglected.

Pharmacology

The brain has a rich blood supply and receives a high concentration of drug shortly after IV injection. When a critical brain concentration is exceeded, unconsciousness occurs. In time, organs less well-perfused than the brain (such as skeletal muscle) begin to take up drug. Plasma levels fall and this creates a diffusion gradient which promotes movement of drug from brain to plasma. Consciousness returns when brain drug levels fall below a critical level. The duration of action of most modern injectable anaesthetics depends on 'redistribution' of drug from brain to less well-perfused tissues; this depends on factors like cardiac output and the mass of tissues available for redistribution of drug.

Most anaesthetics are metabolised in the liver by conversion from lipid to water-soluble molecules. These forms are more easily excreted in bile (appearing later in faeces) or urine. Only very small amounts are excreted unchanged in bile and urine as lipid-soluble drug. The duration of action of drugs which are rapidly metabolised by the liver (e.g. propofol and methohexitone) depends on a combination of redistribution and metabolism.

Practical nursing tip *Label all drugs; this will avoid dangerous mistakes.*

Barbiturates

Barbiturates like thiopentone, methohexitone and pentobarbitone cause unconsciousness but have poor analgesic properties. Muscle relaxation is usually adequate during anaesthesia.

Thiopentone

Thiopentone is available as a sulphurous-yellow powder and requires reconstitution with water. In solution it is highly alkaline (pH of 10.8) and irritant if injected perivascularly. It is highly protein bound and slowly metabolised in the liver, relying primarily on redistribution away from the brain for recovery after administration. Solutions of various strengths may be made. A 1% solution contains 1 g or 1000 mg in 100 ml. A 1% solution, therefore, contains 10 mg/ml and a 2.5% solution of thiopentone contains 25 mg drug/ml. It is reconstituted by adding 100 ml water to 2.5 g of powder.

Thiopentone is a useful anaesthetic agent for short-duration procedures or for induction prior to maintenance with inhalation agents. Doses of 10 mg/kg (intravenously) are used following premedication. Incremental doses should be avoided as they prolong recovery and contribute to 'hangover'.

Mild cardiovascular depression is seen, with hypotension, reduced cardiac output and tachycardia reported. Cardiac dysrhythmias may be seen. Dose-dependent respiratory depression occurs transiently.

The drug is safe in high-risk cases provided the factors which increase patient sensitivity are known (many of these apply to drugs other than thiopentone). Doses are reduced in: hypoalbuminaemia, acidaemia, hypovolaemia, congestive heart failure, azotaemia, toxaemia and obesity. Doses are also reduced when diazepam is injected immediately before or afterwards.

Special precautions Thiopentone causes prolonged recoveries in sight-hounds (e.g. Whippet, Greyhound, Saluki) after otherwise uneventful anaesthesia. The drug should not be used if there is difficulty achieving venous access.

Practical nursing tip *Concurrent administration of a benzodiazepine will significantly reduce the induction agent dose and smooth anaesthetic induction and endotracheal intubation. This is particularly valuable in high-risk cases.*

Methohexitone

Methohexitone is available as a dry powder and is reconstituted to produce a 1% solution. Being twice as potent as thiopentone, its dose is halved to 5 mg/kg. Onset time is similar but its duration of action is shorter; extensive and rapid hepatic metabolism occurs in addition to redistribution. It also is alkaline in solution (pH of 11) but is less irritant when injected outside a vein.

Cardiovascular and respiratory depression are similar to that of thiopentone. Recoveries are not always smooth, especially when pre-anaesthetic medication is withheld. Good premedication prior to methohexitone induction of anaesthesia is recommended. The drug has been favoured in sight-hounds because it produces rapid recoveries.

Pentobarbitone

This once useful drug has been superseded by newer agents except, perhaps, in laboratory animal anaesthesia. Following injection, its onset of action is relatively slow (related to delay in crossing the blood–brain barrier) and recoveries are prolonged. In companion animal practice it is used as an anticonvulsant and for humane destruction.

Steroid anaesthetics – 'Saffan'

'Saffan' is a mixture of alphaxalone (9 mg/kg) and alphadolone (3 mg/kg); the former is the major active component. Induction doses of 3–6 mg/kg (intravenously) are routinely used in the cat. Doses are always expressed in mg of total steroid. The drug has been favoured for some time in cats as it has a high therapeutic index with a wide safety margin. It produces only mild cardiovascular and respiratory depression at clinical doses.

The two steroids are water insoluble and the formulation contains Cremophor EL (polyethoxylated castor oil). This agent causes histamine release in dogs and cannot be used safely in this species. In cats, it causes only mild anaphylactoid reactions with swelling of the pinnae and paws. Normally this is of little consequence but very infrequently cases of fatal pulmonary oedema have been seen. Because the formulation contains no bacteriostat, open ampoules must be discarded.

The intravenous route is preferred because effects are less predictable after intramuscular injection. The solution is viscous but non-irritant. The subcutaneous route is unsuitable; the rate of drug metabolism over absorption is high and so anaesthetic levels are not achieved.

Dissociative anaesthetics – Ketamine

Ketamine is described as a dissociative anaesthetic, producing a unique state of anaesthesia. Protective airway reflexes are maintained, the eyes remain open and the pupils are dilated. Cranial nerve reflexes are less depressed than with other agents, although it cannot be assumed that these will remain entirely protected.

It is presented in an aqueous solution (pH of 3–3.5). It can be given by intravenous, intramuscular, subcutaneous or intraperitoneal injection and is also active when given sublingually. Intramuscular injection is painful although injection volumes are low because the drug is available as a 100 mg/ml solution. Doses of 2–5 mg/kg given intravenously or 5–10 mg/kg, intramuscularly are frequently used.

Heart rate is increased and blood pressure is normally maintained. Breathing is modestly reduced, although at higher doses an apneustic pattern can be seen in which the breath is held after inspiration. Salivation increases. Spontaneous muscle movement unrelated to surgery is a disconcerting feature of ketamine anaesthesia but can be suppressed by concurrently administered drugs. Ketamine is considered to provide good somatic analgesia. Its use to reduce 'wind-up' and central sensitisation to pain has been described.

Poor muscle relaxation is provided and for this reason it is usually given with or after another agent such as an alpha-2 agonist or benzodiazepine. Convulsions are seen in dogs when it is used alone, and its use in this species can only be recommended when combined with a sedative/tranquilliser (e.g. diazepam).

Phenols – Propofol

This water-insoluble phenol derivative (2,6-di-isopropylphenol) forms a characteristic milky-white solution when solubilised in an egg–phosphatidyl–soybean oil emulsion. The solution must not be frozen, though cooling is said to reduce the low incidence of pain on intravenous injection. Perivascular injection does not cause irritation. The solution contains no bacteriostat and so opened ampoules must be discarded.

The drug produces dose-dependent levels of unconsciousness after intravenous injection. Good muscle relaxation is seen. Dogs require 4–6 mg/kg (intravenously), whilst cats require higher doses (6–8 mg/kg, intravenously) for anaesthesia. The drug is also longer-acting in these species, with induction doses lasting up to 20 minutes. Being rapidly metabolised it is a useful agent for total intravenous anaesthesia (TIVA). Maintenance of anaesthesia can be achieved by infusing it at rates of 0.3–0.5 mg/kg/minute.

Cardiovascular and respiratory depression are comparable to those of thiopentone but are generally of longer duration. Occasionally, twitching and spontaneous muscle activity occurs with propofol anaesthesia and excited recoveries have been described.

Propofol has some advantages over thiopentone:

- Recovery is rapid and free from hangover when a single dose is given. This makes it useful in sight-hounds.
- Non-cumulative, maintenance of anaesthesia with top-up injections or by infusion results in less risk of prolonged recoveries.
- Non-irritant when perivascularly administered.

Combinations and neuroleptanalgesia

Minor surgical procedures may be performed using neuroleptanalgesia, benzodiazepine/ketamine and alpha-2-agonist/ketamine mixtures.

Ketamine mixtures

Several drugs are used with ketamine to reduce muscle hypertonicity. These include acepromazine, diazepam, midazolam, xylazine and medetomidine. Some of these also have anticonvulsant effects and render the combinations safe for use in dogs. However, some combinations have adverse physiological effects such as inducing hypoventilation and arrhythmias.

Practial nursing tip – intravenous catheterisation *Adequate physical and/or chemical restraint is a prerequisite. The site must receive surgical preparation. A small skin incision over the vein may facilitate catheter placement in animals with resilient skin (e.g. male cats, dehydrated animals). The catheter is introduced through the skin and directed proximally along the line of the vein. When blood is seen to flow back down the catheter it is advanced a small distance further, to ensure presence of both catheter and stylet within the vein. The catheter is then gently advanced off the stylet whilst stabilising the latter. An obturator or three-way tap is attached to the catheter, the catheter is flushed with heparinised saline and then it is secured to the skin with tape or superglue. Catheters should be bandaged to protect them from the patient when not under direct observation.*

INTRAVENOUS CATHETERISATION

Advantages
- Reduces risk of extravascular injection, ensures full doses are given and prevents tissue damage with irritant drugs.
- Provides rapid intravenous access for emergency drugs.
- Allows fluids to be given rapidly.
- Allows rapid 'deepening' of anaesthesia with injectable anaesthetics.

Disadvantages
- Vein damage: poor catheterisation technique may damage the vein and preclude further access. This occurs when haematoma or thrombosis form.
- Sepsis: in immunosuppressed animals (e.g. diabetics) poor surgical preparation and management of catheters lead to phlebitis.
- More severe conditions like bacteraemia may follow.

KEY POINTS
- Injectable anaesthesia provides rapid onset and good conditions for endotracheal intubation.
- Maintenance of anaesthesia can be achieved by top-up doses or intravenous infusions of an injectable anaesthetic.
- The intravenous route is often preferred though other routes can be used.
- The choice of agent depends on patient consideration, the procedure performed, equipment available, cost and the clinician's experience.

Inhalation anaesthesia

Inhalation, volatile or 'gaseous' anaesthesia refers to the inhalation of anaesthetic vapours or gases delivered into the respiratory tract. Anaesthesia is commonly maintained with inhalation agents, although they can also be used to induce anaesthesia.

Inhaled anaesthetics commonly used in animals include halothane, isoflurane, and nitrous oxide (N_2O). Other agents used include methoxyflurane, enflurane, ether and more recently sevoflurane and desflurane. Oxygen (O_2) and N_2O are known as carrier gases because they 'carry' the volatile anaesthetics.

INHALATION ANAESTHETICS

Advantages

- Recovery depends on respiratory function and is normally rapid and predictable.
- The depth of anaesthesia is readily controlled.
- Single dose rate; minimum alveolar concentration (MAC) is similar in most species.
- Concurrent oxygen delivery; volatile agents are usually 'carried' in oxygen.
- Volatile agent activity is independent of hepatic and renal function.
- Continued administration does not necessarily cause prolonged recoveries.
- Surgery may be prolonged without complication.
- Inhalation drugs have broadly similar effects.
- The airway is usually protected.

Disadvantages

- Induction and recovery may be delayed by inadequate ventilation or lung pathology.
- A considerable range of equipment is required; some items are expensive.
- Intubation is usually necessary.
- Knowledge of breathing systems and anaesthetic machines is required.
- Hazards associated with compressed gas.
- Fire and explosion risks with some agents.
- Possible personnel health risk associated with exposure to volatile agents.

Pharmacokinetics

The behaviour of inhalation anaesthetics can be predicted and compared if two important features are known. These are the blood/gas solubility coefficient and the minimum alveolar concentration.

- *Blood/gas solubility coefficient.* This value describes the solubility of agents in blood. Drugs with low solubility produce rapid induction and recovery rates, and changes in the level of anaesthesia on changing vaporiser settings are more rapid. Values for modern anaesthetics (starting with the most insoluble) are:

  – Desflurane: 0.42
  – N_2O: 0.47
  – Sevoflurane: 0.6
  – Isoflurane: 1.39
  – Enflurane: 1.8
  – Halothane: 2.4
  – Methoxyflurane: 12.0

Hence the use of isoflurane, which is more insoluble than halothane, would be expected to result in a faster induction of anaesthesia, change in depth and recovery.

- *Minimum alveolar concentration (MAC).* MAC of anaesthetics is the alveolar concentration that prevents responses occurring to a specified stimulus (e.g. skin incision) in 50% of patients. It is a measure of potency. Agents with low values have the greatest potency; low inspired concentrations are required for surgery. Many factors alter MAC, the most important being other drugs given during anaesthesia, for instance N_2O, analgesics and pre-anaesthetic medication all reduce MAC of the inhalation agents. Values (starting with most potent) are:

  – Methoxyflurane: 0.23
  – Halothane: 0.8
  – Isoflurane: 1.3
  – Sevoflurane: 2.0
  – Enflurane: 2.2
  – Desflurane: 6.8
  – N_2O: 188–220

Volatile anaesthetics produce anaesthesia when a critical tension is exceeded in the CNS. This tension is achieved by movement of drug molecules down a series of tension gradients, beginning at the anaesthetic machine and ending at the site of action within the CNS. At equilibrium, the tension of drug in the brain mirrors that in arterial blood, which in turn depends on that in the alveoli. Therefore, factors influencing alveolar tensions ultimately determine brain tensions.

Alveolar drug levels depend on those factors that affect delivery to, and removal from, the lung. Factors increasing alveolar delivery include alveolar ventilation rate and the inspired gas concentration. When these are high, induction of anaesthesia is rapid. Removal of anaesthetic from the alveolus depends on blood solubility of the gas, cardiac output and alveolar–venous anaesthetic gradient. Alveolar tensions rise rapidly (and induction is rapid) when cardiac output is low (e.g. in haemorrhagic shock), when insoluble agents (e.g. isoflurane) are used and when the pulmonary venous tension of anaesthetic is high.

Recovery from anaesthesia relies on principles similar to those of induction in the process of removing inhaled agent from the CNS. An added consideration is the presence of a poorly perfused fat-soluble compartment (i.e adipose tissue). During a prolonged period of anaesthesia, a significant uptake of volatile agent into this compartment can occur and this can affect recovery, as release of the inhalation agent from this tissue to the blood will result. Highly fat-soluble agents will produce a greater effect than poorly fat-soluble inhalation agents as more agent will have partitioned within this fatty compartment. Metabolism of the anaesthetic may also play a role in recovery from certain anaesthetics, particularly for drugs undergoing significant hepatic metabolism (e.g. halothane, methoxyflurane).

Individual inhalation agents

Halothane

Currently one of the most common volatile anaesthetic in veterinary anaesthesia in the UK, this halogenated hydrocarbon is a sweet-smelling, clear liquid which decomposes in ultraviolet light (so is stored in amber bottles) and contains an antioxidant (0.01% thymol). It readily evaporates, producing a maximum concentration of 32%. For this reason it must be used from a calibrated vaporiser, or dangerously high levels of anaesthetic could be delivered to the patient. Halothane is a fast-acting anaesthetic. Up to 12–25% of absorbed halothane is metabolised to bromide, trifluroacetate and chloride by the liver.

Halothane affects physiological function of the patient as described below.

Central nervous system effects
Halothane is a potent anaesthetic; concentrations of 1.0–3.0% may be needed for induction but adequate surgical conditions are obtained with inspired concentrations of 0.75–2.0%. Muscle relaxation is modest but analgesia is poor; adrenergic responses occur until deep levels of anaesthesia are reached.

Cardiopulmonary system effects
Halothane lowers blood pressure by depressing cardiac contractility and reducing cardiac output. Heart rate remains unchanged. Halothane produces minimal reduction in systemic vascular resistance, though it causes vasodilatation in capillary beds of the brain, uterus and skin. As a halogenated hydrocarbon, the drug 'sensitises' the myocardium to adrenaline, predisposing the heart to arrhythmias under conditions of high circulating catecholamines (e.g. when stressed).

Halothane depresses ventilation in a dose-dependent manner, causing decreased tidal volume and decreased respiratory rate. It depresses ventilation to a lesser extent than other volatile anaesthetics with the exception of diethyl ether. It is non-irritant to respiratory mucosa and well tolerated for mask induction.

Other effects
In people, halothane-associated hepatitis occurs with repeated halothane anaesthetics. The cause is not fully understood, but seems related to pre-operative enzyme induction caused by smoking and alcohol consumption, as well as intraoperative hypoxia. The condition has not been conclusively demonstrated to occur in animals during surgical anaesthesia.

Halothane lowers body temperature by inhibiting thermoregulatory mechanisms and producing cutaneous vasodilatation.

Special precautions
Halothane triggers malignant hyperthermia in sensitive pigs and this genetically determined condition also occurs in man. It has occurred in dogs, horses and cats but is rare.

Isoflurane

Isoflurane is an isomer of enflurane and a more recently developed volatile agent. Although it is a halogenated ether, it has an unpleasant pungent smell. Its saturated vapour pressure is similar to halothane and the same (cleaned) precision vaporiser may be used for its administration. At room temperature, the maximum concentration possible is 31.5%. It is more expensive than halothane though when delivered via a rebreathing circuit this difference in cost is reduced.

Isoflurane has a low blood/gas solubility coefficient and so inductions and recoveries are rapid, the latter even after prolonged administration. At induction, inspired concentrations of 2–3% are needed. Because it has a higher MAC value than halothane, higher inspired concentrations are needed to maintain anaesthesia (1.5–2.5%).

Central nervous system effects
It is a potent anaesthetic, providing narcosis and muscle relaxation. Recoveries are rapid but may be associated with transient excitatory effects, especially after painful surgery.

Cardiopulmonary system effects
Isoflurane causes dose-dependent hypotension despite non-dose-dependent increases in heart rate. At 1.0 MAC cardiac output is maintained, whilst systemic vascular resistance is reduced. Isoflurane does not sensitise the heart to catecholamine-induced arrhythmias. Isoflurane is a potent respiratory depressant, depressing ventilation to a greater extent than halothane. Because of its pungent odour it is poorly tolerated for mask inductions.

Enflurane

Enflurane, a halogenated ether with a fruity smell, has never gained popularity in veterinary anaesthesia despite some useful features. Chemically it is very stable and contains no preservative. Concentrations of 4–6% are needed for induction, with maintenance requirements of 1–3%. It is relatively expensive. Because it is highly volatile (SVP is 171.8 at 20°C) the maximum concentration achievable is 22% (at that temperature) and so the use of an 'Enfluratec' is advisable.

Central nervous system effects
In humans, deep enflurane anaesthesia causes seizure-type electroencephalographic (EEG) activity which is exacerbated by hypercapnia. Involuntary muscle twitches are seen during anaesthesia and recovery in animals.

Cardiopulmonary system effects
Enflurane depresses blood pressure to the same extent as isoflurane, but less than halothane. Heart rate is increased in a dose-dependent manner. Cardiac output is reduced. It is the most potent respiratory depressant, decreasing rate and depth.

Other effects
Enflurane produces excellent muscle relaxation and markedly potentiates neuromuscular blockers.

Methoxyflurane

This fruity-smelling halogenated ether is the most potent volatile anaesthetic. It is non-reactive but decomposes slowly when exposed to soda–lime and ultraviolet light and so it contains butylated hydroxytoluene. Methoxyflurane evaporates poorly – no more than 3% can be delivered at room temperature. It has high blood-gas (12.0) and rubber-gas (630) solubility coefficients making induction and recovery very slow. This precludes its use in large animals. Induction requires 1.5–2.5% and maintenance 0.2–1.25%.

Central nervous system effects

It is a potent anaesthetic with good muscle relaxant and analgesic properties. Cranial nerve reflexes are lost early and the eye is said to 'centralise' at relatively light levels of anaesthesia.

Cardiopulmonary system effects

Cardiac output is reduced in a dose-dependent manner, causing hypotension. Heart rate tends to slow. It causes more respiratory depression than halothane.

Special precautions

In people, prolonged methoxyflurane anaesthesia causes renal tubular destruction, polyuria and dehydration lasting several days after administration. This is partly due to fluoride and oxalate ions generated from hepatic methoxyflurane metabolism. While the dog kidney is resistant to fluorotoxicosis, acute renal failure has occurred in this species when flunixin has been given peri-operatively. Methoxyflurane should not be used in animals receiving NSAIDs or other potentially nephrotic drugs. Alternatively, these drugs should be withheld from animals in which methoxyflurane anaesthesia is considered desirable.

Ether

Rarely used now in veterinary anaesthesia, it is a pungent irritant vapour. Oxygen–ether mixtures are explosive. It is less potent than halothane though produces sympathetic stimulation providing cardiovascular support. Ether does not sensitise the heart to catecholamine-induced arrhythmias. It has some analgesic activity.

Desflurane

A relatively new agent. Its blood/gas partition coefficient (0.42) is similar to that of nitrous oxide, so it is very insoluble and is associated with rapid induction and recovery. It requires a special temperature-controlled, pressurised vaporiser and is expensive. Its use in veterinary anaesthesia is presently mainly experimental.

Sevoflurane

Popular in human anaesthesia in Japan and veterinary anaesthesia in North America, it has a low blood/gas partition coefficient and also produces rapid induction and recovery. Cardiopulmonary effects are similar to those of isoflurane. It is unstable and degrades in the presence of soda–lime, producing toxic metabolites (i.e. compound A) which have been shown to produce renal pathology in rats.

Nitrous oxide (N_2O)

Nitrous oxide is an odourless relatively inert gas with anaesthetic properties. It is non-flammable, but supports combustion. Nitrous oxide is combined with oxygen as a carrier gas. It must not be used at concentrations greater than 80% as this lowers O_2 below normal levels. Usually no more than 66% is delivered.

The percentage of gas mixtures is calculated on a flow ratio basis. For example, a 50% O_2/N_2O mixture is produced when O_2 and N_2O flows are the same (e.g. 3 l/min O_2 and 3 l/min N_2O). Commonly, 66% or 2:1 N_2O/O_2 mixtures are used. These are produced when N_2O flow is exactly twice that of O_2.

Anaesthetic 'sparing' effect

Nitrous oxide is less potent in animals than in man but does lower the concentration of volatile agent required to produce a given level of anaesthesia. For example, 66% N_2O reduces halothane requirements by about 25%. Because N_2O has minimal effects on cardiac output and ventilation, its inclusion preserves cardiopulmonary performance.

Second gas effect

During induction with N_2O and a volatile agent, the rapid uptake of N_2O from alveoli causes the alveolar concentration of the volatile agent, or second gas, to rise. This accelerates uptake of the second gas and speeds the rate of induction of anaesthesia.

Gas-filled viscous

Because N_2O is 35 times more soluble in blood than Nitrogen, N_2O diffuses into gas filled spaces faster than nitrogen is reabsorbed during denitrogenation of the body. Hence it can accumulate in gas filled spaces, e.g. the dilated stomach of dogs with gastric-dilatation–volvulus complex or the pleural space of animals with closed pneumothorax. Nitrous oxide compromises the animal by enlarging or increasing the pressure within such spaces.

Cardiopulmonary effects

N_2O has a very modest stimulant effect on cardiac output and blood pressure. It has no effect on ventilation; when added to volatile agents, ventilation remains unchanged even though anaesthesia deepens.

Hypoxia

Whenever N_2O is used, the O_2 content of inspired gas is lowered; this increases the possibility of hypoxia arising from other causes like hypoventilation. When used in a rebreathng circuit after the initial stabilisation period, uptake of N_2O from the circuit declines and can build up within the circuit if low flow anaesthesia is being performed. For this reason N_2O should be used with caution in circle or to-and-fro systems.

Diffusion hypoxia

When N_2O delivery is ended, its direction of diffusion reverses – from blood into the alveolar space. The volume evolved in the first few minutes after termination may dilute alveolar O_2. If alveolar oxygen levels are low because the animal is breathing air, not

100% O_2, 'diffusion hypoxia' may occur. Therefore on ending N_2O administration, animals should receive 100% O_2 for at least 3 minutes.

Special precautions   Nitrous oxide should not be used in animals whose arterial oxygen tensions are lowered by disease or where a gas-filled viscous is present.

POLLUTION
Nitrous oxide is relatively odourless and high atmospheric levels are difficult to detect.
There is some evidence that N_2O causes toxic effects like bone-marrow depression after chronic, low-level exposure. It is not absorbed by activated charcoal and so 'canister' scavenging is useless.

Oxygen

Oxygen is an odourless, reactive gas that allows combustion and, in the presence of organic material and activation energy (i.e. sparks or naked flames), explosions.

The gas is given whenever the normal delivery of atmospheric oxygen to active tissue is threatened. This includes anaesthesia (even that produced with injectable agents). Pure oxygen (100%) is usually given to animals which are anaemic, have pulmonary pathology or are hypoventilating. During inhalation anaesthesia, 100% oxygen may be used as the 'carrier gas' but it is frequently diluted to 50% or 33% concentrations by nitrous oxide. Oxygen is also supplied during recovery until the animal is capable of maintaining haemoglobin saturation with room air (20% O_2).

Techniques

Endotracheal intubation

When animals are rendered unconscious by injectable or inhalation drugs, protective airway reflexes are lost. Endotracheal intubation is an important means of ensuring a patent airway and preventing aspiration of fluids and regurgitated food.

Tube selection   Ideally, the tube should extend from the incisor table to a point level with the spine of the scapula. Provided that the cuff lies beyond the glottis, the airway will be secure. Surplus dead-space is minimised by cutting off the projecting tube. The maximum diameter tube appropriate to the patient minimises resistance to air flow.

Intubation   The jaws must be relaxed and laryngeal reflexes suppressed before intubation is attempted. Laryngeal reflexes persist in cats to relatively 'deep' levels of anaesthesia, and laryngospasm is not uncommon following tactile stimulation of the glottis. In this species, laryngeal reflexes may be depressed with topical lignocaine by aerosol.

Laryngoscopy is useful during intubation in cats, in dogs with pigmented oral mucosae or in those with surplus soft tissue in the upper airway.

ENDOTRACHEAL INTUBATION
Advantages
- Airway protection from saliva and gastric contents: if cuffed tubes are not available an oropharyngeal pack – layers of moistened gauze laid in a horseshoe pattern over the tube and 'packed' – may suffice. This is important during dental and oral surgery.
- Allows positive pressure ventilation: a leak-proof cuff allows lung inflation without gas escape.
- Reduces waste-gas pollution.
- Reduces anatomic dead-space.

Disadvantages
- Resistance: cuffs limit the size of tube that can be introduced atraumatically. Small internal diameters critically increase resistance to breathing.
- Kinking or occlusion: overinflated cuffs may compress the underlying tube. Severe occipito-atlantal flexion (e.g. during cisternal puncture) may cause tubes (especially red-rubber types) to kink. If tubes are inadequately cleaned, dried secretions accumulate within the lumen.
- Traumatic laryngitis: poor intubation technique or the use of oversized tubes may physically damage the larynx and/or trachea, causing post-operative respiratory embarrassment.
- Chemical/ischaemic tracheitis: if tubes are inadequately rinsed or irritant sterilants are used, the tracheal mucosa may be irritated. For this reason, tubes must be adequately aired after ethylene oxide sterilisation. Overinflated cuffs left *in situ* for prolonged periods may produce an ischaemic tracheitis and cause post-operative coughing.
- Apparatus dead-space: correctly sized endotracheal tubes reduce anatomic dead-space. However, overlong tubes extending beyond the incisor table constitute apparatus dead-space which should be minimised.
- Endobronchial intubation: excessive advancement of the endotracheal tube down the airway may result in endobronchial intubation. In these circumstances, one lung receives no ventilation and blood deoxygenation may occur.
- False security: the presence of endotracheal tubes does not guarantee a patent airway; they may become kinked, crushed or filled with exudate.
- Interference: conventionally placed (orotracheal) tubes interfere with some types of oral surgery. In such cases pharyngotracheal or tracheostomy placement may be required. In some species nasotracheal intubation is practised.

Mask inductions

Masks are used to provide oxygen in comatose or recovering animals, or for the delivery of volatile anaesthetics when intubation is not performed. Induction of anaesthesia using masks is a useful technique in high-risk cases because animals receive oxygen during induction; if crises develop, switching the vaporiser off may prove life-saving.

MASK INDUCTIONS
Advantages
- Mask inductions do not damage the airway.
- They produce smooth inductions when patients are depressed or heavily sedated.

Disadvantages
- Mask inductions are resisted and cause inelegant inductions in poorly sedated animals.
- Masks increase mechanical dead-space. They do not necessarily add to air-flow resistance but, because the airway is not clear, turbulence or obstruction can occur.
- Ventilation is possible with tightly applied, gas-tight masks. However, some gas inevitably enters the stomach, which inflates and limits diaphragmatic movement.
- Atmospheric pollution is greater with masks. This is reduced by using close-fitting face-masks or eliminating leaks with plasticine.

Chamber inductions

This technique is useful in laboratory animals and can be used in cats and small dogs. Sedation or depression should be present, otherwise inductions may be violent. Pollution is a problem when the chamber is opened. High inspired oxygen levels are present when consciousness is lost; indeed, the chamber usefully serves as an oxygen cage for neonates or small animals.

KEY POINTS
- Inhalation anaesthesia requires more equipment than injectable anaesthesia.
- Greater control and adjustment of depth of anaesthesia exists.
- Recoveries tend to be faster after prolonged procedures.
- A provision of oxygen and IPPV is present.
- Halothane and isoflurane are most commonly used.
- Dose-dependent cardiovascular and respiratory depression are seen.
- Analgesia is rarely provided.

Equipment

Anaesthetic equipment centres on the administration of inhalational anaesthetics. In the past, the 'open method' of administration of inhalational anaesthetics was popular, consisting of the application of liquid anaesthetic to a gauze swab applied to the patient's nose. Ether, chloroform, trichloroethylene and methoxyflurane were used in this system. In modern veterinary practice this system is unacceptable because of pollution and because the inspired gas concentration is difficult to control. The latter is particularly hazardous with anaesthetics like halothane which have high saturated vapour pressures and produce high concentrations at room temperature. Modern techniques require an anaesthetic machine and an anaesthetic breathing system or 'circuit'. The main components include:

- Oxygen source.
- Vaporiser/source of anaesthetic gas.
- Breathing circuit.

Anaesthetic breathing systems

The anaesthetic circuit takes the fresh gas from the common gas outlet of the anaesthetic machine and delivers it to the patient. The functions of the circuit include:

- Removal of exhaled carbon dioxide (CO_2).
- Supply of oxygen (O_2).
- Supply of anaesthetic gases.
- Allow performance of intermittent positive pressure ventilation (IPPV).

Circuit classification varies throughout the world and can be confusing. A simple basis of classification depends on whether expired carbon dioxide is flushed from the system by high gas flow (non-rebreathing circuit) or removed by chemical reaction (e.g. with soda–lime; rebreathing circuit).

Rebreathing systems

Rebreathing circuits (circle and to-and-fro) remove CO_2 from expired gas by chemically absorbing it. Expired breath, in comparison with inspired gas, is low in O_2 and anaesthetic but contains more CO_2 and water vapour and is warm. In rebreathing systems, expired gas passes through soda–lime (absorbent) which removes CO_2. Warm, moist gas is then reinspired and so rebreathing systems conserve heat and moisture. Fresh gas flow requirements are based on the O_2 consumption of the patient. Because this value is low (Table 23.4), rebreathing systems are very efficient.

Absorbent This absorbs CO_2 and consists of granules of:

- 80% sodium hydroxide [NaOH] or 'soda'.
- 18% calcium hydroxide [$Ca(OH)_2$] or 'lime'.
- Silicates.
- pH indicators.

Table 23.4 Respiratory variables in companion animals

Species	Respiratory rate[a] (breaths/min)	Tidal volume[a] (ml/kg)	Minute volume[a] (ml/kg/min)	Oxygen consumption[b] (ml/kg/min)
Dogs				
>30 kg	15–20	12–15	150–250	5.8
<30 kg	20–30	16–20	200–300	6.2
Cats	20–30	7–9	180–380	7.3

[a]During surgery, factors like pain, pyrexia, light versus deep anaesthesia will affect these
[b]Oxygen consumption depends on factors related to metabolic rate: age, temperature, thyroid status, drugs, muscle tone, response to surgery

Carbon dioxide reacts chemically with the soda–lime to produce carbonates and produces heat in the process. Silicates used to be included in medical absorbents to increase the hardness and reduce the formation of irritant dust. pH indicators change colour as soda–lime becomes exhausted. Changes depend on the dyes used. Common absorbents turn from pink to white (although, confusingly, one type turns from white to pink). The container label describes the colour change its contents undergo and should be consulted.

When soda–lime granules are 'spent', they lose their soapy, soft texture and fail to become warm when exposed to CO_2. Spent soda–lime should be replaced, as it will no longer absorb CO_2. If left overnight the surface of the spent granules can return to pink; however, the granules are still exhausted and should be replaced.

Soda–lime is contained in canisters with contents of approximately 50% granules and 50% air space. Efficient absorption requires an air-space volume in excess of tidal volume and so the minimum 'working' canister size is two times the tidal volume of the patient, though generally greater volumes than this are used.

Soda–lime is irritant (alkali) and gloves should be worn when refilling canisters and the dust must not be inhaled or allowed to contact the eyes. Soda–lime reacts with trichloro-ethylene (a once popular volatile agent) to produce phosgene and other toxic gases and should not be used in rebreathing systems. It also reacts with sevoflurane, producing 'compound A'. Detrimental effects of compound A have been demonstrated in rats but not man, or other companion animals.

'Closed' and 'low-flow'
Rebreathing systems are used in one of two ways. In 'closed' systems, gas inflow precisely replaces anaesthetic and O_2 taken up by the patient. Approximately 5–10 ml/kg/min is required. Under these conditions the pressure relief valve is shut. When the system is run in a 'low-flow' fashion, oxygen delivery is in excess of basal requirements (above 10 ml/kg/min) with surplus gas leaking through the open pressure-relief valve. This is the easiest system to operate and therefore the most commonly used in practice.

Nitrous oxide
Once a rebreathing circuit has reached equilibrium the addition of further nitrous oxide can result in its accumulation within the inspired gas, as oxygen continues to be withdrawn from the inspired gas by the patient and CO_2 is removed by the soda–lime. At low flow rates and during long operations this can result in dangerously low oxygen levels developing in the inspired gas, and hypoxia of the patient can result. At higher gas flow rates, i.e. > 30 ml/kg/min of oxygen (and the same of N_2O), this problem can be avoided. A $N_2O:O_2$ ratio of 1:1 is recommended if N_2O is to be used. In general this gas is best used in rebreathing systems only if inspired oxygen content, arterial oxygen saturation or arterial blood-gas analysis can be performed.

Denitrogenation
When connected to breathing systems at the onset of anaesthesia, patients expire considerable volumes of nitrogen (which is present in normal air but not in anaesthetic gas mixtures). This may lower circuit O_2 to hypoxic levels unless purged through the pressure-relief valve (denitrogenation). This is achieved by using high flow rates for the first 10–15 minutes of anaesthesia.

REBREATHING SYSTEMS

Advantages
- Low gas flow requirements.
- Low volatile agent consumption rate.
- 'Closed' or 'low-flow' options.
- Expired moisture and heat conserved.
- Ventilation can be altered (spontaneous to controlled) without changing system performance.
- Low explosion risk (when explosive gases are used).
- Less pollution.

Disadvantages
- Greater resistance to breathing.
- Nitrous oxide must be used cautiously in rebreathing systems.
- Some versions are expensive to purchase.
- Regular soda–lime replacement required.
- Inspired gas content undetermined.
- Denitrogenation required.
- Slow to change level of anaesthesia.
- Cumbersome.

Circle system Circle systems for small dogs and cats are becoming increasingly popular in the UK and modern small-animal circles can be used in patients weighing greater than 5–10 kg. The circle system (Fig. 23.5) has valves causing unidirectional gas movement. With one way flow of gas around the circle, absorption of CO_2 from the soda–lime canister is very efficient. The main components of the circuit are:

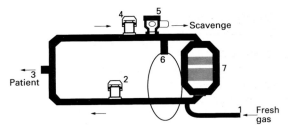

Fig. 23.5 Circle anaesthetic breathing system.

- *Fresh gas inflow* (1). This pipe connects the circuit with the common-gas outlet on the anaesthetic machine.
- *Unidirectional valves* (2 and 4). These are light transparent discs resting on knife-edge valve seats, enclosed within a transparent dome. Units should be easy to disassemble for drying and cleaning.
- *'Y' connector* (3). This connects inspiratory and expiratory limbs with endotracheal tube connectors or masks.
- *Pressure-relief valve* (5). This is opened to release surplus gas from 'low-flow' systems, during denitrogenation, and closed when lung inflation is imposed. Relief valves should be shrouded for attachment to scavenging hoses.
- *Reservoir bag* (6). This allows IPPV; its volume should be 3–6 times the animal's tidal volume. Large bags increase circuit volume, make respiratory movement less obvious and are harder to squeeze. Inadequately sized bags collapse during large breaths and overdistend during expiration.
- *Absorbent canister* (7). Canisters for circle systems may have two compartments. When absorbent in one becomes exhausted, it is discarded; after refilling, the canister is replaced in the reverse direction. This allows optimal use of absorbent.
- *Hoses*. These are corrugated to prevent kinking.

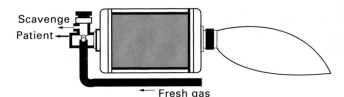

Fig. 23.6 To-and-fro system.

passed through the soda–lime canister. Gas is then exhaled through the soda–lime canister where CO_2 is removed and excess gas is vented out of the expiratory valve. Canisters are designed for either vertical or horizontal use; only the latter are used with companion animals. Features of to-and-fro systems include:

- *Fresh gas inflow*. This is situated adjacent to the endotracheal tube connector allowing dialled concentrations of anaesthetic to be preferentially inspired and, therefore, giving greater control over anaesthesia.
- *Filter*. A metal gauze screen should be sited at the patient end of the canister to limit inhalation of alkaline dust.
- *Scavenging shroud*. Scavenging waste gas from a to-and-fro system relies on a suitable shroud on the pressure-relief valve.
- *Canister*. Transparent canisters allow soda–lime colour and filling adequacy to be checked. Canisters in horizontal to-and-fro systems must be filled to capacity, otherwise the expired gas will 'channel', i.e. take the low resistance path over the absorbent, retaining CO_2.

CIRCLE SYSTEMS

Advantages
- High gas efficiency.
- Mechanical dead-space remains unchanged with use (unlike to-and-fro systems).
- Bronchiolitis unlikely (unlike to-and-fro systems).
- Less circuit inertia than to-and-fro systems.
- Ventilation readily controlled.

Disadvantages
- Some models are expensive.
- Complex, cumbersome and difficult to sterilise.
- Resistance to breathing for animals less than 5–10 kg.
- Unidirectional gas flow is dependent on functioning one-way valves.

To-and-fro (Waters' canister) system In this system (Fig. 23.6) gas oscillates over absorbent in the Waters' canister. The patient breathes in gas from the fresh gas outlet and recycled (CO_2-free) gas that has

---

TO-AND-FRO SYSTEMS

Advantages
- High gas efficiency.
- Bidirectional gas flow improves CO_2 scrubbing efficiency.
- Greater heat conservation (hyperthermia is possible on warm days).
- Lower resistance to breathing than with circle systems (no valves and lower overall circuit length).
- Low circuit volume.
- Denitrogenation achieved rapidly.
- Rapid changes in gas concentration.
- Simple, robust construction.

- Readily sterilised.
- Inexpensive.

Disadvantages
- Valve position is inconvenient for positive-pressure ventilation.
- Mechanical dead-space increases during surgery as absorbent is exhausted.
- 'Channelling' occurs if the canister is not adequately filled.
- Bronchiolitis; aspiration of alkaline dust from canister may cause chemical injury.
- Considerable drag.
- The system has some inertia and is inconvenient during head surgery.

Non-rebreathing systems

Non-rebreathing systems rely on high fresh gas flow rates, based on multiples of minute volume, to flush expired CO_2 from the circuit so that it cannot be rebreathed at the next breath.

NON-REBREATHING SYSTEMS
Advantages
- Low resistance; ideal for small animals and birds.
- Simple construction.
- Inexpensive to purchase.
- Soda–lime not required.
- Inspired gas content similar to that 'dialled' at anaesthetic machine.
- Denitrogenation not required.
- Circuit concentration of anaesthetic can be changed rapidly, allowing more precise control over the patient's level of unconsciousness.

Disadvantages
- High carrier gas flow requirements.
- High volatile agent consumption rate.
- Expired moisture and heat usually lost.
- Ventilatory modes affect system performance for some circuits.
- Different types of non-rebreathing circuits behave differently, and have different flow requirements.

The Magill system The Magill system consists of a reservoir bag and a corrugated hose which ends at an expiratory valve (Fig. 23.7). On inspiration, fresh gas is drawn down the corrugated hose to the patient. On expiration, exhaled gas is pushed back towards the reservoir bag and fresh gas outlet, and when the pressure in the reservoir bag exceeds the pressure to open the expiratory valve subsequently exhaled gas goes out of the valve. The first component of the exhaled gas (dead-space gas) has

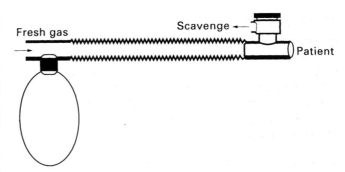

Fig. 23.7 The Magill breathing system.

only been in contact with non-gaseous exchanging tissues (e.g. trachea, primary bronchi) and is CO_2-free gas. This gas passes back up the corrugated hosing. The second component of exhaled gas comes from deep within the lungs and is CO_2-rich (alveolar gas). This CO_2-rich gas is vented out of the expiratory valve. Hence during spontaneous ventilation the Magill circuit is an efficient circuit as it conserves the CO_2-free or dead-space gas. Fresh gas flow rates equal to patient minute volume (approximately 200 ml/kg/min) are required. When N_2O is used, its flow rate is included within this value. For example, a 15 kg dog with a minute volume of 3 litres receives an inspired concentration of 66% N_2O with flows of 1 l/min O_2 and 2 l/min N_2O (3 l/min fresh gas flow rate).

During IPPV the ability of the circuit to conserve dead space gas is lost and higher fresh gas flow rates are required to prevent rebreathing of CO_2. The late inspired gas (fresh gas) is vented through the expiratory valve and the late expired gas (alveolar gas) is reintroduced into the lungs during inspirations rather than expelled through the valve. For longer periods of IPPV this circuit is not recommended.

MAGILL SYSTEM
Advantages
- Efficient general-purpose circuit.
- Readily maintained and sterilised.
- Inexpensive.

Disadvantages
- Expiratory valve resistance precludes its use in animals less than 10 kg.
- Valve location is inconvenient for scavenging and during head and neck surgery.
- Not good for prolonged IPPV.

The coaxial Lack system The inconvenient valve location in Magill circuits is overcome in the coaxial version – the Lack system (Fig. 23.8). In this system, a reservoir bag connects to an outer inspiratory limb; this surrounds an inner expiratory tube which ends at the expiratory valve. Fresh gas flow rates are equivalent to those of the Magill.

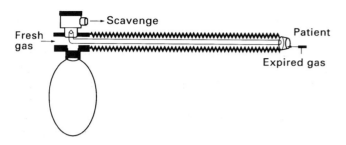

Fig. 23.8 The coaxial Lack breathing system.

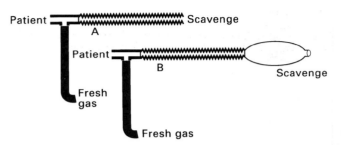

Fig. 23.10 (A) Ayre's T-piece. (B) Jackson–Rees modified Ayre's T-piece.

The parallel Lack system (Fig. 23.9) Problems of coaxial geometry (inner tube disconnection, fracture or kinking of the inner limb) are avoided when the inspiratory and expiratory limbs are placed in a parallel configuration. The system behaves like a Magill circuit and has the same fresh gas flow rate requirements.

LACK SYSTEM

Advantages
- Lightweight and exerts marginally less drag than Magill systems.
- Valve position facilitates surgery on the head and scavenging.
- The system is 1.5 m long, allowing anaesthetic machine positioning away from surgery.
- Lack systems can be used in lieu of the Magill circuit.

Disadvantages
- In coaxial versions the inner hose can become disconnected, causing considerable rebreathing.
- The system is stiffer and inconvenient to use in very small animals.
- Because the Lack system behaves like the Magill, it should not be used for prolonged IPPV.

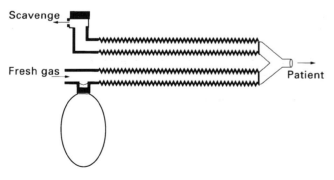

Fig. 23.9 The parallel Lack breathing system.

Ayre's T-piece (Fig. 23.10) This circuit is ideal for small patients under 10 kg as it has no expiratory valve and low expiratory resistance. Gas is inspired from the fresh gas outlet and the expiratory limb (hose). On expiration all expired gas (dead-space and alveolar gas) is exhaled down the expiratory limb where it is vented via a shrouded scavenging port. Hence it is less efficient than the Magill system as dead-space gas is not conserved. Gas flows for T-piece systems must exceed double the minute volume otherwise expired gas is rebreathed (approximately 500 ml/kg/min). Nitrous oxide is included at 50 or 66% of these levels.

The addition of the reservoir bag (Jackson–Rees modification) allows easy IPPV via occlusion of the bag outflow followed by gentle manual compression of the reservoir bag. Gas flow rates remain unchanged during IPPV. The bag also allows observation of respiratory movements.

AYRE'S T-PIECE

Advantages
- Minimal apparatus dead-space and resistance makes the T-piece ideal for cats, small dogs, neonates and birds.
- Simple, inexpensive and easy to sterilise.
- The bag facilitates IPPV and bag movement acts as a useful respiratory monitor.
- Good for IPPV.
- The system is scavenged with appropriate connectors.

Disadvantages
- Fresh gas flow rates are high for larger patients.
- With scavenging shrouds the expiratory connections can twist, obstructing expiratory outflow.

The modified Bain system The modified Bain system (Mapleson D) is a 'co-axial' (tube within a tube) T-piece with an inner inspiratory limb surrounded by an outer expiratory hose (Fig. 23.11). The expiratory limb ends in a reservoir bag and expiratory valve.

It functions like a T-piece and as such requires similar fresh gas flow rates. The presence of an expiratory valve precludes its use in patients less than 10 kg. It is a useful circuit for IPPV as circuit characteristics remain constant under spontaneous and controlled respiration.

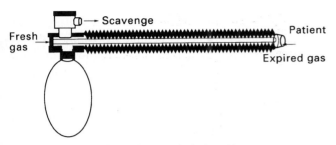

Fig. 23.11 The Modified Bain anaesthetic breathing system.

BAIN SYSTEM
Advantages
- Inexpensive.
- Low drag and mechanical dead-space.
- Good for IPPV.
- The length of the system (1.8 m) allows the anaesthetic machine to be positioned away from surgery, improving access.
- Easily maintained and sterilised.

Disadvantages
- Too much resistance for patients under 10 kg.
- High fresh gas flows in larger patients.
- Rebreathing problems can result from inner limb disconnection.

Anaesthetic machines

The anaesthetic machine functions to produce and deliver safe concentrations of anaesthetic vapour and to provide a means of supplying oxygen and imposing IPPV during apnoea or cardiopulmonary arrest. It also often provides storage for monitoring and other anaesthetic equipment. Understanding the function of anaesthetic machines is needed for the safe administration of volatile anaesthetics and oxygen and for machine maintenance; this prolongs the life of equipment, limits pollution and reduces the risk of equipment failure.

The anaesthetic machine (Fig. 23.12) begins at a carrier gas source (A), passes through a pressure gauge (B), a pressure regulator (C) and flowmeter assembly (D), and ends at the common gas outlet (F), where the anaesthetic breathing system attaches. Vaporisers (E) are usually positioned downstream from the flowmeter assembly. Other features include emergency oxygen valves (a), low oxygen alarms (b), nitrous oxide cut-out devices (c), over-pressure valves (d) and emergency air-intake valves (e).

Gas supply Cylinders are metal containers designed to withstand the pressure of compressed gases. Their size determines the volume of gas contained (in litres) and this is described by letters from AA (very small) to J (large). The volume of oxygen in filled cylinders at room temperature is shown in Table 23.5.

Cylinders are colour-coded in the UK as follows:

- Oxygen cylinders are black with white shoulders.
- Nitrous oxide cylinders are blue.
- Carbon dioxide cylinders are grey.
- Old machines may have a facility for cyclopropane which is delivered in orange cylinders.

Cylinders are opened by anticlockwise rotation of the spindle. Before attachment to the cylinder yoke, the protective cellophane sleeve is removed from the cylinder valve and the spindle briefly opened to flush away the dust that lies in the outlet port. Once connected in the hanger yokes, spindles should be opened slowly two full turns as partially restricted valves may reduce flow when the cylinder pressure falls.

Low-volume cylinders Low-volume 'E' or 'F' cylinders attached to hanger yokes on the machine suit most practices. Machines usually hold two cylinders of O$_2$ and two of N$_2$O. The cylinder valve face has holes which correspond with pins sited within the hanger yoke. The pin and hole pattern constitutes the 'pin-indexing' system and

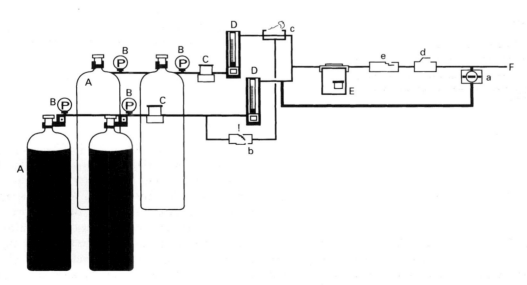

Fig. 23.12 The anaesthetic machine.

Table 23.5 Oxygen cylinder sizes and contents	
Cylinder size	**Content (litres)**
E	680
F	1340
G	3400
J	6800

ensures N_2O or CO_2 cylinders cannot be connected to the O_2 yoke.

Cylinder banks   Vertically standing banks of three to five 'J' or 'G' size cylinders are used in busy practices. Two banks for each gas (oxygen and nitrous oxide) are preferable, with one being 'in use' and the other 'in reserve', gas flows to the operating room through pipes in the wall. These end in wall-mounted Schraeder-type sockets which receive probes from the anaesthetic machine. Pipes are colour-coded and the probes size-coded so that lines cannot be accidentally crossed.

Pressure/contents gauge   The pressure gauge is indispensable for oxygen, because it indicates the gas volume in the cylinder. According to Boyle's law ($PV = k$) the volume of oxygen remaining is directly related to the pressure in the cylinder. A cylinder at half its full cylinder pressure will be half full.

The N_2O pressure gauge is less useful; the full N_2O cylinder contains liquid and gas and the gauge measures the pressure of gaseous N_2O in equilibrium with liquid. This remains constant until all liquid evaporates, after which pressure falls rapidly. Gas volume in N_2O cylinders is found by weighing the bottle and applying the following formula:

Litres N_2O present $=$ (net $-$ tare) weight [grams] 22.4/44

Cylinder tare weight is stamped on the cylinder neck and represents the weight of the empty cylinder. Net weight is the weight of the cylinder and its contents.

Pressure reducing valves or regulators   These produce constant 'downstream' pressure (therefore flow) as cylinder pressure falls with use. Without them, the cylinder valve would need incremental opening to maintain constant flow. They are sited immediately downstream from the hanger yoke, and in modern machines they may be incorporated in the yoke itself and be impossible to find.

Flowmeters   Flowmeters control and measure the rate of gas passing through them. The units are litres per minute (l/min). A freely moving 'float' – either a ball or bobbin – is supported in a transparent, tapered tube by an ascending flow of gas. The flow rate is etched on the tube and read from the top of bobbins and the equator of spheres. The greater the flow, the higher the indicator rises in the glass tube. Flowmeters become inaccurate if dirt or non-vertical positioning makes the float rub against the tube. Flowmeters are calibrated for one gas only and so oxygen flowmeters do not accurately indicate the flow of nitrous oxide. Because of this, flowmeter control knobs are often colour-coded. Flowmeter control knobs must not be over-tightened.

Vaporisers   Vaporisers dilute the saturated vapour of volatile anaesthetics to yield a range of useful concentrations of vaporised liquid. Concentrations leaving the vaporiser depend on:

- Temperature.
- Surface area.
- Gas flow.
- The volatility of the anaesthetic.

As anaesthetic liquid vaporises, the remaining liquid cools and the delivered anaesthetic concentration falls. With increased flow rates, the delivered concentration tends to decrease. Hence ensuring a constant output is not always easy. A number of compensating devices can be employed to maintain output:

- Heat source (or heat sink) – surrounds the liquid anaesthetic to prevent rapid cooling. Heat is transferred from this source to buffer the drop in chamber temperature associated with vaporisation.
- Flow splitting valve – varies the proportion of carrier gas that passes through or bypasses the vaporising chamber allowing control of the percentage of anaesthetic vapour delivered.
- Temperature compensating mechanism – compensates for fall in vaporising temperature and subsequent fall in vapour concentration. Two methods are commonly employed. A bimetallic strip of two dissimilar metals placed back to back, bends in proportion to a given change in temperature. When placed in the flow of the anaesthetic fresh gas it can alter the flow through the vaporising chamber (increasing or decreasing the amount of anaesthetic vaporised) and compensate for a change in anaesthetic vapour pressure caused by a change in temperature. Alternatively, an ether-filled bellows attached to a flow-splitting valve, that expands or contracts in relation to temperature, performs a similar function compensating for variation in vapour concentration with changes in temperature.
- Wicks and baffles – increase the surface area of vaporisation, maximising vaporisation of the inhalation agent.

Draw over vaporisers   Early vaporisers relied on the patient's respiratory efforts to 'draw' carrier gas (often air) over the liquid anaesthetic. They offer relatively little resistance to flow, though are subject to large variations in inspiratory flow, being dependent on the ventilation characteristics of the patient. Compensation for changes in temperature are rarely employed. Consequently, their output is frequently variable and they cannot be reliably calibrated.

They are more commonly used when placed within the anaesthetic circuit, i.e. within a circle circuit. In this position they are termed 'in-circuit vaporisers' (VIC). Anaesthetic machines such as the Stephens machine and the Komezaroff machine incorporate VICs, and work in small animals has demonstrated that they can be safely used. However, caution must be exercised when IPPV is initiated as dangerously high concentrations of anaesthetic gas can be delivered. Some models still in use include:

- Goldman halothane vaporiser – simple, small, inexpensive. It is neither temperature nor flow compensated.
- Oxford miniature vaporiser – used primarily with portable anaesthetic equipment, it is not temperature compensated, though has a heat sink (a sealed water/antifreeze compartment). It can be drained of one anaesthetic and refilled with another and detachable scales of approximate vapour percentage delivered are supplied.
- EMO (Epstein, Macintosh, Oxford) vaporiser – used for ether delivery it has a water-filled compartment as a heat sink.

Plenum vaporisers Plenum vaporisers are designed for use with constant flow of carrier gas and offer greater resistance to flow. Hence they are generally positioned out of the breathing circuit, i.e. they are out-of-circuit vaporisers (VOC). They are mostly calibrated vaporisers with compensatory devices for variations in temperature and flow and are those most commonly used in veterinary practice. Earlier models include uncalibrated types though these are infrequently seen today.

- *Uncalibrated vaporisers.* The Boyle's bottle is simple, inexpensive and easily maintained. It does not have any temperature compensation, though it does have a cowl that can be lowered toward and below the liquid anaesthetic surface to increase vapour uptake for a given control lever position. However, output concentrations are not guaranteed and they 'drift' despite constant control settings. With age the sealing washer (usually cork or rubber) becomes brittle and allows leakage of anaesthetic vapour. The cork stopper placed in the filling orifice is normally retained with a metal chain and often the metal anchor of the chain passes through the cork. If the chain breaks, the cork can act as a sparking plug; if someone charged with static electricity touches the cork–metal top, an explosion may result.
- *Calibrated vaporisers.* Temperature and flow compensation are incorporated as well as a heat sink into these vaporisers. Anaesthetic concentrations from 'Tec and other calibrated vaporisers is similar to that 'dialled' on the spindle, provided that the gas flow through the vaporiser and the temperature of liquid anaesthetic are within ranges specific for the model. In Mark III 'Tecs (Ohmeda), output is constant between 18 and 35°C. Dialled and delivered concentrations are similar

at flows between 0.2 and 15 l/min. In the earlier 'Tec 2, vapour output is reliable from above 2–4 l/min fresh gas flow. Lower flows, as used in low flow anaesthesia, produce delivered concentration different to that displayed on the dial. They come with a performance chart that indicates the delivered vapour concentration for a given dial setting and flow rate. Though obsolete they are still frequently seen in veterinary practice.

Vaporisers are agent-specific. Filling with the wrong anaesthetic is prevented by keyed filling ports. These accept a key-ended tube which only attaches to the corresponding anaesthetic bottle. Used properly, the system also assists pollution control because vaporiser filling occurs without spillage.

Back bar Flowmeters and vaporisers may be joined by tapered connectors and attached to a back bar, producing a series of semi-permanent fixtures. The 'Selectatec SM' manifold allows rapid attachment or removal of 'Tec 3 and 'Tec 4 vaporisers, facilitating vaporiser removal for refilling out of theatre, servicing and rewarming. In accommodating up to three vaporisers, a range of volatile agents may be available.

Common gas outlet (F) This connects the anaesthetic machine to breathing system connectors, ventilators or O_2 supply devices.

O_2 flush Also known as the bypass or purge valve, this receives O_2 from the cylinder and bypasses the vaporiser. Activation produces high flows of pure oxygen to the common gas outlet. The device is used to provide oxygen in emergency situations. It is used to flush anaesthetic from breathing systems before patient disconnection, thus lowering pollution.

Nitrous oxide cut-out devices These devices curtail N_2O flow and sound an alarm when oxygen runs out. These devices are invaluable if N_2O is used, though some older anaesthetic machines do not have them.

Over-pressure valve High pressures downstream from the common gas outlet open this valve and sound an alarm. The device is useful for leak-testing breathing systems; the valve's presence is confirmed by occluding the common gas outlet while pressing the oxygen bypass valve.

Emergency air intake valve When gas flow from the machine accidentally ceases, the patient's inspiratory effort opens an emergency valve which allows room air to enter the breathing system. The valve's opening action is accompanied by a 'whistling' sound. This valve is tested by attaching a pipe to the common gas outlet and applying suction; when sufficient vacuum is present, the valve opens and a whistle is heard.

Checking the anaesthetic machine before use

The anaesthetic machine should receive a major check at the beginning of each working day and a minor check between cases. The major checks include:

- Ensure that flow control valves (at flowmeter) are 'off'.
- Ensure that cylinders are closed and fit securely on the hanger yoke.
- Press the oxygen flush valve until no gas flow is apparent from the common gas outlet.
- Check that flowmeters and pressure gauges read '0'.
- Open the oxygen cylinder valve slowly (anticlockwise) and observe the registered pressure. On machines which carry two O_2 cylinders, test the 'full' or reserve cylinder first.
- Open the oxygen flowmeter control valve to 2–4 l/min to ensure smooth function.
- Whilst this is flowing repeat the procedure for the 'full' N_2O cylinder and open the flowmeter to 2–4 l/min. Close the tested O_2 cylinder. As the oxygen runs out, the low-oxygen alarm should sound and the N_2O cut-off device should trigger, with both bobbins dropping to zero flow.
- The 'full' N_2O cylinder is closed.
- The test is repeated for the 'in use' oxygen and nitrous oxide cylinders.
- Replace bottles that have little remaining gas.
- Open the 'in use' oxygen and nitrous oxide cylinders.
- Ensure that the vaporiser is full, with the filling port tightly closed, that spindle operation is smooth, and that the connection hoses (if appropriate) are connected to the vaporiser.
- Check over-pressure and emergency air-intake valves.

The testing of machines that receive a service supply from banked cylinders requires additional steps. These machines should have an emergency oxygen cylinder attached to the machine and this should be tested with the vaporiser as above. The back-up cylinder is then turned off. The piped source is then connected to the machine and the flowmeter opened to ensure adequate flow.

'Shutting down' the anaesthetic machine

When all surgery is finished, the content status of all cylinders is checked and empty cylinders are removed. If piped gases are present, Schraeder probes are removed from the wall sockets and the pipes neatly coiled. The nitrous oxide and oxygen cylinder valves are closed. The nitrous oxide and oxygen flowmeters are opened to a flow of 2 l/min and closed once the flow indicator has fallen to '0'. The oxygen flush valve is activated until no pressure registers on the pressure gauge. Machine surfaces are wiped down.

Pollution control systems

Exposure to anaesthetic gases has been associated with the development of malignancies, neuropathy, bone marrow toxicity, a higher incidence of abortions and infertility in theatre personnel and congenital abnormalities in their offspring (Corbett et al., 1974; Buring et al., 1985). Though many of the studies reporting these effects have been criticised for poor methodology the risk of chronic exposure remains a serious concern to veterinary staff. Under COSHH (Control of Substances Hazardous to Health) Regulations the employer has a duty to assess the risk of exposure to anaesthetic gases to his employees and take the appropriate measures to protect their health. The Health and Safety Executive have proposed the following occupational exposure standards (OES) based on an 8-hour time-weighted average (TWA), i.e. the average level of anaesthetic gas in the environment if measured over an 8-hour period:

- Nitrous oxide   100 p.p.m.
- Halothane   10 p.p.m.
- Enflurane   50 p.p.m.
- Isoflurane   50 p.p.m.
- Ether   400 p.p.m.

For shorter periods of operation, as more commonly seen in veterinary practice, it is suggested that short-term exposure should not exceed three times this limit. The use of scavenging systems combined with careful anaesthetic techniques can reduce pollution by up to 90% and ensure an environment safely below these OES levels.

Scavenging systems include both passive and active methods. Generally, active methods are more efficient, though in some circumstances passive methods are adequate.

Passive scavenging

This relies on the patient's respiratory efforts to void the waste gases via a wide-bore (22 mm) tube to the outside of the building. To be effective the exit must be protected from significant air currents such that excessive sub-atmospheric or positive pressure could be generated within the tube and effect function. Further scavenging to the roof level would produce a back pressure due to the heavier gases pooling in the tube. Generally, a tube length of no more than 2.6 m is acceptable.

A variation of this method is the active charcoal absorber that chemically absorbs hydrocarbon inhalation anaesthetics. It collects gas via a short tube from the scavenging shroud of the breathing circuit and removes the inhaled anaesthetic. However, it does not absorb nitrous oxide, and confirming that it is not exhausted can only be performed by weighing the absorber; it also adds further resistance to the passive system.

Active–passive scavenging

Similar to the passive system a wide-bore tube scavenges exhaled gas from the expiratory valve of the circuit, but passes the gas to a forced ventilation system rather than outside. It is important to ensure this ventilation system does not dump the gas in another workplace or recirculate the gas.

Active scavenging

This is the preferred method and that most likely to meet COSHH standards. It consists of three main components:

1. *Transfer system.* The transfer system consists of a tube and connector (usually 30 mm) attached to the expiratory port of the circuit.
2. *Receiving system.* The receiving system functions as an air break, preventing excessive positive or negative pressure reaching the breathing system. Often it consists of a simple open-ended reservoir system, allowing venting of excess positive pressure or uptake of atmospheric gas if excess negative pressure develops. Alternatively a reservoir bag and safety valve can be used.
3. *Disposal system to the exterior.* The disposal system delivers the gas to the outside of the building and includes an active suction method. Frequently this consists of a fan unit or a pump system.

Safety procedures

Good anaesthetic technique is also important to ensure minimal exposure to waste gases. Recommended procedures include:

- Check the anaesthetic machine and circuit for leaks.
- Turn on the scavenging system and connect it to the breathing circuit.
- Intubate the patient with an appropriate-sized cuffed endotracheal tube and inflate the cuff.
- Avoid the use of face masks when possible.
- Turn on the anaesthetic gases (other than oxygen) only after the patient is connected to the circuit.
- Avoid disconnecting the patient during anaesthesia.
- Flush the circuit with oxygen for 30 seconds prior to disconnection at the end of procedure and empty the remaining gas in the reservoir bag into the scavenging system.
- Fill the vaporisers at the end of the day in a well-ventilated area.
- Service all equipment annually.
- Annually monitor theatre pollution.

Other anaesthetic equipment

Other equipment required for anaesthesia includes endotracheal tubes, masks, laryngoscopes and suction devices. Proper use and care of these pieces of equipment is invaluable in ensuring safe anaesthesia.

Endotracheal tubes

These connect the patient to the anaesthetic breathing system. Most patterns have cuffs at the distal (patient) end which, when filled with air, produce a gas-tight seal. Construction materials confer different properties on the tube. Red rubber tubes have poor resistance to kinking and conform poorly to airway contours. Tubes made of polyvinyl chloride (PVC) are the softest and least irritating to the tracheal mucosa; they have little tendency to kink and they mould to the curve of the airway at body temperature.

Care, maintenance and storage depend on the material of construction. Red rubber tubes are deteriorated by oil and petroleum-based lubricants. After cleaning and sterilisation, tubes should be dried thoroughly and stored in a cool, dry environment. They should not be exposed to direct sunlight.

Before use, check the tubes for patency and establish the cuffs' ability to hold pressure. The endotracheal tube connector should be tight and fit snugly with the chosen breathing system. The tube should be an appropriate length and a range of tube diameters should be made available.

After use, ensure the tubes are rinsed in running water and leave them to soak in detergent solution. Later they should be scrubbed inside and out to remove residual mucus. Rinsing must be thorough to remove detergent.

Sterilising procedures depend on material. Red rubber tubes are deteriorated by heat sterilisation but can be autoclaved for 10 to 20 times. Alternatively they can be disinfected with chlorhexidine solutions. Polysiloxane tubes can also be autoclaved. While most PVC tubes are designed for single use only, they may be safely re-used after cleaning and sterilising. Ethylene oxide must be used cautiously and adequate aeration allowed afterwards (at least 48 hours). Gamma-irradiated single-use items and PVC tubes should not be sterilised with ethylene oxide.

Masks

These are used for administering oxygen and for volatile anaesthetics when an endotracheal tube is not present. Patterns made of malleable rubber can be shaped to fit the animal's face and minimise apparatus dead-space. Others are made of rigid plastic with a perforated rubber diaphragm; they have high dead-space and so require greater gas flows. However, for birds and laboratory animal species they can be constructed from syringe cases and latex gloves. Customised equipment should have minimum dead space, should be affixable to the animal, should not confer resistance to respiration and should allow the animal to be seen.

Care, maintenance and storage considerations for masks are the same as those for endotracheal tubes. Masks can be sterilised by soaking in a 0.2% chlorhexidine solution.

Laryngoscopes

Laryngoscopes consist of a handle and a blade and are available in several patterns and sizes. They serve to depress the base of the tongue during intubation; in so doing, they evert the epiglottis. A bulb at the tip of the blade illuminates the oropharynx. Ideally, the bulb should only illuminate when the blade is 'fixed' in the working position.

Before use, it is important to ensure that the bulb is firmly positioned and that the batteries are charged. After use, blades should be wiped clean with a swab soaked in alcohol. Laryngoscopes must not be immersed in water.

Suction devices

Connected either to a central vacuum pipeline or to a portable pump unit, these devices allow suction of body secretions and are particularly relevant to anaesthesia. They are probably the most important piece of resuscitation equipment and are used to clear mucus, blood and other debris from the pharynx, trachea and main bronchi. Suction is also used to clear the surgical site of blood, and allow gastrointestinal drainage, wound drainage and pleural drainage. They consist of three essential components:

- Source of vacuum.
- Reservoir or collection vessel.
- Suction tubing.

The vacuum source can be via a central vacuum pipeline or a portable unit. An appropriate-sized collection vessel is one that is large enough to collect the aspirated material but not too large or cumbersome. The interface between the collection vessel and the rest of the unit must be kept clean and free from damage to ensure adequate suction function.

Addition optional features include:

- Cut-off valve – to prevent liquid aspirated entering the pump.
- Bacterial filter – prevents contamination of the room with aspirated bacteria.
- Vacuum control valve – allows adjustment of the degree of vacuum applied.
- Vacuum gauge – indicates the degree of suction.
- Foam prevention – foam may cause closure of the cut-off valve or contaminate the filter or pump.
- Stop valve – to occlude the suction tubing and allow build-up of vacuum.
- Two collection vessels – allowing continuous operation when one vessel is full or non-functional and to provide overflow when the first vessel is full.

KEY POINTS
- Anaesthetic equipment is essential for inhalation anaesthesia.
- All anaesthetic machines consist of similar components.
- A thorough knowledge of the use of the machine will minimise equipment-induced complications.
- A proper anaesthetic equipment check is required each day.
- Anaesthetic circuits deliver oxygen and anaesthetic gas, and remove carbon dioxide from the patient.
- Anaesthetic circuits can be classified on the basis of how they remove exhaled carbon dioxide; rebreathing circuits absorb CO_2 chemically, non-rebreathing circuits remove it with high fresh gas flow rates.
- Scavenging of waste anaesthetic gases is important.

Muscle relaxants

Several types of drug produce muscle relaxation, including general anaesthetics. When absolute relaxation is required, however, neuromuscular blocker agents ('muscle relaxants') are used because they are the most effective and predictable. These drugs, derived from poisons used with blow-darts by indigenous South Americans, act on nicotinic receptors at the neuromuscular junction of skeletal muscle. They have no direct effect on smooth or cardiac muscle.

Neuromuscular blocking drugs do not cross the blood–brain barrier and so do not alter consciousness. However, they eliminate some of the obvious signs of inadequate anaesthesia – movement, ocular position and cranial nerve reflexes – so that monitoring the level of anaesthesia becomes more complicated. Because the animal cannot respond normally to inadequate anaesthesia, the anaesthetist must ensure the animal is unconscious.

The respiratory muscles (external intercostals and diaphragm) are blocked by relaxants and so ventilation stops. Therefore a means of supporting ventilation must be available, e.g. a cuffed endotracheal tube and a suitable breathing system. There are two types of relaxant based on their mechanism of action: depolarising and non-depolarising drugs.

Depolarising drugs

Succinylcholine has a rapid onset time (seconds) and is short-acting (3–5 minutes) in horses, pigs, cats and people. It is used to facilitate endotracheal intubation in humans, and less commonly in pigs and cats, or during induction of anaesthesia in horses.

Non-depolarising drugs

Many types of non-depolarising drug have been used in veterinary practice and some have more or less fallen out of use:

- D-Tubocurarine is seldom used these days because injection causes histamine release in dogs, resulting in vasodilatation, hypotension, tachycardia and bronchial spasm.
- Gallamine became unpopular because of tachycardia and hypertension after injection. Prolonged relaxation occurs with animals in renal failure.
- Alcuronium, a long-acting relaxant, is only occasionally used nowadays.
- Pancuronium has an intermediate onset and long duration of action (more than 30 minutes), causes modest tachycardia after injection, but remains a useful agent.
- Vecuronium, a popular drug, derived from pancuronium, has an intermediate duration of action (20–30 minutes). It has little cumulative effect after repeated doses and little, if any, cardiovascular effect.

- Atracurium is another popular relaxant because of its intermediate duration of action and rapid onset time. It is spontaneously degraded (Hofman degradation) and so the agent is favoured in animals with diseased elimination pathways (liver and kidneys).

Indications for neuromuscular blockade

High-risk cases

Neuromuscular blockers reduce anaesthetic requirements and so cardiopulmonary function is preserved. Positive-pressure ventilation must be imposed.

Thoracic surgery and diaphragmatic hernia repair

For thoracic surgery and repair of diaphragmatic hernias, positive pressure ventilation is required. Positive-pressure ventilation can be imposed without neuromuscular blockade; however, in paralysed animals, reduced rigidity in the thoracic cage (ribs and diaphragm) means lower inflation pressures can be used producing less cardiovascular compromise. Anaesthesia is frequently smoother.

Oesophageal foreign body removal

Oesophageal foreign body removal in dogs is facilitated by neuromuscular blockade as a significant component of oesophageal musculature is skeletal in the dog. Relaxed oesophageal musculature allows retrieval of relatively large objects without the need for thoracotomy.

Laparotomies

During laparotomy, neuromuscular blockers reduce the amount of traction required to produce exposure, causing less tissue trauma on the wound margins with less post-operative inflammation and pain.

Microsurgery

Intraocular and neurological surgery (which is frequently performed under microscopy) requires guaranteed immobility.

Inefficient ventilatory pattern

Joint surgery and other procedures occasionally cause bizarre breathing patterns which are inefficient in terms of gas exchange. In these, relaxants allow positive-pressure ventilation to be imposed without the animal 'fighting the ventilator'.

Monitoring blockade

The degree of relaxation is measured using a peripheral nerve stimulator. Clinical signs must be used when these are unavailable. Because diaphragmatic and respiratory muscles are relatively resistant to neuromuscular blockers, the first sign of a waning block is diaphragmatic 'twitching'.

Neuromuscular blockers paralyse facial skeletal muscle and eliminate normal reflexes; after paralysis, the eyelids are open and the eye is central. There are no corneal or palpebral reflexes. In animals which are paralysed but not unconscious, there may be increased jaw tone and mydriasis, lacrimation, salivation, tachycardia and hypertension. When these signs are present, anaesthesia must be deepened by increasing the vaporiser setting or, by injecting intravenous anaesthetic.

Antagonism

Non-depolarising neuromuscular blockers can be antagonised using a combination of anticholinesterase and antimuscarinic drugs: commonly either edrophonium or neostigmine with atropine or glycopyrrolate.

KEY POINTS
- Muscle relaxants specifically act at the neuromuscular junction.
- Muscle relaxants include depolarising and non-depolarising neuromuscular blockers.
- Indications include ocular, abdominal and thoracic surgery.
- Adequate ability to monitor depth of anaesthesia and ensure unconsciousness is essential for their safe use.
- The provision of IPPV is mandatory if muscle relaxants are used.

Monitoring

Monitoring anaesthesia is an important aspect of safe anaesthesia and is commonly performed by the veterinary nurse. Close attention to the patient allows rapid intervention if the patient is becoming too light or deep or is becoming physiologically compromised. Good monitoring and rapid correction of developing problems prevents minor disturbances from becoming major complications.

The goals of monitoring are to provide an appropriate depth of anaesthesia whilst maintaining normal physiological function of the patient. Central nervous system function is assessed to maintain depth of anaesthesia, whilst cardiovascular and respiratory function are the main systems monitored to ensure normal body function. In addition close attention to body temperature is required.

In performing good monitoring, regular and continuous observation of the patient is required. The maintenance of detailed written records of each anaesthetic is to be recommended in view of the increasing risks of litigation.

Monitoring central nervous system function

Monitoring central nervous system function during anaesthesia is a major component of assessing 'depth' of anaesthesia. Depression of cranial nerve reflexes gives valuable information as to the depth of the patient. Under normal circumstances, the 'deeper' the level of anaesthesia the greater the cardiopulmonary depression. Hence to provide adequate conditions for performing the procedure requested whilst preserving patient physiological function, anaesthesia is generally maintained at a relatively 'light' level. However, the depth required depends on:

- The procedure being performed. Laparotomy requires 'deeper' anaesthesia than cutaneous tumour removal.
- The specific activity during surgery. In orthopaedics, the level of anaesthesia adequate for skin incision may prove inadequate for fracture manipulation.
- Surgical experience.

Consequently, monitoring surgical events is an important aid to monitoring the 'level' of anaesthesia. The 'signs' of anaesthesia are based on:

- Cranial nerve reflexes

  - Palpebral reflex: a 'blink' occurs when the medial canthus of the eye is stroked with a finger. If the test is repeated too frequently, the reflex becomes sluggish.
  - Corneal reflex: 'blinking' also occurs when the cornea is gently touched with a moistened cotton bud. This is not a very sensitive test as during clinical anaesthesia it should always be present.
  - Eye position: during increasing depth of anaesthesia the globe first rocks ventromedially within the orbit and then returns to a more central position with increasing depth.
  - Pupillary diameter: with increasing depth of anaesthesia the pupil dilates.
  - Jaw tone: tension in the jaws indicates light levels of anaesthesia.
  - Tongue curl: during 'light' anaesthesia, the tongue curls when the jaws are opened.
  - Lacrimation: the eye becomes dry at deep levels of anaesthesia.
  - Salivation: profuse salivation can indicate inadequate anaesthesia.

During surgical anaesthesia the eye will be rotated ventromedially (Fig. 23.13) or be just beginning to rotate back dorsally, with a weak or absent palpebral reflex and a constricted pupil.

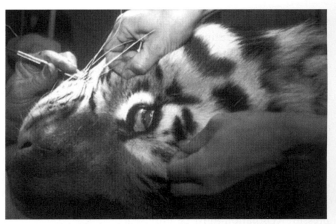

Fig. 23.13 A Siberian tiger with eye rotated ventromedially during anaesthesia for dental surgery.

- Respiratory signs. The rate, depth and pattern of respiration are altered by the level of anaesthesia and the degree of surgical stimulation. Increasing respiratory rate often suggests 'light' anaesthesia but can also be seen when the patient is too deeply anaesthetised, so should be used in conjunction with other signs.
- Cardiovascular signs. Heart rate, blood pressure, and capillary refill time are influenced by the interaction between anaesthetic depth and surgical stimulation. Increasing depth of inhalational anaesthesia is often associated with a dose-dependent decrease in blood pressure with or without a fall in heart rate.
- Skeletomuscular tone and response to toe pinch. Light anaesthesia is associated with greater skeletal muscle tone and limb withdrawal reflexes; however, during clinical anaesthesia these reflexes are generally lost.

Stages in anaesthesia

For convenience, the 'depth' of anaesthesia has been categorised into four stages, although this is somewhat arbitrary because it is based on observations in humans anaesthetised with ether.

Stage I (stage of voluntary excitement or analgesia)
This begins with induction and lasts until unconsciousness is present. The animal resists induction, shows signs of apprehension and fear but later becomes disorientated. Signs reflect a generalised sympatho-adrenal response to threat. Pulse and respiratory rates are elevated, although breath-holding may occur if irritant or pungent vapours are given. The pupil is dilated. Skeletal muscle activity may be marked and hyper-reflexia present. The animal may vocalise, salivate, defecate and urinate

Stage II (stage of involuntary excitement)
This lasts from the onset of unconsciousness until rhythmic breathing is present. All cranial nerve reflexes are present and may be hyperactive. Initially the eye is wide open and the pupil dilated. Later, eyes begin to rotate to a ventromedial position. Responses to toe pinch reflexes

are brisk. Breathing is irregular and gasping may occur but later becomes regular.

Stages I and II are unpleasant for the patient and hazardous for the anaesthetist. They are likely when mask induction is attempted on non-sedated animals or when inadequate doses of injectable anaesthetic are given. An elegant induction passes through these stages rapidly. This is achieved by adequate pre-anaesthetic sedative medication and/or sufficient anaesthetic for induction.

Stage III (surgical anaesthesia)
This is subdivided into three planes:

- *Plane 1*. Respiration is regular and deep. Minute volume is proportional to surgical stimulation. Spontaneous limb movement is absent but pinch reflexes are brisk. Nystagmus, the lateral oscillation of the eyeball, slows and stops by the end of Plane 1; however, it is not always present. Eyeball position in the orbit is ventromedial; opening the eyelids reveals mainly sclera. The third eyelid moves part way across the corneal surface. Palpebral reflexes begin to slow but the corneal reflex is brisk. Cardiovascular function is only slightly depressed. This plane is suitable for abscess lancing and superficial surgery like skin suturing and cutaneous tumour removal.
- *Plane 2*. Eye position is ventromedial and the eyelids may be partially separated. The palpebral reflex is sluggish or absent although corneal reflexes persist. The conjunctival surface is moist and the pupil constricted. Muscle relaxation is more apparent. The pedal reflex becomes sluggish and ultimately is lost. Tidal volume is decreased; rate may be increased or decreased. The heart rate and blood pressure may be modestly reduced. This plane is adequate for most surgery except some laparotomy and thoracotomy.
- *Plane 3*. The eyeball becomes central and the eyelids begin to open. The pupillary diameter increases. Respiratory rate increases; tidal volume is decreased. A pause appears between inspiration and expiration. The pedal reflex is lost and abdominal muscles are relaxed. Heart rate and blood pressure are lowered. This plane is adequate for all procedures.

Stage IV (overdosage)
Characterised by progressive respiratory failure, which begins when ventilation is achieved by diaphragmatic function alone; this eventually ceases. The pulse may be rapid or very slow and becomes impalpable. The eye becomes central, the eyelids open, the pupils are maximally dilated and the corneal surface is dry. Cyanosis progresses to a grey or ashen colour of the mucous membrane. Capillary refill time becomes prolonged. Accessory respiratory muscle activity, indicated by twitching in the throat, represents agonal gasping. This superficially mimics gasping, or inadequate anaesthesia.

Overdosage

Excessive levels of anaesthesia should be avoided because they contribute to prolonged recovery. They also cause unnecessary cardiopulmonary depression, which in turn limits organ perfusion, causing post-operative organ failure. Ultimately it results in cardiac arrest.

Underdosage

Underdosage is equally undesirable. In response to surgery, heart rate increases and respiration becomes rapid and shallow (tachypnoea). Blood pressure rises and increased oozing at the surgical site may be noticed. Capillary refill time may become prolonged and the mucous membranes lose colour. The pupils dilate and spontaneous cranial nerve reflex activity may be seen; lacrimation and salivation may be profuse. Maintaining inadequate levels of anaesthesia because of inexperience or to ensure that the animal 'stays alive' must be avoided because:

- The animal may recover consciousness.
- Movement will compromise delicate surgery, or the animal may extubate itself.
- Catecholamine release may cause arrhythmias, and even cardiac arrest.
- Tachypnoea may impair gas exchange and uptake of anaesthetics. Alternatively, hyperventilation may cause alkalosis.

Monitoring cardiovascular function

Assessing cardiovascular variables continuously, provides information on the depth of anaesthesia, on the effects of surgery (e.g. haemorrhage, inadequate anaesthesia, untoward reflexes) and on cardiovascular function itself. The primary goal is to ensure adequacy of tissue perfusion. In practice there is not one parameter that indicates perfusion absolutely, but rather the veterinary nurse must assess cardiovascular function on the basis of a number of signs. Monitoring of heart rate and pulse characteristics is combined with assessment of the mucous membranes, blood pressure and other parameters to form an overall picture of the state of the cardiovascular system of the patient. The regular direct assessment of pulse character, strength and rate by the veterinary nurse should form the central component of cardiovascular monitoring around which the other aspects and electronic monitoring equipment can be added.

Pulse characteristics, heart rate and rhythm

- *Pulse quality*. The pulse strength gives useful information as to the adequacy of the peripheral circulation. The palpated pulse is the difference between systolic and diastolic arterial blood pressure (i.e. pulse pressure) and though not a direct indicator of blood pressure, it generally gives reliable information as to changes in blood pressure and cardiovascular function. A weak pulse is usually associated with hypotension often due to myocardial depression during anaesthesia, and an increasingly weak pulse suggests cardiovascular depression is increasing.

- *Heart rate.* The absolute rate is important as very high and low heart rates are undesirable. Equally, changes in the rate give information as to the depth of the patient and cardiovascular stability of the patient. For example, tachycardia may be seen during very light anaesthesia due to sympathetic stimulation, or during periods of hypotension following blood loss or during excessively 'deep' anaesthesia and severe cardiovascular depression. The rate is drug dependent, e.g. bradycardia with alpha 2 agonists, so a knowledge of what drugs have been administered is important.
- *Heart rhythm.* The heart rhythm gives an indication as to the presence of arrhythmias. A difference in recorded heart and pulse rate is called the pulse deficit and indicates the failure of a cardiac contraction to result in a palpable pulsation and usually indicates the presence of a significant arrhythmia. Characterisation of such a deficit requires the recording of an ECG (see below).

> **PRACTICAL NURSING TIP**
> Digital palpation of a peripheral pulse is the best method of assessing heart rate and rhythm as it concurrently provides information on pulse strength. Nurses should aim to judge pulse quality using small peripheral arteries (like the lingual and dorsal pedal arteries) because pulsations in these are lost at higher pressures than those in larger vessels like the femoral artery. This gives earlier warning of developing hypotension.

Palpation of the apex beat is useful in very small companion animals and laboratory animals, or when hypotension makes peripheral pulses impalpable. It gives information on heart rate and rhythm but not pulse strength. Similarly, cardiac auscultation allows assessment of heart rate and rhythm but not pulse quality. While heart sounds may be heard with standard (precordial) stethoscopes, these tend to fall off even when adhesive tape is used. Oesophageal stethoscopes are less prone to displacement.

Heart rate monitors detect ECG signal and produce an audible beep or digital readout. This provides limited information as it only indicates the presence of electrical activity and not cardiac output. Such monitors will continue to register a 'beat' long after output from the heart and a palpable pulse have been lost. The electrocardiogram and pulse oximeter can also be used as heart rate monitors (see below).

Mucous membranes and capillary refill time

The general appearance of the mucous membranes can provide valuable indications as to the state of the cardiovascular system. Ideally they should be pink, indicating good tissue oxygenation. However, bright pink suggests hypercapnia. Pale, grey or dry mucous membranes are indicative of poor peripheral perfusion. White can indicate anaemia, peripheral vasoconstriction, or hypovolaemia.

The capillary refill time indicates adequacy of peripheral perfusion. Generally the refill time should be between 1 and 2 seconds. A time of greater than 2 seconds is associated with poor perfusion. It is not absolute though as the refill time may be adequate in some situations of impaired venous return and poor arterial perfusion, as capillaries can refill from engorged veins as well as arteries.

Arterial blood pressure

Arterial blood pressure (ABP) gives information about adequacy of the cardiovascular system. It is not a direct monitor of cardiac output but in the presence of myocardial depressant anaesthetic agents, is a useful indirect indicator. Blood pressure (ABP) is related to cardiac output (CO), right atrial pressure (RAP) and total peripheral resistance (TPR) by the following equation:

$$ABP - RAP = CO \times TPR$$

Most anaesthetics decrease cardiac output and total peripheral resistance (right atrial pressure remains minimally affected). The degree of halothane-induced hypotension is dose dependent, hence blood pressure is an accurate indicator of cardiovascular depression as well as depth of anaesthesia. An exception occurs where vasoconstrictors have been given, producing hypertension without increased CO. This is seen after the administration of an alpha-2 agonist. In general during anaesthesia we aim to maintain mean ABP above 70–80 mmHg.

Direct measurement of blood presssure is the gold standard allowing continuous recording of blood pressure even at low pressures. A catheter is aseptically placed in an accessible artery (e.g. dorsal pedal, femoral, middle auricular arteries). It is connected via a heparin saline column to an anaeroid manometer or to a strain-gauge pressure transducer. The anaeroid manometer is cheap but only indicates mean ABP. The electronic system provides systolic and diastolic pressures as well and a pulse waveform, though is expensive. Arterial catheters allow blood gas analysis and are particularly valuable in high-risk patients.

Indirect methods are based on the use of a cuff applied around a limb/tail and a method of detecting the pulse peripheral to the cuff. The cuff is inflated until the pulse distal to the cuff is no longer detectable, it is then slowly deflated until the pulse is restored. The pressure in the cuff when the pulse is restored is equal to systolic ABP. Cuff width should be about 40% of limb circumference. Wider cuffs transmit pressure more efficiently and underestimate pressure, whilst narrow cuffs overestimate it. Two methods are commonly used:

- *Oscillometric method.* The occluding cuff also senses pulsation. As the cuff is deflated and blood starts to pulse through the cuff, the cuff senses this oscillation. Maximum oscillation corresponds to mean ABP. They are automated and reasonably accurate in small animals, though are less reliable in hypotensive states and are expensive.

- *Doppler flow detection.* A Doppler ultrasound flow detector placed over a peripheral artery senses blood moving in the artery and produces an audible sound for each pulse. The cuff is applied proximally, and inflated and then deflated until the first audible pulsation is detected giving systolic ABP. It is simple and cheap, and reliable in hypotensive states, and is probably the most appropriate method for general practice (see Fig. 23.14).

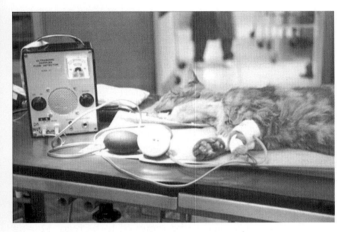

Fig. 23.14 The Doppler flow detector blood pressure monitor used on a cat.

Central venous pressure

Often neglected, central venous pressure (CVP) reflects filling of right heart and provides a valuable indicator of the circulating blood volume. A catheter is introduced into the jugular vein and advanced to the anterior vena cava. The zero point is the pressure of the right atrium or level of the sternal manubrium. It is a useful inexpensive indicator of response to fluid therapy. A change is as important as the actual value, indicating response to therapy and as long as it is within the normal range the risk of overinfusion of fluids is minimal. Normal values are between 3 and 7 cm H_2O in the dog and cat.

Electrocardiogram

The electrocardiogram (ECG) describes the electrical activity of the heart. Changes in rhythm can be associated with systemic abnormalities (hypoxia, electrolyte disturbance) and cardiac pathology. It is not indicative of cardiac output or mechanical activity of the heart and electrical activity can remain normal minutes after onset of cardiac arrest.

Monitoring respiratory function

Assessment of respiratory function is as equally important as monitoring cardiovascular function in ensuring the well-being of the patient during anaesthesia. The veterinary nurse should be continuously observing the respiratory rate and pattern of the animal as well as the extent of reservoir bag inflation and deflation during each breath. In addition there are a number of electronic monitors that can add valuable information to the assessment of ventilation.

Respiration rate, depth and pattern

The rate of respiration gives some information about adequacy of ventilation and depth of anaesthesia. Though only a crude indicator, it alerts to problems when the rate is very slow (bradypnoea) or very fast (tachypnoea). When combined with the assessment of depth of ventilation, a better assessment of ventilation (and depth of anaesthesia) can be made. Observing chest excursion or reservoir bag movement can give the veterinary nurse a good idea of the adequacy of ventilation for the size of the animal. In addition, mechanical and electronic monitors can be used that record the minute volume (i.e. volume of gas inspired per minute) of the patient. An example of a mechanical minute volume recorder is Wright's respirometer.

The pattern of respiration can also provide valuable information. Irregular ventilation can indicate pathology, e.g. Cheyne–Stokes breathing/gasping suggests dangerously 'deep' anaesthesia. Certain drugs are associated with irregular respiratory patterns, for example ketamine anaesthesia in the cat produces an apnoestic pattern with periods of apnoea interspersed with regular bursts of a number of breaths. Very shallow rapid breathing can be seen during inappropriately light planes of anaesthesia.

Pulse oximetry

Pulse oximetry is a non-invasive method of measuring arterial oxygen saturation and gives valuable information about gas exchange and arterial oxygenation. It rapidly responds to falling arterial oxygen saturation and can be life saving in situations such as during airway obstruction and hypoxia. It does not, however, allow accurate assessment of adequacy of ventilation as it does not tell the clinician anything about arterial carbon dioxide, which is the factor mammals primarily regulate their ventilation to. A patient on 100% oxygen during anaesthesia can easily have an arterial oxygen saturation of > 95% even when it is underventilating; however, if ventilation became so reduced as to produce hypoxia the pulse oximeter would then display a reduced oxygen saturation. Primarily, it alerts to hypoxaemia and is particularly valuable when the patient is just being disconnected from the oxygen at the end of a procedure. During this early period of recovery, rapid detection of hypoxia and compromised ventilation can allow early correction of ventilatory problems (e.g. during respiratory obstruction), preventing the development of serious complications and cardiopulmonary arrest (Fig. 23.15).

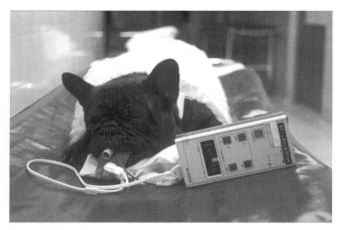

Fig. 23.15 A pulse oximeter being used post-operatively after airway surgery.

The pulse oximeter can be placed anywhere on the patient where there is an area of non-pigmented skin where light can easily be transmitted through tissue. Common sites where it is applied include the tongue, ear pinna, mammary teat and the vulva.

Capnography

Capnography is based on the measurement of exhaled carbon dioxide (end-tidal carbon dioxide) and provides valuable information on respiratory as well as cardiovascular function. Usually it is measured from gas withdrawn from a small tube placed between the circuit and the endotracheal tube. End-tidal carbon dioxide approximates to alveolar carbon dioxide and so gives an excellent indicator of ventilatory adequacy: if the end-tidal carbon dioxide level is high, then it suggests ventilation is inadequate as the body is not blowing off sufficient carbon dioxide, whereas a low level suggests overventilation.

The end-tidal carbon dioxide level is also related to how much carbon dioxide is produced in the tissues and how effectively it is delivered to the lungs. Thus a very high end-tidal carbon dioxide level is seen with malignant hyperthermia due to massively elevated levels of CO_2 production by the tissues (especially muscles). Further, if the heart's ability to pump blood is compromised (e.g. deep anaesthesia), then the amount of CO_2-rich blood (venous blood) delivered to the lungs and exhaled will be reduced. In this situation though blood CO_2 is high the measured end-tidal carbon dioxide will be low.

Capnography is presently relatively expensive so is not seen commonly in practice; however, as the technology becomes cheaper it should begin to find its way into practice anaesthesia.

Blood gas analysis

Blood gas analysis of a blood sample withdrawn from an artery allows the definitive assessment of respiratory gas exchange. The blood gas analyser measures the partial pressure of CO_2 (PCO_2) and O_2 (PO_2) in the sample and pH. It allows the assessment of adequacy of ventilation (PCO_2), arterial oxygenation (PO_2), and acid–base status of the patient (pH). However, blood gas machines are expensive and require regular maintenance. Presently they are found primarily in referral institutions.

Monitoring temperature

General anaesthesia interferes with the animal's ability to regulate temperature and the patient may become hypothermic or hyperthermic. Hypothermia is most commonly seen during anaesthesia. It delays recovery, increases morbidity and at very low temperatures can result in mortality. Though often overlooked during anaesthesia, it is important to monitor temperature peri-operatively. Particular attention should be given to monitoring temperature of very small patients, young and old animals and during prolonged periods of anaesthesia.

Mercury thermometers are the most commonly used thermometers but they need to be removed to be read. During anaesthesia, thermistors or thermocouples are more useful as they allow a continuous record of temperature. Central body temperature ('core' temperature) is the temperature most informative during anaesthesia. It can be estimated by measuring temperature in the thoracic oesophagus or at the tympanic membrane. Rectal temperature is less accurate. In addition, peripheral temperature can be measured at the skin. The difference between 'core' and peripheral temperature gives an indication of the state of peripheral tissue perfusion. During shock the core–peripheral gradient is greater than normal; this is commonly seen in the shocked animal that presents with cold paws and distal limbs.

General monitoring of the patient

Other monitoring activities performed during the anaesthetic period include the following.

Urine output

Catheterising the urinary bladder and measuring the collected urine indicates urine output. This is a simple and valuable method of assessing kidney function. A value in excess of 1 ml/kg/h is held to represent adequate renal perfusion, and therefore vital organ perfusion.

Monitoring fluid administration

If fluids are being given, the administration rates should be checked periodically. If a catheter is in place but fluids are not given, it should be flushed with heparin–saline regularly.

Monitoring surgery

The veterinary nurse should be aware of what surgical activity is occurring throughout anaesthesia. Haemorrhage must be continuously assessed. Liaison with the surgeon is vital during complicated surgery, e.g. thoracotomy.

Monitoring the breathing system

The system must be continuously monitored for behaviour, disconnection, soda–lime, valve action, etc. The pilot balloon of the endotracheal tube must be periodically checked to ensure the cuff remains gas-tight.

Monitoring gas flows and vaporiser settings

Flowmeters may 'drift' with time and should be constantly checked. Vaporiser fluid levels, settings and temperature should also be monitored. Cylinder contents must be continuously assessed.

KEY POINTS
- Careful monitoring is essential for safe anaesthesia.
- Prevention of complications and assessment of intra-operative therapy can be performed.
- Monitoring depth of anaesthesia relies primarily on assessment of indirect signs suggestive of appropriate anaesthesia.
- Monitoring of cardiovascular and respiratory function is used to ensure physiological well-being of the patient.
- Monitoring should continue into the recovery period.

Special anaesthesia

Occasionally, animals with severe physiological disturbances present for procedures requiring general anaesthesia. Each procedure carries its own individual risks; however, the anaesthetic approach should be similar. Careful pre-operative assessment and stabilisation (where possible) are required. Anaesthesia should be smooth with minimal disruption of physiological function and careful attention to the recovery period should be given.

General considerations

Pre-operative assessment

Careful patient evaluation is important (see the beginning of the chapter). Consideration of cardiovascular, respiratory, liver and renal function and concurrent therapy should be given.

Pre-operative stabilisation

Aspects include fluid therapy and electrolyte and acid–base stabilisation, oxygen therapy for hypoxaemia and blood product administration for anaemia, clotting defects, and protein deficits. Also analgesia, antibiosis and specific procedures may be required, e.g. stomach decompression in gastric-dilatation–volvulus (GDV).

General anaesthesia

The high-risk patient is less able to tolerate physiological disturbance. Hence it is important to maintain normal physiological status especially cardiovascular, respiratory and thermoregulatory function. Pre-oxygenation with a face mask prior to induction of anaesthesia can be beneficial. Anaesthetic agents have a more profound effect in the debilitated animal. It is important to reduce drug doses, use drugs that depress cardiopulmonary function less and give induction agents slowly to effect. Careful monitoring is important to alert to dangers and allow rapid correction of problems.

Recovery

Careful attention into the recovery period is often neglected. Monitoring should be continued with fluid therapy, rewarming and analgesia when appropriate.

Anaesthesia of the neonate

Neonates are defined as immature animals less than 12 weeks of age. Significant differences exist from the mature animal. Overestimation of their size often leads to overdose and immature body systems make them more sensitive to anaesthetics and less able to accommodate alterations in their normal function. An understanding of these differences is necessary for safe anaesthetic management.

Physiological considerations

Respiratory system Oxygen consumption is 2–3 times that of the adult, minute ventilation about three times that of the adult, there is a greater risk of airway obstruction, and alveolar collapse is more likely. All these predispose the neonate to hypoxia during anaesthesia.

Careful IPPV may be appropriate but excessive pressure can cause damage. Neonates 4–14 weeks can be allowed to ventilate spontaneously.

Cardiovascular system The myocardium is less contractile, the baroreceptors are immature, and there is a predominance of parasympathetic nervous system activity. Haemoglobin concentrations are lower and the erythrocytes have a shorter life span. Thus neonates are less able to increase force of contraction to meet changes in demand; increases in cardiac output are heart rate dependent. Hence hypotension is a particular problem and neonates are less able to cope with blood loss.

Hepatorenal function Enzyme systems are immature or absent. Hypoglycaemia is likely. Renal function is immature, thus there is poor renal concentrating function and reduced ability to tolerate dehydration. Maximum preparatory starvation of 2–3 hours is suggested. Intraoperative fluids, preferably including glucose, e.g. dextrose–saline, should be given.

Thermoregulation Neonates have immature thermoregulatory control, with reduced shivering ability and reliance on non-shivering thermogenesis. A large surface area to volume ratio and less subcutaneous fat exist. Hence neonates are prone to hypothermia.

Pharmacokinetics Low albumin and a larger percentage body water, lower body fat, and reduced hepatorenal function affect the pharmacology of drugs used. In general the dose of parenteral drugs needs to be reduced in the neonate.

Anaesthesia

The addition of an anticholinergic to maintain heart rate and reduce respiratory secretion is recommended in young neonates. Sedatives should be used sparingly. Benzodiazepines are useful, though often sedation is poor. Below 10 weeks, acepromazine is best avoided. Alpha-2-adrenoceptor agonists are potent sedatives and best avoided. Analgesics such as opioids are useful, though may have a prolonged action and a reduced dose is recommended.

Induction of anaesthesia can be achieved by injectable or inhaled methods. The latter is generally more stressful, but in young neonates can be a valuable technique. With less body fat and reduced metabolic function, prolonged recoveries are likely in the neonate after barbiturate anaesthesia. Propofol produces smooth induction of anaesthesia and a relatively rapid recovery and may be preferred. Dissociative agents, e.g. ketamine, can be used. 'Saffan' can be used in cats but a prolonged recovery may be seen.

Maintenance with inhalation anaesthesia is recommended for all but the shortest procedures. Isoflurane with its lower blood gas solubility than halothane, less reliance on metabolism in the liver, and less myocardial depression is preferred over halothane. Caution is required with endotracheal intubation; the larynx is more susceptible to trauma

and small narrow tubes are more liable to obstruction. Preservation of body temperature is important and these patients should be well insulated and actively warmed during anaesthesia. During recovery, attention to body temperature should be given to encourage a rapid return to consciousness.

Anaesthesia of the geriatric

As for the neonate, ageing affects physiological function and anaesthesia. Age results in a reduced capacity for adaptation and reduced functional reserves of organ systems. Though not a disease itself, it is frequently accompanied by systemic disease.

General considerations

- *Central nervous system.* There are generally reduced requirements for anaesthetics.
- *Respiratory system.* Reduced tidal volume and efficiency of gas exchange, increase the risk of hypoxia.
- *Cardiovascular changes.* The maximum heart rate falls with age and the response to stress/catecholamines is reduced. Geriatrics are poorly tolerant of volume depletion.
- *Hepato-renal function.* Renally excreted drugs are more slowly eliminated. Renal tubular function is reduced, the renin–angiotensin system less responsive and kidneys are less tolerant of hypotension. The older patient may be in chronic renal failure and prolonged periods of reduced renal perfusion (e.g. during hypotensive anaesthesia) may further damage the kidneys resulting in acute renal failure. Hepatic clearance decreases with decreasing liver mass.
- *Thermoregulation.* Geriatrics are prone to hypothermia.
- *Pharmacokinetic considerations.* Contracted blood volume increases plasma concentration of intravenous agents. Protein binding is reduced due to reduced albumen in plasma. Highly protein-bound drugs are more active.

Anaesthesia

There is no one ideal protocol and all drugs should be administered slowly to effect. Avoid heavy premedication as it can significantly compromise the patient and prolong recovery. Caution with alpha-2-adrenoceptor agonists, as they are potent sedatives, causing significant depression of cardiovascular function. Benzodiazepines are valuable and can produce good sedation in the older patient. A rapid smooth induction and calm recovery are preferred. Barbiturates may be associated with a prolonged recovery in patients with significant liver pathology. Propofol ensures a good rapid recovery and 'Saffan' appears acceptable in cats. Inhalation anaesthesia with isoflurane provides a more rapid recovery, but halothane can still be acceptable.

The shorter the procedures the better. Attention to heat loss and fluid therapy are important. Intra-operative fluid therapy is important to maintain renal perfusion and kidney function. Monitoring arterial blood pressure is particularly valuable in ensuring preservation of renal autoregulation and perfusion.

Anaesthesia for caesarean section

Anaesthesia for caesarean section is often an emergency without time for extensive preparation. Both dam and fetal viability are important considerations.

General considerations

Maternal physiology

Pregnancy alters maternal physiology:

- *Central nervous system.* Increased sensitivity to inhalation agents occurs.
- *Respiratory system.* Increased alveolar ventilation, reduced functional residual capacity due to anterior displacement of the diaphragm and increased oxygen consumption are seen. Hence there is increased inhalation agent uptake but also the dam is prone to developing hypoxia and hypercapnia.
- *Cardiovascular system.* Aortocaval compression (compression of the large vessels by the gravid uterus) can occur in dorsal recumbency, compromising venous return from the hindquarters. Increased blood volume (30%), reduced haematocrit and plasma proteins, increased cardiac output (30–50%) and reduced total peripheral resistance occur. There are reduced cardiac reserves and relative anaemia. Thus the dam is less tolerant of cardiovascular compromise.
- *Gastrointestinal system.* Increased gastric acidity, cranial displacement of stomach by the uterus and altered tone in the lower oesophageal sphincter make the dam more prone to regurgitation, vomiting and aspiration pneumonia.

Uteroplacental circulation and fetal viability

Preservation of blood flow to the fetus is essential to prevent hypoxia and acidosis of the fetus developing prior to removal from the placenta. Reduced uterine blood flow reduces placental perfusion and induces fetal hypoxia. This is particularly seen with shock and hypovolaemia, dehydration, and after administration of drugs such as oxytocin and ergotamine. Stress and catecholamines release can vasoconstrict the uterine blood vessels and reduce blood flow to the fetus.

Foetal tissues

The umbilical vein delivers drugs derived from the maternal circulation to the fetal liver and the ductus venosus. The fetal circulation attempts to protect vital tissues from exposure to sudden high concentrations of drugs. However most drugs administered to the dam are transferred rapidly across the placenta and even when diluted, may depress the fetus or neonate.

Pre-operative preparation

This includes clipping if not stressful, to reduce anaesthesia time. Pre-operative fluid therapy is indicated if the patient is shocked. Starvation is rarely possible. Positioning in off-dorsal recumbency reduces aortacaval compression.

Anaesthesia

The goals of anaesthesia are the provision of a smooth induction and maintenance of anaesthesia with a rapid recovery of the dam to consciousness to allow nursing, and delivery of viable alert neonates ready to feed. Minimal sedation is preferred. Induction of anaesthesia should be smooth with rapid endotracheal intubation. Barbiturates inhibit fetal respiration which may be significant if delivered soon after induction. Recovery of the dam and neonate may be delayed. Propofol gives a rapid and smooth induction and recovery and is recommended. 'Saffan' in cats causes minimal respiratory depression, and is also adequate. Ketamine produces minimal fetal depression but may result in disorientated kittens. Inhalation induction is potentially stressful; if used, intubation must be rapid.

For maintenance of anaesthesia, inhalation anaesthesia is recommended, and isoflurane is preferred over halothane for a more rapid recovery. A light plane of anaesthesia should minimise dose-dependent cardiorespiratory depression and reduce the potential for fetal hypoxia. It is important to maintain blood pressure to protect the fetal circulation and intra-operative fluid therapy can be valuable. Post-operative pain relief should be administered.

Neonate resuscitation requires adequate help. Clean mucus from the upper airways, administer oxygen if required, stimulate the skin, and prevent cooling. Aim to get the neonate feeding as soon as possible.

Anaesthesia for the pyometra

The bitch with pyometritis often presents dull and depressed. Closed pyometritis in which the mucopurulent discharge accumulates in the uterus can be life-threatening. Presurgical stabilisation is important; however, complete stabilisation is often impossible prior to removal of the septic focus.

General considerations

- *Shock.* This is a major concern. Hypovolaemia develops via fluid loss to the uterus combined with losses via vomiting and polyuria. Toxaemia can induce septic shock.

- *Renal disease.* Prerenal uraemia due to hypovolaemia, glomerular disease associated with antibody–antigen complexes and tubular disease due to toxins and immune complexes all interfere with the ability to concentrate urine. Concurrent renal disease of the old bitch may be present.
- *Acid–base and electrolyte disorders.* Metabolic acidosis is common with sodium and potassium loss.
- *Bone marrow suppression and clotting disorders.* Reduced erythrocyte and platelet production occurs. Anaemia is common. Clotting disorders may occur.
- *Liver disorders.* Hepatocellular damage develops due to intrahepatic cholestasis and bile pigment retention. Damage can also be secondary to endotoxaemia, dehydration and shock.
- *Arrhythmias* may be present, induced by toxins.

Pre-operative preparation

Fluid therapy is essential to restore circulating blood volume, protect renal function, and correct electrolyte and acid–base disorders. Potassium may need to be supplemented. Broad-spectrum antibiosis should be commenced. Platelet-rich plasma, whole blood or red blood cells may be required if there is thrombocytopaenia, low plasma proteins, clotting disorders or anaemia.

Anaesthesia

Premedication should cause minimal depression. Sedation is often unnecessary, though benzodiazepines may be beneficial to reduce the induction agent dose required. Analgesia is recommended, e.g. morphine or buprenorphine, to reduce intra-operative and post-operative pain. Induction of anaesthesia should be smooth with minimal cardiopulmonary depression. Most injectable anaesthetics are acceptable, though at a reduced dose. Maintenance with inhalation anaesthesia with isoflurane or halothane is preferred. Attention to monitoring and intra-operative fluid therapy are important. Post-operatively, fluid therapy may be required as well as further analgesia with opioids.

Anaesthesia for gastric-dilatation–volvulus (GDV)

GDV is an acute emergency of the large dog with a high incidence of mortality (12–43%). Though complete stabilisation prior to surgery is often impossible, a significant degree of stabilisation dramatically reduces complications and mortality.

General considerations

- *Respiratory compromise.* Ventilation is compromised by the dilated stomach. Endotoxic mediators can disrupt ventilation/perfusion balance compromising gas exchange in the lungs. Pulmonary oedema can occur.
- *Cardiovascular disturbances.* Compression of the caudal vena cava and portal veins, and pooling of blood in splanchnic, renal and capillary beds, reduces venous return and cardiac output. Cellular hypoxia and metabolic acidosis result. Circulating catecholamines, release of myocardial depressant factor and endotoxin, myocardial hypoxia and ischaemia, metabolic acidosis and electrolyte disturbances all predispose to arrhythmias and myocardial depression.
- *Endotoxaemia.* Ischaemic injury to the gut compromises the mucosal barrier, with increased absorption of endotoxin. Liver clearance of endotoxin is reduced. Shock can ensue with disseminated intravascular coagulation and multiple organ failure.
- *Gastric damage.* Increased intraluminal pressure and reduced gastric perfusion result in gastric ischaemia. Mucosal compromise allows leakage of plasma proteins, resulting in hypoproteinaemia and oedema.

Pre-operative preparation

Shock therapy is essential prior to anaesthesia. Aggressive intravenous fluid therapy to restore circulating blood volume is required. Crystalloids, e.g. lactated Ringer's (up to 90 ml/kg/h) can be used alone or combined with colloids and hypertonic saline (7.5% 4 ml/kg). Positive inotropes for hypotension unresponsive to fluids may be required. Correction of acidosis and electrolyte disturbances (especially hyperkalaemia) is necessary. The administration of steroids or NSAIDs remains controversial.

Gastric decompression with an orogastric tube with gastric lavage can dramatically improve cardiopulmonary function. Alternatively, percutaneous trocar placement (18G needle) or a gastrotomy may be required. Oxygen therapy should be given if the patient is hypoxic. Antibiosis is appropriate as the mucosal barrier may be compromised. Antacids, e.g. ranitidine or cimetidine, have been suggested and control of cardiac arrhythmias may be necessary.

Anaesthesia

Premedication again is rarely required. Minimal cardiovascular depression is essential during induction of anaesthesia. Arrhythmias are likely. An opioid/benzodiazepine combination is good, e.g. fentanyl 1–2 µg/kg + diazepam 0.1–0.2 mg/kg (intravenously). Alternatively, a benzodiazepine followed by a reduced dose of propofol given slowly is acceptable. Maintenance of anaesthesia with isoflurane is preferred, it is less arrhythmogenic and causes less cardiovascular depression than halothane. Nitrous oxide should be avoided until the stomach is decompressed as it partitions into gas-filled bodies. Careful monitoring is essential and fluid therapy should be continued.

During recovery, complications are frequent. Monitoring is important. Fluid therapy for shock should be continued. Arrhythmias in the post-operative period are common and may require therapy. Anaemia may result from significant blood loss. Reperfusion injury may occur after derotation of the stomach. Bowel mucosal ischaemia occurs due to gastric torsion and compromise to stomach blood supply. Oxygen free radicals and superoxide ions are produced and can be released to the blood when the volvulus is corrected, resulting in further shock.

KEY POINTS
- Careful pre-operative assessment of the patient is required.
- Pre-operative stabilisation of the systematically ill patient can reduce anaesthetic complications.
- Increased sensitivity to anaesthetic-induced cardiopulmonary depression may occur.
- Continuous monitoring is important.
- Further stabilisation and therapy may be required post-operatively.

Accidents and emergencies

Accidents are frequently avoidable problems, affecting patients or personnel and sometimes involving equipment. Problems may be of minor consequence individually, but collectively they may create emergencies. Emergencies are crises that require rapid responses, as they quickly lead to cardiopulmonary arrest. The most common complications involve respiratory and/or cardiovascular compromise, body temperature abnormalities and delayed return to consciousness. Problems can develop at all stages of anaesthesia, from premedication through to recovery. An understanding of the nature of common complications is important if we are to avoid them and when accidents do occur, rapid and effective therapy is essential if permanent disability or death is to be avoided.

DEFINITIONS
- **Apnoea**: the arrest of breathing.
- **Hypoventilation**: reduced alveolar ventilation.
- **Tachypnoea**: excessive frequency of respiration.
- **Bradypnoea**: excessive slowness of respiration.
- **Hypoxia**: reduced oxygen in the body tissues.
- **Hypercapnia**: excess of carbon dioxide in lungs or blood.
- **Tachycardia**: excessive heart rate.
- **Bradycardia**: excessive slowness of heart rate.
- **Arrhythmia**: irregular heart rhythm.
- **Hypotension**: low arterial blood pressure.
- **Haemorrhage**: bleeding.
- **Hypothermia**: low body temperature.

Respiratory complications

Compromise to ventilation is a significant concern during anaesthesia when the patient is unable to protect its own airway and normal regulation of ventilation is depressed. Apnoea is a particular emergency: severe hypoxia and hypercapnia rapidly cause cardiac arrest. Hypoventilation is less of an acute emergency but if severe may lead to cardiopulmonary arrest also. The circumstances in which apnoea can occur are:

- An acute event that prevents breathing (e.g. pneumothorax, upper airway obstruction, anaesthetic overdose).
- As a sign of cardiac arrest.
- As the end result of progressive hypoventilation.

Signs of apnoea include absence of breathing or irregular gasping with twitching neck muscles and spasmodic diaphragm contractions. In conscious animals the neck is extended, the mouth is wide open, the eyes are staring and the pupils are dilated. Mucous membranes are blue or dirty grey. In anaesthetised animals, only ineffectual breathing attempts, discoloured mucous membranes and signs of overdosage may be present.

There are three main causes of hypoventilation and apnoea (Fig. 23.16) and elements of all three are usually present during surgery:

- Failure of the brain to respond to elevated blood carbon dioxide or reduced blood oxygen levels.
- Airway obstruction (partial or complete).
- Chest-wall fixation and lung collapse.

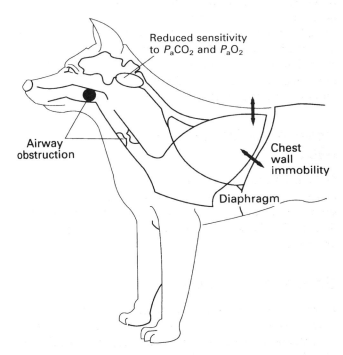

Fig. 23.16 Causes of apnoea and hypoventilation.

Failure of the brain to respond to blood carbon dioxide and oxygen levels

This occurs:

- In severe head trauma.
- When intracranial pressure is raised (e.g. by tumours or by inflammatory processes).
- In anaesthetic overdose.
- In severe hypothermia.

The most common cause of hypoventilation is profound anaesthesia, which reduces medullary sensitivity to carbon dioxide and abolishes chemoreceptor stimulation by hypoxia. The deeper the level of anaesthesia, the greater the degree of respiratory depression. Hypoventilation under anaesthesia is exacerbated by hypothermia. High doses of opioids may induce respiratory depression.

Transient apnoea is common after induction of anaesthesia with propofol and thiopentone. While spontaneous respiration resumes in the course of time, lung inflations should be imposed intermittently until regular ventilation returns.

Reduced alveolar ventilation results from reduced tidal volume and/or reduced respiratory rate. Conversely, very high respiratory rates with low tidal volumes (tachypnoea) also cause hypoventilation because inspired gas does not reach the alveoli effectively.

Airway obstruction

Airway obstruction in the non-intubated animal contributes to hypoventilation because it causes turbulent gas flow, which increases resistance to breathing. Partial or total obstruction is indicated by inspiratory snoring noises and/or paradoxical thoracic wall movement during inspiration (the abdomen moves outwards whilst the chest wall moves inwards). The airway may become obstructed in several ways:

- *Soft-tissue obstruction.* This is likely in brachycephalic breeds when sedatives or anaesthetics depress reflex control of oropharyngeal and nasopharyngeal muscles. Sedated brachycephalics must be observed closely and endotracheal intubation performed once consciousness is lost. During recovery, the return of gag reflexes indicates the need for extubation. Thereafter, surveillance must continue because obstruction remains possible.

  It must be appreciated that oxygen by mask is ineffective during obstruction. Endotracheal intubation, trans-tracheal oxygen or tracheotomy may be required until the obstruction is relieved. During recovery, sustained airway protective reflexes should be restored rapidly in cases at risk of obstruction by using drugs with little residual effect, or by administering an antagonist.
- *Blood and debris.* Obstruction also results from mycotic or neoplastic lesions, or from blood clots after nasal and dental surgery. After surgery involving the oropharynx, nasopharynx or any part of the upper airway, surgical debris must be cleared before the animal recovers and is extubated.
- *Vomit.* Regurgitation. This may occur during induction or post-operatively. Rarely, passive regurgitation occurs during surgery. When there is regurgitation, the animal must be positioned head-down. If it remains conscious, its mouth is gagged and the oropharynx cleared of material. Initially, dry swabs held with towel forceps or haemostats will suffice. Later, moistened swabs may be needed. If consciousness is lost, cursory pharyngeal lavage must be followed by endotracheal intubation and positive pressure ventilation with oxygen. Suction and lavage are then performed.
- *Fluid–pulmonary oedema.* A froth-filled airway indicates pulmonary oedema which results from end-stage left-sided heart failure or, rarely, after use of 'Saffan' in cats. Endobronchial suction should be performed, though the prognosis is poor.
- *Bronchospasm.* Severe bronchospasm (status asthmaticus) is fortunately a rare cause of airway obstruction in companion animals but in theory could occur in response to histamine-releasing drugs, e.g. high doses of pethidine or morphine given intravenously. The administration of adrenaline, beta 2 agonists and steroids may be required.
- *Endotracheal tube complications.* The presence of endotracheal tubes does not guarantee a patent airway. Overinflated cuffs may cause the lumen to collapse, or extreme neck positions may cause kinking. Lightly anaesthetised animals may bite the tube and close the lumen. Cats have particularly sensitive larynxes and are prone to spasm if poor intubation technique is used. Desensitisation of the larynx with local anaesthetic prior to intubation is required in this species. Oesophageal intubation is possible and may result in premature awakening or respiratory compromise.

Chest-wall fixation and lung collapse

Breathing ceases when the chest wall and diaphragm are immobilised or when the lungs are prevented from expanding. In pneumothorax, the lungs are collapsed by thoracic expansion with gas accumulation in the pleural space, resulting in hypoventilation. Similarly, fluid accumulation in the pleural space, in patients with pleural effusions, can compromise ventilation.

Some breathing systems have expiratory valves. If these are inadvertently left closed, there is a rapid build-up in circuit pressure, preventing expiration and causing rapid death. In very small animals, breathing may be suppressed when the chest wall is 'stiffened' by heavy drapes, when surgeons rest heavy instruments on the chest, or when the chest wall is covered by adipose tissue. Breathing is also inhibited by restrictive post-operative bandages and by pain after road traffic accidents or thoracotomy.

Treatment of apnoea or hypoventilation

If the cause of apnoea or hypoventilation is in doubt, the trachea is intubated and a breathing system is connected. The level of anaesthesia is assessed. Anaesthetic administration is ended if cranial nerve signs indicate overdosage.

The lungs are then inflated at a rate of 8–15 breaths per minute. If this is possible without high pressure being needed, the cause is probably upper airway obstruction or central nervous depression. If the lungs feel 'stiff', there is probably pneumothorax, pleural effusion or bronchospasm. If the animal does not breathe after 5 minutes or so, imposed hyperventilation may have caused hypocapnia. In this case the respiratory rate should be reduced.

Opioid antagonists (naloxone) or analeptics (doxapram) may be considered as a last resort. Doxapram stimulates respiration and elevates consciousness but its use is futile when respiratory embarrassment is caused by chest-wall fixation or airway obstruction. Its effects are short-lived and so the drug is only useful for 'buying time'.

Cardiovascular complications

Cardiovascular complications are a major concern during anaesthesia. Most drugs depress cardiovascular function, often in a dose-dependent manner. This combined with pre-existing pathology make such complications relatively common. Alterations in heart rate and rhythm, vacular tone and myocardial contractility can all occur.

Tachycardia and bradycardia

Changes in heart rate are important because they can affect the adequacy of the heart to pump out blood to the organs, they can increase the workload of the heart (especially tachycardia) and they can predispose to serious arrhythmias. Further they may indicate serious underlying pathology or inappropriate depth of anaesthesia. The causes and treatment of these two conditions are given in Table 23.6.

Arrhythmias

Irregularities in heart rhythm may reduce cardiac output and cause hypotension. Without treatment some rhythms may deteriorate into more dangerous forms associated with cardiac arrest (e.g. ventricular fibrillation).

Causes Arrhythmias are caused by inadequate anaesthesia or overdosage, electrolyte and blood-gas abnormalities, certain surgical procedures and pre-existing heart disease. Certain medical conditions like GDV complex are associated with ventricular arrhythmias.

Treatment This depends primarily on diagnosis with electrocardiography and treatment with antiarrhythmic drugs. Often, ensuring an adequate level of anaesthesia and ventilation restores normal rhythm.

Table 23.6 Treating tachycardia and bradycardia

Cause	Treatment
Tachycardia	
Inadequate anaesthesia	Increase vaporiser setting or give intravenous anaesthetic/analgesic
Hypoxia	Ventilate with 100% oxygen, end nitrous oxide administration (if used)
Hypercapnia	Ventilate, reduce anaesthetic depth
Hypotension	Begin fluid infusion at rapid rate, reduce anaesthetic depth, administer inotropes
Hyperthermia	Cool body surfaces, administer cool IV fluids
Drugs	Reversal not generally required
Bradycardia	
Anaesthetic overdose	Reduce vaporiser setting and ventilate. Administer reversal agent (if available)
Terminal hypoxia	Stop anaesthetic and ventilate with 100% oxygen. Initiate CPR
Hyperkalaemia	Instigate fluid therapy, give sodium bicarbonate and or glucose and insulin
Vagal activity	Check surgeon's activity. If this is related to bradycardia then temporarily suspend surgery and give atropine or glycopyrrolate
Drugs	Alpha-2-agonists and high doses of opioids produce bradycardia. Antimuscarinic drugs offset the effects of opioids, but their use with alpha-2-agonist is controversial. Reducing the depth of anaesthesia may increase heart rates reduced by drugs
Hypothermia	Rewarm, and end surgery as soon as possible. Reduce vaporiser setting and ventilate

Hypotension

Prolonged hypotension diminishes perfusion in splanchnic and renal vasculature, ultimately causing tissue damage. When hypotension is severe or prolonged, fatal myocardial and cerebral damage occurs.

Causes Low blood pressure results from several factors. Inadequate cardiac output and reduced systemic vascular resistance cause hypotension. Cardiac output falls because of either extremes of heart rate or inadequate stroke volume. The latter results from poor contractility (e.g. anaesthetic overdose) or reduced preload (hypovolaemia). Alternatively, hypotension can occur from reduced systemic vascular resistance, e.g. when high doses of acepromazine are given.

Treatment If the animal is 'deep' then anaesthetic depth should be reduced and intravenous fluids should be infused rapidly until improvement is seen. If no improvement occurs, inotropes (e.g. dobutamine) may be needed.

Haemorrhage

Blood loss during surgery causes hypotension and ultimately haemorrhagic or hypovolaemic shock. Obvious signs of shed blood at the surgical site combined with tachycardia, pallor and a weak pulse should raise the suspicion of significant haemorrhage. Loss can be estimated by weighing swabs: 1 ml blood weighs 1.3 g. The volume of shed blood can be quantified by deducting the weight of dry swabs from those soaked in blood.

Treatment Lost blood is replaced with either blood, plasma expanders or electrolyte solutions. If blood is used, the volume required equals the volume lost. For blood losses of up to 20% of circulating volume, electrolyte solutions such as Hartmann's can be infused on a 3:1 basis (3 ml fluids are given for each 1 ml of blood lost).

Thermoregulatory complications

Both hypothermia and hyperthermia are seen during anaesthesia. Anaesthetics depress the body's ability to regulate temperature and occasionally can upregulate metabolism, inducing hyperthermia (e.g. malignant hyperthermia). Hypothermia, however, is most common under anaesthesia and results from a number of factors:

- Hypothalamic thermoregulation is impaired by anaesthetics.
- Skin blood vessels vasodilate.
- Skeletal muscle activity ceases.
- Shivering is inhibited during surgical anaesthesia.
- Visceral surfaces are exposed.
- Inspired gases are cold and dry.

Animals most at risk are those with high ratios of surface area to volume (e.g. neonates, birds and small laboratory animals) and those with underdeveloped or impaired thermoregulatory reflexes (the very young and old).

There are important adverse effects of hypothermia:

- Reduced alveolar ventilation.
- Reduced heart rate and cardiac output.
- Haemoglobin binds oxygen more strongly.
- Erythrocytes become stickier; blood viscosity increases.
- During recovery, shivering elevates oxygen consumption and plasma catecholamines.

Consequences Primarily prolonged recovery is seen. This results from reduced elimination of volatile agents, reduced redistribution and retarded metabolism of injectable drugs and may become a self-reinforcing cycle. In human anaesthesia there is evidence that peri-operative hypothermia predisposes to increased morbidity and wound complications (Kurz et al., 1996). If hypothermia is very severe, cardiac arrest may result. Ventricular fibrillation is likely when body temperature falls below 28°C.

Prevention Prevention of hypothermia is better than treatment and can be addressed in a number of ways:

- **Physical factors**:

  - Increase operating room temperature.
  - Do not lay animals on cold, uninsulated surfaces.
  - Do not expose to draughts.
  - Insulate animals with aluminium foil or bubble wrap.
  - Use heated blankets, insulated hot-water bottles and radiant heat lamps.

- **Anaesthetic factors**:

  - Favour the use of short-acting anaesthetics.
  - Avoid deep planes of anaesthesia.
  - Provide adequate but not excessive ventilation.
  - Use rebreathing systems where appropriate.
  - Use warm intravenous fluids.

- **Surgical factors**:

  - During surgical preparation of high-risk animals, do not unnecessarily wet the animal, clip excessively or use volatile preparations such as alcohol.
  - Minimise surgical time.
  - Exposed visceral surfaces must be moistened with warm irrigant fluids. Non-surgical areas must not be allowed to get wet. Incision size must be as small as possible. Viscera should be replaced in body cavities as soon as examination or surgery is completed.

Treatment Post-operatively, the animal should be thoroughly dried using towels and hair dryers. Topical heat may then be applied judiciously using 40 W lightbulbs, radiant infrared lamps or insulated hot-water bottles. Small laboratory animals may be placed in an incubator. If these methods fail, warm-water gastric or rectal lavage may be performed.

Delayed return to consciousness

Prolonged recovery is occasionally seen. Inappropriate depth of anaesthesia, the use of drugs with prolonged durations of action and individual patient sensitivity all contribute to this problem. Acepromazine may cause slow recoveries in certain breeds of dogs and in dogs with diminished liver function. Multiple doses of barbiturates may also delay recovery, particularly in sight-hounds. Drug retention may result from inadequate perfusion or failure of the liver or kidney. Hypothermia causes retarded expiration of volatile agents and the redistribution and reduction of metabolism of injectable agents.

The fundamental approach to prolonged recovery is based on maintaining organ physiological function, providing good nursing (e.g. raising temperature, preventing dependent sore) and creating a diffusion gradient from the drug's site of action to the organ of elimination. Monitoring of the patient should be approached as for the anaesthetised patient. Maintenance of cardiovascular and respiratory function in these cases is vital. Haemodynamic support with intravenous fluids (with or without the use of positive inotropes) may be required. For patients with prolonged periods of unconsciousness, urinary catheterisation and measurement of urine output is valuable. This gives a simple yet excellent indicator of renal perfusion and function and indirectly cardiovascular performance. If the patient is hypoxic, oxygen supplementation is necessary and if hypoventilating, positive pressure ventilation may be required. Rewarming and maintenance of body temperature is also important. Persistent drug activity can be countered if the suspect agent has an antagonist:

Agonist	*Antagonist*
Opioids	Naloxone, nalbuphine
Benzodiazepines	Flumazenil
Alpha-2-agonist	Atipamezole

Miscellaneous accidents

Accidents in recovery

Poor attention to recovering animals contributes to post-operative mortality. Problems are probably more likely at this time because attention relaxes, the perceived high-risk periods of induction and maintenance having passed. Responsibilities during recovery include the following (Fig. 23.17):

- Monitoring vital signs and keeping records.
- Keeping animals calm and dry, and surgical sites and orifices clean.
- Attending to wounds and preventing interference.

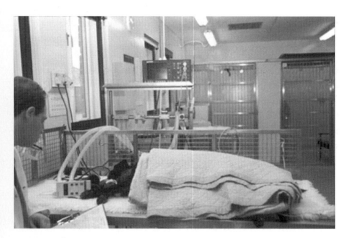

Fig. 23.17 Careful post-operative monitoring following laryngeal surgery.

- Providing post-operative medication.
- Monitoring fluid and energy balance.
- Reporting recovery problems.

Excitation   Bad recoveries characterised by excitation, hyperaesthesia, vocalisation, exaggerated responsiveness and excessive activity may result from pain, emergence, pharmacological phenomena and epilepsy/convulsion.

Pain   This responds to analgesic administration.

Emergence   Some animals recover after non-painful surgery as if in pain. Disconcerting signs are normally short-lived. The incidence is higher with certain drugs (e.g. 'Saffan') but may be reduced if sedative premedications are used and recovery occurs in a quiet environment.

Convulsions/epilepsy   Post-operative convulsions traditionally followed myelographic investigation with certain contrast media. Epileptic patients may be at increased risk of post-operative seizures.

Hypoxia   Although extubation must be performed when gagging, 'bucking' and other cranial nerve reflexes are restored, it is not safe to assume that oxygen delivery may be safely discontinued. Hypothermia, residual anaesthetic drug activity and lung changes may combine to diminish blood oxygenation, while shivering and pain increase oxygen consumption. Oxygen (100%) should be delivered until animals can maintain satisfactory oxygenation on room air. If extubation is necessary before this time, oxygen should be given by mask, intranasal catheter, tracheostomy tube or transtracheal catheter.

Oxygen must be given for at least 3 minutes after the discontinuation of N_2O in order to avoid diffusion hypoxia. Animals incapable of maintaining sternal recumbency should be repositioned every 2–4 hours to prevent hypostatic congestion of the lungs.

Discharge

Animals must not be discharged before full recovery from anaesthesia and surgery. The client must also be forewarned of other anaesthetic and surgery-related complications such as haemorrhage.

Extravascular injections

Extravascular injection of irritant drugs like thiopentone result in tissue sloughs. These are painful, take a long time to heal and leave unsightly blemishes. The risk of this is minimised by:

- Effective patient restraint (physical or chemical) before injection.
- Venous catheterisation.
- Using dilute solutions of drug (e.g. 1.25% for thiopentone) in animals with poorly accessible veins.

- If extravascular injection does occur, the deposition is enthusiastically diluted with sterile saline or water. Large volumes may be safely injected under the skin and massaged. Later a record should be made of the accident.

Burns

Burns occur if excess heat is applied to cold animals. This is more likely when skin blood flow is reduced, as in shock, because poorly perfused skin conducts heat less effectively.

Decubital ulcers

These sores appear when bony prominences remain in prolonged contact with hard surfaces. They are prevented by adequate bedding and frequent turning of the patient.

Hypostatic congestion

Capillaries in the dependent (lowermost) lung fill with blood and alveoli partially collapse when recoveries are prolonged and cardiac output is low. Both changes result in hypoxia. Prevention is based on frequent (2-hourly) turning.

Equipment-based accidents

Cylinders   Cylinders contain gas at high pressure (nearly 1935 p.s.i. or 13 300 kPa) and will explode if mistreated. They must not be dropped or placed in a position where they may fall or become damaged. They should not be exposed to high temperatures (including direct sunlight). They must be stored in dry conditions away from flammable materials.

When a full oxygen cylinder is exposed to elevated temperatures caused, for example, by naked flames, the pressure within it rises and may exceed the test pressure. Eventually the bottle bursts and releases oxygen that fuels further conflagration.

Explosions and fires   Explosions require a source of fuel (usually carbon-based), oxygen and activation energy (a spark or a naked flame). Once initiated, heat released from the reaction provides further activation energy and the reaction proliferates. Explosions are more likely when fuel–oxygen rather than fuel–air mixtures are present.

For these reasons, 'sticking' valves or apparatus involved with pressurised oxygen must never be lubricated or sealed with carbon- or petroleum-based lubricants. In the past, cyclopropane and diethyl ether were commonly used for anaesthesia. They lost popularity because of their flammability and explosive properties, and their redundancy was accelerated by the introduction of thermocautery and electrical monitoring devices in the operating room. Surgical alcohol remains a possible source of fire and explosion.

Risks of fire and explosion are minimised by keeping the three 'components' separate:

- Inflammable agents must not be used when heat, sparks (from static electricity or electrical apparatus) or naked flames are present.
- If thermocautery is required, cyclopropane and ether must be avoided.
- Naked flames, carbon-based fuels and dust must be minimised.

If fires or explosions occur, the emergency services must be informed that supplies of inflammable material and compressed oxygen are within the vicinity of the accident.

Accidents to personnel

Bites and scratches   These are minimised by suitable physical and chemical restraint techniques, by equipment and by common sense precautions. Fingers should not be placed within the mouth of an ungagged, unconscious animal especially during endotracheal intubation: owners should not normally be allowed to restrain animals in case they are injected accidentally or bitten.

When an accident occurs, the appropriate report form must be completed. The injured person should report to hospital for examination and tetanus immunisation. If known, details of the animal's condition should be supplied.

Self-administration of drugs   Risk of self-administration is greatest with Immobilon preparations. There is also risk with sedatives, especially alpha-2-adrenoceptor agonists; toxicity has not yet been reported in humans although the potential is great. Absorption of these drugs across oral mucous membranes is rapid and so placing of needle-caps in mouths is especially hazardous. Ketamine has been inadvertently self-administered, with ensuing toxic signs.

Whenever drug-based accidents occur, the data sheet or NOAH Compendium should be taken to the emergency room with the injured person. Self-administration can be avoided:

- Ensure that the animal is adequately restrained.
- Do not resheath needles but dispose of them immediately after use.
- Do not carry syringes and needles in pockets.
- Do not place syringe caps in the mouth.

When using Immobilon, the manufacturer's guidelines must be followed. If drug splashes into the eye or on to skin, the site must be thoroughly irrigated with copious amounts of fresh water. If injection occurs, or if toxic signs follow 'splashing' accidents, the antagonist protocol must be followed. In any event, hospital services must be notified and the data sheet presented to the attending doctor. Many of the guidelines for the prevention of self-administration of Immobilon are appropriate for other potent injectable drugs:

- The needle used for drug withdrawal from vial should be discarded in a metal container and a new needle used for injection.
- Wear gloves.
- Do not pressurise the vial.
- Have eye and skin washes available.
- An assistant capable of giving the antagonist should be present.

The user should brief the assistant on emergency protocol and whether or not diprenorphine (which has a veterinary product licence only) constitutes part of this protocol. Naloxone and diprenorphine should always be available.

Cardiopulmonary arrest

Cardiopulmonary arrest occurs when cardiopulmonary function fails. Failure to initiate effective cardiopulmonary resuscitation (CPR) under these circumstances leads rapidly to death. Sometimes CPR is not appropriate: it is futile when animals with 'terminal' conditions arrest.

Factors predisposing to arrest can develop rapidly (acute arrests) or more slowly (chronic arrests). 'Acute' arrests result from single devastating events occurring in otherwise normal cases (e.g. thiopentone overdose). 'Chronic' arrests result when many derangements develop slowly and remain unnoticed until the cumulative effect is catastrophic. The latter are probably more common in veterinary practice and indicate that close monitoring and rapid treatment of even mildly deteriorating conditions are important. The axiom 'prevention is better than cure' is most important in the context of CPR.

Causes of arrest

- Myocardial hypoxia (e.g. tachycardia, bradycardia, hypotension, myocardial disease).
- Toxins (e.g. toxaemia, azotaemia, anaesthetic overdose).
- pH extremes (e.g. hypoventilation, shock, diabetic keto-acidosis).
- Electrolyte changes (e.g. hyperkalaemia, hypocalcaemia, hypokalaemia).
- Temperature extremes.

Clinical signs of cardiopulmonary arrest

- Blood at surgical site becomes dark and clots easily.
- Bleeding stops.
- Either 'gasping' ventilation or apnoea is seen (the former resembling 'light' anaesthesia).
- Mucous membranes may become dirty grey, blue or white.
- Capillary refill time becomes prolonged (more than 2 seconds).
- Heart sounds are not audible.
- No palpable pulse.

- Central eye position.
- Pupils dilate.
- Dry cornea.
- Cranial nerve reflexes are lost.
- Generalised muscle relaxation.
- Arrhythmias: those normally associated with arrest include ventricular fibrillation and asystole. However, in electromechanical dissociation there is a near-normal ECG while mechanical cardiac activity is lost. This is a common cause of arrest in dogs.

Treatment

When these clinical signs are recognised, assistance must be summoned immediately. Simultaneously, preparations are made for CPR, the elements of which are remembered with the mnemonic:

- **A**irway.
- **B**reathing.
- **C**irculation.
- **D**rugs.
- **E**lectrical defibrillation.
- **F**ollow-up.

Before these begin, the animal is laid in right lateral recumbency, positioned against a hard surface and if, possible, in a slight head-down position.

Practical nursing tip *Rehearse CPR so that when an emergency occurs everbody knows what to do.*

Airway Effective CPR requires an appropriately positioned, cuffed patent endotracheal tube of suitable size. When assistance is unavailable, tracheal intubation is facilitated by laryngoscopy and is most easily accomplished with the animal in dorsal recumbency. Alternatively, a tracheotomy may be performed or a catheter may be passed to the level of the tracheal bifurcation to allow oxygen insufflation.

Breathing Positive-pressure ventilation with oxygen-enriched gas must be imposed. This can be done using any of the following:

- An anaesthetic machine and appropriate breathing system flushed with 100% oxygen.
- Self-inflating resuscitation bags (e.g. Ambu resuscitator) which connect to endotracheal tubes and allow manual lung inflation with either air (20% oxygen) or 100% oxygen.
- Expired air (containing 16% oxygen).

The lungs are inflated using sufficient volume to produce visibly supranormal chest-wall excursions. The lungs are reinflated immediately expiration is ended, but must be allowed to deflate to the normal end-expiratory position. In single-handed resuscitation attempts, deliver two or three large lung inflations for every 15 chest-wall compressions.

The femoral pulse, mucous membrane colour and heart sounds should be checked within 30 seconds of beginning ventilation. Thereafter they should be monitored continuously, if assistance is available, or at half-minute intervals. Ventilation alone may restore the pulse but in most cases, circulatory support will be required.

Circulation　When the heart stops, cardiac output must be supported by either compressing the rib cage (external cardiac compression) or directly squeezing the surgically exposed heart (internal cardiac compression). Cardiac output produced by either method depends on adequate venous return. This is enhanced by rapid fluid infusion, posture, abdominal compression and adrenaline.

External cardiac compression　There are two forms of external cardiac compression. The first, the 'cardiac pump' method, is most suitable for cats, dogs weighing less than 20 kg, or those with narrow chests (e.g. whippets). The chest wall is compressed in the ventral third of the thorax between the 3rd and 6th rib. This is facilitated if the animal is positioned on a hard surface in right lateral recumbency. For very small dogs, cats and pups, the heart is massaged by compressing the ribs between thumb and forefinger. The compression rate is 80–100 per minute.

The second technique, the 'thoracic pump' method, is suited for larger dogs weighing over 20 kg or lighter dogs with 'barrel' chests (e.g. bulldogs). The rib cage is compressed at the widest point – the junction of the dorsal and middle thirds of the 6th to 7th rib – at 60–120 times per minute. If possible, compressions should be made during peak lung inflation.

The efficiency of this second technique is increased by three manoeuvres:

- *Abdominal binding.* Applying tight bandages to the hind limbs and then the abdomen directs blood flow (generated by external cardiac compression) towards the head.
- *Abdominal counterpulsation (interposed abdominal compression).* The abdomen is manually compressed during the diastolic or relaxation phase of chest compression to increase coronary perfusion and assists venous return.
- *Synchronous lung inflation/chest wall compression.* Cardiac output increases when the chest is compressed.

Because ventilation and cardiac compression must never be suspended, abdominal binding and counterpulsation require the presence of a third resuscitator.

The advantages of external cardiac compression are:

- Reasonably effective in certain patients.
- Requires little preparation.
- Rapidly applied.
- Few hazards.
- Can be performed by lay staff.

The disadvantage is that it is ineffective in some circumstances.

Internal cardiac compression　Internal cardiac compression requires a thoracotomy and direct manual compression of the heart. It is more effective than external cardiac compression and is recommended if the latter is ineffective at generating a palpable pulse within 2–3 minutes of onset of cardiac arrest. Internal cardiac massage allows visualisation of the beating heart and intracardiac drug administration. However, it does require a surgical approach to the thorax and often practitioners are reluctant to perform it or attempt internal massage too late after onset of arrest.

To perform internal thoracotomy a rapid clip of the 3rd to 6th intercostal space on the left side may be needed in long-haired dogs. The appropriate site can be identified by flexing the forelimb so that the olecranon transects the costochondral junction; this point overlies the 5th intercostal space. However, time must not be wasted in surgical preparation. A bold skin incision is made from dorsal to the sternum to ventral to the transverse process of the thoracic vertebrae at intercostal space 5. Scissors are used to cut through the intercostal muscles and the ribs are spread with rib retractors. The heart is then manually compressed.

Signs of effective CPR

Early:

- Palpation of pulse during cardiac compression.
- Constriction of the pupils.
- Ventromedial relocation of the eye.
- Improvement of mucous membrane colour.
- ECG changes.

Late:

- Lacrimation.
- Return of cranial nerve reflexes, e.g. blinking, gagging and coughing.
- Return of spontaneous respiratory activity. Diaphragmatic twitches and irregular breathing appear at first.
- Then regular deep breathing returns; this is a good prognostic sign.
- Return of special senses: response to sound.
- Return of other central nervous function: vocalisation righting reflexes, purposeful movement.

If early signs are not seen within 2 minutes, resuscitative (D)rugs and (E)lectrical defibrillation can be used (D and E of the mnemonic); or an emergency thoracotomy and internal cardiac compression can be undertaken.

Drugs　In cases unresponsive to ventilation and cardiac massage or where a definite diagnosis of an arrhythmia has been made, drug therapy is instituted. The use of a central vein (e.g. jugular vein) is to be recommended as peripheral vein drainage back to the heart is often reduced in these patients. Alternatively, intratracheal drug administration can be used. Commonly used drugs and their doses are included in Table 23.7.

Table 23.7 Drug doses for cardiopulmonary resuscitation

Drug	Route	Indication	Dose
Adrenaline	IV, IT	Asystole, atropine-resistant bradycardia myocardial depression	0.1–0.2 mg/kg
Atropine	IV, IT	Vagal bradycardias, asystole	0.02–0.04 mg/kg
Bicarbonate	IV	Metabolic acidosis	Approx. 1 mEq/kg
Calcium	IV	Hyperkalaemia, hypocalcaemia myocardial depression	10 mg/kg
Dobutamine	IV	Hypotension	1–5 μg/kg/min
Dopamine	IV	Hypotension, renal failure	1–10 μg/kg/min
Electrical defibrillation		Ventricular fibrillation	0.1–0.5 J/kg (internal) 1–5 J/kg (external)
Lignocaine	IV, IT	Ventricular tachycardia	2–4 mg/kg (dog) 40–80 μg/kg (cat)
Dexamethasone	IV	Post-resuscitation	1–2 mg/kg

IV = intravenous, IT = intratracheal

Electrical defibrillation If ventricular fibrillation has occurred, early electrical defibrillation is advised. A fully charged and readily available defibrillator is required.

Follow-up If the patient has been successfully resuscited then careful postoperative intensive care will be required. Maintenance of cardiovascular function may be necessary. Fluid therapy is usually continued into the recovery period and inotropes may be given if blood pressure is not maintained. Attention to renal output is important and some patients may need diuretic therapy in addition to fluid therapy. Those patients inadequately ventilating may require ventilatory support (with or without sedation) into the recovery period. Maintenance of body temperature is often required with the use methods including heated blankets, heat lamps, and warm intravenous fluids. Post-operative attention to neurological status is also often required. Treatment of seizures and brain oedema may be necessary.

Too much practice at resuscitation is not necessarily a good thing, as it suggests more accidents are happening than would be liked. However the veterinary nurse can prepare for such eventualities and can significantly improve the chances for successful resuscitation. A fully stocked and maintained resuscitation box with in-date drugs can be invaluable. Contents of a resuscitation box are described in Table 23.8.

> • Accidents involving veterinary staff should be minimised by vigilance during anaesthesia.
> • The recovery period is a common time during which complications occur.
> • Careful attention to the patient until it has returned to its normal state is required.
> • During an arrest, efficient 'ABC' therapy can prevent long-term organ dysfunction (e.g. brain) whilst the underlying cause is being identified and addressed.

Table 23.8 Drugs and equipment required for cardiopulmonary resuscitation

Drugs	Equipment
Adrenaline	Needles and syringes
Atropine	Urinary catheters for intratracheal
Lignocaine	drug administration
Isoprenaline	Emergency surgical pack
Dopamine	Self-inflating resuscitator bag
Dobutamine	Defibrillator
Propranolol	Internal and external paddles
Frusemide	Intravenous catheters
Mannitol	Endotracheal tubes
Methyl prednisolone	
Procainamide	
Calcium gluconate	
Sodium bicarbonate	
Edrophonium or neostigmine	
Verapamil	
Doxapram	
Naloxone	
Atipamezole	

KEY POINTS
• Complications are potentially numerous during anaesthesia.
• Prevention of anticipated risks is significantly more effective than treatment.
• Rapid identification and corrective measures reduce morbidity and mortality.

Acknowledgements

The author is indebted to Mr R. E. Clutton, the author of the first edition of this chapter from which information and some diagrams have been drawn, to Dr P. M. Taylor for permission to use information from her University of Cambridge Undergraduate Veterinary Anaesthesia lecture notes, and to Ms N. Clifford VN for suggestions for the manuscript.

Further reading

Buring, J. E., Hennekens, C. H., Mayrent, S. L., Rosner, B., Greenberg, E.R. and Colton, T. (1985) Health experiences of operating room personnel. *Anesthesiology*, vol. 62, pp. 325–330.

Capner, C. A., Lascelles, B. D. X. and Waterman-Pearson, A. E. (1999) Current British veterinary attitudes to perioperative analgesia for dogs. *Veterinary Record*, vol. 145, pp. 95–99.

Clutton, R. E. (1993) Management of perioperative cardiac arrest in companion animals part 1. *In Practice*, Nov, pp. 267–277.

Clutton, R. E. (1994) Management of perioperative cardiac arrest in companion animals part 2. *In Practice*, Jan, pp. 3–10.

Corbett, T .H., Cornell, R. G., Endres, J. L. and Lieding, K. (1974) Birth defects among children of nurse anesthetists. *Anesthesiology*, vol. 41, pp. 341–344.

Davey, A., Moyle, J. T. B. and Ward, C. S. (1994) *Ward's Anaesthetic Equipment*, 3rd edn, W. B. Saunders, London.

Hall, L. W., Clarke, K. W. and Trim C. (2000) *Veterinary Anaesthesia*, 10th edn, Baillière Tindall, London.

Hall, L. W. and Taylor, P. M. (1994) *Anaesthesia of the Cat*, Baillière Tindall, London.

Kurz, A., Sessler, D. I. and Lenhardt, R. (1996) Perioperative normothermia to reduce the incidence of surgical-wound infection and shorten hospitalization. *The New England Journal of Medicine*, vol. 334, pp. 1209–1215.

Lascelles, B. D. X., Capner, C. A. and Waterman-Pearson, A. E. (1999) Current British veterinary attitudes to perioperative analgesia for cats and small mammals. *Veterinary Record*, vol. 145, pp. 601–604.

Levick, J. R. (1996) *An Introduction to Cardiovascular Physiology,* 2nd edn, Butterworth-Heinemann, Oxford.

Richmond, C. E., Bromley, L. M. and Woolf, C. J. (1993) Preoperative morphine pre-empts postoperative pain. *The Lancet*, vol. 342, pp. 73–75.

Seymour, C. and Gleed, R. (1999) *Manual of Small Animal Anaesthesia and Analgesia*, BSAVA, Cheltenham.

Thurmon, J. C., Tranquilli, W. J. and Benson, G. J. (1996) *Veterinary Anesthesia*, 3rd edn, Williams & Wilkins, Baltimore.

West, J. B. (1995) *Respiratory Physiology – The Essentials*, 5th edn, Williams & Wilkins, Baltimore.

Woolf, C. J. and Chong, M. (1993) Preemptive analgesia – treating postoperative pain by preventing the establishment of central sensitization. *Anesthesia and Analgesia*, vol. 77, pp. 362–379.

24

Diagnostic imaging

R. Dennis and *C. France*[†]

Learning objectives

After studying this chapter, students should be able to:

• Understand the physical principles of diagnostic radiography.
• Have a sound working knowledge of radiographic equipment, procedures and safety.
• Know how to perform basic radiographic studies and to prepare for and assist in more complex investigations.
• Identify and know how to correct faults in radiography.
• Understand the principles of diagnostic ultrasonography and know how to assist in ultrasound examinations.
• Describe the basic features of MRI, CT and scintigraphy.

Radiography is a fundamental part of veterinary practice and is a procedure in which most nurses become actively involved. The production of diagnostic films requires skill in the use of radiographic equipment, in patient positioning and in the processing of the films. At the same time the procedure must be carried out safely without hazard to the handlers or patient.

This chapter summarises the use of radiography in small animal practice. All parts of the veterinary nursing N/S VQ level 3 standards are covered but it is hoped that the chapter will also prove useful for day-to-day reference.

Basic principles of radiography

X-rays are produced by X-ray machines when electricity from the mains is transformed to a high-voltage current, converting some of the energy in the current to X-ray energy. The intensity and penetrating power of the emergent X-ray beam varies with the size and complexity of the apparatus, and the exposure settings used; portable X-ray machines are capable only of a relatively low output, whereas larger machines are far more powerful.

X-rays travel in straight lines and can be focused into an area called the **primary beam**, which is directed at the patient. Within the patient's tissues some of the X-rays are absorbed; the remainder pass through and are detected by photographic X-ray film producing a hidden image. When the film is processed chemically a permanent picture or radiograph is produced and the image may be viewed.

Production and properties of X-rays

The electromagnetic spectrum

X-rays are members of the **electromagnetic spectrum**, a group of types of radiation which have some similar properties but which differ from each other in their **wavelength** and **frequency** (Fig. 24.1).

The energy in a given type of radiation is directly proportional to the frequency of the radiation and inversely proportional to its wavelength. X-rays and gamma rays are similar types of electromagnetic radiation which have high frequency, short wavelength and therefore high energy. X-rays are produced by X-ray machines and gamma rays by the decay of radioactive materials.

Members of the electromagnetic spectrum have the following common features:

• They do not require a medium for transmission and can pass through a vacuum.
• They travel in straight lines.
• They travel at the same speed – 3×10^8 m/s in a vacuum.
• They interact with matter by being absorbed or scattered.

X-rays have some additional properties which means that they can be used to produce images of the internal structures of people and animals; they are also used in engineering for detecting flaws in pipes and construction materials. Their extra properties are:

• **Penetration**. Because of their high energy they can penetrate substances which are opaque to visible ('white') light. The X-ray photons are absorbed to varying degrees depending on the nature of the substance penetrated and the power of the photons themselves and some may pass right through the patient, emerging at the other side. The shorter its wavelength, the higher the energy of the X-ray photon and the greater its penetrating ability.

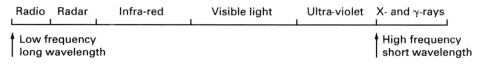

Fig. 24.1 The electromagnetic spectrum.

- **Effect on photographic film**. X-rays have the ability to produce a hidden or latent image on photographic film which can be rendered visible by processing (film in cameras is damaged by exposure to X-radiation).
- **Fluorescence**. X-rays cause crystals of certain substances to fluoresce (emit visible light) and this property is utilised in the composition of intensifying screens which are used in the recording of the image.

X-rays also produce biological changes in living tissues by altering the structure of atoms or molecules or by causing chemical reactions. Some of these effects can be used beneficially in the radiotherapy of tumours, but they are harmful to normal tissues and constitute a safety hazard. Aspects of radiation safety are considered later in the chapter.

Production of X-rays

X-ray photons or quanta are tiny packets of energy which are released whenever rapidly moving electrons are slowed down or stopped. Electrons are present in the atoms of all elements and in order to grasp the fundamentals of simple radiation physics it is necessary to understand the structure of an atom (Fig. 24.2). Atoms contain the following particles:

- **Protons**: positively charged particles contained in the centre or nucleus of the atom.
- **Neutrons**: particles of similar size to protons which are also found in the nucleus but which carry no electrical charge.
- **Electrons**: smaller, negatively charged particles which orbit around the nucleus in different planes or 'shells'.

The number of electrons normally equals the number of protons and so the atom as a whole is electrically neutral. The number of protons and electrons is unique to the atoms of each element and is called the **atomic number**. If an atom loses one or more electrons it becomes positively charged and may be written as X^+ (where X is the symbol for that element). If an atom gains electrons it becomes negatively charged (X^-). Atoms with charges are called **ions** or are said to be ionised. **Compounds** are combinations of two or more elements and usually consist of positive ions of one element in combination with negative ions of another, e.g. silver bromide (in X-ray film emulsion) consists of silver Ag^+ and bromide Br^- ions.

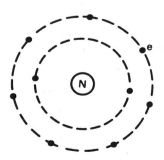

Fig. 24.2 The structure of an atom. N = nucleus (protons and neutrons); e = electron (dotted lines represent electron shells).

In an X-ray tube head, X-ray photons are produced by collisions between fast-moving electrons and the atoms of a 'target' element. Electrons which are completely halted by the target atoms give up all of their energy to form an X-ray photon, whereas those which are merely decelerated give up smaller and variable amounts of energy, producing lower-energy X-ray photons. The X-ray beam produced therefore contains photons of a range of energies and is said to be **polychromatic**. If the number of incident electrons is increased, more X-ray photons are produced, and the intensity of the X-ray beam increases. If the incident electrons are faster-moving then they have more energy to lose and so the X-ray photons produced are more energetic; the X-ray beam's quality is therefore increased and it has greater penetrating power.

The intensity and quality of an X-ray beam can be altered by adjusting the settings on the machine, and the practical effect of this will be discussed in greater detail later.

The X-ray tube head

The X-ray tube head is the part of the machine where the X-rays are generated. A diagram of the simplest type of X-ray tube, a **stationary** or **fixed anode** tube, is shown in Fig. 24.3.

The X-ray tube head contains two electrodes, the negatively charged **cathode** and the positively charged **anode**. Electrons are produced at the cathode, which is a coiled wire filament. When a small electrical current is passed through the filament it becomes hot and releases a cloud of electrons by a process called **thermionic emission**. Tungsten is used as the filament material because:

- It has a high atomic number, 74, and therefore has many electrons.
- It has a very high melting point of 3380°C and so can safely be heated.
- It has helpful mechanical properties which mean that fine, coiled filaments can be made.

The current required to heat the filament is small and so the mains current to the filament is reduced by a **step-down** or **filament transformer** which is wired into the X-ray machine (a transformer is a device for increasing or decreasing an electric current).

Next, the cloud of electrons needs to be made to travel at high speed across the short distance to the target. This is done by applying a high electrical potential difference between the filament and the target so that the filament becomes negative (and therefore repels the electrons) and the target becomes positive (and attracts them). The filament therefore becomes a cathode and the target an anode. The electrons are formed into a narrow beam by the fact that the filament sits in a nickel or molybdenum **focusing cup**, which is also at a negative potential and so repels the electrons. The electron beam constitutes a weak electric current across the tube, which is measured in **milliamperes (mA)**.

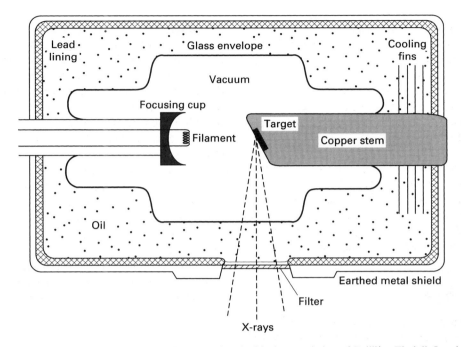

Fig. 24.3 Diagram of a stationary or fixed-anode X-ray tube (reproduced with the permission of Baillière Tindall, London).

The potential difference applied between the filament and the target needs to be very high and many times the voltage of the mains supply, which is 240 volts. In fact it is measured in thousands of volts, or **kilovolts (kV)**, and is created from the mains in a second electrical circuit using a **step-up** or **high-tension transformer**, which is also part of the electrical circuitry of the X-ray machine.

The stream of electrons strikes the target or anode at very high speed. Tungsten or rhenium–tungsten alloy is used as the target material because its high atomic number renders it a relatively efficient producer of X-rays. Unfortunately the process is still very inefficient and more than 99% of the energy lost by the electrons is converted to heat, so the anode must be able to withstand very high temperatures without melting or cracking. Tungsten's high melting point is therefore useful in the target as well as in the filament.

In a simple type of X-ray tube as shown in Fig. 24.3 the target is a small rectangle of tungsten about 3 mm thick set in a copper block. Copper is a good conductor of heat and so the heat is removed from the target by conduction along the copper stem to cooling fins radiating into the surrounding oil bath, which can absorb much heat.

The target is set at an angle of about 20° to the vertical (Fig. 24.4). This is so that the area of the target which the electrons strike (and therefore the area over which heat is produced) is as large as possible. This area is called the **actual focal spot**. At the same time the angulation of the target means that the X-ray beam appears to originate from a much smaller area and this is called the **effective focal spot**. The importance of having a small effective focal spot – ideally a point source – is discussed later in the chapter with regard to image definition.

Some X-ray machines allow a choice of focal spot size using two different-sized filaments at the cathode:

- The smaller filament produces an electron beam with a smaller cross-sectional area and hence smaller effective and actual focal spots. This is known as **fine focus**. The emergent X-ray beam arises from a tiny area and will produce very fine radiographic definition. However, the heat generated is concentrated over a very small area of the target and so the exposure factors that can be used are limited.
- The larger filament produces a wider electron beam with larger effective and actual focal spot sizes – the **coarse** or **broad focus**. Higher exposures can be used but the image definition will be slightly less sharp due to the **penumbra effect**, a blurring of margins related to the geometry of the beam (Fig. 24.5).

In practice, fine focus is selected for small parts when fine definition is required (e.g. the limbs), and coarse focus when thicker areas are to be radiographed (e.g. the chest and

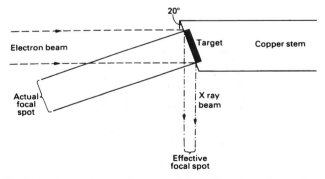

Fig. 24.4 Diagram to show how angulation of target produces a large actual focal spot and a small effective focal spot.

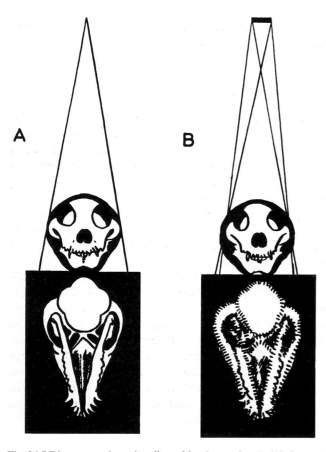

Fig. 24.5 Diagram to show the effect of focal-spot size. In (A) the spot is a pin-point and the projected image is sharp. In (B) the rays from a focal-spot of large dimensions cause a penumbra effect which blurs the projected image. (Reproduced with the permission of Baillière Tindall, London.)

abdomen); these require higher exposure factors and so the heat generated at the target is higher.

The cathode, anode and part of the copper stem are enclosed in a **glass envelope**. Within the envelope is a vacuum, which prevents the moving electrons from colliding with air molecules and losing speed. The glass envelope is bathed in oil which acts both as a heat sink and as an electrical insulator, and the whole is encased in an earthed, lead-lined **metal casing**. X-rays are produced in all directions by the target but only one narrow beam of X-rays is required, and this emerges through a window in the casing, placed beneath the angled target. This beam is called the **primary or useful beam**. X-rays produced in other directions are absorbed by the casing.

Within the X-ray beam are some low-energy or 'soft' X-ray photons which are not powerful enough to pass through the patient but which may be absorbed or scattered by the patient and therefore represent a safety hazard. They are removed from the beam by an **aluminium filter** placed across the tube window; these filters are legally required as a safety precaution and must not be removed.

In stationary anode X-ray tubes the X-ray output is limited by the amount of heat generated at the target. Overheating the target would produce melting and surface irregularity which would reduce the efficiency of the tube; however, in modern machines automatic 'overload' devices prevent such high exposures from being used. Stationary anode X-ray tubes are found in low-powered, portable X-ray machines. These have limited ability to produce short exposure times for thoracic radiography or high output for large patients. More powerful machines require a more efficient way of removing the heat and this is accomplished using a **rotating anode** (Fig. 24.6). In such tubes the target

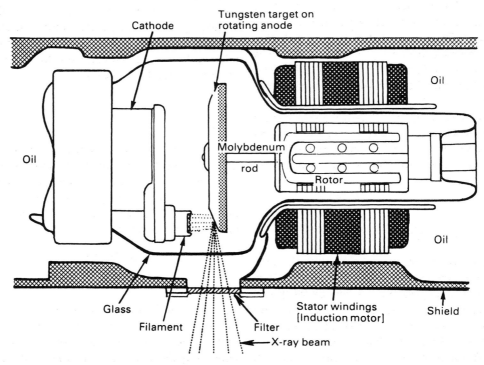

Fig. 24.6 Diagram of a rotating-anode X-ray tube. (Reproduced with the permission of Baillière Tindall, London.)

area is the bevelled rim of a metal disc of about 10 cm diameter whose rim is set at about 20°, as in a stationary anode X-ray tube. The target area is again tungsten or rhenium–tungsten. During the exposure the disc rotates rapidly so that the target area upon which the electrons impinge is constantly changing. The actual focal spot is therefore the whole circumference of the disc and so is many times greater than in a stationary anode X-ray tube. The heat generated is spread over a much bigger area allowing larger exposures to be made, whilst the effective focal spot remains the same. The disc is mounted on a molybdenum rod and is rotated at speeds of up to 10 000 r.p.m. by an induction motor at the other end of the rod. Molybdenum is used because it is a poor conductor of heat and therefore prevents the motor from overheating. Heat generated in the anode is lost by radiation through the vacuum and the glass envelope into the oil bath.

The size of the emerging X-ray beam must be controlled for safety reasons otherwise it will spread out over a very large area. This is achieved using a **collimation device**, preferably a light beam diaphragm. Methods of collimation are described later.

The X-ray control panel

X-ray machine control panels vary in their complexity, but some or all of the following controls will be present.

On/off switch

As well as switching the machine on at the mains socket there will also be an on/off switch or key on the control panel. Sometimes the line voltage compensator (see below) is incorporated into the on/off switch, which therefore performs both functions. When the machine is switched on a warning light on the control panel will indicate that it is ready to produce X-rays or, in the case of panels with digital displays, the numbers will be illuminated. In some old machines the filament is heated continually whilst the machine is on and may burn out. Such machines should always be turned off when the exposure is terminated. X-ray machines must always be switched off when not in use, so that accidental exposure cannot occur when unprotected people are in the room.

Line voltage compensator

Fluctuations in the normal mains electricity output may occur, resulting in an inconsistent output of X-rays. The images produced may appear under- or over-exposed despite using normal exposure factors. In some machines these fluctuations are automatically corrected by an **autotransformer** wired into the circuit, but in others it is controlled manually. A voltmeter dial on the control panel will indicate the incoming voltage which can be adjusted until it

is satisfactory. In such machines the line voltage should be checked before each session of radiography.

Kilovoltage (kV) control

The kilovoltage control selects the **kilovoltage** (potential difference) which is applied across the tube during the instant of exposure. It determines the speed and energy with which the electrons bombard the target and hence the quality or penetrating power of the X-ray beam produced. Depending on the power and sophistication of the X-ray machine, the kilovoltage is controlled in various ways. Ideally it is controlled quite independently of the milliamperage, often in increments of 1 kV, and the kilovoltage meter is either a dial or a digital display.

In smaller machines the kilovoltage is linked to the milliamperage so that if a higher milliamperage is selected only lower kilovoltages can be used. Often there is a single control knob for both kilovoltage and milliamperage and as the kilovoltage is increased the milliamperage available drops. This is not ideal since, for larger patients, a high kilovoltage and high milliamperage may be required at the same time, long exposure times are needed. In very basic machines the kilovoltage and milliamperage are fixed, and only the time can be altered.

Milliamperage (mA) control

The **milliamperage** is a measure of the quantity of electrons crossing the tube during the exposure (the 'tube current') and is directly related to the quantity of X-rays produced. Moving electrons constitute an electrical current which is measured in amperes, but the tube current is very small and is measured in 1/1000 amperes or milliamperes (mA). Adjusting the milliamperage control alters the degree of heating of the filament and hence the number of electrons released by thermionic emission, the tube current and the intensity of the X-ray beam.

Timer

The quantity of X-rays produced depends not only on the milliamperage but also on the length of the exposure, and so a composite term, the milliampere-second or mAs, is often used. A given mAs may be obtained using a high milliamperage with a short time or vice versa; the two numbers are multiplied together, e.g.

$$30 \, \text{mAs} = 300 \, \text{mA for 0.1 s}$$
$$\text{or 30 mA for 1.0 s}$$

The effect on the film is the same except that the longer the exposure the more likely it is that movement blur will occur. One should always therefore use the largest milliamperage allowed by the machine for that kilovoltage setting, in order to minimise the exposure time. It will now be appreciated why the type of machine in which kilovoltage and milli-amperage are inversely linked is less than ideal.

The timer is usually electronic and is usually another dial on the control panel, giving a choice of a wide range of exposure times up to several seconds long. However, release of the exposure button terminates the exposure even when long times have been selected. In larger machines an automatic display of the resulting mAs is also present. At one time, X-ray machines relied on clockwork timers in handsets which also incorporated the exposure button. A dial was 'wound up' to an appropriate time setting and ran back to zero whilst the exposure button was depressed. The time had to be reset between exposures. These timers were not only inaccurate and noisy but also they did not allow the exposure to be aborted if necessary. Some modern machines with a digital display have a single control for mAs which automatically selects the shortest exposure time for the selected mAs.

Exposure button

The exposure button must be at the end of a cable which can stretch to more than 2 m to enable the radiographer to distance himself from the primary beam during the exposure. Alternatively, the button may be on the control panel itself provided that the panel is at least 2 m from the tube head or is separated from it by a lead screen. Most exposure buttons are two-stage devices; depression of the button to a halfway stage ('prepping') heats the filament and rotates the anode if a rotating anode is present; after a brief pause, depression of the button further causes application of the kilovoltage to the tube and an instantaneous exposure to be made. In some machines only a single-stage exposure button is present; in this case there is slight delay between depression of the button and exposure during which time the patient may move. In old machines with single-stage exposure buttons the filament may be constantly heated while the machine is switched on and in these there is a risk of burning out the filament.

Types of X-ray machine

X-ray machines can conveniently be divided into three broad types.

Portable machines (Fig. 24.7)

These are the commonest type of machine found in general practice. As their name suggests they are relatively easy to move from site to site for large animal radiography and many come with a special carrying case. The largest ones weigh about 20 kg. The electrical transformers are located in the tube head which is usually supported on a wheeled metal stand, although some may be wall-mounted. The tube head must never be held for radiography, as this is very hazardous to the person holding. The controls may be either on a

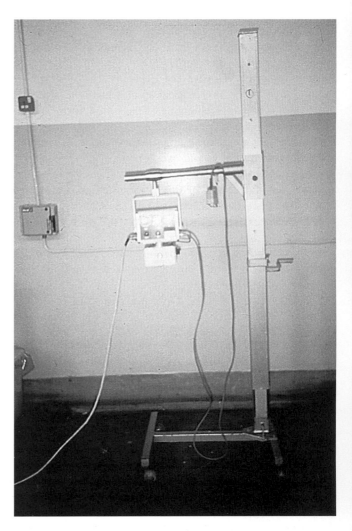

Fig. 24.7 Portable X-ray machine.

separate panel or else on the head itself. Portable machines are low powered, producing only about 20–60 mA and often less. In most the kilovoltage and milliamperage are inversely linked. Although portable machines are widely used their relatively low output means that longer exposure times are needed, and chest and abdomen radiographs of larger dogs are often degraded by the effects of movement blur.

Mobile machines (Fig. 24.8)

These are larger and more powerful than portable machines but can still be moved from room to room on wheels, some having battery-operated motors. The transformers are bulkier and encased in a large box which is an integral part of the tube stand. Mobile machines usually have outputs of up to 300 mA and are likely to produce good radiographs of most small animal patients. Although they are more expensive to buy new, they can sometimes be obtained second-hand from hospitals, where they will have had relatively little use yet been well cared for, having been used mainly for bedridden patients. They are not usually suitable for equine radiography since the tube head will not reach to the floor, although

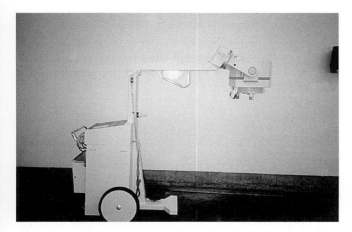

Fig. 24.8 Mobile X-ray machine.

KEY POINTS
Production and properties of X-rays
• X-ray photons are small packets of energy which are produced in an X-ray tube head from the energy of rapidly-moving electrons.
• They can penetrate tissue, affect photographic film and cause fluorescence of phosphor crystals.
• Rotating-anode X-ray machines can produce higher exposures than stationary anode machines.
• X-ray machines may be portable, mobile or fixed.

special tube arm adaptors can be fitted. If used for equine radiography the horse should be restrained in stocks since the X-ray machine cannot be moved away quickly if the patient moves.

Fixed machines (Fig. 24.9)

The most powerful X-ray machines are built into the X-ray room, being screwed to the floor or being mounted on rails or overhead gantries. The tube head is usually quite mobile on its mounting and can be moved in several directions, which is especially valuable for equine radiography. The transformers are situated in cabinets some distance from the machine itself, and connected to it by high-tension cables. The largest fixed machines can produce up to 1250 mA and produce excellent radiographs of all patients, but because of the high cost of purchase, installation and maintenance they are rarely found outside veterinary institutions and large equine practices. However, several companies are now producing smaller, fixed X-ray machines especially for the veterinary market which are much more affordable. Fixed X-ray machines are often linked electronically to a floating table top and moving grid.

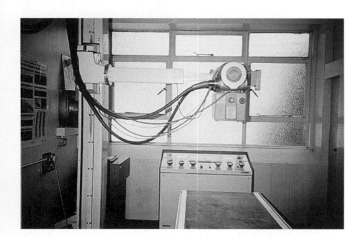

Fig. 24.9 Fixed X-ray machine.

Formation of the X-ray image

The X-ray picture is essentially a 'shadowgraph', or a picture in black, white and varying shades of grey, caused by differences in the amount of absorption of the beam by different tissues and hence in differences in the amount of radiation reaching the X-ray film and causing blackening (Fig. 24.10).

The degree of absorption by a given tissue depends on three factors:

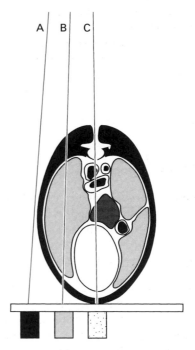

Fig. 24.10 Diagrammatic cross-section of a thorax to show formation of an X-ray shadowgraph. X-ray photons passing along path C are largely absorbed, and result in white areas on the radiograph. X-ray photons passing along path B are partly absorbed and produce intermediate shades of grey on the radiograph. (Reproduced with the permission of Baillière Tindall, London.)

(1) **The atomic number (*Z*) of the tissue**, or the average of the different atomic numbers present (the 'effective' atomic number). Bone has a higher effective atomic number than soft tissue and so absorbs more X-ray photons producing whiter areas on the radiograph. Similarly, soft tissue has a higher effective atomic number than fat.

(2) **The specific gravity of the tissue**. This is the density or mass per unit volume. Bone has a high specific gravity, soft tissue a medium specific gravity and gas a very low specific gravity, hence gas-filled areas absorb few X-rays and appear nearly black on the radiograph.

The combination of effective atomic number and specific gravity produces five characteristic shades to be seen on a radiograph:

* Gas – very dark.
* Fat – dark grey.
* Soft tissue or fluid – mid grey.
* Bone – nearly white.
* Metal – white, as all X-rays absorbed.

Note that solid soft tissue and fluid produce the same radiographic appearance and therefore fluid within a soft tissue viscus (e.g. urine in the bladder or blood in the heart) cannot be differentiated from the tissue that surrounds it. Note also that fat is less radio-opaque (darker) than soft tissue and fluid, so fat in the abdomen is helpful in surrounding and outlining the various organs.

(3) **Thickness of the tissue**. Overlap in the ranges of grey shades on the radiograph occurs due to the fact that thicker areas of tissue absorb more X-ray photons than thinner areas, hence a very thick area of soft tissue may actually appear more radio-opaque (whiter) than a thin area of bone.

Selection of exposure factors

Kilovoltage (kV)

The kilovoltage controls the **quality**, or **penetrating power**, of the X-ray beam. A higher kilovoltage is required for tissues which have a higher atomic number or specific gravity, or which are very thick. Both the nature and depth of the tissue being X-rayed must therefore be taken into consideration when selecting the appropriate kilovoltage setting. A range of about 40 to 100 kV is used in veterinary radiography. The kV affects both the scale of *contrast* on the image (the number of grey shades) and the *radiographic density* (the degree of blackening of the film).

Milliamperage (mA)

The milliamperage setting determines the tube current and therefore the quantity of X-rays per second in the emergent

beam, also known as its **intensity**. Altering the milliamperage will not affect the penetrating power of the beam, i.e. the contrast of the image, but **will** change the degree of blackening of the film under the areas which are penetrated, the radiographic density.

Time

The product of milliamperage and length of the exposure produces the mAs (milliampere-seconds) factor or total quantity of X-rays used for that particular exposure. Normally the maximum mA and shortest time possible are used for the chest, in order to reduce the effects of movement blur (times of less than 0.05s are preferred).

Increasing the kilovoltage will cause greater penetration of all tissues and hence a blacker film. Too high a kilovoltage will overpenetrate tissues, resulting in a dark film with few different shades; this is called a **flat** film or is said to be 'lacking in contrast'. Too low a kilovoltage will underpenetrate tissue (especially bone) which will appear white, on a black or dark grey background. This type of appearance is sometimes called **soot and whitewash**; its contrast is too high. Figure 24.11 shows the effect of alterations in the kilovoltage.

Increasing the mAs will produce more X-ray photons to blacken the film, though they have no more penetrating ability. The contrast between adjacent tissues (the difference in shades of grey) will not change, but the overall picture will be darker. Figure 24.12 shows the effect of alterations in the mAs.

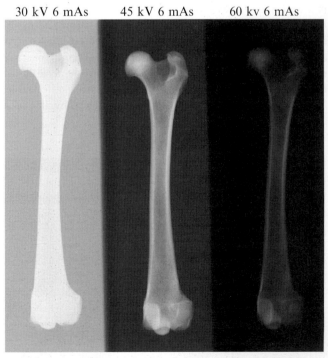

30 kV 6 mAs   45 kV 6 mAs   60 kv 6 mAs

Fig. 24.11 The effect on subject penetration of altering the kilovoltage and keeping the mAs constant. With low kV there is little penetration of the subject and with high kV there is too much.

45 kV 3 mAs   45 kV 6 mAs   45 kV 12 mAs

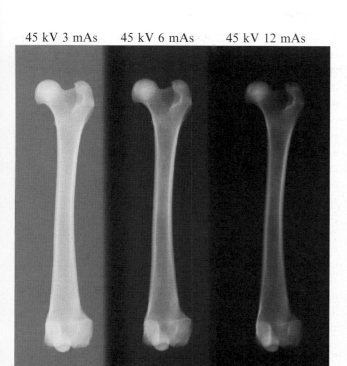

Fig. 24.12 The effect on film blackening of altering the mAs and keeping the kilovoltage constant. The patient penetration (internal detail) is similar in each case but the image is darker with higher mAs.

45 kV 8 mAs   55 kV 4 mAs   65 kV 2 mAs

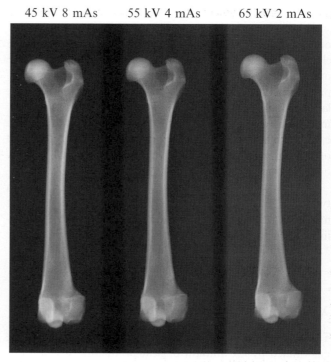

Fig. 24.13 The interplay between kilovoltage and mAs; if the kilovoltage is increased by 10 and the mAs is halved, the effect on the film is almost identical.

Although kilovoltage and mAs can be seen to govern different parameters of the X-ray beam, in the diagnostic range of exposures they are linked, in that pictures which appear similar can be produced by raising the kilovoltage and at the same time lowering the mAs, or vice versa. A useful and simple rule is that for every 10 kV increase, the mAs can be halved (Fig. 24.13). Conversely, if the mAs is doubled, the kilovoltage must be reduced by 10. In practice, the time factor is usually paramount and so it is normal to work with as high a kilovoltage as possible, allowing the mAs to be kept low.

Focal–film distance (FFD)

The FFD is the total distance between the focal spot and the X-ray film. It is important because although the quality of the X-ray beam remains constant as it travels from the tube head, the intensity falls with increasing distance as the beam spreads out over a larger area. Figure 24.14 shows that if the FFD is doubled, the intensity of the beam over a given area is reduced to one-quarter and the film will appear under-exposed unless the mAs is raised. Conversely, if the FFD is reduced the film will appear overexposed. The rule governing this effect is called the **inverse square law**, which states that **the intensity of the primary beam projected on to an X-ray film is reduced to one-quarter by doubling the distance from the X-ray film.** Thus a long FFD requires a higher mAs than a short FFD and the exact figure can be calculated mathematically from the equation:

$$\text{new mAs} = \text{old mAs} \times \frac{\text{new distance}^2}{\text{old distance}^2}$$

Obviously, longer FFDs require a higher mAs to be used, although image definition will be improved due to a reduction in the penumbra effect (see p. 703). It is normal practice to work always at the same FFD for a given X-ray machine; a suitable distance for a portable X-ray machine is 75 cm, whilst 100 cm is normally used for more powerful X-ray machines which produce a higher milliamperage.

Exposure charts

In order to avoid wastage of film and time in repeating radiographs, it is necessary to build up an exposure chart for each machine. An exposure chart is a list of the kV and

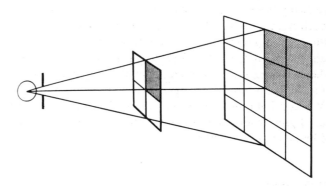

Fig. 24.14 The inverse square law. The intensity of the beam falling on a given area is reduced to one-quarter by doubling the distance from the point of source. (Reproduced with the permission of Baillière Tindall, London.)

mAs required for radiography of various areas of different-sized patients. For the exposure chart to be accurate all other parameters must be kept constant and given on the chart (i.e. line voltage, FFD, film–screen combination, use of a grid and quality of processing). The chart may be compiled for patients of different types (e.g. cats, small, medium, large and giant dogs) or may be made more accurate still by measuring the thickness of the part to be X-rayed using callipers. The exposure chart can be built up over a period of time by recording all exposures made in the X-ray day book, with comments.

Exposure charts are not usually interchangeable between types of machine and may not even be accurate for other machines of the same make and model because of the varying factors listed above.

X-Ray tube rating

The maximum kV and mAs produced by an X-ray tube are determined by the amount of heat production which it can withstand. If this heat production is exceeded the tube is said to be 'overloaded' and damage may occur. The majority of X-ray machines have built-in fail-safe mechanisms which prevent these limits from being exceeded and if too high an exposure combination is selected a warning light will come on and the machine will fail to expose. However, in old machines this may not be the case and so care should be taken to work within the machine's capabilities by consulting the manufacturer's details of maximum safe combinations of kV, mA and time. These details are known as **ratings charts**.

KEY POINTS
Formation of the X-ray image and selection of exposure factors
- An X-ray image is produced by different degrees of beam absorption by the overlying patient's tissues.
- The effective atomic number, the specific gravity and the thickness of a tissue affect its radio-opacity on the image.
- The kV controls the quality or penetrating power of the X-ray beam produced and the mAs controls the quantity or beam intensity.
- Changes in the FFD alter the intensity of the X-ray beam and must be compensated for by changing the mAs according to the inverse square law.
- Exposure charts should be compiled giving details of exposure factors and equipment to be used for various radiographic views.

Scattered radiation

Although most of the X-ray photons entering the patient during the exposure are either completely absorbed or pass straight through, a certain proportion undergo a process known as scattering. Scattering occurs when incident photons interact with the tissues, losing some of their energy and 'bouncing' off in random directions as photons of lower energy (Fig. 24.15). At lower kilovoltages and when thin areas of tissue are being radiographed, the production of **scattered** or **secondary radiation** is small and most is reabsorbed within the patient. Scatter is therefore not a problem when cats, small dogs and the skull and limbs of larger dogs are being radiographed. However, when higher kilovoltages are required in order to penetrate thicker or denser tissues, the amount and energy of the scattered radiation increases and substantial amounts may exit from the patient's body. The problems associated with this scattered radiation are twofold:

- Scatter is a potential hazard to the radiographer, as it travels in all directions and may also ricochet back off the table top or the floor or walls of the room. This remains a problem in the radiographic examination of equine limbs, although it should be less serious in small-animal radiography where patients are usually artificially restrained and the radiographer stands further away.
- Scattered radiation will cause a uniform blackening of the X-ray film unrelated to the radiographic image, and will detract from the film's contrast and definition. The blurring which results is called **fogging.**

Scatter production increases with (a) higher kV used, (b) thicker or denser tissues, and (c) larger field sizes of the primary beam. The amount of scattered radiation produced may be reduced in several ways:

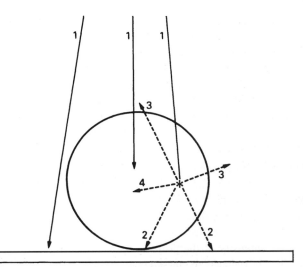

Fig. 24.15 Formation of scattered radiation. (1) Photons of the primary beam. (2) Scatter in a forward direction causing film fogging. (3) Scatter in a backwards direction which is a safety hazard. (4) Some scatter is absorbed by the patient.

- Reduction of the kilovoltage factor will reduce scattered radiation and the lowest practicable kilovoltage should be selected; however, this is not always feasible as in lower-powered X-ray machines the priority is usually to keep exposure time down using a low mAs factor and hence a large kilovoltage.
- Collimation of the primary beam (i.e. restriction in the size of the primary beam using a device such as a light beam diaphragm) has a very large effect on the production of scatter. The primary beam should therefore cover only the area of interest, and tight collimation onto very small lesions (such as areas of bone pathology) will greatly improve the quality of the finished radiograph.
- Reduction of back-scatter from the table top by covering it with a 1 mm thick lead sheet.
- Compression of a large abdomen using a broad radiolucent compression band will reduce the thickness of tissue being radiographed and will also reduce the amount of scattered radiation produced. Compression band devices may be attached to X-ray tables but should be used with caution in animals with abdominal pathology such as uterine or bladder distension. Compression techniques are no longer widely used in veterinary practice.

The use of grids

Even when the above precautions are taken, scattered radiation is still often a significant problem. However, the amount of scatter reaching the film can be greatly reduced by using a device known as a grid, which is a flat plate placed between the patient and the cassette. A grid consists of a series of thin strips of lead alternating with strips of a material which allows X-rays through, such as plastic or aluminium. The whole is encased in a protective aluminium cover. X-ray photons which have passed undeflected through a patient will pass through the radiolucent plastic or aluminium strips ('interspaces') but obliquely moving scattered radiation will largely be absorbed by the lead strips (Fig. 24.16). Thus there will be a reduction in the degree of film fogging and an improvement in the image quality, although with coarse grids the grid lines will be visible. Significant amounts of scattered radiation are produced from depths of solid tissue greater than 10 cm (or a 15 cm depth of chest, which contains much air), and so the use of a grid is usually recommended for areas thicker than this. Various types of grid are available, and there are two broad groups: **stationary** and **moving grids**.

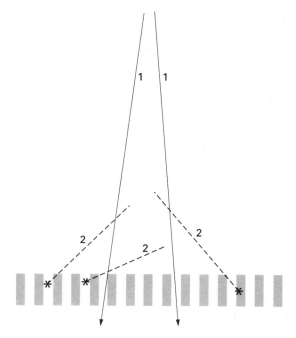

Fig. 24.16 The effect of a grid. (1) Most primary beam X-ray photons pass through the grid. (2) Obliquely moving scattered radiation is absorbed by the strips of lead.

Stationary grids

Stationary grids are either separate pieces of equipment or are built into the front of special cassettes. Various sizes are available, but it is advisable to buy a grid large enough to cover the biggest cassette used in the practice. Grids are expensive and fragile and should be treated with care as the strips may be broken if the grid is dropped.

- *Parallel grids* – a parallel grid is the simplest and cheapest type of grid. The strips are vertical, and parallel to each other (Fig. 24.17a). This means that, since the X-ray beam is diverging from its very small source, the X-ray photons at the edge of the primary beam may also be absorbed by the lead strips, as well as scatter. There may therefore be some reduction in the quality of the film around the edges; this is called **grid cut-off.**
- *Focused grids* – a focused grid should prevent grid cut-off as the central strips are vertical but those on either side slope gradually, to take into account the divergence of the primary beam (Fig. 24.17b). A focused grid must be used at its correct focal–film distance (which is usually written on the front of the grid), and should not be used upside down. The X-ray beam must be centred correctly over the grid and be at right angles to it. Focused grids are considerably more expensive than parallel grids.

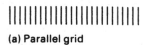

(a) Parallel grid

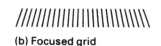

(b) Focused grid

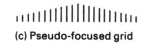

(c) Pseudo-focused grid

Fig. 24.17 Types of stationary grid (diagrammatic cross-sections).

- *Pseudo-focused grids* – a pseudo-focused grid is intermediate between a parallel and a focused grid in efficiency and price. The strips are vertical, but get progressively shorter towards the edges, so reducing the amount of primary beam absorbed (Fig. 24.17c). Pseudo-focused grids should also be used at the correct focal–film distance.
- *Crossed grids* – most grids contain strips aligned only in one direction and therefore scattered radiation travelling in line with the strips will not be absorbed. Crossed grids contain strips running in both directions and so remove much more scattered radiation. The strips may either be parallel or focused. Crossed grids are expensive and are likely only to be used in establishments routinely radiographing equine spines, chests and pelvises.

Moving grids

The use of a stationary grid results in the presence of visible parallel lines on the radiograph. These lines may be eliminated by the use of a grid which oscillates slightly during the exposure. This requires an electronic connection between the X-ray machine and the moving grid or 'Potter–Bucky diaphragm', which is built into the X-ray table. Moving grids are used in larger veterinary institutions and moving grid tables may sometimes be available for purchase second-hand from human hospitals.

Grid parameters

- *Grid factor* – the use of a grid means that as well as scattered radiation the grid will absorb some of the useful, primary beam. The mAs factor must therefore be increased when using a grid (to increase the number of X-ray photons in the beam) by an amount known as the grid factor. This is usually 2.5–3 times, but will be specified for each grid. In most cases it will require that a longer exposure time is used as the X-ray machine will probably be already set at its maximum mA output. The increase in time may increase the risk of movement blur on the film, and the radiographer will have to decide whether or not this is outweighed by the advantages of using a grid.
- *Lines/cm* – the greater the number of lines/cm the finer are the grid lines on the film and the less the disruption to the image; coarse grid lines may be very distracting. The usual number is about 24 lines/cm for grids used in general practice. Grids with finer lines are more expensive.
- *Grid ratio* – the grid ratio is the ratio of the height of the strips to the width of the radiolucent interspace. The larger the grid ratio the more efficient it is at absorbing scatter, but the more expensive the grid and the larger the grid factor. Practice grids usually have a ratio of 5:1 to 10:1. Grids used with more powerful machines may have a ratio of 16:1.

> **KEY POINTS**
> Scattered radiation
> - Scatter is low-energy secondary radiation produced in random directions when photons from the primary beam interact with the patient's tissues and with other objects in their path.
> - Scatter is a safety hazard to operators and will cause fogging of radiographs.
> - It is more significant at higher kVs and when large or denser areas are radiographed.
> - Scatter can be controlled in various ways, most practically by the use of grids.
> - Grids should be used for areas of solid tissue of greater than 10 cm thickness and for chests exceeding 15 cm.

Recording the X-ray image

Once the X-ray beam has passed through the subject and undergone differential absorption by the tissues, it must be recorded in order to produce a visible and permanent image. This is done using X-ray film, which has some properties in common with photographic film, including its sensitivity to white (visible) light. It must therefore be enclosed in a light-proof container (either a metal or plastic cassette or a thick paper envelope) and handled only in conditions of special subdued 'safe-lighting' until after processing.

Structure of X-ray film

The part of the film which is responsible for producing the image is the **emulsion**, which usually coats the film base on both sides in a thin, uniform layer. The emulsion gives unexposed film an apple green, fawn or mauve colour when examined in daylight (obviously an unexposed film examined in this way will then be ruined for X-ray purposes!). The emulsion consists of gelatin in which are suspended tiny grains of silver bromide. The silver bromide molecules are sensitive to X-ray photons and to visible light, both of which change their chemical structure slightly. During a radiographic exposure, X-ray photons passing through the patient will cause this invisible chemical change in the underlying film emulsion, but the picture is not visible to the naked eye and the film will still be spoilt by blackening ('fogging') if exposed to white light. The picture is therefore a hidden or 'latent' image and must be rendered visible to the eye by chemical processing or development. When the film is developed the chemical change in the emulsion continues until those silver bromide grains which were exposed lose their bromine and become grains of pure silver, appearing black when the film is viewed.

The emulsion layers are attached to the transparent polyester film base by a sticky 'subbing' layer and the outer surfaces are protected by a supercoat (Fig. 24.18).

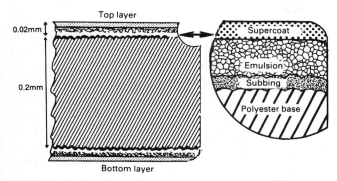

Fig. 24.18 Section of X-ray film, showing emulsion coats bound to the base by subbing layers and protected by supercoats. (Reproduced with the permission of Baillière Tindall, London.)

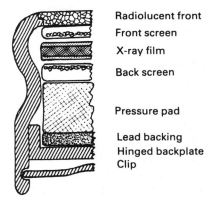

Fig. 24.19 Cross-section through an X-ray cassette. (Reproduced with the permission of Baillière Tindall, London.)

Intensifying screens and cassettes

Unfortunately, X-ray film used alone requires a very large exposure to produce an image and the use of film in this way is unacceptable in most circumstances. However, it was discovered many years ago that the exposure time could be greatly reduced for the same degree of blackening if some of the X-ray photons emerging from the patient were converted into visible light photons using crystals of phosphorescent material coating flat sheets held against the X-ray film. These devices are known as **intensifying screens** (because they **intensify** the effect of the X-rays on the film) and for many years the commonest phosphor used in the construction of intensifying screens was **calcium tungstate** which emits blue light when stimulated by X-rays. More recently a new group of phosphors has been used in intensifying screens; these are the **rare-earth** phosphors which produce blue, green or ultraviolet light. It is important that the X-ray film being used is sensitive primarily to the right colour of light and for this reason some film–screen combinations are incompatible. One advantage of rare-earth screens is that they are more efficient at converting X-radiation into light than are calcium tungstate screens and so exposure factors can be markedly reduced producing less scattered radiation and images with less movement blur. Additionally, they produce finer image definition. Often, the trade name of the screen is embossed along its edge and can be seen on the edge of films exposed in that cassette.

The main benefits of screens are therefore:

(1) They allow much lower mAs settings to be used and so reduce movement blur, scatter production and patient exposure.
(2) They prolong the life of the X-ray tube.
(3) They increase radiographic contrast.

Screens consist of a stiff plastic base covered with a white reflecting surface and then with a layer of the phosphor. Over the top is a protective supercoat layer. The screens are usually used in pairs and are enclosed in a light-proof metal, plastic or carbon fibre box (a **cassette**; Fig. 24.19) with the film sandwiched between. Occasionally a single screen is used together with single-sided emulsion film used for human mammography; such a combination produces higher-definition images but requires slightly larger exposures. These systems are especially popular for equine orthopaedic radiography. For good detail the film and screens must be in close contact and so the cassette contains a thick felt pad between the back plate and the back screen. Poor screen–film contact causes blurring in that part of the film. The top of the cassette must be radiolucent (i.e. allow X-rays through), and the bottom may be lead-lined to absorb remaining X-rays and prevent back-scatter, although this is uncommon with modern cassettes. The cassette must be fully light-proof with secure fastenings and should be robust. Recently, small flexible plastic cassettes containing one or two screens have become available for small animal intra-oral radiography.

Care of intensifying screens and cassettes

Intensifying screens are expensive and fairly delicate and should be treated gently. Scratches or abrasions will damage the phosphor layer permanently, resulting in white (unexposed) marks on all subsequent radiographs produced in that cassette. Screens should not be splashed with chemicals or touched with dirty or greasy fingers. Any dust particles or hairs falling on the screens when the cassette is open in the darkroom will prevent light from reaching the film and will produce fine white specks or lines on the image (even minute particles will prevent the visible light from the intensifying screens from blackening the film in that area although they will not, of course, interfere with the passage of X-rays). Screens should therefore be cleaned periodically by wiping them gently with lint in a circular motion using a proprietary antistatic screen-cleaning liquid. The cassettes are then propped open in a dust-free environment in a vertical position to allow the screens to dry naturally. If they are reloaded whilst the screens are still damp, the film will stick to the screens and damage them.

Cassettes should be handled carefully and never dropped. They should be kept clean, as stains on the front may produce artefactual shadows on the radiograph and fluids seeping in will mark the screens. The catches must not be strained by closing the cassette when a film is trapped along the edges.

Types of X-ray film

Non-screen film

Non-screen film is film designed for use without intensifying screens, i.e. the image is solely due to X-rays. This requires a very large mAs (long exposure time) but produces extremely fine image definition. The film comes wrapped in thick, light-proof paper rather than being used in a cassette. Non-screen film is now only available as small dental film, which is used for dental radiography and other intra-oral views in cats and small dogs. The patient will be anaesthetised for this type of study so the very high exposure required is not a problem as the radiographer can retire to a safe distance and movement blur should not occur. The 13 × 18 cm film which was previously popular for intra-oral radiography of dogs and for radiography of small exotic species is no longer manufactured and has been replaced by flexible plastic cassettes of the same size containing one or two high-detail screens which can be inserted into the mouth of an animal for intra-oral radiography. However, image quality is inferior to that which is obtained with non-screen film. The flexible nature of these cassettes means that image blurring due to poor screen-film contact will occur if the device is bent in the mouth, but they can be reinforced by taping thick cardboard to them. Care should be taken that the patient's teeth do not damage the device and so an appropriate level of anaesthesia is needed.

Screen film

Screen film is designed for use in cassettes and is used for all other studies. The detail produced is less than with non-screen film, as the visible light produced by the phosphor crystals spreads out in all directions and will result in blackening of a larger number of silver halide grains than the initial X-ray photon would have done; an effect called 'screen unsharpness' (Fig. 24.20). **Monochromatic** or blue-sensitive film is for use with calcium tungstate or blue-light-emitting rare-earth screens; it is sensitive only to visible light in the blue part of the spectrum. For use with green-light-emitting rare-earth screens, the sensitivity of the film emulsion is extended to include green as well as blue light; this is called **orthochromatic** film. It can therefore be appreciated that whilst green-sensitive film can be used with blue-light-emitting screens as well (since it is sensitive to both colours), blue-sensitive film can only be used with blue-light-emitting screens. Currently only one manufacturer produces ultra-violet-light-emitting screens which should therefore be used only with the same brand of film.

Most types of film are duplitised or double-sided, that is there is a layer of emulsion on both sides of the base, which doubles the efficiency of the film and the contrast and density of the image. However, this does result in some loss of definition due to the superimposition of two slightly different images, and so single-sided emulsion film has become quite popular, especially for equine limb radiography. Human mammography film is used and gives very finely-detailed images with both good soft tissue and bone detail; it is used in a cassette containing a single green-light-emitting screen. The main disadvantages are that the system requires about five times more exposure and the film cannot be processed in glutaraldehyde-free developer.

Film and screen speed

The **speed** of a film, a screen or a screen–film combination describes the exposure required for a given degree of blackening of the film. The speed is due to the size and shape of the phosphor crystals in the screens and the silver bromide grains in the film emulsion, as well as to the thickness of the layers. Fast film–screen combinations require less exposure but produce poorer image definition (the image is more blurred) whereas slow film–screen combinations produce finer detail and are often called **high definition**. In practice, a medium-speed system is usually the best compromise for keeping exposure times down and still getting reasonable quality images. Rare-earth systems give better definition at the same speed. Different manufacturers describe their various films and screens with different terms, which makes it difficult to make comparisons, but most produce several speeds of film and screen; e.g. slow (high detail), medium and fast. If a choice of speeds of film–screen combinations is available in the practice, then a slow, high-definition combination may be used where exposure times are not a problem (e.g. for bone detail in limbs and skulls) but a faster combination should be used where it is important to keep exposure times short in order to reduce movement blur (e.g. for the chest and abdomen), especially if a grid is used.

Films, screens and cassettes come in a range of sizes from 13 × 18 to 35 × 43 cm. It is wise to have several different sizes available so as not to waste film by radiographing small areas on large plates, although multiple exposures can be made on the same film. Hangers of corresponding size must be available if the films are processed manually.

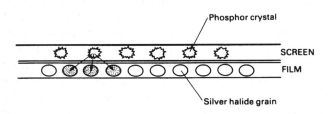

Fig. 24.20 Screen unsharpness. The arrows show how visible light emitted from each phosphor crystal may affect several silver halide grains, resulting in some loss of definition of the image.

Storage of X-ray film

As has already been mentioned, unexposed X-ray film is sensitive to light and so must be stored in a light-proof container. This may be either the original film box or a light-proof hopper. Film boxes and loaded cassettes should be kept away from the X-ray area in case they are fogged by scattered radiation; they may be kept in lead-lined cupboards if stored near a source of radiation.

Films are also sensitive to certain chemical fumes and of course to chemical splashes, so good darkroom technique is essential. They may be damaged by pressure or folding so should be stored upright and handled carefully without being bent or scratched. In hot climates, high temperature or humidity may be a problem and so film should be refrigerated. This is not usually necessary in the UK!

Finally, film has a finite shelf-life which varies with the type of film. It is therefore wise to date the film boxes on arrival and use them in sequence, within the expiry date shown on the box.

KEY POINTS
Recording the X-ray image
- X-rays produce a hidden or 'latent' image on film emulsion, which is rendered visible by chemical processing.
- The efficiency of image production is greatly increased by the use of intensifying screens, which allow a large reduction in exposure factors.
- The film used must be sensitive to the colour of light emitted by the intensifying screens.
- Generally, film and screen speed is inversely related to image definition.

Radiographic processing

The invisible or latent image on the exposed X-ray film is rendered visible and permanent by a series of chemical reactions known as processing. As with photographic film, this must be carried out under conditions of relative darkness as the X-ray film is sensitive to blackening by white light (fogging) until processing is complete.

Although most people now use automatic processors, an understanding of the principles of manual processing is necessary as automatic processors operate on the same principles. This will also permit identification of processing faults, which will appear similar whether caused by problems with manual or automatic processing.

Manual processing

There are five stages in the procedure of manual film processing: development, intermediate rinsing, fixing, washing and drying.

Development

The main active ingredient in the developing solution is either **phenidone-hydroquinone** or **metol-hydroquinone**. These chemicals convert the exposed crystals of silver bromide into minute grains of black, metallic silver whilst the bromide ions are released into the solution. This process is known as **reduction** and the developer acts as a **reducing agent**. The length of time for which the film is immersed in the developer (usually 3–5 minutes) is critical, since longer development times will allow some of the unexposed silver bromide crystals to be converted to black, metallic silver as well, causing uniform darkening of the film (**chemical** or **development fog**: see section on film faults). The developer must also be used at a constant and uniform temperature (usually $20°C/68°F$) and ways of achieving this will be considered later. Precise times and temperatures for developing films are given in the manufacturer's instructions along with some indication of how the development time may be altered to compensate for unavoidable changes in the temperature of the solution.

Other chemicals present in the developing solution include an **accelerator** and a **buffer**, to produce and maintain the alkalinity of the solution necessary for efficient development, and a **restrainer** to reduce the amount of development fog.

X-ray developing solutions are purchased as concentrated liquids. Skin irritation may be observed after handling processing solutions. This may be due to an allergic reaction or due to the alkaline nature of the developer. Gloves should be worn when the chemicals are handled. If the problem is marked, the person's doctor should be consulted and informed of the chemicals involved.

During the development of each film a certain quantity of the developer will be absorbed into the film emulsion and so the level in the developer tank will gradually fall. On no account should the solution be topped up with water as this will cause dilution and subsequent underdevelopment of films. The original developer solution is also unsuitable for topping up, as the proportions of the different chemical constituents of the developer change with each film which is developed and the solution becomes imbalanced. Instead, special **developer replenisher** solutions should be used which take into account, and compensate for, this imbalance. Eventually, however, the developer will become exhausted as the active ingredients are used up and the solution becomes saturated with bromide ions.

Developer will also deteriorate with time by the process of **oxidation**, which will again result in underdevelopment of films. This process can be slowed by keeping the developer tank covered; in larger replenishment tanks there may also be a floating lid on the surface of the solution. Whether or not the developer is used it is therefore unlikely to be fit for use after 3 months, and so the general rule is to change the developer completely either every 3 months or when an equal volume of replenisher has been used, whichever is the sooner.

Rinsing

After the appropriate development time the film and hanger are removed from the solution and quickly transferred to the rinse water tank. Surplus developer should not be allowed to drain back into the developer tank because it will be saturated with bromide ions and will contribute to developer exhaustion. The film should be rinsed for about 10 seconds to remove excess developer solution and prevent carry-over into the fixer tank. Ideally the rinse tank will be situated between the developer and the fixer to prevent splashes of developer falling into the fixer.

Fixing

Following immersion in the developer, development is halted and the image is rendered permanent by a process known as **fixing**. The fixer is acidic, and this neutralises the developer preventing further development of the emulsion. The fixer also removes the unexposed silver halide crystals leaving the metallic silver image which can be viewed in normal light, a process known as 'clearing'. The fixer contains **sodium** or **ammonium thiosulphate** which dissolves the unexposed silver halide causing the emulsion to take on a milky-white appearance until the process is complete. The time taken for the removal of all of the unexposed halide is called the **clearing time** and depends on the thickness of the film emulsion, the temperature and concentration of the solution and the degree of exhaustion of the fixer. The fixer becomes exhausted as the amount of dissolved silver halide builds up within it, and exhaustion of fixer will occur more quickly than exhaustion of developer.

Fixer temperature is not critical but warm fixer will clear a film faster than cold fixer. However, above $21°C/70°F$ staining may occur so the fixer should not be overheated. Fixing can also be speeded up by agitating the film slightly in the fixer. After 30 seconds' immersion in the fixer it is safe to switch on the darkroom light, and the film may be viewed once the milky appearance has cleared. The total fixing time should be at least twice the clearing time, a total of about 10 minutes.

A third function of the fixer bath is to harden the film emulsion (a process known as **tanning**) to prevent the film from being scratched when handled. As well as the fixing agent (thiosulphate) and the **hardener**, the fixer solution also contains a **weak acid**, to neutralise any remaining developer, a **buffer** to maintain the acidity and a **preservative**.

Fixing solutions are normally made up from concentrated liquids by the addition of water according to manufacturer's instructions, as are developing solutions. They should be changed when the clearing time has doubled.

Washing

Following development and fixing, the film must be washed thoroughly to remove residual chemicals which would cause fading and yellow–brown staining of the film. Washing is best achieved by immersion of the film and hanger in a tank with a constant circulation of water using at least 3 litres per minute so that the film is properly rinsed; static water tanks are much less satisfactory. Washing time should be 15–30 minutes.

Drying

Following adequate washing the films should be removed from their hangers for drying. Films left in hangers of the channel type will not dry adequately around the edges. The usual method is to clip the films to a taut line over a sink, taking care that they do not touch each other. The atmosphere should be dust-free with a good air circulation. Drying frames and warm-air drying cabinets are also available and are useful if film throughput is high.

Manual processing procedure

In order to ensure that no mistakes are made a strict protocol should be adhered to and all those involved in film processing must be familiar with it. The following steps should be carried out.

Preparation

(1) Check that the developer and fixer are at the correct level. Check that the developer is at the required temperature and is adequately stirred.
(2) Ensure that hands are clean and dry.
(3) Select a suitable film hanger and check that new films for reloading the cassette are available.
(4) Lock the door, switch on the safe-light and switch off the main light.

Unloading the cassette

Open the cassette and take hold of the film gently in one corner between finger and thumb. Shaking the cassette gently first may help to dislodge the film. Remove the film and close the cassette to prevent dirt falling into it.

Identifying the film

If labelling has not been performed during radiography, label the film using a **light-marker** if available. These are simple devices which allow details written or typed on a thin piece of paper to be imprinted onto the corner of the film before processing, using a small flash of light. Often, cassettes contain small lead blockers in one corner to prevent that part of the film being exposed to X-rays and preserving it for the light-marking identification. The paper slips can be overprinted with the practice's name, which adds a professional touch.

Loading the hanger

Load the film into the hanger, handling it as little as possible and touching it only at the edges. With the channel type of hanger, the film is slid gently down the channels from the top, engaged in the bottom channel and then the top hinge is closed (Fig. 24.21). With the clip type of hanger, the film is attached to the bottom clips first with the hanger upside down, and then the hanger is placed upright and the film attached to the top clips so that it is held taut (Fig. 24.22).

Processing the film (Fig. 24.23)

(1) Remove the developer tank lid, insert the film and hanger and agitate gently to remove air bubbles from the film's surface.
(2) Close the lid and commence timing. The lid is kept on for two reasons: firstly it reduces the amount of oxidation of the developer by the atmosphere, and secondly the developing film is still sensitive to fogging by prolonged exposure to the safe-light.
(3) The film may be agitated periodically during development to bring fresh developer into contact with the film surface and prevent streaking.
(4) At the end of the development period, remove the film and transfer quickly to the rinse tank.
(5) Immerse and agitate the film in the rinse water for about 10 seconds.

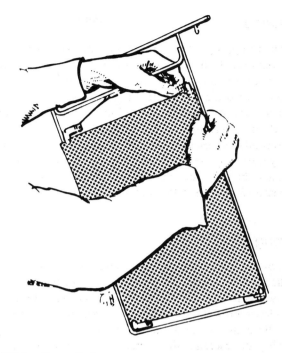

Fig. 24.22 Loading a clip hanger.

(6) Transfer the film to the fixing tank. After 30 seconds the light may be switched on or the door opened. The film may be examined briefly once the milky appearance has cleared but it should be fixed for at least 10 minutes to allow hardening to take place.
(7) Wash in running water for half an hour. (If running water is not available in the darkroom the film may be washed elsewhere.)
(8) Dry the film by hanging it on a taut wire in a dust-free atmosphere. Films in channel hangers must be removed first and hung by clips. Films must not touch each other during drying.

Reloading the cassette

This stage may be performed whilst the film is developing.

(1) Ensure hands are clean and dry.
(2) Open the cassette.
(3) Remove a new film from the film box or hopper. Handle carefully without excessive pressure or bending

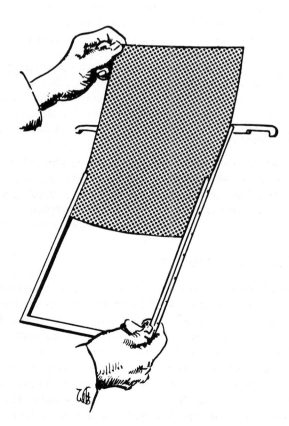

Fig. 24.21 Loading a channel hanger.

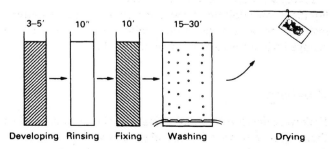

| 3–5′ | 10″ | 10′ | 15–30′ | |
| Developing | Rinsing | Fixing | Washing | Drying |

Fig. 24.23 Processing routine.

as unprocessed films are susceptible to damage by pressure.

(4) Lay the film in the cassette and, with a fingertip, ensure that it is seated correctly and will not be trapped when the cassette is closed.

Manual processing of non-screen film

As the emulsion of non-screen film is thicker than that of screen film it takes longer for the developing and fixing chemicals to penetrate the emulsion and act on the silver halide crystals. Development time should normally be increased by about 1 minute and clearing time in the fixer will be several minutes longer.

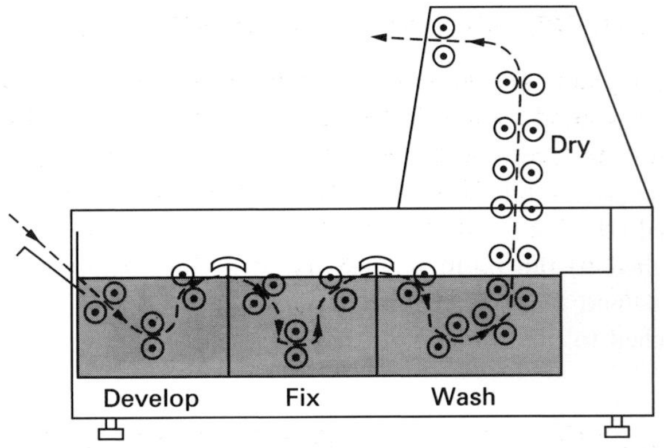

Fig. 24.24 The essential features of an automatic processor. (Reproduced with the permission of Baillière Tindall, London.)

Automatic processing

Automatic film processing has several advantages over systems of manual film development as it saves considerable time and effort and produces a dry radiograph that is ready to interpret in a very short space of time (as low as 90 seconds with some machines). In addition, the films are processed to a consistently high standard.

Automatic processors are now widely used in general practice. A darkroom is still required to unload and reload the cassettes, but only a dry bench is necessary. The processor may be entirely within the darkroom, or the feed tray may pass through the darkroom wall to a processor which is located outside.

An alternative is a daylight processor such as may be used in a human hospital; these do not require a darkroom but require special cassettes and need regular servicing. An alternative which is found in some practices is a small automatic processor with light-proof sleeves into which the forearms are inserted, manipulating the cassette inside a dark area and feeding the film into the machine by feel.

Construction of an automatic processor

An automatic processor consists of a light-proof container enclosing a series of rollers which pass the film through developer, fixer, wash water and warm air (Fig. 24.24). The intermediate rinse is omitted as excess developer is removed from the films by squeegee rollers. The chemicals are used at a higher temperature (about 28°C/82°F) to speed up the process, and the solutions are pumped in afresh for each film at a predetermined rate; there is therefore no risk of poor processing due to the use of exhausted chemicals. A considerable amount of water needs to flow through the unit for the final rinse and so there must be an adequate water supply and adequate drainage. Finally, the films are dried by a flow of warm air. If the film throughput is high, a silver recovery unit may be attached to the processor to retrieve silver from waste chemicals.

Maintenance of the automatic processor

Automatic processors usually require a warm-up period of 10–20 minutes prior to use (longer in cold weather). Films processed before the machine has reached its operating temperature will be underdeveloped. After the warm-up period a piece of unexposed film should be passed through to check the correct functioning of the processor and to remove any dried-on chemicals from the rollers by adherence to the unhardened emulsion. At least 10 films per day should be put through the processor to ensure adequate replenishment of the chemicals in the tanks – if necessary these may be old films. At the end of the working day the machine should be switched off and the superficial rollers wiped or rinsed to remove any chemical scum.

Once a week the machine may be given a more thorough clean according to the manufacturer's instructions. This requires a deep sink so that the whole roller assembly for each of the three tanks can be removed and thoroughly cleaned. An old toothbrush is useful for cleaning around the cogs. The tanks also need to be cleaned once the chemicals have been drained out. An algicide solution (e.g. Milton) can be added to the wash tank to help remove algae from the tank walls and roller assembly.

The chemicals required are produced specially for automatic processors and are not usually interchangeable with solutions for manual processing as they are formulated for use at higher temperatures. Since fresh chemicals are pumped in for each film and then discarded, there is no need for developer replenisher solution. The chemicals are made up by mixing concentrated solutions thoroughly with water; in the case of the developer there are three concentrates, one acting as a 'starter' solution; for fixer there are two. The constituents must be mixed in the correct order and with the correct amount of water.

The automatic processor should be regularly serviced by the manufacturer's engineers as breakdowns can be very inconvenient. Most engineers will also operate an emergency service but nevertheless it may be wise to have the facility to process by hand, should the occasion arise.

Film quality with automatic processing

Although automatic processing will produce films of a consistently good standard, there is always a slight loss of contrast compared with the best that can be achieved by perfect hand processing. However, the latter is not often achieved and so the automatic processor is usually of great benefit to the practice and likely to increase the enthusiasm of the staff for radiography.

Automatic processing of non-screen film

Non-screen film may be put through the automatic processor but will usually require subsequent manual fixing and further washing and drying to finish the clearing process in the thicker enulsion layers. A small amount of the fixer solution placed in a small plastic box is adequate for this. Depending on the size of the film and the nature of the processor, some non-screen film may be too small to pass through the roller system and will need complete manual development.

Film faults

Radiographic quality is often degraded by faults arising during exposure or processing of the film. It is important to be able to recognise the cause of film faults in order to correct them. Sometimes there may be several possible causes for a given fault. Common film faults, their causes and remedies are shown in Table 24.1

Disposal of waste chemicals

Fixer solutions must not be disposed of into the normal mains drainage system as silver in the used fixer is environmentally toxic, and the practice may be fined by their water supplying company. Instead the solution should be collected and disposed of by a company dealing in such waste. An alternative is to pass the solution through a silver recovery system, although the value of this depends on the world price of silver. It may be possible to take fixer to a local hospital to pass through their silver recovery unit. Fixer may be put back into an automatic processor several times, using dipsticks to test it for activity and to show when it is exhausted.

Darkroom design and maintenance

Requirements

The darkroom is an important part of the radiography set-up within each practice. The following factors should be considered in its construction:

- **Size**. Ideally it should be of a reasonable size to allow for satisfactory working conditions, and should not be used for any other purpose.
- **Light-proofing**. The darkroom must be completely light-proof, and this must be checked by standing inside the darkroom for about 5 minutes until the eyes becomes dark-adapted, as small chinks of light entering may otherwise go unnoticed. The room must be lockable from the inside to prevent the door being opened inadvertently whilst films are being processed. Light-proof maze entrances or revolving cylindrical doors are used in busy hospital departments so that radiographers have free access to the darkroom.
- **Services**. There usually needs to be a supply of electricity and mains water and a drain, although some table-top processors use water in bottles rather than mains water. Access to a sink for cleaning the processor also needs to be considered when designing the room.
- **Ventilation**. If the room is used often, some form of light-proofed ventilation is essential.
- **Walls, floor and ceiling**. The walls and ceiling should be painted white or cream (not black) so as to reflect the subdued lighting making it easier for those working inside to see what they are doing. The walls and floor should be washable and resistant to chemical splashes; it may be wise to tile any wall areas likely to be splashed.

Safe lighting

Since X-ray film is sensitive to white light until the fixing stage, illumination must be achieved using light of low intensity and a specific colour from **safe-lights,** which are boxes containing low-wattage bulbs behind brown or dark red filters. The colour of light produced must be safe for the type of film being processed as green-sensitive films require different filters to blue-sensitive films. If the wrong filter is used then the films will become uniformly fogged whilst being handled in the darkroom. Safe-light filters must be checked carefully for flaws and damage as even small pinpricks will allow light leakage; this includes the top filter of an indirect safe-light. The efficiency of the safe-lights may be checked by laying a pair of scissors or a bunch of keys on an unexposed film on the work bench for periods of up to 2 minutes and then processing it. If significant fogging is occurring the metal object will be visible on the film. It should be noted that no safe-light is completely safe if the films are exposed for too long or if the safe-light is too close to the handling area. Film manufacturers will advise on the correct filter colour needed for particular types of film.

Two types of safe-light are available: **direct safe-lights** shine directly over the working area and **indirect safe-lights** produce light upwards which is reflected from the ceiling. The number of safe-lights required varies with the size of the room but should allow efficient film handling without fumbling.

Table 24.1 Common faults and their remedies

Fault	Cause	Remedy
Film too dark	Overexposure	Reduce exposure factors; check thickness of patient; check correct film/screen combination used
	Overdevelopment	Check developer temperature; time development accurately; check automatic processor cycle and thermostat
	FFD too short	Increase FFD
	Fogging	See below for causes and remedies
Film too pale	Underexposure (background black but image too light)	Increase exposure factors; check thickness of patient; check correct film/screen combination used
	Underdevelopment (background pale only)	Check developer temperature; time development accurately; check automatic processor cycle and thermostat; change developer
	FFD too long	Decrease FFD
Patchy film density	Developer not stirred; film not agitated in developer	Correct the development technique
Contrast too high ('soot and whitewash film')	kV too low	Increase kV
Contrast too low ('flat film')	Overexposure	Reduce exposure factors
	Underdevelopment	Correct the development technique
	Overdevelopment	Correct the development technique
	Fogging	See below for causes and remedies
Fogging	Scattered radiation from patient	Collimate the beam; use a grid
	Scattered radiation from elsewhere	Change storage area for films and cassettes
	Exposure to white light before fixing stage	Check darkroom and safe-lights, film hoppers, lids on film boxes, keep lid on developer whilst film in the tank
	Storage fog	Use films before expiry date
	Chemical or development fog	Avoid overdevelopment
Image blurring	Patient movement	
	Tube head movement	
	Cassette movement	Depends on the cause
	Scattered radiation	
	Fogging	
	Poor screen-film contact	
	Large OFD	
	Double exposure	
Extraneous marks:		
small, bright marks	Dirt on the intensifying screens	Clean the screens
black patches	Developer splashes on film	Careful processing
white patches	Fixer splashes onto film	Careful processing
grey patches	Water splashes onto film;	Careful processing
	Chemical splashes on intensifying screens	Careful processing
scratches	Careless handling of unprocessed film guideshoes of automatic processor malaligned	Clean the screens Handle unprocessed film carefully
crescentic black crimp marks	Bending of unprocessed film	Handle unprocessed film carefully
fingerprints	Handling of unprocessed film with dirty hands	Wash and dry hands before processing
branching black marks	Static electricity	Handle unprocessed film carefully; use antistatic screen cleaner
parallel marks on film	Roller marks	Check seating and cleanliness of rollers
scum on surface	Scale or algae in processor	Clean processor; use water softener or anti-algal agents
Chemical stains:		
yellowing/browning on storage	Insufficient fixing or washing	Correct fixing/washing
areas of film supposed to be clear are grey and opaque	Insufficient fixing	Increase fixing time; change fixer
borders around films	Dirty channel hangers	Clean the hangers
Grid lines too coarse	X-ray beam not perpendicular to grid; focused or pseudo-focused grid used upside down	Correct alignment of beam and grid
Damp films for automatic processor	Thermostat malfunction	Call service engineer
	Dryer temperature too low	Call service engineer
	Insufficient fixing	Change fixer

Dry and wet areas

If manual processing is used the darkroom should be divided into two working areas, the **dry area** and the **wet area** (Fig. 24.25). If the room is large enough these areas may be separated by being on opposite sides of the room but where this is not possible they must be separated by a partition to prevent splashes from the wet area reaching the dry bench and damaging the films or contaminating the intensifying screens.

- **Dry area**. In this area the films are stored in boxes (preferably in cupboards) or in film hoppers, loaded into and out of cassettes and placed in the film hangers prior to processing. Sometimes films are also labelled at this stage. Dry film hangers should be stored on a rack above the dry bench and there may also be a storage area for cassettes.
- **Wet area**. The processing chemicals are kept and used here. There should be a viewing box with a drip tray for initial examination of the films, a wall rack for wet hangers and some arrangement for allowing films to dry without dripping over the floor or other working areas.

Usually, the processing solutions are contained in tanks. The developer tank should have a well-fitting lid to slow down the rate of deterioration of the developer due to oxidation by the atmosphere. Ideally the intermediate rinse water is held in a separate tank situated between the developer and the fixer so as to prevent splashes of developer falling into the fixer. The rinse water should be changed frequently. The final wash tank should contain running water if possible and should be at least 4 times the size of the developer tank.

In a busy radiography unit the tanks should be housed together in a larger container filled with water and maintained at a constant temperature (usually $20°C/68°F$) (Fig. 24.26). This water bath ensures that the chemicals are always at the correct, uniform temperature for processing and saves time as well as helping to avoid underdevelopment of films. It is not essential to heat the fixer but inclusion in the water bath will prevent fixing from slowing down in very cold weather. Water bath arrangements may be purchased as special units or may be self-constructed, using an immersion heater and a thermostat.

If a water bath is not available the tanks should sit in a shallow sink to prevent wetting the floor. In this case the developer must be heated prior to use using an immersion heater with a thermostat or a thermometer (the latter requires constant checking) (Fig. 24.27). The solution must not be allowed to overheat and must be thoroughly mixed before the film is placed in the tank, as an uneven temperature in the solution will result in patchy development and a mottled appearance to the film.

If few radiographs are processed, the chemicals may be kept in dark, stoppered bottles and poured into shallow dishes for use (as in photography). It may also be necessary to employ this technique should the automatic processor break down or for small dental film which cannot be put through an automatic processor. Unused cat litter trays

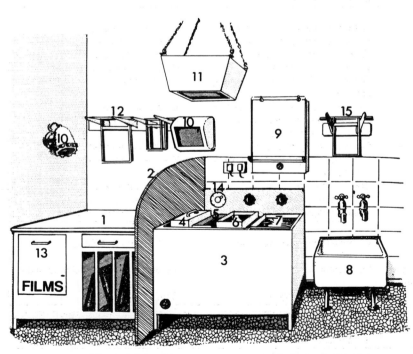

Fig. 24.25 A simple darkroom layout. (1) Dry bench. (2) High partition between dry and wet benches. (3) Wet bench – manual processing unit. (4) Developer tank with lid. (5) Rinse water tank. (6) Fixer tank. (7) Wash tank. (8) Sink. (9) Viewing box. (10) Direct safe-light. (11) Indirect/direct ceiling safe-light. (12) Film hangers on wall rack. (13) Film hopper. (14) Thermostatic control and temperature gauge for processing unit water jacket. (15) Wall rack for wet hangers. (Reproduced with the permission of Baillière Tindall, London.)

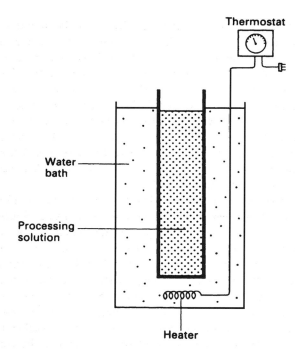

Fig. 24.26 Heating the processing solutions: water bath method.

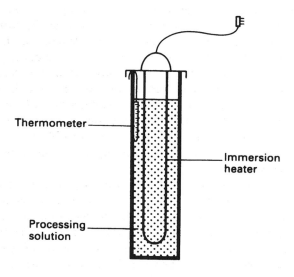

Fig. 24.27 Heating the processing solutions: immersion heater method.

make ideal processing dishes for radiographs. The correct development temperature is achieved either by heating the solution prior to use or by placing the dish on an electric heating pad. The solutions are usually discarded after use as the developer oxidises rapidly.

Other darkroom equipment

Film hangers are required for manual processing and are available in two types: **channel hangers** and **clip hangers**. Each type has its advantages and disadvantages. Channel hangers are easier to load but may result in poor development of the edges of the film. Films must be removed for drying and attached to the drying line using clips. The hangers should be washed after the films are removed as chemicals may otherwise build up in the channels, causing staining of subsequent films. Very large films may not be held securely in channel hangers. Clip hangers avoid these disadvantages but are more fragile and more cumbersome to use and they may tear the films if not used correctly.

A **timer with a bell** should be present in the darkroom so that the period of development can be timed accurately. The timer should ideally be capable of being pre-set to a given time.

A **hand towel** and a **waste-paper bin** are also useful additions to the darkroom.

General care of the darkroom

Most film faults arise during processing and often radiographs which have been carefully taken are spoilt by careless darkroom technique. Competent handling of the films during this stage is therefore vital to the success of radiography within the practice and it is a duty usually delegated to the veterinary nurse. Film faults can also arise during automatic processing.

The darkroom should be kept tidy, clean and uncluttered, with all the equipment in its correct place. Cleanliness is particularly important as undeveloped films handled with fingers which are dirty or contaminated with developer, fixer or water will show permanent fingerprints. Splashes of liquid falling on to undeveloped films result in black (developer), grey (water) or white (fixer) patches on subsequent films due to interference with light emission. Dust and dirt falling into open cassettes will result in small white screen marks on the radiographs.

With manual processing, attention must also be paid to the maintenance of the processing solutions, as underdevelopment is a common film fault. The tanks should be topped up when the fluid levels fall and the chemicals should be changed regularly, with a record being kept of the date on which they are changed. Developer should be renewed every 90 days or when it has been replenished by the same volume as the original solution, whichever is sooner. Whether using manual or automatic processing, separate mixing rods should be used for making up developer and fixer and should be cleaned after use. Chemicals splashing on to the walls or the floor should be wiped up, as they produce dust when dry and they may stain or corrode the surfaces. The chemical solutions may also damage clothing and so aprons should be worn while they are being mixed. The temperature of the solutions for manual processing should be checked regularly and the heater or thermostat adjusted if necessary.

Other important points are to ensure that the cassettes are always reloaded ready for use when the previous film is removed and to check that a sufficient number of film hangers are always clean and dry.

KEY POINTS
Radiographic processing
- Development reduces the exposed silver bromide crystals in the film emulsion to specks of black, metallic silver thereby producing a visible image.
- Fixing has three functions: it stops development, it clears unexposed emulsion from the film base and it hardens the film surface.
- Non-screen film requires longer development and fixing times due to its thick emulsion.
- Automatic processing works on similar principles to manual processing but the chemicals are used at a higher temperature which speeds up the process.
- Careful darkroom technique is important in the production of high quality radiographs.

Viewing the radiograph

Although the radiograph may be examined whilst it is still wet for technical quality, a provisional diagnosis or the need for a contrast study, the image will be somewhat blurred due to swelling of the two layers of wet emulsion. Full examination must be delayed until the film has dried, when the emulsion will have shrunk and the image is clearer. Films should be examined on clean viewing boxes (not held up to a window) in a dim area to allow the eyes to pick out detail on the film without distracting glare from elsewhere. If the film is small, the rest of the viewer may be masked off with a black card – a simple procedure that will allow very much more detail to be appreciated. Relatively overexposed areas should be examined with a special bright light and a magnifying glass may be useful to look for fine detail.

Assessing radiographic quality

Films must be of high technical quality if a radiographic examination is to produce maximum information about the patient. Errors can arise both during radiography and in the darkroom and the radiographer should be able to assess the film for its quality, recognise any faults and know how to correct them.

Before film faults can be recognised, it is necessary to understand the terms **density**, **contrast** and **definition**.

Density

Radiographic **density** is the degree of blackening of the film and is determined by two factors: the **exposure** used and the **processing technique**:

- **Exposure**. Film blackening is affected by the quantity of X-rays passing through the patient and reaching the film. It is influenced by the kilovoltage, the mAs and the FFD. If the patient's image is generally too dark, then the film is **overexposed** and the exposure factors should be reduced or the FFD increased; conversely, if it is too light, then it is **underexposed** and the exposure factors should be increased or the FFD reduced. Usually, corrections are made to the exposure factors; the FFD should remain constant unless it has been inadvertently altered.
- **Processing**. Radiographic density can also be affected by processing. **Underdevelopment**, due to the use of diluted, exhausted or cold developer or development for too short a time, will cause all areas of the film to be too light, including the background. Development can be tested by performing the **finger test**, i.e. putting a finger between the film and the viewer in an area where the film was not covered by the patient and which should therefore be completely black. If the finger is visible, the film is underdeveloped. Underdevelopment is the commonest film fault arising with manual processing, and should be corrected by topping up the developer with replenisher and not water, by changing the solution regularly and by ensuring that it is used at the correct temperature and for the correct length of time. Underdevelopment may also occur with automatic processing, if the machine is not working at the correct temperature. **Overdevelopment** may occur if the developer is too hot or if the film is inadvertently left in the solution for too long. In this case some of the *un*exposed silver halide crystals will be converted to black metallic silver leading to uniform darkening of the film or **development fog**.

Overexposure and **overdevelopment** may be hard to differentiate as both will cause an increased radiographic density. However, areas covered by metal markers during the exposure will remain white if the fault is overexposure but will darken if the film is overdeveloped.

Underexposure and **underdevelopment** can usually be easily differentiated. Underdevelopment will produce a grey background using the finger test; with underexposure the background should still be black but the area covered by the patient will be too pale.

In general, films which are too dark are to be preferred to those which are too light, as they may still yield adequate information when examined under a bright light.

Contrast

Contrast is the difference between various radiographic densities (shades of grey) seen on the radiograph. A medium-contrast film with a reasonable number of grey shades as well as white and black on the image is desirable, as it will yield most information. A film that shows a white image on a black background with few intermediate grey shades has too high a contrast ('soot and whitewash') and is due to the use of too low a kilovoltage with insufficient penetrating power. A film without extremes of density showing mainly grey shades has a very low contrast and is called a 'flat' film. Poor contrast is usually due to underdevelopment, in which case the background will be grey (use the finger test). Overexposure, overdevelopment and various types of fogging will also produce a flat film but in this case the background density will be black and the remainder of the film will also be very dark.

Definition

Definition refers to the sharpness and clarity of the structures visible on a radiograph. Good definition is usually essential if the film is to be diagnostic.

Definition may be affected by a number of factors:

- *Movement blur*. This is the most common cause of poor definition on chest and abdomen radiographs and is usually due to respiration or struggling by the patient. It may also occur if the tube stand is unstable or if the cassette moves (the latter is applicable only to equine radiography). Patient movement is minimised by the use of sedation or general anaesthesia and by adequate artificial restraint using sandbags, etc. The exposure time should be kept as low as possible.
- *Scattered radiation*. Scattered radiation produced when thick or dense areas of tissue are X-rayed will produce random darkening of the film resulting in loss of definition and contrast. Its effects may be reduced by collimating the beam and by the use of a grid.
- *Fog*. Fogging is darkening of the film unrelated to the radiographic image and has a number of causes. These include scattered radiation, accidental exposure of the film to radiation or white light prior to or during processing, the use of an unsuitable safe-light filter, prolonged storage and overdevelopment. The result is a loss of definition and contrast.
- *Poor screen–film contact*. Poor contact between the intensifying screen and the film within the cassette due to shrinkage of the felt pad will cause blurring of the image in the affected area. It will be present in the same place on all films taken in that cassette.
- *Film and screen speed*. Fast film–screen combinations require a lower exposure for a given degree of film blackening than do slower combinations, but the definition of the image is poorer due to the larger size of the phosphor crystals in the intensifying screens and to the characteristics of the film emulsion.
- *Focal spot size*. Some machines allow a choice of focal spot size. **Fine focus** produces finer radiographic detail but the exposure factors available are limited. **Coarse focus** allows higher exposure factors but, since the effective focal spot is larger, some detail is lost by the penumbra effect (Fig. 24.5). The penumbra effect is reduced by

keeping the object–film distance as small as possible and by using a reasonably long focus–film distance.

- *Magnification and object–film distance (OFD)*. Since the X-ray beam diverges from the focal spot, the geometry of the X-ray beam results in some degree of magnification of the image. Magnified images will usually also be blurred because the penumbra effect increases with increasing OFD. In order to reduce this effect, the part being radiographed should always be positioned as close as possible to the film, with the focal–film distance as long as is practicable for that machine (Fig. 24.28).

The more common film faults and their remedies are summarised in Table 24.1.

Labelling of radiographs

All radiographs should be permanently labelled with the case identification (name or number), the date, a right or left marker if appropriate and any other relevant details (e.g. time after administration of a contrast medium). Labelling of the paper sleeve or film envelope only is inadequate and liable to cause mix-ups, especially on busy days. Films can be labelled at one of three stages:

- *Labelling of film during exposure*. Films can be identified during radiography by placing lead letters on the cassette or by writing details on special graphite tape which is then stuck to the cassette. Care should be taken to ensure that the whole of the information appears on the film after processing and is neither lost on the edge of the film nor overexposed. Right or left markers should be used at this stage and not substituted for by the use of personal codes such as scissors or keys!

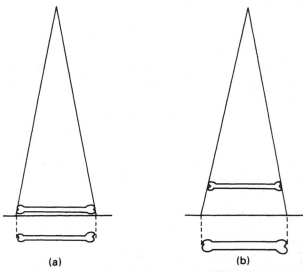

Fig. 24.28 Magnification and object–film distance. (a) Object close to film, so reproduced accurately on radiograph. (b) Object not close to film, so image is magnified.

- *Labelling in the darkroom.* Films may also be identified by labelling in the darkroom prior to processing. The most efficient method is to use a light-marker, which is a small device that prints information, written or typed on paper, on to the corner of the film, using white light. A small rectangular area in the corner of the film must therefore be protected from exposure to X-rays by the incorporation of a piece of lead in the cassette to act as a blocker and leave a space on the film on which these details may be printed. There are also special cassettes available with a movable window which can be inserted into a light-marking camera for imprinting the details; this can be done in daylight outside the darkroom.
- *Labelling of the dry film.* Information may be written on the film after processing using a white 'Chinagraph' pencil, white ink or a black felt-tip pen. Such identification may not be acceptable for films used in legal cases, and so labelling after processing is not good practice.

Identification of radiographs for the BVA/KC Hip and Elbow Dysplasia Scoring Schemes

The requirement for submission of films to the Hip and Elbow Dysplasia Scoring Schemes is that they must be identified with the dog's Kennel Club number during radiography, i.e. using lead letters or tape or by a light-marker before processing. Labelling after processing is not acceptable. The date and right or left markers as appropriate must also be present. If the dog is not registered with the Kennel Club, other identification is acceptable.

Storing and filing radiographs

Radiographs may be required for retrospective study or as legal documents and so should be clearly labelled and carefully filed. Many films can accumulate within a short space of time in a busy practice and the filing system must be simple and fool-proof.

Films processed manually must be completely dry before filing, otherwise they will be damaged by sticking to paper. Films may be stored in their original paper folders or in special X-ray envelopes, with case details (e.g. owner's name, patient information and date) marked clearly on the outside. These may then be kept in film boxes, filing cabinets or on shelving depending on the number of films involved. Films may be stored either chronologically or in alphabetical order of owner's name, with films from each year usually being kept separately. Films of special interest and good examples of normal anatomy should be noted for future reference.

> **KEY POINTS**
> Viewing and storing radiographs
> - Radiographic density (film blackening) is determined by both exposure factors and processing technique.
> - Contrast (the range of grey shades on the image) is also affected by exposure factors and processing technique.
> - There are many causes of reduced film definition, of which the most important are patient motion, scattered radiation and equipment-related factors.
> - Radiographs are legal documents and so they should be carefully labelled and archived.

Radiation protection

The dangers associated with radiography

Exposure of the human or animal body to radiation is not without hazard because of the biological effects which X-rays have on living tissues via cellular chemical reactions. X-rays have four properties which mean that the danger from them may be seriously underestimated:

- They are **invisible**.
- They are **painless**.
- The effects are **latent**, i.e. they are not evident immediately and may not manifest until some time later – even several decades in some cases.
- Their effects are **cumulative**, so that repeated very low doses may be as hazardous as a single large exposure.

Large doses are unlikely to occur in human or veterinary radiography but may be seen after nuclear accidents. It is the danger arising from repeated exposure to small amounts of radiation that concerns people working with veterinary radiography.

The adverse effects of radiation on the body may be divided into three groups: somatic, carcinogenic and genetic.

- *Somatic effects.* These are direct changes in body tissues which usually occur soon after exposure. They include changes such as skin reddening and cracking, blood disorders, baldness, cataract formation and digestive upsets. The latter cause severe dehydration which is the usual cause of death following nuclear accidents or bombs. Different tissues vary in their susceptibility to this type of damage, with the developing fetus being particularly susceptible. The somatic effect is used to advantage in the radiotherapy of tumours since tumour cells are often more sensitive to radiation damage than are normal cells.
- *Carcinogenic effects.* These are the induction of tumours in tissues that have been exposed to radiation. There may be a considerable time lag before these tumours arise,

which may be as long as 20–30 years in the case of leukaemia.

- *Genetic effects.* These occur when gonads are irradiated and mutations are induced in the chromosomes of germ cells. The mutations may give rise to inherited abnormalities in the offspring.

Despite these hazards, it is possible to perform radiography in veterinary practice with no significant risk to any of the people involved, provided that adequate precautions are taken.

Sources of radiation hazard

During an exposure, there are three potential sources of X-rays that may be hazardous to the radiographer (Fig. 24.29).

The tube head

Although the tube head is lead-lined (except at the window where the primary beam emerges), older machines may have suffered cracks in the casing, which allow X-rays to escape in other directions. For this reason the tube head should never be held or touched during an exposure. Checks on the efficiency of the casing can be made by taping envelope-wrapped non-screen film to the tube head, leaving it for a few exposures and then processing it. Any cracks in the casing will cause black lines to appear on the film, where it has been exposed.

The primary beam

The beam of X-rays produced at the anode is directed out of the tube head through the window. This primary beam constitutes the greatest safety hazard, since it consists of high energy X-rays. It may be visualised using a **light beam dia-**phragm, a device attached to the tube head which produces a light over the area covered by the X-ray beam (Fig. 24.30). The light beam diaphragm usually contains crossed wires which produce a shadow in the illuminated area showing the position of the centre of the beam (the **central ray**). Movable metal plates operated by knobs allow the area covered to be adjusted to the size required, a procedure known as **collimation**. Collimation should always be as 'tight' as possible (i.e. to as small an area as possible) and the accuracy of the light beam diaphragm should be checked periodically. This can be done by arranging pairs of coins along each margin of the light beam with their edges touching so that one of each pair lies inside and one outside the light beam and making an exposure. After processing, the image should show four coins inside the black area and the other four coins outside, if the light beam diaphragm was accurate.

An alternative but now uncommon method of collimation is to use conical or cylindrical devices or **cones** attached to the tube window to produce a circular primary beam of varying diameter. Cones are much less satisfactory than light beam diaphragms since the area covered by the primary beam is not seen. Whichever method of collimation is used, the area covered by the primary beam should be no larger than the size of the cassette, and so the borders of the beam should be visible on the processed radiograph.

No part of any handler should come within the primary beam, even if protected by lead rubber clothing. In the rare cases where animals have to be held for radiography, a light beam diaphragm **must** be used to ensure that the primary beam is safely collimated. To prevent the primary beam from passing through the table and scattering off the floor or irradiating the feet of any handlers the table-top should be covered with lead or else a lead sheet placed underneath the cassette.

The use of a horizontal X-ray beam is especially hazardous as the primary beam will pass with little attenuation through doors, windows and thin walls. This procedure should only be performed with great care, with the primary beam directed only towards a thick wall. The procedure for the use of horizontal beam radiography should be described in the Local Rules (see p. 730).

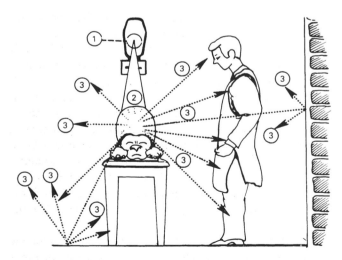

Fig. 24.29 The spread of scattered radiation. (1) The tube head. (2) The primary beam. (3) Scattered radiation. (Reproduced with the permission of Baillière Tindall, London.)

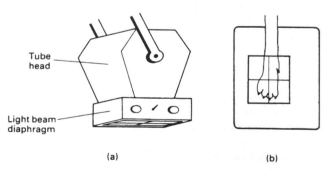

Tube head

Light beam diaphragm

(a)　　　　(b)

Fig. 24.30 (a) Light beam diaphragm. (b) Centring and collimating a paw.

Secondary or scattered radiation

Scattered radiation is produced in all directions when the primary beam strikes a solid object, and so it arises from the patient and the cassette. It is produced by the table or floor if the table-top is not lead-lined and it can also bounce off walls and ceilings and travel in unexpected directions. It is, however, of much lower energy than the primary beam and is absorbed by protective clothing. Its intensity falls off rapidly with distance from the source (due to the inverse square law). The best protection against scatter is to stand as far from the X-ray machine and patient as possible.

Ways of reducing the amount of scatter produced (as already discussed in the section on scattered radiation) include tight collimation of the primary beam, compression of large areas of soft tissue, reduction in the kilovoltage where possible and the use of lead-backed cassettes and a lead-topped table. Protection against scatter is also afforded by protective clothing. In large-animal radiography, rotation of staff involved is advisable, since personnel may of necessity stand closer to the primary beam. With small-animal radiography and non-manual restraint, rotation of staff is less important.

Legislation

In 1985 the law governing the use of radiation and radioactive materials was revised and updated with the publication of The Ionising Radiations Regulations (IRR) 1985, updated as **the Ionising Radiations Regulations (revised) 1999**. This legal document covers all uses of radiation and radioactive materials, including veterinary radiography. As it is written in legal terms and is somewhat lengthy, a second booklet was published at the same time which attempted to explain the Regulations and is called the **Approved Code of Practice for the Protection of Persons against Ionising Radiation arising from any Work Activity**. The Code of Practice does contain some specific references to veterinary radiography but is also rather long-winded and so guidance notes explaining the law as it applies to veterinary radiography were published by the BVA in 2002 **Guidance notes for the safe use of ionising radiations in veterinary practice**. These cover premises, equipment, personnel and procedures and aim to minimise radiation doses received by veterinary staff. A summary of the legislation is given in the following paragraphs.

Principles of radiation protection

Protection follows three basic principles:

(1) Radiography should only be undertaken if there is definite clinical justification for the use of the procedure.

(2) Any exposure of personnel should be kept to a minimum. The three words to remember are **time**, **distance**, **shielding**, i.e. reduce the need for repeat exposures, stand well back and wear protective clothing or stand behind a lead screen.

(3) No dose limit should be exceeded.

The aim is to avoid exposure at all times, but failing this a high standard of protection will exist if the advice contained in the Guidance Notes is followed.

Radiation Protection Supervisor (RPS)

An RPS must be appointed within the practice and will usually be the principal or a senior partner, although may be the head nurse in some practices. The RPS is responsible for ensuring that radiography is carried out safely and in accordance with the Regulations, and that the Local Rules (see p. 730) are obeyed, but the person need not be present at every radiographic examination.

Radiation Protection Adviser (RPA)

Most practices will also need to appoint an external RPA. The qualifications necessary to act as an RPA are laid down in the Approved Code of Practice and may include veterinary surgeons who hold the Diploma in Veterinary Radiology and who have a knowledge of radiation physics, and medical physicists with an interest in veterinary radiography. From January 2005 they will also have to hold a certificate of competence from an appropriate issuing body. The RPA will give advice on all aspects of radiation protection, the demarcation of the controlled area and will draw up the Local Rules and Written Systems of Work.

The controlled area

A specific room should be identified for small-animal radiography and should have sufficiently thick walls that no part of the controlled area extends outside it (single brick is usually adequate; thin walls may be reinforced with lead ply or barium plaster). The room should be large enough to allow people remaining in the room to stand at least 2 m from the primary beam. If this is not possible, a protective lead screen should be provided, unless the radiographer can routinely step outside the room and stand behind a brick wall during the exposure. Unshielded doors and windows may be acceptable if the work load is low and the room is large enough. Special recommendations are made for flooring in cases where there may be an occupied area below the radiography room.

Technically, the **controlled area** is the area around the primary beam within which the average dose rate of exposure exceeds a given limit (laid down in the Regulations). The controlled area for a typical practice is within a 2 m radius from the beam but usually needs to be defined by the RPA. Since the controlled area must be physically demarcated and clearly labelled, it is usually simpler to designate the whole X-ray room as a controlled area and to place warning notices on its doors to exclude people not involved in radiography. When the radiographic examination is completed the X-ray machine must be disconnected from the power supply; the room then ceases to be a controlled area and may be entered freely.

A warning sign should be placed at the entrance to the X-ray room, consisting of the radiation warning symbol and a simple legend (Fig. 24.31). For permanently installed equipment there should also be an automatic signal at the room entrance indicating when the X-ray machine is in a state of readiness to produce X-rays. This signal usually takes the form of a red light or an illuminated sign. Whilst not a legal requirement for portable and mobile X-ray machines (which comprise the majority of practice X-ray machines), many practitioners have installed red lights outside their radiography rooms to warn when radiography is in progress and prevent accidental entry, and this is to be recommended.

In addition, all X-ray machines should have lights visible from the control panel indicating (a) when they are switched on at the mains, and (b) when exposure is taking place. Sometimes (b) is instead a noise such as a beep or buzz.

X-ray equipment

Radiation safety features of the X-ray machine should be regularly checked by a qualified engineer. Leakage radiation from the tube housing must not exceed a certain level and the beam filtration must be equivalent to not less than 2.5 mm aluminium. All machines must be fitted with a collimation device, preferably a light beam diaphragm. The exposure button must allow the radiographer to stand at least 2 m from the primary beam, which means either that it must be at the end of a sufficiently long cable, or that it should be on the control panel which is placed well away from the tube head. The timer should be electronic rather than clockwork, as exposures cannot usually be aborted with the latter, should the patient move.

Suppliers of X-ray machines have a responsibility to ensure that they are safe and functioning correctly, and they should provide a report to this effect when installing the equipment. **Servicing of X-ray machines is a legal requirement and should be carried out at least once a year.**

The X-ray table must be lead-lined, or else a sheet of lead 1 mm thick and larger than the maximum size of the beam should be placed on the table and beneath the cassette to absorb the residual primary beam and reduce scatter. Many practices now use purpose-built X-ray tables which are not only lead-lined but also fitted with hooks to aid in patient positioning.

Practices performing equine radiography also require cassette holders with long handles for supporting cassettes during limb radiography and various types of wooden blocks for positioning the lower limbs with the minimum of manual restraint.

Film and film processing

The Regulations recommend the use of fast film–screen combinations in order to reduce exposure times. They stress the importance of correct processing techniques in order to minimise the number of non-diagnostic films and avoid the need for repeat exposures.

Recording exposures

It is necessary to record each radiographic exposure made and this is done using a daybook for radiography including the following details for each exposure:

- Date.
- Patient identity and description.
- Exposure factors used.
- Quality of image.
- Means of restraint. If the animal has had to be held during radiography then the names of the person(s) doing so must be recorded.

Protective clothing

Protective clothing consists of aprons, gloves and sleeves and is usually made of plastic or rubber impregnated with lead. The thickness and efficiency of the garment is described in millimetres of lead equivalent (LE), i.e. the thickness of pure lead which would afford the same protection. It is important to remember that **protective clothing is only effective against scatter and does not protect against the primary beam.**

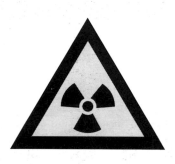
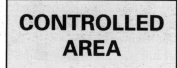

Fig. 24.31 Radiation warning signs.

Lead aprons should be worn by any person who needs to be present in the X-ray room during the exposure. They are designed to cover the trunk (especially the gonads) and should reach at least to mid-thigh level. Their thickness should be at least 0.25 mm LE; many are 0.35 or even 0.5 mm LE, although the latter are rather heavy to wear. Single-sided aprons covering the front of the body but with straps at the back are cheaper but provide less protection than double-sided aprons covering both front and back and are also less comfortable to wear for long periods. Aprons are expensive items and should be handled carefully; when not in use they should be stored on coat hangers or on rails and they must never be folded, as this can lead to undetected cracking of the material (Fig. 24.32).

Lead gloves, open-palm mitts and hand shields must be available for use in those cases where manual restraint of the patient is unavoidable. They are also required for equine radiography when a limb or a cassette holder may need to be held. Lead sleeves are tubes of lead rubber into which the hands and forearms may be inserted as an alternative to gloves. Single sheets of lead rubber draped over the hands are not adequate as they do not protect against back-scatter. Lead rubber neck guards for protection of the thyroid gland may also be used. Gloves, hand shields and sleeves should be at least 0.35 mm LE and must never appear in the primary beam, since they offer inadequate protection against high energy X-rays. It is important to remember that, although a lead glove may appear completely opaque on a radiograph, the film is being protected by two layers of lead rubber but the hand by only one (Fig. 24.33).

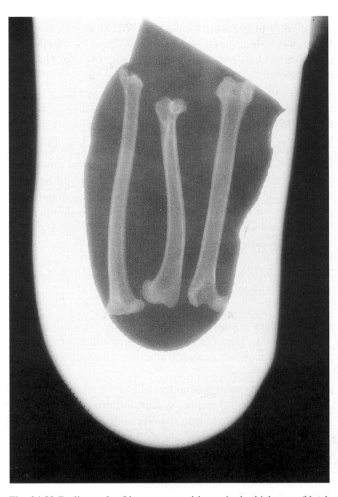

Fig. 24.33 Radiograph of bones covered by a single thickness of lead rubber; compare with the edge where there are two layers of lead rubber.

All items of protective clothing should be checked frequently for signs of cracking. A small defect may not allow many X-rays through but will always be over the same area of skin. If in doubt, the garment may be X-rayed to check for cracks (Fig. 24.34).

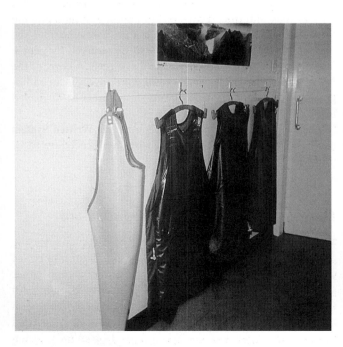

Fig. 24.32 Correct and incorrect storage of lead aprons.

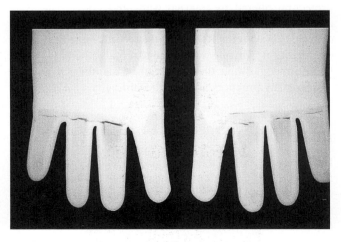

Fig. 24.34 Cracking of the lead rubber at the usual site – the base of the fingers. (Reproduced with the permission of Baillière Tindall, London.)

Mobile lead screens with lead glass windows are also useful as the radiographer can stand behind them during the exposure and still see the patient. Unfortunately they are very expensive.

Dosimetry

All persons who are involved in radiography should wear small monitoring devices or **dosemeters** to record any radiation to which they are exposed. Dosemeters should be worn on the trunk beneath the lead apron, though an extra dosemeter may be worn on the collar or sleeve to monitor the levels of radiation received by unprotected parts of the body. Each dosemeter should be worn only by the person to whom it is issued and it must neither be left in the X-ray room whilst not being worn nor exposed to heat or sunlight. Two types of dosemeter are available:

- **Film badges** contain small pieces of X-ray film and are usually blue. They contain small metal filters which allow assessment of the type of radiation to which the badge has been exposed.
- **Thermoluminescent dosemeters** (TLDs) contain radiation-sensitive lithium fluoride crystals and are usually orange. On exposure to radiation the electrons in the crystals are rearranged, thus storing energy. During the reading process the crystals are heated and give off light in proportion to the amount of energy which they have stored – this gives a quantitative reading.

They are obtained from dosimetry services such as the National Radiological Protection Board (NRPB) and they should be sent off for reading every 1–3 months, depending on the radiographic caseload. If animals are likely to be held for radiography (e.g. equine work), special finger badges may also be worn inside the lead gloves to monitor the dose to the hands.

Dosemeters may also be used to monitor radiation levels in the X-ray room or in adjacent rooms by mounting them on the wall. They can be used to check the adequacy of protection offered by internal walls and doors. The exact arrangement for dosimetry in the practice will be made in consultation with the RPA, and the records must be filed for easy retrieval. Anyone whose badge reveals a reading should be informed, so that the cause can be identified if possible and working practices adjusted accordingly.

Dose limits

Dose limits are amounts of radiation which are thought not to constitute a greater risk to health than that encountered in everyday life. Legal limits have been laid down for various categories of person and for different parts of the body. Dose limits are laid down for the whole body, for individual organs, for the lens of the eye and for pregnancy. 'Classified' persons are those working with radiation who are likely to receive more than 30% of any relevant dose limit. However, in veterinary practice these levels should not be reached and so veterinary workers rarely need to be designated as classified persons, provided that they are working under a Written System of Work (see below).

Staff involved in radiography

The Local Rules will include a list of names of designated persons authorised to carry out exposures. It should be remembered that nurses and other lay staff aged 16 or 17 have a lower dose limit than do adults aged 18 or over and therefore their involvement in radiography should be limited. Young people under 16 years of age should not be present during radiography under any circumstances. Owners should not routinely be present as they are members of the general public and are neither trained in radiography nor wearing dosemeters, although it may be necessary in emergency situations. The Local Rules should ensure that doses to pregnant women are also well within the legal limit, but nevertheless it is wise to avoid the involvement of pregnant women in radiography whenever possible.

The general rule is that the minimum number of people should be present during radiography. When, as is usual, the patient is artificially restrained only the person making the exposure need be present, and this should be the case in the majority of radiographic studies. Often the radiographer will be able to stand outside the room during the exposure.

Local Rules and Written Systems of Work

The **Local Rules** are a set of instructions drawn up by the practice's RPA which set down details of equipment, procedures and restriction of access to the controlled area for that practice. They include the method of restraint of patients for radiography and the precautions to be taken should manual restraint be necessary. They contain an assessment of the maximum dose of radiation likely to be received by people in the practice, and this will normally be zero. A copy of the Local Rules should be given to anyone involved in radiography (including the nurses) and should also be displayed in the X-ray room.

The Local Rules include a subsection, the **Written System of Work**, which describes the step-by-step procedure to be followed for radiography.

Radiographic procedures and restraint

Whenever possible, the beam should be directed vertically downwards on to an X-ray table. The minimum number of people should remain in the room and they should either stand behind lead screens or wear protective clothing. All those present must obey the instructions given by the person operating the X-ray machine. The beam must be collimated to the smallest size practicable, and must be entirely within the borders of the film. Grids should only be used when the part being X-rayed is more than 10 cm thick, as their use necessitates an increase in the exposure.

The method of restraint of the patient is of paramount importance. Many practices previously held all their patients for radiography but this should now be discontinued as it is not only dangerous but also illegal. The Approved Code of Practice states that 'only in exceptional circumstances should a patient or animal undergoing a diagnostic examination be supported or manipulated by hand'. These exceptional circumstances may include severely ill or injured animals for whom a diagnosis requires radiography but for whom sedation, anaesthesia or restraint with sandbags is dangerous (e.g. congestive heart failure; ruptured diaphragm or other severe traumatic injuries). In these cases the animal may be held, provided that those restraining it are fully protected and provided that no part of their hands (even in gloves) enters the primary beam. A light beam diaphragm is essential for manual restraint. The majority of patients may be positioned and restrained artificially under varying degrees of sedation or general anaesthesia, and sometimes with no chemical restraint at all.

Large-animal radiography

Special consideration is given to large-animal radiography using a horizontal beam. The investigation may need to be undertaken outside the X-ray room, when it should preferably take place in a walled or fenced area with the primary beam directed at a wall of double brick. The extent of the controlled area should be identified using portable warning signs, in order to prevent people not involved from being accidentally irradiated. Everyone taking part in radiography must wear protective clothing and dosemeters. The extra hazards posed by the use of a horizontal beam must be remembered and care must be taken not to irradiate the legs of anyone assisting in the procedure. Collimation must be tight and accurate, especially if a limb or cassette holder is being held by a gloved hand close to the primary beam.

KEY POINTS
Radiation protection
- X-rays are hazardous to living tissues, causing harmful effects which may be both immediate and delayed.
- Radiation safety in the UK is governed by the Ionising Radiations Regulations (revised) 1999.
- The RPA advises the practice on radiation safety matters; the RPS is responsible for training and day-to-day safety.
- The three main principles of radiation protection are **time, distance**, and **shielding**.
- Safe radiography involves attention to both equipment and working practices.

Positioning

In order to produce radiographs of maximum diagnostic value it is necessary to position the patient carefully and to centre and collimate the beam accurately. Poor positioning, with rotation or obliquity of the area being radiographed, will result in a film that is hard to interpret or misleading or that fails to demonstrate the lesion.

There are several general rules that should be adhered to when positioning the patient:

- Use a large enough cassette to cover the whole area of interest, such as the chest or abdomen in a large dog – it is very difficult to interpret images which are made up of a mosaic of smaller radiographs.
- Place the area of interest as close to the film as possible in order to minimise magnification and blurring and to produce an accurate image.
- Centre over the area of interest, especially if it is a joint or a disc space.
- Ensure that the central ray of the primary beam is perpendicular to the film otherwise distortion and non-uniform exposure of the structures will result. If a grid is being used, accurate alignment of the primary beam is essential to prevent grid faults.
- Collimate the beam to as small an area as possible, to reduce the amount of scattered radiation produced.
- Since a radiograph is a two-dimensional image of a three-dimensional structure, it is usually necessary to take two radiographs at right angles to each other in order to visualise the area fully.

Oblique views may then be taken to highlight lesions seen on the initial films if appropriate.

Restraint

Small animals should be held for radiography **only in exceptional circumstances**, when a radiograph is essential for a diagnosis but their condition renders other means of restraint unsafe. In practice, patients rarely need to be held and most views may be achieved using a combination of chemical restraint and positioning aids.

Simple lateral views of chest, abdomen and limbs may be possible on placid animals without any form of sedation. Other views require varying degrees of sedation or general anaesthesia and the positioning requirements and the temperament of the patient must be taken into consideration when assessing the depth of sedation required. It is also important to handle patients gently, calmly and firmly during radiography, and to reassure them with touch and voice.

Positioning aids

With the skilful use of positioning aids and the correct degree of chemical restraint, almost any radiographic view may be achieved without the need to hold the animal.

The following positioning aids should be present in the practice:

- *Troughs*. Radiolucent plastic or foam-filled troughs are essential for restraining animals on their backs. They are available in a variety of sizes.
- *Foam wedges*. When lateral views are required, these are placed under the chest, skull or spine to prevent rotation and to ensure that a true lateral view is achieved. They are also useful for accurate limb positioning. They are radiolucent and may therefore be used in the primary beam. It is useful to have several, in different shapes and sizes, and to cover them with plastic for easy cleaning.
- *Sandbags*. Long, thin sandbags of various sizes may be wrapped around limbs or placed over the neck for restraint. They should only be loosely filled with sand, so that they can be bent and twisted. As they are radio-opaque they should not be used in the primary beam. They should be plastic-covered for easy cleaning.
- *Tapes*. Cotton tapes are looped around limbs and may then be tied to hooks on the edge of the table or wrapped around sandbags, for positioning of the limbs. Sticky tape may also be useful at times.
- *Velcro bands*. Fabric bands with velcro fastenings are especially useful for VD hip radiographs, as they can be placed around the stifles to align the femora correctly. Non-stick elasticated bandage can also be used.
- *Wooden blocks*. Wooden blocks are used to raise the cassette to the area of interest, for certain views (e.g. dorso-ventral skull). They are radio-opaque and so should not be placed between the patient and the film.

Nomenclature

Each radiographic projection is named by a composite term describing first the point of entry and then the point of exit of the beam, e.g. a **dorsoventral (DV)** view of the chest involves the X-ray beam entering through the spine (**dorsally**) and emerging through the sternum (**ventrally**). An exception is the lateromedial or mediolateral view, which is commonly just called the **lateral** view. A standardised nomenclature has been devised for veterinary radiology and the naming of the various body regions is shown in Fig. 24.35. Note that the terms 'anterior' and 'posterior' are no longer used in veterinary radiology as they are not appropriate to four-legged creatures. Instead, anteroposterior (AP) and postero-anterior (PA) views of the limbs are called **craniocaudal (CrCd)** or **caudocranial (CdCr)** above the radiocarpal and tibiotarsal joints, and **dorsopalmar (DPa)/palmarodorsal (PaD)** or **dorsoplantar (DPl)/plantarodorsal (PlD)** below. The correct terminology will be used throughout this section. **Dorsal recumbency** describes an animal lying on its back and **sternal recumbency** describes the crouching position.

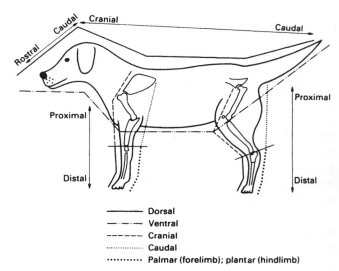

Fig. 24.35 Standardised nomenclature for body regions.

Positioning for common views

The following notes describe in brief the positioning for the more common views performed in veterinary practice. Further details are found in *Principles of Veterinary Radiography* (Douglas et al., 1987). Anatomy texts and radiological atlases should be consulted for identification of normal anatomical structures.

Thorax

The right lateral recumbent position is usually preferred to the left lateral for a single screening film as the heart outline is more consistent in shape. When assessing the lungs it is useful to perform the left lateral view too, as the uppermost lung field is better aerated in lateral recumbency and is therefore more likely to show pathology. When investigating known or suspected lung disease (such as a search for metastases) right and left lateral radiographs, +/− a DV or VD, should always be obtained. For cardiac examination a right lateral and DV are recommended.

If performing radiography under general anaesthesia, the animal should be radiographed as soon as possible after induction, as collapse of the dependent lung area occurs quickly and can mimic pathology. Ideally, the patient should be kept in sternal recumbency until the lateral radiograph is to be taken. Manual inflation of the chest (taking all necessary safety precautions for the person doing this) will be of great benefit in aerating the lungs and improving the image. The kV should be reduced slightly, by about 2–5 kV.

Lateral view (Fig. 24.36)

Place a foam pad under the sternum to raise it to the same height above table-top as the spine. Draw the forelimbs forwards with tapes or sandbags to prevent them from obscuring the cranial thorax. Restrain the hindlimbs with a sandbag and place a further sandbag carefully over the neck. Centre on the middle of the fifth rib and level with the caudal border of

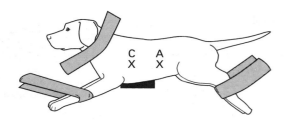

Fig. 24.36 Positioning for lateral chest/abdomen views.

the scapula. Collimate to include lung fields and expose on inspiration for maximum aeration.

Identify the trachea, heart, aorta, caudal vena cava, diaphragm, bronchovascular lung markings and skeletal structures. The oesophagus is not normally visible on plain films.

Dorsoventral view (Fig. 24.37)   The dorsoventral view and not the ventrodorsal must be used for assessment of the heart because in the latter position the heart may tip to one side. Position the patient in sternal recumbency, crouching symmetrically. Push the elbows laterally to 'prop' up the dog or cat. Drape a sandbag over the neck to keep the head down, shaking the sand into either end to produce a sparsely filled area in the middle of the sandbag. It may be useful to rest the patient's chin on a foam pad or wooden block. Centre in the midline between the tips of the scapulae. Collimate to include the lung fields and expose on inspiration.

Identify the structures visible on the lateral view.

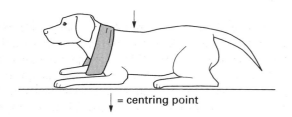

↓ = centring point

Fig. 24.37 Positioning for dorsoventral chest view.

Ventrodorsal view (Fig. 24.38)   Patients must never be placed on their backs if pleural fluid, pneumothorax or a ruptured diaphragm is suspected as this may cause respiratory embarrassment.

Position in dorsal recumbency using a radiolucent trough or sandbags around the hind end. Ensure that the patient is

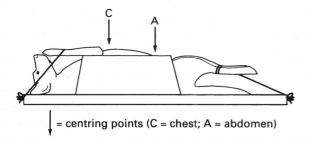

↓ = centring points (C = chest; A = abdomen)

Fig. 24.38 Positioning for ventrodorsal chest/abdomen.

lying straight and not tipped to one side. Draw the forelimbs forwards with tapes or by placing a sandbag gently over them. Secure the hindlimbs too if necessary. Centre on the mid-point of the sternum, collimate to the lung field and expose on inspiration.

Identify the same structures as on the lateral and DV views.

Abdomen

Lateral view (Fig. 24.36)   Position the patient in lateral recumbency and pad up the sternum if necessary. Restrain the fore- and hindlimbs with sandbags, ensuring that the hindlimbs are pulled well back so that they do not obscure the caudal abdomen. Place a further sandbag over the neck (sometimes one end of the sandbag placed around the forelimbs can be used for this). Centre over the area of interest and collimate as necessary. Expose on expiration to give a more 'spread out' view of the abdominal viscera.

Identify the liver, spleen, kidneys, bladder, stomach, small and large intestine and skeletal structures.

Ventrodorsal view (Fig. 24.38)   Position in dorsal recumbency using a trough, or by placing sandbags on either side of the chest. Sandbag or tape the fore- and hindlimbs if necessary. Centre and collimate as required and expose on expiration. **Dorsoventral** views of the abdomen are rarely performed as the viscera are usually compressed and distorted but may be all that is possible if the patient is dyspnoeic and cannot be placed on its back.

Identify the same structures as on the lateral view.

Skull

Skull views generally require general anaesthesia, as accurate positioning cannot otherwise be achieved.

Lateral view   Position the animal in lateral recumbency, using foam wedges under the nose and mandible to ensure that the line between the eyes is vertical and that the midline is horizontal and parallel to the table. The degree of padding depends on the shape of the patient's skull. It may also be necessary to pad the neck and sternum. Centre and collimate as required.

Identify the cranium, frontal sinuses, nasal chambers, teeth, mandibles and tympanic bullae.

Dorsoventral view   Place the animal in a crouching position, with the chin resting on a wooden or foam block, on which is placed the cassette. Secure the head with a sandbag over the neck if necessary. Ensure that the line between the eyes is horizontal. Centre and collimate as required. If an endotracheal tube is being used, it may require removal before exposure so as not to obscure any structures in the midline.

Ventrodorsal view   Place the animal in dorsal recumbency in a trough, with the head and neck extended. Put foam pads under the neck and nose. Hold the nose down using a tape placed behind the upper canine teeth, or using sticky tape.

Lateral oblique view for tympanic bullae
Place the animal in lateral recumbency with the side to be radiographed down. Using foam pads, rotate the skull about 20° around its long axis, towards the VD position (this will skyline the tympanic bulla nearest the table). Centre and collimate by palpation of the bulla. It is usually necessary to repeat the procedure for the other bulla, either to give a normal for comparison or to check if it is also affected. Care should be taken to ensure that the positioning is the same for the two sides.

Intra-oral DV (occlusal) view for nasal chambers   This view always requires general anaesthesia. Place the animal in sternal recumbency with the chin resting on a wooden or foam block. Insert a non-screen film or flexible plastic cassette into the mouth above the tongue, placing it corner first so as to get it as far back in the mouth as possible. Ensure that the head is level. Centre and collimate over the nasal chambers.

Many other views of the skull are possible but their description is beyond the scope of this chapter. They include the intra-oral VD for the mandibles, special obliques for temporomandibular joints, obliques for dental arcades and the frontal sinuses, skyline views of the frontal sinuses and cranium and the open-mouth view for tympanic bullae and the odontoid peg of C2.

Vertebral column

Spinal pathology is often undramatic and therefore requires particularly careful positioning, especially if disc spaces are under scrutiny. General anaesthesia is usually required in order to obtain diagnostic radiographs. Great care should be taken with patients that may have spinal fractures or dislocations in case positioning for radiography causes displacement of the fragments; in such cases the use of a horizontal beam for VD views could be considered as this will remove the need to roll the patient onto its back.

It is not possible to get an accurate picture of the entire spine on one film, since the X-ray beam is diverging and will not equally penetrate all disc spaces, and so it is usually necessary to take serial radiographs of small areas. In medium and large dogs, up to six films may be required for a spinal survey as follows:

- Cervical C1–C6.
- Cervico-thoracic C6–T3.
- Thoracic T3–T11.
- Thoraco-lumbar T11–L3.
- Lumbar L1–L7.
- Sacral and caudal (coccygeal) L6–Cd4.

Once a lesion is suspected, collimated views taken over the area of interest should be made. For disc disease, only the few disc spaces in the centre of the film are fully assessable (Fig. 24.39).

Lateral view   Ample use of foam pads is required to prevent the spine sagging or rotating (Fig. 24.40) and to ensure that it forms a straight line parallel to the table-top. Centre and collimate to the area of interest by the palpation of bony landmarks (in obese animals the spine may be some distance below the skin surface).

Ventrodorsal (VD) views   The patient is positioned in symmetrical dorsal recumbency using a trough or sandbags. The limbs are secured as appropriate. Centre and collimate over the area of interest. For VD views of the cervical spine and cervicothoracic junction, the X-ray beam must be angled 15° to 20° towards the patient's head in order to pass through the disc spaces.

The forelimbs

Although many diagnoses may be possible from a single view (usually the mediolateral) it is often necessary to obtain the orthogonal view too (i.e. the view at right-angles to this). For investigation of suspected joint disease centre over the joint of interest. Some joint diseases, such as osteochondrosis (OCD) are commonly bilateral and so the opposite limb should be radiographed as well. For long bones, centre over the middle of the bone but include the joints above and below, with the long bone parallel to the film. If there is any doubt about the significance of a lesion or if the normal length of a bone must be known for fracture repair, then the opposite limb will serve as a useful control.

Mediolateral (ML) scapula   Lie the animal on the side to be radiographed. Pull the lower limb caudally and the upper limb cranially, flexing it towards the head and securing it with a tape. It may also be pushed slightly dor-

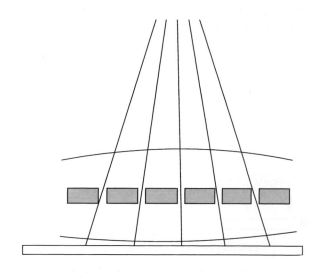

Fig. 24.39 Radiography of disc spaces.

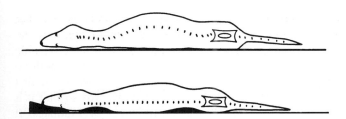

Fig. 24.40 Use of foam pads for spinal radiography.

sally so that it lies above the level of the spine. Centre and collimate to the lower scapula by palpation.

Caudocranial (CdCr) scapula   Lie the animal on its back in a trough, tipping it slightly over to the side not under investigation. Draw the limb cranially and secure in maximum extension with a tape. Centre and collimate by palpation.

Mediolateral shoulder (Fig. 24.41)   Lie the animal on the side to be radiographed. Draw the lower limb cranially and secure it; pull the upper limb well back out of the way. Extend the head and neck. Centre and collimate to the shoulder joint by palpation.

Caudocranial shoulder   As for caudocranial scapula but centre on the shoulder joint.

Cranioproximal–craniodistal (CrPr–CrDi) shoulder   This special oblique view is used to skyline the bicipital groove in cases of suspected shoulder tenosynovitis. With the patient in sternal recumbency (as for a DV chest) the affected forelimb is flexed at the shoulder and elbow, the opposite side of the body being raised on a sandbag and the head displaced away from the shoulder under investigation. The cassette is supported on the forearm beneath the shoulder joint. Centre and collimate to the shoulder joint.

Mediolateral humerus (Fig. 24.41)   As for the lateral shoulder but centre on the humerus.

Caudocranial humerus   As for the caudocranial scapula, but centre on the humerus.

Craniocaudal humerus   An alternative view. Lie the animal on its back and pull the affected limb caudally, securing with a tape. The humerus should lie parallel to the film. It may not be possible to use a trough for this view.

Mediolateral elbow   **Extended view** is as for mediolateral shoulder, but centre on the elbow (Fig. 24.41).

Flexed view (more useful for assessing degenerative joint disease) is as for mediolateral shoulder, but flex the lower limb at the elbow so that the paw comes up to the patient's chin. Secure with a tape or sandbag (Fig. 24.42a).

Craniocaudal elbow   Position the animal in sternal recumbency with both forelimbs extended and pulled cranially. Turn the head and neck to the non-affected side and restrain by draping a sandbag over the neck. Take care that the affected elbow does not slide sideways. Centre on the elbow joint, angling the beam about 10° towards the patient's tail (Fig. 24.42b).

Caudocranial elbow   An alternative view. As for caudocranial shoulder, but centre on the elbow joint.

Mediolateral forearm (radius and ulna), carpus and paw (Fig. 24.41)   Lie the animal on the affected side, drawing the lower limb cranially and the upper limb caudally out of the way. Ensure that a lateral position is achieved using foam pads or sticky tape. Centre and collimate to the appropriate area.

For individual toes, it may be useful to separate them by drawing the affected one forwards and the others backwards with tapes.

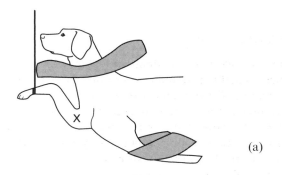

(a)

X = centring point

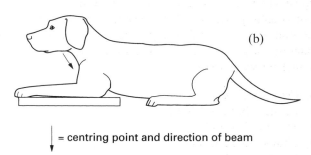

(b)

↓ = centring point and direction of beam

Fig. 24.42 (a) Positioning for flexed lateral elbow. (b) Positioning for craniocaudal elbow view.

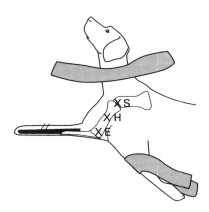

Fig. 24.41 Positioning for lateral forelimb views. X = centring points; S = shoulder; H = humerus; E = elbow.

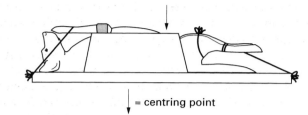

↓ = centring point

Fig. 24.43 Positioning for assessment of hip dysplasia.

Craniocaudal forearm and dorsopalmar (Dpa) carpus and paw   As for craniocaudal elbow, but centre and collimate to the appropriate area and use a vertical beam.

The hindlimbs

Lateral pelvis   Position the patient on its side, using foam pads under the spine and sternum to achieve a true lateral position. Centre on the hip joints.

Ventrodorsal (VD) pelvis   The **extended hip position** will be described in some detail as it is required for official assessment of hip dysplasia in dogs. It requires general anaesthesia or a reasonable degree of sedation.

Place the patient on its back in a trough, ensuring that it is perfectly upright and not tipped to either side. Extend the forelimbs cranially and secure them with tapes; a sandbag may also be draped over the sternum, taking care not to impair respiration. Extend the hindlimbs caudally using tapes looped just above the hocks and tied to hooks on the edge of the table. The femora should be parallel to each other and to the table-top, and the stifles should be rotated inwards by means of a further tape or Velcro/Vetrap band tied firmly around them (Fig. 24.43). Centre on the pubic symphysis. Perfect positioning may be achieved in this way without the need for manual restraint.

For submission to the BVA/Kennel Club Hip Dysplasia Scoring Scheme the film must be permanently identified with the patient's Kennel Club number, the date and a right or left marker before processing. Radiographs labelled after processing will not be accepted by the scheme.

Identify the various anatomical areas of the hip joint assessed under the scoring scheme.

The **flexed or frog-legged view** allows some assessment of the hips but is not as satisfactory as the extended view. The hindlimbs are flexed and allowed to fall to either side. Sandbags may be used to steady the hindpaws.

The **dorsal acetabular rim (DAR) view** is used to provide measurements prior to triple pelvic osteotomy surgery. The dog lies in sternal recumbency with a trough under its chest. The hindlimbs are pulled forwards so that the pelvis is rotated towards a more vertical position and the hocks are raised on sandbags. The pelvis is palpated to ensure that it is symmetrical and the tail is extended caudally. Centring is at the base of the tail. The exposure needs to be increased

about 5–10 kV from that used for the extended VD projection.

Mediolateral femur   Two methods are used, both requiring the patient to lie on the affected side. In the first method the uppermost limb is pulled upwards so that it is roughly vertical, and secured with tapes or sandbags. It may be difficult to prevent superimposition of part of this limb over the femur under investigation and so an alternative is to pull the lower hindlimb cranially and the upper hindlimb back. In this case the lower femur is radiographed through the soft tissues of the abdomen.

Craniocaudal femur   As for the extended view of the hips, but centring and collimating to the femur. It may help to tilt the patient slightly away from the side being radiographed. Centre to the mid-femur and include the hip and stifle.

Caudocranial femur   An alternative to the CrCd projection. With the dog in dorsal recumbency, the thorax is supported in a trough and sandbags are draped over the forelimbs. Using a tie around the hock of the affected leg, the leg is pulled cranially and the tie is secured around cleats at the head of the table. The femur should be parallel to the table top, and may be held away from the dog's body using a foam wedge. This projection shows the head of the femur very well with no superimposition of the pelvis or tail.

Mediolateral stifle (Fig. 24.44)   Position the animal with the affected side down. Move the other hindlimb upwards or caudally so that it is not superimposed over the lower stifle. Ensure that a true lateral projection is obtained by placing a small pad under the hock. In obese animals, the mammary tissue or sheath may obscure the stifle joint; this may be prevented by tying a tape around the caudal abdomen to act like a corset. Centre and collimate on the stifle by palpation.

Craniocaudal stifle   Similar to ventrodorsal pelvis (extended view) by positioning in dorsal recumbency and extending the affected limb. The other hindlimb may be left free. It may be useful to tilt the patient slightly away from the affected side to ensure a true craniocaudal view.

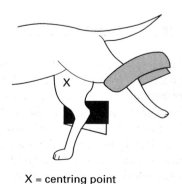

X = centring point

Fig. 24.44 Positioning for lateral stifle view.

Caudocranial stifle An alternative view. Position in sternal recumbency and extend the affected limb caudally. The opposite side of the patient may need to be raised on sandbags to obtain a true CdCr position.

Mediolateral tibia, hock and paw Lie the patient with the affected side down. Draw the upper limb cranially or caudally to prevent superimposition. Use sandbags to achieve a true lateral position if necessary. Centre and collimate to the required area.

Craniocaudal tibia and dorsoplantar hock As for craniocaudal stifle, but centre and collimate to the appropriate area. For the hock, the tape is looped around the paw. To reduce the object–film distance for the hock view, it may be necessary to raise the cassette from the table with a wooden block.

Dorsoplantar paw Two methods are available. Firstly, the patient may be positioned as for craniocaudal stifle, but with the paw held down to the cassette with strong radiolucent tape. Alternatively, the animal may crouch, with the affected paw pulled slightly outwards and resting on the cassette.

KEY POINTS
Positioning
- Manual restraint must be avoided whenever possible, and positioning instead achieved using sedation/anaesthesia and appropriate positioning aids.
- The geometry of the X-ray beam must be taken into account in order to produce accurate and clear images.
- Place the area of interest as close to the film as possible.
- Centre over the region of interest and collimate to the smallest area possible.
- Two views at right-angles to each other are often required, and further projections may be necessary in some cases.

Radiographic contrast studies

Although much information about soft tissues can be gained from good-quality radiographs, certain structures may be unclear either because they are radiolucent or because they are masked by other structures. In addition, the inner lining (the mucosal surface) of hollow, fluid-filled organs cannot be assessed because it is of the same radiographic density as the fluid contained within the organ. A good example is the urinary bladder, which appears simply as a homogeneous pear-shaped structure of soft tissue/fluid density.

Contrast studies aim to render these structures and organs more apparent and to outline the mucosal surface where appropriate, either by changing the radio-opacity of the structure itself or by altering that of the surrounding tissue. Both procedures increase the contrast between the structure of interest and the surrounding tissues, allowing assessment of its **position, size, shape** and **internal architecture**. If serial films are taken over a period, it may also be possible to gain some idea of the **function** of the organ (e.g. rate of stomach emptying).

Many contrast techniques are possible, but only those of most relevance to veterinary radiography will be discussed.

Types of contrast media

Two broad groups of contrast media exist: positive and negative. **Positive contrast agents** contain elements of high atomic number which absorb a large proportion of the X-ray beam and are therefore relatively radio-opaque, appearing whiter on radiographs than do normal tissues. They are said to provide **positive contrast** with soft tissues. The agents most commonly used are compounds of barium (atomic number 56) and iodine (atomic number 53).

- **Barium sulphate preparations**. Barium sulphate is a white, chalky material which may be mixed with water to produce a fine colloidal suspension. It is available as a liquid, a paste or a powder which is made up to the desired thickness by the addition of water. It is used almost exclusively in the gut and is not suitable for injection into blood vessels. Being inert, it is non-toxic and well-tolerated by the patient and it produces excellent contrast. Its main disadvantages are that if it is aspirated it may cause pneumonia and if it leaks through a perforated area of gut into the thoracic or abdominal cavities it may provoke the formation of granulomas or adhesions. Barium should not be given to constipated patients as it will exacerbate the condition.
- **Water-soluble iodine preparations**. The iodine compounds are water-soluble and may therefore be injected into the bloodstream. However, anaphylaxis is a possibility (although extremely rare) and so an emergency protocol for such an eventuality should be in place. They are then excreted by the kidney and outline the upper urinary tract. They are also safe to use in many other parts of the body. Intravascular injection of these media usually causes nausea and retching and so the patient must be heavily sedated or anaesthetised. Despite being radio-opaque, they appear as clear solutions to the eye (unlike barium).

  Being water-soluble, the iodine preparations are absorbed by the body and so should be used in the gut in preference to barium if there is a possibility of perforation. However, due to the high osmotic pressure of most of these media they absorb fluid during their passage through the gut with the result that they become progressively diluted, so that the pictures they produce have much less contrast than those obtained using barium and there is a risk of collapse in a dehydrated patient. They are therefore not routinely used for gut studies.

Many different water-soluble iodine preparations are available but most contain diatrizoate, metrizoate or iothalamate as the active ingredients. For myelography, special iodine media with lower osmotic pressures must be used to avoid irritation of the spinal cord, and these are iohexol and iopamidol.

Negative contrast agents are gases which, because of their low density, appear relatively radiolucent or black on radiographs, providing **negative contrast** with soft tissues. Room air is usually used in veterinary radiography.

Studies on hollow organs may utilise both a positive and a negative agent in a **double-contrast study**. In these cases a small amount of positive contrast agent is used to coat the inner lining of the organ, which is then distended with gas. This provides excellent mucosal detail and prevents the obliteration of small filling defects, such as calculi, by large volumes of positive contrast. Examples of commonly performed studies are double-contrast cystography (bladder) and double-contrast gastrography (stomach).

Patient preparation

Adequate patient preparation is essential before many of the contrast studies. Prior to a barium study of the stomach or small intestine, the animal must be starved for at least 24 hours to empty the gut of residual ingesta. If food remains in the gut it will mix with the barium, mimicking pathology. Patients should also be starved prior to studies on the kidneys, as a full stomach may obscure the renal shadows. However, most patients are anaesthetised for kidney studies and so will have been starved anyway.

The presence of faeces in the colon will also obscure much abdominal detail and so an enema is often required prior to the contrast study. This is particularly important before investigations of the urinary tract as faeces may obscure or distort the kidneys, ureters, bladder or urethra. The colon must be completely empty of faeces if a barium enema is to be performed as even a small amount of faecal material will produce filling defects, giving the appearance of severe pathology. The patient should therefore be starved for 24 hours and the colon must be thoroughly washed out with tepid saline or water.

Plain radiographs must **always** be taken and examined before the contrast study commences. They are assessed for the following factors:

- Any pathology previously overlooked.
- Correct exposure factors, to avoid the need to repeat films after the contrast study has begun.
- Adequacy of patient preparation.
- Assessment of the amount of contrast medium required.
- Comparison with subsequent radiographs (to show whether any shadows on the images are due to contrast media or were already present).

A brief description of common contrast studies is given below. More detailed information can be found in Chapter 13 of *Principles of Veterinary Radiography* (Douglas et al., 1987) and in Chapter 7 of the *Manual of Small Animal Diagnostic Imaging* (Lee, 1995) produced by the BSAVA.

Gastrointestinal tract

Oesophagus (barium swallow)

- **Indications**. Regurgitation, retching, dysphagia (difficulty in swallowing).
- **Preparation**. No patient preparation required; plain radiographs.
- **Equipment**. Barium paste is usually preferred, since it is sticky and adheres to the oesophageal mucosa for several minutes. Barium liquid may be used if paste is not available (5–50 ml depending on patient size). Oral water-soluble iodine preparations should be used if a perforation is suspected. Liquid barium mixed with tinned meat should be used if a megaoesophagus is suspected clinically or on plain radiographs, as paste or liquid alone may fail to demonstrate the full extent of the oesophagus.
- **Restraint**. Moderate sedation; heavy sedation or general anaesthesia is contraindicated because of the possibility of regurgitation and aspiration.
- **Technique**. Barium paste is deposited on the back of the tongue. Barium or iodine liquids should be given slowly by syringe into the buccal pouch, allowing the patient to swallow a small amount at a time to avoid aspiration. Barium/meat mixture is usually eaten voluntarily as animals with megaoesophagus tend to be hungry.

Radiographs are taken immediately after administration of the contrast medium. Lateral views are usually sufficient but ventrodorsal views may also occasionally be indicated. Two separate radiographs may be needed to cover the cervical and thoracic areas of the oesophagus.

Stomach (gastrogram)

Two techniques are used: barium only or barium and air (double-contrast gastrogram). The latter gives better mucosal detail.

- **Indications**. Persistent vomiting, haematemesis, displacement of stomach, assessment of liver size.
- **Preparation**. 24 hours of starvation; enema if necessary; plain radiographs.
- **Equipment**. Barium liquid (20–100 ml depending on patient size). NB: Barium paste and barium/meat mixtures are not suitable and oral water-soluble iodine preparations should be used if a perforation is suspected. Syringe or stomach tube plus three-way tap.
- **Restraint**. Moderate sedation (to allow positioning); acepromazine has least effect on gut.

- **Technique**. (i) *Barium only*. Administer the required dose of barium liquid by syringe or stomach tube. Roll the patient to coat the gastric mucosa. Take four radiographs; DV, VD, left and right lateral recumbency. Take further radiographs as indicated, e.g. to follow stomach emptying.

  (ii) *Double-contrast gastrogram*. Stomach tube the patient. Give liquid barium, using the syringe and three-way tap, roll the patient (with the stomach tube still in place) and then distend the stomach with room air. Remove the stomach tube and immediately take four views of the stomach as above.

Method (ii) is preferred if a definite gastric lesion is suspected, but follow-up radiographs of the small intestine may be hard to interpret because of the presence of the air.

Small intestine (barium series)

- **Indications**. Persistent vomiting, haematemesis, abdominal masses, weight loss, malabsorption, intestinal dilatation (usually unrewarding in cases of chronic diarrhoea).
- **Preparation**. As for stomach.
- **Equipment**. As for stomach.
- **Restraint**. As for stomach.
- **Technique**. Administer liquid barium by syringe or stomach tube. Take serial lateral and VD radiographs to follow the passage of barium through the small intestine (usually at intervals of 15–60 minutes, plus a 24-hour radiograph) depending on any pathology seen.

Large intestine

Three techniques are used: air only (pneumocolon), barium only (barium enema) and barium and air (double-contrast enema). A pneumocolon will outline soft tissue masses within the colon and the use of barium alone will demonstrate displacement or compression of the colon; but for most purposes a double-contrast enema is indicated as it yields maximum information about the colonic mucosa.

- **Indications**. Tenesmus, melaena, colitis, identification of certain abdominal masses.
- **Preparation**. 24 hours of starvation; thorough enema, using tepid water or saline until no faecal matter returns; plain radiographs.
- **Equipment**. Cuffed rectal catheter or Foley catheter. For pneumocolon: three-way tap and large syringe. For barium and double-contrast enemas: gravity feed can and hose or a proprietary barium enema bag; barium sulphate liquid diluted 1:1 with warm water.
- **Restraint**. Moderate to deep sedation (to allow positioning) or general anaesthesia.
- **Technique**. (i) *Pneumocolon*. Position the rectal catheter and inflate the colon with room air, using the syringe and three-way tap, until air leaks out around the catheter.

Take lateral and VD radiographs without removing the catheter.

(ii) *Barium enema*. Position the rectal catheter and allow barium to flow into the colon under gravity, until it just begins to leak out around the catheter (usually 10–20 ml/kg is required). Take lateral and VD radiographs without removing the catheter.

(iii) *Double-contrast enema*. As (ii) for initial radiographs. Then allow excess barium to drain out and reinflate with air. This can be a very messy procedure unless a special barium enema bag is used; when the bag is lowered to the floor the barium drains back down the tube from the colon into the bag. If the bag is then compressed, the air within it will inflate the colon (Fig. 24.45). Repeat the lateral and VD radiographs after the introduction of the air.

Urogenital tract

Kidneys and ureters (intravenous urography (IVU), excretion urography)

Contrast radiography of the upper urinary tract involves the intravenous injection of a water-soluble iodine preparation which is subsequently excreted by, and opacifies, the kidneys and ureters. Two methods are used: rapid injection of a small volume of a very concentrated solution (**bolus intravenous urogram**) and a slow infusion of a large volume of a weaker solution (**infusion intravenous urogram**). The bolus

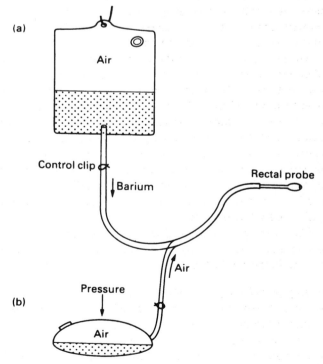

Fig. 24.45 Barium enema bag. In position (a) barium flows under gravity into the colon. In position (b) barium empties from the colon into the bag and then pressure on the bag will distend the colon with air for the double-contrast effect.

IVU produces excellent opacification of the kidneys. The infusion IVU is preferred for investigation of the ureters, as it produces more ureteric distension by inducing a greater degree of osmotic diuresis.

- **Indications**. Identification of kidney size, shape and position, haematuria, urinary incontinence.
- **Preparation**. 24 hours of starvation; enema; plain radiographs.
- **Equipment**. Intravenous catheter (perivascular leakage of contrast medium is irritant).

    For bolus IVU: syringe and three-way tap; concentrated contrast medium (300–400 mg iodine/ml) at a dose of up to 850 mg iodine/kg bodyweight, i.e. about 50 ml for a 25 kg dog (if there is poor renal function, the dose may be increased by up to 50% more).

    For infusion IVU: drip giving set; weaker contrast medium (150–200 mg iodine/ml) at a dose rate of up to 1200 mg iodine/kg bodyweight, i.e. about 200 ml for a 25 kg dog. Concentrated solutions may be diluted with saline for this study if necessary.
- **Restraint**. General anaesthesia to prevent patient nausea and allow positioning.
- **Technique**. (i) *Bolus IVU*. Warm the contrast medium to body temperature to reduce its viscosity and make it easier to inject. Inject the whole amount as quickly as possible. Take lateral and VD radiographs immediately and at 2, 5, 10 minutes and so on as indicated by the initial pictures.

    (ii) *Infusion IVU*. If the patient has urinary incontinence and the position of the ureteric endings is being assessed, a pneumocystogram should be performed first to produce a radiolucent background. Infuse the total dose over 10–15 minutes. Take lateral and VD radiographs once most of the contrast medium has run in. Oblique radiographs are also useful for ureteric endings.

Bladder (cystography)

Direct or retrograde cystography may be performed in three ways: using negative contrast (**pneumocystogram**), positive contrast (**positive contrast cystogram**) or a combination of the two (**double-contrast cystogram**). Pneumocystography is quick and easy but gives poor mucosal detail and will fail to demonstrate small bladder tears, as air leaking out will resemble intestinal gas. Positive contrast cystography is ideal for the detection of bladder ruptures but will mask small lesions and calculi. Double-contrast cystography is usually the method of choice as it produces excellent mucosal detail and will demonstrate all types of calculi. A positive contrast cystogram will also be seen following an IVU, if the patient cannot be catheterised for any reason. Excreted contrast should be mixed with urine already present in the bladder by rolling the animal. This type of cystogram is not ideal as adequate bladder distension cannot be ensured.

- **Indications**. Haematuria, dysuria, urinary incontinence, urinary retention, suspected bladder rupture, identification of the bladder if not visible on the plain radiograph, assessment of prostatic size.
- **Preparation**. Enema, if faeces are present; plain radiographs.
- **Equipment**. Appropriate urinary catheter; syringe and three-way tap; dilute water-soluble iodine contrast medium for positive and double-contrast cystogram.
- **Restraint**. Sedation or general anaesthesia to allow catheterisation and positioning.
- **Technique**. Catheterise bladder and drain completely of urine (obtaining sterile urine sample if required).

    (i) *Pneumocystogram*. Inflate the bladder slowly with room air, using a syringe and three-way tap. The bladder should be inflated until it is felt to be moderately firm by abdominal palpation (usually requires 30–300 ml air depending on patient size).

    (ii) *Positive contrast cystogram*. As for (i), but using diluted iodine contrast medium instead of air. However, for detection of bladder rupture, a much smaller quantity is required.

    (iii) *Double-contrast cystogram*. Inject 2–15 ml iodine contrast medium at a concentration of about 150 mg iodine/ml into the empty bladder via the catheter. Palpate the abdomen or roll the patient to coat the bladder mucosa. Inflate with air until the bladder feels turgid. The bladder wall will be lightly coated with positive contrast, and residual contrast will pool in the centre of the bladder shadow, highlighting calculi and other filling defects.

Lateral radiographs are usually more informative, but VD and oblique views may be taken if required.

Urethra (retrograde urethrography – dogs; retrograde vaginourethrography – bitches)

- **Indications**. Haematuria, dysuria, urinary incontinence, urinary retention, prostatic disease, vaginal disease.
- **Preparation**. Enema, if faeces are likely to obscure the urethra on either view; plain radiographs.
- **Equipment**. Appropriate urinary catheter; syringe; dilute iodine contrast medium (150 mg iodine/ml) (may be mixed with equal amount of KY jelly for studies on male dogs, to increase urethral distension); gentle bowel clamp (for bitches).
- **Restraint**. Sedation (dogs) or general anaesthesia (bitches).
- **Technique**. (i) *Retrograde urethrography (males)*. Insert the urinary catheter into the penile urethra. Occlude the urethral opening manually, to prevent leakage of contrast. Inject 5–15 ml contrast or contrast/KY jelly mixture slowly. Release the urethral occlusion and stand back prior to exposure (or make the injection wearing lead mittens and an apron, and ensuring tight collimation to exclude the hands). Lateral views are most useful and should be taken with the hindlegs pulled forwards for the ischial arch and backwards for the penile urethra.

(ii) *Retrograde vaginourethrography (females)*. Snip off the tip of a Foley catheter, distal to the bulb. Insert the catheter just inside the vulval lips, inflate the bulb and clamp the vulval lips together with the bowel clamp to hold the catheter in place. Inject up to 1 ml/kg bodyweight of iodine contrast medium carefully (vaginal rupture has been reported). Lateral views are most informative, and demonstrate filling of the vagina and urethra.

In cats these studies are rarely performed, but may be carried out using simple cat catheters.

Spine (myelography)

A narrow space surrounds the spinal cord as it runs along the vertebral column; this is called the **subarachnoid space** and it contains **cerebrospinal fluid (CSF)**. It may be opacified by the injection of positive contrast medium and will then demonstrate the spinal cord, showing areas of cord swelling (e.g. tumours) or cord compression (e.g. prolapsed intervertebral discs) not evident on plain radiographs. This technique, which is called **myelography**, requires the use of special water-soluble iodine preparations which have lower osmotic pressures than do the other iodine media and which are therefore less irritant to nervous tissue. The two low osmolar contrast media currently in use in human and veterinary myelography are iohexol and iopamidol.

Two approaches may be made to the subarachnoid space: the one most commonly used in veterinary radiology is the **cisternal puncture**, where the needle is inserted into the cisterna magna – the cranial end of the subarachnoid space just behind the skull. Myelography may also be performed by injection in the lumbar area via a **lumbar puncture**, which is more commonly used in humans. Lumbar myelography involves passing the needle through the spinal cord and injecting into the ventral subarachnoid space. Both techniques involve practice and skill and the patient must be anaesthetised to prevent movement during needle placement or injection.

- **Indications.** Spinal pain, spinal neurological signs (ataxia, paralysis), identification of prolapsed intervertebral discs prior to surgery.
- **Preparation.** Clip relevant area, i.e. caudal to skull or over lumbar spine.
- **Equipment.** Spinal needle of suitable length depending on patient size; contrast medium, warmed to body temperature to reduce viscosity and ease injection (dose rate 0.25–0.45 ml/kg of 200–350 mg iodine/ml solution – dose administered depends on size of patient and expected site of lesion, but no more than a maximum of 15 ml); syringe; sample bottles for CSF if required for analysis; some means of elevating the head end of the table for cisternal punctures, to aid flow of contrast along the spine.
- **Restraint.** General anaesthesia.

- **Technique.** (i) *Cisternal puncture*. Elevate the table to about 10° tilt with the head at the raised end. Clip and surgically cleanse the injection site. Flex the head to a 90° angle with neck. Insert the needle carefully into the cisterna magna, between the skull and atlas (Fig. 24.46), advancing the needle slowly until CSF drips out of the hub. Collect several millilitres of CSF then inject warmed contrast medium slowly. Remove the needle and extend the head again. Take several lateral radiographs until either contrast reaches the lesion or the whole spine is shown well. VD and oblique views may also be taken, especially if a lesion is found. Improved filling of the subarachnoid space in the lower neck area can be ensured by obtaining DV rather than VD views of this area. When the animal is on its back for the VD view, this area is furthest from the table and contrast medium runs cranially and caudally away from the area of interest, but with the dog in sternal recumbency, this area is closest to the table and therefore contrast pools here.

(ii) *Lumbar puncture*. Clip and surgically cleanse the injection site. Flex the vertebral column by pulling the hindlimbs forwards. Insert the needle carefully (usually at L5–6); as it passes through the cauda equina the animal's hindlegs and anus will usually twitch slightly. Little or no CSF may appear from this site, and if this is the case a small test injection is required to check needle placement. Inject contrast medium. Remove the needle, extend the spine and take radiographs as above.

N.B. Keep the head raised during the recovery period, since contrast medium entering the brain may precipitate fits.

Other contrast techniques

Some other contrast techniques occasionally performed in veterinary practice are described briefly.

Angiocardiography

Angiocardiography is used to demonstrate both congenital and acquired cardiac disease. It involves the opacification of the heart chambers and major vessels by the injection of a

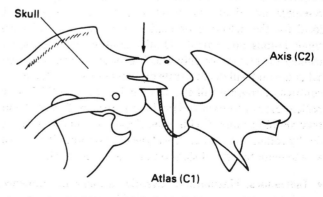

Fig. 24.46 Myelography: site for cisternal puncture.

bolus of concentrated water-soluble iodine contrast medium. The procedure requires general anaesthesia to prevent patient discomfort or movement. The contrast medium may be injected into the jugular or cephalic vein (**non-selective angiocardiography**) or deposited directly into the heart chambers and major vessels via catheters inserted surgically into the jugular vein and carotid or femoral arteries (**selective angiocardiography**). The latter will also allow blood pressure and blood-gas measurements to be made if the appropriate high-technology equipment is available.

Although a single image may provide a diagnosis, it is desirable to obtain a number of radiographs taken over a very short space of time in order to follow the bolus of contrast around the heart and lungs. This is performed using a special rapid film-changing angiography table with serial exposures made at predetermined time intervals.

Angiocardiography is performed much less often than it used to be, since similar information can usually be obtained by cardiac ultrasound (echocardiography), which is safe and non-invasive.

Portal venography

Portal venography is used to diagnose certain types of liver disease (e.g. congenital porto-systemic shunts, cirrhosis) by demonstration of the vascular system within the liver parenchyma. Under general anaesthesia a laparotomy is performed and a splenic or mesenteric vein catheterised. A small quantity of concentrated iodine contrast medium is injected as a bolus and a single radiograph taken at the end of the injection. The contrast medium enters the liver via the hepatic portal vein and in the normal animal shows branching and tapering portal vessels throughout the liver.

Bronchography

Bronchography is opacification of part of the bronchial tree using specially prepared iodine-containing medium, propyliodone. This medium is rather thicker than the other iodine media, to prevent alveolar flooding. Each study may only demonstrate the left or the right bronchial tree; if both sides are to be investigated then two studies must be performed several days apart. The patient is anaesthetised and placed in lateral recumbency with the side to be investigated down. The contrast medium is injected down the endotracheal tube via a dog urinary catheter. The patient is manipulated to ensure that the contrast has entered all of the bronchi on the side of interest and several radiographs are taken over about 10 minutes.

Bronchography may demonstrate bronchial foreign bodies, *Oslerus osleri* nodules, bronchial tumours, lung lobe torsion and bronchiectasis. It has, however, been largely superseded by bronchoscopy.

Arthrography

Arthrography is the demonstration of a joint space using negative contrast (air), positive contrast (iodine) or double-contrast techniques injected under sterile conditions. The joints most amenable to arthrography in small animals are the shoulder and stifle. General anaesthesia is required as the procedure is uncomfortable. Arthrography will demonstrate joint capsule distension or rupture and defects in the articular cartilage, which is normally radiolucent.

Fistulography

Fistulography is the opacification of sinus tracts and fistulae using water-soluble or oily iodine contrast media. Fistulography will demonstrate the extent and course of these lesions and may outline radiolucent foreign bodies such as pieces of wood.

KEY POINTS
Radiographic contrast studies
- Contrast studies allow assessment of the position, size, shape, internal architecture and occasionally the function of certain soft tissue organs.
- Contrast media can be divided into two main groups: positive and negative contrast agents.
- Positive and negative agents can be used together as double contrast studies to show the inside surface of hollow organs.
- Barium is used for most gastrointestinal studies.
- Water-soluble iodine compounds are administered intravascularly for a range of studies, and can also be used in a variety of other ways.
- Myelography requires the use of special low-osmolarity iodinated contrast agents to avoid damage to nervous tissue.

Other imaging techniques

Diagnostic ultrasound

Diagnostic ultrasound is being increasingly used in small-animal practice as a complementary imaging tool to radiography. Ultrasound has the advantage that it is painless and safe to both patient and operators and can therefore be used in the conscious patient without the need for sedation or anaesthesia (Fig. 24.47). It can differentiate between soft tissue and fluid, which radiography cannot, and it produces a 'real-time' or moving picture which is invaluable in the assessment of cardiac function and of peristalsis. Its main disadvantage is that it does not penetrate bone or air so it cannot be used for investigations of the skeletal system or lungs. Bone reflects all of the incident ultrasound, resulting

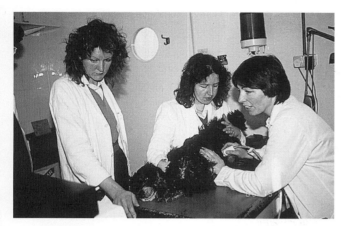

Fig. 24.47 Ultrasonography of a conscious patient.

in 'acoustic shadows' or radiating black streaks in deeper tissues (Fig. 24.48).

Ultrasonography is a difficult technique to master, since experience is required both to obtain and interpret the images. However, some simple diagnoses may be made even by relatively inexperienced operators, such as pregnancy diagnoses.

Ultrasound is sound energy at a higher frequency than can be detected by the human ear. In the diagnostic range, the frequencies used range from about 2.5 to 15 megahertz (MHz). Ultrasound of higher frequency produces better image resolution but cannot penetrate so far into the body, and so the highest frequency compatible with the type of study and patient is selected. For most small-animal ultrasonography, a 5 MHz transducer is used. For cats and very small dogs, 7.5 MHz may be preferred and for very superficial examinations such as of the eye or tendons, transducers of 10 MHz or higher are needed.

In an ultrasound machine the sound waves are created by the vibrations of special crystals in the probe or transducer which alter their shape when an electrical current is applied to them. This is known as the 'piezo-electric effect'. When the probe is applied to the patient's skin the sound waves are passed through the patient's soft tissues as pressure waves,

and at interfaces between organs or between clusters of different cells within an organ a certain percentage of the sound waves are reflected and may return to the transducer. Returning sound waves in turn create a vibration of the tissues and of the crystals in the probe and this is converted back into electrical impulses which are quickly converted by a computer into an image. The image is basically built of many tiny dots of different brightnesses depending on the strength of the returning pulses of ultrasound and the location in the body from which they have been reflected. It is a cross-sectional picture of the internal architecture of the tissues under investigation. The basic principle of ultrasound is shown in Fig. 24.49.

Ultrasound equipment consists of one or more transducers, a TV monitor and a control panel (Figs 24.50 and 24.51). There is also likely to be some sort of printer for recording the images. Ultrasound transducers are of two main types. In linear array transducers, the piezo-electric crystals are arranged in a line and the image is rectangular (Fig. 24.52). Although a wide image of the tissues close to the transducer is obtained, linear array transducers need a long contact area with the patient which is hard to achieve in small animals (remember that ultrasound does not pass through air). Linear array transducers are mainly used for rectal investigations in large animals. Sector scanning transducers are much more suitable for small-animal work, since the crystals are arranged close together so that only a small area of contact with the patient is required (Fig. 24.53). The ultrasound beam fans out to produce a triangular image which shows as much of the deeper tissues as possible. The image can be altered in depth, brightness and contrast using the ultrasound machine's controls, and measurements can be made on a frozen image. In dogs and cats the fur must usually be clipped to allow good contact between the

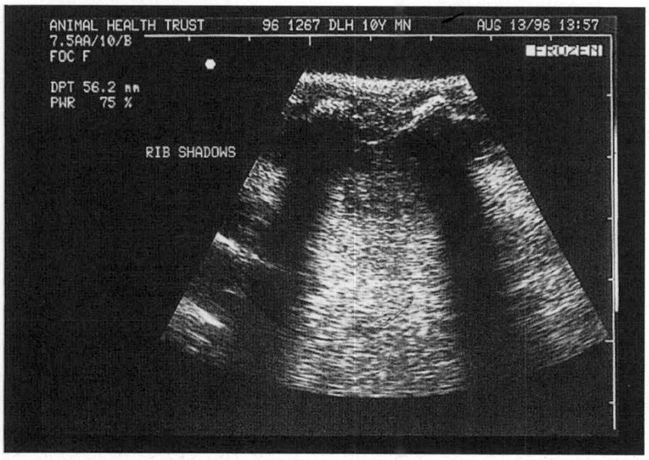

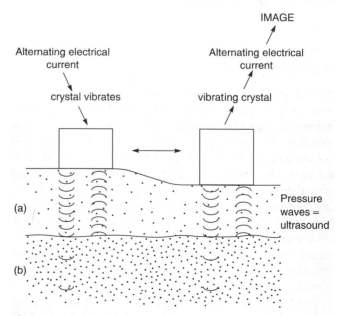

Fig. 24.49 Diagrammatic representation of the production of ultrasound waves by the transducer and the detection of returning sound waves.

Fig. 24.48 Acoustic shadows created by ribs.

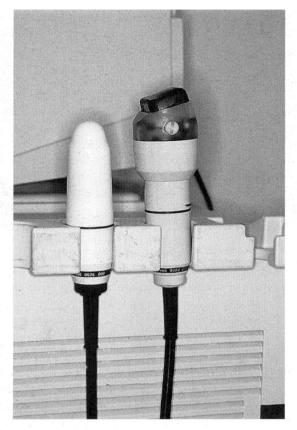

Fig. 24.50 Ultrasound transducers.

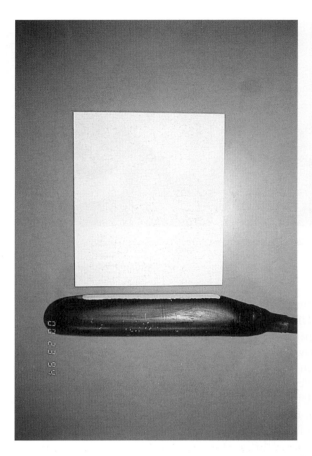

Fig. 24.52 Linear array transducer and image field.

transducer and the skin, since small air bubbles trapped in hair will greatly degrade the image. A special coupling gel is then applied to improve contact further (Fig. 24.54). In long-haired animals, it may be possible simply to part the hair and hold it aside using gel.

Most ultrasound examinations are performed with the animal in lateral or dorsal recumbency, scanning from the ventral surface of the body or through the uppermost body wall. However, echocardiography (ultrasonography of the heart) is best performed from beneath through a cut-out in a special table-top. In lateral recumbency the heart sinks towards the dependent chest wall and therefore the

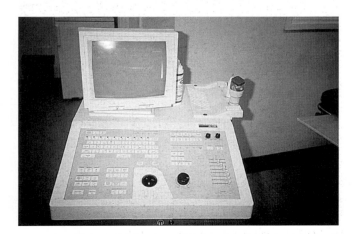

Fig. 24.51 Ultrasound TV monitor and control panel.

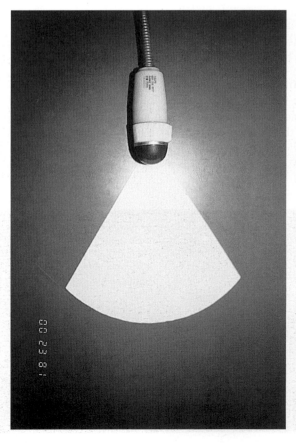

Fig. 24.53 Sector scanner transducer and image field.

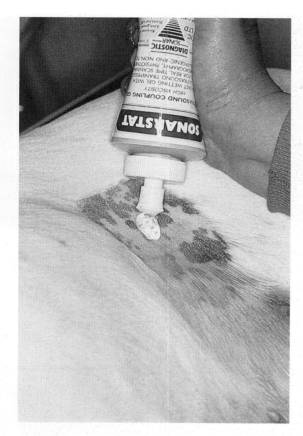

Fig. 24.54 Clipping of hair and gel application for good transducer–skin contact.

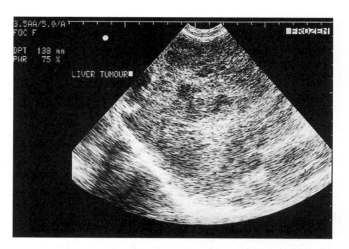

Fig. 24.56 Liver tumour in a dog, giving rise to a mottled, irregular pattern to the liver.

best acoustic window (the least intervening lung) is on the underneath side.

Most ultrasound performed uses B-mode ('brightness' mode ultrasound) as described above, to create a two-dimensional image of the tissues. Small sound reflections within tissues create a fine, granular pattern to organs, with different organs producing different brightnesses on the image (Fig. 24.55). Pathology within an organ can often be recognised as a change in the overall brightness or **echogenicity** of the organ or a mottled appearance disrupting normal architecture (Fig. 24.56). Areas of altered echogenicity are said to be anechoic (black), hypoechoic (dark) or hyperechoic (bright). Fluid is usually seen as an anechoic area because it gives rise to very few ultrasound reflections. Thus, free abdominal fluid can be seen as a black background surrounding abdominal organs (Fig. 24.57). One of the main advantages of ultrasound is that it allows examination of the abdominal structures when free fluid renders radiography unhelpful by obscuring the organs.

In November 2000 the Feline Advisory Bureau launched an ultrasonographic screening scheme for the detection of polycystic kidney disease (PKD) in cats. This follows similar schemes in a number of other countries. PKD is an inherited disease which affects mainly Persian cats, with an incidence of over 50% in the UK. Certain other pedigree breeds, such as the Exotic Shorthair, may also be affected. Although severely affected cats eventually develop renal failure, this is not usually until after their breeding life, and therefore detection of the cysts when they are subclinical means that these cats can be excluded from breeding, which should eventually eradicate the disease.

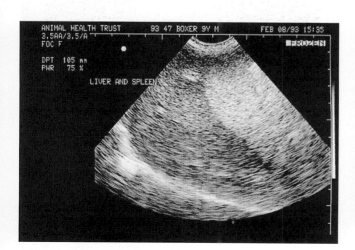

Fig. 24.55 Normal ultrasound image of liver and spleen.

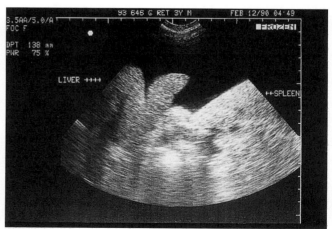

Fig. 24.57 Free abdominal fluid seen as a black area, outlining abdominal organs.

Ultrasound is increasingly used for biopsy or fine-needle aspiration of small diseased areas within organs. Since the internal organ architecture and the needle can both be seen, the needle can be guided into the affected area without damaging other structures (Fig. 24.58). This technique can often be performed with the patient conscious and avoids the need for surgical biopsy.

A further refinement of ultrasound is the use of M-mode ('movement' mode) to quantify heart motion. First, a B-mode image is obtained and a cursor (line of dots) is placed on it and moved right or left until it passes through the heart in the required position. At the touch of a button the ultrasound beam produced by the transducer is converted into a thin line which produces a vertical band of dots indicating reflections at tissue interfaces along that line. This is rapidly updated with the movement of the heart and the image scrolled along a horizontal axis with time. The resultant image shows the degree of heart motion and can be frozen to allow measurements of the heart chambers and walls in systole and diastole. Figure 24.59 shows a combined B-mode and M-mode image of a heart.

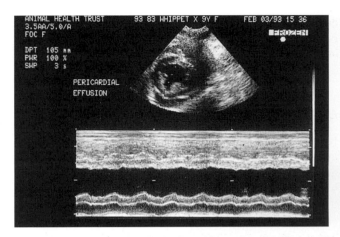

Fig. 24.59 M-mode ultrasound of a dog with a pericardial effusion. The top image is a B-mode image of the heart and the line of dots indicates the position of the fine ultrasound beam used for the M-mode study. The lower image shows the M-mode image with time along the horizontal axis. Blood in the left ventricle and pericardial fluid are seen as black areas on both images.

Computed tomography (CT scanning)

CT involves the production of a highly detailed cross-sectional radiograph of the patient's tissues. The CT scanner is a large piece of apparatus with a central orifice; the X-ray tube head moves quickly around the circumference during the exposure. The patient lies on a movable table-top which is advanced a few millimetres between exposures so that each image shows a different 'slice' of the tissues. Naturally, veterinary patients must be anaesthetised for CT scanning because of the very high doses of radiation involved (Fig. 24.60).

Although essentially a radiographic technique, CT images produce much more tissue definition than radiography and will differentiate between different types of soft tissue and between fluid and soft tissue. CT is especially valuable for imaging the skeletal system (Fig. 24.61). The images can be manipulated on a computer after acquisition to enhance

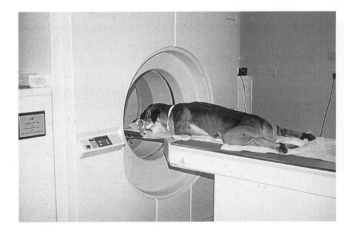

Fig. 24.60 CT scanner and patient.

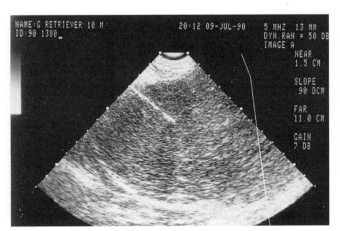

Fig. 24.58 Fine-needle aspirate of an abdominal mass, the needle being seen as a bright line entering the mass.

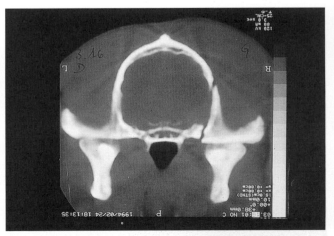

Fig. 24.61 CT scan of a skull fracture; bone appears white as in radiography. This image has been processed by the computer to 'flatten' the soft tissues into a single grey shade to emphasise bone better.

detail, a procedure known as 'post-processing'. Iodinated radiographic contrast media can be given intravenously or into the subarachnoid space to enhance the images further.

Magnetic resonance imaging (MRI scanning)

MRI is the newest diagnostic imaging technique and involves completely different physical principles, combining magnetism and radio energy. Because it does not use ionising radiation (unlike radiography and CT) it is thought to be completely safe, although veterinary patients must still be anaesthetised to keep them still during the scanning time, which may sometimes be up to an hour in complex cases. The scanner itself is a very powerful magnet, which is usually long and cylindrical, the patient lying in the centre of the magnet's bore (Fig. 24.62). The tissues within the magnet become magnetised, which has an effect on the protons of the hydrogen atoms in the body. The patient is then subjected to a series of radio waves, each lasting for several minutes; these have the effect of disorientating the protons so that they emit tiny radio signals themselves. The emitted signals are detected and converted to an image by a computer.

As with CT, the images are cross-sectional slices through the patient's tissues, but the soft tissue information produced is even greater and the images yield fantastic detail about the tissues. MRI is used particularly in the diagnosis of brain and spinal conditions in small animals (Fig. 24.63) but it can also be used to investigate many other disease processes, such as neoplasia, soft tissue foreign bodies and orthopaedic conditions. The use of MRI and to a lesser extent CT have meant that surgery and radiotherapy of brain tumours in cats and dogs can now be performed successfully. They are also very helpful in planning surgery or radiotherapy as the full extent of a disease process is often not evident on radiographs. MRI and CT are becoming increasingly used in veterinary diagnostic imaging as referral centres gain access to human scanners or even obtain their own machines, and as owner expectations and the number of insured animals continue to rise.

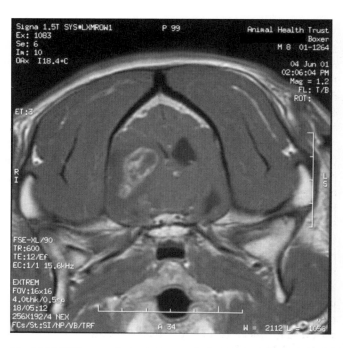

Fig. 24.63 MRI scan of a brain tumour in an 8-year-old Boxer. This scan has been obtained following intravenous injection of MRI contrast medium, which shows the tumour as a bright, ring-like structure in the brain. Head muscles are grey and bones are either black (cortical bone) or white (bone marrow). This tumour responded well to radiotherapy.

Nuclear medicine (scintigraphy)

Scintigraphy is used mainly in horses for the diagnosis of bony orthopaedic problems. A gamma ray-emitting radioactive substance which will be taken up by the tissue under investigation (usually bone) is injected into the bloodstream under conditions which protect the handler from irradiation and the horse is returned to an isolation stable. Several hours later the radioactivity will have become concentrated in areas of increased bone turnover, creating 'hot spots', which are emitting more gamma radiation than are the surrounding tissues. The emitted photons can be detected either by a hand-held radioactivity counter or by a large detector known as a gamma camera (Fig. 24.64). A pattern of emitted radioactivity is produced which allows the source

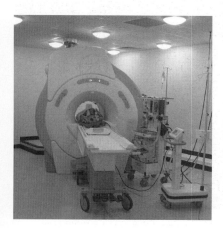

Fig. 24.62 MRI scanner and anaesthetised patient.

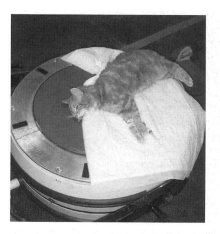

Fig. 24.64 A sedated cat and gamma camera during scintigraphy.

of the lameness to be diagnosed. Although the 'image' itself is rather crude since it reflects metabolism rather than anatomical detail, the technique is very sensitive to early bone changes which cannot be seen with radiography. In small animals, scintigraphy is used mainly for the detection of thyroid tissue in hyperthyroid cats, for diagnosis of porto-systemic shunts and in a widespread search for bone metastases.

KEY POINTS
Other imaging techniques
- Diagnostic ultrasound is increasingly used in general practice for soft tissue imaging and is complementary to radiography.
- Ultrasonography can be performed on conscious patients with manual restraint and is safe and painless.
- Ultrasonography permits guided fine needle aspiration or biopsy of lesions within soft tissue structures.
- CT and MRI produce cross-sectional images of the patient in very fine detail – their main use in veterinary imaging is for neurological diagnosis.
- Scintigraphy is most often used for the investigation of lameness in horses and involves intravenous injection of a radioactive material.

Further reading

Dennis, R. (1992) Practice tip – choosing an X-ray machine. In *Practice*, vol. 14, pp. 181–184.

Dennis, R. (1997) Veterinary diagnostic imaging – into a new era. *The Veterinary Nursing Journal*, vol. 12, pp. 43–52.

Douglas, S. W., Herrtage, M. E. and Williamson, H. D. (1987) *Principles of Veterinary Radiography*, 4th edn, Baillière Tindall, London.

HMSO (2002) Guidance notes for the safe use of ionising radiations in veterinary practice. B.V.A. June 2002.

Lee, R. ed. (1995) *Manual of Small Animal Diagnostic Imaging*, BSAVA, Cheltenham.

Paugh Partington, B. (1998) Diagnostic imaging. In McCurnin, D. M. (ed.), *Clinical Textbook for Veterinary Technicians*, pp. 183–215, 4th edn, W. B. Saunders, Philadelphia.

Ryan, G. D. (1981) *Radiographic Positioning of Small Animals*, Baillière Tindall, London.

Ticer, J. W. (1975) *Radiographic Technique in Small Animal Practice*, W. B. Saunders, Philadelphia.

25

Problem behaviour and its management

D. S. Mills and *C. B. Mills*

Learning objectives

After studying this chapter, students should be able to:

- Explain the extent of behaviour problems in pet cats and dogs and their fundamental nature.
- Identify the factors influencing the development and expression of behaviour and state the knowledge base required for managing behaviour problems.
- Support a client with a potential problem and state the most appropriate course of initial action given the available expertise.
- Provide advice on the methods used to prevent behaviour problems in puppies.
- Describe the four main techniques and four key strategies used to bring about a change in behaviour.
- Discuss the difference between reward- and punishment-based training, distinguish between positive and negative reinforcement and punishment, define and implement a programme of counter-conditioning and systematic desensitisation.
- Identify how the risks associated with owning an aggressive animal can be reduced.
- State the difference between treating a presenting complaint versus the cause of that complaint and the skills required for each.

Introduction

A survey of the veterinary nursing profession (Atkinson, 2001) reported that more than 80% of veterinary nurses are involved in educating and advising clients on issues of pet behaviour. However, 91% felt that their training did not provide them with sufficient knowledge of companion animal behaviour. Unwanted behaviour remains a common reason for euthanasia, especially in the dog. It is therefore essential that the compulsory element of education required for success in professional qualifications is supplemented with further reading and education, if the level of service desired by clients is to be met. Whatever the circumstances, it is important that individuals do not offer advice beyond their own knowledge base as this can have disastrous consequences for the client, patient and practice. A behaviour problem may be defined as any behaviour which causes concern to an owner, for which they do not suspect a medical cause. The owner's perception of the situation is therefore an integral part of the problem. The behaviour is not the diagnosis but a sign of the problem and may be normal or a genuine disorder of behaviour. There are therefore two integral parts to understanding a behaviour problem:

- The owner's views and beliefs.
- The animal's behaviour.

Every situation is unique, since it is the situation rather than the animal per se which needs treating. However, we can provide a framework for analysing that situation in a methodical way: first we must make an initial assessment of the situation and support the client in the most appropriate way. Then we may make a more detailed assessment of the animal's behaviour.

Initial assessment

Initial assessment should balance the significance of the animal's behaviour and the owner's perception of it, then identify the most efficient strategy for managing them appropriately. For example, the puppy which is chewing the furniture when it has never been trained to chew on specific toys is behaving perfectly normally. Successful treatment will involve educating the client about the normal behaviour of puppies and how to train their puppy to chew on toys in preference to anything else. On the other hand, an animal which has recently become aggressive may be suffering from a medical condition to make it more irritable. This will require prompt attention by a veterinary surgeon in the first instance.

Accepting and admitting that a pet has a behaviour problem is often very difficult and stressful for clients. They may feel like failed parents and so may be very sensitive to whatever advice you give them and how it is given. Their embarrassment may mean that they delay in seeking advice for a relatively minor problem until it has become a major issue of concern. Unfortunately the longer a problem has been going on the longer, and often harder, it is to treat. Nonetheless, clients should never be criticised or made to feel stupid because they do not understand their pet's behaviour. They should always be regarded with respect and consideration and time taken to listen to their problem without making a judgement on their competence as a pet owner.

The first priority is then to determine what level of advice is most appropriate. The range of services offered by the practice should include informal advice, specialist consultation within the practice and referral. All of this should be explained to clients in the beginning so they can make an informed decision about the preferred option of treatment.

Informal advice may be the initial preferred option in many cases, but practice staff must be aware that they are still liable for the content of this advice. **If casual advice is given which results in injury or further distress to the owner, legal proceedings could follow and so a note must always be made on the client's records when such advice is given.** An alternative is to use professional handouts (e.g. Landsberg et al., 2001). We have a duty to provide a professional service and that includes explaining the limitations of informal advice and the value of specialist consultations. Behaviour clinics are run by members of staff or individuals from outside the practice with particular knowledge, expertise and skill in the area of concern. Explaining the option of a specific consultation on the matter also helps reassure the clients that they are right to take their problem seriously and that they are not alone. Voith (1984, 1985) reported that 42% of dog owners and 47% of cat owners in the USA indicated that their pet engaged in some form of problem behaviour. However, more recent surveys in the UK on dogs (Mills, 1997) and cats (Bradshaw, 2000) suggest that the prevalence of potentially problematic behaviour may be much higher with over 95% of dog owners and up to 89% of cat owners describing potentially problematic behaviours. Amongst dogs it was found that 76% had shown some form of aggression, 70% had occasional house-soiling problems, 57% pulled on the lead, 57% chased cats, 48% became easily overexcited, 29% had tried to escape from the home area, 27% run away when off lead, 23% were restless when travelling and 20% difficult to medicate. However, when asked to describe any complaints about these animals, owners rated aggression highest followed by obedience, barking, excitability, nervousness, house-soiling and destructiveness. The difference between these lists demonstrates the importance of the owner in determining what is presented as a problem. The data also show the extent of possible assistance required by owners from those keen to develop this area of practice. Amongst cats, excluding scratching of furnishings which is ubiquitous, the most common concerns relate to fear of unfamiliar people (49%), aggression to other cats (48%), fear of cats (40%), fear and aggression to household members (12%), inappropriate elimination of some form (19%), bonding problems (12%) and anxiety-related disorders (11%).

Assessment of animal behaviour

In order to assess a behaviour problem fully, a broad history is necessary (Overall, 1997). An animal's behaviour at any given moment is a response to certain influences otherwise known as motivational factors. These can be divided into external and internal factors (Askew, 1996). External factors include the general management of the animal and the specific environment at the time the behaviour is shown. Internal factors include the genetic composition of the individual, its physiological and psychological state. If we wish to address the cause of a problem (rather than simply contain the problem), then we need to be aware of how these factors interact and influence behaviour. The knowledge base for dealing with behaviour problems therefore draws on very disparate fields including just about every branch of zoology as well as various branches of psychology, veterinary medicine, animal management and nutrition. Individuals may know more about one particular area, e.g. using training rather than medical intervention, but whatever our preference we must recognise our limitations and appreciate the value of other treatment options. The problem must be defined fully – not only what is happening but where, when, with whom and why. Some owners will hold back information either because they think it is not important or because they feel guilty about some aspect of it. It is essential to establish a bond of trust with the client. Both the trainer and the client must be relaxed.

Genetic influences

These provide the blueprint for the behaviour of the individual. Genetic factors not only determine what is normal but may also set certain limits. This can be seen at three levels.

Species typical behaviour

This describes those behaviours that define a dog as a dog and a cat as a cat. Many popular texts will often make analogies to wild relatives, such as the wolf in the case of the dog, but dogs are not wolves, and their behaviour is quite different as they have evolved to survive in a very different environment, so the value of such analogies is limited and can lead to inaccurate advice (Coppinger and Coppinger, 2001). It is essential to be well versed in the normal behaviours of the species in order to appreciate if something is genuinely abnormal (e.g. an owner thinking that the cat in oestrus, rolling on the floor, is abnormal or in pain). It is not possible to go into detail here about the species typical behaviour patterns of companion animals, so the reader is referred to the list of further reading at the end of the chapter.

Breed characteristics

Just as the dog is not a wolf, neither are all breeds of dog or cat alike. Thus breed characteristics also determine what is normal (e.g. vocalisation of the Siamese or fixed eye in the Border Collie). Breed behaviour may indicate what problems may be likely in a given breed (e.g. noise phobias in Bearded Collies, urine spraying in Siamese cats). An understanding of the breed is also important when trying to advise a potential owner about a new pet. Again the reader should refer to breed specific texts as appropriate.

Individual characteristics

In any population there is a variation and some of this has a genetic basis. Thus even within a breed, some animals are predisposed to being more fearful than others, for example nervousness has been reported to have a heritability of 0.58 in potential Guide Dog Labradors (Goddard and Beilharz, 1983). This information is particularly important when considering the prevention of behaviour problems through selective breeding as well as appreciating the limits of behavioural modification for a given individual.

Physiological and psychological influences

Behaviour is physiology that you can see with the naked eye and psychology reflects the ongoing physiology of the brain. So an understanding of physiological processes and how they affect behaviour and the mind is essential (Carlson, 2001). Normal physiology can bring about changes in behaviour associated with development and life stage. For example, some forms of aggression seen during false pregnancy are intimately associated with the hormonal changes in the bitch at the same time, which bring about perceptual changes that encourage protective aggression.

Physiological rather than genetic differences between the sexes also tend to underlie the difference seen at this level. For example, urine spraying in cats is more common in males, but neutering usually helps in the prevention and treatment of the problem in both sexes, by altering their physiological state. The relationship between internal physiology and behaviour is usually complex and generalisations should be avoided. Aggression is neither a male-typical nor steroid-dependent behaviour, but influenced by numerous physiological factors (Brain and Haug, 1992). These need to be assessed so that rational treatment options can be offered. Castration may even be contraindicated in some cases.

The physiology of an animal also changes with disease and this may result in an apparent behaviour problem, e.g. aggression in the hyperthyroid cat or rabid animal. Chronic lead poisoning in farm dogs may be seen as a result of animals licking or chewing items treated with old-fashioned lead paint. This can present as anxiety and/or a reduction in the working dog's obedience (Nicholls, 1983).

Drug therapy also affects an animal's physiological state, since it alters the balance of nerve transmitters in the brain. Whilst there are some drugs like the antidepressants and anxiolytics which are specifically designed for this purpose (Dodman and Shuster, 1998), other drugs may produce behaviour changes as a secondary affect, for example, phenylpropanolamine is used to control urinary incontinence in dogs but may also cause aggression in some cases (Anon, 2001).

Diet can also influence behaviour through its physiological effects. This ranges from the ingestion of stimulants which result in overactivity and the problem associated therein to the manipulation of diet to maximise the availability of precursors of neurotransmitters (Strong, 1999).

Current external environment

A problem may arise with an animal's behaviour because of the situation in which it finds itself. In these cases, altering the environment may avoid the problem. Such measures include rehoming a dog with separation related problems to a family where it will not be left on its own or muzzling the aggressive dog. Whilst this may resolve the situation, and save the animal's life, it is important to realise the behaviour still exists although it is no longer expressed. Alternatively, the environment can be temporarily changed, by bringing in a dog-sitter for the dog that howls when left alone, so that the problem does not arise whilst the behaviour is modified through careful training and behaviour therapy.

Previous environment

In early life, dogs and cats have 'sensitive phases' when they learn more rapidly or form impressions which will affect their behaviour and temperament. Animals reared in impoverished environments also do not develop as well intellectually and may have difficulty in regulating their emotions. These not only predispose an individual to a variety of problems but also reduce the prognosis for treatment.

Sensitive phases

During the socialisation period, the way the animal will tend to respond to both the physical and social elements of its environment are largely determined. This period appears to be between the 4th and 10th week of age in the puppy (Scott and Fuller, 1965) and between the 2nd and 7th week in the kitten (Karsh, 1983). It is vital that pets receive pleasant experiences at this time associated with things that are to be accepted later. For example they should be handled gently by a range of handlers, old and young, so they do not shy away from people later in life. Overstressing, for example by early weaning, should be avoided as this interferes with the animal's learning ability and appears to result in fundamental emotional changes (Neville, 1996). Around this life stage, most temperament problems develop: damage done at this time is much harder to undo later.

During the juvenile period, the animal matures sexually and later matures socially. Social maturation influences the role the animal will assume within its social group (instigator or follower). At this time, problems may become apparent with other members of the household, both human and animal, as the young adult tries to assert itself. Cats and dogs are capable of forming strong attachments to new owners at this time if they have been socialised to people previously.

Many problems arise because the animal has not been properly socialised or trained when young. It is far easier to teach appropriate behaviour from the outset than it is to correct problems later. The veterinary practice has an important role in this aspect of preventive medicine.

Preventing problems

Advice should be given to breeders and potential new owners on suitable weaning, handling and exposure procedures. An outline programme is given for the first 6 weeks in Fig. 25.1.

Practices should consider running 'puppy' classes, where the expertise exists to manage them appropriately. These classes combine basic obedience training with socialisation, plenty of handling and lots of novel stimuli provided in a controlled and pleasant environment. Puppies are taught what is acceptable and what is not (e.g. biting). All vaccinated puppies can be invited to the classes and given the opportunity to mix with puppies of their own age and new people. A recommended 4-week programme is given below. These are not only an important service, but excellent PR for the practice, as well as a lot of fun for all involved.

Four-week puppy class programme

The whole family should be encouraged to attend the classes and take part in the exercises. The principles of training (see later) should also be described as part of the course, so owners understand not only what they should do but also why.

Each week new skills are taught and established ones reinforced. It is important to explain the principles behind the tasks and to provide handouts, since the owners will inevitably be distracted by their puppies some of the time. If classes are to be run outside normal surgery hours or at a different venue to the normal site of the veterinary practice, it is important to check that the practice insurance still covers the work.

Week 1 exercises

- **Sit**: With the puppy standing move a small food treat back over its head and then slightly lower it. The nose should follow the treat and the backlegs naturally fold underneath as the treat is lowered. Try to avoid putting pressure on the hind quarters.
- **Stand**: Move the food lure slightly up and forward in front of the sitting puppy.
- **Down**: Move the food to the floor just in front of the puppy and keep it there.
- **Recalls**: Take the puppy away from the owners and get them to encourage it towards them. Make sure that there are no distractions for the puppy when you do this for the

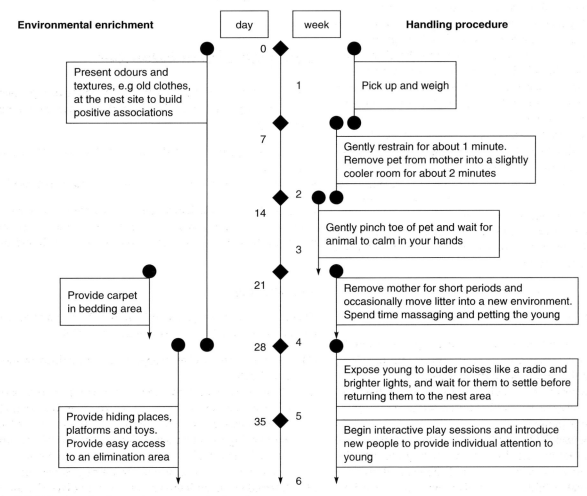

Fig. 25.1 Behaviour development programme for breeders.

first time and tell the owners to always be pleased to see the puppy and bend down to greet it.

- **Chew control**: Select a range of toys for the puppy and either smear an edible reward on them like peanut butter or load hollow toys with treats which fall out as the puppy chews on them.
- **Bite control**: Whilst playing calmly with the puppy, slip your hand into his mouth, as the teeth make contact with your skin and well before it hurts, let out a scream, withdraw your hand and walk away. After a short time repeat the exercise. Soon the puppy will learn to inhibit its bite towards people. This is one of the most important lessons a dog can learn.
- **Handling exercises**: Ask someone to reward the puppy with gentle praise and small treats as the dog is handled all over. Make sure you include an examination of the ears, under the tail, between the toes and in the mouth. This will need to be done in stages initially.

Week 2 exercises

- **Off and take it**: Show the puppy some food in your hand and say 'off' loudly to interrupt its investigation. If the puppy persists then close your hand around the treat and repeat the command even louder. When the puppy stops trying to get it, ask it to take it and give the reward.
- **Stay**: Steadily increase the time the puppy has to wait for a reward once the command word has been given.
- **Recall from play**: Ask all the owners in the class, other than the one who will be giving the recall command, to grab their dogs when the owner doing the training calls their dog. The dog should be given lots of praise as it approaches the owner.
- **Off lead heel**: Hold a treat (toy or favourite food) by your side approximately level with the puppy's head. Encourage the puppy to heel as you move forward just a few steps. As you stop, ask the puppy to sit. When you turn for the first time turn towards the puppy so your leg will guide him round if necessary.
- **Food bowl exercise**: Remove the food bowl from the puppy and offer him a preferred treat before returning it with an added titbit.

Week 3 exercises

- **Relax**: Quietly and gently reassure the puppy as a suitable command word like 'time out' is softly repeated. Keep going until the puppy is totally relaxed.
- **Heeling on lead:** If enough off-lead practice has been given you only need to add the lead to have a dog that heels without pulling.
- **Greeting people:** Whilst walking the dogs on lead, stop as you meet other owners. Each owner then gives the other person's dog a 'sit' command, bends down, and gives the puppy a treat. Children must also learn how to behave around dogs. They should not encourage mouthing, chas-

ing or clothes chewing, but should give treats when the puppy is well behaved.

- **Socialisation**: Encourage owners to get out and about with their puppies. The idea is to expose the puppy to every situation we may want it to accept in its adult life in the next few weeks, without getting it overexcited, scared or overtired. So do not let owners do too much in one go.

Week 4 exercises

- **Tricks**: The principles of learning are explained earlier in the course and all owners are asked to teach their dog a trick in preparation for this week. This helps them demonstrate their understanding of training. Certificates can be given to all making it this far. These might include a picture of the puppy taken earlier in the course and make a great souvenir.

General considerations

All visits to the practice at this time should be made as pleasant as possible. When injections need to be given, as for vaccination, distract the animal during the procedure and then reward it afterwards. Overindulging the crying animal will make it more fearful.

Modifying current behaviour

There are two important elements to behaviour problem treatment, beyond the skills of good communication and counselling:

- The techniques to be used – i.e. what level of intervention is to be used.
- The treatment strategy – i.e. how the goal is achieved.

Both need to be considered before treatment commences. When talking about any treatment, talk about what 'we' will do, rather than telling the owner what *they* should do.

Techniques

There are four techniques available for the management of animal behaviour (Mills and Nankervis, 1999).

(1) **Training and psychotherapy**. This is described in more detail below.
(2) **Environmental manipulation**. This involves changing the environment in such a way as to alter the animal's behaviour, e.g. providing scratch posts for cats which are clawing the furniture, using a commercial preparation of feline facial pheromones in the home to calm the anxious cat or a muzzle on an aggressive dog.
(3) **Internal chemical intervention**. This involves the use of dietary manipulation or the prescription of drugs to

alter behaviour. Under the terms of the Veterinary Surgeons Act 1966, pharmacological recommendations should only be made by a veterinary surgeon. There are a number of antidepressants (clomipramine and selegiline) and other drugs which modify behaviour (e.g. progestogens) now licensed for use in animals.

(4) **Physical intervention**: This includes the use of surgery, such as castration of the urine-marking cat or dog and the use of massage and physiotherapy to help an animal relax, which may be part of a counterconditioning programme (see below).

Principles of animal training and psychotherapy

Improving success

One of the keys to successful problem resolution is an understanding of the nature of the problem by both the therapist and the client. The situation should be viewed and explained from the animal's point of view. Learning is greatest when motivation is highest, therefore the nature of the bond between owner and pet should be considered and modified accordingly. The owner should be in control but force is not necessary to establish this.

As with other aspects of the consultation, judgemental comments should be avoided. Rather than criticise an owner for using an ineffectual technique, suggest that it may be better to try an alternative method, explaining what the chosen method is expected to achieve and why. Do not let the client expect too much too soon, as unrealistic expectations often lead to abandonment of the plan when these goals are not reached. The requirements set must also be realistic for the owners in question, as they will not commit themselves to something they do not really believe in.

Client compliance is essential, as it is they who will train the animal using the techniques you demonstrate. Two facts beyond an understanding of the problem and trust in the therapist help in the early stages:

- An initial, early follow-up of a week or two.
- The use of a relatively small number of simple exercises which you predict will bring about noticeable change in the animal's behaviour.

The thought that it is only a temporary measure helps to motivate the owner to break previous habits or to follow what may be an inconvenient plan of action. Once this has been done it is much easier to continue and extend the programme. If owners are given too much, they are more likely to abandon the programme. Training or retraining an animal often requires a vivid imagination and a flexible approach by the trainer. What may be suitable for one client and their pet may not be appropriate for another with the same problem.

Training techniques

Learning focuses on how an animal's potential for a behaviour changes with experience of the external environment, whilst training describes the techniques used to ensure that this comes about in a predictable way in response to human intervention (Mills, 2002). The term reinforcement is often used to refer to the consequences of an action. Any process which increases the likelihood of an associated behaviour recurring in similar circumstances is called appetitive reinforcement. Two types of appetitive reinforcement are commonly described: positive and negative. With positive reinforcement it is the presentation of a pleasant event (e.g. food) which reinforces the behaviour, whereas in negative reinforcement it is the removal of an unpleasant event (e.g. the pressure from a check chain) which has the effect of encouraging the desired behaviour. Punishment is also a form of reinforcement (aversive reinforcement) and describes any process which decreases the likelihood of an associated behaviour recurring in similar circumstances. A common source of problems in training is the difference between the intended reinforcement and the actual reinforcement provided. Reinforcement is defined by its effect, and not by its intended function. If a dog is whining for attention and the owner tells it to be quiet, they are probably encouraging the behaviour as they have inadvertently allowed the behaviour to achieve its goal, i.e. attention from the owner.

Many owners of problem pets focus on what they do not want (i.e their pet to do such and such); one of the skills of a good trainer is to turn this situation around, so that the owner focuses not on what they do not what, but rather on what they do want. The desired behavioural goal can then be worked towards. This also helps break the vicious cycle of ineffective punishment that has often developed and may be exacerbating the problem. Other points to note when training are:

- The subject must be attentive to the trainer. This may require the use of a whistle or other aids to interrupt the animal's current activity. It is also important not to train for so long that you exceed the animal's attention span.
- In order to encourage the animal to comply, any reward must be truly rewarding compared with available alternatives. There is no point in offering a food reward just after the animal's main meal.
- Initially, do not give commands that cannot be enforced. This may mean leaving a long training lead or lead and head-collar attached if it is safe to do so.
- Training sessions should always finish on a positive note, even if it means returning to a basic command.

The use of positive reinforcement and reward-based training

This involves encouraging an animal to perform a desired behaviour by means of pleasant lures and rewards. Positive reinforcement should always be used if appropriate since it teaches the animal precisely what is required, is relatively easy to apply, is humane, helps to strengthen the trainer–animal bond and helps clients to break out of an ineffective punishment mentality. Initially every correct response is rewarded (continuous reinforcement), but as the animal learns what is required a more reliable response can be established by only rewarding the better 50% of responses (differential intermittent reinforcement). In this way the animal's behaviour will not only continue to improve, but it will remain reliable when the owner has no rewards to hand.

The teaching of basic obedience, if not already present in the problem dog, is to be recommended, as it helps provide consistency in the pet–owner relationship, which, if missing, may be a source of considerable stress that underlies many problems.

It is not always possible to train the exact goal straight away, but rather it may only be achieved in stages. The steps involved must be identified and explained explicitly to the client. There are a number of ways that positive reinforcement can be used in this way:

- **Behaviour chaining** involves teaching each behaviour with a command word in the normal way. A new command word is then introduced before the old instructions are given in a set order. Soon the dog will learn, through a process known as **classical conditioning**, that the first command is always followed by the set sequence and so will perform the whole act without the need for the individual commands. This is the behaviour chain. The individual commands can then be dropped and a single reward given at the end of the chain. Sometimes it is necessary to construct several short chains before bringing them together to form a longer sequence.
- **Counterconditioning**. This involves training a behaviour which is incompatible with the problem behaviour (e.g. a dog is taught to sit to greet rather than jumping up). The new behaviour is initially taught away from the problem situation until it is reliable; distractions may then be introduced (these should be graded according to the problem). When the behaviour has become reliable even in these situations, it may be used when the problem would normally arise. So long as the association with the new acceptable behaviour is stronger than the motivation to engage in the problem behaviour, the new behaviour will be expressed in preference to the problem one which is not associated with a reward.
- **Successive approximation**. This is also known as behavioural shaping and involves the incremental reinforcement of a behaviour towards the final goal. This process underpins the widely used technique of **systematic desensitisation**. Systematic desensitisation is used to reduce an animal's excitement or fear to a given situation. This situation is broken down into component stimuli which do not produce a response on their own. For example, in the case of an animal that is scared of the vet, it may be possible to safely expose the animal to people in white coats or the disinfectant used in the clinic off site, the vet

in a different overalls on site and so forth. Acceptance can be improved if the animal is distracted during the process, a counterconditioned command used or some form of relaxation exercise applied such as massage. The animal is rewarded as long as it does not show an inappropriate response. The process is then repeated and the stimuli gradually made more similar to the final goal. It is essential not to rush this process but to do it at a pace that the animal can accept.

Other techniques

Behavioural habituation
This may be used if a response is inappropriate to a given situation and is not self-rewarding but it is safe and humane to allow the animal to express it. The response is neither rewarded nor punished but allowed to run its course, in the hope that it will pass away, since it achieves nothing. This can be used for certain forms of hysterical behaviour, so the animal learns that there is nothing to be gained from this response.

Punishment
The use of **punishment** is associated with many problems and its misuse is an abuse. Punishment does not teach an animal what it should be doing; punishment only signals that what the animal is doing is wrong. It is therefore a much less efficient training tool than positive reinforcement. The overuse of punishment by owners may not only result in a dog which is fearful of them, but possibly people in general. It also creates an animal that is less responsive and able to learn. If an animal is fearful or nervous, punishment must *never* be used as it reinforces the fear, i.e. it signals to the animal that it was appropriate to be scared of what was going on. However, punishment may be useful and necessary in certain circumstances to discourage a behaviour. In these situations an alternative behaviour which can be expressed by the animal must be identified and encouraged with positive reinforcement at the same time. If punishment seems to be needed a lot of the time, the trainer should always ask: 'Where have I gone wrong?'

Non-reward – extinction: The withholding of a reward which is normally in association with a behaviour is actually a form of punishment, since it ultimately reduces the chance of a behaviour recurring. It is not, however, a simple technique to use as the behaviour will often intensify before it starts to wane. The technique may be used to treat certain attention-seeking behaviour problems, since these are behaviours that have been regularly rewarded in the past. In such cases, any attention (good or bad) rewards and reinforces the behaviour. Attempts at physical punishment are contra-indicated as these are also a form of attention, which may worsen the behaviour in the longer term. Doing nothing is not necessarily very easy, especially if an owner enjoys stroking the pet. Owners should also be warned that the behaviour will become more intense before it disappears. It is critical that they do not give in at this time otherwise they will make matters worse, having just reinforced a more extreme form of the behaviour.

Punishment is effective if it is associated with the problem behaviour rather than a given person. For this reason, remote punishments like booby traps are preferable to ones which are obviously delivered by the trainer. One of the most widely used booby traps is a drinks can with a few coins inside. When the animal starts to misbehave, this is thrown close to (but not directly at the animal), without warning and without attracting attention to the trainer. The animal then learns that this behaviour has this unpleasant consequence. For example the dog that tries to chase people passing by when on the lead, can have the behaviour interrupted in this way. As soon as the can lands, the owners should encourage the dog to come towards them and reward it for doing so. If a booby trap is used in the home like a noise alarm linked to an out of bounds area, it is worth using a discriminatory signal, like a drop of essential oil on the threshold of the area to warn the animal. In this way the animal will soon learn to avoid wherever the scent it placed. Avoidance of these areas is then reinforced by negative reinforcement, so the booby traps can be removed.

Further details on the skilful implementation of behaviour therapy can be found in Martin and Pear (1992).

Pheromone therapy   Pheromone therapy involves the use of chemicals normally used in intraspecific communication for the modification of problem behaviour. There has been great interest in the facial secretions of the cat and the mammary secretions of the bitch, both of which appear to have anxiolytic effects in specific contexts. The exact mechanism remains unclear as the efficacy of these products appears to relate to specific contexts. Undoubtedly this area of science will grow further in future and so nurses should keep up to date on developments (see Mills 2002b for a current review). At present these products are only available through veterinary practices and it is important that their sale is accompanied by sound and relevant behaviour advice.

Treatment strategies

There are usually several strategies whereby a problem behaviour may be managed and more than one may be employed at the same time, but sometimes this is unnecessary or counterproductive. It is therefore important to recognise the strategies in use and best to apply those which are most likely to bring success with the minimum of discomfort to both the pet and owner, in the first instance. Broadly speaking four strategies which are recognised which use the techniques described above (Mills and Nankervis, 1999):

(1) **Prevention** of expression of the problem. For example a dog can be prevented from biting by muzzling it. This does not address the causal factors, but may offer short-term relief or reduce immediate risk.
(2) Address the **causal factors**. These may be eliminated or their perception altered. For example, when one dog is rehomed in a case of inter-dog rivalry in the house or the thyroid removed from an aggressive, hyperthyroid cat,

the causes of the problem have been removed. Alternatively the phobic dog may be desensitised or prescribed anxiolytics (anti-anxiety medication). This alters the animal's perception of the cause of the problem.
(3) **Behavioural redirection**. In this case the behaviour is still allowed, but it may only be directed towards things that do not cause a problem. For example the cat which scratches the furniture may be trained to scratch only on a scratching post and scratching elsewhere discouraged.
(4) **Increased behavioural competition**. In this case a behaviour is introduced which competes with the problem behaviour. This is the principle behind counterconditioning and the use of toys to prevent problems associated with lack of stimulation.

First aid for common behaviour problems

Many problems are amenable to retraining using the principles discussed above; however, common problems, such as aggression, house-soiling and house destruction, represent complaints for which there are many causes. The specific cause for a given case therefore needs to be identified if it is to be treated effectively and this will often require special evaluation. The veterinary nurse should explain this clearly to the client and also give behavioural first aid to contain the problem in the meantime.

Aggression

Aggression in the dog is a serious concern for all involved and should only be tackled by skilled handlers. True behavioural aggression, which is associated with defence or control of resources, must be distinguished from medical disorders, play and predation, which are functionally very different behaviours. Medical assessment is essential as pain will often present as increased irritability. Animals often assume an aggressive stance when there is uncertainty or frustration in the environment; again this relates to a form of defence, and punishment is likely to exacerbate the situation. Prior to special evaluation, the risks to others from an aggressive animal should be minimised. This involves the following:

- Owners must be informed of their responsibility to prevent injury to others.
- Owners should aim to avoid situations which are likely to exacerbate the condition. This may include identifiable trigger stimuli, like other dogs, children, etc., and/or incidences of competition, uncertain, frustrating or fearful situations.
- The animal should not be approached when it has no opportunity to retreat.
- If it is safe to do so, the owner should be encouraged to muzzle-train an aggressive dog away from arousing or dangerous environments. A basket muzzle is preferable

to a nylon one, as it allows the dog to pant and drink but not bite while it is on. When it accepts the muzzle being slid on and off, the muzzle may be held on for a while by hand and a reward given when it is removed. With time the dog will soon accept the muzzle for longer periods, at which time it can start to be fastened. The most common problem with muzzles is that they are only used when the dog is already showing aggression and will resent restraint. This is why training should begin away from distractions and the trained dog should be muzzled before a problem arises.

- A special appointment should be made to discuss the problem further.

House-soiling

When asked about a house-soiling problem it is important to establish what form of elimination is involved and if it involves urine, whether the animal is scent marking (spraying in the cat or spot marking in the dog) as these represent fundamentally different behaviours to urinary and faecal elimination. A urinalysis should be requested in all cases of inappropriate urination to eliminate lower urinary tract disease.

It is then important to establish that the animal has been properly housetrained:

- Feline urine spraying, which is not due to cystitis, is most effectively treated with a commercial preparation of feline facial pheromone and may not require any additional retraining advice. However, marked areas should be cleaned with a solution of biological washing powder followed by surgical spirit. They are then rinsed with water and wiped dry with paper towels (Mills and White, 2000).
- Cats which have been urine marking for some time may also stop using the litter box. Other reasons for indiscriminate elimination include lower urinary tract disease, litter box and litter aversions, an emotional problem or substrate preferences. It should be checked that the litter box is in a quiet, secluded area where the cat cannot be disturbed, that the box is cleaned regularly and completely and that there have been no changes to the normal routine, e.g. change of litter, etc. Bleach, ammonia-based disinfectants or strong-smelling cleaners are not recommended as the smell may be aversive to the cat. If the cause is not readily identifiable and the animal is healthy, then expert advice should be sought.
- In the dog, house-soiling is most commonly a result of loss of housetraining, scent marking, excitement, disease, fear or separation distress. Any disease must be recognised promptly, but in all cases the pet will need retraining. This is most effectively achieved by ensuring that the dog is taken out regularly to a particular toilet area and returned if it does not eliminate. When it does, it should be given lots of praise and a treat. This might be a longer walk or titbit. Owners should always clear up after their pet. The recommended treatment for scent marking is

chemical (steroidal) or surgical neutering as this will eliminate the problem in the majority of cases.

- Dogs may eliminate when they feel threatened; this is a normal appeasement gesture. Owners often get annoyed at this reaction and so may make matters worse by telling their dog off. Eye contact alone may be sufficient to set off this appeasement behaviour in some dogs. Owners should be encouraged not to appear threatening in any way towards their pet but should jolly it along with praise and without eye contact. Confidence-building exercises and possibly psychopharmacy (serotonin reuptake inhibitors) may be necessary to allow these animals to lead a normal life.
- Dogs also eliminate when they are scared, e.g. during thunderstorms, or distressed in some other way such as by the departure of the owner (Landsberg et al., 1997). This latter problem is considered further below.

Soiling in the owner's absence

The term separation 'anxiety' or separation-related problem is often used to describe any problem which arises in the owner's absence. It therefore describes the presenting complaint rather than identifies any specific cause. There are many reasons why an animal may not be able to cope with the absence of its owner. These include overattachment to the owner, in which case treatment must focus on reducing this attachment, or developing an owner substitute. Alternatively, the animal may be fearful of the isolation experienced when left alone. In this case a companion may help or the animal trained to gradually cope with steadily increasing periods of isolation. A third cause of the problem relates to the stress of confinement or barrier frustration and results in primary attempts at escape. These cases often carry a poorer prognosis. Whatever the cause, behaviour modification advice is generally essential for the long-term resolution of the problem, but this should be tailored to address the factors underlying the behaviour for maximum success (Takeuchi et al., 2000). Drugs like clomipramine may help speed up the rate of response in certain cases. Current research also suggests that commercial preparations of dog pheromones may be just as helpful in this respect.

Dogs with such separation-related problems may also be extremely destructive at this time, howl or vomit and any of these signs may be the main presenting complaint.

House destruction

Dogs that destroy when left alone may be doing so because of some form of distress associated with the owners' absence (see above), because of a lack of stimulation at this time or be trying to escape from the house because something attracts them from outside or scares them from within the house.

- All dogs should be provided with stimulating toys when left alone for long periods of time. These can be made attractive at the time of leaving by smearing them with food paste or filling them with food. The toy can be taken up when the owner returns so access is limited and its value to the dog increased.

- Dogs should also be trained to chew on appropriate items when left alone and it should not be assumed that they will naturally stop chewing on things when they stop teething.
- Further advice on this and other behaviour problems is given in the reading list below.

Conclusion

All problems of behaviour in the dog and cat reported to the veterinary nurse should be considered seriously and, if necessary, referred to a more experienced colleague, but often some initial advice can be given.

Counterconditioning is a technique which involves the training of a behaviour which is incompatible with the problem, so the problem is no longer expressed. Systematic desensitisation involves bringing about a change in the animal's perception of a problem stimulus, so that it no longer reacts in an undesirable way to it.

- Individual ability, legal liability and insurance matters must always be considered. A veterinary practice may be responsible for all advice given, including casual comments on a problem. If in doubt or if an animal responds in an unexpected way to a given treatment, seek help from a more experienced colleague. Only a veterinary surgeon should advise on the potential use of medication for a behaviour problem.

KEY POINTS

- Behaviour problems reflect a problem in the relationship between owner and pet at some level. They are very common and range from behaviours that are a minor inconvenience to those which threaten the life of the pet. It is important to identify rapidly the level of advice and intervention required for safe and successful resolution of the problem.
- A thorough history and specific knowledge of both breed and species typical behaviour are essential prerequisites to dealing with any case. In addition, knowledge of the fundamentals of physiology, ethology and learning are essential.
- A given response reflects a pet's perceived priorities at that time. Reinforcement which encourages the behaviour to recur may be positive (pleasurable) or negative (relieving). The use of rewards in training inevitably focuses on directing the animal towards the desired goal. Punishment only discourages an undesired response without necessarily guiding the creation of the correct behaviour.
- Behaviour develops throughout life and the aim of behaviour therapy is to structure the experiences of the patient so that undesired behaviour is modified into a more acceptable form. Puppy and kitten classes seek to structure the animal's early experiences in a controlled way so that it responds appropriately to the environment and is able to cope with future change.
- Behaviour may be modified by preventing its expression, redirecting it onto a different focus, encouraging an alternative behaviour or addressing the causal factors.

Further reading

Anon. (2001) *NOAH Compendium of Data Sheets of Veterinary Products*, National Office of Animal Health Ltd, Enfield, Middx.

Askew, H. R. (1996) *Treatment of Behaviour Problems in Dogs and Cats*, Blackwell Scientific, Oxford.

Atkinson, T. (2001) VN training is insufficient, *Veterinary Practice Nurse*, vol. 13, no. 13 (2), pp. 8–10.

Bradshaw, J. W. S. (1992) *The Behaviour of the Domestic Cat*, CAB International, Wallingford, Oxford.

Bradshaw, J. W. S. (2000) The occurrence of unwanted behaviour in the pet cat population. In Casey, R. (ed.), *Proceedings of the 2000 CABTSG Annual Study Day*, pp. 41–42.

Brain, P. F. and Haug, M. (1992) Hormonal and neurochemical correlates of various forms of animal 'aggression', *Psychoneuroendocrinology*, vol. 17, pp. 537–551.

Carlson, N. R. (2001) *Physiology of Behavior*, 7th edn, Allyn and Bacon, London

Coppinger, R. and Coppinger, L. (2001) *Dogs*, Scribner, New York.

Dodman, N. H. and Shuster, L. (1998) *Psychopharmacology of Animal Behavior Disorders*. Blackwell Science, Malden, MA.

Goddard, M. E. and Beilharz, R. G. (1983) Genetics of traits which determine the suitability of dogs as guidedogs for the blind. *Applied Animal Ethology*, vol. 9, pp. 229–315.

Horwitz, D., Mills, D.S. and Heath, S. E. (2002). *BSAVA Manual of Canine and Feline Behavioural Medicine*, BSAVA Publications, Gloucester.

Karsh, E. B. (1983) The effects of early handling on the development of social bonds between cats and people. In Katcher A. H. and Beck A. M. (eds), *New Perspectives on Our Lives with Companion Animals*, pp. 22–28, University of Pennsylvania Press, Philadelphia.

Landsberg, G., Hunthausen, W. and Ackerman, L. (1997) *Handbook of Behaviour Problems of the Dog and Cat*, Butterworth-Heinemann, Oxford.

Landsberg, G., Horwitz, D., Heath, S. and Mills D. (2001) *Client Information Handouts, Behaviour*, Lifelearn Ltd, Newmarket.

Lindsay, S. R. (2000) *Handbook of Dog Behaviour and Training*. Oiwa State University Press, Ames.

Martin, G. and Pear, J. (1992) *Behaviour Modification: What It Is and How to Do It*, Prentice-Hall, Englewood Cliffs.

Mills, D. S. (1997) Unpublished survey of 502 dog owners for Sanofi Animal Health Ltd.

Mills, D.S. (2002a) Learning, training and behaviour modification techniques. In Horwitz, D., Mills D. S. and Heath S. E. (eds), *BSAVA Manual of Canine and Feline Behavioural Medicine*, BSAVA, Gloucester, pp 37–48.

Mills, D.S. (2002b) Pheromone therapy – an integral part of modern companion animal practice, *UK Vet*, vol. 7. pp 61–63.

Mills, D. S. and Nankervis, K. J. (1999) *Equine Behaviour – Principles and Practice*, Blackwell Science, Oxford.

Mills, D. S. and White, J. C. (2000) Long-term follow up of the effect of a pheromone therapy on feline spraying behaviour, *Veterinary Record*, vol. 147, pp. 746–747.

Neville, P. (1996) The behavioural impact of weaning on cats and dogs. In Raw, M. E. and Parkinson, T. J. (ed), *The Veterinary Annual*, vol. 36, pp. 98–108, Blackwell Science, Oxford.

Nicholls, T. J. (1983) Behavioural changes associated with chronic lead poisoning in working dogs. *Veterinary Record*, vol. 112, pp. 607.

Overall, K. L. (1997) *Clinical Behavioral Medicine for Small Animals*, Mosby, St Louis.

Scott, J. P. and Fuller, J. L. (1965) *Genetics and the Social Behavior of the Dog*, Chicago University Press, Chicago.

Serpell, J. (1995). *The Domestic Dog: Its Evolution, Behaviour and Interactions with People*, Cambridge University Press: Cambridge.

Strong, V. (1999) *The Dog's Dinner*, ALPHA, Windsor.

Takeuchi, Y., Houpt, K. A. and Scarlett, J. M. (2000) Evaluation of treatments for separation anxiety in dogs, *Journal of the American Veterinary Medical Association*, vol. 217, pp. 342–345.

Turner, D. C. and Bateson, P. (2000) *The Domestic Cat: The Biology of its Behaviour*, Cambridge University Press, Cambridge.

Voith, V. L. (1984) Why should veterinarians study animal behavior? *Modern Veterinary Practice*, vol. 65, pp. 363–364.

Voith, V. L. (1985) Human–Animal Relationships. In Anderson R. S. (ed.), *Nutrition and Behaviour of Dogs and Cats*, pp. 147–156, Pergamon Press, Oxford.

26

Managing animal death: helping clients through pet loss

L. Jones and *M. F. Stewart*

Learning objectives

After studying this chapter, students should be able to:

- Be aware of the factors which influence the reaction people experience when losing a pet.
- Understand the process of grieving and the different manifestations of grief.
- Become skilled in the sensitive management of euthanasia and animal death.
- Develop personal strategies for dealing with the emotional aspects of their job.

The reputation of a veterinary practice is often based on the way that animal death is handled. Compassionate and competent nurses have a crucial role in this as well as in the smooth and pleasant running of the practice. Along with their clinical nursing duties, they are expected to be a source of emotional support. They often have to spend time listening to clients' anxieties and complaints, while always remaining loyal to the practice.

This chapter aims to encourage nurses to develop a familiarity and ease with the emotional side of their work, and to establish good practices that increase their own and their clients' confidence and satisfaction.

Factors influencing owners' reactions to pet death

Special animals

If you have had many animals, you will know that while each has been unique, there may have been one that you felt most attached to, a special one. Some of the things that make animals special:

- **Character, personality**. Some animals are just outstanding individuals, and even a short relationship with them can leave a lasting impression.
- **Length of time involved in the relationship**. The longer we live with an animal adapting to each other's ways, the more we become attached.
- **Links with past events or life transitions**. This may have been our very first animal, or a gift on an important occasion. It may have helped us through troubled times, a bereavement or other major trauma.

- **Links with other people**. An animal may represent some sort of link with a person who has died or disappeared from our lives.
- **Assistance animals**, or those who are partners in some shared activity, such as mountain rescue, police work, competitions.
- **Rescued animals, orphans, chronically ill**. The more nurturing and care invested, the stronger the attachment.

Though every animal is different and special in its own way, some are special over and above others. When clients indicate the importance of animals in their lives, it is helpful to acknowledge that you have heard and appreciate what they are saying.

Human factors/vulnerable people

- The age, stage in life, life circumstances.
- Personal coping mechanisms – some people seem to have difficulty in adjusting to loss generally.
- Dependence on the animal – this can happen whenever people are lonely or feeling isolated for any reason, such as the death of loved ones, a family break-up or some illness or debility.
- For those who have no children, the animal may actually be their little family.

Being aware of these important issues, nurses can be alerted to the possibility of intense reactions should critical illnesses or accidents occur. When interviewing a new client a few simple questions such as, 'How long have you had Sandy?' will often let you know quite a lot about the background picture and what the animal represents in the owner's life. In a very short time you can get a feeling about the relationship as well as establishing a rapport with the owner.

The circumstances of the death

The cause and circumstances of a death have an impact on the immediate reaction and the grieving process that follows. Some of the most difficult are:

- Sudden unexpected deaths, especially anaesthetic deaths of animals undergoing minor procedures.
- Acute medical conditions.
- Violent deaths, road accidents, shootings.
- Euthanasia of healthy animals is upsetting for the staff as well as the owners. The reasons may be family

disputes, housing regulations, persistent behaviour problems. Owners are often grateful for suggestions about options other than death. Be well informed about behavioural therapists and animal rescues in your area. Imposed euthanasias of dogs that have attacked people or livestock are devastating for the owners, so never be judgemental.

- Problematic euthanasias – making the decision about euthanasia is tough enough. When anything goes wrong, especially if distressed animals die struggling, owners may be severely traumatised.

  It is wise to enter details of difficult euthanasias in the case records, dated and signed, for later reference.

Be prepared for some extra commitment on your part if a special animal, belonging to a vulnerable owner dies under distressing circumstances.

Phase 1   **Numbness**. Close to the time of loss a period of numbness and unreality helps the mourner to disregard the truth of the loss for a short time. Reality gradually seeps in.

Phase 2:   **Yearning**. There is pining, grieving and sorrowing, a longing for the lost one to return. There may be a tendency to deny the loss at some level, although the real knowledge is there too. There may be vivid dreams, and seemingly catching glimpses of the lost one. Guilt and anger are often experienced at this time.

Phase 3:   **Disorganisation, despair**. There may be difficulty in functioning or getting involved in normal activities.

Phase 4:   **Readjustment**. Life starts getting back together again and emotional energy can be reinvested.

Manifestations of grief: bereavement

All of us will experience losses during our lives, and we will learn from those. Having a general understanding of loss and grief provides a framework for understanding the feelings and reactions that may accompany animal death. As well as giving us an insight for helping others, it prepares us for our own emotional responses to loss and gives us an insight for helping others.

Grief associated with the death of a significant human

Bereavement at the loss of a significant person can be devastating and may take 3 years or more to work through. Some aspects of life may be permanently changed.

Although the following material describes bereavement for a significant human, vet staff will recognise many aspects that clients may display concerning the illness and death of an animal.

Anticipatory grief begins before death; this affects both the dying person and their loved ones and begins on hearing bad news about a terminal condition. At first there may be **denial**, **shock**, **numbness**. The person may not hear, may not be able to assimilate or may not believe what is being said. Then **anger**. Once they have acknowledged the situation, they may feel angry, 'It's not fair! Why me?' Then **bargaining**. A person may try to make a deal with fate, to extend time, to try and change things. 'Please God, just let me stay alive until my son comes home'. Then follows **preparatory grief**; **depression**, then **acceptance of the situation**, and **preparation for death**.

After the death, reactions of grieving people are often described as involving four phases. Though these are useful in understanding the process, there is great individual variation and these are only indicators of what may happen.

Animal death

Veterinary nurses who have owned and loved animals will be aware not only of the pleasures of their company, but also of the anxiety that comes when things go wrong. This is a good starting place for building up an empathy with your clients, keeping in mind that each of us is distinct, and each relationship is different. You will never know just how another person is feeling, but you can have some understanding of their situation. **Never say 'I know just how you feel'**, because you don't. If, however, they ask if you've lost a pet, you can indicate that you also have 'been there'. When an animal dies, people often say, 'It's like a death in the family' and in a way it is, since our animals are family members.

Though the basic process of bereavement (including anticipation) may be similar, there are usually great differences in the magnitude of the grief, the time span involved, the long-term effect on life. The whole process could involve just days or weeks, though it may be months before feeling ready to take on another animal.

Occasionally when feelings of guilt or anger are unresolved, the grief may be intense and protracted.

The client's reactions

Nurses should be prepared for all kinds of reactions; the most usual are:

On hearing bad news

Initial responses are often alarm, shock and disbelief. People may actually not hear what is being said, and even if they can hear, they may not take in what they are told.

Owners' needs: **Time** to accept the reality and adjust to the situation, **Encouragement** to ask questions. **Confirmation** that the situation has been correctly assessed, and **explanations** given that they can understand. **Confidence** that the vet staff care about them and their animal.

When the outlook is increasingly serious, an anxious client needs reassurance that all options have been explored and that everything possible has been done.

At the time of death

Shock Disbelief at the swift transition from life to death.

Owners' needs: Support appropriate for that person. A few moments to adjust.

Tears and sobs People often say 'I cried more for (Daisy) than I did for my (mother)'. This doesn't mean they cared less for their mother, but that with an animal death, the shock is less, the implications simpler, and the emotions are more immediately on the surface. Be aware of the possibility that tears for an animal have opened the floodgates to a deeper grief that is still being worked through.

Owners' needs: Acknowledgement of their grief, encouragement to feel bad and to cry. 'Don't apologise, its appropriate and good to cry, and a real tribute to Zack that you care so much.'

Guilt This is often immediate and powerful.

Owners' needs: To be reassured that nearly everyone feels guilty, even while accepting that they did their best. When making life and death decisions, some degree of guilt is almost inevitable.

Anger This is a recognised component in grief. It is, however, not as common a reaction to animal death as it is to human death. It may be triggered by poor communication, or careless treatment.

Owners' needs: To be heard and their anger acknowledged. Never argue or get defensive. Listen to their complaints with patience and suggest an opportunity to have a calm discussion about it with the vet that was involved.

On reflection afterwards, ask yourself if something was done or not done that could have compounded the anger. Remember that something that seems trivial to you may have been magnified in the owners' perceptions.

Good practice is built on acknowledging and learning from mistakes.

Unless there are follow-up visits or contacts for a special reason, in many cases the practice will not be aware of the grieving process that continues after a client leaves the surgery.

Management of euthanasia

Pre-euthanasia discussion

If possible, it is helpful to arrange a quiet time for an informal talk about the impending euthanasia, and explore options:

- **Where?** Home-based euthanasia may be easier for the client and the animal, but more difficult for the vet staff. If at the surgery, the appointment should be arranged so that a client doesn't have to sit in a waiting room with other clients.
- **Who should be present?** Does the owner (and other family members) want to attend? As long as things go smoothly and the death is peaceful, most clients feel good about having stayed.
- **What will happen?** Explain the procedure, how long it will take, and what the animal will experience.
- **Arrangements for the body.** Though it feels awkward, it is important to help clients decide what they want beforehand. Be prepared with information about local services.
- **Other people.** When the final decisions about euthanasia of a family pet are being discussed, confirm that the rest of the family, and especially the children, are being involved in an appropriate way, and will be given the opportunity to say goodbye.

Always refer to the animal by name and get the sex right.

Euthanasia procedure

Ensure:

- That the client doesn't have to spend time in a crowded waiting room.
- That the staff are aware of the impending euthanasia and act sensitively (no laughter or joking).
- That anyone handling the animal speaks kindly to it, using the animal's name.
- That the consent form is presented sensitively, acknowledging the difficulty.

Confirm the clients' decision whether or not to stay. Give them a chance to change their mind. They may decide to go in with the animal, give it a last cuddle, then go out and wait while the injection is being given, coming back in afterwards to say a final goodbye.

When the client is present

Ensure:

- That a staff member who is familiar to the client is dealing with the euthanasia. If the client's usual vet cannot be there, it is essential that the attending nurse is someone with whom the client has built up a rapport.

- That in the room there are chairs, a box of tissues, a mat for sliding under the animal, absorbent wipes, and a blanket if the owner has not brought one.
- That there should be no interruptions (turn off pagers).

Inform the owner:

- Explain the procedure again: 'We'll just clip a little hair so we can see the vein better. He will feel a pin prick when he gets the injection of concentrated anaesthetic. Then he'll take a few deep breaths as he becomes unconscious.' Prepare them for the rapid change from life to death; warn them of the reflex gasps, and that the eyes will remain open.
- Show the owner where to stand and what to do.
- Tell them their voice and touch will comfort the animal as it dies.

WARNING
Around the euthanasia process, an owner will experience a sense of heightened awareness. Everything that is said and done becomes MAGNIFIED. Little things become highly significant. The reactions of other people, their understanding and support, or lack of it, will be remembered forever.

Nurses' action:

- While holding the animal before the injection, try to reassure it by gently stroking it, and speaking its name softly. After the injection, slip it into a comfortable-looking position. If a muzzle had to be used, remove it immediately. (Avoid muzzles if possible.)
- Gently tidy the animal, and put absorbent material in place in case of sphincter relaxation.
- Remove all equipment, swabs, hair clippings, etc.
- Make sure the animal looks peaceful, maybe covering the body (not the head), with a small blanket.
- Say something appropriate, like 'That's it, she's peaceful now'.

Then give your attention to the owner.

Find out:

- If they want a few minutes alone to say goodbye.
- If they just want to leave (preferably by an exit other than the waiting room).

Make sure that the owner's last image is of the animal looking comfortable.

Further action:

Offer appropriate support. Some may want comforting, others may just want acknowledgement.

- If owners are crying and very distressed, pass them a tissue, letting them know it's OK to cry. Offer them a seat. They may want you to sit with them for a moment. If you feel it's appropriate a touch on the forearm is a kind gesture (not the hands). They may want to talk about their animal. Even when you are busy, just a few moments are very helpful for the owner.
- Acknowledge their sadness, and warn them that they may also feel guilty, and that is normal.
- If arrangements for the body have not been made beforehand, this will have to be broached sensitively. Avoid words like 'dispose', 'incinerate'. Provide them with information, and let them know that the body will be retained if they need time to think about it.
- If they are taking the body home, make sure to express the bladder. Slip a plastic sheet or folded bag under the body before wrapping it in a blanket, explaining why. Warn that there may be a little muscle twitching, and suggest they arrange the body in the desired position before rigor mortis sets in.
- Have available BSAVA leaflets, and details about SCAS/ Blue Cross Pet Bereavement Support Service Helpline.
- Suggest reading material; this is useful for emphasising the shared aspects of grieving for pets.
- If an owner is very distressed and will be driving home, settle them in a quiet spot, maybe with a cup of tea. Unless they seem to want to be alone, you might walk them to their car and let them know by your manner that you care. You will soon develop a sense of what is appreciated.
- Unless the owner is new to the practice, or wants to pay on the spot, don't suggest they settle the account at such a sensitive time. The bill, for services rendered, should be sent two weeks later, unless advance payment has already been made.

After death

- Label and retain any of the animals' possessions, like collars or leads, that were left at the surgery. Owners may remember and want them later.
- Send a personalised card or letter soon after the death. (Not with the bill!) Acknowledge that this must be a sad time for them, and that you are thinking of them. If the owner wasn't present, reassure them that the death had been peaceful.

Where the practice has arranged cremation, the way ashes are returned is almost as important to some people as the actual euthanasia.

- The nurse whom the client knows best should make the phone call that the ashes are ready for collection. Never leave that message on an answer phone. Don't hand the ashes over the counter in a busy waiting room. Best to carry them out to the car for the owner.
- If you are very concerned about a distressed client who lives alone, it is good practice to give them a ring in a day

or two. This lets them know someone cares about them, and gives them an opportunity to talk about things that are on their mind. They may need to be reassured about something or may just want to share their sadness.

- If clients let you know they are having difficulty in coping, refer them to the Pet Bereavement Support Helpline (0800 096 6606). Femail support available at pbssmail@bluecross.org.uk.

Some practices have set up their own pet loss support group, while others have a staff member who has done some training in pet bereavement work.

WARNING

If a 'specialist in pet bereavement counselling' has advertised a service in your area, get someone to check them out before recommending them.

It should be policy and the aim of the practice that animal deaths are managed in such a skilful and sensitive way that the client won't need the help of a counsellor to handle what is an understandable grief. What may be needed is someone to just listen to them, and to assure them that what they are experiencing is normal. The responsibility of the practice is not to provide a personal bereavement counselling service, unless someone has been specifically trained for that. Even in that case, boundaries must be established, and dependency avoided.

Records Ensure that the animal's death has been entered in the records, that all the staff know, and that no automatic reminders are sent out.

Things clients have expressed appreciation about

- A warm reception and friendly attitude.
- The staff recognising owner and animal, especially when they remember the animal's name.
- Being treated with respect. Not being patronised.
- Handling the animal gently and competently, speaking its name.
- Making appreciative comments about the animal, giving the impression that it is valued.
- Being encouraged to ask questions, and given useful explanations. Being listened to.
- Management of euthanasia in a sensitive way: helping the animal have a peaceful death.
- Allowing time with the dead animal, and giving the client privacy.
- The body being treated with respect.
- Receiving a condolence card or letter.

Coping with personal emotions

Animal death, especially by euthanasia, is potentially the greatest source of stress in veterinary practice. Paradoxically, if handled well, it can also be the greatest source of satisfaction and the aspect of your work that is most appreciated by your clients.

It is important to ensure a balanced approach between over- and under involvement. Getting too personally involved and swamped by clients' grief is not helpful to anyone. The grief belongs to the client, but you can be touched by it and respond to it. On the other hand, cultivating a cool detached attitude may seem like protection from emotional overload, but it might be interpreted by the owner as being cold and uncaring. Detachment also deprives a nurse of one of the most rewarding aspects of the job. This is hard to define but it's something like sharing sadness as well as joy, and gets people in touch with their own humanity. The gratitude of clients when they have been moved by the kindness of nurses, is well evidenced by the cards, letters and gifts they send in after an animal has died. In a simple way, it's acknowledgement of a job well done.

Strategies for coping with and enjoying the emotional aspects of veterinary nursing

- Have some sort of mutual support system with colleagues, or a friend, so that you can 'off-load' and share experiences (best not involve a partner).
- Take an active interest in client/animal relationships.
- Get a life outside of the practice, look after yourself.
- Keep a sense of humour.
- Do your best, but don't expect to work miracles.
- Do some training in pet bereavement support, which will allow you to explain and explore your own reactions, as well as helping grieving clients (see further reading list).

KEY POINTS

- Awareness of the heightened sensitivity experienced by clients at the time of their animals' death, and appreciation that the events of that day can remain with them for a long time, should dictate your approach.
- Your skilful and compassionate management of animal death reflects on your professional abilities and the reputation of the practice.

Further reading and support material

For Veterinary Nurses

Adams, C. and Cohen, S. *Pet Loss and Client Grief.* CDrom. e-mail: sales@Lifelearn.com.

Stewart, M. F. (1999) *Companion Animal Death: A Comprehensive Guide for the Veterinary Practice*, Butterworth-Heinemann, Oxford.

Books for clients:

Ironside, V. (1994) *Goodbye Dear Friend*, Robson Publications, UK.

Lee, L. and Lee, M. (1991) *Absent Friend, Coping with the Loss of a Treasured Pet*, Heston, High Wycombe.

Materials for client support

The following are available from Pet Bereavement Support Service, Blue Cross Shilton Road, Burford Oxon OX18 4PF (01993 825 539).

When a Pet Dies, a distance-learning pack for people who want to support grieving owners.

Pet loss poster and leaflets detailing Blue Cross/SCAS Pet Bereavement Support Service Helpline.

Death of an Animal Friend, SCAS booklet for owners.

A Kind Goodbye, SCAS video.

Children and Pet Bereavement. Useful tips for supporting children when their pet dies.

Guide to professional conduct for veterinary nurses

Introduction

(1) Under the Veterinary Surgeons Act 1966, the Royal College of Veterinary Surgeons (RCVS) is responsible for all ethical matters relating to veterinary practice within the United Kingdom. That responsibility encompasses the work of both veterinary surgeons and veterinary nurses.

(2) This code is issued to assist veterinary nurses in maintaining acceptable professional standards. Matters of concern should be raised first with their employer and thereafter if not satisfactorily resolved, with the British Veterinary Nursing Association (BVNA).

General standards

(3) Veterinary nurses should be mindful that they are only permitted to act under the supervision or direction of a veterinary surgeon.

(4) They should be familiar with and work within the RCVS 'Guide to Professional Conduct'.

(5) They are personally responsible for their own professional standards and negligence.

(6) They shall act at all times in the best interests of the animal while taking into consideration the wishes of the owner/keeper and employer and in such a manner as to justify the trust and confidence of the public and to uphold the good standing of the veterinary profession.

Acknowledgement of limitations

(7) Veterinary nurses are expected to maintain their professional knowledge and competence.

(8) They are equally expected to acknowledge any limitations in knowledge or competence, and, where relevant, to make these known to their employer.

(9) Similarly an employer should not ask a veterinary nurse to undertake any task above and beyond their known level of competence.

Relationship with veterinary colleagues

(10) Veterinary nurses should cooperate fully with veterinary surgeons, assisting them in the provision of veterinary care.

(11) They should encourage and help colleagues to develop their professional skills.

Conscientious objections

(12) Veterinary nurses should discuss with any employer and/or prospective employer any conscientious objection which they may have to any treatment of any species of animal. Nevertheless it must be recognised that the welfare of the animal is always paramount and that there will be circumstances when this overrides any conscientious objection.

Confidentiality

(13) Veterinary nurses must keep confidential any information relating to an animal or owner, an employer or fellow employee, acquired in the course of their work.

(14) Such information must not be disclosed to anyone except where:

(a) They are required to do so in a court of law or

(b) Where animal welfare or the wider public interest would be endangered by non-disclosure.

Health and safety

(15) Veterinary nurses should be mindful of their responsibility to report to their employer any circumstances where the health and safety of staff or animals is put at risk.

Promotion of products or services

(16) Veterinary nurses employed in veterinary practice should not permit their professional qualification to be used as a means of promoting commercial animal related products or services to the public, nor should they allow commercial considerations to override their professional judgement.

Index

Page numbers in *italic* refer to figures and those in **bold** to tables.